Gerontology and Geriatrics for NPs and PAs

An Interprofessional Approach

Gerontology and Geriatrics for NPs and PAs

An Interprofessional Approach

Jill Beavers-Kirby, DNP, MS, ACNP-BC, ANP-BC

Retired
Formerly:
Associate Professor and Coordinator of NP Programs
Mount Carmel College of Nursing
Columbus, Ohio
Visiting Professor
Chamberlain University
Columbus, Ohio

Freddi Segal-Gidan, PA, PhD

Associate Professor
Clinical Neurology and Family Medicine
Keck School of Medicine of USC
Los Angeles, California
Director of USC/Rancho California Alzheimer's Disease Center
Rancho Los Amigos National Rehabilitation Center
Downey, California

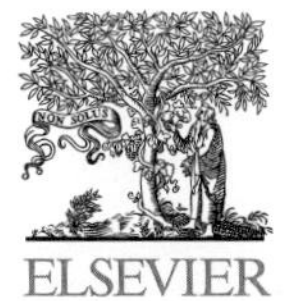
ELSEVIER

Elsevier
3251 Riverport Lane
St. Louis, Missouri 63043

GERONTOLOGY AND GERIATRICS FOR NPs AND PAs: AN INTERPROFESSIONAL APPROACH

ISBN: 978-0-323-60845-9

Notice

Practitioners and researchers must always rely on their own experience and knowledge in evaluating and using any information, methods, compounds or experiments described herein. Because of rapid advances in the medical sciences, in particular, independent verification of diagnoses and drug dosages should be made. To the fullest extent of the law, no responsibility is assumed by Elsevier, authors, editors or contributors for any injury and/or damage to persons or property as a matter of products liability, negligence or otherwise, or from any use or operation of any methods, products, instructions, or ideas contained in the material herein.

Executive Content Strategist: James Merritt
Content Development Manager: Danielle Frazier
Senior Content Development Specialist: Sarah Vora
Publishing Services Manager: Julie Eddy
Senior Project Managers: Abigail Bradberry / Cindy Thoms
Design Direction: Margaret Reid

Printed in India

Last digit is the print number: 9 8 7 6 5 4 3 2 1

To my family who loves and supports me all the time even when I've bitten off more than I can chew. I wouldn't be here without you.

Jill Beavers-Kirby

Dedicated to all the patients and families who have allowed me into their lives, taught me so much, and helped to make me a better provider.

Freddi Segal-Gidan

Reviewers

Leslee D'Amato-Kubiet, PhD, ARNP
Associate Lecturer/Campus Coordinator
College of Nursing
University of Central Florida
Daytona Beach Regional Campus
Daytona Beach, Florida
Florida Hospital Hospice and Palliative Care
Palm Coast, Florida

Dawn Carpenter, DNP, ACNP-BC, CCRN
Nurse Practitioner, Trauma and Surgical ICU
Guthrie Healthcare System
Sayre, Pennsylvania

Karen Dick, PhD, GNP-BC, FAANP
Associate Professor
UMASS Chan Medical School
Tan Chingfen Graduate School of Nursing
University of Massachusetts Medical School
Worcester, Massachusetts

Roseann S. Dust, MS, PA-C
Clinical Instructor
School of Allied Health Sciences
Baylor College of Medicine
Michael E. DeBakey VA Medical Center
Houston, Texas

Christine M. Everett, PhD, MPH, PA-C
Associate Professor
Department of Community and Family Medicine
Physician Assistant Division
Duke University School of Medicine
Durham, North Carolina

Jennifer Gilhooly, MS, PA-C
Physician Assistant
Emergency Department
Mount Carmel Hospital/ESI
Columbus, Ohio

Robert Lee Grabowski DNP, MBA, APRN-CNP, AGACNP-BC, CPNP-AC, CEN, CCRN, CFRN, CMTE, EMT-P
Chief Flight Nurse Practitioner
Special Faculty
Metro Life Flight, The MetroHealth System
Frances Payne Bolton School of Nursing
Case Western Reserve University
Cleveland, Ohio

Aruba Jahangir, MSc, BSc (Hons)
Physician Associate
Primary Care Doncaster
Doncaster, United Kingdom

Kathleen S. Jordan, DNP, MS, FNP-BC, ENP-BC, ENP-C, SANE-P, FAEN
Clinical Associate Professor
Nurse Practitioner
School of Nursing, Emergency Department
The University of North Carolina at Charlotte
Mid-Atlantic Emergency Medicine Associates
Charlotte, North Carolina

†Kathy Kemle, MS, PA-C, DFAAPA
Physician Assistant
Assistant Professor
Family Medicine
Medical Center of Central Georgia/Navicent Health
Macon, Georgia

Senthilkumaran Lakshmanan, PA (Texas), MPAS, NCCPA (Cert), BLS (Cert)
Director of Didactic Education
South University
Austin, Texas

Terri Lipps, DNP, CNE, APRN, FNP-BC
Associate Professor, FNP Program Director
Saint Francis Medical Center College of Nursing
Peoria, Illinois

Jan Victoria Scott, MHS, PA-C
Associate Consulting Professor
Community and Family Medicine, Physician Assistant Program
Duke University
Durham, North Carolina

†Deceased

Jennifer K. Sofie, DNP, FNP, ANP
Associate Clinical Professor & Nurse Practitioner
College of Nursing
Montana State University & Three Rivers Medical Clinic
Bozeman, Montana

Laura Steadman, EdD, CRNP, MSN, RN
Assistant Professor/Family Nurse Practitioner
Specialty Track Coordinator of the Nurse Educator Masters Program
School of Nursing
Adult/Acute Health, Chronic Care and Foundations
The University of Alabama at Birmingham
Birmingham, Alabama

Grace Ellen Urquhart DNP, FNP-C
Family Nurse Practitioner, Assistant Professor
Frontier Nursing University
Versailles, Kentucky

Daryle Wane, PhD, APRN, FNP-BC
BSN Program Director – Professor of Nursing
Pasco-Hernando State College
New Port Richey, Florida

Contributors

Phyllis Atkinson, RN,MS,GNP-BC,WCC
Gerontological Nurse Practitioner
Wright State Physicians
Dayton, Ohio

Janet Cho, PharmD, BCGP
Clinical Pharmacist
School of Pharmacy
University of Southern California
Los Angeles, California

Laura Corrales-Diaz Pomatto, MS, PhD
Post-Doctoral Research Fellow
National Institute on Aging (NIA)
National Institute of Health (NIH)
Baltimore, Maryland
PRAT Fellow
National Institute of General Medical Sciences (NIGMS)
National Institute of Health (NIH)
Bethesda, Maryland

Jennifer Cox, MSW, LICSW
Director of Behavioral Health
Psychiatry
Baystate Medical Center
Springfield, Massachusetts
Instructor
Social Work
Westfield State University
Westfield, Massachusetts

Lauren Diegel-Vacek, DNP, APRN, FNP-BC, CNE, FAANP
Clinical Associate Professor
Biobehavioral Nursing Science
University Illinois Chicago College of Nursing
Chicago, Illinois

Sarah Endicott, DNP, APNP, PMHNP-BC, GNP-BC
Clinical Professor
Nursing
University of Wisconsin
Madison, Wisconsin

Leslie Chang Everston, DNP, RN, GNP-BC
Geriatric Nurse Practitioner
Geriatrics
UCLA Health
Los Angeles, California

Kerry S. Fankhauser, DNP, RN, AHN-BC, UZIT
Associate Professor, Director of the Prelicensure Program
Mount Carmel College of Nursing
Columbus, Ohio

Rory B. Farrand, MS, MA, MSN, APRN-BC
Vice President Palliative and Advanced Care
Palliative Care
National Hospice and Palliative Care Organization
Finleyville, Pennsylvania

Denise Gobert, PT, PhD, NCS, CEEAA
Professor
Physical Therapy
Texas State University
Round Rock, Texas

Valerie Gruss, PhD, APRN, CNP-BC, FAAN
Clinical Professor
Project Co-Director, ENGAGE-IL
AAN, Edge Runner
University of Illinois at Chicago
College of Nursing (CON)
BioBehavioral Nursing Science
Chicago, Illinois

Tatyana Gurvich, PharmD, BCGP
Assistant Professor of Clinical Pharmacy
Dept of Clinical Pharmacy
USC School of Pharmacy
Manhattan Beach, California
Adjunct Assistant Professor of Family Medicine
Family Medicine
UCI Medical Center
Orange, California

Abiola Keller, MPAS, MPH, PhD
Assistant Professor
College of Nursing
Marquette University
Milwaukee, Wisconsin

†Kathy Kemle, MS, PA-C, DFAAPA
Physician Assistant
Assistant Professor
Family Medicine
Medical Center of Central Georgia/Navicent Health
Macon, Georgia

Soo Jung Kim, MSN, ANP, AGPCNP-BC
Nurse Practitioner
Geriatrics Service
Memorial Sloan Kettering Cancer Center
New York, New York

Maripat DiGioia King, DNP, ACNP, RN
Clinical Assistant Professor
Biobehavioral Nursing Sciences
University of Illinois–Chicago
Chicago, Illinois

Teresa Kiresuk, DNP
Program Director, Adult Gerontologic Primary Care Nurse Practitioner Program
Graduate Nursing, Online Programs
South University
Savannah, Georgia
Clinical Nurse Practitioner
Premise Health
Minneapolis, Minnesota

Tracy McClinton, DNP, AGACNP-BC, APRN, EBP-C
Assistant Professor
College of Nursing
University of Tennessee Health Science Center
Memphis, Tennessee

Debra McDowell, BS, MSHP, PhD
Doctor of Physical Therapy
Texas State University
Round Rock, Texas

Lisa Ruth McLean, MMS, PA-C
President
Geriatric Medicine PAs
American Academy of PAs
Plymouth, Michigan
PA-C
Occupational Medicine
Detroit, Michigan

Sincere Simone McMilan, DNP, MS, BSN
Nurse Practitioner
Geriatric Medicine
Memorial Sloan Kettering Cancer Center
New York, New York

Yuen Man Ng, PharmD, APh
Former Adjunct Clinical Instructor of Pharmacy Practice
School of Pharmacy
University of Southern California
Los Angeles, California

Daniel Podd, BS, MPAS
Associate Professor
Clinical Health Professions
St. John's University
Queens, New York

Kris T. Pyles-Sweet, DMSc, PA-C
Medical Director/ Owner
Modern Medical Aesthetics and Wellness
Morganton, North Carolina
Director-at-Large
American Academy of Physician Associates
Alexandria, Virginia

Kemi Iyabo Reeves, RN, BSN, MSN, GNP-BC
Supervisor-Nurse Practitioner
Geriatric Medicine
HealthCHEC Comprehensive Health Evaluation Center
Long Beach, California
Dementia Care Specialist
UCLA Alzheimer's and Dementia Care Program
UCLA Department of Medicine: Division of Geriatrics
Los Angeles, California
Assistant Clinical Professor-Volunteer
UCLA Adult-Gerontologic Nurse Practitioner Program
UCLA School of Nursing
Los Angeles, California
INTERACT Training Coach
California Association of Long-Term Care Medicine
Santa Clarita, California

Eden D. Ruiz-Lopez, MPA
Assistant Deputy Director
Department of Family Medicine
Keck School of Medicine of the University of Southern California
Los Angeles, California
Director
Rancho/USC California Alzheimer's Disease Center (CADC)
Rancho Los Amigos National Rehabilitation Center
Downey, California

†Deceased

C. Kim Stokes, DMSc, MHS, PA-C
Associate Professor
Physician Assistant Studies
Elon University
Elon, North Carolina

Lorie L. Weber, MS, PA-C
Assistant Professor
Physician Assistant Studies
A.T. Still University
Mesa, Arizona

Sharon Woods, BS, MPAS, PA-C
Physician Assistant
Department of Medicine
Division of Geriatrics and Palliative Care
Baystate Medical Center
Springfield, Massachusetts

Heidi Yulico, RN, MS
GNP
Geriatrics
Memorial Sloan Kettering Cancer Center
New York, New York

Evolve Writers

Daniel Vetrosky, BA, BHS, MEd, PhD
Retired Director of Didactic Education
Department of Physician Assistant Studies
University of South Alabama
Mobile, Alabama

Bridget C. Calhoun, DrPH, PA-C
Associate Dean for Academic Affairs and Research
John G. Rangos Sr. School of Health Sciences
Duquesne University
Pittsburgh, Pennsylvania

Preface

The idea for this book was born before the COVID pandemic and, as such, took several years to complete. At the onset, we knew that health care in the 21st century requires a team approach. The COVID pandemic only proved our hypothesis.

Throughout the COVID pandemic nurse practitioners (NPs) and physician associates (PAs) came together to provide various levels of care to millions of people affected by COVID. For some NPs and PAs this was a new concept. For the two of us this was a concept that we knew would be the best for all patients regardless of setting, from home to clinic to hospital to long-term care.

Nurse practitioners and physician associates are health care providers whose roles in the health care system are similar, and in some places interchangeable. However, our initial training is different. The unique differences in our trainings help us work together to provide the best care for everyone.

This book focuses on taking an interdisciplinary approach to care for the older adult population while incorporating best practices from Healthy People goals and standards of care from various national and international organizations. It incorporates evidence-based outcomes, which is the cornerstone of patient care for all medical providers.

Providing care to the geriatric population has always been a passion of ours. People of advanced age aren't simply just "older people." They are someone's child, someone's parent, someone's sibling, and they are the future for each of us who is fortunate enough to live a full life span. Each older adult patient is a person who has a lifetime of experiences to share. They possess a wealth of information about themselves and their history. They provide innumerable information that is essential for the NP or PA professional to understand and appreciate in order to provide appropriate care and obtain desired outcomes.

This text provides NP and PA health care providers with information about how to assess and treat the older patient and to provide the best care for them that also fits with their goals. It is designed to meet the needs of the student learning the basic tenets of geriatric medicine and for the provider wanting to enhance their understanding and improve care for the aging adult patients they care for.

Features

- Evidence-based approach (with levels of evidence) to both gerontology and geriatrics incorporates the latest national and international guidelines and protocols, as well as research evidence.
- Covers both primary care and acute care of older adults.
- Fully addresses the graduate-level core competencies for care of older adults.
- Interprofessional collaborative approach incorporates the IPEC core competencies and the unique perspectives that nurse practitioners and physician assistants each bring to the core competency of teamwork and collaboration.
- Strong emphasis on wellness (including nutrition and the Healthy People 2030 targets), normal aging, common syndromes of aging, disease management, patient safety (particularly in acute care settings), and patient-centered care.
- Richly illustrated in full color and featuring a full-color design with graduate-level learning features, including Key Points at the end of each chapter for quick reference and exam preparation.
- Tools Appendix that provides examples and further details on the professional tools relevant to each chapter.
- An Evolve site that provides a Test Bank and access to the Image Collection.

Jill Beavers-Kirby, DNP, MS, ACNP-BC, ANP-BC
Freddi Segal-Gidan, PA, PhD

Contents

Appendix 1: Tools Contents

1 Biological and Physiological Change Theories

LAURA POMATTO, PHD

OBJECTIVES

Student Learning Objectives

After completing this chapter, the student should be able to do the following:

1. List the major evolutionary and biologic theories of aging.
2. Describe the role inflammation plays in the aging process.
3. Describe dietary interventions to longevity.

Practitioner Objectives

After completing this chapter, the practitioner should be able to do the following:

1. Describe how evolutionary and biologic theories of aging inform the clinical care of older adults.
2. Outline clinical applications of dietary interventions to longevity in the care of older adults.
3. Describe how evolutionary and biologic theories of aging can explain the development of age-associated disease or accelerate a patient's disease state.

Introduction: The Evolutionary "Why" of Aging

Aging. It is a universal experience, but one for which we have the least biologic understanding. Almost every component of our biologic selves is deleteriously impacted by age (Gulsvik et al., 2011; Niccoli & Partridge, 2012). Moreover, aging increases our vulnerability to environmental insults and elevates our risk of morbidity and mortality. Due to the widespread physiologic decline that results from aging, a vast number of theories (more than 300) have emerged to explain the complexity that causes aging (Medvedev, 1990).

Yet to ask why we age requires an evolutionary framework. Evolutionary pressures (natural selection) diminish with age. Weisman was the first to posit a link between natural selection and cellular aging (cytogerontology), beginning at the cellular level (Weismann et al., 1891). In his original work, he argued that aging was a beneficial trait, one necessary to rid the population of nonreproductive individuals, and hence his reasoning and prediction for the finite replicative potential (and repair) of somatic tissue (Kirkwood & Cremer, 1982; Vijg & Kennedy, 2016). However, even Weisman came to question his own theories, as aging, itself, served no evolutionary fitness advantage (Kirkwood & Cremer, 1982). Later work by Haldane and Hamilton mathematically suggested that the forces driving natural selection decline with age (Charlesworth, 2000). This is because the selective pressures of natural selection can only work at the biologic fitness of *reproductively able* organisms. Past reproductive prime, natural selection is useless.

These pivotal keystones set the groundwork for Peter Medawar's "mutation accumulation" theory of aging, wherein he suggests that aging results from the gradual accumulation of mutations in the germline. These mutations, though beneficial early in life (when reproductive value is high), become detrimental with increasing age, and reproductive value decreases (Medawar, 1952; Mueller, 2022). Medawar's theory was the basis for the concept of "antagonistic pleiotropy" presented by Michael Rose, which argues that because natural selection is unable to act beyond reproductive capability, any changes in the genetic makeup that are favorable to reproduction can become deleterious with age. The age-specific duality of these genes, being beneficial in young to becoming deleterious with age, occurs after the reproductive period and renders natural selection unable to eliminate these deleterious age-associated genes (Rose, 1982). Rose, recognizing the relationship between aging and reproductive fitness, was the first to demonstrate, in the invertebrate model *D. melanogaster*, that by delaying reproduction, it was possible to delay aging (Rose & Charlesworth, 1980). This was a seminal finding because it suggested a potentially definitive cause (and, consequently, pathways) driving aging. Another clear example of antagonistic pleiotropy is growth hormone (GH), a peptide hormone that signals cells and tissues to promote growth and metabolic function. It is essential for bone growth, nutrient balance, and muscle mass, and it has pleiotropic effects on the cardiovascular, nervous, and immune systems (Lu et al., 2019). Though low levels of GH can be harmful early in life, due to delayed growth, muscle-to-fat imbalance and, in some cases, hypoglycemia (Lu et al., 2019; Soto-Rivera et al., 2018), it can prove beneficial in later life. Indeed, the analysis of a subset of the Ecuadorian population with a mutation in the growth hormone receptor shows abnormally low levels of GH, but members of this population are resistant to the majority of age-related diseases, including cancer and type 2 diabetes (Guevara-Aguirre et al., 2011), suggesting the duality of GH depending on the life stage.

A key caveat linking many of these evolutionary theories is the assumption that evolutionary pressures are driven by the cost and benefit to the *individual*. Specifically, any trait must benefit the reproductive fitness of an individual (or its offspring). As aging represents a decline in reproductive fitness, it could not be beneficial to the organism. However, if evolutionary pressures are widened to benefit the species, aging may serve a beneficial purpose by increasing resources available to the reproductively fit portion of the population. For example, menopause, which eliminates the reproductive abilities of an individual, may serve a broader purpose by allowing that individual to care for the young (Rose & Charlesworth, 1980). Thus programmed aging theories evolved, suggesting the individual life span was finite, because it was necessary and beneficial for the well-being of the population (Goldsmith, 2014; Skulachev, 2002).

The frame in which we view aging, whether at the population or individual level, reshapes our perception of whether aging is viewed in a beneficial (programmed) or detrimental (nonprogrammed) perspective. However, it is important to recognize the driving force behind natural selection: to improve reproductive fitness. Thus mechanisms that improve growth and reproduction may be detrimental to the aged soma. Indeed, many of the age-associated genes identified are tied to our reproductive trade-off: growth/reproduction or somatic repair. For example, under high nutrient conditions, the mammalian target of the rapamycin (mTOR) cascade is activated, which promotes cell proliferation (Shanley & Kirkwood, 2001). The mTOR signaling pathway is an essential means to ensure growth and, more important, reproductive fitness. Conversely, limiting mTOR signaling (and hence dampening growth) was found to extend the life span in mice, but at the cost of small body size (Lamming et al., 2012; Wu et al., 2013). Hence the trade-off between reproduction and somatic repair is a crucial variable in our quest to understand why we age.

Evolutionary Theories of Aging

Mutation Accumulation Theory of Aging

From an evolutionary perspective, the mutation accumulation theory of aging postulates that aging results from the inability of natural selection to remove deleterious alleles, which only manifest later in life (following reproductive fitness) (Medawar, 1952). The concept originated from Medawar's recognition of the similarities between aging and Huntington disease: both are deleterious, yet natural selection, which favors traits beneficial to the individual, had not eliminated them. Huntington disease, an autosomal neurodegenerative disease, though crippling to health had no impact on reproductive success due to its occurrence late in life, post-reproduction (Haldane, 1941). Thus from the perspective of natural selection, the deleterious mutation was immune to elimination. Other diseases have since been identified, including familial Parkinson disease (Lill, 2016), the APOE4 allele in Alzheimer disease (Liu et al., 2013), and other late-onset dominant mutations (Wright et al., 2003), all of which further demonstrate that genes that may be relatively neutral early in life can quickly become deleterious.

Studies in humans offer support in favor of the mutation accumulation theory. For example, genetic variants linked to 120 genetic diseases were identified at higher rates of clustering within variants associated with late-onset diseases compared to those associated with early-onset diseases (Rodríguez et al., 2017), suggesting that small, relatively neutral genetic mutations, free from evolutionary pressures, can accumulate at higher frequencies later in life. Another study assessed the heritable patterns of DNA methylation. Age-dependent changes in DNA methylation patterns, strongly linked to biologic age (Hannum et al., 2013), were identified to be heritable and increase with age (Robins et al., 2017). Moreover, work looking across mammalian species and their respective tissues identified genes that not only contributed to aging phenotypes but were found to contain only slightly deleterious alleles (Turan et al., 2019), adding further support to the mutation accumulation theory of aging.

Antagonistic Pleiotropy Theory of Aging

Antagonistic pleiotropy, a term originally coined by George Williams, extended the work of Medawar's mutation accumulation theory. Specifically, Williams hypothesized that genes that are beneficial to reproductive success early in life may outweigh their deleterious consequences caused in post-reproductive organisms (Williams, 1957). When he first proposed his theory in 1957, Williams presented a hypothetical scenario: a gene, though beneficial to developmental arterial calcification early in life, later in life could accelerate arterial calcification and, consequently, increase the risk of cardiovascular disease (Austad & Hoffman, 2018; Williams, 1957). His scenario highlights the duality of an allele: beneficial early in life only to become deleterious in later life. This phenomenon is dubbed antagonistic pleiotropy due to the temporal roles it plays (pleiotropy) depending on an organism's stage in the life span (antagonistic). Thus aging is the result of a biologic tradeoff between early and late-life fitness. The yeast reproductive cycle is highly linked to nutrient availability, as under high nutrient conditions, yeast undergo exponential asymmetric division.

Comparing Evolutionary Theories

This begs the question, which theory (mutation accumulation or antagonistic pleiotropy) is conserved across species? Addressing this concern requires the recognition of a key underlying difference between how these deleterious genetic variants accumulate. As Austed and Hoffman noted, mutation accumulation requires random, spontaneous mutations to occur in one genetic line. Yet these spontaneous mutations will differ across lineages and even more so across species, suggesting aging (and how it manifests) is lineage specific (Austad & Hoffman, 2018). Conversely, if natural selection finds only a small portion of alleles beneficial early in life but detrimental later in life, it would demonstrate that the mechanisms of aging are conserved across species (Austad & Hoffman, 2018). Ample evidence favors the latter.

The Biologic Trade-Off: Yeast to Mice

Many genes have been identified that can extend survival when their activity is modulated (i.e., activated, suppressed, or inhibited). The unicellular budding yeast (*Saccharomyces cerevisiae*) was a crucial model in the early discovery of longevity genes. Approximately 30% of the yeast genome is shared with humans, many of which are the aging-centric pathways (Zimmermann et al., 2018), including nutrient cycling (Slavov et al., 2012), DNA repair mechanisms (Ulrich, 2007), stress response (Longo & Fabrizio, 2002), and regulated cell death (Eisenberg & Buttner, 2014). These pathways are so well conserved that half (and in some cases, 90%) of key yeast proteins can be replaced with their human equivalent, or orthologs, and still function (Kachroo et al., 2015). As well, many of the yeast-aging phenotypes show similar traits to those in human postmitotic cellular aging (Longo & Fabrizio, 2011). Two forms of aging are evident in yeast: replicative and chronologic aging. Replicative aging is measured by the number of progeny (or "buds") a mother yeast is able to generate before she dies. As yeast divide by asymmetric division, the "mother" cell retains damaged cellular material to ensure the maximal fitness of her progeny, and after 20 to 25 cycles, the mother bud dies (Steinkraus et al., 2008). In contrast, chronologic aging is a low-nutrient environment (to prevent division) wherein a subset of cells is switched back to a high-nutrient environment and assessed for the ability to reenter the cell cycle. The inability to do so is termed *terminal life span* (Fig. 1.1). Because nutrient availability plays such an important role in yeast replication, it is not surprising many of the first-discovered aging-centric pathways involved nutrient sensing mechanisms. Mutants lacking key enzymes within the glucose-dependent pathways, such as *RAS2, PKA*, and *SCH9*, show a dramatic increase (~300%) in chronologic life span (Fabrizio et al., 2001; Pichová et al., 1997), mediated by many stress-protective pathways (Fabrizio et al., 2003).

Although yeast was the first organism to identify many aging-related genes, concurrent genetic work in invertebrate

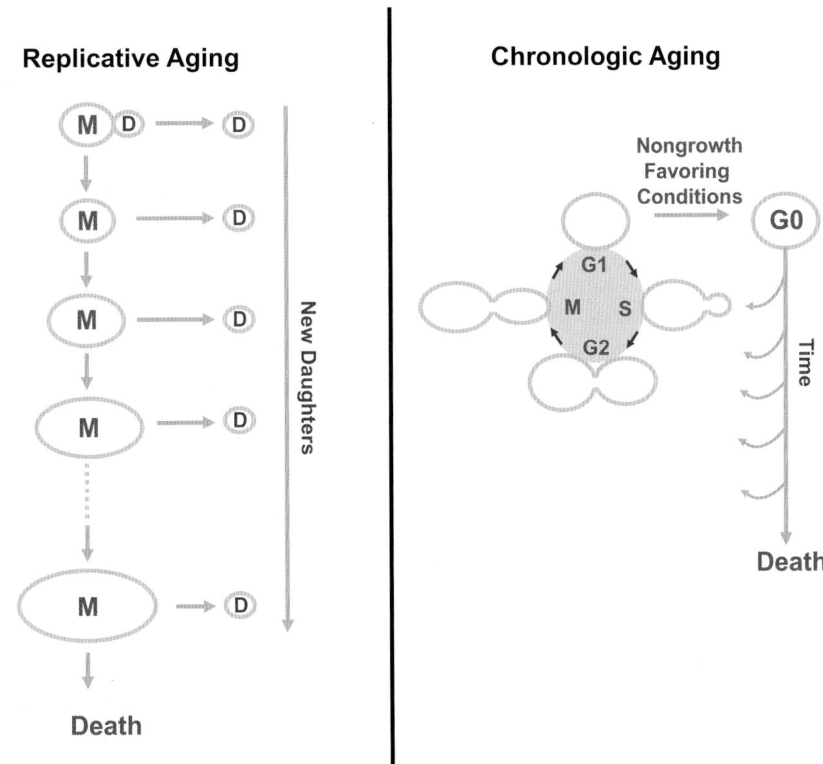

• **Fig. 1.1** Chronologic Versus Replicative Aging in Yeast. Replicative aging refers to the number of daughter buds a mother cell produces over her lifetime (mitotic divisions) before she enters senescence. Concurrently, as mothers age they accumulate damaged proteins and organelles. Replicative viability is calculated as the average number of daughter buds produced from a single mother cell. Chronologic aging is the amount of time yeast remain viable in the postreplicative phase (G0). Chronologic viability is calculated by the fraction of the yeast culture that is capable of reentering the cell cycle after an extended period in the stationary phase.

model organisms, namely, the nematode worm (*Caenorhabditis elegans*) and fruit fly (*Drosophila melanogaster*), was used to determine if single genetic mutations could bestow a similar life span extension in higher organisms. Much of our understanding about longevity pathways was first identified in the worm. One of the most notable was the robust life span extension evident in worms lacking the insulin/insulin growth factor IGF receptor, *daf-2* (Dorman et al., 1995). Mutants lacking *daf-2* lived threefold longer than their wild-type counterparts (Dorman et al., 1995). Similarly, *age-1* mutants (a kinase critical in the insulin/IGF pathway) showed on average a 50% increase in survival (Friedman & Johnson, 1988).

Many of the genes originally identified in worms were found to be conserved in fruit flies. Flies lacking the insulin receptor (InR) substrate, dubbed *chico* due to their small size, showed dramatic life span extension (Clancy et al., 2001). A similar life span extension was evident upon the loss of the insulin receptor (InR) (Chen et al., 1996; Tatar et al., 2001). Furthermore, simply selecting for *D. melanogaster* strains prone to later-life reproduction showed increased survival when compared to controls (Luckinbill & Clare, 1985). However, exploration of larval fitness found larvae from shorter-lived, early reproducing lines to outcompete larvae from longer-lived, delayed reproducing lines (Partridge & Fowler, 1992). Moreover, early comparisons assessing starvation resistance were negatively correlated to early life reproduction (Chippindale et al., 2004), suggesting the trade-off between limited nutritional resources is being directed toward either reproduction or maintenance of the soma.

A consistent trend arose from findings in yeast and invertebrate models: nutrient signaling pathways, necessary for growth and reproduction, were the key mediators in determining an organism's longevity. Therefore it is not too much of a stretch to hypothesize that a decrease in nutrient signaling pathways, many of which were conserved across lower organisms, would bestow a similar outcome in the mammalian mouse model. The Ames and Snell dwarf mouse strains showcased the duality between longevity and growth. In both instances, both strains have impaired pituitary function, leading to reduced levels of growth hormone production (Bartke, 2000; Flurkey et al., 2001), but a near doubling in life span. Within the nutrient sensing pathway, mice lacking either the insulin receptor (InR), crucial in energy metabolism (Kulkarni et al., 1999), or the insulin growth factor type 1 receptor (IGF-1R), the mediator of growth (Lupu et al., 2001), showed a dramatic increase in longevity (Blüher et al., 2003; Holzenberger et al., 2003; Selman et al., 2008). Other pathways have been identified that include the positive health benefits resulting from ablation of the growth and stress-responsive p66shc adaptor protein, including atherosclerosis and obesity resistance (Ramsey et al., 2013). However, much less is known about the reproductive trade-offs in these longevity mutants.

But the proverbial saying "nothing in life is free" is evident in these genetic manipulations. Specifically, genes beneficial to longevity are likely to be detrimental early in life (i.e., reduced reproductive fitness). In yeast, direct competition assays between longevity mutants and their wild-type counterparts show that mutants have lower reproductive fitness, resulting from slower growth rates (Delaney et al., 2011). In the case of the *daf-2* and *age-1* mutants, fecundity is dramatically suppressed. Mutant *daf-2* worms show a 20% decrease in reproductive capabilities compared to wild-type worms, which under nutrient-rich conditions are eliminated within four generations (Chen et al., 2007). Moreover, under sporadic food conditions, *age-1* is unable to compete, suggesting an explanation for why wild-type alleles still persist in the population (Walker et al., 2000). A similar trend is evident in flies, with *chico* mutant females being sterile (Clancy et al., 2001). It is important to note that this phenomenon (at least in terms of the survival/reproductive tradeoff) is not universal, as evident in other genetic manipulations found to extend invertebrate life span (Hwangbo et al., 2004; Rogina et al., 2000). In the Ames and Snell dwarf mice, due to a negligent expression of pituitary hormones (the growth-promoting signal), these mutants are sterile, highly sensitive to cold, and smaller than wild-type mice (Bartke et al., 2001). Another example is the decreased reproductive fitness evident in $p66^{shc}$ homozygous or heterozygous mice when compared to laboratory wild-type strains, suggested to occur because of their reduced stress tolerance and lowered fecundity (Giorgio et al., 2012). Additionally, it is important to highlight that much of our understanding of aging in mouse models is slightly skewed. This is in part because many of the commonly utilized strains have been heavily bred to favor accelerated reproductive maturity and production of large litter sizes (Yuan et al., 2012). Interestingly, due to these selective pressures, many laboratory strains are shorter lived than their wild-type counterparts (Miller et al., 2002). Together, these are just a few examples from our long-lived mutants that provide support for antagonistic pleiotropy as an evolutionary driver of aging.

The Naked Mole Rat: An Evolutionary Wrench to the Antagonistic Pleiotropy Theory of Aging

Reproduction versus survival is the underlying principle driving evolutionary aging theories. Under most conditions, animals with high reproductive fitness face a shorter life expectancy. The high energetic cost of reproduction comes with inadequate maintenance of the soma. Conversely, animals with delayed reproduction have longer life expectancy. Yet the naked mole rat is an evolutionary anomaly. The longest-lived rodent species (up to 30 years in captivity), the naked mole rat can outlive its laboratory counterpart approximately nine-fold (Buffenstein et al., 2012). They have exceptionally long health spans and no age-associated acceleration in mortality risk, evident by the maintenance of bone health (Pinto et al., 2010), lean mass (O'Connor et al., 2002), metabolic rate, and enzymatic activities (Ungvari et al., 2008), all of which are ordinarily negatively impacted with aging. In terms of reproduction, the majority of females within a colony do not reproduce, with each colony having only one breeding female and two to three breeding males (Jarvis, 1981). Interestingly, breeding females show *no differences* in life span (Buffenstein, 2005, 2008). Moreover, breeding females not only are capable of reproducing for most of their life span, but their reproductive fitness (litter size) increases with age. In the wild, breeding females reportedly live at least four times longer than nonbreeding ones. Together, these findings are exceptional, especially in the context of the metabolic cost necessary for reproduction, suggesting that these animals evolved to circumvent many of the evolutionary trade-offs associated with reproduction and survival.

Let's Talk About Sex: The Genetic Trade-Off Between the Sexes

A key aspect often overlooked in aging is the impact of sex. Women live longer than men (Austad, 2006), a finding starkly evident during the final stages of life (Finch & Tower, 2014). Moreover, many chronic diseases associated with aging, including cardiovascular disease (Regitz-Zagrosek & Kararigas, 2016), cancer (Cook et al., 2011), and neurodegenerative diseases (Mazure & Swendsen, 2016), are sex specific. Yet the underlying cause of sexual dimorphism is not well understood. From an evolutionary perspective, antagonistic pleiotropy argues that aging is a result of alleles, which are beneficial in younger life but become detrimental in later life, but overlooks the genetic nuances of sex. Because males and females share the same autosomal makeup but their respective sex-linked genes are different (i.e., X/X versus X/Y), varying (and potentially deleterious) selective pressures result. Hence sexual antagonistic pleiotropy is the selection of certain alleles that benefit one sex but are deleterious to the other (Rice, 1992). This is in part because males have only one X chromosome, whereas females have two. As a result, genes on the X chromosome have had a longer evolutionary history under female-favored selection. Indeed the X chromosome shows high levels of sexual antagonistic variations, including reproductive success and female fertility (Gibson et al., 2002). Indeed, evidence highlights the X-favored benefit in longevity. In mice and humans, the Y chromosome contains the *sry* gene, which controls the development of testes and perinatal masculinization. Utilization of the four core genotypes (FCG) mice (De Vries et al., 2002) results in a genetic manipulation to place the *sry* gene so that it is located on an autosomal chromosome, allowing the inheritance of *sry* (and consequently testes) to occur with or without the presence of the Y chromosome and thus generating four sex phenotypes: XX (ovaries), XX (tests), XY (ovaries), and XY (testes). Interestingly, the XX female sex chromosome complement increases survival in both male and female mice, which is further extended in combination with ovaries (Davis et al., 2019), suggesting that sex-linked genes play a larger determining factor in longevity than the sex-specific hormonal effect. Moreover, studies using the FCG mouse model have shown that sex chromosomes also contribute to an array of sexually dimorphic disease presentations, including atherosclerosis (Link et al., 2015) and ischemia-reperfusion injury in the heart (Li et al., 2014).

Abnormalities in sex chromosomes also negatively impact health in humans. Women with Turner syndrome (XO) show an elevated body mass index, a four-fold higher risk of developing type 2 diabetes, and are more susceptible to dying from cardiovascular disease–related complications (Mavinkurve & O'Gorman, 2015). In a similar vein, men with Klinefelter syndrome (XXY) are also more likely to develop cerebrovascular disease and type 2 diabetes, both of which are linked to metabolic irregularities (Calogero et al., 2017). Beyond these rare genetic abnormalities, sex differences are highly persistent, especially in the context of inflammation and autoimmunity. Many key genes involved in the innate and adaptive immune responses are located on the X chromosome. One such is forkhead box protein P3 (FoxP3), which plays an important role in T-cell activation. Subpopulations of T cells are strong predictors of sex outcomes in disease. For example, in cardiovascular disease, T-cell subpopulations in men and women show a disproportional bias between proinflammatory and antiinflammatory cytokine production: women have a higher production of IFNY, whereas men have a higher propensity to produce IL-17, a proinflammatory cytokine (M. A. Zhang et al., 2012). Conversely, women have nearly a 10-fold higher risk of developing systemic lupus nephritis (SLE), a severe autoimmune disease capable of leading to deleterious kidney damage. In this scenario, women with SLE show a change in the T-cell subpopulation toward elevated proinflammatory circulating T cells (Tedeschi et al., 2013). Therefore the role of sex chromosomes on our health and survival is highly sexually dimorphic and may serve as a strong predictor of male and female survival.

Mitochondrial inheritance is another example of sexual selective pressures. Though most genes are nuclear encoded, 13 are directly encoded in the mitochondria. As mitochondria are maternally transmitted, selective pressures on mitochondrial DNA mutations are female favored (Finch & Tower, 2014). Therefore it is conceivable that over evolutionary time, males may have a higher mitochondrial mutation load, aptly dubbed "mother's curse" (Gemmell et al., 2004). Evidence from fruit flies demonstrates that numerous mutations in the mitochondria negatively impact male aging (Camus et al., 2012). In higher organisms, the mitochondria are key players in physiologic responses. For example, studies on mitochondrial transplantation in mice wherein the nuclear genome is maintained but the mitochondria are switched indicate that it is a strong predictor in terms of health span and life span (Latorre-Pellicer et al., 2016). Moreover, numerous studies have explored the physiologic and functional differences between male and female mitochondria. In cardiac tissue, females have a higher number of functionally intact mitochondria and their associated DNA compared to males (Khalifa et al.,

2017). More intriguing, sex-specific differences in the mitochondria are evident early in the fetus. For example, maternal nutrient restriction, which can predispose offspring to kidney dysfunction and hypertension (Pereira et al., 2015), finds females to be more protected than males, partially due to differences in genes involved in mitochondrial respiration (Kett & Denton, 2011). In humans, much less work has focused on uncovering sex-dependent differences in mitochondrial-linked diseases. One prominent example is Leber's hereditary optic neuropathy (LHON), which shows a higher prevalence in males (Rosenberg et al., 2016). Overall, selective pressures that favor one sex over the other will result in higher risk of disease and mortality in a sex-specific pattern.

Sex differences are also not limited to genes solely found on the sex chromosomes. Moreover, as most mitochondrial genes are nuclear encoded, they also demonstrate a sex-specific signature. A wide array of autosomal genes has been identified to be differentially expressed in male and female tissue (Winkler et al., 2015). The liver was the first to suggest sexual dimorphism in gene expression, and these differences are amplified with age (Kwekel et al., 2010). Analyses of male and female brains (Berchtold et al., 2008) and cardiac tissue (Vijay et al., 2015) show a greater downregulation in mitochondrial genes in males compared to females. However, much more work is necessary to fully understand the role of sex on our health and survival.

Biologic Theories of Aging

The Benefit and Plight of Aerobic Organisms

Because we are aerobic organisms, oxygen is central to our existence; we rely on aerobic respiration to sustain life. Molecular oxygen is critical in adenosine-triphosphate (ATP) generation, the cell's biologic currency for energy production. Unlike anerobic respiration, which yields only two ATPs for every glycolytic reaction, mitochondrial oxidative phosphorylation, the primary source of ATP generation in aerobic respiration, produces 15 times that amount (~30 ATPs), highlighting the cellular efficiency of maximizing energy capture from one molecule of glucose. In consequence, more efficient energy production led to the transition from single cell to multitissue organisms.

In simplistic terms, oxidative phosphorylation (OXPHOS) is the flow of electrons through an electron transport chain, resulting in the unequal accumulation of positive charge (hydrogen protons, H^+) on one side of the mitochondrial membrane, forming a proton motive force. In turn, ATP synthase, the enzyme responsible for generating ATP, relies on the movement of hydrogen protons down their electrochemical gradient for ATP production. Oxygen is crucial during this process, so much so that the process consumes 80% of the oxygen we breathe. In turn, oxygen serves as the final electron acceptor in the electron transport chain (Fig. 1.2).

Our reliance on oxygen is largely due to its chemical properties. As a singular atom, oxygen is highly unstable, due

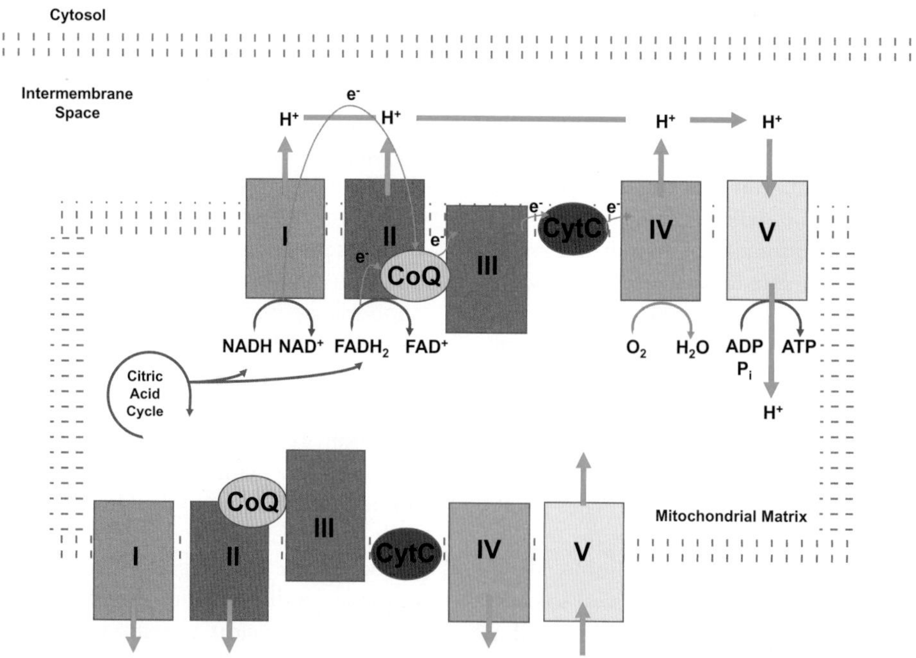

• **Fig. 1.2** Mitochondrial Electron Transport Chain. The mitochondrial electron transport chain (ETC) is located within the membrane of the mitochondrial matrix and comprises four complexes (I–IV) and electron transporters (coenzyme Q [CoQ] and cytochrome C [CytC]). The citric acid cycle generates two electron donors, NADH and $FADH_2$, which transfer their electrons to electron acceptors within complexes I and II. These electrons are passed through the ETC until they reach the final electron acceptor (O_2) to generate water. Concurrently, an electrochemical gradient is formed, with a higher concentration of protons sequestered within the intermembrane space compared to the concentration of protons in the mitochondrial matrix. As a result, the imbalance in protons enables them to flow down the proton gradient through complex V (ATP synthase), which drives the formation of ATP, the energy currency of the cell.

to an unpaired electron. Instead, it tends to bind to another molecule of oxygen to form molecular oxygen (O_2) or, in the case of the electron transport chain, two molecules of hydrogen. However, to maximize energy generation, movement of hydrogen to oxygen is not immediate. Rather, hydrogen molecules are moved via electron carriers (such as nicotinamide adenine dinucleotide, NAD^+, and the flavins [flavin mononucleotide, FMN, and flavin adenine dinucleotide, FAD]), which are continually cycled between oxidized (having a positive charge and being capable of accepting electrons) and reduced states (meaning neutral charge and being unable to accept electrons) until they reach the terminal electron acceptor, oxygen.

It is important to highlight, due to the instability of oxygen's chemical makeup, its desire to gain an electron. To overcome this, multiple enzymes of the electron transport chain, primarily cytochrome oxidase (Belevich et al., 2006), have evolved to chaperone oxygen as it moves from a partially reduced state (highly reactive and unstable) to its fully reduced and stable state. Yet no system is perfect. Approximately, 1% to 3% of semireduced, highly unstable oxygen (primarily in the form of the superoxide radical or hydroxyl radical) will escape. In turn, these highly unstable oxygen radicals will seek to gain an electron, pulling it from any neighboring protein, lipid, or molecule and initiating the radical chain reaction (Fig. 1.3).

Due to the high reliance of aerobic organisms on oxygen for energy production, it is no surprise that oxygen radicals represent the most abundant radical species generated in living organisms. Collectively termed *reactive oxygen species (ROS)*, which include both oxygen radicals and certain nonradicals, such as hydrogen peroxide, they can be easily converted into radicals (Miller et al.,1990). Though we have focused mainly on the mitochondria, other endogenous cellular sources—such as cytochrome P450 (Bondy & Naderi, 1994), peroxisomes (Del Río & López-Huertas, 2016), enzymes involved in inflammatory pathways (Biswas et al., 2017), and any "free" metals released from metalloprotein complexes and enabling Fenton chemistry (Fridovich, 2013; Miller et al., 1990)—contribute to ROS generation. As well, exogenous sources, such as ionizing radiation, pollution, heavy metals, and tobacco, can further contribute to the cellular ROS load.

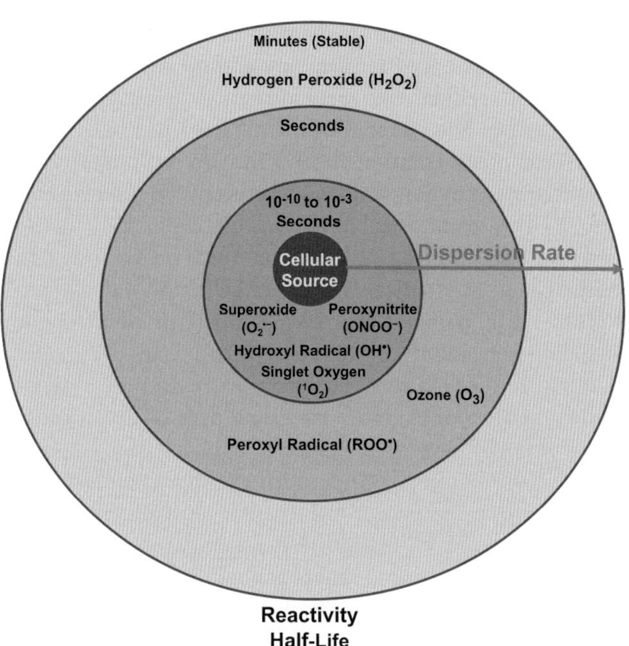

• **Fig. 1.3** Cellular Dispersion Rate of Free Radicals. Highly reactive free radicals (such as superoxide and the hydroxyl radical) are unstable and destructive but have a short half-life and, as a result, a limited radius for damage. In contrast, more stable species, such as hydrogen peroxide, have much less damage but have a much longer half-life; consequently they can disperse a greater radius within the cell.

Fortunately, we have evolved multiple cellular defense pathways to combat oxidative cellular damage. Within the mitochondria, superoxide dismutase reduces the highly reactive superoxide radical to hydrogen peroxide, which in turn is further reduced to water by catalase. Within the cytosol, multiple enzymes serve to maintain the cellular redox balance, including glutathione reductase. Moreover, secondary repair and removal systems, such as protein turnover mediated by the ubiquitin-proteasome-system (UPS), autophagy, DNA repair systems, and mitochondrial biogenesis, are all instrumental in cellular homeostasis.

The Free Radical Theory of Aging: Is It Relevant?

In general, aging describes the deleterious decline in the efficacy of physiologic processes necessary to maintain homeostasis. Aging represents not only the leading risk factor for the development of age-associated pathologies, including cardiovascular disease (Paneni et al., 2017), type 2 diabetes (Jaacks et al., 2016; Ligthart et al., 2016), cancer (Shay, 2016), and neurodegenerative decline (Baker & Petersen, 2018), but it is the driving force behind geriatric syndromes such as frailty, immobility, and incontinence (Hazzard & Halter, 2009). Though multiple theories have been developed and tested, there is no known definitive cause of aging. At the cellular level, aging is manifested by the gradual accumulation of molecular damage, resulting from a decline/failure of repair/clearance pathways (Kirkwood, 2005), in turn leading to an unfavorable homeostatic imbalance between damage clearance and aggregation, becoming highly evident in the last one-third of life (Levine & Stadtman, 2001). However, the mechanism by which this damage is initiated is not clear. Multiple theories have been proposed to help fill this gap, one of the most notable being the free radical theory of aging.

The free radical theory of aging, first hypothesized by Denham Harman (Harman, 1956), has greatly shaped the direction of aging research. The free radical theory of aging is based on Harman's observational findings linking the similarities between aerobic respiration and irradiation. In both processes, highly reactive free radicals are generated, the most notable being the hydroxyl (·OH) and superoxide ($O_2^{\cdot-}$) radicals (Harman, 1956), and the less reactive nonradical, hydrogen peroxide (H_2O_2). Harman postulated that if these highly unstable and reactive molecules are not removed or neutralized, they damage cellular macromolecules (proteins, lipids, and DNA) either directly or indirectly (via Fenton chemistry) (Fridovich, 2013). Hence his theory, when first proposed, was believed to be the driving force of aging:

Deleterious side attacks of free radicals (which are normally produced in the course of cellular metabolism) on cell constituents and on the connective tissues (Harman, 1956, p. 298). Harman's hypothesis was highly appealing because if "harmful" molecules were removed, their deleterious impact on cellular integrity would be blunted, and thus too the aging process. Several lines of evidence lend support to Harman's hypothesis, including the age-dependent rise in DNA, lipid, and protein damage, which is consistent across multiple species and tissues (Bokov et al., 2004). Skin fibroblasts from a wide-array of rodents demonstrate a correlation between increased life span and increased resistance to H_2O_2 (Harper et al., 2007) and maintenance of protein quality control (Pickering et al., 2014, 2015). Studies in longer-lived species also indicate lower levels of oxidative damage or increased resistance; for example, mutations in the insulin/IGF-1 signaling pathway are shown to increase survival in worms (Ishii et al., 2002), flies (Kabil et al., 2007; M. C. Wang et al., 2003), and mice (Holzenberger et al., 2003). Similarly, longevity-promoting dietary interventions, such as chronic caloric restriction, have also been implicated to lower levels of oxidative stress (Redman et al., 2018). Studies of muscle tissue from rhesus monkeys have demonstrated that elevated 4-hydroxynonenal (4-HNE), a marker of lipid peroxidation, occurs with increasing age, which was blunted under caloric restriction (Zainal et al., 2000). Conversely, genetic manipulations, which deleteriously impact DNA repair systems and are necessary to remove damage, show signs of accelerated aging and shortened life span (Vermeij et al., 2016). These findings all lend evidence to support the free radical theory—lowering chronic oxidative stress promotes longevity.

Along with this, much of the early work in free radical biology concentrated efforts on the removal of all potentially damaging free radicals. Antioxidants, either formed in vivo or obtained from the diet, are broadly defined as "any substance that, when present at low concentrations compared with those of an oxidizable substate (protein, lipid, DNA), significantly delays or prevents oxidation of the substrate" (Halliwell & Gutteridge, 2015, p. 3–20). They work by a variety of mechanisms, including catalytically removing reactive species, preventing their formation, or serving as enzymes that protect biomolecules from oxidative damage. Copper-zinc superoxide dismutase (CuZnSOD, also known as SOD1) is probably one of the most well-studied enzymes to protect against free radical damage. CuZnSOD is highly efficient at catalyzing the very reactive superoxide radical (primarily generated from the electron transport leak) into the less reactive hydrogen peroxide, which is subsequently further reduced by catalase into water. As the majority of superoxide is derived from the mitochondria (electron transport chain leak), an additional variant known as manganese superoxide dismutase (MnSOD, also known as SOD2 due to the substitution of manganese as its cofactor) also serves to directly eliminate this strong oxygen radical (Zelko et al., 2002). Another important antioxidant enzyme is glutathione peroxidase (GPx), which removes hydrogen peroxide by coupling its reaction with water and reduced glutathione (GSH). Under homeostatic conditions the ratio between reduced and oxidized glutathione is high, which is not surprising as GSH serves as an antioxidant because it can directly reduce highly reactive radicals, including the hydroxyl radical (Halliwell & Gutteridge, 2015).

Following the discovery of the mitochondrial genome, an offshoot of the free radical theory of aging was developed in the form of the mitochondrial free radical theory of aging, which suggests the mitochondria (more specifically, subunits of the mitochondrial electron transport chain) are the central source of reactive oxygen species and the primary source for mitochondrial DNA damage. As a result, the accumulation of damaged mitochondrial DNA can perpetuate this cycle by leading to the formation of defective electron transport chain components and further elevating reactive oxygen species (Miquel et al., 1980). To counteract damage, a major approach focused on using antioxidants as a means of eliminating all free radicals. In the 1970s, Linus Pauling first proposed high intake of the antioxidant vitamin C to promote health and prevent common viral infections (Pauling, 1976), based on the assumption that high levels of antioxidants could remove any and all free radicals and thus prevent cellular damage. However, systemic reviews and meta-analyses have since shown a different conclusion: antioxidant supplementation has no impact on longevity, nor does it prevent major cardiovascular events (Bjelakovic et al., 2007). This paradoxical outcome highlights the nuances between cells and free radicals. Too much or too long of an onslaught in free radicals can overwhelm and damage multiple cellular systems. However, short-term nondamaging signaling is necessary to activate a broad array of pathways and repair mechanisms. For example, exercise training, a known inducer of oxidative stress and necessary to stimulate mitochondrial biogenesis, is shown, upon exogenous administration of vitamin C, to dampen the mitochondrial turnover and repair pathways and to lower antioxidant enzymes (Gomez-Cabrera et al., 2008). Together, these examples highlight three points: (1) more is not always better, as complete elimination of free radicals eliminates cellular signaling; (2) free radicals serve as signaling molecules within the cell; and (3) free radical generation is a component of the transient homeostatic response. Thus a limitation of the free radical theory of aging is the assumption of an all-or-nothing approach—that is, that all free radicals are detrimental and are the primary drivers behind aging.

Yet no system is perfect. Many of these cellular protective pathways, though efficient, are unable to eliminate all cellular damage. With age, the ability to maintain balance between cellular damage accrual and removal diminishes, resulting in an accumulation of oxidized, nonfunctioning macromolecules. Early work has demonstrated that with increasing age is a linear increase in 8-hydroxy-2'-deoxyguanosine (8-OHdG), a marker of DNA oxidation (de La Asunción et al., 1996). Protein homeostasis is also crucial in preventing a wide range of age-related diseases because protein misfolding and aggregation are associated with cellular toxicity and disease pathology (Balch et al., 2008). Interestingly, protein aggregation is not a linear process throughout the life span but rather shows an exponential rise in the final one-third of life (Levine & Stadtman, 2001). A key enzyme in protein homeostasis is the 20 S proteasome, which is necessary for the turnover of oxidized proteins. However, increasing age is accompanied by a diminished pool of enzymatically active 20 S proteasome, tilting the scale in favor of protein aggregation. In contrast, the disaggregation of protein clumps has been shown to restore proteasome activity in aged cells (Andersson et al., 2013).

It is important to note that the loss of protein homeostasis is not a universal trait in aged animals. Specifically, many long-lived species, such as the naked mole rat, seem to contradict the free radical theory of aging. Unlike most laboratory mouse or rat species, which have an average life span of 3 to 4 years, the naked mole rat reportedly can live up to 25 years but has a higher rate of oxidative damage (Hekimi et al., 2011). Additionally, evidence from nematode worms show mutations in complex 1 of the mitochondrial electron transport chain, which leads to increased oxidative stress and results in an *increased* life span compared to controls (Yang & Hekimi, 2010). Both examples demonstrate opposition to the free radical theory of aging, suggesting a more nuanced and dynamic hypothesis is necessary.

Adaptive Homeostasis

A shortcoming in the free radical theory of aging is its static perspective on a dynamic system. Much research has focused on manipulating levels of stress-protective enzymes. For example, transgenic and knockout mouse lines are used to overexpress or knock out these stress-responsive enzymes, respectively, in order to ascertain if a key antioxidant enzyme is important to overall survival. These studies have yielded mixed results, either in support of or against the free radical theory of aging. For example, the majority of studies using genetic manipulations of oxidative stress genes showed that few had an effect on life span (Pérez et al., 2009). Only enzymes that are necessary for transcriptional activation, such as nuclear factor erythroid 2-related factor 2 (Nrf2) (Pomatto et al., 2020), or those that lack cellular redundancy in their activity, such as superoxide dismutase (SOD1) (Elchuri et al., 2005), or those that serve multiple roles in the cell, such as cytochrome B5 reductase (Martin-Montalvo et al., 2016), showed a significant impact on survival.

However, a major limitation in all these studies is a lack of system perturbation. Specifically, the primary role of many stress-responsive enzymes is to respond to short-term and transient cellular insults. For example, under oxidative stress, Nrf2 translocates into the nucleus, wherein it binds to antioxidant response elements (ARE) and activates a plethora of phase II and stress-protective enzymes (L. C. D. Pomatto & Davies, 2018; H. Zhang et al., 2015). In turn, increased levels of stress-responsive enzymes protect against any oxidative damage. Once any associated damage is cleared, levels of stress-protective enzymes return to baseline (L. C. D. Pomatto & Davies, 2018; L. C. D. Pomatto, Sun, & Davies, 2019). Thus a limitation in many of these earlier studies exploring the necessity of stress-protective enzymes on life span were completed in nonperturbed states.

Adaptive homeostasis, which is a modification of the free radical theory of aging, aims to address this gap and is described as "the transient expansion or contraction of the homeostatic range in response to exposure to sub-toxic, non-damaging, signaling molecules or events, or the removal or cessation of such molecules or events" (Davies, 2016, p. 1–7). Unlike the free radical theory of aging, which takes a binary viewpoint toward free radicals (all are negative), adaptive homeostasis utilizes the concept that low, nondamaging levels of free radicals serve as signaling molecules that are necessary and vital for intracellular communication. For example, nondamaging doses of H_2O_2 (in the picomolar to micromolar range) have been shown in yeast (Davies et al., 1995), mammalian cells (Pickering et al., 2012), nematode worms (Pickering et al., 2013; Raynes et al., 2017), and fruit flies (Pickering et al., 2013; L. C. Pomatto et al., 2017) to stimulate upregulation of various stress-protective enzymes, including the 20 S proteasome. In turn, upregulation of multiple cellular repair and stress-protective pathways enables these organisms to better withstand a semilethal exposure to the same oxidant (typically in the millimolar to molar range, a ~1000-fold higher concentration). Moreover, this response is transient, typically lasting up to 16 hours before downstream targets return to basal levels (Pickering et al., 2012). Yet with age, the adaptive homeostatic response becomes more sluggish and compressed. Specifically, studies in aged worms and flies show a loss in the ability to activate the stress response, evident by no change in the 20 S proteasome levels or activity (Pomatto, Sun, Yu, et al., 2017; Raynes et al., 2017). Similarly, mammalian cells exposed to chronically high levels of oxygen (the in vitro "accelerated aging" model) demonstrate an inability to upregulate stress protective enzymes (Pomatto, Sun, Yu, et al., 2019). In both instances, basal levels of multiple stress responsive enzymes increase, but upon transient stimulation, they cannot be induced further, suggesting the adaptive response is compressed. These findings are important because they highlight the dynamic response evident in young organisms, which becomes nonexistent with age. Moreover, it extends upon the free radical theory of aging, which simply argues that aging is a result of accumulated oxidative damage, without taking into consideration the necessity for transient and short-term responses to cope with day-to-day variations in the cellular environment.

Inflammaging

A major hallmark of aging is elevated and persistent inflammation, largely attributed to poor diet, increased adiposity, advanced age, reduced sex hormones, and sedentary lifestyle (Freund et al., 2010). Three of the most prevalent proinflammatory markers are interleukin-6 (IL-6), tumor necrosis factor (TNFα), and C-reactive protein (CRP). In turn, these biomarkers of inflammation are highly predictive of an individual's risk for morbidity and mortality (Franceschi et al., 2017), as many age-related diseases, such as type 2 diabetes, cardiovascular disease, and cancer, have a higher prevalence in individuals with chronic low-grade inflammation. Indeed, in neurologic diseases, such as Alzheimer disease (AD), which is largely characterized by chronic inflammation, many of these proinflammatory cytokines are involved in the production and processing of the insoluble and pathologic form of the amyloid-beta peptide, which is a hallmark of AD (Giunta et al., 2008). Moreover, increasing age is accompanied by increased concentrations of inflammatory markers, with older adults showing a much higher level compared to younger individuals (Singh & Newman, 2011).

Despite its negative perception, the ability to activate a robust inflammatory response is necessary for our survival from infancy to child-bearing years because the immune system is our primary defense against pathogenic infections and antigens. However, over the life course the continual challenge to a wide array of stressors (including infections, exogenous damage, and poor clearance of cellular molecules), all of which can induce an immune response, can eventually push the immune system toward a proinflammatory state. This perpetual state of chronic, low-grade inflammation, evident with age, was first coined by Claudio Franceschi as "inflamm-aging" (Franceschi et al., 2000). This was originally introduced as an offshoot of the remodeling theory of aging, which argues there is a continual push-pull between internal and external stressors and the repair and removal systems necessary to combat them; however, with age these defense pathways wane, causing us to age. More specifically, inflammaging is the result of excessive stimulation of the proinflammatory pathways over the lifetime and ineffective means of dampening these responses with age, leading to chronic inflammation, and these are the driving forces behind age-related diseases (Morrisette-Thomas et al., 2014). According to Franceschi, two criteria must be reached before inflammation turns into disease. He proposed a "two-hit hypothesis," which suggests an individual's susceptibility toward inflammation is highly dependent on chronic exposure of inflammatory stimuli over the lifetime (the "first hit"), which when coupled with poor gene variants (the "second hit") will accelerate chronic inflammation into an inflammatory-based disease (atherosclerosis, type 2 diabetes, cancer, and AD) (Franceschi et al., 2017). Paradoxically, centenarians have been identified to have high serum levels of proinflammatory markers (the first hit), including IL-6, IL-18, and CRP, but unlike their counterparts who fall susceptible to frailty and disease, they show high levels of antiinflammatory molecules including TGF-β1 and cortisol (Franceschi et al., 2007). This suggests that it is not so much the level of proinflammatory markers but rather that balance maintenance between these pro- and antiinflammatory markers that makes the difference.

Fortunately, dietary modifications and increased physical activity can slow the age-related inflammatory state. Indeed, many chronic proinflammatory diseases are also linked to a sedentary lifestyle, wherein physically inactive adults show higher basal levels of inflammatory markers. In part, this is due to increased adipose tissue. Originally thought to be an inert organ, adipose tissue is highly proinflammatory and has been shown to have increased production of TNFα and IL-6 and secretion of immune cell attracting factors (Fried et al., 2018). Moreover, physical inactivity is linked to elevated glucose and hyperinsulinemia, as inflammatory cytokines can interfere with insulin signaling, resulting in insulin resistance, a hallmark of type 2 diabetes (T2D) (Lumeng & Saltiel, 2011). Yet despite the ability of exercise to delay Franceschi's first-hit criteria for inflammaging, only 50% of US adults achieve the recommended amount of daily physical activity, which sharply declines upon increasing age, with less than 5% of US adults over age 60 reaching this mark (Macera et al., 2005). In contrast, increased exercise in aged adults is shown to markedly lower CRP levels. In the National Health and Nutrition Examination Survey III of more than 13,000 adults, participants showed an age-adjusted odds ratio for an elevated CRP of 0.78, 0.59, and 0.3 for light, moderate, and vigorous physical activity (Ford, 2002), respectively. Moreover, a period of only 12 weeks of moderate exercise was found to lower levels of the proinflammatory marker, TNFα (Onambélé-Pearson et al., 2010). Additionally, changes in dietary intake, such as caloric restriction (Kalani et al., 2006) or time-restricted feeding (Longo & Panda, 2016; Sutton et al., 2018), have also been shown to help lower the inflammatory burden.

Dietary Interventions to Longevity

Caloric Restriction

Chronic caloric restriction (CR) is the leading and most well-studied nonpharmaceutical intervention to promote longevity and improve the health span. A seemingly simple approach, CR is a dietary intervention wherein an organism reduces its total caloric intake chronically throughout its life span, while maintaining sufficient intake of essential micronutrients. In the early 1900s, Francis Peyton Rous was the first to demonstrate that reduced food consumption led to lower spontaneous tumorigenesis in rats (Rous, 1914), a finding highly relevant to the gerontology field as it presented a means of slowing carcinogenesis, which is largely an age-dependent disease (Rozhok & DeGregori, 2016). Subsequently, Osborne and Mendel demonstrated that caloric and nutrient restriction not only increased life span in female rats but consequently delayed sexual maturity, providing early evidence for the antagonistic pull between growth versus survival and repair pathways (Osborne et al., 1917).

Yet it was not until the work of McCay and colleagues wherein CR was largely recognized for its ability to extend life span. More important, unlike earlier studies, their findings were the first to demonstrate increased survival that was solely the result of decreasing total calories, rather than a combination of nutrient and caloric reduction, which had been previously employed and resulted in premature death and shortened life span (Drummond et al., 1938). In their studies, the researchers divided rats into three treatment groups: the first group had unlimited food access (ad libitum), and the second two groups were either restricted from weaning or weaned and allowed to grow for 2 weeks before restriction. In both instances, rats on the restricted diets survived significantly longer than their ad libitum controls (McCay et al., 1935). A key finding from their studies was the unequal survival across the sexes: though male rats showed significant increase in life span, females, when subjected to the same CR regime, showed no change in survival (McCay et al., 1935). Later studies have since shown that the beneficial gains in CR-mediated survival are highly contingent on the sex and strain of the rodent (Forster et al., 2003; Mitchell et al., 2016). Additionally, McCay thought the combination of nutrient deficiency coupled with reduced caloric intake would cause not only delayed growth but metabolic deficiencies. Concurrent studies demonstrated McCay's point, as a combination of reduced overall calories coupled with inadequate levels of vitamin B, calcium, or protein led to premature death and shortened life spans in rats (Drummond et al., 1938; Sherman et al., 1937).

Since these influential studies, CR has consistently been shown to improve survival in yeast, worms, flies, and rodents. However, as an organism's complexity increases (i.e., from yeast upward to humans), the gain in longevity decreases. Yeast and worms show the greatest life span gain (1000% increase in survival), whereas flies show only a maximum of 60% to 70% improved longevity, which is further compressed in mice, demonstrating only a 30% to 50% increased life span in response to CR (Fontana et al., 2010). Even less is known about whether chronic CR is capable of increasing life span in humans (or the least-stringent level of CR that is beneficial); however, studies in humans who practice CR (at an approximately 18% restriction) show a reduced risk for cardiovascular disease, type 2 diabetes, and cancer.

Work in nonhuman primates paints a more nuanced picture of the relationship between CR and longevity. Two concurrent studies in nonhuman primates (NHPs), one conducted at the National Institute on Aging (NIA) and the other at the University of Wisconsin, found drastically different results in CR-mediated life span improvement. The NIA study found no increase in survival in NHPs subjected to 30% CR (Mattison et al., 2012), whereas the Wisconsin study showed increased life span and overall reduction in all-cause mortality (Colman et al., 2009). Though highly controversial at the time, seemingly minor differences in study design have come to the forefront as potential causes for these opposing outcomes. Genetic differences (the Wisconsin primates originated from India, whereas the NIA primates originated from China and India) along with timing and food access (Fig. 1.4) highlight the importance of consistency in implementing the CR regime (Mattison et al., 2017). In-depth comparison found the Wisconsin feeding protocol implemented unrestricted food access (ad libitum) to better represent human eating habits. In contrast, the NIA approach regulated portioning of the ad libitum group in order to prevent stomach complications due to gorging. Additionally, further investigation into these two studies found that upon exclusion of animals that died from acute non–age-related conditions, control animals had nearly a threefold increased likelihood of death compared to CR animals (Mattison et al., 2017), suggesting that CR can delay age-associated death.

One of the most highly contested differences in the study was dietary composition. Though both diets contained 60% carbohydrates, the NIA diet was higher in protein (17.3% versus 13.1% in the Wisconsin study) and fiber (6.5% to 9.0% NIA versus 5% Wisconsin), and lower in fat (5% NIA versus 10.6% Wisconsin) and sucrose (3.9% NIA versus 28.5% Wisconsin). Moreover, unlike the NIA diet, which was naturally sourced, the Wisconsin diet was semipurified, which contributed to differences in macronutrient content (Mattison et al., 2017; Mitchell et al., 2019). This finding was highly insightful, as it reopened the question of whether dietary composition, rather than simply blanket reduction in overall caloric intake as originally postulated by McCay, was the driving force behind increased life span. To address this finding, male C57BL/6J mice were fed either the NIA or the Wisconsin chow diets and subdivided into three treatment groups: ad-libitum (AL) controls, 30% chronic CR, and meal-fed (MF). The mice on MF received the same amount of food as the mice on AL, but instead of constant food access they received all their food once per day. Paradoxically, dietary composition (NIA versus Wisconsin) had no impact on survival. In both dietary groups, AL mice had the shortest life span, followed by MF, and the longest in chronic CR (Mitchell et al., 2019). These findings were important because they emphasized that, at least in mice, CR-mediated longevity was independent of dietary composition. These findings highlight a confounding variable with many CR-studies: time-restricted feeding. For example, most CR protocols provide the food allotment once per day. As a result, mice rapidly consume the allotted food and, consequently, undergo a large fasting period (~18 to 21 hours). Accordingly, we face a crossroads in deducing whether it is the overall reduction in CR or its accompanying fasting period that serves as the predominant driving force behind life span extension. Interestingly, work exploring the

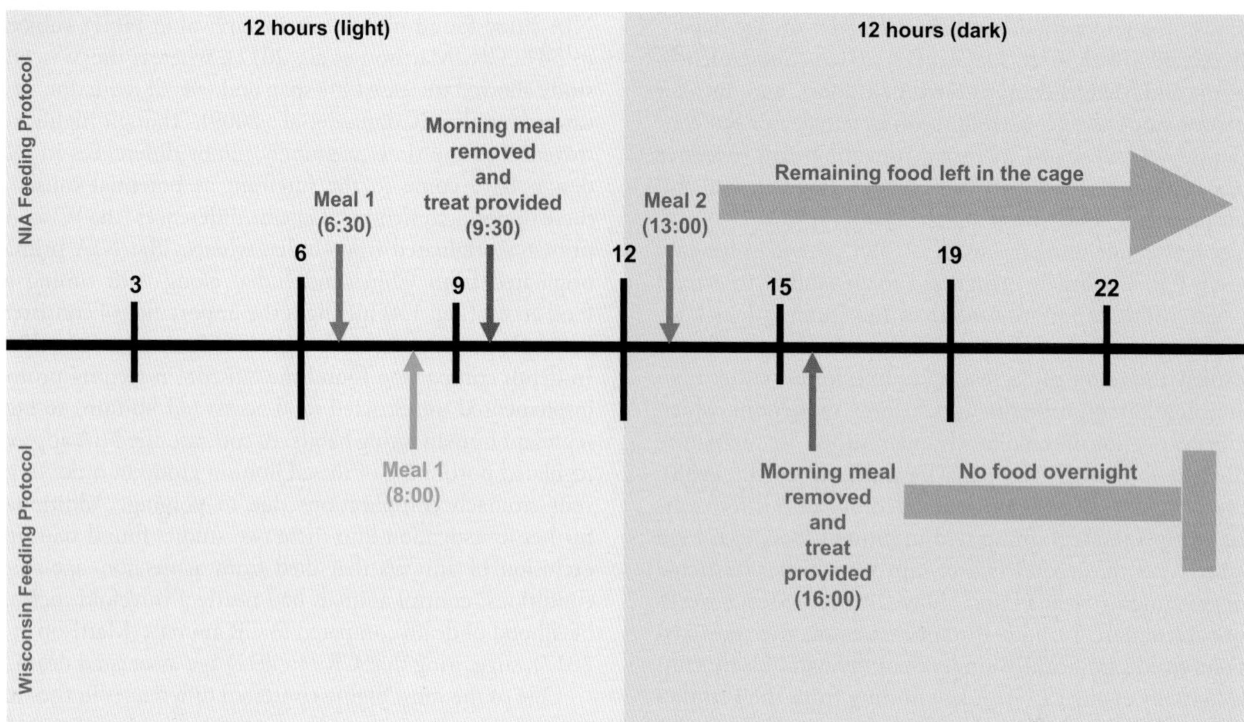

• **Fig. 1.4** Caloric Restriction (CR) Feeding Protocols Used at the National Institute on Aging (NIA) and University of Wisconsin in Nonhuman Primates (NHP). A major controversy within the aging field occurred from the opposing results from the NIA (no differences in life span in CR-fed NHP compared to controls) versus those obtained in the University of Wisconsin CR study in NHP (increased life span in CR-fed NHP compared to controls). Since publication, identification of dietary composition, genetic heterogeneity in founding NHP populations, and feeding protocol were the leading variables to account for these differences. Specifically, within the feeding protocol the major difference was food access. The NIA feeding protocol *(top panel)* left any remaining food after the second meal. As a result, animals could continually snack on this food until their morning feeding. In contrast, the Wisconsin feeding protocol *(bottom panel)* removed any remaining food, imposing a 16-hour fasting period on the animals.

role of nutrient composition on survival, wherein CR was inadvertently introduced into the study due to dietary dilution, found no increase in survival, as mice had the ability to continually eat (thus eliminating the time-restricted feeding component) (Solon-Biet et al., 2014).

Alternatives to Caloric Restriction

Though seemingly novel, interest in alternatives to CR began as early as the 1930s. Whereas McCay and his colleagues sought to use chronic CR as a means of understanding the driving mechanisms behind CR-mediated life span extension, others were focused on the practicality of chronic CR in humans. For example, the broadly termed *intermittent fasting (IF)*, first demonstrated in rats subjected to repeated cycles of 1 day fasting and 2 days refeeding and subsequent increased survival (Carlson & Hoelzel, 1946), sparked the quest to identify less stringent and feasible alternatives to CR. Since then, multiple forms of IF have evolved, the most popular of which included alternate day fasting, whole day fasting, and time-restricted feeding (Fig. 1.5). It is important to note there is no uniform experimental regime, as some studies allowed for a small caloric intake during fasting days (approximately 25% baseline daily caloric consumption), whereas others allowed for water-only fasting, study duration, and participant characteristics, including body weight, age, and sex. Yet even with all these variabilities, improvements were notable.

Alternate Day Fasting

Alternate day fasting (ADF) refers to 1 fasting day (consisting of water-only fasting or the consumption of ~25% baseline calories) followed by 1 day of unrestricted eating. Studies in mice show improvement in life span (Goodrick et al., 1990) but little impact on improving markers of health (Xie et al., 2017). In humans, studies using short-term alternate day fasting (water-only) for 22 days showed a 0.5% and 1% loss in body weight and fat mass, respectively, and a drop in serum triglycerides (males only) (Heilbronn et al., 2005). In overweight or obese premenopausal women, a 6-month, randomized clinical trial found fasting for 2 nonconsecutive days per week showed improved physiologic measures (reduced body weight, fat mass, and waist circumference) and reduced serum concentration of total and low-density lipoprotein (LDL) cholesterol, triglycerides, C-reactive protein, and arterial blood pressures (Harvie et al., 2011). Additional studies utilizing alternate-day fasting or intermittent fasting showed similar drops in body weight (Eshghinia & Mohammadzadeh, 2013; Johnson et al.,

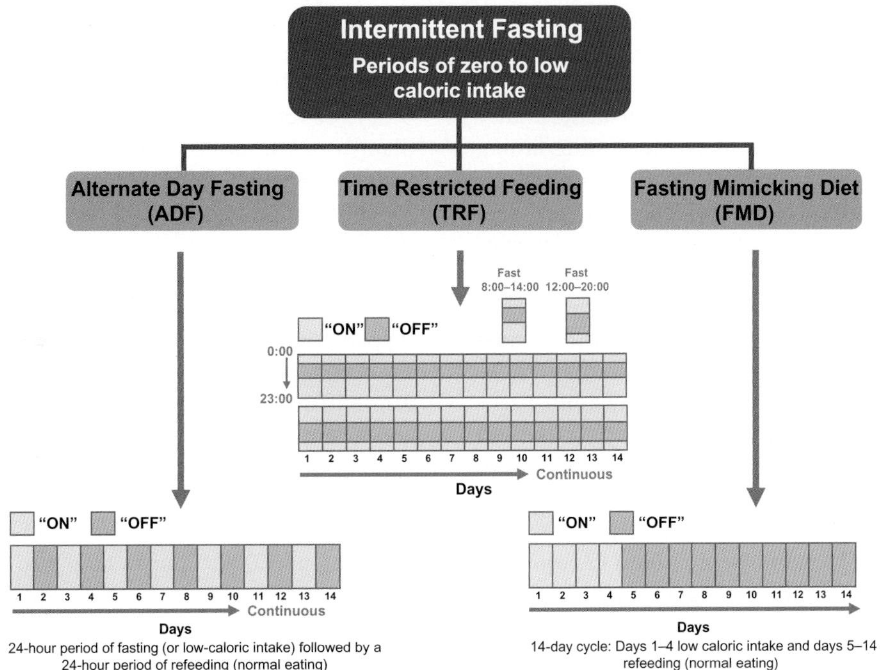

• **Fig. 1.5** Different Forms of Intermittent Fasting. Intermittent fasting (IF) is a broadly defined term used to encompass dietary interventions that combine periods of low caloric intake followed by periods of ad libitum eating. Alternative day fasting (ADF) refers to a 48-hour cycle wherein the first 24-hour period consists of low-to-zero caloric intake (dubbed the "ON" portion of the cycle) and the following 24-hour period consists of refeeding (ad libitum eating). The cycles can be repeated continuously. Time restricted feeding (TRF) occurs over a 24-hour cycle wherein food is consumed only within an 8-hour (or shorter) feeding window. The typical windows tested are 0800 to 1400 and 1200 to 2000 (dubbed "OFF"). The remaining 16-hours are spent fasting (dubbed "ON"). The cycles can be repeated continuously. The fasting mimicking diet (FMD) refers to a 14-day cycle wherein subjects consume a very low calorie, plant-based diet for the first 4 days (dubbed "ON"), followed by 10 days of refeeding/ad libitum eating (dubbed "OFF").

2007; Varady et al., 2013). Comparison studies exploring the impact of chronic CR (25% reduction in total daily caloric intake), ADF (alternating days of 25% baseline caloric intake or unlimited food intake), or moderate exercise (three times per week) found all three showed similar reductions in body weight (Varady et al., 2011). Further studies found ADF alone or in combination with moderate exercise could significantly lower body weight and improve markers of cardiovascular health (Bhutani et al., 2013). Similar benefits were evident with whole-day fasting (which consists of 1 to 2 days per week of water-only or severe caloric restriction), with improvements matching those undergoing chronic CR (Harvie et al., 2011; Teng et al., 2013). It is important to note that the variability in study design, including participant characteristics (age, weight, and sex), along with the number of fasting days per week and consecutive versus nonconsecutive days, makes it difficult to pinpoint which experimental modification would maximize the greatest health gains.

Time-Restricted Feeding

Time-restricted feeding (TRF), which is another form of IF, consists of 12 to 20 hours of daily food restriction. The first clinical trial of TRF showed the beneficial gains in restricting food access to one meal per day during a 4-hour timeframe in the evening, without limiting caloric intake. After 8 weeks, the treatment group showed decreased body weight and fat mass, with mixed results on markers of cardiovascular health, compared to controls, which consumed three meals per day (Tinsley & La Bounty, 2015). Interestingly, though the study was designed to have no limitation on calories consumed, the treatment group showed an average decrease in caloric intake. However, a limitation of the study was the large attrition rate (26%) because of the limited eating window or other health related issues independent the study.

Less-stringent forms of TRF, specifically a wider feeding window, have garnered increasing interest, specifically the 8-hour eating and 16-hour fasting paradigm. Studies in mice found that limiting food access to an 8-hour daily window reduced weight gain when subjected to a high-fat diet (Hatori et al., 2012). In humans much less is known, especially as some individuals inadvertently practice the 8-hour feeding/16-hour fasting by skipping breakfast and not eating after dinner. This approach, though much less stringent than the one meal per day option (4-hour eating window), was predicted to be relatively feasible in healthy adults. However, intriguing findings from Panda and company debunked our conventional belief that healthy adults consume all their calories within a 12-hour span (three meals per day). Instead, they found eating patterns were erratic and varied between weekdays and weekends, with only a short time frame (5 hours between 1 a.m. and 6 a.m.) when food was not consumed (Gill & Panda, 2015; Gupta et al., 2017). These findings were important because they demonstrated the inability for a metabolic resting/fasting state due to the high frequency of food consumption, tilting the metabolic phase toward a constant postprandial state. More recent studies have demonstrated the beneficial gains in practicing TRF in patients with metabolic dysfunction. For example, participants with metabolic syndrome showed improved physiologic and cardiovascular markers (decreased body weight, waist circumference, blood pressure, and LDL cholesterol) when limiting food consumption within a self-selected 10-hour daily window for 12 weeks (Wilkinson et al., 2020). Men diagnosed with type 2 diabetes showed improved glucose and insulin response following 7 days of TRF, irrespective of whether the eating phase was in the morning (8 a.m. to 5 p.m.) or evening (12 p.m. to 8 p.m.). Fasting blood glucose was significantly improved only in the 8 a.m. to 5 p.m. eating window. These findings, irrespective the feeding window (morning versus evening), show a significant improvement in the glycemic response (Hutchison et al., 2019). A similar outcome was evident in a shorter feeding window (8 a.m. to 2 p.m.) (Jamshed et al., 2019), coupled with a reduction in appetite and increased fat utilization in overweight adults (Ravussin et al., 2019). Other studies have also shown that TRF is a feasible intervention in overweight, sedentary older adults (≥ 65 years). Eight weeks of 8-hour feeding/16-hour fasting cycles showed decreased body weight and improved gait speed (decreased gait speed is a clinical marker of frailty) (Anton et al., 2019).

TRF may also serve as a practical approach for weight loss and other metabolic markers in young healthy adults. Young women (mean age 21) who completed 4 weeks of TRF (using an 8-hour eating window between 12 p.m. to 8 p.m.) showed a decrease in body weight (~0.5 kg), and when coupled with strength training, these subjects experienced an additional decrease in fat mass (~0.7 kg) (Smith et al., 2017). A significant increase in gut microbiota diversity was also evident in healthy males undergoing 16 hours of daily fasting for 25 days (Zeb et al., 2020). Interestingly, studies using TRF in pediatric mice (younger than 4 weeks) with subsequent shifting to AL feeding in adulthood showed detrimental effects, including increased body weight, increased blood glucose levels, poor immune function, and retarded growth (Hu et al., 2019). These findings highlight the importance (and lack of our current understanding) of the age of intervention and the level of fasting necessary to maximize the health and longevity benefits from TRF.

The Fasting Mimicking Diet

The fasting mimicking diet (FMD) is a plant-based diet designed to mimic the benefits of fasting (i.e., lowered serum levels of IGF-1 and glucose and increased levels of ketone bodies) (Brandhorst et al., 2015; Wei et al., 2017), without the burden of fasting by providing necessary micro- and macronutrients through specially designed meal substitutes. During the "on" cycle of the intervention, which consists of 5 days of very low caloric intake, participants are provided plant-based meal substitutes: the first day provides approximately 4600 kJ, which is subsequently lowed to 3000 kJ for the remaining 4 days. During the "off" cycle following the 5-day reduced caloric intake, participants can resume their normal food consumption for 20 days, at which point the cycle is repeated. A phase 2 clinical trial in healthy participants who completed three cycles of the FMD regime showed a decrease in physiologic markers (body weight, waist circumference, body mass index [BMI], and body fat) and serum IGF-1 levels. Additionally, a 3-month follow-up study found the beneficial gains were retained (Wei et al., 2017). The FMD regime has also been tested and shown to be beneficial in mice for resisting autoimmune diseases (Choi et al., 2016; Rangan et al., 2019), slowing primary tumor growth (when coupled with chemotherapy) (Di Biase et al., 2016), and promoting longevity (Brandhorst et al., 2015). However, much more research is necessary to fully elucidate if the FMD regime is a viable and long-term approach to promote longevity in humans.

Can We Drug Our Way to Longevity?

The use of chronic caloric restriction (CR) offers researchers not only a method to increase life span and delay age-associated diseases, but a means of uncovering longevity-promoting pathways. In turn, activation of these nutrient-sensing cascades is evident at the physiologic level, leading to notable improvements in body weight loss (predominantly fat mass), lowered blood glucose levels, and improved insulin sensitivity. Concurrently, evidence suggests CR leads to a significant decrease in proinflammatory signals (including tumor necrosis factor alpha) and a reduction in cardiometabolic risk factors (lower systolic blood pressure, triglycerides, and cholesterol) (Most et al., 2018; Ravussin et al., 2015), with the beneficial effects further amplified in obese individuals (Dube et al., 2011). Overall, studies ranging from yeast to humans indicate the beneficial improvement to health and longevity that can be derived from simply continually reducing how much we eat (Bishop & Guarente, 2007; Fontana et al., 2010).

However, the major limitation of CR is that it is impractical for humans. Lack of compliance and long-term adherence have shown that CR is difficult for most people to implement (Phelan & Rose, 2005). As a result, much effort has focused on developing alternative, less cumbersome approaches that will lead to the same improvement in health. Caloric restriction mimetics (CRMs) are characterized as pharmacologic approaches that exert the same physiologic improvements as CR but without the burden of a continual reduction in caloric intake.

The need to rapidly identify successful CRMs is crucial. By 2030 the US Census Bureau estimates 1 in 5 Americans will be over the age of 65 (Colby & Ortman, 2015), leading to a concurrent rise in the prevalence of costly chronic diseases, including cancer, cardiovascular and cognitive diseases. The need to have a pharmacologic intervention that can delay aging and the burden of long-term disease-associated costs is crucial. However, the chasm to overcome this hurdle is large. Many pharmacologic interventions tested in animal models extend life span, but unfortunately, most of these drugs are untested and unapproved for use in humans. Translatable approaches are further delayed because we lack reliable biomarkers of aging and hence measurable targets to assess a drug's efficacy. To overcome these many hurdles, researchers rely on understanding the pathways activated by CR and rather than develop novel pharmacologic therapies, repurpose drugs approved by the Food and Drug Administration (FDA) that target these same pathways.

Nutrient Sensing Pathways

Glucose is the predominant energy source for most organisms, but excess intake is identified as a leading cause of age-associated diseases such as type 2 diabetes and cardiovascular disease. Under homeostatic conditions, elevated blood glucose levels stimulate insulin secretion, binding, and subsequent activation of the insulin/IGF signaling cascade, a growth-promoting response that is crucial in early-life development. In turn, this leads to PI3K/Akt/Ras growth and proliferation signaling with concurrent repression of Forkhead box O (FOXO), a key stress-responsive and cellular repair transcription factor (Hemmings & Restuccia, 2012; Salih & Brunet, 2008). Conversely, mutations decreasing or blocking the insulin/IGF-1 signaling lead to increased life span in nematode worms (Murphy et al., 2003) and fruit flies (Clancy et al., 2001). However, it is still unclear whether CR-mediated life span extension is fully dependent on the insulin/IGF pathway, as mutations in the long-lived Ames dwarf mice, which are deficient in growth hormone, prolactin, and thyroid-stimulating hormone, are still capable of positively responding to caloric restriction (Brown-Borg et al., 1996).

Another crucial evolutionarily conserved nutrient-sensing pathway is the target of rapamycin (TOR, mTOR in mammals). The TOR kinase is composed of the TOR complex (TORC) 1 and 2, wherein TORC1 is responsible for protein synthesis, mediated by S6 kinase activation. Conversely under nutrient restriction, TORC1 promotes autophagy and protein turnover (Bjedov & Partridge, 2011). Downregulation of TOR or its downstream targets is linked to increased life span in worms (Jia et al., 2004), flies (Kapahi et al., 2004), and rodents (Selman et al., 2009; Wu et al., 2013), but the dependency of the life-extending benefit of CR on the TOR pathway is unclear (Sharma et al., 2012), as implementation of CR does not cause downregulation of mTOR pathway proteins (Sharma et al., 2012).

Activation of the primary energy sensor, 5' AMP-activated protein kinase (AMPK), is emerging as another potential nutrient-sensing enzyme crucial in CR life span improvement. Under limited nutrients, AMPK is activated by LKB phosphorylation, leading to the generation of ATP and inhibition of mTOR (Cantó & Auwerx, 2011). In nematode worms, overexpression of AMPK leads to increased life span, which is further extended under glucose restriction (Schulz et al., 2007). Conversely, removal of AMPK in nematode worms eliminates CR-mediated life span extension (Greer et al., 2007). However, studies in higher organisms do not provide as clear a link between AMPK and CR life span extension.

Lastly, sirtuins have been identified as a potential mediator of the CR effect. Sirtuins are evolutionary-conserved nicotine amide (NAD)–dependent histone deacetylases, with seven identified in mammals (SIRT1-7) after originally identified in *S. cerevisiae* as a silent information regulator 2 protein (Sir2). The most-well studied is SIRT1, which has been identified to serve a wide-range of regulatory roles, including nutrient sensing, energy metabolism, and genome stability. Sirtuin function is dependent on the metabolic state of the cell or tissue, specifically on the levels of NAD^+ because it is a necessary substrate for its deacetylase activity (Imai et al., 2000) and one that declines with age (Imai & Guarente, 2016).

Overexpression of Sir2 homologues in yeast (Kaeberlein et al., 1999), worms (Tissenbaum & Guarente, 2001), and flies (Rogina & Helfand, 2004) leads to increased survival. In mice, the picture is less clear. Overexpression of SIRT1 specific to pancreatic beta-cells (Moynihan et al., 2005), or brain and adipose tissue (Bordone et al., 2007), leads to improved glucose tolerance. Similarly, whole-body overexpression of SIRT1 is protected against diet (Pfluger et al., 2008), genetically induced obesity (Banks et al., 2008), and associated diabetes. Conversely, one report has shown that Sirt1 deletion in proopiomelanocortin (POMC) neurons, which regulate food intake and energy expenditure, results in increased susceptibility to diet-induced diabetes (Ramadori et al., 2010), whereas other reports show that Sirt1 deletion protects against glucose intolerance and fatty liver disease (Bordone et al., 2005). It is important to note that results obtained from Sirt1-deletion studies in mice are difficult to interpret, as the majority of pups die in the perinatal period, with survivors showing developmental defects (Cheng et al., 2003). The role of Sirt1 in mediating the beneficial effects of CR are less clear in mice. Sirt1 expression increases in multiple tissues in response to CR (Cohen et al., 2004). Studies using Sirt1-null mice find CR has no impact on life span (Boily et al., 2008), but whether this effect is dampened due to the associated-development defects associated with this strain or because Sirt-1 is necessary for CR-life span extension is difficult to discern.

Together, these four nutrient-sensing pathways (insulin/IGF-1, mTOR, AMPK, and sirtuins) are the current targets of CRMs. The most notable CRMs are metformin, rapamycin, and resveratrol. Multiple translational studies are underway to examine the effect of using these drugs to delay the onset of diseases in humans.

Caloric Restriction Mimetics: A Pill for Caloric Restriction?

Metformin

Metformin (dimethylbiguanide) is currently the most widely prescribed glucose-lowering agent for type 2 diabetes worldwide (Bailey, 2017). As well, it is one of only a handful of drugs capable of extending life span in mice (Anisimov, Berstein, et al., 2011; Martin-Montalvo et al., 2013). Metformin serves as a great alternative to other antidiabetic drugs for older patients because of the reduced risk of hypoglycemia and nonfatal cardiovascular events (Schlender et al., 2017). Additional research suggests the therapeutic potential of metformin to delay age-associated diseases, including impaired glucose tolerance (Hostalek et al., 2015), obesity, hypertension, atherosclerosis (Zhou et al., 2017), and cancer (Heckman-Stoddard et al., 2017), as well as to lower the risk for frailty (Sumantri et al., 2016). Long-term treatment with metformin is shown to not only slow cognitive decline in older adults with type 2 diabetes (Ng et al., 2014), but it also helps to lower chronic inflammation (Saisho, 2015), a precursor to age-associated diseases. Specifically, metformin is able to lower high-sensitivity C-reactive protein (Haffner et al., 2005), a predominant marker of inflammation, and improve endothelial function (Vitale et al., 2005). Furthermore, a study found metformin lowers the risk of cardiovascular disease in otherwise healthy males by 6%, which is further increased in those diagnosed as frail to 18%, and by 48% in those with high cardiovascular risk (C.-P. Wang et al., 2017).

However, the most intriguing outcome results from an observational retrospective study from the UK Clinical Practice Research Datalink, which sets the groundwork of metformin as a potential CRM. The study found that long-term use of metformin in type 2 diabetes patients leads to longer overall survival compared to sex- and age-matched, nondiabetic controls (Bannister et al., 2014). This study offered the first evidence that metformin has the potential to delay age-associated diseases in nondiabetic individuals. Large-scale randomized clinical trials were initiated, with the same goal of assessing whether metformin can delay the onset of age-associated diseases. In 2018, the Investigation of Metformin in Pre-Diabetes on Atherosclerotic Cardiovascular outcomes (VA-IMPACT) set out to determine whether metformin could slow the morbidity and cardiovascular mortality in patients with prediabetes and established cardiovascular diseases (Clinical Trials Identifier: NCT02915198). Additionally, a multicenter randomized clinical trial to assess the efficacy of metformin in delaying microvascular complications and cognitive decline in individuals with nondiabetic intermediate hyperglycemia is currently underway (Clinical Trials Identifier: NCT03222765) (Gabriel et al., 2020).

The last trial, Targeting Aging with Metformin (TAME), is geared toward healthy older adults, who have previously not been diagnosed with any age-associated condition to assess whether metformin can delay or prevent the onset and progression of aging-related pathologies (Barzilai et al., 2016). The TAME trial is novel because unlike singular disease pathologies, which have associated physiologic markers, aging does not have a defined physiologic endpoint marker(s) to determine effectiveness (Vaiserman & Lushchak, 2017). Thus if the trial is successful, it will set the groundwork for future testing and evaluation of novel age-targeting molecules.

Rapamycin

Rapamycin (sirolimus) is one of the first pharmaceutical agents found to specifically inhibit mTOR1 activation. It was originally FDA-approved to prevent organ-transplant rejection and as a treatment option for certain rare forms of cancer. Since then, low doses of rapamycin have been shown to extend life span in yeast, worms, and flies (Johnson et al., 2013); delay many age-associated markers in mice, including cancer incidence (Anisimov, Berstein, et al., 2011); restore stem cell (Chong Chen et al., 2009) and muscle function (Bitto et al., 2016); and improve oral health (An et al., 2017). However, some studies have found that long-term use in mice leads to defective spermatogenesis, poor performance on glucose tolerance tests, and increased risk of cataracts (Lamming et al., 2012). Intermittent rapamycin administration may potentially overcome some of the negative effects associated with long-term rapamycin treatment (Arriola Apelo, Neuman, et al., 2016; Bitto et al., 2016).

Furthermore, rapamycin is the first pharmacologic agent shown to extend the life span of heterogenous mice, irrespective of whether it is fed early or late in life (Harrison et al., 2009; Miller et al., 2010), and showed a sex- and dose-dependent effect (Miller et al., 2014), a finding consistent when tested in additional inbred strains (Anisimov, Zabezhinski, et al., 2011; Neff et al., 2013) and primarily attributed to delaying tumorigenesis. More recent studies have shown that transient treatment is also capable of extending rodent life span (Arriola Apelo, Pumper, et al., 2016; Bitto et al., 2016). Rapamycin is currently being tested in companion dogs to assess whether long-term treatment is beneficial at delaying canine-specific aging pathologies (Urfer et al., 2017). As no study has been conducted on rapamycin in humans, the use of companion dogs serves as a good alternative. Unlike most mouse studies, which are conducted in a homogenous strain and in uniformed environments, studies on companion dogs enable an assessment of rapamycin efficacy across a heterogenic population and in diverse backgrounds.

Due to concerns about safety associated with rapamycin, much less is known as to whether or not lower doses of rapamycin are capable of delaying aging in humans. However, some limited evidence suggests that rapamycin and, more recently, its analogs ("rapalogs") may be beneficial (Wagner & Dancey, 2016). For example, the Sarcoma Multicenter Clinical Evaluation of the Efficacy of Ridaforolimus (SUCCEED) found that patients with advanced sarcomas showed significant improvement in progression-free survival with the rapalog, ridaforolimus (Demetri et al., 2013). However, much more work and exploration of rapamycin in human clinical trials are necessary to understand if it will be a viable CRM.

Resveratrol

The first SIRT1 activator to be widely studied was resveratrol, a polyphenol most notably found in grape skins and originally identified in a screen to extend the life span of *S. cerevisiae* (Howitz et al., 2003). Since its discovery, resveratrol has been credited for providing the beneficial effects of the "French Paradox," a diet that is high in saturated fat and moderate wine consumption but results in lower rates of cardiovascular disease (Catalgol et al., 2012). Resveratrol has since been identified to induce the same effects as SIRT1 activation, evident by improved markers of health, including insulin sensitivity, inhibition of tumor growth, and improved cardiovascular health. As well, studies in yeast (Timmers et al., 2012), worms, and flies (Bass et al., 2007) have shown that resveratrol increases life span.

Studies in mice fed resveratrol over the majority of the life span led to transcriptional changes that mimic dietary restriction but do not lead to life span extension in nonobese inbred male mice (Pearson et al., 2008) or genetically heterogenous mice (Miller et al., 2010). Under metabolic stress, such as under a high-fat diet, resveratrol leads to life span extension in inbred male mice (Baur et al., 2006).

Clinical studies show resveratrol is potentially beneficial in humans with metabolic disorders, including diabetes, obesity, and cardiovascular disease (Crandall et al., 2012), but it is highly dose-dependent (Poulsen et al., 2013; Timmers et al., 2011; Zordoky et al., 2015). Due to the positive outcomes from preclinical findings, resveratrol was touted as a means for primary prevention of age-associated diseases.

However, in healthy nonobese adults, resveratrol appears to have limited to no metabolic benefit. In nonobese postmenopausal women with normal glucose tolerance (Yoshino et al., 2012), resveratrol had no impact on metabolic markers and inconsistent metabolic improvements in obese individuals (Poulsen et al., 2013). These findings question the use of resveratrol as a supplement to combat metabolic disorders or suggests it may only be beneficial in individuals with abnormal metabolic baseline parameters. For example, one study suggests resveratrol is potentially protective in individuals who are considered to be at low risk for atherosclerosis based on present screening measures (Agarwal et al., 2013). Taken together, these instances highlight the need for further exploration to understand the specific disease and dosage necessary to maximize the benefit from resveratrol.

NAD^+ and NAD^+ Precursors

More recently, interest in nicotinamide adenine dinucleotide (NAD^+) supplementation is being explored as an alternative for sirtuin activation. NAD^+ and its reduced form NADH facilitate hydrogen transfer in key metabolic pathways. As sirtuins are NAD^+-dependent deacetylases, they are crucial for mediating cellular responses to environmental and metabolic perturbations and regulation of the circadian clock. Multiple studies have suggested an age-dependent decline in sirtuin activity and concurrent reduction in NAD^+ levels (Gomes et al., 2013; Ramsey et al., 2008). The age-dependent decline in sirtuin activity/ NAD^+ levels could be overcome with supplementation of an NAD^+ intermediate, nicotinamide mononucleotide (NMN), which is converted to NAD^+ by NMN adenylyltransferase. Supplementation studies of NMN were found to restore NAD^+ levels and prevent diet- and age-induced type 2 diabetes in mice (Yoshino et al., 2011) and to restore age-dependent fertility decline in retired female breeders (Bertoldo et al., 2020). Similarly, another NAD^+ precursor, nicotinamide riboside (NR), which is converted first to NMR and then to NAD^+, was shown to boost NAD^+ levels and counteract the age-dependent decline evident in worms (Mouchiroud et al., 2013) and mice fed a high-fat diet (Cantó et al., 2012). Less is known about NAD^+ and its precursors' (NMR and NR) supplementation in humans. One double-blind placebo-controlled study showed chronic NR supplementation was well tolerated and raised NAD^+ levels in older adults over a 6-week period (Martens et al., 2018). Similarly, administration of oral NR over a 3-week period to healthy 70- to 80-year-old men increased the available pool of NAD^+ levels in skeletal muscle and lowered circulating inflammatory cytokines (Elhassan et al., 2019). Overall, much work is still needed to assess the viability of NAD^+ or its precursors to help invigorate sirtuin activity and serve as a feasible supplement to prevent age-associated diseases.

Key Points

- Multiple theories of why we age have been proposed, but none have been capable of explaining all biologic outcomes associated with aging.
- Multiples theories of how we age have been proposed, with the free radical theory of aging being the most attractive. However, since its inception multiple modifications to the free radical theory of aging have ensued.
- Dietary intervention (primarily chronic caloric restriction) is the leading nonpharmaceutical approach for improved health and survival across multiple model organisms.
- Dietary interventions delay many of the deleterious age-associated markers of the free radical theory of aging and its offshoots.
- Caloric-restriction mimetics (CRMs) offer a pharmaceutical approach to gaining some of the benefits of chronic caloric restriction.
- More work is necessary to determine whether CRMs will offer a viable antiaging approach in humans.

More information about tools and Interprofessional Education Collaborative (IPEC) competencies mentioned in this chapter can be found in Appendix 1: Tools and Appendix 2: IPEC Competencies.

References

Agarwal, B., Campen, M. J., Channell, M. M., Wherry, S. J., Varamini, B., Davis, J. G., & Smoliga, J. M. (2013). Resveratrol for primary prevention of atherosclerosis: Clinical trial evidence for improved gene expression in vascular endothelium. *International Journal of Cardiology, 166*(1), 246–248. https://doi.org/10.1016/j.ijcard.2012.09.027.

An, J. Y., Quarles, E. K., Mekvanich, S., Kang, A., Liu, A., Santos, D., & Kaeberlein, M. (2017). Rapamycin treatment attenuates age-associated periodontitis in mice. *GeroScience, 39*(4), 457–463.

Andersson, V., Hanzén, S., Liu, B., Molin, M., & Nyström, T. (2013). Enhancing protein disaggregation restores proteasome activity in aged cells. *Aging (Albany NY), 5*(11), 802.

Anisimov, V. N., Berstein, L. M., Popovich, I. G., Zabezhinski, M. A., Egormin, P. A., Piskunova, T. S., & Kovalenko, I. G. (2011). If started early in life, metformin treatment increases life span and postpones tumors in female SHR mice. *Aging (Albany NY), 3*(2), 148.

Anisimov, V. N., Zabezhinski, M. A., Popovich, I. G., Piskunova, T. S., Semenchenko, A. V., Tyndyk, M. L., … Blagosklonny, M. V. (2011). Rapamycin increases lifespan and inhibits spontaneous tumorigenesis in inbred female mice. *Cell Cycle, 10*(24), 4230–4236.

Anton, S. D., Lee, S. A., Donahoo, W. T., McLaren, C., Manini, T., Leeuwenburgh, C., & Pahor, M. (2019). The effects of time restricted feeding on overweight, older adults: A pilot study. *Nutrients, 11*(7), 1500.

Arriola Apelo, S. I., Neuman, J. C., Baar, E. L., Syed, F. A., Cummings, N. E., Brar, H. K., … Lamming, D. W. (2016). Alternative rapamycin treatment regimens mitigate the impact of rapamycin on glucose homeostasis and the immune system. *Aging Cell, 15*(1), 28–38.

Arriola Apelo, S. I., Pumper, C. P., Baar, E. L., Cummings, N. E., & Lamming, D. W. (2016). Intermittent administration of rapamycin extends the life span of female C57BL/6J mice. *The Journals of Gerontology: Series A, 71*(7), 876–881. https://doi.org/10.1093/gerona/glw064.

Austad, S. N. (2006). Why women live longer than men: Sex differences in longevity. *Gender Medicine, 3*(2), 79–92.

Austad, S. N., & Hoffman, J. M. (2018). Is antagonistic pleiotropy ubiquitous in aging biology. *Evolution, Medicine, and Public Health, 2018*(1), 287–294. https://doi.org/10.1093/emph/eoy033.

Bailey, C. J. (2017). Metformin: Historical overview. *Diabetologia, 60*(9), 1566–1576. https://doi.org/10.1007/s00125-017-4318-z.

Baker, D. J., & Petersen, R. C. (2018). Cellular senescence in brain aging and neurodegenerative diseases: Evidence and perspectives. *Journal of Clinical Investigation, 128*(3), 1208–1216.

Balch, W. E., Morimoto, R. I., Dillin, A., & Kelly, J. W. (2008). Adapting proteostasis for disease intervention. *Science, 319*(5865), 916–919.

Banks, A. S., Kon, N., Knight, C., Matsumoto, M., Gutiérrez-Juárez, R., Rossetti, L., & Accili, D. (2008). SirT1 gain of function increases energy efficiency and prevents diabetes in mice. *Cell Metabolism, 8*(4), 333.

Bannister, C., Holden, S., Jenkins-Jones, S., Morgan, C. L., Halcox, J., Schernthaner, G., & Currie, C. (2014). Can people with type 2 diabetes live longer than those without? A comparison of mortality in people initiated with metformin or sulphonylurea monotherapy and matched, non-diabetic controls. *Diabetes, Obesity and Metabolism, 16*(11), 1165–1173.

Bartke, A. (2000). Delayed aging in Ames dwarf mice. Relationships to endocrine function and body size. In S. Hekimi (Ed.), *The molecular genetics of aging* (pp. 181–202). Springer.

Bartke, A., Brown-Borg, H., Mattison, J., Kinney, B., Hauck, S., & Wright, C. (2001). Prolonged longevity of hypopituitary dwarf mice. *Experimental Gerontology, 36*(1), 21–28.

Barzilai, N., Crandall, J. P., Kritchevsky, S. B., & Espeland, M. A. (2016). Metformin as a tool to target aging. *Cell Metabolism, 23*(6), 1060–1065.

Bass, T. M., Weinkove, D., Houthoofd, K., Gems, D., & Partridge, L. (2007). Effects of resveratrol on lifespan in Drosophila melanogaster and Caenorhabditis elegans. *Mechanisms of Ageing and Development, 128*(10), 546–552.

Baur, J. A., Pearson, K. J., Price, N. L., Jamieson, H. A., Lerin, C., Kalra, A., & Sinclair, D. A. (2006). Resveratrol improves health and survival of mice on a high-calorie diet. *Nature, 444*(7117), 337–342. https://doi.org/10.1038/nature05354.

Belevich, I., Verkhovsky, M. I., & Wikström, M. (2006). Proton-coupled electron transfer drives the proton pump of cytochrome c oxidase. *Nature, 440*(7085), 829–832.

Berchtold, N. C., Cribbs, D. H., Coleman, P. D., Rogers, J., Head, E., Kim, R., & Trojanowski, J.Q. (2008). Gene expression changes in the course of normal brain aging are sexually dimorphic. *Proceedings of the National Academy of Sciences, 105*(40), 15605–15610.

Bertoldo, M. J., Listijono, D. R., Ho, W.-H. J., Riepsamen, A. H., Goss, D. M., Richani, D., & Habibalahi, A. (2020). NAD+ repletion rescues female fertility during reproductive aging. *Cell Reports, 30*(6), 1670–1681. e1677.

Bhutani, S., Klempel, M. C., Kroeger, C. M., Trepanowski, J., Phillips, S. A., Norkeviciute, E., & Varady, K. A. (2013). Alternate day fasting with or without exercise: Effects on endothelial function and adipokines in obese humans. *e-SPEN Journal, 8*(5), e205–e209.

Bishop, N. A., & Guarente, L. (2007). Genetic links between diet and lifespan: Shared mechanisms from yeast to humans. *Nature Reviews Genetics, 8*(11), 835–844.

Biswas, S., Das, R., & Banerjee, E. R. (2017). Role of free radicals in human inflammatory diseases. *AIMS Biophysics, 4*(4), 596.

Bitto, A., Ito, T. K., Pineda, V. V., LeTexier, N. J., Huang, H. Z., Sutlief, E., … Smith, K. (2016). Transient rapamycin treatment can increase lifespan and healthspan in middle-aged mice. *eLife, 5*, e16351.

Bjedov, I., & Partridge, L. (2011). A longer and healthier life with TOR down-regulation: Genetics and drugs. *Biochemical Society Transactions, 39*(2), 460–465. https://doi.org/10.1042/BST0390460.

Bjelakovic, G., Nikolova, D., Gluud, L. L., Simonetti, R. G., & Gluud, C. (2007). Mortality in randomized trials of antioxidant supplements for primary and secondary prevention: Systematic review and meta-analysis. *Journal of the American Medical Association, 297*(8), 842–857.

Blüher, M., Kahn, B. B., & Kahn, C. R. (2003). Extended longevity in mice lacking the insulin receptor in adipose tissue. *Science, 299*(5606), 572–574.

Boily, G., Seifert, E. L., Bevilacqua, L., He, X. H., Sabourin, G., Estey, C., & Jardine, K. (2008). SirT1 regulates energy metabolism and response to caloric restriction in mice. *PLoS One, 3*(3), e1759. https://doi.org/10.1371/journal.pone.0001759.

Bokov, A., Chaudhuri, A., & Richardson, A. (2004). The role of oxidative damage and stress in aging. *Mechanisms of Ageing and Development, 125*(10–11), 811–826.

Bondy, S. C., & Naderi, S. (1994). Contribution of hepatic cytochrome P450 systems to the generation of reactive oxygen species. *Biochemical Pharmacology, 48*(1), 155–159.

Bordone, L., Cohen, D., Robinson, A., Motta, M. C., Van Veen, E., Czopik, A., ... Luo, J. (2007). SIRT1 transgenic mice show phenotypes resembling calorie restriction. *Aging Cell, 6*(6), 759–767.

Bordone, L., Motta, M. C., Picard, F., Robinson, A., Jhala, U. S., Apfeld, J., & Szilvasi, A. (2005). Sirt1 regulates insulin secretion by repressing UCP2 in pancreatic β cells. *PLoS Biology, 4*(2), e31.

Brandhorst, S., Choi, In. Y., Wei, M., Cheng, Chia W., Sedrakyan, S., Navarrete, G., & Longo, Valter D. (2015). A periodic diet that mimics fasting promotes multi-system regeneration, enhanced cognitive performance, and healthspan. *Cell Metabolism, 22*(1), 86–99. https://doi.org/10.1016/j.cmet.2015.05.012.

Brown-Borg, H. M., Borg, K. E., Meliska, C. J., & Bartke, A. (1996). Dwarf mice and the ageing process. *Nature, 384*(6604), 33–33. https://doi.org/10.1038/384033a0.

Buffenstein, R. (2005). The naked mole-rat: A new long-living model for human aging research. *The Journals of Gerontology Series A: Biological Sciences and Medical Sciences, 60*(11), 1369–1377.

Buffenstein, R. (2008). Negligible senescence in the longest living rodent, the naked mole-rat: Insights from a successfully aging species. *Journal of Comparative Physiology B, 178*(4), 439–445. https://doi.org/10.1007/s00360-007-0237-5.

Buffenstein, R., Park, T., Hanes, M., & Artwohl, J. E. (2012). Chapter 45: Naked mole rat. In M. A. Suckow, K. A. Stevens, & R. P. Wilson (Eds.), *The laboratory rabbit, guinea pig, hamster, and other rodents* (pp. 1055–1074). Academic Press.

Calogero, A., Giagulli, V., Mongioì, L., Triggiani, V., Radicioni, A., Jannini, E., & Pasquali, D. (2017). Klinefelter syndrome: Cardiovascular abnormalities and metabolic disorders. *Journal of Endocrinological Investigation, 40*(7), 705–712.

Camus, M. F., Clancy, David J., & Dowling, Damian K. (2012). Mitochondria, maternal inheritance, and male aging. *Current Biology, 22*(18), 1717–1721. https://doi.org/10.1016/j.cub. 2012.07.018.

Cantó, C., & Auwerx, J. (2011). Calorie restriction: Is AMPK a key sensor and effector? *Physiology, 26*(4), 214–224.

Cantó, C., Houtkooper, R. H., Pirinen, E., Youn, D. Y., Oosterveer, M. H., Cen, Y., & Cettour-Rose, P. (2012). The NAD+ precursor nicotinamide riboside enhances oxidative metabolism and protects against high-fat diet-induced obesity. *Cell Metabolism, 15*(6), 838–847.

Carlson, A. J., & Hoelzel, F. (1946). Apparent prolongation of the life span of rats by intermittent fasting: One figure. *Journal of Nutrition, 31*(3), 363–375.

Catalgol, B., Batirel, S., Taga, Y., & Ozer, N. (2012). Resveratrol: French paradox revisited. *Frontiers in Pharmacology, 3*(141). https://doi.org/10.3389/fphar.2012.00141.

Charlesworth, B. (2000). Fisher, Medawar, Hamilton and the evolution of aging. *Genetics, 156*(3), 927–931.

Chen, C., Jack, J., & Garofalo, R. S. (1996). The Drosophila insulin receptor is required for normal growth. *Endocrinology, 137*(3), 846–856.

Chen, C., Liu, Y., Liu, Y., & Zheng, P. (2009). mTOR regulation and therapeutic rejuvenation of aging hematopoietic stem cells. *Science Signaling, 2*(98), ra75–ra75.

Chen, J., Senturk, D., Wang, J.-L., Müller, H.-G., Carey, J. R., Caswell, H., & Caswell-Chen, E. P. (2007). A demographic analysis of the fitness cost of extended longevity in Caenorhabditis elegans. *The Journals of Gerontology Series A: Biological Sciences and Medical Sciences, 62*(2), 126–135.

Cheng, H.-L., Mostoslavsky, R., Saito, S. I., Manis, J. P., Gu, Y., Patel, P., ... Chua, K. F. (2003). Developmental defects and p53 hyperacetylation in Sir2 homolog (SIRT1)-deficient mice. *Proceedings of the National Academy of Sciences, 100*(19), 10794–10799.

Chippindale, A. K., Hoang, D. T., Service, P. M., & Rose, M. R. (2004). The evolution of development in Drosophila melanogaster selected for postponed senescence. In M. R. Rose, H. B. Passananti, & M. Matos (Eds.), *Methuselah flies: A case study in the evolution of aging* (pp. 370–389). World Scientific.

Choi, I. Y., Piccio, L., Childress, P., Bollman, B., Ghosh, A., Brandhorst, S., ... Morgan, T. E. (2016). A diet mimicking fasting promotes regeneration and reduces autoimmunity and multiple sclerosis symptoms. *Cell Reports, 15*(10), 2136–2146.

Clancy, D. J., Gems, D., Harshman, L. G., Oldham, S., Stocker, H., Hafen, E., ... Partridge, L. (2001). Extension of life-span by loss of CHICO, a Drosophila insulin receptor substrate protein. *Science, 292*(5514), 104–106. https://doi.org/10.1126/science.1057991.

Cohen, H. Y., Miller, C., Bitterman, K. J., Wall, N. R., Hekking, B., Kessler, B., ... Sinclair, D. A. (2004). Calorie restriction promotes mammalian cell survival by inducing the SIRT1 deacetylase. *Science, 305*(5682), 390. https://doi.org/10.1126/science.1099196.

Colby, S. L., & Ortman, J. M. (2015). Projections of the size and composition of the US population: 2014 to 2060. Population estimates and projections. *Current Population Reports* P25–1143. US Census Bureau.

Colman, R. J., Anderson, R. M., Johnson, S. C., Kastman, E. K., Kosmatka, K. J., Beasley, T. M., ... Kemnitz, J. W. (2009). Caloric restriction delays disease onset and mortality in rhesus monkeys. *Science, 325*(5937), 201–204.

Cook, M. B., McGlynn, K. A., Devesa, S. S., Freedman, N. D., & Anderson, W. F. (2011). Sex disparities in cancer mortality and survival. *Cancer Epidemiology and Prevention Biomarkers, 20*(8), 1629–1637.

Crandall, J. P., Oram, V., Trandafirescu, G., Reid, M., Kishore, P., Hawkins, M., ... Barzilai, N. (2012). Pilot study of resveratrol in older adults with impaired glucose tolerance. *The Journals of Gerontology Series A: Biomedical Sciences and Medical Sciences, 67*(12), 1307–1312.

Davies, J. M., Lowry, C. V., & Davies, K. J. (1995). Transient adaptation to oxidative stress in yeast. *Archives of Biochemistry and Biophysics, 317*(1), 1–6.

Davies, K. J. (2016). Adaptive homeostasis. *Molecular Aspects of Medicine, 49*, 1–7. https://doi.org/10.1016/j.mam.2016.04.007.

Davies, K. J. (2016). Adaptive homeostasis. *Molecular aspects of medicine, 49*, 1–7. https://doi.org/10.1016/j.mam.2016.04.007.

Davis, E. J., Lobach, I., & Dubal, D. B. (2019). Female XX sex chromosomes increase survival and extend lifespan in aging mice. *Aging Cell, 18*(1), e12871.

de La Asunción, J. G., Millan, A., Pla, R., Bruseghini, L., Esteras, A., Pallardo, F., ... Vina, J. (1996). Mitochondrial glutathione oxidation correlates with age-associated oxidative damage to mitochondrial DNA. *The FASEB Journal, 10*(2), 333–338.

De Vries, G. J., Rissman, E. F., Simerly, R. B., Yang, L.-Y., Scordalakes, E. M., Auger, C. J., ... Arnold, A. P. (2002). A model system for study of sex chromosome effects on sexually dimorphic neural and behavioral traits. *Journal of Neuroscience, 22*(20), 9005. https://doi.org/10.1523/JNEUROSCI.22-20-09005.2002.

Del Río, L. A., & López-Huertas, E. (2016). ROS generation in peroxisomes and its role in cell signaling. *Plant and Cell Physiology, 57*(7), 1364–1376.

Delaney, J. R., Murakami, C. J., Olsen, B., Kennedy, B. K., & Kaeberlein, M. (2011). Quantitative evidence for early life fitness defects from 32 longevity-associated alleles in yeast. *Cell Cycle, 10*(1), 156–165.

Demetri, G. D., Chawla, S. P., Ray-Coquard, I., Le Cesne, A., Staddon, A. P., Milhem, M. M., ... Cranmer, L. D. (2013). Results of an international randomized phase III trial of the mammalian target of rapamycin inhibitor ridaforolimus versus placebo to control metastatic sarcomas in patients after benefit from prior chemotherapy. *Journal of Clinical Oncology, 31*(19), 2485–2492.

Di Biase, S., Lee, C., Brandhorst, S., Manes, B., Buono, R., Cheng, C.-W., ... Wei, M. (2016). Fasting-mimicking diet reduces HO-1 to promote T cell-mediated tumor cytotoxicity. *Cancer Cell, 30*(1), 136–146.

Dorman, J. B., Albinder, B., Shroyer, T., & Kenyon, C. (1995). The age-1 and daf-2 genes function in a common pathway to control the lifespan of Caenorhabditis elegans. *Genetics, 141*(4), 1399–1406.

Drummond, J., Baker, A. Z., Wright, M. D., Marrian, P. M., & Singer, E. M. (1938). The effects of life-long subsistence on diets providing suboptimal amounts of the "vitamin B complex." *Epidemiology & Infection, 38*(3), 356–373.

Dube, J., Amati, F., Toledo, F., Stefanovic-Racic, M., Rossi, A., Coen, P., & Goodpaster, B. (2011). Effects of weight loss and exercise on insulin resistance, and intramyocellular triacylglycerol, diacylglycerol and ceramide. *Diabetologia, 54*(5), 1147–1156.

Eisenberg, T., & Buttner, S. (2014). Lipids and cell death in yeast. *FEMS Yeast Research, 14*(1), 179–197. https://doi.org/10.1111/1567-1364.12105.

Elchuri, S., Oberley, T. D., Qi, W., Eisenstein, R. S., Roberts, L. J., Van Remmen, H., ... Huang, T.-T. (2005). CuZnSOD deficiency leads to persistent and widespread oxidative damage and hepatocarcinogenesis later in life. *Oncogene, 24*(3), 367–380.

Elhassan, Y. S., Kluckova, K., Fletcher, R. S., Schmidt, M. S., Garten, A., Doig, C. L., ... Lavery, G. G. (2019). Nicotinamide riboside augments the aged human skeletal muscle NAD+ metabolome and induces transcriptomic and anti-inflammatory signatures. *Cell Reports, 28*(7), 1717–1728.e1716. https://doi.org/10.1016/j.celrep.2019.07.043.

Eshghinia, S., & Mohammadzadeh, F. (2013). The effects of modified alternate-day fasting diet on weight loss and CAD risk factors in overweight and obese women. *Journal of Diabetes & Metabolic Disorders, 12*(1), 4.

Fabrizio, P., Liou, L.-L., Moy, V. N., Diaspro, A., Valentine, J. S., Gralla, E. B., & Longo, V. D. (2003). SOD2 functions downstream of Sch9 to extend longevity in yeast. *Genetics, 163*(1), 35–46.

Fabrizio, P., Pozza, F., Pletcher, S. D., Gendron, C. M., & Longo, V. D. (2001). Regulation of longevity and stress resistance by Sch9 in yeast. *Science, 292*(5515), 288–290.

Finch, Caleb E., & Tower, J. (2014). Sex-specific aging in flies, worms, and missing great-granddads. *Cell, 156*(3), 398–399. https://doi.org/10.1016/j.cell.2014.01.028.

Flurkey, K., Papaconstantinou, J., Miller, R. A., & Harrison, D. E. (2001). Lifespan extension and delayed immune and collagen aging in mutant mice with defects in growth hormone production. *Proceedings of the National Academy of Sciences, 98*(12), 6736–6741.

Fontana, L., Partridge, L., & Longo, V. D. (2010). Extending healthy life span—from yeast to humans. *Science, 328*(5976), 321–326.

Ford, E. S. (2002). Does exercise reduce inflammation? Physical activity and C-reactive protein among US adults. *Epidemiology*, 561–568.

Forster, M. J., Morris, P., & Sohal, R. S. (2003). Genotype and age influence the effect of caloric intake on mortality in mice. *The FASEB Journal, 17*(6), 690–692.

Franceschi, C., Bonafè, M., Valensin, S., Olivieri, F., De Luca, M., Ottaviani, E., & De Benedictis, G. (2000). Inflamm-aging: An evolutionary perspective on immunosenescence. *Annals of the New York Academy of Sciences, 908*(1), 244–254.

Franceschi, C., Capri, M., Monti, D., Giunta, S., Olivieri, F., Sevini, F., ... Scurti, M. (2007). Inflammaging and anti-inflammaging: A systemic perspective on aging and longevity emerged from studies in humans. *Mechanisms of Ageing and Development, 128*(1), 92–105.

Franceschi, C., Garagnani, P., Vitale, G., Capri, M., & Salvioli, S. (2017). Inflammaging and "Garb-aging." *Trends in Endocrinology & Metabolism, 28*(3), 199–212.

Freund, A., Orjalo, A. V., Desprez, P.-Y., & Campisi, J. (2010). Inflammatory networks during cellular senescence: Causes and consequences. *Trends in Molecular Medicine, 16*(5), 238–246.

Fridovich, I. (2013). Oxygen: How do we stand it? *Medical Principles and Practice, 22*(2), 131–137.

Fried, S. K., Bunkin, D. A., & Greenberg, A. S. (1998). Omental and subcutaneous adipose tissues of obese subjects release interleukin-6: Depot difference and regulation by glucocorticoid1. *Journal of Clinical Endocrinology & Metabolism, 83*(3), 847–850. https://doi.org/10.1210/jcem.83.3.4660.

Friedman, D. B., & Johnson, T. E. (1988). A mutation in the age-1 gene in Caenorhabditis elegans lengthens life and reduces hermaphrodite fertility. *Genetics, 118*(1), 75–86.

Gabriel, R., Boukichou Abdelkader, N., Acosta, T., Gilis-Januszewska, A., Gómez-Huelgas, R., Makrilakis, K., ... On behalf of the e, P. C. (2020). Early prevention of diabetes microvascular complications in people with hyperglycaemia in Europe. ePREDICE randomized trial. Study protocol, recruitment and selected baseline data. *PLoS One, 15*(4), e0231196. https://doi.org/10.1371/journal.pone.0231196.

Gemmell, N. J., Metcalf, V. J., & Allendorf, F. W. (2004). Mother's curse: The effect of mtDNA on individual fitness and population viability. *Trends in Ecology & Evolution, 19*(5), 238–244.

Gibson, J. R., Chippindale, A. K., & Rice, W. R. (2002). The X chromosome is a hot spot for sexually antagonistic fitness variation. *Proceedings of the Royal Society of London. Series B: Biological Sciences, 269*(1490), 499–505.

Gill, S., & Panda, S. (2015). A smartphone app reveals erratic diurnal eating patterns in humans that can be modulated for health benefits. *Cell Metabolism, 22*(5), 789–798.

Giorgio, M., Berry, A., Berniakovich, I., Poletaeva, I., Trinei, M., Stendardo, M., ... Migliaccio, E. (2012). The p66Shc knockout mice are short lived under natural condition. *Aging Cell, 11*(1), 162–168.

Giunta, B., Fernandez, F., Nikolic, W. V., Obregon, D., Rrapo, E., Town, T., & Tan, J. (2008). Inflammaging as a prodrome to Alzheimer's disease. *Journal of Neuroinflammation, 5*(1), 51.

Goldsmith, T. C. (2014). Modern evolutionary mechanics theories and resolving the programmed/non-programmed aging controversy. *Biochemistry (Moscow), 79*(10), 1049–1055. https://doi.org/10.1134/S000629791410006X.

Gomes, A. P., Price, N. L., Ling, A. J., Moslehi, J. J., Montgomery, M. K., Rajman, L., … Hubbard, B. P. (2013). Declining NAD+ induces a pseudohypoxic state disrupting nuclear-mitochondrial communication during aging. *Cell, 155*(7), 1624–1638.

Gomez-Cabrera, M.-C., Domenech, E., Romagnoli, M., Arduini, A., Borras, C., Pallardo, F. V., … Vina, J. (2008). Oral administration of vitamin C decreases muscle mitochondrial biogenesis and hampers training-induced adaptations in endurance performance. *American Journal of Clinical Nutrition, 87*(1), 142–149.

Goodrick, C., Ingram, D., Reynolds, M., Freeman, J., & Cider, N. (1990). Effects of intermittent feeding upon body weight and lifespan in inbred mice: Interaction of genotype and age. *Mechanisms of Ageing and Development, 55*(1), 69–87.

Greer, E. L., Dowlatshahi, D., Banko, M. R., Villen, J., Hoang, K., Blanchard, D., … Brunet, A. (2007). An AMPK-FOXO pathway mediates longevity induced by a novel method of dietary restriction in C. elegans. *Current Biology, 17*(19), 1646–1656. https://doi.org/10.1016/j.cub.2007.08.047.

Guevara-Aguirre, J., Balasubramanian, P., Guevara-Aguirre, M., Wei, M., Madia, F., Cheng, C.-W., … Longo, V. D. (2011). Growth hormone receptor deficiency is associated with a major reduction in pro-aging signaling, cancer, and diabetes in humans. *Science Translational Medicine, 3*(70), 70ra13. https://doi.org/10.1126/scitranslmed.3001845.

Gulsvik, A. K., Thelle, D. S., Samuelsen, S. O., Myrstad, M., Mowé, M., & Wyller, T. B. (2011). Ageing, physical activity and mortality—a 42-year follow-up study. *International Journal of Epidemiology, 41*(2), 521–530.

Gupta, N. J., Kumar, V., & Panda, S. (2017). A camera-phone based study reveals erratic eating pattern and disrupted daily eating-fasting cycle among adults in India. *PLoS One, 12*(3), e0172852. https://doi.org/10.1371/journal.pone.0172852.

Haffner, S., Temprosa, M., Crandall, J., Fowler, S., Goldberg, R., Horton, E., … Barrett-Connor, E. (2005). Intensive lifestyle intervention or metformin on inflammation and coagulation in participants with impaired glucose tolerance. *Diabetes, 54*(5), 1566–1572. https://doi.org/10.2337/diabetes.54.5.1566.

Haldane, J. B. S. (1941). *New paths in genetics*. London: George Allen and Unwin, Ltd., 1941.

Halliwell, B., & Gutteridge, J. M. (2015). *Free radicals in biology and medicine*. USA: Oxford University Press.

Hannum, G., Guinney, J., Zhao, L., Zhang, L., Hughes, G., Sadda, S., … Gao, Y. (2013). Genome-wide methylation profiles reveal quantitative views of human aging rates. *Molecular Cell, 49*(2), 359–367.

Harman, D. (1956). Aging: A theory based on free radical and radiation chemistry. *Journal of gerontology, 11*(3), 298–300. https://doi.org/10.1093/geronj/11.3.298.

Harper, J. M., Salmon, A. B., Leiser, S. F., Galecki, A. T., & Miller, R. A. (2007). Skin-derived fibroblasts from long-lived species are resistant to some, but not all, lethal stresses and to the mitochondrial inhibitor rotenone. *Aging Cell, 6*(1), 1–13. https://doi.org/10.1111/j.1474-9726.2006.00255.x.

Harrison, D. E., Strong, R., Sharp, Z. D., Nelson, J. F., Astle, C. M., Flurkey, K., … Carter, C. S. (2009). Rapamycin fed late in life extends lifespan in genetically heterogeneous mice. *Nature, 460*(7253), 392–395.

Harvie, M. N., Pegington, M., Mattson, M. P., Frystyk, J., Dillon, B., Evans, G., … Cutler, R. G. (2011). The effects of intermittent or continuous energy restriction on weight loss and metabolic disease risk markers: A randomized trial in young overweight women. *International Journal of Obesity, 35*(5), 714–727.

Hatori, M., Vollmers, C., Zarrinpar, A., DiTacchio, L., Bushong, E. A., Gill, S., … Fitzpatrick, J. A. (2012). Time-restricted feeding without reducing caloric intake prevents metabolic diseases in mice fed a high-fat diet. *Cell Metabolism, 15*(6), 848–860.

Hazzard, W. R., & Halter, J. B. (2009). *Hazzard's geriatric medicine and gerontology*. Univerza v Ljubljani, Medicinska fakulteta.

Heckman-Stoddard, B. M., DeCensi, A., Sahasrabuddhe, V. V., & Ford, L. G. (2017). Repurposing metformin for the prevention of cancer and cancer recurrence. *Diabetologia, 60*(9), 1639–1647.

Heilbronn, L. K., Smith, S. R., Martin, C. K., Anton, S. D., & Ravussin, E. (2005). Alternate-day fasting in nonobese subjects: Effects on body weight, body composition, and energy metabolism. *American Journal of Clinical Nutrition, 81*(1), 69–73.

Hekimi, S., Lapointe, J., & Wen, Y. (2011). Taking a "good" look at free radicals in the aging process. *Trends in Cell Biology, 21*(10), 569–576.

Hemmings, B. A., & Restuccia, D. F. (2012). Pi3k-pkb/akt pathway. *Cold Spring Harbor Perspectives in Biology, 4*(9), a011189.

Holzenberger, M., Dupont, J., Ducos, B., Leneuve, P., Géloën, A., Even, P. C., … Le Bouc, Y. (2003). IGF-1 receptor regulates lifespan and resistance to oxidative stress in mice. *Nature, 421*(6919), 182–187. https://doi.org/10.1038/nature01298.

Hostalek, U., Gwilt, M., & Hildemann, S. (2015). Therapeutic use of metformin in prediabetes and diabetes prevention. *Drugs, 75*(10), 1071–1094.

Howitz, K. T., Bitterman, K. J., Cohen, H. Y., Lamming, D. W., Lavu, S., Wood, J. G., … Zhang, L.-L. (2003). Small molecule activators of sirtuins extend Saccharomyces cerevisiae lifespan. *Nature, 425*(6954), 191–196.

Hu, D., Mao, Y., Xu, G., Liao, W., Ren, J., Yang, H., … Wang, W. (2019). Time-restricted feeding causes irreversible metabolic disorders and gut microbiota shift in pediatric mice. *Pediatric Research, 85*(4), 518–526.

Hutchison, A. T., Regmi, P., Manoogian, E. N., Fleischer, J. G., Wittert, G. A., Panda, S., & Heilbronn, L. K. (2019). Time-restricted feeding improves glucose tolerance in men at risk for type 2 diabetes: Arandomized crossover trial. *Obesity, 27*(5), 724–732.

Hwangbo, D. S., Gersham, B., Tu, M.-P., Palmer, M., & Tatar, M. (2004). Drosophila dFOXO controls lifespan and regulates insulin signalling in brain and fat body. *Nature, 429*(6991), 562.

Imai, S.-i, Armstrong, C. M., Kaeberlein, M., & Guarente, L. (2000). Transcriptional silencing and longevity protein Sir2 is an NAD-dependent histone deacetylase. *Nature, 403*(6771), 795–800. https://doi.org/10.1038/35001622.

Imai, S.-i, & Guarente, L. (2016). It takes two to tango: NAD+ and sirtuins in aging/longevity control. *NPJ Aging and Mechanisms of Disease, 2*(1), 16017. https://doi.org/10.1038/npjamd.2016.17.

Ishii, N., Goto, S., & Hartman, P. S. (2002). Protein oxidation during aging of the nematode Caenorhabditis elegans. *Free Radical Biology and Medicine, 33*(8), 1021–1025.

Jaacks, L. M., Siegel, K. R., Gujral, U. P., & Narayan, K. V. (2016). Type 2 diabetes: A 21st century epidemic. *Best Practice & Research Clinical Endocrinology & Metabolism, 30*(3), 331–343.

Jamshed, H., Beyl, R. A., Della Manna, D. L., Yang, E. S., Ravussin, E., & Peterson, C. M. (2019). Early time-restricted feeding improves 24-hour glucose levels and affects markers of the circadian clock, aging, and autophagy in humans. *Nutrients, 11*(6), 1234.

Jarvis, J. U. (1981). Eusociality in a mammal: Cooperative breeding in naked mole-rat colonies. *Science, 212*(4494), 571–573. https://doi.org/10.1126/science.7209555.

Jia, K., Chen, D., & Riddle, D. L. (2004). The TOR pathway interacts with the insulin signaling pathway to regulate C. elegans larval development, metabolism and life span. *Development, 131*(16), 3897–3906. https://doi.org/10.1242/dev.01255.

Johnson, J. B., Summer, W., Cutler, R. G., Martin, B., Hyun, D.-H., Dixit, V. D., … Maudsley, S. (2007). Alternate day calorie restriction improves clinical findings and reduces markers of oxidative stress and inflammation in overweight adults with moderate asthma. *Free Radical Biology and Medicine, 42*(5), 665–674.

Johnson, S. C., Martin, G. M., Rabinovitch, P. S., & Kaeberlein, M. (2013). Preserving youth: Does rapamycin deliver? *Science Translational Medicine, 5*(211), 211fs240.

Kabil, H., Partridge, L., & Harshman, L. G. (2007). Superoxide dismutase activities in long-lived Drosophila melanogaster females: Chico 1 genotypes and dietary dilution. *Biogerontology, 8*(2), 201–208.

Kachroo, A. H., Laurent, J. M., Yellman, C. M., Meyer, A. G., Wilke, C. O., & Marcotte, E. M. (2015). Evolution. Systematic humanization of yeast genes reveals conserved functions and genetic modularity. *Science, 348*(6237), 921–925. https://doi.org/10.1126/science.aaa0769.

Kaeberlein, M., McVey, M., & Guarente, L. (1999). The SIR2/3/4 complex and SIR2 alone promote longevity in Saccharomyces cerevisiae by two different mechanisms. *Genes & Development, 13*(19), 2570–2580.

Kalani, R., Judge, S., Carter, C., Pahor, M., & Leeuwenburgh, C. (2006). Effects of caloric restriction and exercise on age-related, chronic inflammation assessed by C-reactive protein and interleukin-6. *The Journals of Gerontology Series A: Biological Sciences and Medical Sciences, 61*(3), 211–217.

Kapahi, P., Zid, B. M., Harper, T., Koslover, D., Sapin, V., & Benzer, S. (2004). Regulation of lifespan in Drosophila by modulation of genes in the TOR signaling pathway. *Current Biology, 14*(10), 885–890. https://doi.org/10.1016/j.cub.2004.03.059.

Kett, M. M., & Denton, K. M. (2011). Renal programming: Cause for concern? *American Journal of Physiology-Regulatory, Integrative and Comparative Physiology, 300*(4), R791–R803.

Khalifa, A. R. M., Abdel-Rahman, E. A., Mahmoud, A. M., Ali, M. H., Noureldin, M., Saber, S. H., … Ali, S. S. (2017). Sex-specific differences in mitochondria biogenesis, morphology, respiratory function, and ROS homeostasis in young mouse heart and brain. *Physiological Reports, 5*(6), e13125.

Kirkwood, T. B. (2005). Understanding the odd science of aging. *Cell, 120*(4), 437–447. https://doi.org/10.1016/j.cell.2005.01.027.

Kirkwood, T. B. L., & Cremer, T. (1982). Cytogerontology since 1881: A reappraisal of August Weismann and a review of modern progress. *Human Genetics, 60*(2), 101–121. https://doi.org/10.1007/BF00569695.

Kulkarni, R. N., Brüning, J. C., Winnay, J. N., Postic, C., Magnuson, M. A., & Kahn, C. R. (1999). Tissue-specific knockout of the insulin receptor in pancreatic β cells creates an insulin secretory defect similar to that in type 2 diabetes. *Cell, 96*(3), 329–339.

Kwekel, J. C., Desai, V. G., Moland, C. L., Branham, W. S., & Fuscoe, J. C. (2010). Age and sex dependent changes in liver gene expression during the life cycle of the rat. *BMC Genomics, 11*(1), 675.

Lamming, D. W., Ye, L., Katajisto, P., Goncalves, M. D., Saitoh, M., Stevens, D. M., … Ahima, R. S. (2012). Rapamycin-induced insulin resistance is mediated by mTORC2 loss and uncoupled from longevity. . *Science, 335*(6076), 1638–1643.

Latorre-Pellicer, A., Moreno-Loshuertos, R., Lechuga-Vieco, A. V., Sánchez-Cabo, F., Torroja, C., Acín-Pérez, R., … Enríquez, J. A. (2016). Mitochondrial and nuclear DNA matching shapes metabolism and healthy ageing. *Nature, 535*(7613), 561–565. https://doi.org/10.1038/nature18618.

Levine, R. L., & Stadtman, E. R. (2001). Oxidative modification of proteins during aging. *Experimental Gerontology, 36*(9), 1495–1502.

Li, J., Chen, X., McClusky, R., Ruiz-Sundstrom, M., Itoh, Y., Umar, S., … Eghbali, M. (2014). The number of X chromosomes influences protection from cardiac ischaemia/reperfusion injury in mice: One X is better than two. *Cardiovascular Research, 102*(3), 375–384.

Ligthart, S., van Herpt, T. T., Leening, M. J., Kavousi, M., Hofman, A., Stricker, B. H., … Dehghan, A. (2016). Lifetime risk of developing impaired glucose metabolism and eventual progression from prediabetes to type 2 diabetes: A prospective cohort study. *The Lancet Diabetes & Endocrinology, 4*(1), 44–51.

Lill, C. M. (2016). Genetics of Parkinson's disease. *Molecular and Cellular Probes, 30*(6), 386–396.

Link, J. C., Chen, X., Prien, C., Borja, M. S., Hammerson, B., Oda, M. N., … Reue, K. (2015). Increased high-density lipoprotein cholesterol levels in mice with XX versus XY sex chromosomes. *Arteriosclerosis, Thrombosis, and Vascular Biology, 35*(8), 1778–1786.

Liu, C.-C., Liu, C.-C., Kanekiyo, T., Xu, H., & Bu, G. (2013). Apolipoprotein E and Alzheimer disease: Risk, mechanisms and therapy. *Nature Reviews. Neurology, 9*(2), 106–118. https://doi.org/10.1038/nrneurol.2012.263.

Longo, V., & Fabrizio, P. (2002). Visions & reflections: Regulation of longevity and stress resistance: A molecular strategy conserved from yeast to humans? *Cellular and Molecular Life Sciences, 59*(6), 903–908.

Longo, V. D., & Fabrizio, P. (2011). Chronological aging in Saccharomyces cerevisiae. In M. Breitenbach, S. M. Jazwinski, & P. Laun (Eds.), *Aging research in yeast* (pp. 101–121). Springer.

Longo, V. D., & Panda, S. (2016). Fasting, circadian rhythms, and time-restricted feeding in healthy lifespan. *Cell Metabolism, 23*(6), 1048–1059.

Lu, M., Flanagan, J. U., Langley, R. J., Hay, M. P., & Perry, J. K. (2019). Targeting growth hormone function: Strategies and therapeutic applications. *Signal Transduction and Targeted Therapy, 4*(1), 3. https://doi.org/10.1038/s41392-019-0036-y.

Luckinbill, L. S., & Clare, M. J. (1985). Selection for life span in Drosophila melanogaster. *Heredity, 55*(1), 9.

Lumeng, C. N., & Saltiel, A. R. (2011). Inflammatory links between obesity and metabolic disease. *Journal of Clinical Investigation, 121*(6), 2111–2117.

Lupu, F., Terwilliger, J. D., Lee, K., Segre, G. V., & Efstratiadis, A. (2001). Roles of growth hormone and insulin-like growth factor 1 in mouse postnatal growth. *Developmental Biology, 229*(1), 141–162.

Macera, C. A., Ham, S. A., Yore, M. M., Jones, D. A., Kimsey, C. D., Kohl III, H. W., & Ainsworth III, B. E. (2005). Prevalence of physical activity in the United States: Behavioral risk factor surveillance system, 2001. *Preventing Chronic Disease, 2*(2), A17.

Martens, C. R., Denman, B. A., Mazzo, M. R., Armstrong, M. L., Reisdorph, N., McQueen, M. B., … Seals, D. R. (2018). Chronic nicotinamide riboside supplementation is well-tolerated and elevates NAD+ in healthy middle-aged and older adults. *Nature Communications, 9*(1), 1286. https://doi.org/10.1038/s41467-018-03421-7.

Martin-Montalvo, A., Mercken, E. M., Mitchell, S. J., Palacios, H. H., Mote, P. L., Scheibye-Knudsen, M., … Blouin, M.-J.

(2013). Metformin improves healthspan and lifespan in mice. *Nature Communications*, *4*, 2192.

Martin-Montalvo, A., Sun, Y., Diaz-Ruiz, A., Ali, A., Gutierrez, V., Palacios, H. H., & Abulwerdi, G. A. (2016). Cytochrome b 5 reductase and the control of lipid metabolism and healthspan. *NPJ Aging and Mechanisms of Disease*, *2*(1), 1–12.

Mattison, J. A., Colman, R. J., Beasley, T. M., Allison, D. B., Kemnitz, J. W., Roth, G. S., ... Anderson, R. M. (2017). Caloric restriction improves health and survival of rhesus monkeys. *Nature Communications*, *8*, 14063.

Mattison, J. A., Roth, G. S., Beasley, T. M., Tilmont, E. M., Handy, A. M., Herbert, R. L., ... Bryant, M. (2012). Impact of caloric restriction on health and survival in rhesus monkeys from the NIA study. *Nature*, *489*(7415), 318–321.

Mavinkurve, M., & O'Gorman, C. S. (2015). Cardiometabolic and vascular risks in young and adolescent girls with Turner syndrome. *BBA Clinical*, *3*, 304–309.

Mazure, C. M., & Swendsen, J. (2016). Sex differences in Alzheimer's disease and other dementias. *The Lancet. Neurology*, *15*(5), 451.

McCay, C. M., Crowell, M. F., & Maynard, L. A. (1935). The effect of retarded growth upon the length of life span and upon the ultimate body size: One figure. *Journal of Nutrition*, *10*(1), 63–79.

Medawar, P. (1952). Uniqueness of the individual. In P. B. Medawar (Ed.), *An Unsolved Problem of Biology*. HK Lewis.

Medvedev, Z. A. (1990). An attempt at a rational classification of theories of ageing. *Biological Reviews*, *65*(3), 375–398.

Miller, D. M., Buettner, G. R., & Aust, S. D. (1990). Transition metals as catalysts of "autoxidation" reactions. *Free Radical Biology and Medicine*, *8*(1), 95–108.

Miller, R. A., Harper, J. M., Dysko, R. C., Durkee, S. J., & Austad, S. N. (2002). Longer life spans and delayed maturation in wild-derived mice. *Experimental Biology and Medicine*, *227*(7), 500–508.

Miller, R. A., Harrison, D. E., Astle, C. M., Baur, J. A., Boyd, A. R., de Cabo, R., ... Strong, R. (2010). Rapamycin, but not resveratrol or simvastatin, extends life span of genetically heterogeneous mice. *The Journals of Gerontology: Series A*, *66A*(2), 191–201. https://doi.org/10.1093/gerona/glq178.

Miller, R. A., Harrison, D. E., Astle, C. M., Fernandez, E., Flurkey, K., Han, M., & Nelson, J. F. (2014). Rapamycin-mediated lifespan increase in mice is dose and sex dependent and metabolically distinct from dietary restriction. *Aging Cell*, *13*(3), 468–477.

Miquel, J., Economos, A. C., Fleming, J., & Johnson, J. E. (1980). Mitochondrial role in cell aging. *Experimental Gerontology*, *15*(6), 575–591. https://doi.org/10.1016/0531-5565(80)90010-8.

Mitchell, S. J., Bernier, M., Mattison, J. A., Aon, M. A., Kaiser, T. A., Anson, R. M., & de Cabo, R. (2019). Daily fasting improves health and survival in male mice independent of diet composition and calories. *Cell Metabolism*, *29*(1), 221–228. e223.

Mitchell, S. J., Madrigal-Matute, J., Scheibye-Knudsen, M., Fang, E., Aon, M., González-Reyes, J. A., & Patel, B. (2016). Effects of sex, strain, and energy intake on hallmarks of aging in mice. *Cell Metabolism*, *23*(6), 1093–1112.

Morrisette-Thomas, V., Cohen, A. A., Fülöp, T., Riesco, É., Legault, V., Li, Q., ... Ferrucci, L. (2014). Inflamm-aging does not simply reflect increases in pro-inflammatory markers. *Mechanisms of Ageing and Development*, *139*, 49–57.

Most, J., Gilmore, L. A., Smith, S. R., Han, H., Ravussin, E., & Redman, L. M. (2018). Significant improvement in cardiometabolic health in healthy nonobese individuals during caloric restriction-induced weight loss and weight loss maintenance. *American Journal of Physiology-Endocrinology and Metabolism*, *314*(4), E396–E405.

Mouchiroud, L., Houtkooper, R. H., Moullan, N., Katsyuba, E., Ryu, D., Cantó, C., & Schoonjans, K. (2013). The NAD+/sirtuin pathway modulates longevity through activation of mitochondrial UPR and FOXO signaling. *Cell*, *154*(2), 430–441.

Moynihan, K. A., Grimm, A. A., Plueger, M. M., Bernal-Mizrachi, E., Ford, E., Cras-Méneur, C., ... Imai, S.-I (2005). Increased dosage of mammalian Sir2 in pancreatic β cells enhances glucose-stimulated insulin secretion in mice. *Cell Metabolism*, *2*(2), 105–117.

Mueller, L. D. (2022). Mutation accumulation aging theory. In *Encyclopedia of Gerontology and Population Aging* (pp. 3360–3365). Cham: Springer International Publishing.

Murphy, C. T., McCarroll, S. A., Bargmann, C. I., Fraser, A., Kamath, R. S., Ahringer, J., ... Kenyon, C. (2003). Genes that act downstream of DAF-16 to influence the lifespan of Caenorhabditis elegans. *Nature*, *424*(6946), 277–283.

Neff, F., Flores-Dominguez, D., Ryan, D. P., Horsch, M., Schröder, S., Adler, T., & Garrett, L. (2013). Rapamycin extends murine lifespan but has limited effects on aging. *Journal of Clinical Investigation*, *123*(8), 3272–3291.

Ng, T. P., Feng, L., Yap, K. B., Lee, T. S., Tan, C. H., & Winblad, B. (2014). Long-term metformin usage and cognitive function among older adults with diabetes. *Journal of Alzheimer's Disease*, *41*(1), 61–68.

Niccoli, T., & Partridge, L. (2012). Ageing as a risk factor for disease. *Current Biology*, *22*(17), R741–R752.

O'Connor, T. P., Lee, A., Jarvis, J. U., & Buffenstein, R. (2002). Prolonged longevity in naked mole-rats: Age-related changes in metabolism, body composition and gastrointestinal function. *Comparative Biochemistry and Physiology Part A: Molecular & Integrative Physiology*, *133*(3), 835–842.

Onambélé-Pearson, G. L., Breen, L., & Stewart, C. E. (2010). Influence of exercise intensity in older persons with unchanged habitual nutritional intake: Skeletal muscle and endocrine adaptations. *Age*, *32*(2), 139–153.

Osborne, T. B., Mendel, L. B., & Ferry, E. L. (1917). The effect of retardation of growth upon the breeding period and duration of life of rats. *Science*, *45*(1160), 294–295.

Paneni, F., Cañestro, C. D., Libby, P., Lüscher, T. F., & Camici, G. G. (2017). The aging cardiovascular system: Understanding it at the cellular and clinical levels. *Journal of the American College of Cardiology*, *69*(15), 1952–1967.

Partridge, L., & Fowler, K. (1992). Direct and correlated responses to selection on age at reproduction in Drosophila melanogaster. *Evolution*, *46*(1), 76–91.

Pauling, L. (1976). Vitamin C, the common cold, and the flu. WH Freeman & Co.

Pearson, K. J., Baur, J. A., Lewis, K. N., Peshkin, L., Price, N. L., Labinskyy, N., ... de Cabo, R. (2008). Resveratrol delays age-related deterioration and mimics transcriptional aspects of dietary restriction without extending life span. *Cell Metabolism*, *8*(2), 157–168. https://doi.org/10.1016/j.cmet.2008.06.011.

Pereira, S. P., Oliveira, P. J., Tavares, L. C., Moreno, A. J., Cox, L. A., Nathanielsz, P. W., & Nijland, M. J. (2015). Effects of moderate global maternal nutrient reduction on fetal baboon renal mitochondrial gene expression at 0.9 gestation. *American Journal of Physiology-Renal Physiology*, *308*(11), F1217–F1228.

Pérez, V. I., Bokov, A., Remmen, H. V., Mele, J., Ran, Q., Ikeno, Y., & Richardson, A. (2009). Is the oxidative stress theory of aging dead? *Biochimica et Biophysica Acta (BBA)—General Subjects*, *1790*(10), 1005–1014. https://doi.org/10.1016/j.bbagen.2009.06.003.

Pfluger, P. T., Herranz, D., Velasco-Miguel, S., Serrano, M., & Tschöp, M. H. (2008). Sirt1 protects against high-fat diet-induced metabolic damage. *Proceedings of the National Academy of Sciences, 105*(28), 9793–9798.

Phelan, J. P., & Rose, M. R. (2005). Why dietary restriction substantially increases longevity in animal models but won't in humans. *Ageing Research Reviews, 4*(3), 339–350. https://doi.org/10.1016/j.arr.2005.06.001.

Pichová, A., Vondráková, D., & Breitenbach, M. (1997). Mutants in the Saccharomyces cerevisiae RAS2 gene influence life span, cytoskeleton, and regulation of mitosis. *Canadian Journal of Microbiology, 43*(8), 774–781.

Pickering, A. M., Lehr, M., Kohler, W. J., Han, M. L., & Miller, R. A. (2014). Fibroblasts from konger-lived species of primates, rodents, bats, carnivores, and birds resist protein damage. *The Journals of Gerontology: Series A, 70*(7), 791–799. https://doi.org/10.1093/gerona/glu115.

Pickering, A. M., Lehr, M., & Miller, R. A. (2015). Lifespan of mice and primates correlates with immunoproteasome expression. *Journal of Clinical Investigation, 125*(5), 2059–2068. https://doi.org/10.1172/JCI80514.

Pickering, A. M., Linder, R. A., Zhang, H., Forman, H. J., & Davies, K. J. (2012). Nrf2-dependent induction of proteasome and Pa28αβ regulator are required for adaptation to oxidative stress. *Journal of Biological Chemistry, 287*(13), 10021–10031.

Pickering, A. M., Staab, T. A., Tower, J., Sieburth, D., & Davies, K. J. (2013). A conserved role for the 20S proteasome and Nrf2 transcription factor in oxidative stress adaptation in mammals, Caenorhabditis elegans and Drosophila melanogaster. *Journal of Experimental Biology, 216*(4), 543–553.

Pinto, M., Jepsen, K., Terranova, C., & Buffenstein, R. (2010). Lack of sexual dimorphism in femora of the eusocial and hypogonadic naked mole-rat: A novel animal model for the study of delayed puberty on the skeletal system. *Bone, 46*(1), 112–120.

Pomatto, L. C., Dill, T., Carboneau, B., Levan, S., Kato, J., Mercken, E. M., & de Cabo, R. (2020). Deletion of Nrf2 shortens lifespan in C57BL6/J male mice but does not alter the health and survival benefits of caloric restriction. *Free Radical Biology and Medicine, 152*, 650–658. https://doi.org/10.1016/j.freeradbiomed.2020.01.005.

Pomatto, L. C., Sun, P. Y., Yu, K., Gullapalli, S., Bwiza, C. P., Sisliyan, C., & Oliver, P. L. (2019). Limitations to adaptive homeostasis in an hyperoxia-induced model of accelerated ageing. *Redox Biology, 24*, 101194.

Pomatto, L. C., Wong, S., Carney, C., Shen, B., Tower, J., & Davies, K. J. (2017). The age-and sex-specific decline of the 20s proteasome and the Nrf2/CncC signal transduction pathway in adaption and resistance to oxidative stress in Drosophila melanogaster. *Aging (Albany NY), 9*(4), 1153.

Pomatto, L. C. D., & Davies, K. J. A. (2018). Adaptive homeostasis and the free radical theory of ageing. *Free Radical Biology and Medicine, 124*, 420–430. https://doi.org/10.1016/j.freeradbiomed.2018.06.016.

Pomatto, L. C. D., Sun, P. Y., & Davies, K. J. A. (2019). To adapt or not to adapt: Consequences of declining adaptive homeostasis and proteostasis with age. *Mechanisms of Ageing and Development, 177*, 80–87. https://doi.org/10.1016/j.mad.2018.05.006.

Poulsen, M. M., Vestergaard, P. F., Clasen, B. F., Radko, Y., Christensen, L. P., Stødkilde-Jørgensen, H., … Jørgensen, J. O. L. (2013). High-dose resveratrol supplementation in obese men. *An Investigator-Initiated, Randomized, Placebo-Controlled Clinical Trial of Substrate Metabolism, Insulin Sensitivity, and Body Composition, 62*(4), 1186–1195. https://doi.org/10.2337/db12-0975.

Prattichizzo, F., De Nigris, V., Spiga, R., Mancuso, E., La Sala, L., Antonicelli, R., & Ceriello, A. (2018). Inflammageing and metaflammation: The yin and yang of type 2 diabetes. *Ageing Research Reviews, 41*, 1–17. https://doi.org/10.1016/j.arr.2017.10.003.

Ramadori, G., Fujikawa, T., Fukuda, M., Anderson, J., Morgan, D. A., Mostoslavsky, R., & Nillni, E. A. (2010). SIRT1 deacetylase in POMC neurons is required for homeostatic defenses against diet-induced obesity. *Cell Metabolism, 12*(1), 78–87.

Ramsey, J. J., Tran, D., Giorgio, M., Griffey, S. M., Koehne, A., Laing, S. T., & Lloyd, K. K. (2013). The influence of Shc proteins on life span in mice. *The Journals of Gerontology Series A: Biomedical Sciences and Medical Sciences, 69*(10), 1177–1185.

Ramsey, K. M., Mills, K. F., Satoh, A., & Imai, S. i (2008). Age-associated loss of Sirt1-mediated enhancement of glucose-stimulated insulin secretion in beta cell-specific Sirt1-overexpressing (BESTO) mice. *Aging Cell, 7*(1), 78–88.

Rangan, P., Choi, I., Wei, M., Navarrete, G., Guen, E., Brandhorst, S., & Ocon, V. (2019). Fasting-mimicking diet modulates microbiota and promotes intestinal regeneration to reduce inflammatory bowel disease pathology. *Cell Reports, 26*(10), 2704–2719.

Ravussin, E., Beyl, R. A., Poggiogalle, E., Hsia, D. S., & Peterson, C. M. (2019). Early time-restricted feeding reduces appetite and increases fat oxidation but does not affect energy expenditure in humans. *Obesity, 27*(8), 1244–1254.

Ravussin, E., Redman, L. M., Rochon, J., Das, S. K., Fontana, L., Kraus, W. E., … Villareal, D. T. (2015). A 2-year randomized controlled trial of human caloric restriction: Feasibility and effects on predictors of health span and longevity. *The Journals of Gerontology: Series A, 70*(9), 1097–1104.

Raynes, R., Juarez, C., Pomatto, L. C., Sieburth, D., & Davies, K. J. (2017). Aging and SKN-1-dependent loss of 20S proteasome adaptation to oxidative stress in C. elegans. *The Journals of Gerontology Series A: Biomedical Sciences and Medical Sciences, 72*(2), 143–151.

Redman, L. M., Smith, S. R., Burton, J. H., Martin, C. K., Il'yasova, D., & Ravussin, E. (2018). Metabolic slowing and reduced oxidative damage with sustained caloric restriction support the rate of living and oxidative damage theories of aging. *Cell Metabolism, 27*(4), 805–815. E804.

Regitz-Zagrosek, V., & Kararigas, G. (2016). Mechanistic pathways of sex differences in cardiovascular disease. *Physiological Reviews, 97*(1), 1–37.

Rice, W. R. (1992). Sexually antagonistic genes: Experimental evidence. *Science, 256*(5062), 1436–1439.

Robins, C., McRae, A. F., Powell, J. E., Wiener, H. W., Aslibekyan, S., Kennedy, E. M., & Visscher, P. M. (2017). Testing two evolutionary theories of human aging with DNA methylation data. *Genetics, 207*(4), 1547–1560.

Rodríguez, J. A., Marigorta, U. M., Hughes, D. A., Spataro, N., Bosch, E., & Navarro, A. (2017). Antagonistic pleiotropy and mutation accumulation influence human senescence and disease. *Nature Ecology & Evolution, 1*(3), 0055.

Rogina, B., & Helfand, S. L. (2004). Sir2 mediates longevity in the fly through a pathway related to calorie restriction. *Proceedings of the National Academy of Sciences, 101*(45), 15998–16003.

Rogina, B., Reenan, R. A., Nilsen, S. P., & Helfand, S. L. (2000). Extended life-span conferred by cotransporter gene mutations in Drosophila. *Science, 290*(5499), 2137–2140.

Rose, M., & Charlesworth, B. (1980). A test of evolutionary theories of senescence. *Nature, 287*(5778), 141–142.

Rose, M. R. (1982). Antagonistic pleiotropy, dominance, and genetic variation. *Heredity*, *48*(1), 63.

Rosenberg, T., Nørby, S., Schwartz, M., Saillard, J., Magalhaes, P. J., Leroy, D., & Duno, M. (2016). Prevalence and genetics of Leber hereditary optic neuropathy in the Danish population. *Investigative Ophthalmology & Visual Science*, *57*(3), 1370–1375.

Rous, P. (1914). The influence of diet on transplanted and spontaneous mouse tumors. *Journal of Experimental Medicine*, *20*(5), 433–451.

Rozhok, A. I., & DeGregori, J. (2016). The evolution of lifespan and age-dependent cancer risk. *Trends in Cancer*, *2*(10), 552–560.

Saisho, Y. (2015). Metformin and inflammation: Its potential beyond glucose-lowering effect. *Endocrine, Metabolic & Immune Disorders-Drug Targets (Formerly Current Drug Targets-Immune, Endocrine & Metabolic Disorders)*, *15*(3), 196–205.

Salih, D. A., & Brunet, A. (2008). FoxO transcription factors in the maintenance of cellular homeostasis during aging. *Current Opinion in Cell Biology*, *20*(2), 126–136. https://doi.org/10.1016/j.ceb.2008.02.005.

Schlender, L., Martinez, Y. V., Adeniji, C., Reeves, D., Faller, B., Sommerauer, C., & Renom-Guiteras, A. (2017). Efficacy and safety of metformin in the management of type 2 diabetes mellitus in older adults: A systematic review for the development of recommendations to reduce potentially inappropriate prescribing. *BMC Geriatrics*, *17*(1), 227. https://doi.org/10.1186/s12877-017-0574-5.

Schulz, T. J., Zarse, K., Voigt, A., Urban, N., Birringer, M., & Ristow, M. (2007). Glucose restriction extends Caenorhabditis elegans life span by inducing mitochondrial respiration and increasing oxidative stress. *Cell Metabolism*, *6*(4), 280–293. https://doi.org/10.1016/j.cmet.2007.08.011.

Selman, C., Lingard, S., Choudhury, A. I., Batterham, R. L., Claret, M., Clements, M., & Blanc, E. (2008). Evidence for lifespan extension and delayed age-related biomarkers in insulin receptor substrate 1 null mice. *The FASEB Journal*, *22*(3), 807–818.

Selman, C., Tullet, J. M., Wieser, D., Irvine, E., Lingard, S. J., Choudhury, A. I., … Ramadani, F. (2009). Ribosomal protein S6 kinase 1 signaling regulates mammalian life span. *Science*, *326*(5949), 140–144.

Shanley, D. P., & Kirkwood, T. B. (2001). Evolution of the human menopause. *Bioessays*, *23*(3), 282–287.

Sharma, N., Castorena, C. M., & Cartee, G. D. (2012). Tissue-specific responses of IGF-1/insulin and mTOR signaling in calorie restricted rats. *PLoS One*, *7*(6), e38835–e38835. https://doi.org/10.1371/journal.pone.0038835.

Shay, J. W. (2016). Role of telomeres and telomerase in aging and cancer. *Cancer Discovery*, *6*(6), 584–593.

Sherman, H., Campbell, H., & Rice, P. (1937). Nutritional well-being and length of life as influenced by different enrichments of an already adequate diet: One figure. *The Journal of Nutrition*, *14*(6), 609–620.

Singh, T., & Newman, A. B. (2011). Inflammatory markers in population studies of aging. *Ageing Research Reviews*, *10*(3), 319–329.

Skulachev, V. P. (2002). Programmed death phenomena: From organelle to organism. *Annals of the New York Academy of Sciences*, *959*(1), 214–237.

Slavov, N., Airoldi, E. M., van Oudenaarden, A., & Botstein, D. (2012). A conserved cell growth cycle can account for the environmental stress responses of divergent eukaryotes. *Molecular Biology of the Cell*, *23*(10), 1986–1997.

Smith, S. T., LeSarge, J. C., & Lemon, P. W. (2017). Time-restricted eating in women: A pilot study. *Western Undergraduate Research Journal: Health and Natural Sciences*, *8*(1). https://doi.org/10.5206/wurjhns.2017-18.3.

Solon-Biet, S. M., McMahon, A. C., Ballard, J. W. O., Ruohonen, K., Wu, L. E., Cogger, V. C., … Melvin, R. G. (2014). The ratio of macronutrients, not caloric intake, dictates cardiometabolic health, aging, and longevity in ad libitum-fed mice. *Cell Metabolism*, *19*(3), 418–430.

Soto-Rivera, C. L., Romero, C. J., & Cohen, L. E. (2018). Childhood growth hormone deficiency and hypopituitarism. In S. Radovick & M. Misra (Eds.), *Pediatric endocrinology: A practical clinical guide* (pp. 3–29). Springer International.

Steinkraus, K. A., Kaeberlein, M., & Kennedy, B. K. (2008). Replicative aging in yeast: The means to the end. *Annual Review of Cell and Developmental Biology*, *24*, 29–54. https://doi.org/10.1146/annurev.cellbio.23.090506.123509.

Sumantri, S., Setiati, S., Purnamasari, D., & Dewiasty, E. (2016). Relationship between metformin and frailty syndrome in elderly people with type 2 diabetes. *Acta Medica Indonesiana*, *46*(3), 183–188.

Sutton, E. F., Beyl, R., Early, K. S., Cefalu, W. T., Ravussin, E., & Peterson, C. M. (2018). Early time-restricted feeding improves insulin sensitivity, blood pressure, and oxidative stress even without weight loss in men with prediabetes. *Cell Metabolism*, *27*(6), 1212–1221. e1213.

Tatar, M., Kopelman, A., Epstein, D., Tu, M.-P., Yin, C.-M., & Garofalo, R. (2001). A mutant Drosophila insulin receptor homolog that extends life-span and impairs neuroendocrine function. *Science*, *292*(5514), 107–110.

Tedeschi, S. K., Bermas, B., & Costenbader, K. H. (2013). Sexual disparities in the incidence and course of SLE and RA. *Clinical Immunology*, *149*(2), 211–218.

Teng, N. I. M. F., Shahar, S., Rajab, N. F., Manaf, Z. A., Johari, M. H., & Ngah, W. Z. W. (2013). Improvement of metabolic parameters in healthy older adult men following a fasting calorie restriction intervention. *The Aging Male*, *16*(4), 177–183.

Timmers, S., Auwerx, J., & Schrauwen, P. (2012). The journey of resveratrol from yeast to human. *Aging (Albany NY)*, *4*(3), 146.

Timmers, S., Konings, E., Bilet, L., Houtkooper, , Riekelt, H., van de Weijer, T., Goossens, , Gijs, H., & Schrauwen, P. (2011). Calorie restriction-like effects of 30 days of resveratrol supplementation on energy metabolism and metabolic profile in obese humans. *Cell Metabolism*, *14*(5), 612–622. https://doi.org/10.1016/j.cmet.2011.10.002.

Tinsley, G. M., & La Bounty, P. M. (2015). Effects of intermittent fasting on body composition and clinical health markers in humans. *Nutrition Reviews*, *73*(10), 661–674.

Tissenbaum, H. A., & Guarente, L. (2001). Increased dosage of a sir-2 gene extends lifespan in Caenorhabditis elegans. *Nature*, *410*(6825), 227–230.

Turan, Z. G., Parvizi, P., Dönertaş, H. M., Tung, J., Khaitovich, P., & Somel, M. (2019). Molecular footprint of Medawar's mutation accumulation process in mammalian aging. *Aging Cell*, *18*(4), e12965. https://doi.org/10.1111/acel.12965.

Ulrich, H. (2007). Conservation of DNA damage tolerance pathways from yeast to humans. *Biochemical Society transactions*, *35*(Pt 5), 1334–1337. https://doi.org/10.1042/BST0351334.

Ungvari, Z., Buffenstein, R., Austad, S. N., Podlutsky, A., Kaley, G., & Csiszar, A. (2008). Oxidative stress in vascular senescence: Lessons from successfully aging species. *Front Bioscience*, *13*, 5056–5070.

Urfer, S. R., Kaeberlein, T. L., Mailheau, S., Bergman, P. J., Creevy, K. E., Promislow, D. E. L., & Kaeberlein, M. (2017). A randomized controlled trial to establish effects of short-term rapamycin treatment in 24 middle-aged companion dogs. *GeroScience, 39*(2), 117–127. https://doi.org/10.1007/s11357-017-9972-z.

Vaiserman, A., & Lushchak, O. (2017). Implementation of longevity-promoting supplements and medications in public health practice: Achievements, challenges and future perspectives. *Journal of Translational Medicine, 15*(1), 160.

Varady, K. A., Bhutani, S., Klempel, M. C., & Kroeger, C. M. (2011). Comparison of effects of diet versus exercise weight loss regimens on LDL and HDL particle size in obese adults. *Lipids in Health and Disease, 10*(1), 119.

Varady, K. A., Bhutani, S., Klempel, M. C., Kroeger, C. M., Trepanowski, J. F., Haus, J. M., & Calvo, Y. (2013). Alternate day fasting for weight loss in normal weight and overweight subjects: A randomized controlled trial. *Nutrition Journal, 12*(1), 146.

Vermeij, W., Dollé, M., Reiling, E., Jaarsma, D., Payan-Gomez, C., Bombardieri, C. R., & Van Der Eerden, B. (2016). Restricted diet delays accelerated ageing and genomic stress in DNA-repair-deficient mice. *Nature, 537*(7620), 427–431.

Vijay, V., Han, T., Moland, C. L., Kwekel, J. C., Fuscoe, J. C., & Desai, V. G. (2015). Sexual dimorphism in the expression of mitochondria-related genes in rat heart at different ages. *PLoS One, 10*(1), e0117047. https://doi.org/10.1371/journal.pone.0117047.

Vijg, J., & Kennedy, B. K. (2016). The essence of aging. *Gerontology, 62*(4), 381–385. https://doi.org/10.1159/000439348.

Vitale, C., Mercuro, G., Cornoldi, A., Fini, M., Volterrani, M., & Rosano, G. (2005). Metformin improves endothelial function in patients with metabolic syndrome. *Journal of Internal Medicine, 258*(3), 250–256.

Wagner, S., & Dancey, J. E. (2016). Potential future indication of rapamycin analogs for the treatment of solid tumors. In M. Mita, A. Mita, & E. K. Rowinsky (Eds.), *mTOR inhibition for cancer therapy: Past, present and future* (pp. 229–249). Springer Paris.

Walker, D. W., McColl, G., Jenkins, N. L., Harris, J., & Lithgow, G. J. (2000). Natural selection: Evolution of lifespan in C. elegans. *Nature, 405*(6784), 296.

Wang, C.-P., Lorenzo, C., Habib, S. L., Jo, B., & Espinoza, S. E. (2017). Differential effects of metformin on age related comorbidities in older men with type 2 diabetes. *Journal of Diabetes and Its Complications, 31*(4), 679–686.

Wang, M. C., Bohmann, D., & Jasper, H. (2003). JNK signaling confers tolerance to oxidative stress and extends lifespan in Drosophila. *Developmental Cell, 5*(5), 811–816.

Wei, M., Brandhorst, S., Shelehchi, M., Mirzaei, H., Cheng, C. W., Budniak, J., & Longo, V. D. (2017). Fasting-mimicking diet and markers/risk factors for aging, diabetes, cancer, and cardiovascular disease. *Science Translational Medicine, 9*(377), eaai8700. https://doi.org/10.1126/scitranslmed.aai8700.

Weismann, A., Poulton, E. B., & Shipley, A. E. (1891). *Essays upon heredity and kindred biological problems* (Vol. 1). Clarendon Press.

Wilkinson, M. J., Manoogian, E. N., Zadourian, A., Lo, H., Fakhouri, S., Shoghi, A., & Panda, S. (2020). Ten-hour time-restricted eating reduces weight, blood pressure, and atherogenic lipids in patients with metabolic syndrome. *Cell Metabolism, 31*(1), 92–104. E105.

Williams, G. C. (1957). Pleiotropy, natural selection, and the evolution of senescence. *Evolution*, 398–411.

Winkler, T. W., Justice, A. E., Graff, M., Barata, L., Feitosa, M. F., Chu, S., Kilpeläinen, T. O., Lu, Y., Mägi, R., Mihailov, E., Pers, T. H., Rüeger, S., Teumer, A., Ehret, G. B., Ferreira, T., Heard-Costa, N. L., Karjalainen, J., … Loos, R. J. (2015). The influence of age and sex on genetic associations with adult body size and shape: A large-scale genome-wide interaction study. *PLoS Genetics, 11*(10), e1005378. https://doi.org/10.1371/journal.pgen.1005378.

Wright, A., Charlesworth, B., Rudan, I., Carothers, A., & Campbell, H. (2003). A polygenic basis for late-onset disease. *TRENDS in Genetics, 19*(2), 97–106.

Wu, J. J., Liu, J., Chen, E. B., Wang, J. J., Cao, L., Narayan, N., … Springer, D. A. (2013). Increased mammalian lifespan and a segmental and tissue-specific slowing of aging after genetic reduction of mTOR expression. *Cell Reports, 4*(5), 913–920.

Xie, K., Neff, F., Markert, A., Rozman, J., Aguilar-Pimentel, J. A., Amarie, O. V., … Henzel, K. S. (2017). Every-other-day feeding extends lifespan but fails to delay many symptoms of aging in mice. *Nature Communications, 8*(1), 1–19.

Yang, W., & Hekimi, S. (2010). A mitochondrial superoxide signal triggers increased longevity in Caenorhabditis elegans. *PLoS Biology, 8*(12), e1000556. https://doi.org/10.1371/journal.pbio.1000556.

Yoshino, J., Conte, C., Fontana, L., Mittendorfer, B., Imai, S., Schechtman, K. B., & Klein, S. (2012). Resveratrol supplementation does not improve metabolic function in nonobese women with normal glucose tolerance. *Cell Metabolism, 16*(5), 658–664. https://doi.org/10.1016/j.cmet.2012.09.015.

Yoshino, J., Mills, K. F., Yoon, M. J., & Imai, S.-I. (2011). Nicotinamide mononucleotide, a key NAD+ intermediate, treats the pathophysiology of diet-and age-induced diabetes in mice. *Cell Metabolism, 14*(4), 528–536.

Yuan, R., Flurkey, K., Meng, Q., Astle, M. C., & Harrison, D. E. (2012). Genetic regulation of life span, metabolism, and body weight in Pohn, a new wild-derived mouse strain. *The Journals of Gerontology Series A: Biomedical Sciences and Medical Sciences, 68*(1), 27–35.

Zainal, T. A., Oberley, T. D., Allison, D. B., Szweda, L. I., & Weindruch, R. (2000). Caloric restriction of rhesus monkeys lowers oxidative damage in skeletal muscle. *The FASEB Journal, 14*(12), 1825–1836.

Zeb, F., Wu, X., Chen, L., Fatima, S., Haq, I.-u, Chen, A., & Li, M. (2020). Effect of time restricted feeding on metabolic risk and circadian rhythm associated with gut microbiome in healthy males. *British Journal of Nutrition, 123*(11), 1216–1226. https://doi.org/10.1017/S0007114519003428.

Zelko, I. N., Mariani, T. J., & Folz, R. J. (2002). Superoxide dismutase multigene family: A comparison of the CuZn-SOD (SOD1), Mn-SOD (SOD2), and EC-SOD (SOD3) gene structures, evolution, and expression. *Free Radical Biology and Medicine, 33*(3), 337–349.

Zhang, H., Davies, K. J., & Forman, H. J. (2015). Oxidative stress response and Nrf2 signaling in aging. *Free Radical Biology and Medicine, 88*, 314–336.

Zhang, M. A., Rego, D., Moshkova, M., Kebir, H., Chruscinski, A., Nguyen, H., & Steinman, L. (2012). Peroxisome proliferator-activated receptor (PPAR) α and-γ regulate IFNγ and IL-17A production by human T cells in a sex-specific way. *Proceedings of the National Academy of Sciences, 109*(24), 9505–9510.

Zhou, L., Liu, H., Wen, X., Peng, Y., Tian, Y., & Zhao, L. (2017). Effects of metformin on blood pressure in nondiabetic patients: A meta-analysis of randomized controlled trials. *Journal of Hypertension, 35*(1), 18–26.

Zimmermann, A., Hofer, S., Pendl, T., Kainz, K., Madeo, F., & Carmona-Gutierrez, D. (2018). Yeast as a tool to identify anti-aging compounds. *FEMS Yeast Research, 18*(6), foy020. https://doi.org/10.1093/femsyr/foy020.

Zordoky, B. N. M., Robertson, I. M., & Dyck, J. R. B. (2015). Preclinical and clinical evidence for the role of resveratrol in the treatment of cardiovascular diseases. *Biochimica et Biophysica Acta (BBA)—Molecular Basis of Disease, 1852*(6), 1155–1177. https://doi.org/10.1016/j.bbadis.2014.10.016.

2 Normal Aging

LISA MCLEAN, MMS, PA-C

OBJECTIVES

Student Learning Objectives

After completing this chapter, the student should be able to do the following:

1. Appreciate that the normal aging process of an older adult is mutually exclusive from the pathologies and diseases of humankind.
2. Identify the normal phenotypic expressions of aging per organ system.

Practitioner Objectives

After completing this chapter, the practitioner should be able to do the following:

1. Appreciate the social biases against aging and keep oneself—and one's patients—from perpetuating them.
2. Appreciate the value of older adults in the workforce and community.
3. Appreciate the value of an interdisciplinary team to optimize the routine care of normal older adults.

Introduction

From conception to age 18, normal developmental changes are considered milestone accomplishments. There is an innate, evolutionary love for pediatric patients and their rapid progression into adulthood. As the rate of change becomes more subtle and the person becomes more independent, the social view of aging changes from accomplishment to burden, a sign of impending and unwelcome frailty, death, or both. The markets of the Western world capture this concern clearly, as a significant segment of the global economy is dedicated to antiaging products, books, procedures, and services of all kinds. In 2019 the global antiaging industry closed at $54.2 billion USD (Anti-Aging Market Size, Share, Trends and Forecast 2020–2025, n.d.). Even amid the 2020 global pandemic, the stock market forecasters anticipated growth in the antiaging market. This is likely due to the spectacular job of marketing and advertising, which links antiaging services and products to desired words such as *youth, vitality, smooth, treatment, prevention*, and *dermatologist approved*, with a side-by-side picture of a highly wrinkled version of an older woman against her impossibly unblemished younger self.

Although the antiaging market overtly advertises to female consumers with spending power, the male ego is also passively attacked. Men are quietly addressed by advertisements that identify age-related experiences—such as thinning hair or delayed erection time—as easy, necessary corrections to maintain confidence and sex appeal.

At present, societal trends all over the globe are confusing advertisements for medical truths: Many adults live in a dynamic where wrinkles are considered a treatable condition, but knee pain and memory loss are a part of "just aging." In other words, the general public is miseducated about which features of aging are physiologic versus pathologic.

Practitioners must be aware that they are—and have been—subject to social and marketing pressures throughout their own lives. They are therefore subject to the same implicit bias against aging (see Chapter 4). It is imperative that physician assistants (PAs) and nurse practitioners (NPs) acknowledge this implicit bias in order to fulfill the professional competencies of social justice, leadership, and systems-based practice (PAEA et al., 2005; Position Statements & White Papers—National Organization of Nurse Practitioner Faculties [NONPF], n.d.). Providers must intentionally refine their practical and evidence-based recommendations regarding normal aging. This chapter reviews that knowledge base by providing a current, complete evaluation of how the human being develops into and through the phenotype of the older adult. In addition, this chapter emphasizes various practical tips and resources by body system.

Let us first review the practical benefit of the older adult in society, as well as the practical benefit of understanding normal aging processes and the varying members of an interdisciplinary team.

The increasing average life span and the financial pressures of society have kept older adults in the workforce. In the United States, older adults are incentivized to stay in the workforce as long as possible to maximize the retirement money received from the federal government (Social Security). For instance, a person at the minimum age to request Social Security benefits (age 62) would receive $500 USD per month for the rest of her or his life, whereas a person at who starts receiving payments at age 70 would receive $1000 USD per month (Benefits Planner: Retirement, n.d.). This effectively keeps more older adults in the workforce.

CASE STUDY

A 74-year-old man presents to his PA or NP provider requesting a medical clearance note to start employment. The patient was hoping to work as a part-time assembly worker for a company "just 5 minutes from my house." He is not sure what the work will entail, but he is "sure I can do it. I used to do all kinds of things." He presents a note from a workplace health practitioner requesting medical clearance to lift/push/pull objects greater than 50 pounds in order to satisfy the employer's job description. The workplace health provider is requesting medical clearance due to the patient's history of low back pain treated with occasional opioid use. The patient states that the opioid use is "only at night to help me sleep" and his back pain is "only bad when I'm lifting wrong." The medical provider is also requesting medical clearance for the man's blood pressure, which was 174/94 on three readings in the workplace health office. His readings are 165/92 in your office today. How should the practitioner guide this office visit?

All practitioners should be mindful that age does not preclude a person from being a functional and low-risk employee; however, there are practical considerations a practitioner must objectively evaluate when medically clearing an older adult to start or continue employment. Organ-specific functional declines may interfere with a particular job—such as vision or reflex impairment as risks to a truck driver—and the provider may have a clear-cut benchmark to allow or disqualify the patient only from the job that would cause medical harm to the patient or fellow employees. The practitioner should also inquire about recreational and financial motives for employment. The older adult who once attempted retirement but missed being employed is likely to add value to the workforce. An older adult who appears demoralized or bound by financial hardship may be inclined to omit medical information that could reduce the chances of passing a preemployment medical physical. Practitioners will do justice to both the patient and the employer by presenting themselves as kind, unbiased agents for workplace safety. The practitioner's role is to make sure that the employee is medically capable of performing the tasks the employer is requesting. Therefore, the person's physiology, the consequences of any cumulative pathologies, and the nature of the job are all important components for a successful office visit and safe employment.

Practitioners outside of workplace health practices are often confused about how to approach a patient's request for medical clearance to work. Unlike the typical "off work/off school" note, a medical clearance note is simply an honest assessment about what the patient can safely perform on a daily basis. Here are some suggestions about how to satisfy the requests of older adult employees who are looking to enter, alter, or maintain their position in the workforce:

- Requesting job descriptions from the employer's human resource department is an easy, rapid, and Health Insurance Portability and Accountability Act (HIPPA)–compliant way for the provider to quickly understand the demands of the desired job. The employee does not need to sign a release of medical information for the practitioner to request it.
- If there is a medical concern or contraindication for a particular job function, that itself does not exclude that employee from gainful employment. As much as possible, practitioners should avoid labeling an employee as "disqualified" from being hired into a facility, and favor the practice of "pending medical clearance" from the primary care practitioner or specialist. The specialist can give either full medical clearance or a restriction note stating the maximum functional capacity of the patient. It may be reasonable to refer the patient for a *functional capacity exam*, which is often performed by a physical therapist.

A restriction note should comment on the upper limit of the patient's physical capacity. If the condition is temporary, the practitioner should list the duration or the date of the next patient-provider follow-up visit. For instance, a pregnant employee's obstetrician may restrict her to "no lifting more than 20 pounds from [these listed dates]." In the case of the case presented in the case study, the primary care practitioner could use restrictions such as "no lifting over 30 pounds, no lifting below waist or above shoulder height" to accommodate the patient's back pain and hypertension and "no safety-sensitive tasks" to accommodate the patient's use of opioids. The employer only needs to know what the person should not do so that injury can be avoided.

If the provider is uncertain of the employee's true functional capacity, the practitioner could consider the following:

- Reviewing other specialist imaging studies, such as the Bruce protocol treadmill stress tests or pulmonary function tests.
- Reviewing other interdisciplinary team member notes, such as range of motion and strength capacity from physical therapy notes.
- Referring the patient for a functional capacity evaluation.
- Requesting medical clearance or guidance from one of the patient's specialists. The employer may find that the employee's restrictions easily fall within the functional parameters of the job. If not, the employer may find a more suitable job for the older adult within the company.

Practitioners must be the reassuring guides between the aging workforce and employers. Practitioners in all disciplines must work with their patients to help them balance the demands of the workforce and the needs of the body. Practitioners should remember that the benefit of gainful employment in the right job yields much reward to both employee and employer.

Normal Phenotypic Expressions of Aging

Although it is understood that "parts wear out over time," and that the individual's blend of genetic disposition and life story can hasten or delay that fate, the discussion that follows is an evidence-based review of how each organ system evolves with the aging process. The scientific community continues to deepen the pool of fundamental knowledge of human anatomy and physiology. Organs that are easily biopsied and visualized—such as the integumentary system, heart, lungs, and kidneys—have well-understood physiologic processes. As a result, the normal phenotype of aging has been appreciated for decades. With the development and increased availability of advanced imaging techniques, many areas of the body have been rediscovered. For instance, functional magnetic resonance imaging (fMRI) has allowed significant areas of the brain to be mapped and associated with different regions of the body. This capacity has added a completely new approach to data collection and, ultimately, the understanding about how normal aging is experienced in each organ and systemic function.

Sleep: Normal Changes in the Older Adult

Despite popular belief, sleep changes very little in older adulthood compared to the changes that occurred earlier in life (Li et al., 2018; Fig. 2.1). Adults of all ages appear to maintain their ability to initiate or reinitiate sleep, in keeping with their baseline (Obayon et al., 2004). Total sleep time appears to reduce by 10 minutes per decade between childhood to age 60, then it plateaus into later adulthood (Campbell & Murphy, 2007; Li et al., 2018; Obayon et al., 2004). Sleep efficiency drops dramatically between adolescence to adulthood, with a steady decline into older adulthood. However, once at age 60, sleep efficiency remains stable or declines only very slowly (Obayon et al., 2004).

Deep sleep appears to reduce with age, though there is no significant change between middle adulthood and older age. More specifically, there is a slow and stable reduction of rapid-eye-movement (REM) sleep compared to nonrapid eye movement sleep (Floyd et al., 2007).

Sleep is intimately intertwined with the circadian rhythm. The circadian rhythm monitors the physiologic interplay among several body systems, including body temperature; excretion of melatonin, thyroid-stimulating hormone (TSH), and cortisol; heart rate; blood pressure; bone remodeling; sleep wake-pattern; and rest-activity pattern (Wright & Frey, 2008). The suprachiasmatic nucleus (SCN), which regulates this rhythm, appears to atrophy with age and offers less robust control over the circadian rhythm's active phase. In addition, atrophy of the SCN leads to less robust expression and speed when switching between the 24-hour cycles. As a result, the normal aging adult will experience melatonin release and body temperature changes earlier in the evening than a younger adult, and the older adult may also wake earlier in the morning (Duffy et al., 2015; Mattis & Sehgal, 2016; Fig. 2.2).

Melatonin, the hormone responsible for inducing sleepiness in response to darkness, is excreted in smaller volumes with aging (Copinschi & Caufriez, 2013). The Endocrine System section, presented next, offers a more complete review of major hormone variances in TSH, levothyroxine (T4), glucocorticoid, and sex steroids and their influence with sleep.

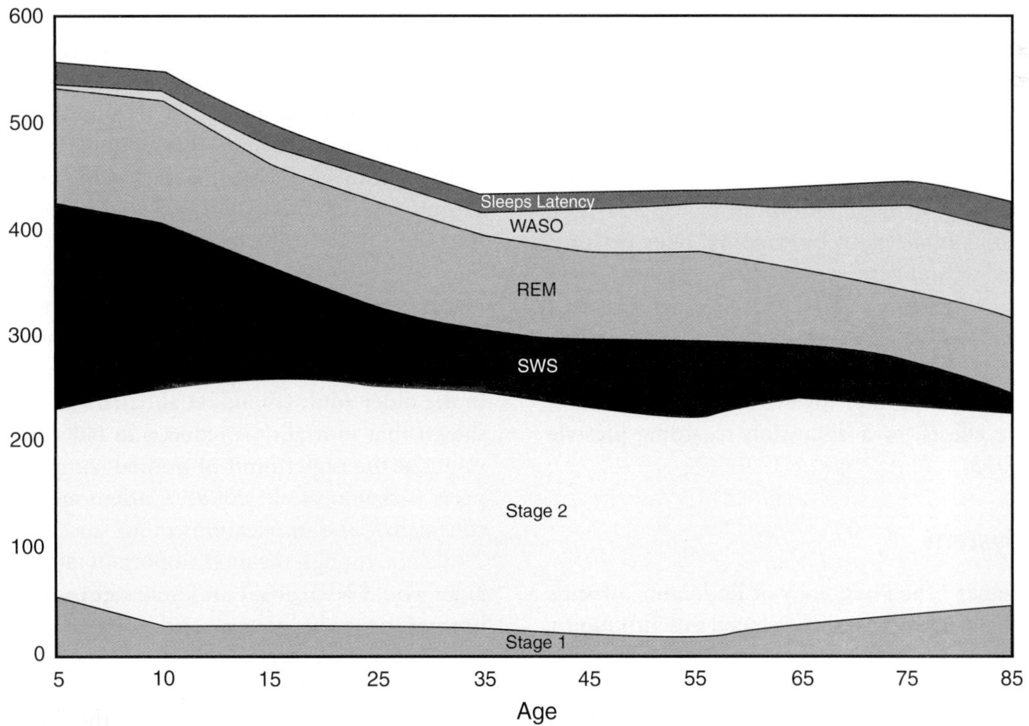

• **Fig. 2.1** Changes in Sleep Architecture Throughout Normal Aging. REM, rapid eye movement; SWS, slow wave sleep; WASO, wake after sleep onset. (From Obayon, M. M., Carskadon, M. A., Guilleminault, C., et al. [2004]. Meta-analysis of quantitative sleep parameters from childhood to old age in healthy individuals: Developing normative sleep values across the human life span. *Sleep, 27*[7], 1255–1273.)

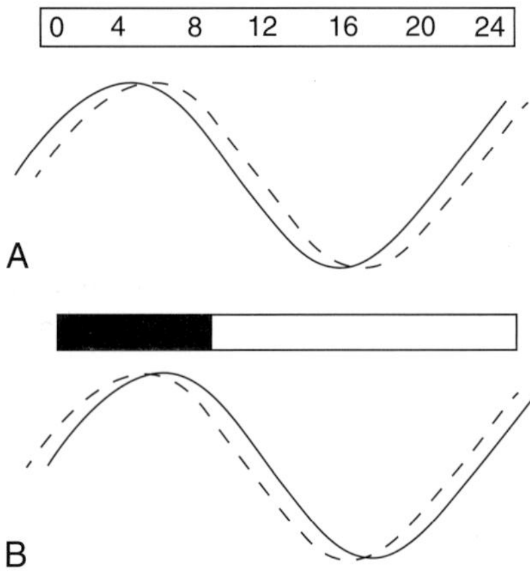

• **Fig. 2.2** Circadian Phase in Older Adults as Compared to Younger Adults. The solid line represents older adults' body temperature and plasma melatonin circadian profile. The dashed line represents young adults' body temperature and plasma melatonin circadian profile. The bar across the top of (A) represents the clock time. The horizontal black bar denotes the sleep or dark period. The horizontal white bar denotes wake or light period. (A) When compared with clock time, the phase of both core body temperature and plasma melatonin is earlier in older adults *(solid line)* than it is in young adults *(dashed line)*. (B) When compared with their usual sleep–wake and dark–light timing, the phase of both core body temperature and plasma melatonin is later with respect to sleep/darkness in older adults *(solid line)* than it is in young adults *(dashed line)*. (Redrawn from Duffy, J. F., Zitting, K. M., & Chinoy, E. D. [2015]. Aging and circadian rhythms. *Sleep Medicine Clinics, 10*[4], 423–434.)

Daytime napping and excessive daytime sleepiness is not, per se, a behavior predicted by normal physiology. Older adults admit to taking more naps than younger adults, but objective studies have determined that older adults do not nap longer or more frequently than younger adults (Obayon et al., 2004). Several confounding factors promote the perception of increased napping in normal aging. For instance, retirement renders more time for napping; increased pathologies, medications, or demoralization can increase daytime somnolence, which is alleviated by napping; one's personal desire for a schedule and pattern may affect napping behavior; and cultural adherence to napping schedules may be a factor. Thus, the healthy older adult does not physiologically require a nap (Obayon et al., 2004), and excessive daytime sleepiness should prompt investigation for pathology, medication side effects, or a discussion regarding lifestyle (Lopes et al., 2013).

Endocrine System

In their 2018 paper "The Physiology of Endocrine Systems With Ageing," Van Den Beld et al. developed a useful graphic to surmise the physiologic changes of normal aging (van den Beld et al., 2018; Fig. 2.3). Normal aging of endocrine axes manifest as less-robust hormone volume and delayed time to homeostasis. Not only does the cyclical time between phases elongate, but the reaction time to a stressing event elongates (van den Beld et al., 2018). These effects may be due to atrophy of a target organ (such as with the ovaries and testes), changes in the epigenetics of local mRNA that cause a shift in local tissue enzyme activity (such as with aromatase, 5-alpha-reductase, and 11-beta-hydroxysteroid dehydrogenase), or changes to receptor expression in target tissues.

Glucocorticoids and the Adrenal Axis

The adrenal axis regulates glucocorticoid expression in a negative-feedback pattern among the hypothalamus, pituitary, and adrenal glands. Homeostatic cortisol levels are influenced by a diurnal circadian rhythm. In a normal rhythm, cortisol is released at its peak shortly after awakening, then declines throughout the day and into the evening. As discussed previously, the sleep rhythm for an older adult is shifted earlier into the evening and of a slightly reduced duration (10 minutes lost per decade). Because sleep inhibits cortisol secretion and cortisol secretion disturbs sleep, the older adult's misaligned cortisol-to-sleep pattern increases the likelihood of nighttime awakenings and early morning awakenings (Copinschi & Caufriez, 2013; Fig. 2.4).

Despite the reduced pulsations and amplitude of cortisol expression, the older adult actually experiences an increase in bioactive cortisol in certain organs, most importantly the skin. The Skin section, presented later in the chapter, discusses this further.

Thyroid Axis and Hormones

The thyroid-stimulating hormone follows a circadian cycle as well. It peaks at the initiation of sleep, then stays low throughout the day. It is not usually secreted during sleep, as a sudden spike will cause awakening. Studies suggest that the timing and concentration of TSH's peak and nadir remain stable (or increase slightly) throughout life, though the overall amount of T4 secreted by the thyroid reduces slowly and steadily throughout adulthood and into older adulthood (Fig. 2.5) (Copinschi & Caufriez, 2013; Li et al., 2018). However, evidence suggests that isolated T4 supplementation is not clinically beneficial in an otherwise healthy older adult, and, in fact, subclinical hyperthyroidism (low TSH and elevated T4) has more worrisome clinical consequences in the older adult (Biondi et al., 2015) Several studies have shown that mortality is reduced in older adults with TSH values at the upper limit of normal compared to euthyroid peers (Atzmon et al., 2009). Current areas of research are considering the implications of age-specific TSH, T4, and T3 values, though the most important takeaway for the provider would be to avoid unnecessary treatment with thyroid hormones—even for suspected subclinical hyper- or hypothyroidism—until more evidence is available.

Somatostatins

Somatostatin, also called growth hormone, achieves its peak during puberty and then declines steadily with age.

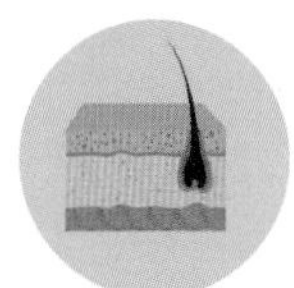

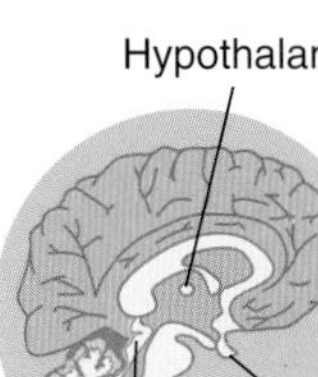
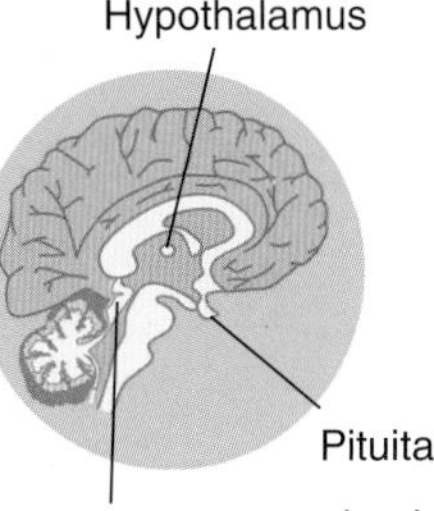
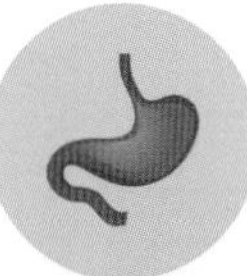
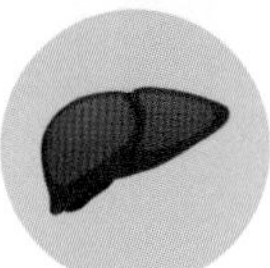
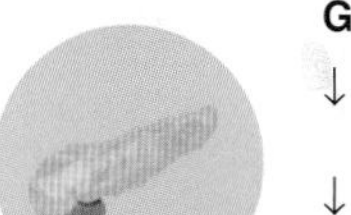
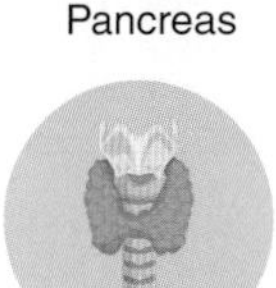
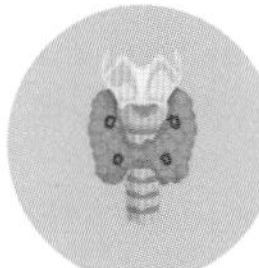
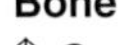
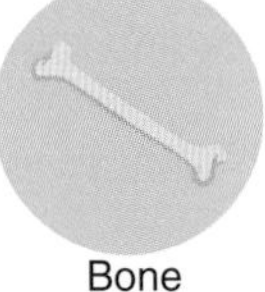
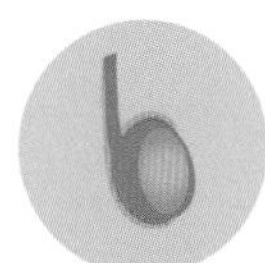
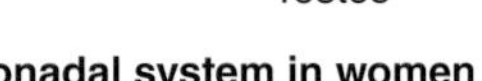

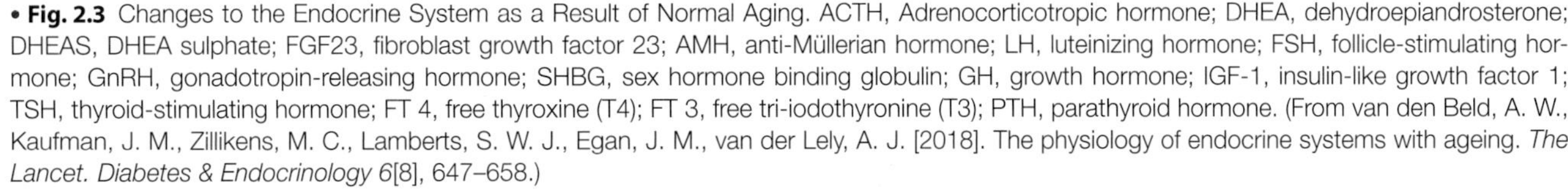

• **Fig. 2.3** Changes to the Endocrine System as a Result of Normal Aging. ACTH, Adrenocorticotropic hormone; DHEA, dehydroepiandrosterone; DHEAS, DHEA sulphate; FGF23, fibroblast growth factor 23; AMH, anti-Müllerian hormone; LH, luteinizing hormone; FSH, follicle-stimulating hormone; GnRH, gonadotropin-releasing hormone; SHBG, sex hormone binding globulin; GH, growth hormone; IGF-1, insulin-like growth factor 1; TSH, thyroid-stimulating hormone; FT 4, free thyroxine (T4); FT 3, free tri-iodothyronine (T3); PTH, parathyroid hormone. (From van den Beld, A. W., Kaufman, J. M., Zillikens, M. C., Lamberts, S. W. J., Egan, J. M., van der Lely, A. J. [2018]. The physiology of endocrine systems with ageing. *The Lancet. Diabetes & Endocrinology* 6[8], 647–658.)

Curiously, growth hormone is interlocked in a negative-feedback axis with insulin-like growth factor-1 (IGF-1) during puberty, though both hormones slowly decline over time. This is unlike the thyroid axis and the adrenal axis discussed earlier, which will maintain their negative-feedback relationships throughout the person's life. The reduction of growth hormone and circulating IGF-1 is called *somatopause* and is clinically associated with increased adipose tissue (Di Somma et al., 2011). However, much in the way that reduced T4 (and thus increased TSH) promotes healthy longevity, somatopause also demonstrates longevity in animal studies (Junnila et al., 2013).

There are benefits and detriments to the loss of growth hormone. Lower levels of growth hormone and IGF-1 have

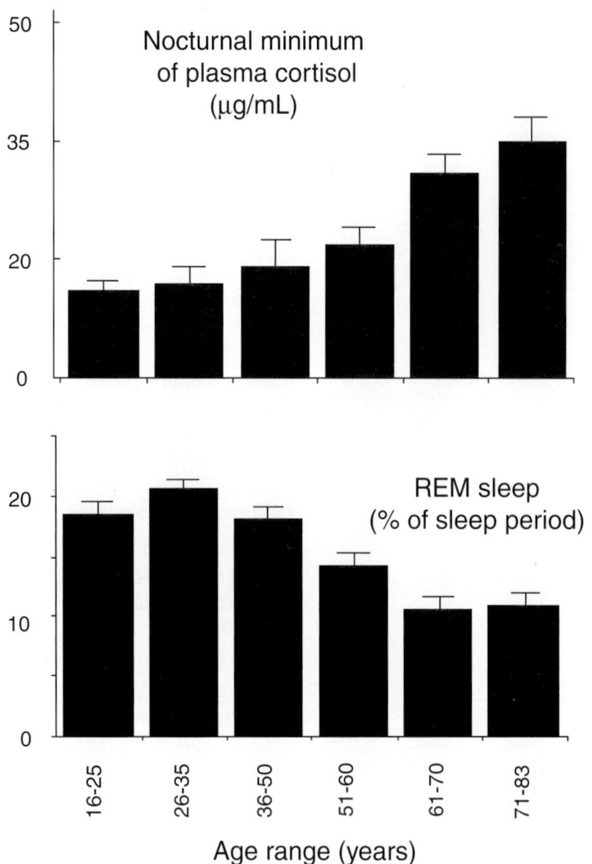

• **Fig. 2.4** Percentage of REM Sleep Compared to the Nocturnal Minimum Plasma Cortisol in Healthy Adults per Decade. (From Copinschi, G., & Caufriez, A. [2013]. Sleep and hormonal changes in aging. *Endocrinology and Metabolism Clinics of North America, 42*[2], 371–389.)

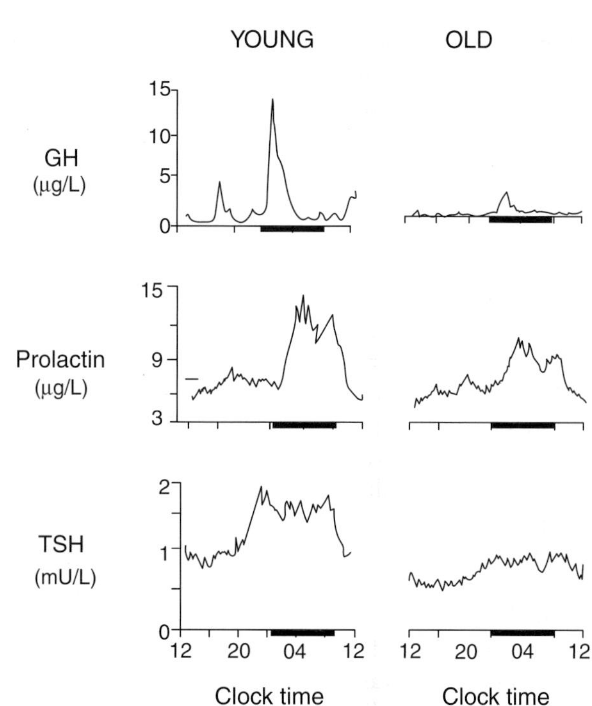

• **Fig. 2.5** Age-Related Changes to the Rhythmic Release of GH, Prolactin, and TSH. Mean values of plasma growth hormone (GH), prolactin, and thyrotropin (TSH) in eight young (20–27 years) and eight old (67–84 years) healthy men. The mean sleep time is demonstrated by the thick black bars in the Clock Time axis. (From Copinschi, G., & Caufriez, A. [2013]. Sleep and hormonal changes in aging. *Endocrinology and Metabolism Clinics of North America, 42*[2], 371–389.)

been shown to reduce the development of diabetes mellitus and cancer (Junnila et al., 2013). As a tradeoff, low-levels of IGF-1 mean that the person has low levels of nitrous oxide in the vascular smooth tissues, reduced plasticity within the vessels, reduced muscle strength, and less stimulation for neuron growth (Ceda et al., 2005). These results show that the tradeoff of neurologic slowness, reduced vascular compliance, and adiposity are preferred to muscle strength, rapid growth, and thus replication of imperfect cellular structures. This concept of cellular senescence will be pervasive throughout this section, though a complete review is beyond the scope of this chapter. More information can be found in Parikah et. al.'s review of cellular senescence (Parikh et al., 2019).

Gonadotropins: Estrogen and Testosterone

The gonadotropin axis, as well as the ultimate expression and use of the expressed hormones, can be complex for both genders. The pituitary-gonad axis includes the ebb and flow of sex hormones over the life span and changes dramatically throughout life to accommodate prepubescence, puberty, fertile stages, and post/reduced fertility stages. The features of reduced robustness explained in the introduction of the Endocrine System section apply strongly to gonadotropins.

Estrogen for Aging Men and Women

In women, estrogen is synthesized directly by the ovaries for local and systemic use. In men, the gonads produce a precursor androgen (testosterone) that is then subjected to conversion depending on the target tissue. In target organs such as the brain and internal genitalia, spermatogenesis relies on the conversion of testosterone into estrogen by an enzyme called aromatase. Aromatase is tightly regulated. It is located in a handful of tissues that convert just enough testosterone into estrogen for local tissue use (Stocco, 2012). Atrophy of the gonads reduces the amount of estrogen available for local and systemic use, causing tissue to upregulate production of aromatase. Multiple studies have described how estrogen binding to tissue affects cognition, brain function and memory (Rosenfeld et al., 2018), sexual drive, local urogenital vitality, ovary function, sperm fertility and mobility, bone density, muscle mass, and adiposity (Stocco, 2012). The phenotypic effects will be discussed per organ system and throughout the textbook.

The reduced circulating and local estrogen for both men and women will cause bone reabsorption in women and reduced bone formation in men (Compston et al., 2019), and osteopenia is the natural consequence. More discussion related to estrogens and the musculoskeletal system can be found in the Musculoskeletal System section presented later in the chapter.

Estrogen in Women

In women, the years of fertility between puberty and menopause are marked by a 28-day cycle of hormone fluctuations with ovulation. As women's ovaries have finite numbers of follicles, the onset of menopause is subject to the individual's rate of follicle depletion, as determined by the length of ovulatory and anovulatory menstrual cycles. The latter can be affected by follicle number at birth, stress, disease, or simply multiparity. Thus, the ovulatory menstrual cycles can continue until age 40 to 60, with a shift to anovulatory cyclical hormone fluctuations once menopause is achieved (Stocco, 2012).

In this brain-gonad endocrine axis, the neurochemical that stimulates the ovaries to mature a follicle are follicle-stimulating hormone (FSH) and luteinizing hormone (LH), which are suppressed by the hormones (androgens, inhibin A, and inhibin B) released by the ovaries during ovulation (Broekmans et al., 2009). As the woman ages beyond menopause, it is important to appreciate that a woman's neurologic axis will continue to secrete increased amounts of FSH and luteinizing hormone in an attempt to stimulate a follicle that is no longer present. Once the follicles are no longer present, the increased circulating luteinizing hormone stimulates the ovaries to secrete more testosterone instead of estrogens. The shift toward increasing testosterone causes the variety of symptoms associated with the perimenopausal years, including vasomotor dysregulation, changes in bone metabolism, virilization, and changes in the urogenital system (Cannarella et al., 2019).

In addition, the loss of ovarian estrogen production means that the woman is no longer producing her major source of estrogen, forcing the body to rely on the aromatase enzyme in adipose tissue to convert androgens into estrogens (Stocco, 2012). Therefore, it is an apparent physiologic mechanism that women maintain or increase adipose tissue after menopause: it is now the primary means of estrogen creation.

Testosterone for Aging Men and Women

In addition to a reduced stimulation of testosterone, the normal aging process for men and women is associated with an increase in a sex-hormone binding glycoprotein, a substance that binds to the circulating testosterone, making it less bioavailable for tissue use (Fabbri et al., 2016). As a result, longitudinal studies show that free testosterone steadily declines in both sexes steadily from age 30, with a pronounced reduction for males at age 70 and for women in the peri- and postmenopausal time frames (Fabbri et al., 2016).

Testosterone in Men

Testosterone excretion in men and women reduces starting at age 30 and drops steadily with age. Testosterone is expressed by the pulsatile release of gonadotropin-releasing hormone from the hypothalamus onto the pituitary gland, which then releases luteinizing hormone and follicle-stimulating hormone to stimulate the Leydig cells and Sertoli cells, respectively. Androgens are released into circulation, and the high volumes of aromatase enzyme in the testes convert testosterone into estrogens to maintain spermatogenesis (Institute of Medicine US Committee on Assessing the Need for Clinical Trials of Testosterone Replacement Therapy, 2004). As discussed in the Sleep: Normal Changes in the Older Adult and Endocrine System sections presented earlier, normal aging disposes all circadian and pulsatile rhythms to lose both robustness of expression and resilience to changes in homeostasis. Thus, older adult men still produce sperm, but at a lower concentration and reduced viability.

In addition, the circulating testosterone must be converted into an active substrate to enact change to the target tissue. The 5-alpha-reductase enzymes convert testosterone into dihydroxytestosterone (DHT), and aromatase enzymes convert testosterone into estrogens (Institute of Medicine [US] Committee on Assessing the Need for Clinical Trials of Testosterone Replacement Therapy, 2004). Downregulation or upregulation of either enzyme will alter the phenotype of the target organ. Testosterone conversion into DHT is critical for internal and external genitalia development, libido, red blood cell production, and musculoskeletal maintenance (Institute of Medicine [US] Committee on Assessing the Need for Clinical Trials of Testosterone Replacement Therapy, 2004). Testosterone conversion into estrogen is critical for spermatogenesis in the gonads (Stocco, 2012). as well as copulation urges in the brain (Azcoitia et al., 2011; Beyer et al., 1976). See Table 2.1 for a summary of the tissues that rely on DHT and estrogen for local regulation in the healthy middle-aged adult.

Body Shape: Normal Changes in the Older Adult

Body shape and musculoskeletal composition changes with age are related to a variety of factors. For both men and women, the volume of systemically circulating testosterone compared to estradiol determines the degree of abdominal adiposity compared to bone and muscle density (Elraiyah et al., 2014; Harman et al., 2001). As reduced circulating estrogens alter patterns in bone reabsorption and synthesis for women and men, respectively, body mass composition shifts toward increased adipose tissue and less lean muscle mass. However, this increase in adiposity is a beneficial in situ means of sex hormone production: far from a passive nuisance, adipose tissue is a thermal insulator and local estrogen producer. It is suspected that the decrease in muscle mass is a reflection of cellular senescence: as the DNA telomeres shorten, the mitochondria are unable to efficiently generate

TABLE 2.1 Organ Systems That Rely on the Final Products of Testosterone Conversion for Normal Function

Organ System	5 Alpha-Reductase-p Redominant (i.e., DHT—Dependent Tissues)	Aromatase-Predomin ant (i.e., Estrogen-Dependent Tissues)
Hair pattern: axillary, pubic, facial, scalp[a,b]	X	
Red-blood cell stimulation[a,b]	X	
Prostate[a,b]	X	
External genitalia formation* (penis, scrotum, testis) and internal genitalia formation (vas deferens, seminal vesicles, epididymis)[a,b]	X	
Vocal cord (enlargement)[a,b]	X	
Libido[c,d,e]		X
Spermatogenesis[a,b,c,d,e]	X	X
Nonreproductive regions of brain: amygdala, preoptic/septal areas, cerebellum, brainstem[e]		X

The enzyme 5-apla-reductase converts testosterone into dihydrotestosterone (DHT). The enzyme aromatase converts testosterone into estrogen.
*Concentration of DHT and formation of external genitalia is most significant during stages of in vivo development.
[a]Data from Azzouni, F., Godoy, A., Li, Y., & Mohler, J. (2012). The 5 alpha-reductase isozyme family: a review of basic biology and their role in human diseases. *Advances in Urology, 2012*, 530121.
[b]Data from Randall, V. A. (1994). Role of 5 alpha-reductase in health and disease. *Bailliere's Clinical Endocrinology and Metabolism, 8*(2), 405–431.
[c]Data from Institute of Medicine (US) Committee on Assessing the Need for Clinical Trials of Testosterone Replacement Therapy, Liverman, C. T., & Blazer, D. G. (2004). *The 5 alpha-reductase isozyme family: A review of basic biology and their role in human diseases*. National Academies Press (US).
[d]Data from Stocco, C. (2012). Tissue physiology and pathology of aromatase. *Steroids, 77*(1–2), 27–35.
[e]Data from Azcoitia, I., Yague, J. G., & Garcia-Segura, L. M. (2011). Estradiol synthesis within the human brain. *Neuroscience, 191*(September), 139–147.

enough energy and replicate at the speed necessary to maintain the muscle mass of youth (Parikh et al., 2019). Part of the systemic response of normal aging includes an epigenetic chemical environment shift, which ultimately reduces the amount of heavy and energy-requiring organ (muscle) and converts it into a steroid-generating organ (adipose tissue). The estrogen from the adipose tissue supplies local muscle, bones, and visceral tissue with enough regulatory steroids to maintain basic endocrine and regulatory functions. Although clinical studies with long-term cohorts are underway, this concept underscores the mechanism for evolutionary preservation of osteopenia, sarcopenia, and shifts toward adipose tissue in normal aging.

The net effect of these changes can be monitored in organ-specific testing, but also in the body mass index (BMI). At present, BMI classifications are not age specific and include "underweight" (BMI < 18.5), "normal weight" (BMI 18.5 to 24.9), "overweight" (BMI 25.0 to 29.9), and "obesity" (BMI > 30.0). Despite no formal changes to guidelines, there appears to be a significant benefit to optimizing the weight of an older adult in the "overweight" category instead of the "normal weight" category. A large, multiethnic study of older adults ages 70 to 75 with a 10-year follow-up regarding morbidity and mortality over the following 10 years concluded that there was a 13% reduction in mortality for older adults who maintained their body mass index in the "overweight" category compared to the "normal" category (Flicker et al., 2010). Thankfully, these data were consistent between men, women, and health status for adults ages 70 to 75 (Fig. 2.6). Similarly, Winter et al. demonstrated that all-cause mortality for adults ages 65 and older was greatly reduced when the BMI reached 27.5 (Fig. 2.7). Though a healthy weight and lifestyle is the ultimate goal, the conclusions of several studies have recommended an age-adjusted BMI chart that encompasses the "overweight" figures into the "normal weight" category (Murphy et al., 2014; Winter et al., 2014; Zaslavsky et al., 2016).

SAFETY ALERT

There is no clinical benefit to supplementation of steroid precursors, such as dehydroepiandrosterone (DHEA), during normal aging to prevent low estrogen or low testosterone side effects. The effect of high-circulating steroids not only is useless to cells that are unable to use or process the steroids, but the side effects are significantly more dangerous than the conditions that precipitated the treatment (Elraiyah et al., 2014). Treatment of osteoporosis or sarcopenia should be offered only to prevent or to correct pathology, and the treatment goal should be modified to achieve the normal bone density of patients by gender and age.

The Brain

Gray matter and white matter reduce with aging. For gray matter, it is postulated that the mass reduction is predominantly caused by reductions in neuron density (Harada et al., 2013). Neuron density reduction is a slow and steady

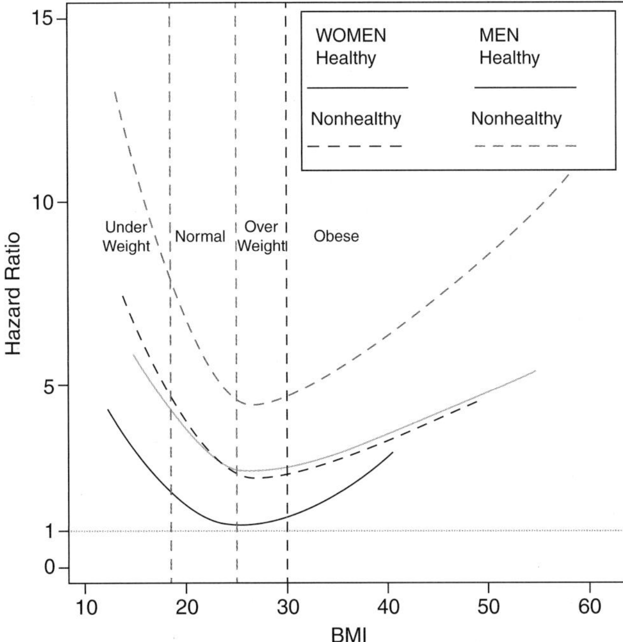

• **Fig. 2.6** "Overweight" Adults Ages 70 to 75 Have Reduced Risk of All-Cause Mortality. The hazard ratios of all-cause mortality for older adults ages 70–75, striated by health status and gender. A BMI of 25 is in the category of overweight and demonstrates the lowest risk of all-cause mortality for all groups. (From Flicker, L., McCaul, K. A., Hankey, G. J., Jamrozik, K., Brown, W. J., Byles, J. E., & Almeida, O. P. [2010]. Body mass index and survival in men and women aged 70 to 75. *Journal of the American Geriatrics Society, 58*[2], 234–241.)

progression throughout the life span, that leads, it is hypothesized, to a nonpathologic "primary senile dementia" when a healthy adult reaches age 130 (Terry & Katzman, 2001). Therefore, until the average human life span reaches ages closer to 130, overt dementia should never be considered a feature of normal aging. Such symptoms should prompt the clinician to investigate for reversible or pathologic causes of the dementia.

Although it is inappropriate to consider overt dementia as a feature of normal aging, there are still clinically significant phenotypes that occur as a consequence of normal density loss and brain shrinkage. For one, previously robust and independently functional regions of the brain lose their ability to *differentiate*, which is the ability to complete tasks in isolation of other regions of the brain. Function MRI (fMRI) has been used to demonstrate that the normal aging brain will accommodate dedifferentiation by employing other parts of the brain to assist in task completion (Cabeza, 2002; Cabeza et al., 2002). Thus, it can be extrapolated that the steady rate of neuron density loss allows the brain sufficient time to compensate, and that the cognition of the older adult should vary only slightly from the patient's younger self. The phenotype of the aging brain will clinically manifest in the patient's cognition, which is described next.

Cognition

Appreciable cognitive decline of older adulthood occurs at different life stages and progresses at different rates. The domains of age-associated cognitive decline include fluid intelligence (problem solving and reasoning of nonfamiliar concerns); processing speed of cognitive and motor responses;

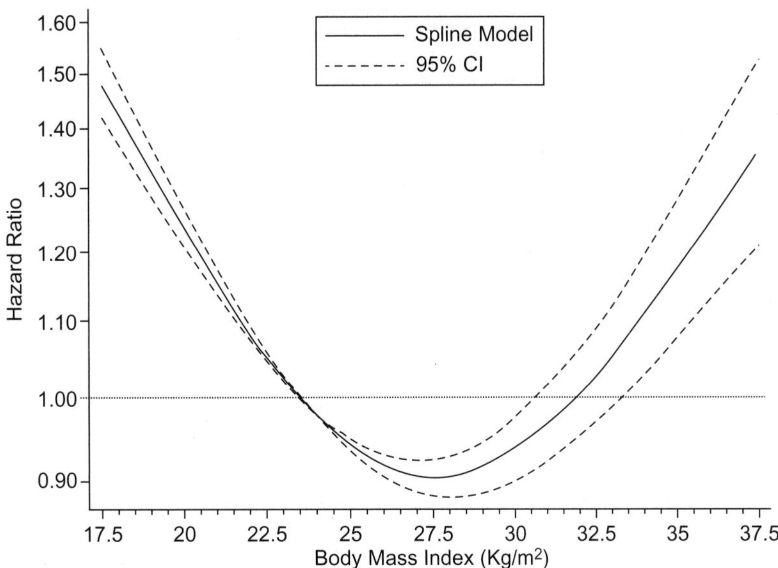

• **Fig. 2.7** "Overweight" Older Adults (All Ages) Have Reduced Risk of All-Cause Mortality. The solid line is the projected hazard ratio (spline model) comparing all-cause mortality to body mass index in adults aged 65 and older. The dashed lines represent the 95% confidence intervals (CIs) in their model. A body mass index of 27.5 was associated with the lowest risk of all-cause mortality. (From Winter, J. E., MacInnis, R. J., Wattanapenpaiboon, N., & Nowson, C. A. [2014]. BMI and all-cause mortality in older adults: A meta-analysis. *American Journal of Clinical Nutrition, 99*[4], 875–890.)

TABLE 2.2 **Rate and Initiation Age of Cognitive Decline**

Cognitive Function	Age When Cognition Function Reduces	Rate of Change	Source
Crystalized intelligence	50 s through 60 s	Stable or increase by 0.003 to 0.02 standard deviations per year	(Salthouse, 2012)
Fluid intelligence	30 s	Reduce by 0.02 standard deviations per year	(Salthouse, 2012)
Processing speed	20 s	Continuous decline through life	(Carlson et al., 1995)
Immediate memory/auditory attention span	Late life	"Slight decline" per year	(Presbyopia: Overview, 2020)
Selective attention	Unknown age	Unknown rate of decline	
Divided attention	Unknown age	Unknown rate of decline	
Declarative memory, semantic	60 s or later	Unknown rate of decline	(Rönnlund et al., 2005)
Declarative memory, episodic	Unknown age, suggested that rate of decline begins in 20 s	Stable rate of decline through life	(Rönnlund et al., 2005)
Rate of acquisition of learning	Initial drop in 40 s with second large drop in 70 s.	Steady decline between ages 40–70, then 70+	(Haaland et al., 2003)

complex attention tasks, including simple concentration of a sound amid other stimuli as well as multitasking; declarative/explicit memory, including episodic memory (one's self-story) and semantic memory (knowledge of practical application, such as language use and skill); visual construction of a three-dimensional object; and finally, the entire domain of executing functioning (independent and purposeful behavior, inhibition control, verbal and mathematical reasoning skills).

It should be noted that the rate of decline does not begin at age 65 when the term "older adult" is defined, but each cognitive ability begins to decline at much earlier life stages (Harada et al., 2013). Nondeclarative/procedural memory, crystallized intelligence (including memory and components of language), and visuospatial abilities do not change throughout adulthood (Lezak et al., 2004; Salthouse, 2012). Table 2.2 compares the normal timing and progression of functional decline, if applicable, per cognitive task. Clinical deviation from this chart—either premature symptoms for age or evidence of inappropriate symptoms—should alert the clinician to investigate for pathology. Table 2.3 presents common clinical vignettes of normal and pathologic changes related to memory (Harada et al., 2013).

Hematology

Red Blood Cells

A significant amount of preventative care, medication management decisions, and pathology investigation is predicated on the blood work, or the ratio of products in the blood in vascular circulation. The result of such testing is often an essential component that will affect a practitioner's clinical decision making and recommendations.

Hematology is a field of medical study that relies heavily on the concentrations of blood-borne products. Thus, it is a field that must establish number-based values that classify certain product concentrations as "normal" or "abnormal" per person based on age, ethnicity, and comorbid condition. One of the most controversial medical discussions in hematology is defining anemia in normal aging. "Anemia of older age" describes the phenomenon whereby large percentages of otherwise healthy (and unhealthy) adults present with hemoglobin levels below the World Health Organization's threshold for acceptable values. At present, the World Health Organization defines the phenotype of hemoglobin for normal adults to be at or above 130 g/L (13 g/dL) in men and 120 g/L (12 g/dL) in women (Chaves et al., 2002), without, it should be noted, any recommended adjustment for age. Available research at the time concluded that patients within these target ranges experienced reduced morbidity and mortality in the setting of severe or chronic disease (Izaks et al., 1999).

After the definition was established and venipuncture became a staple of primary care management, "anemia" became a pervasive diagnosis of females ages 17 to 49, though the trend was explained by menses and iron deficiency. The prevalence for anemia also drastically increased for men at ages 75+ and women at ages 85+, regardless of health status. In fact, roughly 33% to 50% of older adults have "unexplained anemia," which is defined by the inability to determine a pathologic cause of anemia based on serum blood samples (Stauder et al., 2018). More research is occurring to determine if a "lower baseline lab value" is more appropriate

TABLE 2.3 Normal Changes and Preserved Functions of Memory in Aging

Declines With Age	Remains Stable With Age
Delayed free recall: Spontaneous retrieval of information from memory without a cue Example: Recalling a list of items to purchase at the grocery store without a cue	Recognition memory: Ability to retrieve information when given a cue Example: Correctly giving the details of a story when given yes/no questions
Source memory: Knowing the source of the learned information Example: Remembering if you learned a fact because you saw it on television, read it in the newspaper, or heard it from a friend	Temporal order memory: Memory for the correct time or sequence of past events Example: Remembering that last Saturday you went to the grocery store after you ate lunch with your friends
Prospective memory: Remembering to perform intended actions in the future Example: Remembering to take medicine before going to bed	Procedural memory: Memory of how to do things Example: Remembering how to ride a bike

From Harada, C. N., Natelson Love, M. C., & Triebel, K. L. (2013). Normal cognitive aging. *Clinics in Geriatric Medicine, 29*(4), 737–752.

than supplementation (Guralnik et al., 2004), and investigations are still underway (Rosko et al., 2018). Additional and equally important information is the consideration of ethnicity and gender, which may lead clinicians toward developing a matrix of acceptable values between men and women. Until the evidence is generated and the conclusions are implemented into clinical practice, the American Geriatric Society and the American Society of Hematology advise providers to monitor clinical symptoms as well as the gap between the patient value and the lower limit of normal: a continued hemoglobin decline into the ranges of "moderate anemia" or "severe anemia" onset of symptoms justifies pathologic investigation, as would symptomatic anemia (Salive et al., 1992).

White Blood Cells

Much like the red blood cell count, the white blood cell (WBC) count also reduces progressively during the normal process of aging. Men have more white blood cells than women at a baseline, though women have more platelets at a baseline. Between adulthood and older adulthood, the total WBC count remains between the established values of "normal," though the ratio of the component parts changes significantly: Neutrophils increase significantly with normal aging, whereas the lymphocyte and eosinophil counts decrease proportionally with aging. Basophils and monocytes remain stable throughout aging (Nah et al., 2018; Fig. 2.8).

Immune System

The effects of aging in adaptive immunity are well-understood based on results of vaccine studies. Vaccine studies monitor the temporary simulation of the immune system, the speed of response, and the speed of return to homeostasis with newly acquired humoral immunity. With aging, higher antigen circulation is required to stimulate a cytokine response sufficient to trigger the immune system cascade. Effector memory T-cell production in older adults is therefore quite delayed relative to younger adults and children. Wagner et al. demonstrated that there is a significant difference in vaccine concentration efficacy starting at age 60 (Wagner et al., 2018). The latter is a well-understood phenomenon, as it is the primary justification for providing a high-dose vaccine (i.e., high viral antigen) for adults ages 65 and older. Practitioners should consider this when recommending catch-up schedules for vaccines or travel vaccines for older adults. The adult should likely have his or her first vaccine before age 60 with high-dose boosters to follow into older adulthood.

Alterations to adaptive immunity also predispose an older adult to conditions seldom considered by practitioners. Saliva, for example, carries antimicrobial properties as part of humoral immunity and growth factor for taste bud rejuvenation (Mese & Matsuo, 2007). As discussed in the Gustation section presented later in the chapter, concomitant reductions in circulating saliva and saliva antimicrobial potency predispose the patient to the clinical consequences of dental caries, gingival infections, and mucosal infection with delayed recovery.

Aging also causes changes and delays in innate immunity. Evidence suggests that there is a shift in macrophage type from a vibrant, circulating macrophage to a slower, more dormant version (Gibon et al., 2016).

Eyes and Vision

The complex nature of the human eye and its proximity to the brain has granted a significant amount of research money toward anatomy research. The Choroidal Vascularity Index (CVI) is the most modern metric to discuss and track the health of the human eye. The CVI captures the overall integrity of the eye's main vascular network, the choroid, by describing the ratio between the lumen of the choroid vessels and the total eye surface reached by these vessels (Iovino et al., 2020). It has been demonstrated that CVI reduction starts in the mid-30s with a depreciation rate of −0.7% to 2.4% per decade (Nivison-Smith et al., 2020). Not only does the ratio of lumen to total vessel volume decrease, but the individual components decrease as well. Finally, it has also been appreciated that the rate of depreciation in different

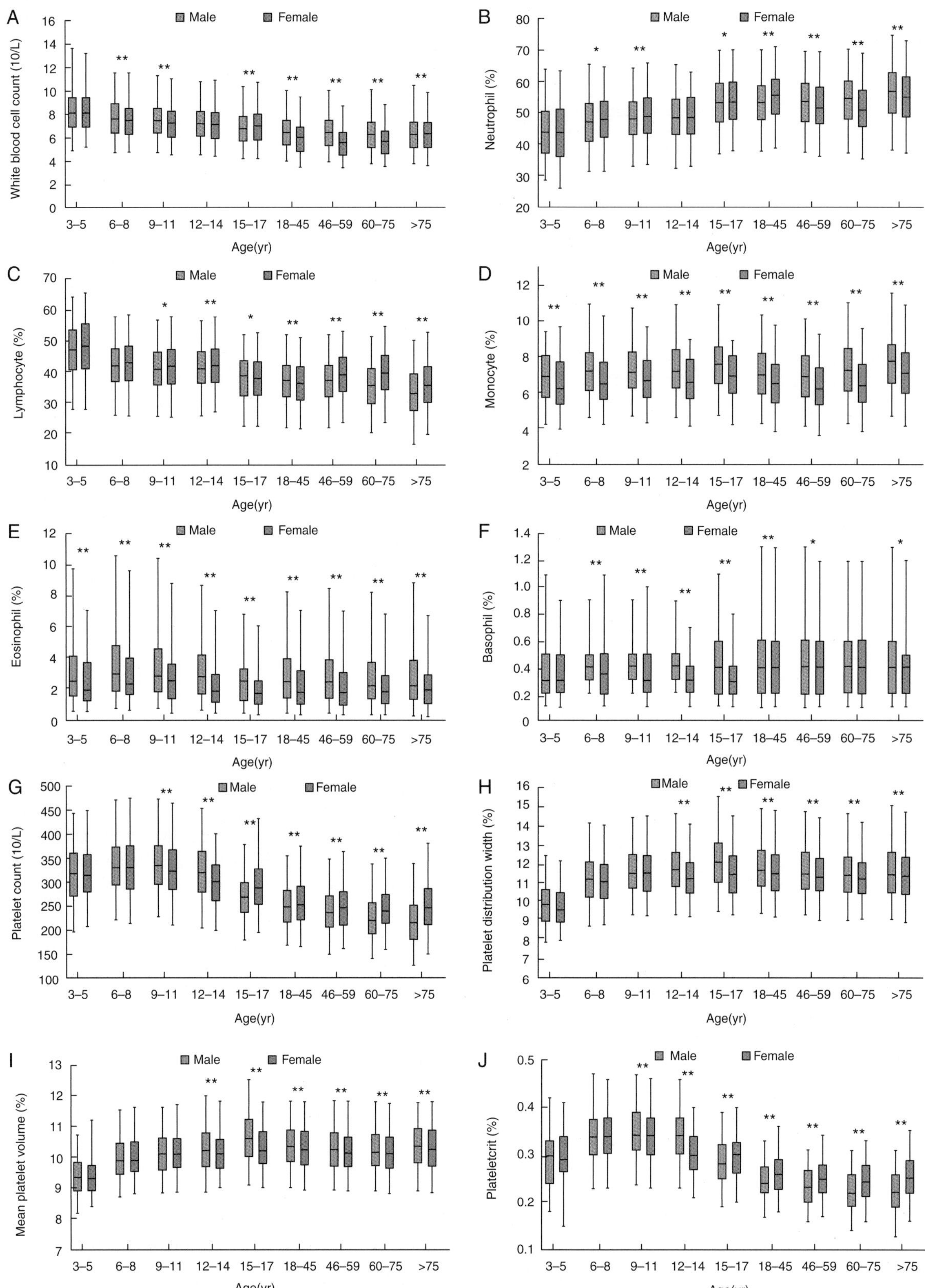

• **Fig. 2.8** Age and Gender Effects on White Blood Cell and Platelet Parameters. (A) White blood cell count. (B) Neutrophil count. (C) Lymphocyte count. (D) Monocyte count. (E) Eosinophil count. (F) Basophil count. (G) Platelet count. (H) Platelet distribution width. (I) Mean platelet volume. (J) Plateletcrit. Box limits and horizontal lines within boxes represent interquartile ranges and the median, respectively. The upper and lower whiskers indicate the 97.5th and 2.5th percentiles, respectively. The difference in median values between sexes in each age group was determined using the Wilcoxon rank sum test: *P<0.05. The median values among age groups for each sex differed significantly (P < 001, Kruskal-Wallis test). (Redrawn from Nah, E. H., Kim, S., Cho, S., & Cho, H. I. [2018]. Complete blood count reference intervals and patterns of changes across pediatric, adult, and geriatric ages in Korea. *Annals of Laboratory Medicine, 38*[6], 503–511.)

branches of the choroid is asymmetric, with most consistent vascular compromises occurring in the structures that nourish the retina, internal macula (spatial appreciation), and rods of the eyes (Nivison-Smith et al., 2020). Thus, the normal ocular changes of aging are related to light reception for neural transmission, depth perception, and the ability to see in low lighting, all of which are affected by the vascular changes in the choroid.

Presbyopia describes the visual acuity loss that results from aging. The exact cause is multifactorial and is likely a combination of well-documented changes such as lens thickening and reduced contractile power of the ciliary muscles (Presbyopia: Overview, 2020); reduced pupillary reflexes, pupillary reactivity, and difficulties coordinating refraction with extraocular motor control (ocular pursuit and up-gazing) (Seraji-Bzorgzad et al., 2019); and the vascular changes described previously. Thus, the clinician should be mindful that normal age-related changes to vision begin to occur in the fourth and fifth decades of life and are usually symmetric. Rapid deceleration or asymmetric changes should prompt investigation for pathology.

SAFETY ALERT

Safe Showers Without Glasses

Although reading glasses can achieve adequate visual acuity, glasses are never brought into the shower. To improve visual recognition of common bathroom objects, practitioners should encourage the older adult to choose two plastic bottles with different colors to make it easier to distinguish between products. For instance, the shampoo can be in a bright pink container and the conditioner can be in a blue container. Maintaining the same pattern will improve independence and safety. Family members performing the shopping should be mindful of any color keys that have been established and adhere to them.

Ears and Hearing

Presbycusis is defined as the symmetric, sensorineural hearing loss of aging, though the clinical presentation is quite variable. The traditional and objective definition describes hearing loss frequencies above 2 Hz with eventual difficulties in the speaking frequencies (0.5 to 2 Hz) (Gates & Mills, 2005). However, otolaryngologists further classify presbycusis into seven categories: sensory, neural, strial (metabolic), cochlear, conductive, mixed, and indeterminate (Tu & Friedman, 2018). These types can be combined to offer greater descriptions, such as "sensorineural" and "cochlear conductive" to describe the problematic area and the type of hearing loss. The variants of presbycusis are clinical and distinct. For instance, nerve sensitivity (sensory) distortions of the auditory nerve (neural) may result in pure-tone hearing reductions (sensorineural), whereas the reduced synapse space between the end of the cochlea and the auditory nerve may result in the inability to distinguish speech in a noisy environment (i.e., conduction deficit at the cochlea) (Ralli et al., 2019; Tu & Friedman, 2018).

These changes manifest slowly and are often seldom appreciated by the person experiencing the deficit. Therefore, concerns for hearing loss are often reported by family, friends, or employers that monitor hearing status as part of their occupational health and safety requirements. The clinician should be mindful to ask family members and other members of the interdisciplinary team about changes in the patient's attention in noisy conditions, changes in volume control, or even changes to emotional stimuli, which may appear to indicate a frontal cortex pathology. Regardless of sex, hearing loss at any age and normal hearing after age 60 causes significant delays and misinterpretations in the emotional tonality of language. Auditorily intact older adults, men and women, have been shown to have reduced accuracy when asked to decipher the type of verbal emotion expressed. Older adult listeners also had reduced reaction time and difficulty interpreting emotion in the male voice. Finally, the age and gender of the speaker does play a large role in the older adult listener's success in interpreting the emotion (Christensen et al., 2019). Essentially, a younger adult who speaks more quickly and at a higher pitch will overwhelm the basic word-processing function of the older adult listener. By the time the words are appreciated, the tone and emotions cannot be reassociated with the spoken words. Unfortunately, it is difficult for the typical speaker to deliver the same spoken words with the original tone and emotional cantor, and repeating the same words does not typically mean that the same associated emotions have been repeated. Therefore, an important practitioner takeaway is to speak slowly enough and with enough body gestures to articulate both the words and the emotion of the words the first time they are spoken.

Olfaction

The normal aging process is associated with reduced quantity and quality of neuroepithelium in the nasal cavity, as well as the interneurons of the olfactory bulb. In fact, the olfactory neuroepithelium is slowly replaced with respiratory epithelium, reducing smell perception (Kondo et al., 2020). It is therefore common for the older adult to have a diminished perceived and objective sense of smell during normal aging.

The phenotype of loss of olfaction can manifest in a variety of ways: the patient may simply describe a loss of taste, or there may be more dramatic manifestations of malnutrition, unintentional weight loss, or social disconnect present as distracting sequelae (Kondo et al., 2020). Although these symptoms are often associated with clinical depression, the practitioner may be able to differentiate depression from primary loss of olfaction by a mood assessment. A cheerful mood, appropriate affect, and normal energy levels are less common in depressed or demoralized older adults.

Gustation

In addition to the relationship between olfaction and gustation, a significant number of age-related changes affect gustation. Saliva is a major contributor to the sense of taste, and age-associated loss of taste is closely linked to the composition and volume of saliva. Even though the parotid gland function and saliva production remain unchanged with aging, total saliva excretion and volume reduce with aging, particularly in the submandibular and submental salivary glands, which are responsible for 70% of resting salivation flow and 50% of active salivation flow (Affoo et al., 2015). Reduced saliva reduces one's ability to dissolve and disperse food to appropriate receptors (Pushpass et al., 2019a, 2019b), and older adults slowly lose sensitivity to different tastes.

Age-related changes in salivary protein and mucin concentration appear to reduce the sensitivity of bitter tastes, making greater volumes of bitters more palatable (Pushpass et al., 2019a, 2019b). Additional reports have noted that the perceived taste of umami was reduced by 15% between young adulthood (mean age 24) and older adulthood (mean age 72), with objective reductions in active salivation by 17%. Interestingly, the sensation of chemical heat on the transient receptor potential (TRP) is unchanged with age, indicating that older adults preserve full sensitivity to spicy foods (Pushpass et al., 2019a, 2019b). Thus, using chemical heat or spicy seasoning may be a reliable, affordable way to improve salivation in the older adult.

Oral Cavity, Mastication, and Deglutition

To date, there is no evidence that the mucosa in the oral cavity changes significantly during the process of normal aging (Abu Eid et al., 2012). The process of mastication does appear to change with time. The temporalis and masseter muscles thicken in adolescence, causing progressive increases in contractile power and bite-force throughout aging (Kang et al., 2016; Palinkas et al., 2013). Interestingly, the power and mobility of the tongue reduces with age, and the older adult will chew more times with increased bite force before feeling the confidence to swallow the food bolus (Kang et al., 2016). The coordination of mastication, glottis coordination between breaths and chewing, and eventual food bolus progression through the esophagus takes more time in the older adult as a result, though there is no loss of voluntary or involuntary muscle synchronization (Shaw et al., 1995). As always, the practitioner should be mindful of the delicate balance between a slight slowing in mastication and deglutition versus pathologic losses of muscle control and coordination.

Musculoskeletal System

One of the most notable changes of aging is the physical change of the musculoskeletal system. The more overt changes present as height loss, loss of lean muscle mass, and a more pronounced conversion from muscle to fat. Unseen changes in the musculoskeletal system reach the cellular level (sarcopenia and osteopenia), which will also be reviewed later as organ-specific effects of previously discussed conditions of normal aging.

Reductions in circulating estrogens and increased circulation of parathyroid hormone directly promote both osteoclast ("bone reabsorber") and osteoblast ("bone builder") activity, though the net combination results in faster bone turnover than overall remodeling (Wein & Kronenberg, 2018). Estrogen affects two processes that overall enhance bone strength: It suppresses osteoblast apoptosis as well as the cytokines that promote macrophage differentiation into osteoclasts (Florencio-Silva et al., 2015). When estrogen concentrations are reduced, there is faster destruction of osteoblasts and more rapid production of osteoclasts. As men maintain sufficient volumes of aromatase enzyme in appropriate local tissues throughout their lives (see the Gonadotropins: Estrogen and Testosterone section), older women without a secondary reserve of aromatase enzyme tend to experience bone thinning within years of menopause. The bone thinning can be slowed by increasing adiposity (see the Body Shape: Normal Changes in the Older Adult section presented earlier).

In contrast to common belief, joint disease and functional loss is not a normal condition of aging. Loss of cartilage quality and rate of production is not associated with aging (Aurich et al., 2002). There is also no evidence to show that the normal immune system changes associated with aging influence the joints of the older adult. Therefore, osteoarthritic joint pain or stiffness should be considered a pathologic imbalance between the rate of deterioration and the normal rate of regeneration.

Muscle mass changes are also multifactorial, though the same processes that affect the bone tend to influence the muscle tissue as well. Tissue biopsies of older adult skeletal muscle show that aging bone marrow leads to changes in the circulating macrophages, which in turn cause muscle fibrosis and collagen deposition in functional contractile muscle (Florencio-Silva et al., 2015; Wang et al., 2015).

Muscle contraction response to neural and environmental stimulation also changes over time, causing changes in balance and proprioception. A comparison of the neurologic and muscular responses of physically similar older adults and younger adults concluded that older adults require drastically more stimuli for the brain to attempt postural and balance correction than do younger adults (Walker et al., 2020). Once the brain was alerted to correct the posture (i.e., from falling), the reflexive response time to postural correction was delayed in the older adult. Finally, because muscular contractile power contraction of healthy muscle was not significantly reduced in the older adult, the brain and reflexive response may trigger unintentional and unrefined muscular corrections too late in the phase of postural correction. These findings are consistent with the themes discovered in other areas of the brain (see the Cognition section). Multiple organ-specific studies demonstrate that the rich vascular and innervation networks of youth atrophy in varying degrees with aging, causing delayed time to organ activation, task completion, and prolonged time to hemostasis. However, the net effects of these normal changes do not cause symptomatic clinical or functional disturbances during normal aging.

Vascular System

Normal vascular aging includes the replacement of elastic fibers with stiff collagen fibers; the fraying of older elastic fibers; and a striking variety of smooth muscle endothelial changes that not only affect the integrity of the organ but also the endocrine-like homeostasis of vasoconstriction/dilation and anti-/pro-angiogenic factors (Xu et al., 2017). Biopsy studies demonstrate that collagen fibers replace elastic fibers as early as the first day of birth (Iurciuc et al., 2017), though significant changes in arterial compliance are noted at age 10, age 80, and most drastically at age 55 in the otherwise healthy European adult (Reference Values for Arterial Stiffness' Collaboration, 2010). The structural changes to the elastic vascular structures thereby cause both a slight widening of the lumen (pressed open due to systolic pressure) and an overall widening of the artery (Fig. 2.9) (Xu et al., 2017). In contrast, the smaller, thin-walled capillaries are literally only a single endothelial layer thick. Endothelial damage and oxidative stress occlude the lumen of these structures with aging, causing the obliteration of these fine structures. The consequent reduction in microvascular density causes relative hypoperfusion to structures in the skin, brain, intestines, kidneys, and gonads (Xu et al., 2017). Interestingly, age-related hypoperfusion appears to unfold in a fairly predictable pattern that can help the practitioner to delineate pathology from normal aging. For instance, decreased blood flow in the anterior and posterior cerebral arteries is most notable at age 40 (Ackerstaff et al., 1990), though hypoperfusion to the cortical brain initiates and progresses at age 60 (Chen et al., 2011). Hypoperfusion to the cortical brain is most pronounced in the left hemisphere relative to the right (Pagani et al., 2002), and the frontal, parietal, and temporal lobes take the greatest reductions in regional blood flow and velocity (Chen et al., 2011). These patterns are consistent with the patterns of cognitive decline described earlier in this chapter. In contrast to the fate of elastic arteries and capillaries noted previously, the muscular arteries and arterioles do not appear to lose compliance or experience collagen deposition with normal aging (van der Heijden-Spek et al., 2000). Recall that muscular arteries are the medium-sized vessels lined with smooth muscle, with the function of titrating the bolus of blood from the large elastic arteries into the high-resistance vascular structures approaching the target organs. Famous examples of muscular arteries include the brachial artery, radial artery, and femoral artery. Also recall that arterioles are almost exclusively made of smooth muscle; connect the vascular system to large organs; and are under regulatory control of the endocrine system (Tucker et al., 2020).

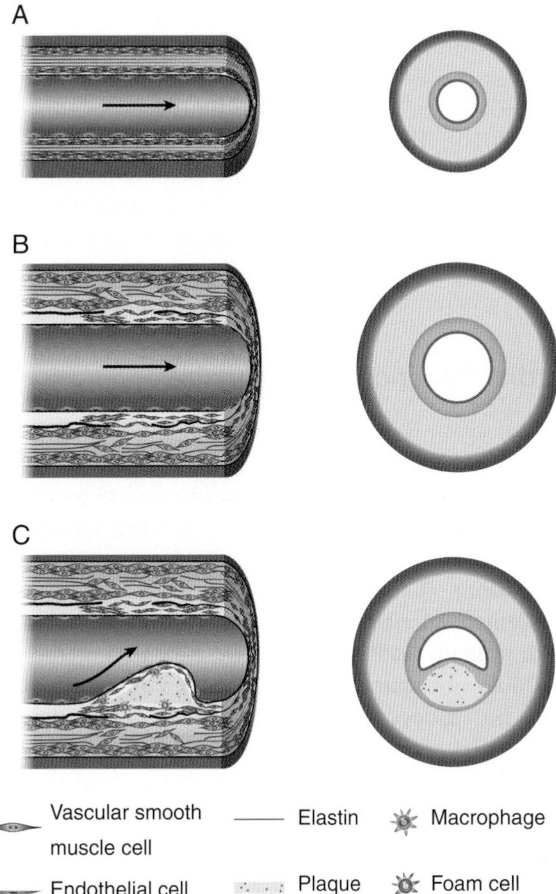

• **Fig. 2.9** Effects of Vascular Aging. The artery of a healthy adult up to age 60 (A) is the normal artery of an adult after age 60 (B). (C) A pathologic variant called atherosclerosis. This is not associated with normal aging, though it is a common pathology associated with aging. (Redrawn from Xu, X., Wang, B., Ren, C., Hu, J., Greenberg, D. A., Chen, T., Xie, L., & Jin, K. [2017]. Age-related impairment of vascular structure and functions. *Aging and Disease, 8*[5], 590–610.)

A significant number of studies use the term *arterial aging* or *vascular aging* to describe the phenomenon of progressive stiffening and widening of the vascular structures (Laurent, 2012). Though studies have determined the timing and rate of the normal arterial aging process, most articles use the term *vascular aging* to describe early or accelerated arterial aging as a result of disease. Thus, practitioners should consider using the term *early vascular aging* or *biologic age* to describe the status of the vascular system due to pathology. Further, the practitioner should closely review literature describing vascular aging or arterial aging and determine if their sample population is healthy or morbid.

Venous System

The venous system is a remarkably simple and elegant structure compared to the vascular system. It accommodates over three-quarters of circulating blood at all times yet maintains a low-pressure system and is composed of a three-layer vessel system with one-way valves (Tucker et al., 2020).

Age-related changes to the venous system are related to the progressive thickening of the one-way valves. Although valve thickness is associated with poor valve function, age is not directly associated with poor valve function (van Langevelde et al., 2010). The venous system, like the vascular system, responds to substrates that promote dilation or constriction. Pharmacologic studies demonstrate that venoconstriction remains unchanged with aging, though there is conflicting evidence as to whether the effects of venodilators are maintained or reduced with aging (Moore et al., 2003).

Cardiac Function and Structure

Normal aging is associated with structural changes to the myocardium as well as reduced valve compliance. In addition to the ubiquitous cellular and DNA changes of aging, aging cardiac cells lose the ability to efficiently remove accumulated waste proteins, causing an accumulation in the myocardium (Leon & Gustafsson, 2016). Similar to the replacement of elastic with collagen, the accumulation of waste proteins leads to progressive stiffening of the heart. This does not appear to influence the contractility of the heart, but it does appear to increase diastolic pressure by reducing myocardium diastolic recoil; reduce the available preload that navigates through the chambers of the heart; and slightly upend the synchrony between the systole and diastole (Vancheri & Henein, 2018).

The valves of the heart also undergo steady and continuous changes from birth to death. The lumen diameter of all four valves increases, slowly separating the margins between the closing leaflets. It should be noted that the effect is more pronounced in women than in men. Interestingly, only the leaflets of the aortic and pulmonic valves appear to both thicken and elongate to cover the increased lumen diameter (Gumpangseth et al., 2019). Calcium deposition also increases leaflet thickening, though the rate of deposition is likely genetic (Waller, 1988). One of the greater concerns for reduced valve function is not necessarily valve leaflet thickening, but the stiffness and shortening of papillary muscles and chordae tendineae. Progressive stiffening can lead to retraction of the leaflets, thereby causing incomplete closure and incomplete opening (Schenk & Heinze, 1975). The increased risk of turbulent blood flow is not, per se, a normal function of cardiac aging, but it is a significant risk factor for thrombosis development. It has not gone unnoticed by practitioners that some features of normal aging mimic—or occasionally cause—common cardiac pathologies of the older adult. See Table 2.4 for common clinical associations between normal aging and pathologic changes.

Despite the significant changes noted here, there are features of the heart that remain constant in adults of all ages. In regard to the electrical conductivity of the heart, the sinoatrial node pace and efficiency remain stable, and fundamental features on an electrocardiogram remain unchanged in normal aging. The functional capacity of the left ventricle remains the same throughout adulthood, specifically regarding left ventricular fill-volume and ejection fraction (Vancheri & Henein, 2018).

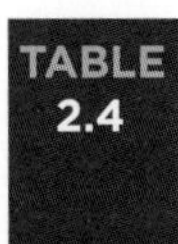

TABLE 2.4 Comparison Between the Normal Processes of Aging to Clinically Significant, Pathologic Look-Alikes

Normal Function of Aging That Can Mimic Pathology	Pathology
Aortic valve calcium	Aortic stenosis
Mitral valve annular calcium	Mitral stenosis
Amyloid deposits	Amyloid heart disease
Thickening of ventricular septum	Hypertrophic cardiomyopathy
Valve leaflet "buckling"	Floppy valve
Retraction of papillary muscles and chordae tendineae	Valve insufficiency, regurgitation

From Waller, B. F. (1988). The old-age heart: Normal aging changes which can produce or mimic cardiac disease. *Clinical Cardiology, 11*(8), 513–517.

Pulmonary Function

The lungs are particularly sensitive to both biologic and chronologic aging. Lung function is affected by a variety of factors: parenchyma and alveolar integrity, gas-exchange capacity, volume capacity as allowed within the confines of the boney borders, and adequate receptor response to hypercapnia or hypoxia (Sharma & Goodwin, 2006). The adult lung fully matures around age 20 to 25, then functionally declines from age 35 onward (Sharma & Goodwin, 2006). The normal aging process leads to notable tissue changes around age 50, causing a progressive picture of *senile emphysema*, described as homogenous enlargement of alveolar air spaces (and, thus, air trapping in "dead space"), though airway contractility is maintained (Parikh et al., 2019). Clinically, increased dead space limits the amount of oxygen-exchange with the bloodstream, though carbon dioxide diffusion is unchanged. Therefore, the deconditioned patient may find it more difficult to respond to physiologic stress (pathologic or elective exercise) without experiencing shortness of breath.

Older adults will continue to breathe at the same rate as younger adults, though the involuntary response to lower oxygen or elevated carbon dioxide is delayed in older adults (Kronenberg & Drage, 1973). However, adults older than age 70 have more intense bronchospasm in response to methacholine chemicals than middle-aged adults. In fact, the intensity of the bronchospasm as related to the methacholine dose is similar to a child's dose response (Hopp et al.,

1985). Further, older adults will have delayed recovery from bronchospasms even with the use of beta-adrenergic therapy (Connolly et al., 1995).

Even in normal aging, older adults are at high risk of pulmonary infection. Delayed and weak responses to hypercapnia or hypoxia, reduced systemic immunity, and reduced forced expiratory volume (FEV1) in the setting of a hyperreactive airway increases the risk for a delayed presentation of pulmonary pathology. Oxygen saturation is a cost-effective, noninvasive, and rapid modality for families, patients, and practitioners to monitor pulmonary function.

SAFETY ALERT

Monitor oxygen saturation as part of a routine assessment of the patient's vital signs. Even asymptomatic deviations from baseline may require close monitoring.

Gastrointestinal System

As reviewed earlier in the Oral Cavity, Mastication, and Deglutition section, normal aging is associated with changes to the power and control of food in the oral cavity that will slow the person's overall eating time. However, the coordination between deglutition, glottis closure over the trachea, and bolus passage into the esophagus and toward the sphincter is preserved. The response time for complete opening of the cardiac sphincter is delayed only slightly, though the entire bolus of food will be able to transit into the stomach without residual in the esophagus (Shaw et al., 1995).

The stomach, however, is an organ with a significant array of specialized cells and functions. As with all other cells in the body, these cells are also predisposed to reduced proliferation and reduced function over time. Thus, the older adult is less able to produce high volumes of digestive enzymes on demand (Shaw et al., 1995), though the production of acid appears to remain stable in normal aging (McCloy et al., 1995). Not only does this cause food to break down more slowly, but it has the potential to create an imbalance between the nutrients consumed and the ability to absorb those nutrients. To allow for prolonged saturation of the food bolus in the stomach, gastric emptying time is reduced, causing prolonged satiety with smaller food volumes. Normal aging is also associated with reduced robustness of gastrointestinal hormones, lessening the adult's perception of hunger and thirst as well as reduced connectivity between ingested food and appropriate enzyme production from the liver and pancreas (Shaw et al., 1995).

The small and large intestines undergo changes in structure, function, and even content during normal aging. Over the course of a person's lifetime, the surface area of the intestine increases with the growth of the intestinal villa. With advancing age, the villa appears to increase, then decrease nearly to the level of a newborn (Thomson & Keelan, 1986). The flatter intestinal wall also becomes more thin and less resilient to bolus pressure, increasing the risk for diverticula (Shaw et al., 1995). The function of the intestines is to regulate the absorption of water and nutrients, which is mediated by the brush border. The brush border continues to absorb nutrients and glucose during normal aging, yet absorption of cholesterol and fatty acids is reduced (Thomson & Keelan, 1986). The large intestine maintains its function of water absorption by osmosis as well as small ion regulation throughout the aging process (Azzouz & Sharma, 2020). Finally, the intestines must peristalsis the food through the gastrointestinal tract by coordinating mechanosensory and chemosensory stimulation. Biopsy studies show that there is reduced innervation throughout the intestines, causing inefficient delays in colonic transit and bolus stagnation. The effect is exacerbated by laxity in the pelvic floor muscles (Keating & Grundy, 2016).

SAFETY ALERT

Double-check the diagnosis. Many older adults will report constipation when they are truly experiencing progressive slowing of their colonic transit time. Establish realistic expectations through patient education and quantifying the acceptable timings between stools, avoid overmedication, and monitor for true pathology.

Other than food stuff, the gastrointestinal tract is home to billions of microbiota, which also see alterations through normal aging. Studies regarding the gut microbiome have demonstrated that biologic and chronologic aging is associated with reduced diversity in the gut microflora (Maffei et al., 2017), with particular reductions in the ubiquitous gut bacteria, bifidobacteria (Arboleya et al., 2016). The gut microbiome of healthy adults shows that at least 4% to 16% of bifidobacteria is maintained throughout the chronologic aging process, and these cultures can be replenished with fermented milk and probiotics. The reductions of microbiota in normal aging are due to assaults from one's lifestyle (antibiotics or the introduction of pathogenic bacteria) as well as changes to the lumen of the gastrointestinal tract (general thickening of mucus causing poor mucosal adhesion and fewer villi available for surface area adhesion) (Arboleya et al., 2016). The significance of this response is linked to the condition of low-grade inflammation and immune senescence in the older adult.

Renal System

Large-sample comparison studies of healthy individuals 20 to 70 years of age have demonstrated that kidney parenchyma decreases at a rate of 10% per decade (Glodny et al., 2009). Total kidney volume reduces by a rate of 16.3 cm^3 per decade, with more rapid deceleration at age 60 (Roseman et al., 2017).

The cortex of the kidney decreases with age, and the medulla increases (Wang et al., 2014). The medulla increases due to nephron hypertrophy (Emamian et al., 1993).

Because the cortex of the kidney is the highly vascular space that connects the nephrons, the reduced volume of the cortex has a postulated association with the systemic arteriosclerosis of aging (Denic et al., 2016). The nephron tubules also appear to become more riddled with diverticula as aging progresses (Baert & Steg, 1977), leading to an acceptable increase of asymptomatic parenchymal cysts (Rule et al., 2012).

Glomerulosclerosis is a condition that relates to the permeability and flexibility of the glomeruli, and it is usually caused by the filling or thickening of the glomeruli. Biopsy studies demonstrate that a completely sclerosed glomeruli is reabsorbed by the kidney, with an average loss of 6200 to 6800 glomeruli per year per kidney (Denic et al., 2017; Hoy et al., 2003). This reduces the glomerular density. Because the glomeruli progress toward complete sclerosis gradually, nephrologists have established an age-adjusted level for the acceptable range of sclerosed glomeruli per biopsy (Kremers et al., 2015). Biopsy studies have also demonstrated that the mechanism of the sclerosis of the glomeruli is different in normal aging versus that of pathologic glomerulosclerosis; in the former, a collagenous material fills the Bowman capsule, and in the latter, the glomeruli solidify completely (Marcantoni et al., 2002).

Although there are many studies to suggest that aging is associated with glomerular hypertrophy, more recent studies of healthy kidney donors have demonstrated that the glomeruli remain the same size in normal aging (Denic et al., 2016, 2017; Hayslett et al., 1968). Therefore, albuminuria, which is associated with glomerular hypertrophy, is also not associated with normal healthy aging.

The glomerular filtration rate (GFR) reduces as part of the normal aging process—a result of the collective changes listed here. Although GFR identifies the speed of filtration, creatinine clearance monitors the function, or accuracy, of renal filtration. Studies have determined that renal function begins to reduce around the time people are in their 30s and 40s, with a rapid rate of decline with each passing decade (Fig. 2.10) (Baba et al., 2015; Cohen et al., 2014; Muntner, 2009). Although numerous human studies have demonstrated that aging women preserve more renal function for more years of life, there is not a dramatic enough change in rate to portend age-adjusted and gender-adjusted norms for renal function (Erdely et al., 2003).

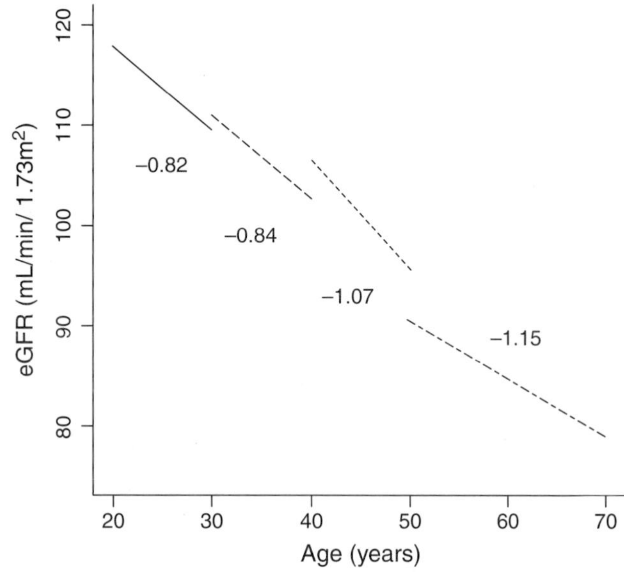

• **Fig. 2.10** Decline of Estimated Glomerular Filtration Rate (eGFR, ml/min/year/1.73 m2) per Year in Healthy Adults. Different dashes indicate the rate of change between decades. (From Cohen, E., Nardi, Y., Krause, I., Goldberg, E., Milo, G., Garty, M., & Krause, I. [2014]. A longitudinal assessment of the natural rate of decline in renal function with age. *Journal of Nephrology, 27*[6], 635–641.)

Urinary System: Normal Changes in the Older Adult

The older adult experiences progressive functional decline of the urinary system, though clinical burden varies from person to person. Evidence derived from functional magnetic resonance imaging (fMRI) demonstrates that the brain and bladder have reduced connectivity with aging. This reduced sensitivity reduces the older adult's awareness for when voiding should occur (Griffiths et al., 2009). Structural changes of the urinary smooth muscles (detrusor and urethral) show that normal aging is associated with slight collagen deposition between smooth muscles cells. The new layer of collagen material sandwiched between the contractile smooth muscle cells allows the urinary bladder to hold more volume before reaching sufficient stretch to stimulate micturition. Thus, the urinary system of the older adult experiences a significant increase in tolerated detrusor volume, increased ureter luminal volume, and reduced contractile force. As a result, there is some urine retention even in otherwise asymptomatic older adults (Liu et al., 2019).

The difference between symptoms and no symptoms of detrusor dysfunction appears to be associated with the amount and location of collagen deposition throughout the smooth muscle. For example, large collagen-induced gaps between cells cause hypocontraction in nonspecific regions of the detrusor muscle. Simultaneously, smooth muscle cells displaced by boluses of collagen will overlap with neighboring contractile cells, causing pockets of hypercontraction (Haferkamp & Elbadawi, 2004). Therefore, the net effect of asymmetric detrusor movement depends on the location of these structural changes. (See Fig. 2.11.)

Genitourinary System: Changes in Women

A woman's genitourinary system changes drastically between pre-, mid-, and post-fertile years. Circulating estrogens maintain not only functional vaginal moisture, but cell fullness and elasticity. With the ovarian exhaustion of estrogen, only low-volume estrogens and testosterones are readily available for basic cellular maintenance. Local tissue effects include a thinning of epithelial tissue, making it appear dehydrated; reabsorption of the vaginal rugae that

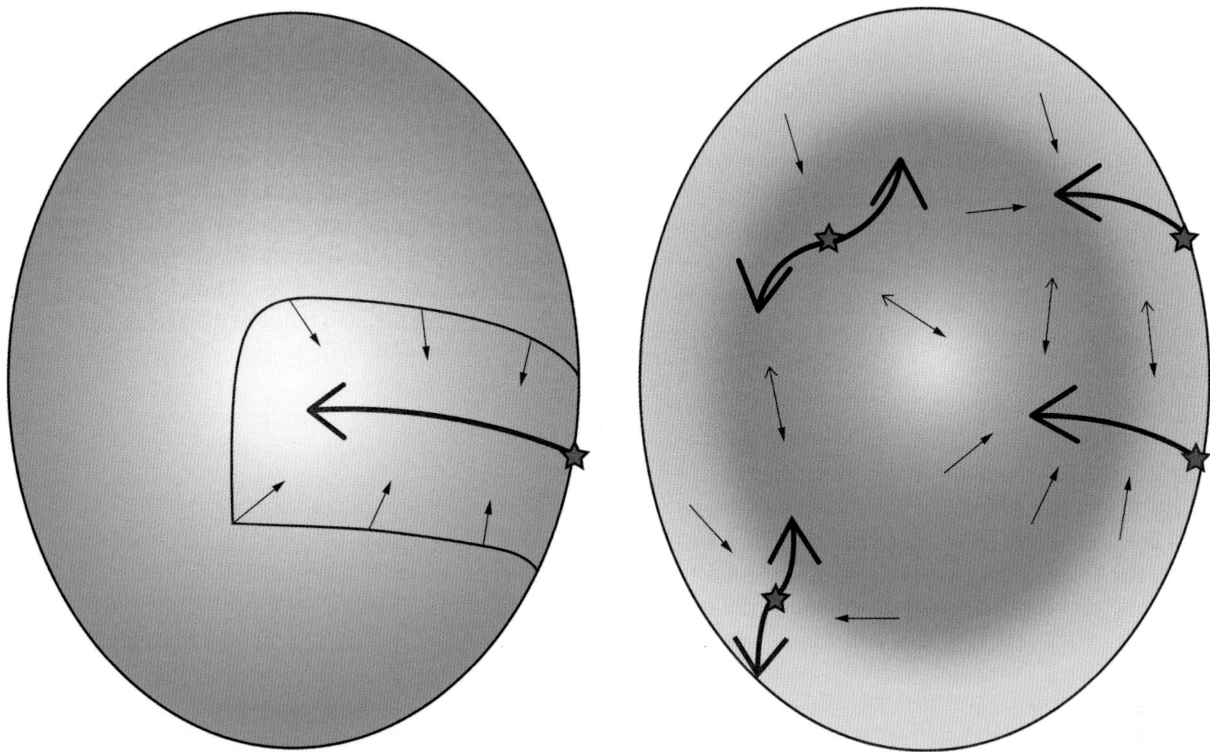

• **Fig. 2.11** Detrusor Wall Contraction in Youth and Older Adulthood. *(Left)* Normal contractile movement along a normal bladder wall, where the star represents the single point of contraction and its energy spans over a limited region of the bladder wall. The remainder of the bladder wall does not contract. *(Right)* Contractile cells that have been physically displaced by collagen fibers now overlap with other contractile cells, creating multiple foci of contractility. Contraction of one site is likely to trigger contraction of other sites, causing asymmetric stimulation of the whole bladder wall. (From Reynolds, W. S., & Cohn, J. A. [2021]. Overactive bladder. *Campbell-Walsh-Wein Urology, 117*, 2637–2649.e4.)

accommodate distention of the vagina during intercourse; and reduced vascular support of the region overall, leading to reduced production of secretions (Sturdee et al., 2010) and reduced neurovascular support of pelvic floor muscles (Mannella et al., 2013). This is a significant change to the genital region. Instead of rebounding to the cells' original state after intercourse, penetration through a thinned, shorted, nonelastic, and mal-lubricated vaginal introitus becomes more similar to a blunt-force trauma to the genital structures. Fibrosis and stricture are pathologic results of this physiologic change in the vaginal and urethral meatus (Nappi et al., 2019). In addition, changes to the moisture and cell composition alters the acidity of the region from 5.0 to 7.4, which in turn changes the local flora of the vagina from predominantly lactobacilli to opportunistic skin bacteria (streptococci & staphylococci) (Nappi et al., 2019).

Genitourinary System: Changes in Men

The prostate enlarges with aging, though the exact mechanism is not fully understood. As a smooth muscle, the prostate is subject to collagen deposition and reduced intercellular coordination. Animal models suggest that aromatase enzyme volumes are preserved in the prostate with normal aging, though free-circulating testosterone decreases. Thus, available testosterone is more likely converted into estrogen before finding a receptor on the prostate, and highly available estrogens are able to stimulate available estrogen receptors. Estrogen's local effect on the prostate causes a change in local epigenetics and increased prostate cell proliferation and cell size (Cooke et al., 2017; Morais-Santos et al., 2018). However, additional studies suggest that normal prostate growth rate (as measured by weight and density) does not particularly accelerate at any stage after puberty (Liu et al., 2019). This stable rate of growth is more likely to cause clinical burden if local estrogens cause hypertrophy to local cells, causing an increase in organ size without increasing the density. The take-away messages from these studies are that local and systemic changes with normal aging do affect the prostate, though their precise combination causes a unique expression per individual. There are no studies to suggest the urinary penis changes with normal aging, though other integrated processes subject to atrophy or dysfunction may influence the appearance and function.

Integumentary System

The integumentary system is the complete organ system that includes hair, skin, nails, and sweat glands. More than simply cosmetic changes to the hair and skin, the integumentary system as a whole also undergoes changes that affect thermoregulation, immune system response, and organ integrity.

Structural changes within the integumentary system itself are caused by progressive atrophy of component size and function, and also the atrophy of intercellular networking between components. This organ-wide atrophy is intimately linked with the normal aging of the vascular system and endocrine systems. The following sections address these changes by the component parts (skin, sweat glands, hair, and nails), with special attention paid to the downstream, organ-wide functional changes that occur as a result.

Skin

The thinned and xerotic appearance of aged skin is a result of the reduced proliferation of basal keratinocytes, the progenitors of the varying layers of skin (Rittié & Fisher, 2015). Reduced vascular architecture in the dermis and hypodermis as well as telomere shortening are the major suspected causes for keratinocyte degradation. The imbalance between continued environmental assaults and delayed the production of new skin cells results in progressive thinning of the lipid-rich, waterproof layer of stratum corneum. The effect is equally distributed throughout the surface area of the body, and normal aging skin still maintains a layer of stratum corneum sufficient to prevent water loss from the body and prevent microbiologic invasion (Rittié & Fisher, 2015). Thinned and wrinkled skin is still highly functional as a barrier when left intact. Pathology occurs as a feature of cancer or interruption of skin integrity.

SAFETY ALERT

Delayed skin recovery due to delayed immune system presence and response are the conditions that may predispose an older adult to opportunistic diseases. The layers of the skin are also affected by changes in systemic endocrine function. As explained in the Endocrine System section, reduced circulating cortisol triggers an increase in cortisol receptors in the skin, with increased local conversation of cortisone into bioavailable cortisol (Tiganescu et al., 2011). Increased cortisol redistributes fat away from the skin and toward the visceral organs (Tiganescu et al., 2011; van den Beld et al., 2018), thereby thinning the layer of subcutaneous fat and adherence between skin layers. Older adults experience this phenomenon as intolerance to cold environments.

Sweat Glands

Heat dissipation is regulated by eccrine sweat glands, which also degrade as vascular connections are lost and the skin layers separate. Thus, an older adult is more susceptible to overheating than a younger adult, and the condition should be managed accordingly (Rittié & Fisher, 2015). The apocrine sweat glands assist in the expression of skin-produced hormones, which ultimately saturate the region-specific hairs to express maturation and mating preparedness (Zouboulis et al., 2007).

Hair

Another common phenotype of normal aging is reduced pigmentation in hair. The pigment of hair, lentigines, and overall skin tone is maintained by melanin, a product of melanocytes. Biopsy studies have demonstrated that melanocytes reduce their production by 10% to 20% per decade after age 25, with the effect of graying scalp and body hair (Ortonne, 1990). Although the skin is functionally affected by the reduction of pigment—melanin is protective of ultraviolet solar exposure, and reduced melanin increases the risk of skin cancers—the hair is most cosmetically affected by the loss of melanocytes.

Trichogram studies of scalp hair density demonstrate a very insignificant change to average hair thickness, though the density of hairs per area does change significantly. Hair density appears to peak in the early 20 s, plateau until the 50 s, and then progressively decrease after age 50 (Kim et al., 2013). Leerunyakul and Suchonwanit's diversity-minded studies have added that Africans and Caucasians have a greater initial hair density than Asians (Leerunyakul & Suchonwanit, 2020).

Although there is some progressive decline in hair density in other body areas, there does not appear to be a significant reduction in body hair or hairs that distribute pheromones and scents (axillary and genital) (Astore et al., 1979). In contrast, hair thickness and length appear to increase in expressive/identification hairs (eyebrows) (Papageorgiou et al., 2012) and hair that protect orifices (eyelashes, ears, and nares in men, upper lip/chin in women) (Ali & Wojnarowska, 2011; Fenske & Lober, 1986).

Nails

The function of fingernails and toenails is preserved throughout aging, though the rate of growth is reduced. Starting at age 25, the rate of growth is reduced by 0.5% per year from the baseline rate of 3 mm/month for fingernails and 1 mm/month for toenails (Abdullah & Abbas, 2011). In addition, the nail plate of an older adult is generally more thin, brittle, and has more rugae than that of a younger adult (Fenske & Lober, 1986).

Behavior and Relationships: Psychological and Emotional

Other than organ-specific features that may alter a person's perception of the world, the older adult still feels and understands the same emotions expressed in young adulthood. A normal aging adult is still interested in feeling pro-ego emotions such as happiness, gratitude, fulfillment of self, and satisfaction with living circumstances. These pro-ego emotions are the net effects of societal expectations, the health of peers, one's own sense of physical function, one's own sense of societal utility, and, of course, personality.

Each older adult is able to tolerate a unique threshold of disruptions and still maintain a positive perception. This is likely due to the older adult's ability to consciously and unconsciously compare a lifelong repertoire of pro-ego and anti-ego experiences. Consciously, a normal aging adult may feel gratitude for health superior to his or her peers as well as frustration for health that is perceived as inferior to one's younger self (Bennett et al., 2017, 2020). The provider should be sensitive that many older adults are unable to communicate the overwhelming and complex balance of gratitude, fear, frustration, uncertainty, and other responses that accompanies aging and nearing the end of life. Profound and sustained deviations from pro-ego emotions and behaviors should prompt investigation for primary or secondary demoralization or depression. (See)

Behavior and Relationship Between the Older Adult and Health

Older adults place greater emphasis on improving or maintaining their state health compared to younger adults. It is pervasive in their conversations and decision-making processes. This may be due to more frequent and ubiquitous rumination about how one wants to live one's remaining days.

Interestingly, the very definition of "health" and how to accomplish this is drastically different between individuals. This phenomenon can be captured scientifically in the general trend for annual wellness visit attendance. Requests for an annual wellness visit increase with age and one of the following features: increased access to medical services (urban), higher socioeconomic class, marriage, female gender, and ethnicity that matches the dominant culture (Dryden et al., 2012; Sun et al., 2014). These are the older adults who seek to understand themselves and their bodies with the guidance of a medical practitioner and social support. They tend to follow through with medical recommendations. They are interested in understanding what a medical provider has to say about their condition. These older adults believe that a medical provider is the ultimate consultant for health-related norms and issues, and they are comfortable requesting the services of medicine. These individuals see benefit in paying for these services; they follow practitioner recommendations as an active way to maintain or improve health and, thus, their goals in older adulthood. Essentially, these adults are ready to enter a service that they believe was designed for them by people like them.

In contrast, older adults of low socioeconomic income status, male gender, single status, or from marginalized ethnic groups tend to cope with the changes of older adulthood without the guidance of a medical practitioner (Dryden et al., 2012). These older adults still ruminate on their mortality and health status just as any older adult, but they greet every aspect of the aging experience with the perception that "it's just aging; nothing to do," find the financial and time cost of medicine overwhelming, or ultimately conclude that they "may as well enjoy life" in whatever form that may take. These adults have never felt welcome to utilize a medical service operated by highly educated, high-income individuals who could possibly chastise them for present or lacking characteristics. These adults will thus not enter a service that they feel was not designed for them.

These older adults fear what a medical provider will do or say regarding their health, so avoiding the practitioner preserves their sense of well-being and happiness. They are more likely to articulate their disdain for the world of medicine or frequently reiterate that "life is short," and they will, therefore, continue with the behaviors that would incite discussion in a medical office.

Within and between these two groups is a new generation of older adults who not only found health advice from blogs, advertisements, and vitamin stores during young adulthood, but also found antiaging advice. The great difficulty of understanding oneself during aging is similar to how the adolescent experiences puberty: as change approaches or occurs, it is frightening. There is an overwhelming desire to seek understanding from social constructs and trusted sources. As mentioned in the introduction of this chapter, the "antiaging" stock market capitalizes on the vulnerable balance of our ego and our desire to understand the complexities of our lives. It inserts itself more frequently, boldly, attractively, and (most important) effortlessly to a person's life. Further, marketing and antiaging sentiments insert their most unshakable impressions when the adults cease to receive care from the pediatrician, offering new and tailored-for-you products to address every ailment in one's life.

This practice is not, per se, an enemy to medicine, but it is competing with traditional medicine. It is a potent social influence that helps the person anticipate what's coming next and how to fix or treat it. Practitioners must appreciate this powerful tool with reverence, realizing that patients are forming opinions and behaviors about their health—consciously or unconsciously—because of these influences. Practitioners can and should compete in the same marketing space as the antiaging market by offering services with competitive affordability, inclusivity, targeted marketing, and future consumer marketing. To use more patient-centric terms, practitioners can and should offer anticipatory guidance and support legislation that makes their services both affordable and socially welcomed throughout communities.

Interdisciplinary Teamwork

Everyone Is a Member of the Interdisciplinary Team

Recall the 74-year-old employee from the beginning of this chapter. Recall all of the facts that surprised you throughout this chapter. To best guide a normal adult through the normal aging process, the practitioner must have a strong grasp of these processes as well as a cross-discipline network from which to learn and refer. In addition to the variety of valuable team members listed throughout the chapter, the following sections describe only a few more of the many team members that can be of high value for all aging adults. It is important to consider family members, religious leaders, community services, insurance companies, home health services, and housing authorities as potentially valuable members of the interdisciplinary team.

Counselors on the Interdisciplinary Team

Counselors can be valuable for both the individual and the family. They can perform simple and beneficial assessments, such as hosting a counseling session between the patient and family with and without hearing aids to determine if the patient would benefit from consistent use. They can encourage family members to use additional physical cues to express emotions, such as slow lip motions, eye contact, body language, and hand gestures. Their office setting offers an ideal place for family members to practice techniques of modified communication, such as sitting face to face for enhanced emotional response between talker and listener, encouraging discussions in quiet environments, and encouraging the use of phrases that reinforce understanding, such as "I did not understand you" or "Did I hear you correctly when you said...?"

Nutritionists in the Interdisciplinary Team

Nutritionists appreciate the older adult's cultural, social, and personal relationship to food and drink, then they refine their recommendations down to a dose, potency, and quantity of nutrients for the older adult to follow. For example, nutritionists can prevent issues related to reduced gustation—anorexia, weight loss, poor salivation—by recommending the precise type and amount of spice to add to a diet. Refer the Gustation section, presented earlier, to review the systemic cascade of taste receptors.

Though practitioners believe that they could or would make such suggestions in the office, it is often difficult for the clinical practitioner to give customized dietary guidance without clinical time and exquisite insight into the older adult's cultural and personal preferences regarding "spicy" or "hot" food. That latter part is especially critical for success. For instance, Indian cuisine has significant amounts of heat and seasoning, whereas British cuisine tends to be very bland. Without proper dosing, the older adult may use an ineffective volume of the spice—too much or too little—to achieve the desired effect. A nutritionist will be mindful of these circumstances when prescribing the ideal diet for the patient.

Encourage Cultural Sensitivity Within the Interdisciplinary Team

Practitioners should utilize colleagues of different cultures, socioeconomic backgrounds, ethnicities, and genders to improve their own cultural empathy and patient rapport. When the practitioner understands the nuances of a culture, it is easier for the practitioner to bridge gaps in understanding or anticipate a patient's hesitation to a recommendation. A practitioner's misunderstanding of a patient's basic cultural norms could cause a sense of confusion or mistrust. For instance, culturally appropriate gestures of affirmation would be nodding in North America and a head wobble in India. In both cultures, increasing the cadence of the head gesture suggests increased understanding. A simple lack of familiarity with the head wobble as a gesture of affirmation may appear as shaking the head, which is a gesture of disapproval in North America.

Maintaining social savviness can alleviate unforeseen barriers before they arise. If cultural barriers do arise, practitioners should tactfully double-check the patient's understanding throughout the office visit. A patient—especially an older adult—may feign comprehension for a variety of reasons. When working with a patient of an unfamiliar cultural background, the practitioner would benefit from a proactive admission of ignorance and can remind patients of their intention to help. Practitioners can identify the barriers in the office visit (language, eye contact, etc.) and then ask members of that community what is normal behavior. When working with a patient of a familiar cultural background, a practitioner could determine patient comprehension by assessing patient response. Signs of patients' comprehension may include the use of expressions such as "Oh, I see," repeating the practitioner's metaphor using their own words, maintaining eye contact, or changing their posture into a relaxed or attentive pose.

If these signs are not present in the office, it would be valuable to ask other members of the interdisciplinary team if the patient appeared to understand their condition(s). The practitioner could ask the patient, "What did the counselor and the physical therapist tell you at your most recent office visits?" to reinforce the benefit of those visits. All members of the interdisciplinary team could then ensure that their messages were completely received by the patient, family, and colleagues on the interdisciplinary team.

Key Points

1. PAs and NPs in all fields of medicine must consider the nuances of normal aging to promote the health of the patient, community, and economy.
2. The normal aging process of an older adult is mutually exclusive from the pathologies and diseases of humankind. Practitioners must educate the community about the acceptable symptoms of aging.
3. Practitioners must acknowledge preexisting the social biases against aging. They can be overcome with intentional self-education and the utilization of cross-cultural, cross-disciplinary teams.

More information about tools and the Interprofessional Education Collaborative (IPEC) competencies mentioned in this chapter can be found in Appendix 1: Tools and Appendix 2: IPEC Competencies.

References

Abdullah, L., & Abbas, O. (2011). Common nail changes and disorders in older people: Diagnosis and management. *Canadian Family Physician Medecin de Famille Canadien*, *57*(2), 173–181.

Abu Eid, R., Sawair, F., Landini, G., & Saku, T. (2012). Age and the architecture of oral mucosa. *Age*, *34*(3), 651–658.

Ackerstaff, R. G., Keunen, R. W., van Pelt, W., Montauban van Swijndregt, A. D., & Stijnen, T. (1990). Influence of biological factors on changes in mean cerebral blood flow velocity in normal ageing: A transcranial Doppler study. *Neurological Research*, *12*(3), 187–191.

Affoo, R. H., Foley, N., Garrick, R., Siqueira, W. L., & Martin, R. E. (2015). Meta-analysis of salivary flow rates in young and older adults. *Journal of the American Geriatrics Society*, *63*(10), 2142–2151.

Ali, I., & Wojnarowska, F. (2011). Physiological changes in scalp, facial and body hair after the menopause: A cross-sectional population-based study of subjective changes. *British Journal of Dermatology*, *164*(3), 508–513.

Anti-Aging Market Size, Share, Trends and Forecast 2020–2025. (n.d.). https://www.imarcgroup.com/anti-aging-market

Arboleya, S., Watkins, C., Stanton, C., & Ross, R. P. (2016). Gut bifidobacteria populations in human health and aging. *Frontiers in Microbiology*, *7*, 1204.

Astore, I. P., Pecoraro, V., & Pecoraro, E. G. (1979). The normal trichogram of pubic hair. *British Journal of Dermatology*, *101*(4), 441–445.

Atzmon, G., Barzilai, N., Surks, M. I., & Gabriely, I. (2009). Genetic predisposition to elevated serum thyrotropin is associated with exceptional longevity. *Journal of Clinical Endocrinology and Metabolism*, *94*(12), 4768–4775.

Aurich, M., Poole, A. R., Reiner, A., Mollenhauer, C., Margulis, A., Kuettner, K. E., & Cole, A. A. (2002). Matrix homeostasis in aging normal human ankle cartilage. *Arthritis and Rheumatism*, *46*(11), 2903–2910.

Azcoitia, I., Yague, J. G., & Garcia-Segura, L. M. (2011). Estradiol synthesis within the human brain. *Neuroscience*, *191*, 139–147.

Azzouz, L. L., & Sharma, S. (2020). *Physiology, large intestine*. StatPearls Publishing.

Baba, M., Shimbo, T., Horio, M., Ando, M., Yasuda, Y., Komatsu, Y., Masuda, K., Matsuo, S., & Maruyama, S. (2015). Longitudinal study of the decline in renal function in healthy subjects. *PloS One*, *10*(6), e0129036.

Baert, L., & Steg, A. (1977). Is the diverticulum of the distal and collecting tubules a preliminary stage of the simple cyst in the adult? *Journal of Urology*, *118*(5), 707–710.

Benefits Planner: Retirement. (n.d.). https://www.ssa.gov/benefits/retirement/planner/agereduction.html

Bennett, E. V., Clarke, L. H., Kowalski, K. C., & Crocker, P. R. E. (2017). "I'll do anything to maintain my health": How women aged 65-94 perceive, experience, and cope with their aging bodies. *Body Image*, *21*, 71–80.

Bennett, E. V., Hurd, L. C., Pritchard, E. M., Colton, T., & Crocker, P. R. E. (2020). An examination of older men's body image: How men 65 years and older perceive, experience, and cope with their aging bodies. *Body Image*, *34*, 27–37.

Beyer, C., Morali, G., Larsson, K., & Söderstein, P. (1976). Steroid regulation of sexual behavior. *Journal of Steroid Biochemistry*, *7*(11-12), 1171–1176.

Biondi, B., Bartalena, L., Cooper, D. S., Hegedüs, L., Laurberg, P., & Kahaly, G. J. (2015). The 2015 European Thyroid Association guidelines on diagnosis and treatment of endogenous subclinical hyperthyroidism. *European Thyroid Journal*, *4*(3), 149–163.

Broekmans, F. J., Soules, M. R., & Fauser, B. C. (2009). Ovarian aging: Mechanisms and clinical consequences. *Endocrine Reviews*, *30*(5), 465–493.

Cabeza, R. (2002). Hemispheric asymmetry reduction in older adults: The HAROLD model. *Psychology and Aging*, *17*(1), 85–100.

Cabeza, R., Anderson, N. D., Locantore, J. K., & McIntosh, A. R. (2002). Aging gracefully: Compensatory brain activity in high-performing older adults. *NeuroImage*, *17*(3), 1394–1402.

Campbell, S. S., & Murphy, P. J. (2007). The nature of spontaneous sleep across adulthood. *Journal of Sleep Research*, *16*(1), 24–32.

Cannarella, R., Barbagallo, F., Condorelli, R. A., Aversa, A., La Vignera, S., & Calogero, A. E. (2019). Osteoporosis from an endocrine perspective: The role of hormonal changes in the elderly. *Journal of Clinical Medicine Research*, *8*(10). https://doi.org/10.3390/jcm8101564.

Carlson, M. C., Hasher, L., Connelly, S. L., & Zacks, R. T. (1995). Aging, distraction, and the benefits of predictable location. *Psychology & Aging*, *10*, 427–436.

Ceda, G. P., Dall'Aglio, E., Maggio, M., Lauretani, F., Bandinelli, S., Falzoi, C., Grimaldi, W., Ceresini, G., Corradi, F., Ferrucci, L., Valenti, G., & Hoffman, A. R. (2005). Clinical implications of the reduced activity of the GH-IGF-I axis in older men. *Journal of Endocrinological Investigation*, *28*(11 Suppl. Proceedings), 96–100.

Chaves, P. H. M., Ashar, B., Guralnik, J. M., & Fried, L. P. (2002). Looking at the relationship between hemoglobin concentration and prevalent mobility difficulty in older women. Should the criteria currently used to define anemia in older people be reevaluated? *Journal of the American Geriatrics Society*, *50*(7), 1257–1264.

Chen, J. J., Rosas, H. D., & Salat, D. H. (2011). Age-associated reductions in cerebral blood flow are independent from regional atrophy. *NeuroImage*, *55*(2), 468–478.

Christensen, J. A., Sis, J., Kulkarni, A. M., & Chatterjee, M. (2019). Effects of age and hearing loss on the recognition of emotions in speech. *Ear and Hearing*, *40*(5), 1069–1083.

Cohen, E., Nardi, Y., Krause, I., Goldberg, E., Milo, G., Garty, M., & Krause, I. (2014). A longitudinal assessment of the natural rate of decline in renal function with age. *Journal of Nephrology*, *27*(6), 635–641.

Compston, J. E., McClung, M. R., & Leslie, W. D. (2019). Osteoporosis. *The Lancet*, *393*(10169), 364–376.

Connolly, M. J., Crowley, J. J., Charan, N. B., Nielson, C. P., & Vestal, R. E. (1995). Impaired bronchodilator response to albuterol in healthy elderly men and women. *Chest*, *108*(2), 401–406.

Cooke, P. S., Nanjappa, M. K., Ko, C., Prins, G. S., & Hess, R. A. (2017). Estrogens in male physiology. *Physiological Reviews*, *97*(3), 995–1043.

Copinschi, G., & Caufriez, A. (2013). Sleep and hormonal changes in aging. *Endocrinology and Metabolism Clinics of North America*, *42*(2), 371–389.

Denic, A., Alexander, M. P., Kaushik, V., Lerman, L. O., Lieske, J. C., Stegall, M. D., Larson, J. J., Kremers, W. K., Vrtiska, T. J., Chakkera, H. A., Poggio, E. D., & Rule, A. D. (2016). Detection and clinical patterns of nephron hypertrophy and nephrosclerosis among apparently healthy adults. *American Journal of Kidney Diseases: The Official Journal of the National Kidney Foundation*, *68*(1), 58–67.

Denic, A., Lieske, J. C., Chakkera, H. A., Poggio, E. D., Alexander, M. P., Singh, P., Kremers, W. K., Lerman, L. O., & Rule, A. D. (2017). The substantial loss of nephrons in healthy human kidneys with aging. *Journal of the American Society of Nephrology: JASN*, *28*(1), 313–320.

Di Somma, C., Brunelli, V., Savanelli, M. C., Scarano, E., Savastano, S., Lombardi, G., & Colao, A. (2011). Somatopause: State of the art. *Minerva Endocrinologica*, *36*(3), 243–255.

Dryden, R., Williams, B., McCowan, C., & Themessl-Huber, M. (2012). What do we know about who does and does not attend general health checks? Findings from a narrative scoping review. *BMC Public Health, 12*, 723.

Duffy, J. F., Zitting, K. -M., & Chinoy, E. D. (2015). Aging and circadian rhythms. *Sleep Medicine Clinics, 10*(4), 423–434.

Elraiyah, T., Sonbol, M. B., Wang, Z., Khairalseed, T., Asi, N., Undavalli, C., Nabhan, M., Altayar, O., Prokop, L., Montori, V. M., & Murad, M. H. (2014). Clinical review: The benefits and harms of systemic dehydroepiandrosterone (DHEA) in postmenopausal women with normal adrenal function: A systematic review and meta-analysis. *Journal of Clinical Endocrinology and Metabolism, 99*(10), 3536–3542.

Emamian, S. A., Nielsen, M. B., Pedersen, J. F., & Ytte, L. (1993). Kidney dimensions at sonography: Correlation with age, sex, and habitus in 665 adult volunteers. *American Journal of Roentgenology, 160*(1), 83–86.

Erdely, A., Greenfeld, Z., Wagner, L., & Baylis, C. (2003). Sexual dimorphism in the aging kidney: Effects on injury and nitric oxide system. *Kidney International, 63*(3), 1021–1026.

Fabbri, E., An, Y., Gonzalez-Freire, M., Zoli, M., Maggio, M., Studenski, S. A., Egan, J. M., Chia, C. W., & Ferrucci, L. (2016). Bioavailable testosterone linearly declines over a wide age spectrum in men and women from the Baltimore longitudinal study of aging. *The Journals of Gerontology. Series A, Biological Sciences and Medical Sciences, 71*(9), 1202–1209.

Fenske, N. A., & Lober, C. W. (1986). Structural and functional changes of normal aging skin. *Journal of the American Academy of Dermatology, 15*(4 Pt 1), 571–585.

Flicker, L., McCaul, K. A., Hankey, G. J., Jamrozik, K., Brown, W. J., Byles, J. E., & Almeida, O. P. (2010). Body mass index and survival in men and women aged 70 to 75. *Journal of the American Geriatrics Society, 58*(2), 234–241.

Florencio-Silva, R., Sasso, G. R., da, S., Sasso-Cerri, E., Simões, M. J., & Cerri, P. S. (2015). Biology of bone tissue: Structure, function, and factors that influence bone cells. *BioMed Research International, 2015*, 421746.

Floyd, J. A., Janisse, J. J., Jenuwine, E. S., & Ager, J. W. (2007). Changes in REM-sleep percentage over the adult lifespan. *Sleep, 30*(7), 829–836.

Gates, G. A., & Mills, J. H. (2005). Presbycusis. *The Lancet, 366*(9491), 1111–1120.

Gibon, E., Lu, L., & Goodman, S. B. (2016). Aging, inflammation, stem cells, and bone healing. *Stem Cell Research & Therapy, 7*, 44.

Glodny, B., Unterholzner, V., Taferner, B., Hofmann, K. J., Rehder, P., Strasak, A., & Petersen, J. (2009). Normal kidney size and its influencing factors—a 64-slice MDCT study of 1.040 asymptomatic patients. *BMC Urology, 9*, 19.

Griffiths, D. J., Tadic, S. D., Schaefer, W., & Resnick, N. M. (2009). Cerebral control of the lower urinary tract: How age-related changes might predispose to urge incontinence. *NeuroImage, 47*(3), 981–986.

Gumpangseth, T., Mahakkanukrauh, P., & Das, S. (2019). Gross age-related changes and diseases in human heart valves. *Anatomy & Cell Biology, 52*(1), 25–33.

Guralnik, J. M., Eisenstaedt, R. S., Ferrucci, L., Klein, H. G., & Woodman, R. C. (2004). Prevalence of anemia in persons 65 years and older in the United States: Evidence for a high rate of unexplained anemia. *Blood, 104*(8), 2263–2268.

Haferkamp, A., & Elbadawi, A. (2004). Ultrastrukturelle Veränderungen der Altersblase. *Der Urologe, Ausgabe A, 43*(5), 527–534.

Harada, C. N., Natelson Love, M. C., & Triebel, K. L. (2013). Normal cognitive aging. *Clinics in Geriatric Medicine, 29*(4), 737–752.

Harman, S. M., Metter, E. J., Tobin, J. D., Pearson, J., Blackman, M. R., & Baltimore Longitudinal Study of Aging, (2001). Longitudinal effects of aging on serum total and free testosterone levels in healthy men. Baltimore longitudinal study of aging. *The Journal of Clinical Endocrinology and Metabolism, 86*(2), 724–731.

Hayslett, J. P., Kashgarian, M., & Epstein, F. H. (1968). Functional correlates of compensatory renal hypertrophy. *Journal of Clinical Investigation, 47*(4), 774–799.

Hopp, R. J., Bewtra, A., Nair, N. M., & Townley, R. G. (1985). The effect of age on methacholine response. *Journal of Allergy and Clinical Immunology, 76*(4), 609–613.

Hoy, W. E., Douglas-Denton, R. N., Hughson, M. D., Cass, A., Johnson, K., & Bertram, J. F. (2003). A stereological study of glomerular number and volume: Preliminary findings in a multiracial study of kidneys at autopsy. *Kidney International. Supplement, 83*, S31–S37.

Institute of Medicine (US) Committee on Assessing the Need for Clinical Trials of Testosterone Replacement Therapy, (2004). In C. T. Liverman & D. G. Blazer (Eds.), *Testosterone and aging: Clinical research directions*. National Academies Press.

Iovino, C., Pellegrini, M., Bernabei, F., Borrelli, E., Sacconi, R., Govetto, A., Vagge, A., Di Zazzo, A., Forlini, M., Finocchio, L., Carnevali, A., Triolo, G., & Giannaccare, G. (2020). Choroidal vascularity index: An in-depth analysis of this novel optical coherence tomography parameter. *Journal of Clinical Medicine Research, 9*(2). https://doi.org/10.3390/jcm9020595.

Iurciuc, S., Cimpean, A. M., Mitu, F., Heredea, R., & Iurciuc, M. (2017). Vascular aging and subclinical atherosclerosis: Why such a "never ending" and challenging story in cardiology? *Clinical Interventions in Aging, 12*, 1339–1345.

Izaks, G. J., Westendorp, R. G., & Knook, D. L. (1999). The definition of anemia in older persons. *Journal of the American Medical Association, 281*(18), 1714–1717.

Junnila, R. K., List, E. O., Berryman, D. E., Murrey, J. W., & Kopchick, J. J. (2013). The GH/IGF-1 axis in ageing and longevity. *Nature Reviews. Endocrinology, 9*(6), 366–376.

Kang, A. J., Kim, D. -K., Kang, S. H., Seo, K. M., Park, H. S., & Park, K. -H. (2016). EMG activity of masseter muscles in the elderly according to rheological properties of solid food. *Annals of Rehabilitation Medicine, 40*(3), 447–456.

Keating, C., & Grundy, D. (2016). Ageing and gastrointestinal sensory function. *Advances in Experimental Medicine and Biology*. https://doi.org/10.1007/978-3-319-27592-5_8.

Kim, J. E., Lee, J. H., Choi, K. H., Lee, W. -S., Choi, G. S., Kwon, O. S., Kim, M. B., Huh, C. -H., Ihm, C. -W., Kye, Y. C., Ro, B. I., Sim, W. -Y., Kim, D. W., Kim, H. O., & Kang, H. (2013). Phototrichogram analysis of normal scalp hair characteristics with aging. *European Journal of Dermatology, 23*(6), 849–856.

Kondo, K., Kikuta, S., Ueha, R., Suzukawa, K., & Yamasoba, T. (2020). Age-related olfactory dysfunction: Epidemiology, pathophysiology, and clinical management. *Frontiers in Aging Neuroscience, 12*, 208.

Kremers, W. K., Denic, A., Lieske, J. C., Alexander, M. P., Kaushik, V., Elsherbiny, H. E., Chakkera, H. A., Poggio, E. D., & Rule, A. D. (2015). Distinguishing age-related from disease-related glomerulosclerosis on kidney biopsy: The aging kidney anatomy study. *Nephrology, Dialysis, Transplantation, 30*(12), 2034–2039.

Kronenberg, R. S., & Drage, C. W. (1973). Attenuation of the ventilatory and heart rate responses to hypoxia and hypercapnia with aging in normal men. *Journal of Clinical Investigation, 52*(8), 1812–1819.

Laurent, S. (2012). Defining vascular aging and cardiovascular risk. *Journal of Hypertension*, *30*(Suppl), S3–S8.

Leerunyakul, K., & Suchonwanit, P. (2020). Evaluation of hair density and hair diameter in the adult thai population using quantitative trichoscopic analysis. *BioMed Research International*. https://doi.org/10.1155/2020/2476890.

Leon, L. J., & Gustafsson, Å. B. (2016). Staying young at heart: Autophagy and adaptation to cardiac aging. *Journal of Molecular and Cellular Cardiology*, *95*, 78–85.

Li, J., Vitiello, M. V., & Gooneratne, N. S. (2018). Sleep in normal aging. *Sleep Medicine Clinics*, *13*(1), 1–11.

Liu, T. T., Thomas, S., Mclean, D. T., Roldan-Alzate, A., Hernando, D., Ricke, E. A., & Ricke, W. A. (2019). Prostate enlargement and altered urinary function are part of the aging process. *Aging*, *11*(9), 2653–2669.

Lezak, M. D., Howieson, D. B., Loring, D. W., & Fischer, J. S. (2004). *Neuropsychological Assessment*. Oxford University Press.

Lopes, J. M., Dantas, F. G., & de Medeiros, J. L. A. (2013). Excessive daytime sleepiness in the elderly: Association with cardiovascular risk, obesity and depression. *Revista Brasileira de Epidemiologia [Brazilian Journal of Epidemiology]*, *16*(4), 872–879.

Maffei, V. J., Kim, S., Blanchard, E., 4th, Luo, M., Jazwinski, S. M., Taylor, C. M., & Welsh, D. A. (2017). Biological aging and the human gut microbiota. *The Journals of Gerontology. Series A, Biological Sciences and Medical Sciences*, *72*(11), 1474–1482.

Mannella, P., Palla, G., Bellini, M., & Simoncini, T. (2013). The female pelvic floor through midlife and aging. *Maturitas*, *76*(3), 230–234.

Marcantoni, C., Ma, L. -J., Federspiel, C., & Fogo, A. B. (2002). Hypertensive nephrosclerosis in African Americans versus Caucasians. *Kidney International*, *62*(1), 172–180.

Mattis, J., & Sehgal, A. (2016). Circadian rhythms, sleep, and disorders of aging. *Trends in Endocrinology and Metabolism*. https://www.sciencedirect.com/science/article/pii/S1043276016000205.

McCloy, R. F., Arnold, R., Bardhan, K. D., Cattan, D., Klinkenberg-Knol, E., Maton, P. N., Riddell, R. H., Sipponen, P., & Walan, A. (1995). Pathophysiological effects of long-term acid suppression in man. *Digestive Diseases and Sciences*, *40*(2 Suppl), 96S–120S.

Mese, H., & Matsuo, R. (2007). Salivary secretion, taste and hyposalivation. *Journal of Oral Rehabilitation*, *34*(10), 711–723.

Moore, A., Mangoni, A. A., Lyons, D., & Jackson, S. H. D. (2003). The cardiovascular system. *British Journal of Clinical Pharmacology*, *56*(3), 254–260.

Morais-Santos, M., Werneck-Gomes, H., Campolina-Silva, G. H., Santos, L. C., Mahecha, G. A. B., Hess, R. A., & Oliveira, C. A. (2018). Basal cells show increased expression of aromatase and estrogen receptor α in prostate epithelial lesions of male aging rats. *Endocrinology*, *159*(2), 723–732.

Muntner, P. (2009). Longitudinal measurements of renal function. *Seminars in Nephrology*, *29*(6), 650–657.

Murphy, R. A., Patel, K. V., Kritchevsky, S. B., Houston, D. K., Newman, A. B., Koster, A., Simonsick, E. M., Tylvasky, F. A., Cawthon, P. M., & Harris, T. B. (2014). Weight change, body composition, and risk of mobility disability and mortality in older adults: A population-based cohort study. *Journal of the American Geriatrics Society*, *62*(8), 1476–1483.

Nah, E. H., Kim, S., Cho, S., & Cho, H. I. (2018). Complete blood count reference intervals and patterns of changes across pediatric, adult, and geriatric ages in Korea. *Annals of Laboratory Medicine*, *38*(6), 503–511.

Nappi, R. E., Martini, E., Cucinella, L., Martella, S., Tiranini, L., Inzoli, A., Brambilla, E., Bosoni, D., Cassani, C., & Gardella, B. (2019). Addressing vulvovaginal atrophy (VVA)/genitourinary syndrome of menopause (GSM) for healthy aging in women. *Frontiers in Endocrinology*, *10*, 561.

Nivison-Smith, L., Khandelwal, N., Tong, J., Mahajan, S., Kalloniatis, M., & Agrawal, R. (2020). Normal aging changes in the choroidal angioarchitecture of the macula. *Scientific Reports*, *10*(1), 10810.

Obayon, M. M., Carskadon, M. A., Guilleminault, C., & Vitiello, M. V. (2004). Meta-analysis of quantitative sleep parameters from childhood to old age in healthy individuals: Developing normative sleep values across the human lifespan. *Sleep*, *27*(7), 1255–1273.

Ortonne, J. P. (1990). Pigmentary changes of the ageing skin. *British Journal of Dermatology*, *122*(Suppl. 35), 21–28.

PAEA, AAPA, ARCPA, & NCCPA. (2005). Competencies for the PA Profession. 2, 4. https://www.aapa.org/wp-content/uploads/2017/02/PA-Competencies-updated.pdf

Pagani, M., Salmaso, D., Jonsson, C., Hatherly, R., Jacobsson, H., Larsson, S. A., & Wägner, A. (2002). Regional cerebral blood flow as assessed by principal component analysis and (99m) Tc-HMPAO SPET in healthy subjects at rest: Normal distribution and effect of age and gender. *European Journal of Nuclear Medicine and Molecular Imaging*, *29*(1), 67–75.

Palinkas, M., Cecilio, F. A., Siéssere, S., Borges, T. F., de Carvalho, C. A. M., Semprini, M., de Sousa, L. G., & Regalo, S. C. H. (2013). Aging of masticatory efficiency in healthy subjects: Electromyographic analysis—Part 2. *Acta Odontologica Latinoamericana*, *26*(3), 161–166.

Papageorgiou, K. I., Mancini, R., Garneau, H. C., Chang, S. -H., Jarullazada, I., King, A., Forster-Perlini, E., Hwang, C., Douglas, R., & Goldberg, R. A. (2012). A three-dimensional construct of the aging eyebrow: The illusion of volume loss. *Aesthetic Surgery Journal/The American Society for Aesthetic Plastic Surgery*, *32*(1), 46–57.

Parikh, P., Wicher, S., Khandalavala, K., Pabelick, C. M., Britt, R. D., Jr, & Prakash, Y. S. (2019). Cellular senescence in the lung across the age spectrum. *American Journal of Physiology. Lung Cellular and Molecular Physiology*, *316*(5), L826–L842.

Position Statements & White Papers—National Organization of Nurse Practitioner Faculties (NONPF). (n.d.). https://www.nonpf.org/page/16

Presbyopia: Overview. (2020). Institute for Quality and Efficiency in Health Care (IQWiG).

Pushpass, R. -A. G., Daly, B., Kelly, C., Proctor, G., & Carpenter, G. H. (2019a). Altered salivary flow, protein composition, and rheology following taste and trp stimulation in older adults. *Frontiers in Physiology*, *10*, 652.

Pushpass, R. -A. G., Pellicciotta, N., Kelly, C., Proctor, G., & Carpenter, G. H. (2019b). Reduced salivary mucin binding and glycosylation in older adults influences taste in an in vitro cell model. *Nutrients*, *11*(10). https://doi.org/10.3390/nu11102280.

Ralli, M., Greco, A., De Vincentiis, M., Sheppard, A., Cappelli, G., Neri, I., & Salvi, R. (2019). Tone-in-noise detection deficits in elderly patients with clinically normal hearing. *American Journal of Otolaryngology*, *40*(1), 1–9.

Reference Values for Arterial Stiffness' Collaboration, (2010). Determinants of pulse wave velocity in healthy people and in the presence of cardiovascular risk factors: "Establishing normal and reference values. *European Heart Journal*, *31*(19), 2338–2350.

Rittié, L., & Fisher, G. J. (2015). Natural and sun-induced aging of human skin. *Cold Spring Harbor Perspectives in Medicine*, *5*(1), a015370.

Rönnlund, M., Nyberg, L., Bäckman, L., & Nilsson, L. -G. (2005). Stability, Growth, and Decline in Adult Life Span Development of Declarative Memory: Cross-Sectional and Longitudinal Data From a Population-Based Study. *Psychology and Aging, 20*(1), 3–18. https://doi.org/10.1037/0882-7974.20.1.3.

Roseman, D. A., Hwang, S. -J., Oyama-Manabe, N., Chuang, M. L., O'Donnell, C. J., Manning, W. J., & Fox, C. S. (2017). Clinical associations of total kidney volume: The Framingham Heart Study. *Nephrology, Dialysis, Transplantation, 32*(8), 1344–1350.

Rosenfeld, C. S., Shay, D. A., & Vieira-Potter, V. J. (2018). Cognitive effects of aromatase and possible role in memory disorders. *Frontiers in Endocrinology, 9*, 610.

Rosko, A. E., Olin, R. L., Artz, A., Wildes, T. M., Stauder, R., & Klepin, H. D. (2018). A call to action in hematologic disorders: A report from the ASH scientific workshop on hematology and aging. *Journal of Geriatric Oncology, 9*(4), 287–290.

Rule, A. D., Sasiwimonphan, K., Lieske, J. C., Keddis, M. T., Torres, V. E., & Vrtiska, T. J. (2012). Characteristics of renal cystic and solid lesions based on contrast-enhanced computed tomography of potential kidney donors. *American Journal of Kidney Diseases, 59*(5), 611–618.

Salive, M. E., Cornoni-Huntley, J., Guralnik, J. M., Phillips, C. L., Wallace, R. B., Ostfeld, A. M., & Cohen, H. J. (1992). Anemia and hemoglobin levels in older persons: Relationship with age, gender, and health status. *Journal of the American Geriatrics Society, 40*(5), 489–496.

Salthouse, T. (2012). Consequences of age-related cognitive declines. *Annual Review of Psychology, 63*, 201–226.

Schenk, K. E., & Heinze, G. (1975). Age-dependent changes of heart valves and heart size. *Recent Advances in Studies on Cardiac Structure and Metabolism, 10*, 617–624.

Seraji-Bzorgzad, N., Paulson, H., & Heidebrink, J. (2019). Neurologic examination in the elderly. *Handbook of Clinical Neurology, 167*, 73.

Sharma, G., & Goodwin, J. (2006). Effect of aging on respiratory system physiology and immunology. *Clinical Interventions in Aging, 1*(3), 253–260.

Shaw, D. W., Cook, I. J., Gabb, M., Holloway, R. H., Simula, M. E., Panagopoulos, V., & Dent, J. (1995). Influence of normal aging on oral-pharyngeal and upper esophageal sphincter function during swallowing. *American Journal of Physiology, 268*(3 Pt 1), G389–G396.

Stauder, R., Valent, P., & Theurl, I. (2018). Anemia at older age: Etiologies, clinical implications, and management. *Blood, 131*(5), 505–514.

Stocco, C. (2012). Tissue physiology and pathology of aromatase. *Steroids, 77*(1–2), 27–35.

Sturdee, D. W., Panay, N., & International Menopause Society Writing Group, (2010). Recommendations for the management of postmenopausal vaginal atrophy. *Climacteric: The Journal of the International Menopause Society, 13*(6), 509–522.

Sun, X., Chen, Y., Tong, X., Feng, Z., Wei, L., Zhou, D., Tian, M., Lv, B., & Feng, D. (2014). The use of annual physical examinations among the elderly in rural China: A cross-sectional study. *BMC Health Services Research, 14*, 16.

Terry, R. D., & Katzman, R. (2001). Life span and synapses: Will there be a primary senile dementia? *Neurobiology of Aging, 22*(3), 347–348. discussion 353–354.

Thomson, A. B., & Keelan, M. (1986). The aging gut. *Canadian Journal of Physiology and Pharmacology, 64*(1), 30–38.

Tiganescu, A., Walker, E. A., Hardy, R. S., Mayes, A. E., & Stewart, P. M. (2011). Localization, age- and site-dependent expression, and regulation of 11β-hydroxysteroid dehydrogenase type 1 in skin. *Journal of Investigative Dermatology, 131*(1), 30–36.

Tu, N. C., & Friedman, R. A. (2018). Age-related hearing loss: Unraveling the pieces. *Laryngoscope Investigative Otolaryngology, 3*(2), 68–72.

Tucker, W. D., Arora, Y., & Mahajan, K. (2020). *Anatomy, blood vessels*. StatPearls Publishing.

Vancheri, F., & Henein, M. (2018). The impact of age on cardiac electromechanical function in asymptomatic individuals. *Echocardiography, 35*(11), 1788–1794.

van den Beld, A. W., Kaufman, J. -M., Zillikens, M. C., Lamberts, S. W. J., Egan, J. M., & van der Lely, A. J. (2018). The physiology of endocrine systems with ageing. *The Lancet. Diabetes & Endocrinology, 6*(8), 647–658.

van der Heijden-Spek, J. J., Staessen, J. A., Fagard, R. H., Hoeks, A. P., Boudier, H. A., & van Bortel, L. M. (2000). Effect of age on brachial artery wall properties differs from the aorta and is gender dependent: A population study. *Hypertension, 35*(2), 637–642.

van Langevelde, K., Srámek, A., & Rosendaal, F. R. (2010). The effect of aging on venous valves. *Arteriosclerosis, Thrombosis, and Vascular Biology, 30*(10), 2075–2080.

Wagner, A., Garner-Spitzer, E., Jasinska, J., Kollaritsch, H., Stiasny, K., Kundi, M., & Wiedermann, U. (2018). Age-related differences in humoral and cellular immune responses after primary immunisation: Indications for stratified vaccination schedules. *Scientific Reports, 8*(1), 9825.

Walker, S., Monto, S., Piirainen, J. M., Avela, J., Tarkka, I. M., Parviainen, T. M., & Piitulainen, H. (2020). Older age increases the amplitude of muscle stretch-induced cortical beta-band suppression but does not affect rebound strength. *Frontiers in Aging Neuroscience, 12*, 117.

Waller, B. F. (1988). The old-age heart: Normal aging changes which can produce or mimic cardiac disease. *Clinical Cardiology, 11*(8), 513–517.

Wang, X., Vrtiska, T. J., Avula, R. T., Walters, L. R., Chakkera, H. A., Kremers, W. K., Lerman, L. O., & Rule, A. D. (2014). Age, kidney function, and risk factors associate differently with cortical and medullary volumes of the kidney. *Kidney International, 85*(3), 677–685.

Wang, Y., Wehling-Henricks, M., Samengo, G., & Tidball, J. G. (2015). Increases of M2a macrophages and fibrosis in aging muscle are influenced by bone marrow aging and negatively regulated by muscle-derived nitric oxide. *Aging Cell, 14*(4), 678–688.

Wein, M. N., & Kronenberg, H. M. (2018). Regulation of bone remodeling by parathyroid hormone. *Cold Spring Harbor Perspectives in Medicine, 8*(8). https://doi.org/10.1101/cshperspect.a031237.

Winter, J. E., MacInnis, R. J., Wattanapenpaiboon, N., & Nowson, C. A. (2014). BMI and all-cause mortality in older adults: A meta-analysis. *American Journal of Clinical Nutrition, 99*(4), 875–890.

Wright, K. P., & Frey, D. J. (2008). *Geriatric sleep medicine* (1st edition). CRC Press.

Xu, X., Wang, B., Ren, C., Hu, J., Greenberg, D. A., Chen, T., Xie, L., & Jin, K. (2017). Age-related impairment of vascular structure and functions. *Aging and Disease, 8*(5), 590–610.

Zaslavsky, O., Rillamas-Sun, E., LaCroix, A. Z., Woods, N. F., Tinker, L. F., Zisberg, A., Shadmi, E., Cochrane, B., Edward, B. J., Kritchevsky, S., Stefanick, M. L., Vitolins, M. Z., Wactawski-Wende, J., & Zelber-Sagi, S. (2016). Association between anthropometric measures and long-term survival in frail older women: Observations from the women's health initiative study. *Journal of the American Geriatrics Society, 64*(2), 277–284.

Zouboulis, C. C., Chen, W. -C., Thornton, M. J., Qin, K., & Rosenfield, R. (2007). Sexual hormones in human skin. *Hormone and Metabolic Research—Hormon-Und Stoffwechselforschung—Hormones et Metabolisme, 39*(2), 85–95.

3

Principles of Care

ABIOLA KELLER, PA-C AND SARAH ENDICOTT, DNP, RN GNP-BC

OBJECTIVES

Student Learning Objectives

After completing this chapter, the student should be able to do the following:

1. Explain unique attributes of older adult patients.
2. List and describe principles of care for older adults.
3. Explain why an interprofessional, team-based approach to older adults is essential in optimizing health outcomes.
4. Describe how social determinants of health affect health outcomes for older adults.

Practitioner Objectives

After completing this chapter, the practitioner should be able to do the following:

1. Differentiate the roles and responsibilities of professionals from health and other fields in assessing and addressing the health care needs of older adults.
2. Describe the cultural considerations for caring for an older adult.
3. Explain the health outcomes and health disparities using a social determinants approach.
4. Compare and contrast the different settings where older adults receive care.

Introduction

The older adult population of the United States is in a rapid expansion due to the aging of baby boomers, which started turning 65 in 2011 (Roberts et al., 2018). The US Census Bureau predicts that by 2034, older adults will outnumber children, when those over the age of 65 reach 77 million (Vespa, 2019). In 2030, when all baby boomers reach the age of 65, older adults will represent 21% of the population, compared to 15% of the population today (Vespa, 2019). Although many older adults have few interactions with the health care system, they already account for a substantial proportion of inpatient stays, outpatient and home care visits, and nursing home residents. Despite the size of the older adult population and high health care usage by this population subgroup, the health care system is poorly equipped to meet the diverse health care needs of such a heterogenous group. It is important for any health care provider to understand the unique needs of older adults and work to meet them within the current limitations of the system.

Due to advances in sanitation, social services, and medicine, global life expectancy for humans has increased since the 1800s (Aunan et al., 2016). Life span is longer, but for many people, the period of life spent in good health is not (World Health Organization, 2015). The challenge for health care providers working with older adults is to provide high-quality care based on individual needs and preferences, and to do so in systems not designed for this task. The two overarching goals of health care for older adults are to maximize the ability to function as independently as possible and to enhance quality of life. Providers should consider whether any given intervention will work toward or against these goals (Ferrucci et al., 2018).

In this chapter, we aim to lay the foundation of knowledge you will need to care for older adults. Although older adults are a heterogenous group, they share risk factors for diseases and health care conditions largely influenced by the physiology of aging as well as social determinants of health. When older adults face health challenges, their conditions are considered complicated or complex, often requiring models of care that extend beyond a single discipline or setting of care. While the health care system evolves to meet the needs of this group, individual providers can rely on basic tenants of geriatric care to provide high-quality care in any setting.

Chronologic Age Is Only a Guideline

Aging, Health, and Life Span Are Not Genetically Predetermined but Can Be Modulated

Aging is a highly individual process that can be measured in both subjective and objective ways. An individual's chronologic age gives us one objective measure of aging, but it is not always clinically useful. Those who have experience in health care can easily recall situations in which, for example, an 85-year-old patient who recovers easily from the same illness that leads to complications for a 60-year-old with functional impairments, multiple chronic conditions, and poor social support. The definition of successful aging is a more subjective measure than chronologic age. There are multiple theories of successful aging (see Chapter 1), but

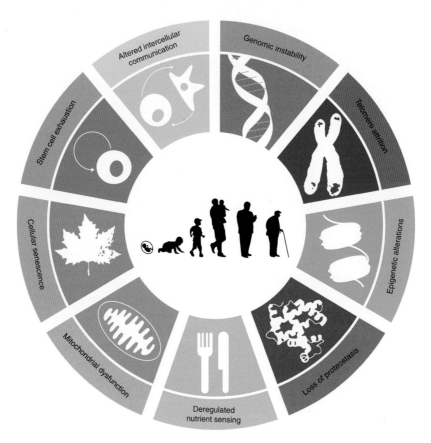

• **Fig. 3.1** Hallmarks of Aging. (From Aunan, J. R., Watson, M. M., Hagland, H. R., & Soriede, K. [2016]. Molecular and biological hallmarks of ageing. *British Journal of Surgery*, *103*[2], e29–46. https://doi.org/10.1002/bjs.10053.)

common components include longevity, absence of disease and disability, high physical and cognitive function, social engagement, productive involvement in society, life satisfaction, and well-being (Finkenzeller et al., 2019). As technology and medical advances enhance our ability to increase years of life lived, it is important to consider quality of life and how our interventions enhance successful aging.

As a biologic process, aging is a time-dependent progressive loss of physiologic functioning that leads to functional disability, increased risk of disease, and eventual death (Lopez-Otin et al., 2013; World Health Organization, 2018). Aging is caused by damage to molecules, cells, and organs over time. This damage is the result of multiple factors that scientists are still striving to understand. Lopez-Ortin and colleagues identified hallmarks of aging at a molecular level (Fig. 3.1) including genomic instability, telomere attrition, epigenetic alterations, loss of proteostasis, deregulated nutrient sensing, mitochondrial dysfunction, cellular senescence, stem cell exhaustion, and altered intercellular communication (Lopez-Otin et al., 2013). The interaction and interconnectedness of these hallmarks are not fully understood, but researchers are showing that counteracting them extends life span (Berger et al., 2018).

Aging Occurs at Different Rates

Differences Among Individuals

How quickly a person ages is dependent on several factors, many within an individual's control. Genetic factors certainly play a role in aging. In studies of super-seniors, the oldest-old who live without chronic disease or major functional decline, scientists have found strong genetic similarities (Sebastiani et al., 2017; Tindale et al., 2019). We also know there is a genetic component to many diseases that shorten life expectancy, such as bipolar disorder, cardiovascular disease, breast cancer, and diabetes. Chronic disease, lifestyle, and environmental factors have a significant impact on biologic changes related to age (Zhang et al., 2017). Telomere length, a widely accepted biomarker for aging, is shortened due to alcohol use, obesity, stressful life events, and exposure to ultraviolet radiation. Conversely, optimal body weight, physical activity, vitamins and dietary additives, the Mediterranean diet, and statin treatment have all been shown to lengthen telomeres (Fyhrquist, 2016). Longitudinal studies show that not smoking and maintaining a healthy weight at midlife increase survival (Franzon et al., 2015; Muezzinler et al., 2014). Although exact mechanisms are still being explored, it is clear that genetics and lifestyle factors contribute to aging. The important message for providers and patients is that preventive care matters.

Differences Within a Person

Organs and tissues within an individual show signs of biologic aging at different rates (Zhang et al., 2017). This is true even within an organ system or from tissue to tissue in the same location (Zhang et al., 2017). Scientists have discovered that there are many cells within the body as old as the organism itself. For example, most neurons do not divide during adulthood, but similarly, some cells within the pancreas, heart, and liver are nondividing and show extreme longevity (Arrojo et al., 2019). Certain tissues that do divide show signs of being biologically older than other tissues. In one study, researchers found that breast tissue in a group of women with an average age of 46 was 3 years older than actual age (Horvath, 2013). Conversely, heart tissue was found to be 9 years younger than groups with average ages of 55 and 60 (Horvath, 2013). Cancerous tissue was found to be significantly older than healthy tissue, as much as 36 years older. Tissues may age or become pathologic due to repeated hormone exposure, whereas heart tissue is constantly regenerated by stem cells (Horvath, 2013).

Older Adults Are a Heterogenous Population

There is no typical older adult. Of all age demographics, older adults may be the most heterogenous. Health care providers can agree on the health priorities of a typical 6-year-old girl, but this same exercise is impossible when imagining a typical 75-year-old woman. Many older adults enjoy good health, live independently, and have few unplanned interactions with the health care system. Although a much smaller proportion of older adults have frequent interactions with the health care system, the needs of this group are highly individual and dependent on the specific health conditions, cognition, social support, financial resources, and an individual's goals and values.

Advanced Age Is the Single Biggest Risk Factor for a Variety of Conditions

More than 90 diseases can be classified as age related (Chang et al., 2019). Cardiovascular disease, cancer, Alzheimer disease, and diabetes are among the leading causes of death and disability in the United States (Centers for Disease Control and Prevention, 2017). Age is the most significant risk factor for these conditions. Physiologic reserve is the ability of an organ or system to withstand recurring stress and return to normal homeostatic baseline within a short period of time (Atamna et al., 2018). Although physiologic reserve declines starting around age 25, the decline accelerates after age 50 (Atamna et al., 2018; Clegg et al., 2013). Reduced reserve plays a major role in the increased risk for disease, infection, and functional decline in old age.

Cardiovascular disease remains the leading cause of death in the United States (Heron, 2019). Over 90% of cardiovascular disease occurs in middle-aged or older adults (Santos-Parker, et al., 2014). Among older adults, cardiovascular disease accounts for 40% of all deaths (North & Sinclair, 2012). Pathologic changes to the cardiovascular system associated with age include hypertrophy, altered left ventricular diastolic function, and impaired endothelial function (North & Sinclair, 2012). Importantly, with age, large arteries such as the aorta and carotid arteries stiffen, leading to increased systolic blood pressure and increased pulse pressure (Santos-Parker et al., 2014). The increased pulse pressure leads to microvascular tissue damage in the heart, brain, and kidneys. Maximum heart rate and heart rate variability change due to the loss of cells in the sinoatrial node and structural changes secondary to hypertrophy and fibrosis. The net result of these changes leads to an increased incidence of atherosclerosis, hypertension, myocardial infarction, and stroke (North & Sinclair, 2012).

The risk of common cancers increases exponentially with age, consequently over half of all cancers are diagnosed in those over the age of 65 (Zhang et al., 2017). This is thought to be due to the accumulation of cell mutation, chronic low-level inflammation, or immune system dysregulation associated with aging (Zhang et al., 2017). Once older adults initiate treatment for cancer, their age and general health greatly affect prognosis (Atamna et al., 2018). Older adults are particularly susceptible to treatment toxicities, but the likelihood of incidence is dependent on pretreatment health. Measures of physiologic age, such as comorbid conditions and functional status, are more important than chronologic age alone in determining treatment strategies (Bond, 2010).

Alzheimer disease and related dementias (ADRD) constitute the sixth leading cause of the death in the United States. Whereas deaths from the other leading causes have decreased since the early 2000s, deaths from ADRD have increased by 145% (Alzheimer's Association, 2019). Age remains the greatest risk factor for ADRD. Most people with ADRD are over age 65, and the prevalence increases with age. Just 3% of people ages 65 to 74 have Alzheimer disease, whereas one in three people over the age of 85 have the condition (Alzheimer's Association, 2019). Alzheimer disease (AD) is recognized as the most common form of dementia, but we know that pure AD is rare, and most people with any form of dementia have multiple comorbidities that worsen outcomes (Power et al., 2018). Multiple age-related neuropathologies are linked to ADRD, but how they interrelate or account for risk is still unknown (Power et al., 2018).

Older adults have the highest prevalence of diabetes among any age group, with over 25% of those over age 65 living with the disease (Centers for Disease Control and Prevention, 2020). The aging of the American population, coupled with the rise in obesity, has largely driven the diabetes epidemic (Centers for Disease Control and Prevention, 2020). Older adults with diabetes have reduced functional status, higher risk of mortality, increased risk of nursing home placement, and are at higher risk of acute and chronic diabetes complications (Kirkman et al., 2012). The higher prevalence in type 2 diabetes among older adults is attributed to insulin resistance and declines in pancreatic islet function. Insulin resistance in older adults is caused by age-related pathologic changes such as adiposity and decreased muscle mass, but also lifestyle factors like decreased physical activity. Declines in pancreatic islet cell function and islet proliferation capacity are age related (Kirkman et al., 2012). The American Diabetes Association's guidelines recommend that providers individualize treatment for older adults based on risk factors, comorbid conditions, cognitive abilities, and functional capacity (Kirkman et al., 2012).

Implications for Practice

A common saying is that age is just a number. In other words, age is a marker of chronology alone and does not signify maturity, health, physical ability, societal role, or quality of life (World Health Organization, 2002). Chronologic age is a factor in important clinical decisions, such as when to screen for certain health conditions, provide vaccinations, or prescribe a medication. Clinical guidelines often use the age of 65 to classify older adults and base treatment recommendations on that age (American Diabetes Association, 2020; US Preventive Services Task Force, 2012). When applying these guidelines, clinicians need to account for variation in the individual. For example, the US Preventive Services Task Force recommends screening for colon cancer in adults from age 50 to 75 years (US Preventive Serivces Task Force, 2013). This recommendation is based on existing evidence and the relatively low risk of complications compared to life-years gained. The decision whether and how often to screen is not just based on family history and prior results, but also on the overall relative health of the individual and whether the older adult would benefit from the test. The decision whether to screen might differ when considering a 65-year-old with multiple serious health problems, poor functional status, and a limited life expectancy versus a 65-year-old who is still working, living independently, and managing a single chronic health issue with ease.

Multimorbidity

What Is Multimorbidity?

Chronic conditions are the leading causes of disability and death in the United States (Centers for Disease Prevention and Control, 2019a). A chronic condition is a physical or mental health condition that lasts 1 year or more and causes functional restrictions or requires ongoing monitoring or treatment (Centers for Disease Prevention and Control, 2019a). Multimorbidity, also known as multiple chronic conditions (MCC), refers to situations in which an individual suffers from two or more chronic conditions, which has a high prevalence in the older population (Buttorff et al., 2017; Johnston et al., 2019) (Fig. 3.2). As part of its chronic care payment system introduced in 2015, the Centers for Medicare and Medicaid Services has defined individuals with multimorbidity/MCC as those with two or more chronic conditions who are at significant risk of death, acute exacerbation or decompensation, or functional decline (Edwards & Landon, 2014). The most common chronic condition dyads in MCC are hypertension in combination with arthritis, diabetes, cancer, or coronary heart disease, and arthritis with diabetes or cancer. The most frequently occurring triads are hypertension and arthritis in combination with diabetes, cancer, or cardiovascular disease (Edwards & Landon, 2014). Although the most frequently occurring disease dyads and triads are made up of physical health conditions, mental health conditions, such as depression and anxiety, are often part of multimorbidity disease patterns (Prados-Torreset et al., 2014).

Multimorbidity is associated with many adverse outcomes, including death (Tisminetzky, et al., 2016), disability (Buttorff et al., 2017), and poorer quality of life (Buck et al., 2015). Multimorbidity also increases the risk for adverse drug events and medical complications (Panagioti et al., 2015). The economic burden of multimorbidity is high. Adults with multimorbidity utilize more health services and spend more on health care. However, they are also more likely to delay

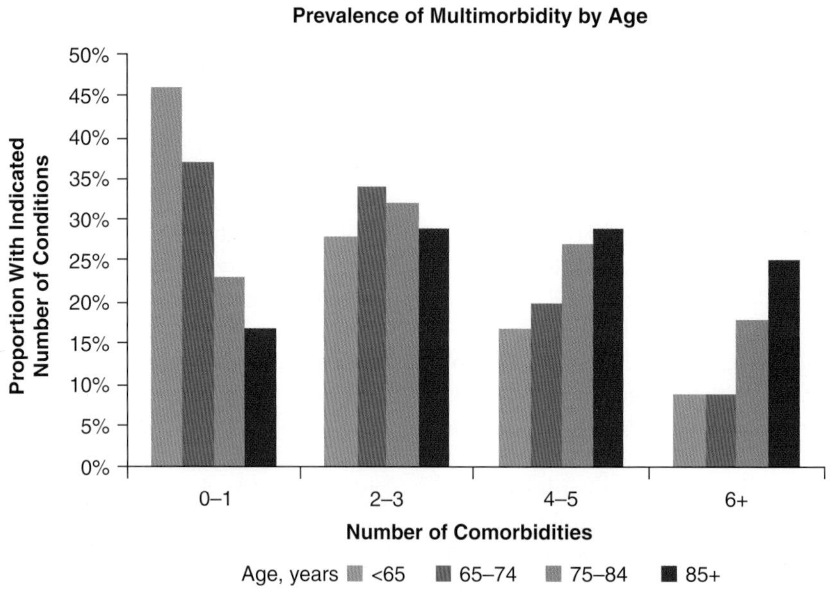

• **Fig. 3.2** Prevalence of Multimorbidity by Age. (From Forman, D. E., Maurer, M. S., Boyd, C., Brindis, R., Salive, M. E., Horne, F. M., Bell, S. P., Fulmer, T., Reuben, D. B., Zieman, S., & Rich, M. W. [2018]. Multimorbidity in older adults with cardiovascular disease. *Journal of the American College of Cardiology, 17* [19], 2149–2161. https://doi.org/10.1016/j.jacc.2018.03.022)

or forego health care because of cost- and non-cost-related reasons (Bucknall et al., 2020).

Demographic Trends of Multimorbidity

By Age

The prevalence of multimorbidity is higher among older adults. Although the prevalence of multimorbidity among all US adults is around 42%, it is estimated to be 81% for adults 65 years and older (Fig. 3.3) (Buttorff et al., 2017).

By Gender

Among older adults, the incidence and prevalence of multimorbidity are similar between men and women (Buttorff et al., 2017; St Sauver et al., 2015); however, the prevalence of five or more conditions is higher among men (Rocca et al., 2014).

By Race and Ethnicity

The burden of multiple chronic conditions is not equally shared among racial and ethnic groups. The overall risk of multimorbidity is higher among African Americans compared to Whites and lower in Asian Americans compared to Whites (St Sauver et al., 2015). Among older adults, the greatest racial and ethnic differences are seen in diabetes and cancer. The prevalence of diabetes alone or diabetes in combination with cardiovascular disease in non-Hispanic Blacks and Hispanics is two times that of non-Hispanic Whites. Additionally, the occurrence of diabetes with cancer is more common among non-Hispanic Black older adults than their Hispanic or non-Hispanic White counterparts (Davis et al., 2017).

Care of Older Adults With Multimorbidity

The heterogeneity and complexity of multimorbidity make it particularly challenging for clinicians to optimally manage care for many older adults. Although evidence-based clinical practice guidelines exist for many chronic conditions, their emphasis on the management of a single disease limits their applicability to individuals with multimorbidity. In recognition of the need for an approach to care that

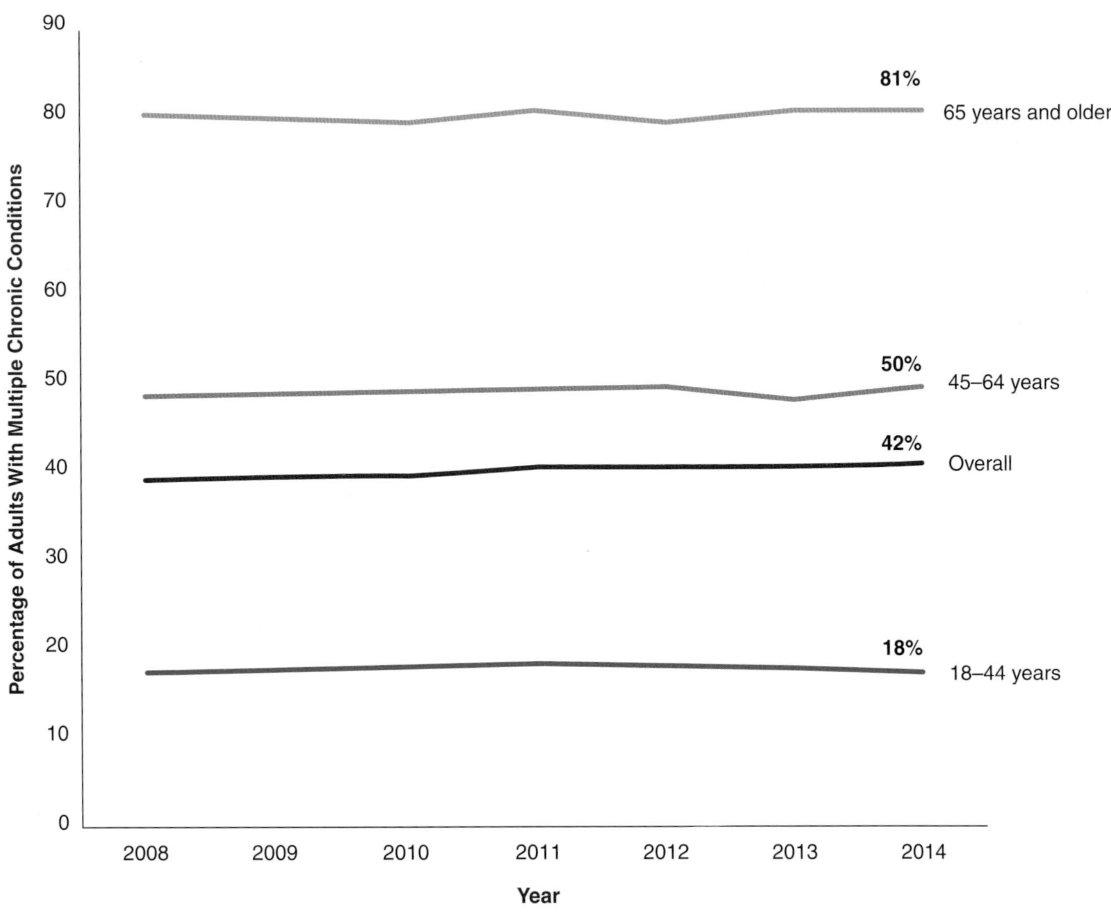

• **Fig. 3.3** Prevalence of Multiple Chronic Conditions, by Age (2008–2014). (From Buttorff, C., Ruder, T., & Bauman, M. [2017]. *Multiple chronic conditions in the United States, RAND Corporation*, TL-221-PFCD. www.rand.org/t/TL221.)

TABLE 3.1 Guiding Principles for the Care of Older Adults With Multimorbidity

Domain I	Incorporate Patient Preferences—Elicit and incorporate patient preferences into the clinical decision-making process.
Domain II	Interpret the Evidence—Interpret and apply the medical literature specific to older adults with multimorbidity.
Domain III	Incorporate Prognosis—Consider clinical decisions in the context of burdens, risks, benefits, and prognosis.
Domain IV	Consider Clinical Feasibility—Acknowledge and address the complexities and burden of treatment options.
Domain V	Prioritize Treatments and Interventions—Choose treatments and interventions that optimize quality of life and maximize benefit while minimizing harm.

Adapted from Guiding principles for the care of older adults with multimorbidity: An approach for clinicians. (2012). American Geriatrics Society Expert Panel on the Care of Older Adults with Multimorbidity. *Journal of the American Geriatrics Society*, *60*(10), E1–E25. https://doi.org/10.1111/j.1532-5415.2012.04188.x.

accounts for the multiple health concerns particular to older adults with multimorbidity, the American Geriatric Society recommends five domains that should be considered in the clinical management of older adults with multiple chronic conditions: patient preferences, interpreting the evidence, prognosis, clinical feasibility, and optimizing therapies and care plans (American Geriatric Society, 2012). These five domains (Table 3.1) can be incorporated into a stepwise approach for evaluating and managing the older adult with multimorbidity (Fig. 3.4).

Incorporate Patient Preferences

Patient preferences should be elicited and incorporated into the clinical decision-making process. Making decisions about the care of older adults with multimorbidity often involves complex situations with numerous options. To determine the best treatment approach, clinicians must create opportunities for patients and their families and caregivers to express their opinions about the treatment options along with their values and priorities. However, before attempting to garner information about preferences and priorities, clinicians should make certain that individuals participating in the decision-making process are appropriately informed about the expected outcomes, including the anticipated benefits and potential harms (e.g., side effects), of all treatments and interventions.

Interpret the Evidence

Evidence-based practice (EBP) involves integrating the clinical setting, patient preferences, health care resources, and the best available research evidence to make a decision that is informed by clinical expertise (Ganann et al., 2018). Thoughtful EBP requires the availability of clinical evidence from research that is valid and relevant. With regard to study designs, randomized controlled trials have the greatest potential for producing high-quality evidence. Yet these studies are less likely to include older adults with multimorbidity in the study sample. Therefore the evidence from high-quality studies may not be directly relevant or applicable to older adults with multimorbidity. When assessing health-related research studies, clinicians must examine the extent to which older adults with multimorbidity were included as there may be a need to balance study quality with applicability.

Incorporate Prognosis

Clinical decisions for older adults with multimorbidity should be considered within the context of burdens, risks, and benefits. Although efforts to understand and communicate information about prognosis and prognostic factors often focus on mortality and life expectancy (Yourman et al., 2012), more proximal outcomes such as pain, fatigue, sleep, physical function, anxiety, and depression should also be considered (Working Group on Health Outcomes for Older Persons with Multiple Chronic, 2012). As described by the American Geriatric Society, clinical decisions can be prioritized based on life expectancy and proximal outcomes of relevance to the patient and categorized as short-term (within the next year), midterm (within the next 5 years), and long-term (beyond 5 years) (American Geriatric Society, 2012). Conversations with patients with limited life expectancy and their families should be guided to focus on relevant short-term decisions, which might include decisions around intensifying or discontinuing medications or transitions in living arrangements. Midterm or long-term decisions such as cancer screening would have lower priority.

Although clinicians recognize the importance of incorporating prognosis into clinical decisions, they often face challenges to doing so (Finkenzeller et al., 2019). Notably, there are limited tools for estimating prognosis in older adults with multimorbidity (Yourman et al., 2012), and there continues to be uncertainty about the use of these measures in clinical practice. Nonetheless, patients and their caregivers value having conversations about prognosis and life expectancy with their health care providers (Cagle et al., 2016).

Consider Clinical Feasibility, and Prioritize Treatments and Interventions

An essential component of caring for older adults with multimorbidity is recognizing and addressing the complexities and burden of managing multiple chronic conditions. Clinicians need to ensure that both the tasks required and the frequency at which they must occur are in alignment with the ability of the patient, the patient's family, and caregivers. Efforts to minimize treatment burden should begin with attempting to identify medications that may be inappropriate (American Geriatrics Society, 2012). Tools

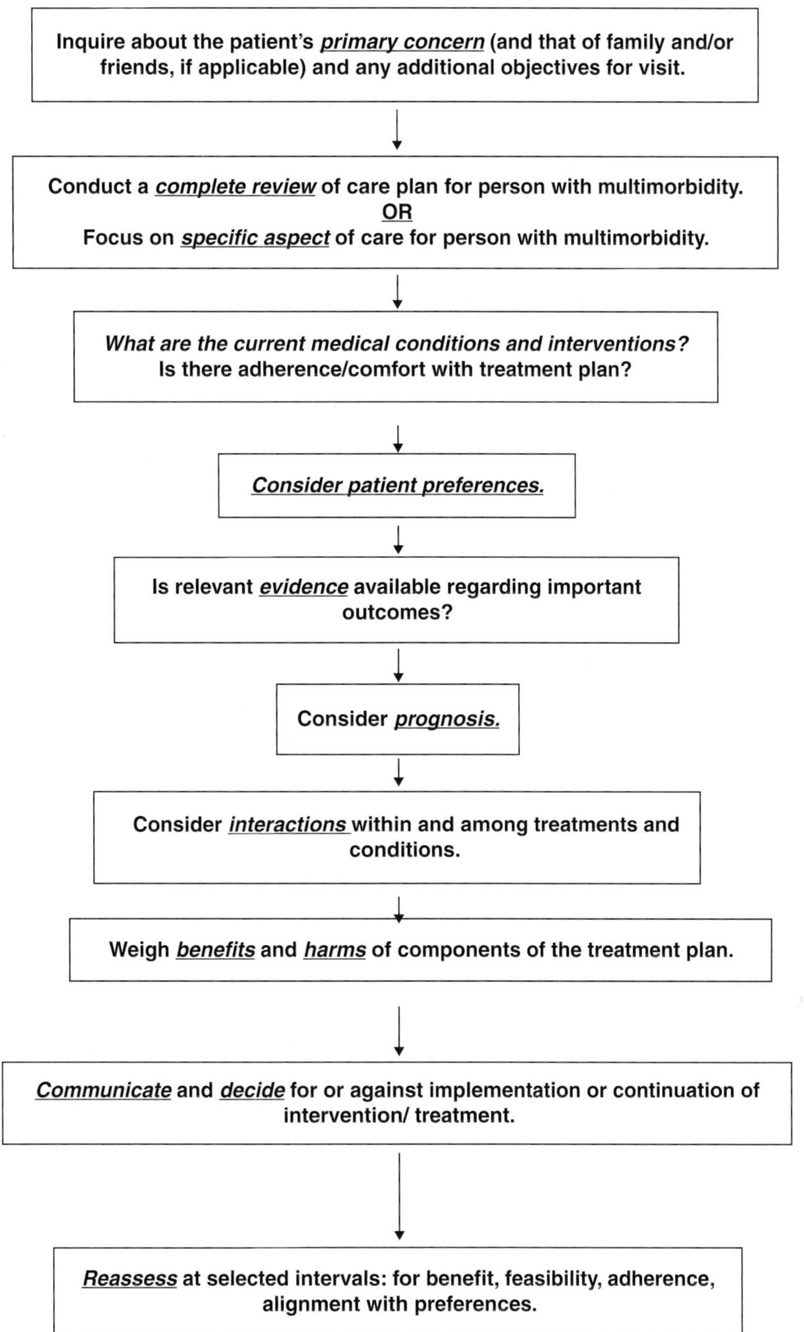

• **Fig. 3.4** Approach to the Evaluation and Management of the Older Adult With Multimorbidity. (From American Geriatrics Society Expert Panel on the Care of Older Adults With Multimorbidity, Fig. 1. Guiding principles for the care of older adults with multimorbidity: An approach for clinicians. [2012]. American Geriatrics Society Expert Panel on the Care of Older Adults with Multimorbidity. *Journal of the American Geriatrics Society*, *60*[10], E1–E25. https://doi.org/10.1111/j.1532-5415.2012.04188.x)

such as the Beers Criteria (American Geriatrics Society, 2019), the Screening Tool of Older People's Prescriptions (STOPP), and Screening Tool to Alert to Right Treatment (START) criteria, version 2 (O'Mahony et al., 2015) can be used to identify potentially inappropriate medications and guide the process of choosing treatments and interventions that optimize quality of life and maximize benefit while minimizing harm.

Cultural Issues

Racial and Ethnic Diversity of Older Adults in the United States

In 2016, over three-fourths of adults ages 65 and older in the United States were White, approximately 9% were African American, and 8% were Hispanic. Less than 5% were Asian

Population by Race and Hispanic Origin: 2012 and 2060
(Percent of total population)

	2012	2060
White alone	78	69
Black alone	13	15
AIAN alone	1.2	1.5
Asian alone	5.1	8.2
NHPI alone	0.2	0.3
Two or More races	2.4	6.4
More races Hispanic White alone	63	43
Hispanic (of any race)	17	31

AIAN = American Indian and Alaska Native; NHPI = Native Hawaiian and Other Pacific Islander

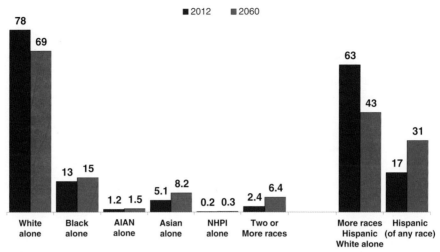

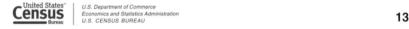

• **Fig. 3.5** Population by Race and Hispanic Origin: 2012 and 2060. (From U.S. Census Bureau. *Population by race and Hispanic origin: 2012 and 2060*. https://www.census.gov/newsroom/cspan/pop_proj/20121214_cspan_popproj_13.pdf.)

and less than 1% identified as American Indian and Alaska Native or Native Hawaiian and Other Pacific Islander (Hogan et al., 2017). By 2060, it is projected that the percentage of older African Americans, Hispanics (any race), and Asians will increase to 15%, 31%, and 8.2%, respectively. American Indian and Alaska Natives are also expected to increase to 1.5%, whereas Native Hawaiian and Other Pacific Islanders will remain under 1% (Fig. 3.5) (Arbesman et al., 2014). As the racial and ethnic diversity of the older adult population in the United States increases, in order to achieve the Healthy People 2030 overarching goal of building a healthier future for all (Office of Disease Prevention and Health Promotion, 2020a), health care providers must remain committed to providing culturally appropriate and accessible care.

Ethnogeriatrics

Ethnogeriatrics, defined as the influence of culture, race, and ethnicity on health care for older adults from diverse ethnoracial populations, was developed in response to the need for clinicians and educators to have a distinct term to describe the unique issues encountered when caring for the increased number of older adults from diverse backgrounds (Skinner et al., 2017)—namely, that some minority groups experience a disproportionate burden of diseases, morbidity, and premature mortality. Health disparities are "preventable differences in the burden of disease, injury, violence, or in opportunities to achieve optimal health experienced by socially disadvantaged racial, ethnic, and other population groups, and communities" (Centers for Disease Control & Prevention, 2019b). Racial and ethnic disparities exist across the life course but compound with age. Hispanic and African American older adults have a higher incidence and prevalence of diabetes than Whites (Centers for Disease Control & Prevention, 2017). Additionally, although the death rate for heart disease is decreasing for all racial and ethnic groups, African American adults continue to be more likely to die of heart disease than their White non-Hispanic counterparts (Centers for Disease Control & Prevention, 2019c).

Although the term *health disparity* often refers to racial and ethnic minorities, any population that has experienced systematic social, economic, or environmental disadvantage or have other characteristics historically linked to discrimination or exclusion can experience health disparities. Therefore approaches to improving the health and well-being of older adults must utilize an intersectional lens (Calasanti & Giles, n.d.) whereby individuals' experiences, resources, and outcomes are examined in the context of the intersecting identities of their lives such as age, race and ethnicity, gender, socioeconomic status, sexual orientation, and disability (Bowleg, 2008; Crenshaw, 1991).

Health Literacy

To improve health and achieve equity, older adults must be able to understand and use the health information they see, hear, and read from numerous sources. Health literacy—defined as the degree to which individuals have the capacity to obtain, process, and understand basic health information and services needed to make appropriate health decisions

(Institute of Medicine [US] Committee on Health Literacy, 2004)—is an important determinant of health. Yet 36% of adults in the United States have difficulty using everyday health information (Kutner, 2006). Adults ages 65 years and older, racial and ethnic minorities, and individuals with less than a high school education or with limited English proficiency are more likely to have limited health literacy (Kutner, 2006). The health literacy level of older adults can be negatively impacted by cognitive, vision, and hearing challenges and limited health literacy has been associated with poorer health outcomes, including higher health care utilization and expenditures, receipt of preventive services (MacLeod et al., 2017), hospital readmission (Jaffee et al., 2016), and mortality (Baker et al., 2008).

Health literacy comprises numerous skills including numeracy, oral literacy, and print literacy (i.e., the ability to read, write, and understand written language), and it depends on cultural and conceptual knowledge (Institute of Medicine [US] Committee on Health Literacy, 2004); yet efforts focus primarily on assessing print literacy. Among older adults, the Short Test of Functional Health Literacy in Adults (S-TOFHLA) (Baker et al., 1999) and the Rapid Estimate of Adult Literacy in Medicine (Bass et al., 2003) are widely used health literacy assessment tools in research (Chesser et al., 2016). The amount of time required to administer these tools has limited their use in clinical practice. Research has shown that a single item literacy screener (SIL) can be easily incorporated into a clinical visit and can identify individuals at risk for limited health literacy (Morris et al., 2006). Despite the available assessment tools and screeners, identifying individuals with limited health literacy remains a challenging task. Moreover, older adults of all literacy levels are likely to benefit from strategies and interventions designed to make health-related information easier to read and comprehend, and there is the potential that health literacy screening and limited health literacy-specific interventions could potentially harm patients by perpetuating fear and feelings of stigma (Paasche-Orlow & Wolf, 2008). As such, the Agency for Healthcare Research and Quality (AHRQ) advocates for clinicians to treat all patients as though they were at risk for not understanding health information. To support this universal approach, AHRQ developed a Health Literacy Universal Precautions Toolkit (Dewalt et al., 2010) to assist primary care practices with assessing and implementing the necessary changes to improve communication with and support for patients. The toolkit includes evidence-based guidance and 21 tools for improving spoken communication, written communication, self-management and empowerment, and supportive systems.

The ability to understand and use health information is also influenced by language spoken. English is the language most frequently used within the health care system in the United States. Yet in 2011, nearly 15% of adults 60 years and older spoke a language other than English in their home. Over half of those who spoke another language in the home reported that they spoke English less than very well (Ryan, 2013). These individuals often have limited English proficiency (LEP) (i.e., limited ability to read, write, speak, or understand English), which places them at an increased risk for adverse health outcomes (Divi et al., 2007; Keller et al., 2014; Wilson et al., 2005). Professional medical interpreters are frequently used within the health care system to increase language access, and using them has been associated with positive benefits on clinical care and satisfaction with care (Karliner, 2007).

Implications for Practice

Cultural Competence

Although often viewed as an event, cultural competence refers to a process where health care providers are continuously working to enhance their ability to effectively provide care within the cultural context of their patients and their families (Campinha-Bacote, 2002). Within this lens, providers are becoming culturally competent as opposed to being culturally competent. As described in the model for the Process of Cultural Competence in the Delivery of Healthcare, the cultural competence process is composed of five constructs: (1) cultural awareness, (2) cultural knowledge, (3) cultural skill, (4) cultural encounters, and (5) cultural desire.

Cultural awareness involves "being aware of one's strengths, limitations, values, beliefs, behavior, and appearance to others" (Foronda et al., 2016, p. 2) and examination of one's own cultural and professional background. When working with individuals from diverse backgrounds, providers must be cognizant of their own beliefs, values, and biases. Without this awareness, there is a greater risk for engaging in the ethnocentric approach of treating others the way you would want to be treated as opposed to the way they would want to be treated (Bennett, 2013).

Cultural knowledge is the process of obtaining and integrating information about diverse cultural and ethnic groups. A key component of this process is obtaining understanding about patients' health-related beliefs or worldviews. Although one of three major health belief systems or worldviews (the magico-religious paradigm, the scientific paradigm, and the holistic health paradigm) (Andrews, 2003) typically dominates a cultural group, aspects of all three are often present. An individual's health belief system will guide how one thinks about his or her health and well-being, especially as it relates to the etiology of disease. It is imperative that providers possess the ability to gather complete and accurate information from patients of diverse backgrounds in a nonjudgmental way (cultural skill) so they are better able to incorporate the patients' health beliefs appropriately. Providers must also have the cultural knowledge and skill to address differences in disease incidence and prevalence among diverse groups as well as recognize how physical variations such as skin color might impact physical examination findings.

Growth in the process of cultural competency requires exposure to cultural encounters that provide opportunities for health care providers to interact with patients who have culturally diverse backgrounds. These cultural encounters are most beneficial for all participants when health care providers are motivated by a desire to engage in the process of cultural competence and approach each encounter with cultural humility (Foronda et al., 2016).

Language Access

Providing access to professional medical interpreters for older adults with LEP is a key component to addressing disparities in the quality-of-care system-wide interventions to promote culturally and linguistically appropriate services. Specifically, the National Standards for Culturally and Linguistically Appropriate Services in Health and Health Care (US Department of Health and Human Services Health Resources and Services Administration, 2018) advocates for providing patient education materials in the languages of the groups represented in the service areas, collecting and updating information about patient spoken and written language preferences, and providing ongoing education and training in culturally and linguistically appropriate service delivery for personnel (US Department of Health and Human Services Health Resources and Services Administration, 2018).

Addressing Limited Health Literacy

Using a health literacy universal precautions approach avoids opportunities for misunderstandings. Communication strategies within this approach include using plain language, drawing pictures, using models, and repeating and summarizing information. Additional strategies are often necessary to address the cognitive, vision, and hearing challenges unique to older adults (Table 3.2).

In addition to clear and concise communication, it is also essential to confirm that patients understand the information that has been provided. Patient comprehension can be evaluated using methods such as the teach-back method, which allows providers to check understanding by asking patients to share in their own words what they need to know or do about their health. Similarly, the show-me method can be used to ensure that patients can follow specific instructions (as noted in the AHRQ Health Literacy Universal Precautions Toolkit).

TABLE 3.2 Strategies for Developing Materials to the Match Health Literacy Skills of Older Adults

Challenge	Strategies
Cognitive	• Repeat essential information. • Focus on the important meaning of the information (3–5 key points). • Use plain language. • Use reminders to aid memory (i.e., brochures, pamphlets). • Include skill building with information activities to reinforce meaning.

Visual	• Make information easy to see and read:
	  • *Contrast:* Print text with the highest possible contrast. For example, black text on a white background.
	  • *Font size:* 16-to-18-point size font or larger is best for materials for older adults.
	  • *Spacing between lines of text:* People with low vision may have difficulty finding the beginning of the next line when reading, so it is preferable for space between lines of text to be at least 25% of the point size.
	  • *Paper finish:* Avoid a glossy finish because it can cause problems with glare.
	• Provide audio information when possible.
	• Limit the amount of text.

Hearing	• Always talk face to face. • Limit background noise. • Speak clearly with more volume. • Do not chew gum or eat while speaking.

Adapted from the Centers for Disease Control and Prevention. (n.d.) https://www.cdc.gov/healthliteracy/developmaterials/audiences/olderadults/understanding-challenges.html

Social Determinants of Health

Understanding the Social Determinants of Health

The social determinants of health represent the many factors outside of the health care system that affect an individual's health and the ability to engage in healthy behaviors. The World Health Organization (WHO) defines the social determinants of health as "the conditions [in the environment] in which people are born, grow, live, work and age" (World Health Organization, 2020). Similarly, Healthy People 2020 expands on this definition by stating that these conditions "affect a wide range of health, functioning, and quality-of-life outcomes and risks" (Office of Disease Prevention and Health Promotion, 2020a). The importance of addressing the social determinants of health as a mechanism for improving the health of all Americans is demonstrated by the inclusion of "Create social, physical, and economic environments that promote attaining full potential for health and well-being for all" as a Healthy People 2030 goal. As part of its approach to addressing the social determinant of health, Healthy People 2030 emphasizes five key areas or determinants, including (see Fig. 3.4) (1) economic stability, (2) education, (3) social and community context, (4) health care, and (5) neighborhood and built environment (Office of Disease Prevention and Health Promotion, 2020b) (See Healthy People 2030 Box).

Although each of the social determinants contributes greatly to the health and well-being across the life course, for older adults, economic stability, neighborhood and built environment, and social and community context are of particular importance (Fig. 3.6).

Economic Stability	Education	Social and Community Context	Health and Health Care	Neighborhood and Built Environment
• Employment • Food insecurity • Housing instability • Poverty • Debt	• Early childhood education and development • Higher education • High school graduation • Language and literacy • Vocational training	• Civic participation • Discrimination • Incarceration • Social cohesion • Support systems	• Access to health care • Access to primary care • Health literacy • Provider linguistic and cultural competency • Quality of care	• Access to healthy foods • Crime and violence • Environmental conditions • Quality of housing • Transportation

• **Fig. 3.6** Social Determinants of Health. (Data from US Census Bureau Public Information Office. [2016, May 19]. *U.S. Census Bureau projections show a slower growing, older, more diverse nation a half century from now - population - newsroom - U.S. Census Bureau. United States Census Bureau*. https://www.census.gov/newsroom/releases/archives/population/cb12-243.html)

Economic Stability

Economic stability refers to the connection between the financial resources available to individuals and their families and their health. Critical issues within this determinant for older adults include food insecurity and job loss.

Food Insecurity

The US Department of Agriculture (USDA) defines food insecurity as a social or economic condition, at the household-level, where there is limited or uncertain access to enough food (US Department of Agriculture, 2020). This is differentiated from hunger, which the USDA defines as a physiologic condition occurring at the individual-level that may result from food insecurity. Food insecurity is an important consideration when caring for older adults. Currently, nearly 6 million older adults experience food insecurity (Ziliak & Gundersen, 2019), and about 8 million will experience food insecurity by 2050 (Ortman & Velkoff, 2014). Older adults belonging to a racial or ethnic minority group and those with lower incomes are more likely to experience food insecurity (Ziliak & Gundersen, 2019). When experiencing food insecurity, older adults may face spending tradeoffs that can increase their risk for poor outcomes. They frequently must choose between paying for food and paying for other necessities such as housing, medical care, utilities, and transportation (Feeding America, 2014). Food insecurity also adversely affects the health of older adults. Specifically, older adults experiencing food insecurity are more likely to have chronic conditions such as diabetes, depression, hypertension, congestive heart failure, and asthma. They are also more likely to report being in fair or poor general health (Ziliak & Gundersen, 2017).

Although there are several federally funded programs available to assist with meeting the nutritional needs of older adults, many of these programs, such as the Supplemental Nutrition Assistance Program (SNAP), are underutilized (US Department of Agriculture, 2018). Health care providers can play a critical role in addressing food insecurity among older adults by identifying those at risk and connecting them to available federal and community resources. The AARP recommends systematic food security screening for all older adults (Pooler, 2016) with valid screening tools such as the two-item food insecurity screen (Hager et al., 2010). However, before initiating efforts to systematically identify older adults at risk for food insecurity, health care systems must ensure that they have developed the appropriate partnerships with senior services and antihunger organizations to allow for a robust and comprehensive referral and follow-up system.

Job Loss

Among older adults still participating in the paid workforce, the loss of a job can be particularly problematic, as older adults often encounter more challenges with securing new employment and replacing lost earnings and savings (Chan & Stevens, 1999). Although retirement can improve mental health outcomes for older adults (Van et al., 2013), involuntary job loss can increase the risk for poor mental health (Mandal & Roe, 2008) and mortality (Noelke & Beckfield, 2014).

Neighborhood and Built Environment

The determinant of neighborhood and built environment refers to the connections between the physical environment (natural and built) and health and well-being. For older adults, one of the most crucial aspects of their environment is the space in which they reside. As adults age, most prefer to stay in their own homes (Binette & Vasold,

2018), also known as "aging in place" (National Institute on Aging, 2017). Yet the majority of housing units occupied by older adults were built before the year 2000 and are likely ill-equipped to allow older adults to successfully age in place (Johnson & Appold, 2017). The ability for older adults to continue to live independently is often impeded by the increased need for support and assistance that results from the physical disabilities and cognitive impairments that occur with aging. Among older adults between 65 and 79 years of age, approximately 40% have at least one mobility disability (e.g., difficulty walking, climbing stairs, and getting in and out of bed), self-care disability (e.g., difficulty eating, toileting, bathing, or dressing), or household activity disability (e.g., difficulty preparing meals, doing housework, driving, and shopping). By the age of 80, the prevalence of a disability that affects an individual's independent living skills rises to nearly 71% (Joint Center for Housing Studies of Harvard University, 2016). Assistive devices such as canes, walkers, adapted utensils, grab bars, and researchers can help older adults overcome some limitations. Moreover, emerging technologies including wearable and home environment sensors may also increase safety and facilitate independence among older adults. Despite their potential benefits, older adults may be reluctant to use assistive devices and technologies due to concerns about stigma, privacy, or perceived need and suitability (Yusif et al., 2016). Health care providers are well equipped to provide counseling related to lifestyle changes (Noordman et al., 2012); as such, patient-provider communication that validates patient concerns while emphasizing the benefits and versatility of available assistive devices and technologies may increase the likelihood of adoption.

The built environment can also affect the health of older adults by influencing their ability to engage in health-promoting behaviors like physical activity. The US Department of Health and Human Services recommends that older adults engage in at least 150 minutes of moderate-intensity aerobic activity per week and highlights the relationship between this recommended amount of physical activity and reduced mortality and improved functioning. In cases where older adults are limited by chronic conditions, the US Department of Health and Human Services recommends that older adults be as physically active as their ability and conditions allow (US Department of Health and Human Services, 2018). Despite the benefits of physical activity, nearly one in four adults age 50 years and older are inactive, with the prevalence of inactivity increasing with age (Watson et al., 2016). For older adults, aspects of the neighborhood and build environment, including concerns about safety from traffic and crime, sidewalk conditions, and street connectivity, can present challenges to outdoor walking (Yen, 2014). Health care providers must be prepared to continue to promote the benefits of physical activity to their older adult patients and facilitate discussion regarding strategies to overcome barriers to engaging in physical activity.

Social and Community Context

The determinant of social and community context refers to the connections between social relationships (i.e., interactions with family, friends, coworkers and other community members), cultural attitudes, norms, and expectations and health and well-being (Office of Disease Prevention and Health Promotion, 2014). Social network involvement (i.e., having a family member, friend, or other social network member who provides assistance and facilitates care) may be particularly important for older adults, given the role of family caregivers in their overall well-being. Moreover, older adults who lack social connections are at increased risk for premature mortality (Holt-Lunstad et al., 2015).

Social Networks

Social ties can be conceptualized based on structure and function. Social networks represent the structure or pattern of social relationships that surround an individual. Networks can be described based on the characteristics of the network as a whole (e.g., size, homogeneity, geographic dispersion) as well as by the characteristics of the individual relationships within the network (e.g., intensity, reciprocity, formality) (Gallant, 2013). Social networks can provide a variety of social functions that influence health, including companionship, social support, and social control (Heaney & Israel, 2008). Although these three functions are conceptually different and capable of affecting the health of older adults in different ways, social relationships often provide more than one function simultaneously.

Companionship

Companionship refers to the day-to-day interactions that occur through engaging in social and recreational activities with other network members. Companionship is an integral part of daily life. Core concepts related to companionship include friendship, intimacy, and loneliness. In this context, friendship is defined as the availability of network members with whom older adults can interact or affiliate with. Intimacy refers to the availability of network members to whom an older adult feels close or emotionally connected, and loneliness is the feeling that one is isolated from others (Cyranowski et al., 2013). Among older adults, having companionship can decrease distress and also positively influence overall well-being (Newsom et al., 2005). Conversely, the lack of companionship, either because of too few social contacts or feeling isolated from existing contacts, has been associated with an increased risk of adverse cardiovascular outcomes (Valtorta et al., 2016) as well as premature mortality (Holt-Lunstad et al., 2015).

Social Support

Receiving social support from family and friends has been associated with positive health outcomes (DiMatteo, 2004; Franks et al., 2006; Rosland, 2015). Generally, social support refers to the psychological and material resources and

• BOX 3.1 Interprofessional Education Collaborative (IPEC) 2016 Core Competencies

Competency 1

Work with individuals of other professions to maintain a climate of mutual respect and shared values. (Values/Ethics for Interprofessional Practice.)

Competency 2

Use the knowledge of one's own role and those of other professions to appropriately assess and address the health care needs of patients and to promote and advance the health of populations. (Roles/Responsibilities.)

Competency 3

Communicate with patients, families, communities, and professionals in health and other fields in a responsive and responsible manner that supports a team approach to the promotion and maintenance of health and the prevention and treatment of disease. (Interprofessional Communication.)

Competency 4

Apply relationship-building values and the principles of team dynamics to perform effectively in different team roles to plan, deliver, and evaluate patient/population-centered care and population health programs and policies that are safe, timely, efficient, effective, and equitable. (Teams and Teamwork.)

From Interprofessional Education Collaborative (2016). *Core competencies for interprofessional collaborative practice: 2016 update.* https://ipec.memberclicks.net/assets/2016-Update.pdf

aid provided to help another person cope with a stressor (Cohen, 2004). Social support can be categorized into four supportive behaviors: emotional, instrumental, informational, and appraisal. Emotional support involves providing expressions such as love, trust, caring, empathy, sympathy, and concern. Instrumental support, sometimes referred to as tangible support, is when an individual physically provides goods and services that directly assist a person in need. Informational support refers to the provision of messages that include advice, suggestions, and knowledge or facts that a person can use to address problems. Appraisal support is defined as the provision of constructive feedback and affirmation that the recipient can use for self-evaluation purposes (Heaney & Israel, 2008; Ko et al., 2013).

Social Control

There is often great concern about the amount of social support available to older adults as evidenced by Healthy People 2030 Health Social and Community Context Goal: Increase social and community support (see Box 3.1) (Office of Disease Prevention and Health Promotion, 2020b). Another pathway through which social network members can affect health is by influencing and monitoring older adults' health behaviors. This social function is referred to as social control (Franks et al., 2006; Helgeson, 2004). Although often treated as a unidimensional construct, social control can be positive (persuasion or reinforcement) or negative (pressure) (Okun, 2007; Tucker, 2002). Compared to negative control, positive social control is more likely to encourage healthy behaviors (Craddock, 2015). Alternatively, negative control has been associated with engaging in fewer self-care behaviors (Fekete et al., 2009). Yet experiencing either positive or negative control has been associated with more oppositional behaviors (e.g., doing the opposite of what is desired or hiding unhealthy behavior) (Craddock, 2015). Among older adults, positive social control has been associated with better adherence and negative control with poorer adherence to a recommended diet (Stephens et al., 2010).

Along with the amount of social support available to older adults, consideration must be given to the *who* and *what* of social networks (Heaney & Israel, 2008). Health-related social functions can be performed by a variety of people, including members of an older adult's informal network (e.g., family and friends) or the person's formal network (e.g., health care professionals). The effectiveness of the social function and behavior will likely be influenced by the type of network member providing it. The *what* of social network involvement refers to the distinction between received and perceived health-related social functions. *Received* reflects the quality and quantity of health-related social functions given, and *perceived* refers to the types and adequacy of health-related social functions that individuals believe is available to them from their social network (Vangelisti, 2009). The distinction between received and perceived health-related social functions is of great importance, as perceptions about health-related social functions have been shown to have a greater positive effect on health than do received functions (Eagle et al., 2019). When considering the social network of older adults, efforts should be made to assess their beliefs about the types of social relationships they have and their functions.

Strategies to Address the Social Determinants of Health in Clinical Practice

There are multiple ways clinicians can engage in addressing patients' social determinants of health. Kovach et al. identified five clinical engagement strategies and three population-based engagement strategies (Kovach et al., 2019).

Clinical engagement strategies include the following:

- Screening patients for social determinants of health
- Referring patients to community-based resources to address social determinants of health
- Capturing data about social determinants of health in the electronic health record
- Using community health workers to address patient's social determinants of health
- Using community health data to complement patient information

Population-based engagement strategies include the following:

- Communicating with elected officials to support public policies aimed at addressing social determinants of health

- Providing testimony at a hearing to support public policies aimed at addressing social determinants of health
- Participating in community health needs assessment or other collaborative initiatives aimed at improving community health

To facilitate the health care system's ability to address the social determinants of health, the National Academy of Medicine (NAM, formerly the Institute of Medicine) recommends capturing social and behavioral domains in the patient electronic health record (EHR). Specifically, they recommend that measures related to 11 domains be routinely collected and made available in the EHR. Four of these domains (alcohol use, race and ethnicity, residential address, and tobacco use/exposure) are commonly collected during health care encounters; however, NAM advocates for information about census tract-median income, symptoms of depression, educational attainment, financial strain, intimate partner violence, physical activity, social connections and social isolation, and stress to also be collected (Institute of Medicine Board on Population Health Public Health Practice: Committee on the Recommended Social Behavioral Domains Measures for Electronic Health Records, 2015). Incorporating information about the social determinants of health into the EHR provides a mechanism for routinely and systematically collecting the data and also ensures that the data will be available at the right time and place to encourage clinicians to engage in activities to address patients' social determinants of health (DeVoe et al., 2016).

Interprofessional Teams

What Is an Interprofessional Team?

An interprofessional team consists of multiple health care professionals who share common goals, have clear roles, and work together to provide care (Table 3.3). The composition of an interprofessional team will vary based on the setting, needs of the patient or population, and available resources or programs. Teams organized around a setting include home care, rehabilitation, and acute care for the elderly (ACE) units. Patients with a diagnosis of congestive heart failure may receive care from an interprofessional team designed to treat that specific condition. Some programs require unique interprofessional teams, such as hospice or geriatric assessment clinics. Regardless of the organizing factor, the goal of the interprofessional team is to provide patient-centered care. This requires a clear understanding of team-member roles, ongoing communication and coordination, and shared responsibility for desired outcomes (Interprofesional Education Collaborative, 2016).

Significance to Care of the Older Person

The health care needs of older adults are complex and transcend the education and training of any single discipline (Advisory Committee on Interdisciplinary Community-Based Linkages [ACICBL], 2019). Chronic disease is associated with significant functional decline, especially among the oldest old (Fong, 2019). Chronic disease and functional disability can lead to the need for specialty health services, community-based support programs, or long-term care. Fixed incomes and transportation challenges experienced by many older adults can limit access to these services (Advisory Committee on Interdisciplinary Community-Based Linkages [ACICBL], 2019). Geriatric specialists are best prepared to provide the tailored approach required to meet complex health and psychosocial needs for older adults, but clinicians certified in geriatrics are in short supply. In 2018, there were 49.2 million adults over the age of 65 in the United States, but just 3940 practicing geriatricians (American Geriatric Society, 2018). The numbers of geriatric specialists in other disciplines like nursing and pharmacology are also low, as only 5% are licensed to provide geriatric care (Institute of Medicine, 2011). Although the numbers of geriatric specialists are rising, it is not a rate proportional to the rise in the older adult population (American Geriatric Society, 2018). Teams of qualified professionals with varied areas of expertise can meet the needs of the older adult population in the absence of a health care system that adequately addresses varied needs, goals, preferences, and resources.

Innovative models of interprofessional collaborative practice (IPCP) show promise for increasing the quality of care older adults receive and improving key outcomes. Interprofessional collaborative practice is "when multiple health workers from different professional backgrounds work together with patients, families, [careers], and communities to deliver the highest quality of care" (World Health Organization, 2010). Models of IPCP in geriatrics span the health care continuum and vary in composition of team members based on the setting and goals of care. Although researchers have yet to demonstrate clearly that these models simultaneously improve population health, reduce health care costs, and improve the quality of care delivered to patients (Brandt et al., 2014), a variety of positive outcomes for geriatric patients have been demonstrated. Interprofessional teams in primary care have been able to reverse both physical and cognitive frailty measures for older adults (Romera-Liebana et al., 2018). In acute care, the use of ACE teams and ACE units have resulted in greater adherence to geriatric care guidelines, shorter hospital stays for older adults, improved functional status on discharge, and reduced costs associated with hospitalizations (Flood et al., 2018).

Interprofessional Education Collaborative (IPEC) Competencies

The Institute of Medicine and the World Health Organization recognized interprofessional teams as one solution for a health care system poorly structured to care for a growing older adult population in seminal reports on quality and safety in health care (Institute of Medicine Committee on Quality of Health Care in America, 2001; World Health Organization, 2010). The Robert Wood Johnson Foundation, John A.

TABLE 3.3 Members of the Interprofessional Geriatric Care Team

Essential Members	Primary Role	Potentially Useful Members	Primary Role
Patient	Express preferences for treatment, communication, and involvement of family members	Family member	Coordinate appointments Communicate with insurance companies, health care providers, and community-based service providers Provide assistance with ADLs and IADLs Provide emotional support to the patient
Primary care provider	Assess, manage, and treat health problems Coordinate care with other medical providers Consult with specialists Refer for services in the community Educate patients and families about medical conditions and self-management	Physical therapist	Diagnose and treat mobility problems
Nurse	Assess the patient response to illness and disability Implement PCP orders Serve as patient advocate	Occupational therapist	Optimize ADLs and IADLs
Social worker	Conduct psychosocial assessments Provide referrals for community-based services Coordinate transitions of care Provide counseling for patients and family members Assess for and coordinate completion of advance care planning documents	Speech pathologist	Assess and manage communication and swallowing problems
Pharmacist	Optimize medications Assess for adverse drug effects Counsel patients and families about medications Recommend cost-effective pharmacologic treatment options	Registered dietician	Identify nutritional needs Plan and implement nutritional interventions
		Psychiatrist/ psychologist	Comanage psychiatric disorders Administer and interpret neuropsychological tests Provide therapy
		Attorney	Counsel patients and families about legal and financial concerns Draft advance care planning documents

ADLs, Activities of daily living (ADLs); IADLs, instrumental activities of daily living; PCP, primary care provider.

Hartford Foundation, and other influential organizations have strongly supported interprofessional education (Flaherty & Bartels, 2019). In 2011, a panel representing six education associations of multiple disciplines came together as the Interprofessional Education Collaborative (IPEC) to develop and report on the core competencies for interprofessional practice (Interprofessional Education Collaborative Expert Panel, 2011). In 2016, the panel expanded to include 15 education associations. The more inclusive IPEC panel was tasked with reorganizing the core competencies under the single domain of interprofessional collaboration and aligning the competencies with the Triple Aim (Interprofesional Education Collaborative, 2016). The Institute for Healthcare Improvement, recognizing the challenges of aging populations, increased longevity, and chronic health problems, developed the Triple Aim framework to optimize health system performance (Institute for Healthcare Improvement, 2020). The Triple Aim includes improving the patient experience, improving the health of populations, and reducing per capita cost of health care (Institute for Healthcare Improvement, 2020).

There are four core competencies for interprofessional collaboration according to the 2016 IPEC update (Box 3.1) (Interprofesional Education Collaborative, 2016). The competencies speak directly to values and ethics for interprofessional practice, roles and responsibilities of the team, effective interprofessional communication, and teams and teamwork (Interprofesional Education Collaborative, 2016). Subcompetencies for each of the core competencies further illustrate desired principles for patient-centered, team-based care. The panel's intention is for the core and subcompetencies to apply to all health professions across the learning continuum (Interprofesional Education Collaborative, 2016).

The second core competency of interprofessional collaborative practice calls for team members to understand their own role, as well as the role of other members of the team. This allows team members to capitalize on the knowledge, skills, and abilities of each team member, as well as communicate these roles and responsibilities to patients and families (Interprofesional Education Collaborative, 2016). Geriatric interprofessional care teams have core members, as well as other team members that may join the team as needed based on patient needs (Table 3.2).

Typical Team Members

Patient

The older adult is the center of the interprofessional care team. According to the American Geriatric Society Expert Panel on Person-Centered Care, "person-centered care means that individuals' values and preferences are elicited and, once expressed, guide all aspects of their health care, supporting their realistic health goals" ("Person-Centered Care: A Definition and Essential Elements," 2016). Patient autonomy is crucial, but it is important to recognize that based on patient preferences, values, cultural norms, and cognitive ability, the patient may rely on significant others, family members, or the health care team to drive decision making.

Primary Care Providers

No single team member is more qualified than others to direct the interprofessional care team. Among providers for an older adult patient, it is important for one provider to coordinate the care of providers in other care settings and specialties. This role often falls to the primary care provider (PCP), who could be a physician, physician assistant, or advanced practice registered nurse.

Physicians are highly skilled clinicians with extensive training. The practice of medicine includes the diagnosis, treatment, correction, advisement, or prescription for any human disease, ailment, injury, infirmity, deformity, pain, or other condition, physical or mental, real or imaginary. After receiving a bachelor's degree, medical students attend either an allopathic program resulting in a doctor of medicine (MD) degree or an osteopathic program that confers a doctor of osteopathic (DO) degree. Physicians complete a residency in a particular field of medicine. Primary care physicians complete either an internal medicine or family practice residency. Residencies are clinical training programs that can last 3 to 5 years and involve rotations in both the hospital and clinic settings. Physicians are licensed by the state. Board certification is an optional way for physicians to demonstrate expertise through rigorous ongoing professional development, testing, and peer evaluation (American Geriatric Society, 2020). Physicians pursuing a specialty in geriatrics can complete a 1- or 2-year geriatric fellowship following residency or after practicing for 1 or more years. Geriatrics is recognized as a specialty with a board certification (American Geriatric Society, 2018).

Physician assistants (PAs) are practitioners who practice in every area of medicine, including primary care. Physician assistants diagnose illness, develop, and manage treatment plans and prescribe medications (American Academy of PAs, 2019). Physician assistants complete a bachelor's degree, specific prerequisite courses, and direct patient contact hours before enrolling in a master's level PA program. A program typically lasts 2 to 3 years and includes more than 2000 hours of clinical rotations in various settings. Physician assistants are trained in general medicine and may practice in any health care setting. State regulations dictate licensing requirements for PAs, which typically involve an agreement with a specific physician to practice (American Academy of PAs, 2019). The degree of geriatric education PAs receive will vary by program. Although less than 2% of PAs specialize in geriatrics, 27% work in primary care and 92.1% see patients over the age of 65 (Smith et al., 2019). Physician assistants, skilled in collaborative care, have been shown to be highly effective in long-term care settings, reducing annual hospital admissions in one study by 38% (Ackermann & Kemle, 1998).

Advanced practice registered nurses (APRNs) are registered nurses with advanced education and training to practice at the highest scope of clinical practice in the profession. Nurse practitioners, clinical nurse specialists, nurse anesthetists, and nurse midwives are all APRNs (American Nurses Association, n.d.). Nurse practitioners (NP) are the largest group of APRNs. Of the more than 270,000 licensed NPs in the United States, 87.1% work in primary care (American Association of Nurse Practitioners, 2019). Nurse practitioners receive one or more certifications for both a specific population and setting. To be eligible for licensing in most states, NPs must pass a national certification exam in a specialty area, like adult-gerontology acute care or adult-gerontology primary care. Some states allow APRNs to practice independently, whereas others require either collaborative or supervisory agreements with physicians. Nurse practitioners prescribe medications, perform exams, diagnose and treat illnesses, and deliver a wide range of other services from care coordination to quality assurance (American Geriatric Society, 2020). As nurses, NPs receive education organized around the nursing model that focuses on preventive care, health promotion, and the human response to illness.

The education, training, and licensing requirements for physicians, physician assistants, and advanced practice nurses vary, but often these health care providers serve similar roles on the interprofessional team as the primary care provider. There are various ways each can pursue additional education, training, or specialty certification in geriatrics (American Geriatric Society, 2020).

Nurse

Nurses make up the largest component of the health care workforce, practicing in every setting where older adults receive care. According to the American Nurses Association (ANA), nursing is "the protection, promotion and optimization of health and abilities, prevention of illness and injury, alleviation of suffering and treatment through the diagnosis and treatment of human response, and advocacy in the care of individuals, families, communities, and populations." Licensed practical nurses/vocational nurses (LPNs/LVNs) typically have 1 year of vocational or technical college. LPN/LVNs can work in any setting, but the majority, 54%, work in long-term care (National League for Nursing, 2014). An LPN/LVN administers medications, delivers treatments, delegates to nursing assistants, and participates in care planning (American Geriatric Society, 2020). Registered nurses (RNs) have a broader scope of practice than LPNs/LVNs and have either an associate degree or bachelor's degree. There are currently 3.8 million licensed RNs in the United States, with just over half practicing in hospital settings on general medical and surgical units (Rosseter, 2019). Registered nurses provide most of the care in long-term care settings, from care coordination and direct care, to administration and training (American Geriatric Society, 2020). The American Nurses Credentialing Center provides a Gerontological Nursing Certification (RN-BC) to recognize nurses with expertise in the care for older adults.

Social Worker

Care for older adults requires consideration of financial, social, legal, and psychological issues that can impact the overall health of an individual. In interprofessional geriatric care teams, social workers help assess and manage the social and behavioral health needs of older adults (Donelan et al., 2019). There are more than 680,000 social workers in the United States, and that number is expected to grow in the coming decade (National Association of Social Workers, n.d.). Although social work education starts with preparing generalists in undergraduate programs, master's prepared social workers choose a specialty focus (American Geriatric Society, 2020). Graduate programs may allow a student to choose either a clinical or nonclinical focus, typically last 2 years, and include practicums. In most states, a master's degree is a requirement for licensure. The National Association of Social Workers (NASW) offers both a specialty certification and credentialing for gerontology (American Geriatric Society, 2020).

Pharmacist

Older adults have a higher risk of adverse drug events (ADEs) due to physiologic aging that affects drug metabolism, frequent transitions of care, and polypharmacy. Most practitioners have limited time with patients, despite complex medical conditions and multimorbidity. Pharmacists are particularly suited to optimize medications for the older adult patient and to provide education on evidence-based pharmacologic treatments to patients and other team members. In 2019, there were 387,000 licensed pharmacists in the United States (National Association of Boards of Pharmacy, 2019). Pharmacists hold a doctoral degree that requires 2 to 4 years of prerequisite training and takes 4 years to complete. Pharmacists may complete a residency, and geriatrics is one possible residency experience (American Geriatric Society, 2020). After graduation and passing an exam through the National Association of Boards of Pharmacy, pharmacists are licensed through individual states. There are a number of roles for pharmacists in the care of older adult patients, from in-patient settings and primary care clinics to retail pharmacies and long-term care. There is a board-certification for pharmacists in geriatrics. Having a pharmacist on the interprofessional geriatric care team can decrease unplanned health care visits, hospital admissions, and long-term care transitions and can reduce health care costs (Campbell et al., 2018).

Additional Optional Team Members

The older adult population is diverse, with a variety of health care needs. Although primary care providers, nurses, social workers, and pharmacists make up the core interprofessional team, there are many others who should be brought into the team depending on the needs of the individual older adult. It is important for the team to establish who is responsible for communicating with others outside the core team.

Family Members

Either by patient preference or necessity, family members may be part of the care team. When an older adult can no longer make her or his own health care decisions, a family member often becomes the decision maker. This person is proxy for the patient and charged with making decisions based on the values and preferences of the patient. Even when the older adult can make medical decisions, family members are often intimately involved in the care, providing varied tasks from assisting with medications, making appointments, and communicating with insurance companies, to providing transportation and doing housework, to bathing, dressing, and delivering toileting help (Riffin et al., 2017). In a 2019 report on family caregiving by the Founders of the Home Alone Alliance, researchers found that health care coordination among providers and systems falls to a family caregiver 44.8% of the time (Reinhard et al., 2019). By comparison, 24.8% of older adult patients took on that responsibility, whereas just 7% of health care professionals coordinated care (Reinhard et al., 2019). It is good practice to assess for social support systems and obtain consents to speak with a trusted family member when necessary to coordinate care.

Physical Therapists

Physical therapists diagnose and manage the care for individuals with health-related problems that limit their ability to move and function in their daily life. Older adults might work with a physical therapist in the hospital, skilled nursing facility, rehabilitation unit, or the home. Health problems that are common to older adults, such as stroke, osteoarthritis, fractures, falls, and pain, can result in mobility and functional limitations.

Occupational Therapists

Occupational therapists help older adults with occupations, or daily activities. Occupational therapy is evidence based and person centered, focusing on how to adapt environments or tasks to fit the individual (The American Occupational Therapy Association, n.d.). Studies show that occupational therapists can assist older adults in independent living, fall reduction, safe driving, limitations due to a stroke, cognitive impairment, and chronic care management (Arbesman et al., 2014).

Speech Pathologists

Speech-language pathologists are the primary providers for all aspects of communication and swallowing (American Speech-Language-Hearing Association, 2016). Working with a speech-language pathologist could benefit older adults with cerebral vascular accident, Alzheimer disease and related dementias, Parkinson disease, dysphagia, respiratory problems, as well as other disorders (American Speech-Language-Hearing Association, 2016).

Dieticians

Older adults are high risk for malnutrition (Severin et al., 2019). Malnutrition can lead to significant poor outcomes for older adults, including functional decline and increased mortality (Severin et al., 2019). Patients at risk for malnutrition should be referred to a registered dietician for assessment and management of nutritional needs. Registered dieticians work in hospitals, outpatient settings, long-term care, and the community (Wilkinson et al., 2017).

Psychiatrists/Psychologists

Older adults are at high risk for mental health problems due to social isolation, chronic illness, physical and psychological pain, and neurocognitive impairment (Conejero et al., 2018). Psychiatric disorders are prevalent among older adults. A study with a nationally representative sample cited estimates of anxiety and mood disorders at 11.4% and 6.8%, respectively (Reynolds et al., 2015). Although suicide attempts are highest among adolescents and young adults, suicide rates are proportionally highest among older adults (World Health Organization, 2019). There are other serious consequences such as increased disability and health care utilization (World Health Organization, 2017). Psychiatrics and psychologists can be important members of the interprofessional team to address the mental health care of older adults.

Attorneys

There are several legal issues that can affect an older adult. Attorneys who specialize in elder law can assist with the completion of advance directives, guardianships, estate planning, housing concerns, and insurance matters.

Aging and Disability Resource Center Managers

Aging and disability resource centers (ADRCs) are in every county and state in the United States. An ADRC serves as a resource for community members to get reliable information and counseling regarding access to services and supports (Administration for Community Living, 2017). Long-term supports and services (LTSS) for older adults are dependent on a daunting matrix of financial considerations and bureaucratic requirements that can be difficult for older adults and their families to navigate. Managers and staff of ADRCs are invaluable resources for both older adults and health care providers. An ADRC is a one-stop shop for navigating services for veterans, care transitions from nursing home back to the community and the reverse, and access to both public and private programs to support older adults. Staff of ADRCs can also include adult protective service professionals.

Dementia Care Specialists

Some states and counties employ social workers and other nonmedical personnel who have specialized training in the care of people living with dementia. These individuals, sometimes called dementia care specialists, are a community-based resource for caregivers of people living with dementia. Dementia care specialists might run support groups, meet individually with caregivers struggling with different aspects of care, or provide community lectures and classes to educate caregivers and other people in the community about dementia care.

As a nonprofit organization, the Alzheimer's Association is a valuable resource for people living with dementia, their caregivers, and health care professionals (Box 3.2). The Alzheimer's Association website has links to local resources, studies recruiting participants, research findings, and patient and practitioner education materials. The Alzheimer's Association also staffs a 24-hour, 7-days-a-week helpline. Many states have regional nonprofit organizations to support people living with dementia and their caregivers. Practitioners should seek out local resources when establishing a practice.

Private Patient Navigators

Private patient advocates, also known as health advocates or health managers, are unlicensed professionals who focus on care and cost of health care (The Alliance of Professional Health Advocates, 2020). Private patient advocates provide

• BOX 3.2 Alzheimer's Association Website and Hotline

Alzheimer's Association
www.alz.org
24/7 Helpline
800-272-3900

several nonmedical services to their clients. They are typically paid directly by clients, although some employers do provide these services through employee assistance programs. As of 2018, private patient advocates complete a certification exam through the Patient Advocate Certification Board (PACB) (The Alliance of Professional Health Advocates, 2020). This is a relatively small but growing profession (Nemko, 2007).

Direct Care Workers

Direct care workers (DCWs) provide the bulk of care for older adults who need long-term service and support (LTSS) (US Department of Health and Human Services, 2017). Direct care workers include nursing assistants, home health aides, personal care aides, and psychiatric assistants or aids (US Department of Health and Human Services, 2017). They represent 71% of the LTSS workforce (US Department of Health and Human Services, 2017). The demand for these occupations is growing rapidly. Despite this, DCW pay remains low, at or near minimum wage (Kelly et al., 2020), and turnover is high (Hamadi et al., 2016; Yeatts et al., 2018). The federal government requires training for nursing assistants and home health aides who work in Medicare- and Medicaid-certified nursing homes and home health agencies. The training requirements of other DCWs are dependent on institution and setting. Most of the training for all DCWs is short-term, on-the-job training (Bureau of Labor Statistics, 2022).

Care Coordination Across Care Settings

Care Settings for Older Adults

Unless a provider specializes in pediatrics or obstetrics, most physician assistants and nurse practitioners will work extensively with older adults. Care for older adults occurs in many settings, including hospitals, ambulatory primary and specialty care practices, long-term care facilities, home health, and rehabilitation facilities. In the United States, older adults account for 40% of hospitalized patients (Hamidi & Joseph, 2019). After infants, hospitalization rates are highest among the oldest old, those over the age of 85 (Weiss, 2014). After hospitalization, older adults may need additional care or monitoring at home with a home care agency or in a rehabilitation or long-term care facility. Over 80% of home health agency patients are older adults (Harris-Kojetin et al., 2016). Although only 3% of people over the age of 65, or 1.2 million people, live in nursing homes (Administration for Community Living, 2018), a much higher percentage will utilize nursing homes only to be discharged back to the community. Older adults make up 84% of nursing home residents (Harris-Kojetin et al., 2016), and they are high users of ambulatory care, second only to infants (Ashman, 2019). These transitions happen frequently, but the health care team rarely follows the older adult from one setting of care to another. As a result, older adults are cared for in multiple settings, by multiple providers (Fig. 3.7).

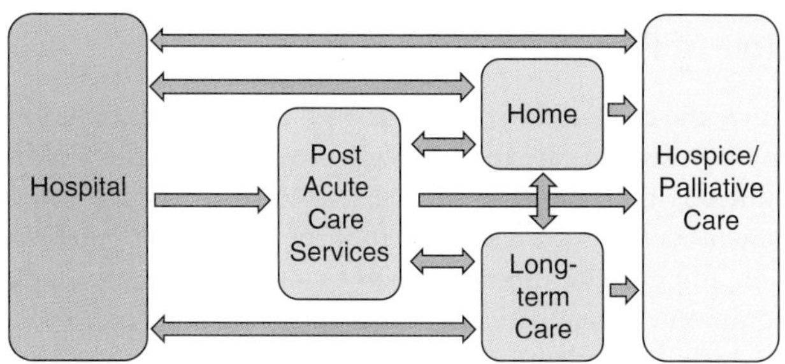

• **Fig. 3.7** Common Transitions in Care Across and Between Settings and Providers. (From Hirschman, K. B., & Hodgson, N. A. [2018]. Evidence-based interventions for transitions in care for individuals living with dementia. *Gerontologist*, *58*[Suppl. 1], S129–S140. https://doi.org/10.1093/geront/gnx152.)

Adverse Health Outcomes for Uncoordinated Care

Poorly coordinated care can lead to negative outcomes for older adults. Most of the research has focused on adverse outcomes as older adults move from the hospital setting to long-term care or outpatient settings. Poor outcomes during this transition include drug-related adverse events, readmission to the hospital, and pending test results not being monitored by outpatient providers (Snow et al., 2009). Other consequences of poor care transitions include mistrust, anxiety, and confusion among patients and families, and these issues can precipitate family conflict (Mitchell et al., 2018). At its worst, poorly coordinated care increases morbidity and mortality among older adults (Moore et al., 2003).

Factors that contribute to problematic care transitions include poor cross-site communication and collaboration, lack of knowledge of patients' wishes, preferences and goals of care, and errors in medication reconciliation (Sheikh et al., 2018). In many health care systems, hospitalists provide acute care, rather than primary care providers who are often not informed that their patient has been hospitalized. Providers in all settings might discharge a patient or approve transfer to a setting that they are unfamiliar with. For example, a hospitalist or primary care provider might not be aware of treatments and services available at a skilled nursing facility. When patients move across care settings, there is evidence to suggest that providers communicate across sites less than 30% of the time (Sheikh et al., 2018). Goals of care discussions are rare outside of an acute illness. Without knowledge of an older adult's wishes, patients might be transferred and receive care inconsistent with their wishes and values. Medication errors are more likely during a care transition. Older adults are a group at high risk for adverse drug events, making transitions a particularly dangerous time. Interventions designed to improve care transitions aim to improve communication, incorporating patient preferences, and medication reconciliation. After examining successful care transition interventions, the Joint Commission identified eight elements for effective care transitions (The Joint Commission, 2012).

Role of Providers

Since the early 2000s, there has been an emphasis on creating transitional care models to improve outcomes for older adults as they move from one setting to the other. These care models require the support of the health care organization and are intentional in their practices and goals. Some common characteristics of successful transitional care models include discharge planning and instructions, tools for health care professionals, patient and family education, and patient-centered care (Enderlin et al., 2013).

In the absence of an organized transitional care model, individual providers can practice in a way that enhances successful care transitions. In qualitative studies, patients and family members identified factors that are valuable to them during care transitions:

- Assistance with medication self-management
- A patient-centered record owned and maintained by the patient to facilitate the transfer of information across care settings
- Timely follow-up with primary or specialty care
- A list of red flags indicative of a worsening condition and instructions on how to respond to them
- A clear point of contact to turn to for advice or medical care during the transition (Coleman et al., 2006; Mitchell et al., 2018)

Patients and family members were able to identify specific provider behaviors that led them to feel care for and cared about by medical providers and to feel capable of implementing the plan of care:

- Empathic language and gestures
- Anticipating patient needs to support self-care at home
- Collaborative discharge planning
- Providing actionable information
- Providing uninterrupted care with minimal hand-offs (Mitchell et al., 2018)

As leaders on health care teams, providers should advocate for patient-centered processes for care transitions. Patient-centered care includes being available to providers at the next setting of care to offer valuable information that is often more effectively communicated by a simple phone call. Poor communication between health care providers during patient hand-offs can result in poor outcomes for patients (see Safety Alert) (Horwitz et al., 2006). Although there are numerous evidence-based strategies for safe and effective patient hand-offs, there are several key factors to ensure quality communication between providers.

SAFETY ALERT

Effective communication during provide-to-provider patient hand-offs is essential for safe transfers of care.

1. Communicate verbally to allow for dialogue between providers.
2. Provide a standardized written transition record that includes key pieces of information.
3. Prioritize crucial information in the verbal hand-off:
   - Current health status
   - Code status
   - Decision-making capacity
   - Current level of function for activities of daily living (ADLs) and instrumental activities of daily living (IADLs)
   - Last living situation and previous level of functioning
   - Key patient contact
4. Provide anticipatory guidance to the next provider (task-based, if-then statements)

Care Coordinators and Discharge Planners

Members of the interprofessional team, such as nurses and social workers, are utilized in specific roles to assist patients in transitions of care. The role of care coordinators and discharge planners is to identify and engage with patients during hospitalization in order to anticipate postacute care needs and follow those patients through to the next care setting (Kripalani et al., 2019). Key activities of care coordinators include individualized needs assessments, medication reconciliation, patient and caregiver education, anticipatory guidance for postdischarge, scheduling postdischarge appointments, communicating with the primary care provider, and follow-up phone calls (Kranker et al., 2018; Kripalani et al., 2019). When care coordinators are involved in transitions of care, patients have improved outcomes (Conway et al., 2019), decreased health care costs (Kranker et al., 2018), and fewer readmissions (Kripalani et al., 2019).

Common Preventable and Reversible Conditions

Definition of the Problem

Older adults are susceptible to preventable and reversible conditions that are often underdiagnosed and undertreated. This susceptibility stems from an overall reduction in physiologic reserve, but the conditions are frequently caused or complicated by medical interventions. Comprehensive geriatric care requires a focus on preventing common problems among older adults, identifying reversible conditions early, and choosing individualized treatment strategies that maintain physical function, independence, and quality of life.

Examples of Preventable and Reversible Conditions

Delirium

Delirium is an acute neuropsychiatric syndrome commonly caused by a medical illness, medical complication, or adverse drug event (T. G. Fong et al., 2009). Prevalence estimates vary between 115% and 42% (Kukreja et al., 2015), depending on the setting. Delirium is characterized by inattention and acute cognitive dysfunction. The greatest risk factors for delirium are dementia and age 65 or older (Fong et al., 2009). The most common underlying conditions that lead to delirium include pain, dehydration, infections, stroke, metabolic disturbances, and surgery (Kukreja et al., 2015). Although the prevalence of delirium is relatively rare in the community, being hospitalized increases the risk significantly. During hospitalization, older adults are usually acutely ill and may be exposed to new drugs, new environments, stress, and functional impairment, all predisposing factors for the condition. Prevention of delirium requires a tailored multicomponent approach that includes assessment of risk, prevention of dehydration, immobility, hypoxia, pain, and sleep disturbance, and careful consideration of medications, particularly those known to cause adverse drug effects in older adults.

Falls

Falls are the leading cause of death and disability in older adults (Centers for Disease Control and Prevention, 2019d). The greatest risk factors for falls are a history of falls, decreased strength, gait and balance impairment, and use of psychoactive medications (Lee et al., 2013). Polypharmacy is a common risk factor for falls, but individual classes of drugs are also implicated in falls, such as tricyclic antidepressants, benzodiazepines, and opioid analgesics (American Geriatrics Society Beers Criteria Update Expert, 2019; Park et al., 2015). Effective fall prevention interventions are usually interprofessional and have multiple components. For a provider, the most important steps to take include asking about a history of falls to determine risk, reviewing medications with special consideration for those on the Beers List (American Geriatrics Society Beers Criteria Update Expert, 2019), and assessing functional abilities, particularly gait (Lee et al., 2013).

Depression

Major depressive disorder (MDD) in adults age 60 and older is called late life depression (LLD) (Melrose, 2019). Major depressive disorder or associated symptoms that are still clinically relevant affect up to 49% of adults over the age of 65 (Melrose, 2019). The consequences of LLD are significant and include development of cognitive impairment, premature death, chronic course of illness, functional impairment, and increased risk of suicide (Brown et al., 2018). The etiology of LLD is complex, with biologic age-related changes likely playing a role (Brown et al., 2018). Other underlying causes of LLD include medical conditions, polypharmacy, or substance use. Loneliness and cognitive impairment increase susceptibility to LLD or depressive symptoms (Melrose, 2019). Providers should be alert to atypical depressive symptoms in older adults, such as depression without sadness, which presents as withdrawal or apathy (Melrose, 2019). One of the classic signs of MDD, a loss of interest is pronounced in LLD and should not be attributed to losses associated with aging alone. Signs such as weight loss and early morning awakenings resulting in sleep loss are also important indicators of LLD (Melrose, 2019). In evaluating an older adult with depressive symptoms, metabolic causes, such as hypothyroidism and medication effects, should be ruled out.

Implications for Practice

Age-friendly health systems proactively structure services to provide care that matches patient and family goals, ensures older adults live as long as possible in the community, and decreases the number of in-patient days and readmissions (Pelton et al., 2018). In 2017, the John A. Hartford Foundation supported an initiative in partnership with the Institute for Healthcare Improvement (IHI), American Hospital Association, and the Catholic Health Association of the Unites States to create an age-friendly health system ("NICHE and Age-Friendly Health Systems: An Interview With Dr. Terry Fulmer, PhD, RN, FAAN President, The John A. Hartford Foundation," 2019). The result of this collaboration is the "4Ms" (Box 3.3). The "4Ms" are a framework for providing excellent care for older adults: what matters, medication, mentation, and mobility. Interventions that focus on the 4Ms have been shown to reduce inpatient and intensive care unit stays, decrease costs and length of stay, decrease morbidity and mortality, and prevent iatrogenic complications (Fulmer, 2019).

Palliative Care and Hospice

Definitions

The World Health Organization defines palliative care as "an approach that improves the quality of life of patients and their families facing the problems associated with life-threatening illness, through the prevention and relief of suffering by means of early identification and impeccable assessment and treatment of pain and other problems, physical,

• BOX 3.3 The "4Ms" of an Age-Friendly Health Systems

What Matters

Know what matters: health outcome goals and care preferences for current and future care, including end of life. Act on what matters for current and future care, including end of life.

Medication

Implement standard processes for age-friendly medication reconciliation. Prescribe and adjust doses to be age-friendly.

Mentation

Implement an individualized mobility plan. Create an environment that enables mobility.

Mobility

Ensure adequate nutrition, hydration, sleep, and comfort. Engage and orient to maximize independence and dignity. Identify, treat, and manage dementia, delirium, and depression.

From Mate, K. S., Berman, A., Laderman, M., Kabcenell, A., & Fulmer, T. (2018). Creating age-friendly health systems—A vision for better care of older adults. *Healthcare (Amsterdam), 6*(1), 4–6. https://doi.org/10.1016/j.hjdsi.2017.05.005

psychosocial and spiritual" (World Health Organization, 2013). Palliative care is appropriate for any older adult who could benefit from the management of physical and psychological symptoms related to a serious illness. Palliative care does not replace a patient's primary treatment team, is not time limited, and does not prevent a patient from pursing curative treatment (National Hospice and Palliative Care Organization, 2019). Patients can receive palliative care in any care setting.

Hospice is a philosophy of care for people with a terminal diagnosis and life expectancy of 6 months or less (Centers for Medicare & Medicaid Services, 2017). Hospice care focuses on treating the individual rather than the disease. To enroll in hospice, a treatment provider or hospice medical director must certify that the older adult is terminally ill, and the older adult or her or his proxy decision maker must choose for the individual to receive hospice care. Hospice is a comprehensive benefit offered by Medicare Part A (Box 3.4). Individuals who enroll in hospice care waive the right for Medicare to pay for any other services to treat the terminal illness (Centers for Medicare & Medicaid Services, 2017). Medicare offers four levels of hospice care for patients: routine, inpatient, continuous, and respite care. An interprofessional team provides hospice care in most care settings (National Hospice and Palliative Care Organization, 2019).

Palliative and hospice care exist on a continuum (Fig. 3.8). Most seriously ill patients should be offered palliative care services at the time of diagnosis. Not all patients will be ready to accept services at that time, so the issue can be readdressed as appropriate over the course of the illness. When a patient approaches the terminal stages of the disease, with a general life expectancy of less than 6 months, a hospice referral is appropriate. The palliative care team can aid in the transition from treatment focused on a cure to a hospice care plan where quality of life is the principal goal.

• BOX 3.4 Hospice Benefits

- Physician services
- Nursing services
- Medical equipment ([durable medical equipment] DME)
- Medical supplies
- Physical and occupational therapy
- Speech-language pathology services
- Medical social services
- Dietary counseling
- Home health aide and homemaker services
- Grief and loss counseling services
- Short-term inpatient care for pain and symptoms management
- Prescription drugs for symptom control or pain relief

From Centers for Medicare & Medicaid Services. (2017). *Medicare hospice benefits*. https://www.medicare.gov/Pubs/pdf/02154-Medicare-Hospice-Benefits.PDF

Significance

The prevalence of frailty, multimorbidity, dementia, and cancer increases with age. The symptom burden associated with these conditions can result in increases in long-term care placement, hospitalizations, and mortality (Deardorff et al., 2019, 2020; Kamitani et al., 2020; Maxwell et al., 2018). Older adults are significantly burdened by symptoms from their medical problems (Patel et al., 2019). In a sample representative of older adults in the United States, Patel et al. found that nearly half of older adults have two or more co-occurring symptoms. Symptom burden led to functional limitations and increased the risk for slow gait speed, falls, hospitalizations, disability, and mortality (Patel et al., 2019).

Palliative care and hospice care can improve the quality of care and quality of life for older adults. Palliative care can also substantially decrease health-care-related costs

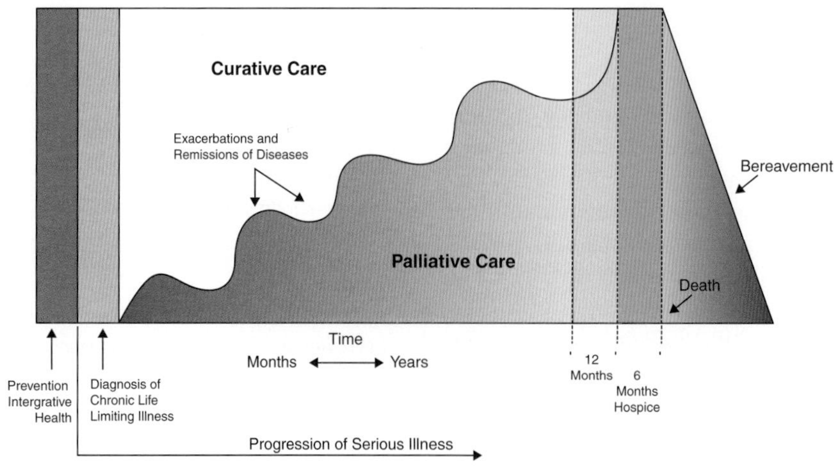

• Fig. 3.8 Introduction to Hospice and Palliative Care. (Adapted from Lynn, J., & Adamson, D. M. [2003]. *Living well at the end of life: Adapting health care to serious chronic illness in old age*. RAND, with permission.)

(May et al., 2016; Triplett et al., 2017). In a study of Medicare beneficiaries with advanced cancer, those who received palliative care had lower rates of hospitalization, received fewer invasive procedures, and were less likely to have chemotherapy administration than those who did not receive palliative care (Triplett et al., 2017). Most Americans express a preference for dying at home (Gruneir et al., 2007). Enrolling in hospice care increases the likelihood that this will happen (Shepperd et al., 2016).

Implications for Practice

Although the numerous benefits of palliative and hospice care have been demonstrated, they are both underutilized services. Although the Medicare benefit allows for 6 months or more of hospice care, in the United State, in 2017, approximately 40% of Medicare beneficiaries were enrolled in hospice for less than 2 weeks before death (National Hospice and Palliative Care Organization, 2018). There are also significant geographic and racial differences in use of hospice services. African American and Hispanic older adults are much less likely than Whites to enroll in hospice (LoPresti et al., 2014). In a review of data from the Dartmouth Atlas of Healthcare, geographic differences included much higher rates of hospice utilization in Ogden, Utah, compared to Miami, Florida or Los Angeles, California (MacPherson & Parikh, 2017). Researchers continue to explore why these significant differences exist. When a consult is made for palliative or hospice care, it often comes late in the illness trajectory and the patient has limited time to benefit from this care (Saracino et al., 2018). Evidence suggests that the longer patients have to benefit from palliative care, the lower their overall health care utilization at end of life (Triplett et al., 2017).

HEALTHY PEOPLE 2030 SOCIAL DETERMINANTS OF HEALTH GOALS

Social determinant of economic stability
Goal: Help people earn steady incomes that allow them to meet their health needs
Social determinant of education access and quality
Goal: Increase educational opportunities and help children and adolescents do well in school
Social determinant of health care access and quality
Goal: Increase access to comprehensive, high-quality health care services
Social determinant of neighborhood and built environment
Goal: Create neighborhoods and environments that promote health and safety
Social determinant of social and community context
Goal: Increase social and community support

Summary

As leaders and providers at the front lines of health care across the spectrum of care delivery models, physician assistants and nurse practitioners need to be prepared to care for older adults. Globally, health care systems are experiencing an influx of older adult patients, and the number is poised to grow dramatically. In many settings in the United States, we have sophisticated diagnostic tools and treatments that extend life, but we still struggle as a system to provide a high quality of life for all adults in their advanced years. Although age alone is a risk factor for many serious health conditions and older adults share risk factors for chronic disease and multimorbidity, much of what determines quality of life in later years is attributed to social determinants of health. Health and well-being are largely dependent on social support, financial security, access to health care, and the lived environment. Health literacy plays a major role in an older adult's ability to self-manage health conditions. Due to the complex medical and social factors, the health care of older adults requires excellent interprofessional care across diverse care settings. Providers caring for older adults need to understand the individual needs of the patient, the patient's family members, and caregivers, and the limitations of the health care system in its current state to provide high-quality care. An astute understanding of what different settings of care, as well as specialty services like palliative and hospice care, will aid a practitioner in providing patient-centered care to older adults.

Key Points

- The older adult population is heterogeneous. Although chronologic age is a factor in guiding assessment and treatment, level of function, multiple health conditions, and patient values are essential considerations for tailoring care to the individual patient.
- The aging populations is increasingly racially and ethnically diverse, requiring health care providers to embrace culturally appropriate and accessible care.
- Individual health care providers should recognize and address social determinants of health in the care plan for older adults, including financial concerns, social support, and the neighborhood and built environment.
- Comprehensive geriatric care requires skilled, high-functioning, interprofessional teams, in which each member is valued and contributes to patient care.
- Effective communication is key to ensure high-quality attention during transitions of care.

More information about tools and Interprofessional Education Collaborative (IPEC) competencies mentioned in this chapter can be found in Appendix 1: Tools and Appendix 2: IPEC Competencies.

References

2019 American Geriatrics Society Beers Criteria Update Expert Panel. (2019). American Geriatrics Society 2019 updated AGS Beers criteria for potentially inappropriate medication use in older adults. *Journal of the American Geriatric Society, 67*(4), 674–694. https://doi.org/10.1111/jgs.15767.

Ackermann, R. J., & Kemle, K. A. (1998). The effect of a physician assistant on the hospitalization of nursing home residents. *Journal of the American Geriatric Society, 46*(5), 610–614. https://doi.org/10.1111/j.1532-5415.1998.tb01078.x.

Administration for Community Living. (2017). *Aging and disability resource centers program/no wrong door system.* https://acl.gov/programs/connecting-people-services/aging-and-disability-resource-centers-programno-wrong-door.

Administration for Community Living. (2018). *2018 Profile of older Americans.* https://acl.gov/aging-and-disability-in-america/data-and-research/profile-older-americans.

Advisory Committee on Interdisciplinary Community-Based Linkages (ACICBL). (2019). *Preparing the current and future health care workforce for interprofessional practice in sustainable, age-friendly health systems.* https://www.hrsa.gov/sites/default/files/hrsa/advisory-committees/community-based-linkages/reports/seventeenth-2019.pdf.

Alzheimer's Association. (2019). Alzheimer's disease facts and figures. *Alzheimer's and Dementia Journal, 15*(3), 321–387.

The Alliance of Professional Health Advocates. (2020). *An overview of the professional of patient advocacy.* https://aphadvocates.org/profession-overview/.

American Academy of PAs. (2019). *What is a PA?* https://www.aapa.org/what-is-a-pa/#:~:text=For%20full%20methodology%20visit%20aapa,in%20every%20specialty%20and%20setting.

American Association of Nurse Practitioners. (2019). NP fact sheet.https://www.aanp.org/about/all-about-nps/np-fact-sheet.

American Diabetes Association. (2020). Standards of medical care in diabetes. *Journal of Clinical and Applied Research and Education,* 43. care.diabetesjournals.org/content/43/Supplement_1.

American Geriatric Society. (2018). *State of the geriatrician workforce.* https://www.americangeriatrics.org/geriatrics-profession/about-geriatrics/geriatrics-workforce-numbers.

American Geriatric Society. (2020). *Training for geriatricians.* https://www.americangeriatrics.org/geriatrics-profession/training-requirements/training-geriatricians.

American Geriatric Society Expert Panel on the Care of Older Adults with Multimorbidity. (2012). Guiding principles for the care of older adults with multimorbidity: An approach for clinicians. *Journal of the American Geriatric Society, 60*(10), E1–E25. https://doi.org/10.1111/j.1532-5415.2012.04188.x.

American Nurses Association. (n.d.). *Advance practitioner registered nurse.* https://www.nursingworld.org/practice-policy/workforce/what-is-nursing/aprn/.

The American Occupational Therapy Association. (n.d.). *What is occupational therapy?* https://www.aota.org/Conference-Events/OTMonth/what-is-OT.aspx.

American Speech-Language-Hearing Association. (2016). *Scope of practice in speech-language-pathology* [scope of practice]. www.asha.org/policy/.

Andrews, M. (2003). The influence of cultural and health belief systems on health care practices. In M. M. Andrews, J. S. Boyle, & T. J. Carr (Eds.), *Transcultural concepts in nursing care* (pp. 73–91). Lippincott Williams & Wilkins.

Arbesman, M., Lieberman, D., & Metzler, C. A. (2014). Using evidence to promote the distinct value of occupational therapy. *American Journal of Occupational Therapy, 68*(4), 381–385. https://doi.org/10.5014/ajot.2014.684002.

Arrojo, E. D. R., Lev-Ram, V., Tyagi, S., Ramachandra, R., Deerinck, T., Bushong, E., & Hetzer, M. W. (2019). Age mosaicism across multiple scales in adult tissues. *Cell Metabolism, 30*(2), 343–351. e343. https://doi.org/10.1016/j.cmet.2019.05.010.

Ashman, J. J., Rui, P., & Okeyode, T. (2019). Characteristics of office-based physician visits, 2016. *NCHS data brief*(331), 1–8.

Atamna, H., Tenore, A., Lui, F., & Dhahbi, J. M. (2018). Organ reserve, excess metabolic capacity, and aging. *Biogerontology, 19*(2), 171–184. https://doi.org/10.1007/s10522-018-9746-8.

Aunan, J. R., Watson, M. M., Hagland, H. R., & Soreide, K. (2016). Molecular and biological hallmarks of ageing. *British Journal of Surgery, 103*(2), e29–e46. https://doi.org/10.1002/bjs.10053.

Baker, D. W., Williams, M. V., Parker, R. M., Gazmararian, J. A., & Nurss, J. (1999). Development of a brief test to measure functional health literacy. *Patient Education and Counseling, 38*(1), 33–42. https://doi.org/10.1016/s0738-3991(98)00116-5. [pii].

Baker, D. W., Wolf, M. S., Feinglass, J., & Thompson, J. A. (2008). Health literacy, cognitive abilities, and mortality among elderly persons. *Journal of General Internal Medicine, 23*(6), 723–726. https://doi.org/10.1007/s11606-008-0566-4.

Bass, P. F., Wilson, J. F., & Griffith, C. H. (2003). A shortened instrument for literacy screening. *Journal of General Internal Medicine, 18*(12), 1036–1038. https://doi.org/10.1111/j.1525-1497.2003.10651.x. [pii].

Bennett, M. J. (2013). *Basic concepts of intercultural communication: Paradigms, principles, & practice: Selected readings* (2nd ed.). Intercultural Press.

Berger, S., Escher, A., Mengle, E., & Sullivan, N. (2018). Effectiveness of health promotion, management, and maintenance interventions within the scope of occupational therapy for community-dwelling older adults: A systematic review. *American Journal of Occupational Therapy, 72*(4), 1–10. https://doi.org/10.5014/ajot.2018.030346.

Binette, J., & Vasold, K. (2018). 018 Home and community preferences: A national survey of adults age 18-plus. In AARP Research. https://www.aarp.org/research/topics/community/info-2018/2018-home-community-preference.html.

Bond, S. M. (2010). Physiological aging in older adults with cancer: Implications for treatment decision making and toxicity management. *Journal of Gerontological Nursing, 36*(2), 26–37. https://doi.org/10.3928/00989134-20091103-98.

Bowleg, L. (2008). When Black + lesbian + woman ≠ Black lesbian woman: The methodological challenges of qualitative and quantitative intersectionality research. *Sex Roles, 59*(5), 312–325. https://doi.org/10.1007/s11199-008-9400-z.

Brandt, B., Lutfiyya, M. N., King, J. A., & Chioreso, C. (2014). A scoping review of interprofessional collaborative practice and education using the lens of the Triple Aim. *Journal of Interprofessional Care, 28*(5), 393–399. https://doi.org/10.3109/13561820.2014.906391.

Brown, P. J., Wall, M. M., Chen, C., Levine, M. E., Yaffe, K., Roose, S. P., & Rutherford, B. R. (2018). Biological age, not chronological age, is associated with late-life depression. *The Journals of Gerontology Series A: Biological Sciences & Medical Sciences, 73*(10), 1370–1376. https://doi.org/10.1093/gerona/glx162.

Buck, H. G., Dickson, V. V., Fida, R., Riegel, B., D'Agostino, F., Alvaro, R., & Vellone, E. (2015). Predictors of hospitalization and quality of life in heart failure: A model of comorbidity, self-efficacy and self-care. *International Journal of Nursing Studies, 52*(11), 1714–1722. https://doi.org/10.1016/j.ijnurstu.2015.06.018.

Bucknall, T. K., Hutchinson, A. M., Botti, M., McTier, L., Rawson, H., Hitch, D., & Chaboyer, W. (2020). Engaging patients and families in communication across transitions of care: An integrative review. *Patient Education and Counseling* https://doi.org/10.1016/j.pec.2020.01.017.

Bureau of Labor Statistics, US Department of Labor. (September 08, 2022). *Occupational outlook handbook, home health aides and personal care aides.* https://www.bls.gov/ooh/healthcare/home-health-aides-and-personal-care-aides.htm.

Buttorff, C., Ruder, T., & Bauman, M. (2017). *Multiple chronic conditions in the United States.* https://www.rand.org/content/dam/rand/pubs/tools/TL200/TL221/RAND_TL221.pdf

Cagle, J. G., McClymont, K. M., Thai, J. N., & Smith, A. K. (2016). "If you don't know, all of a sudden, they're gone": Caregiver perspectives about prognostic communication for disabled elderly adults. *Journal of the American Geriatrics Society, 64*(6), 1299–1306. https://doi.org/10.1111/jgs.14137.

Calasanti, T., & Giles, S. (n.d.). The challenge of intersectionality. https://www.asaging.org/blog/challenge-intersectionality.

Campbell, A. M., Coley, K. C., Corbo, J. M., DeLellis, T. M., Joseph, M., Thorpe, C. T., & Sakely, H. (2018). Pharmacist-led Drug Therapy problem management in an interprofessional geriatric care continuum: A subset of the PIVOTS Group. *American Health & Drug Benefits, 11*(9), 469–477. Retrieved from http://search.ebscohost.com/login.aspx?direct=true&AuthType=ip,uid&db=rzh&AN=133620253&site=ehost-live&scope=site.

Campinha-Bacote, J. (2002). The Process of cultural competence in the delivery of healthcare services: A model of care. *Journal of Transcultural Nursing, 13*(3), 181–184. https://doi.org/10.1177/10459602013003003. 25.

Centers for Disease Control and Prevention. (2017). Deaths: Leading causes for 2017. *National Vital Statistics Reports, 68*(6), 1–77.

Centers for Disease Control and Prevention. (2017). *National diabetes statistics report,* 2017. https://www.cdc.gov/aging/disparities/index.htm.

Centers for Disease Control and Prevention. (2019a). *About chronic disease.* https://www.cdc.gov/chronicdisease/about/index.htm.

Centers for Disease Control and Prevention. (2019b). *Health disparities.* https://www.cdc.gov/aging/disparities/index.htm.

Centers for Disease Control and Prevention. (2019c). *Health, United States: Infographics.* https://www.cdc.gov/nchs/hus/spotlight/2019-heart-disease-disparities.htm.

Centers for Disease Control and Prevention. (2019d). *Home and recreational safety.* https://www.cdc.gov/homeandrecreationalsafety/falls/fallcost/deaths-from-falls.html.

Centers for Disease Control and Prevention. (2020). *National diabetes statistics report,* 2020. https://www.cdc.gov/diabetes/data/statistics/statistics-report.html.

Centers for Medicare & Medicaid Services. (2017). *Medicare hospice benefits.* https://www.medicare.gov/Pubs/pdf/02154-Medicare-Hospice-Benefits.PDF.

Chan, S., & Stevens, A. H. (1999). Employment and retirement following a late-career job loss. *The American Economic Review, 89*(2), 211–216. http://www.jstor.org/stable/117108.

Chang, A. Y., Skirbekk, V. F., Tyrovolas, S., Kassebaum, N. J., & Dieleman, J. L. (2019). Measuring population ageing: An analysis of the global burden of disease study 2017. *Lancet Public Health, 4*(3), e159–e167. https://doi.org/10.1016/s2468-2667(19)30019-2.

Chesser, A. K., Keene Woods, N., Smothers, K., & Rogers, N. (2016). Health literacy and older adults: A systematic review. *Gerontology & Geriatric Medicine, 2* https://doi.org/10.1177/2333721416630492. 2333721416630492-Dec.

Clegg, A., Young, J., Iliffe, S., Rikkert, M. O., & Rockwood, K. (2013). Frailty in elderly people. *Lancet (London, England), 381*(9868), 752–762. https://doi.org/10.1016/S0140-6736(12)62167-9.

Cohen, S. (2004). Social relationships and health. *American Psychologist, 59*(8), 676–684. https://doi.org/10.1037/0003-066X.59.8.676.

Coleman, E. A., Parry, C., Chalmers, S., & Min, S. (2006). The care transitions intervention: Results of a randomized controlled trial. *Archives of Internal Medicine, 166*(17), 1822–1828. http://search.ebscohost.com/login.aspx?direct=true&AuthType=ip,uid&db=rzh&AN=106019826&site=ehost-live&scope=site.

Conejero, I., Olié, E., Courtet, P., & Calati, R. (2018). Suicide in older adults: Current perspectives. *Clinical Interventions in Aging, 13,* 691–699. https://doi.org/10.2147/CIA.S130670.

Conway, A., O'Donnell, C., & Yates, P. (2019). The effectiveness of the nurse care coordinator role on patient-reported and health service outcomes: A systematic review. *Evaluation & the Health Professions, 42*(3), 263–296. https://doi.org/10.1177/0163278717734610.

Craddock, E., vanDellen, M. R., Novak, S. A., & Ranby, K. W. (2015). Influence in relationships: A meta-analysis on health-related social control. *Basic and Applied Social Psychology, 37*(2), 118–130. https://doi.org/10.1080/01973533.2015.1011271.

Crenshaw, K. (1991). Mapping the margins: Intersectionality, identity politics, and violence against women of color. *Stanford Law Review, 43*(6), 1241–1299. https://doi.org/10.2307/1229039.

Cyranowski, J. M., Zill, N., Bode, R., Butt, Z., Kelly, M. A., Pilkonis, P. A., & Cella, D. (2013). Assessing social support, companionship, and distress: National Institute of Health (NIH) toolbox adult social relationship scales. *Health Psychology: Official Journal of the Division of Health Psychology, American Psychological Association, 32*(3), 293–301. https://doi.org/10.1037/a0028586.

Davis, J., Penha, J., Mbowe, O., & Taira, D. A. (2017). Prevalence of single and multiple leading causes of death by race/ethnicity among US adults aged 60 to 79 years. *Preventing Chronic Disease, 14,* E101. https://doi.org/10.5888/pcd14.160241.

Deardorff, W. J., Liu, P. L., Sloane, R., Van Houtven, C., Pieper, C. F., Hastings, S. N., & Whitson, H. E. (2019). Association of sensory and cognitive impairment with healthcare utilization and cost in older adults. *Journal of the American Geriatric Society, 67*(8), 1617–1624. https://doi.org/10.1111/jgs.15891.

DeVoe, J. E., Bazemore, A. W., Cottrell, E. K., Likumahuwa-Ackman, S., Grandmont, J., Spach, N., & Gold, R. (2016). Perspectives in primary care: A conceptual framework and path for integrating social determinants of health into primary care practice. *Annals of Family Medicine, 14*(2), 104–108. https://doi.org/10.1370/afm.1903.

Dewalt, D. A., Callahan, L. F., Hawk, V. H., Broucksou, A., Hink, R., & Rudd, R. (2010). Health literacy universal precautions toolkit. *Agency for Healthcare Research and Quality*

DiMatteo, M. R. (2004). Social support and patient adherence to medical treatment: A meta-analysis. *Health Psychology: Official Journal of the Division of Health Psychology, American Psychological Association, 23*(2), 207–218. https://doi.org/10.1037/0278-6133.23.2.207.

Divi, C., Koss, R. G., Schmaltz, S. P., & Loeb, J. M. (2007). Language proficiency and adverse events in US hospitals: A pilot study. *International Journal for Quality in Health Care, 19*(2), 60–67. https://doi.org/10.1093/intqhc/mzl069.

Donelan, K., Chang, Y., Berrett-Abebe, J., Spetz, J., Auerbach, D. I., Norman, L., & Buerhaus, P. I. (2019). Care management for older adults: The roles of nurses, social workers, and physicians. *Health Affairs (Millwood), 38*(6), 941–949. https://doi.org/10.1377/hlthaff.2019.00030.

Eagle, D. E., Hybels, C. F., & Proeschold-Bell, R. (2019). Perceived social support, received social support, and depression among clergy. *Journal of Social & Personal Relationships, 36*(7), 2055–2073. https://doi.org/10.1177/0265407518776134.

Edwards, S. T., & Landon, B. E. (2014). Medicare's chronic care management payment--payment reform for primary care. *The New England Journal of Medicine*, *371*(22), 2049–2051. https://doi.org/10.1056/NEJMp1410790.

Enderlin, C. A., McLeskey, N., Rooker, J. L., Steinhauser, C., D'Avolio, D., Gusewelle, R., & Ennen, K. A. (2013). Review of current conceptual models and frameworks to guide transitions of care in older adults. *Geriatric Nursing*, *34*(1), 47–52. https://doi.org/10.1016/j.gerinurse.2012.08.003.

Feeding America. 2014. Hunger in America 2014. https://www.feedingamerica.org/sites/default/files/research/hunger-in-america/hia-2014-executive-summary.pdf.

Fekete, E., Geaghan, T. R., & Druley, J. A. (2009). Affective and behavioural reactions to positive and negative health-related social control in HIV+men. *Psychology & Health*, *24*(5), 501–515. https://doi.org/10.1080/08870440801894674.

Ferrucci, L., Levine, M. E., Kuo, P. L., & Simonsick, E. M. (2018). Time and the metrics of aging. *Circulation Research*, *123*(7), 740–744. https://doi.org/10.1161/circresaha.118.312816.

Finkenzeller, T., Potzelsberger, B., Kosters, A., Wurth, S., Amesberger, G., Dela, F., & Muller, E. (2019). Aging in high functioning elderly persons: Study design and analyses of behavioral and psychological factors. *Scandinavian Journal of Medicine & Science in Sports*, *29*(Suppl. 1), 7–16. https://doi.org/10.1111/sms.13368.

Flaherty, E., & Bartels, S. J. (2019). Addressing the community-based geriatric healthcare workforce shortage by leveraging the potential of interprofessional teams. *Journal of the American Geriatrics Society*, *67*(S2), S400–S408. https://doi.org/10.1111/jgs.15924.

Flood, K. L., Booth, K., Vickers, J., Simmons, E., James, D. H., Biswal, S., & Bowman, E. H. (2018). Acute care for elders (ACE) team model of care: A clinical overview. *Geriatrics (Basel)*, *3*(3). https://doi.org/10.3390/geriatrics3030050.

Fong, J. H. (2019). Disability incidence and functional decline among older adults with major chronic diseases. *BMC Geriatrics*, *19*(1), 323. https://doi.org/10.1186/s12877-019-1348-z.

Fong, T. G., Tulebaev, S. R., & Inouye, S. K. (2009). Delirium in elderly adults: Diagnosis, prevention and treatment. *Nature Reviews. Neurology*, *5*(4), 210–220. https://doi.org/10.1038/nrneurol.2009.24.

Foronda, C., Baptiste, D. L., Reinholdt, M. M., & Ousman, K. (2016). Cultural humility: A concept analysis. *Journal of Transcultural Nursing: Official Journal of the Transcultural Nursing Society*, *27*(3), 210–217. https://doi.org/10.1177/1043659615592677.

Franks, M. M., Stephens, M. A., Rook, K. S., Franklin, B. A., Keteyian, S. J., & Artinian, N. T. (2006). Spouses' provision of health-related support and control to patients participating in cardiac rehabilitation. *Journal of Family Psychology*, *20*(2), 311–318. https://doi.org/10.1037/0893-3200.20.2.311.

Franzon, K., Zethelius, B., Cederholm, T., & Kilander, L. (2015). Modifiable midlife risk factors, independent aging, and survival in older men: Report on long-term follow-up of the uppsala longitudinal study of adult men cohort. *Journal of the American Geriatrics Society*, *63*(5), 877–885. https://doi.org/10.1111/jgs.13352.

Fulmer, T., Berman, A., Mate, K., & Pelton, L. (2019). Age-friendly health systems: The 4Ms: *Try this: Best practices in nursing care to older adults* (pp. 1–2). The Hartford Institute for Geriatric Nursing, New York University Rory Meyers College of Nursing.

Fyhrquist, F. Y., & Saijonmaa, O. J. (2016). Modifiable factors influencing telomere length and aging. In A. C. S. C. Bondy (Ed.), *Inflammation, aging, and oxidative stress. oxidative stress in applied basic research and clinical practice* (pp. 67–80). Springer, Cham.

Gallant, M. P. (2013). Social networks, social support, and health-related behavior: *The Oxford handbook of health communication, behavior change, and treatment adherence* (pp. 305–322). Oxford University Press.

Ganann, R., McAiney, C., & Johnson, W. (2018). Engaging older adults as partners in transitional care research. *Canadian Medical Association Journal*, *190*(Suppl.), S40–S41. https://doi.org/10.1503/cmaj.180396.

Gruneir, A., Mor, V., Weitzen, S., Truchil, R., Teno, J., & Roy, J. (2007). Where people die: A multilevel approach to understanding influences on site of death in America. *Medical Care Research and Review*, *64*(4), 351–378. https://doi.org/10.1177/1077558707301810.

Hager, E. R., Quigg, A. M., Black, M. M., Coleman, S. M., Heeren, T., Rose-Jacobs, R., & Frank, D. A. (2010). Development and validity of a 2-item screen to identify families at risk for food insecurity. *Pediatrics*, *126*(1), 26. https://doi.org/10.1542/peds.2009-3146.

Hamadi, H., Probst, J. C., Khan, M. M., Bellinger, J., & Porter, C. (2016). Home-based direct care workers. *Workplace Health & Safety*, *64*(6), 249–261. https://doi.org/10.1177/2165079916630554.

Hamidi, M., & Joseph, B. (2019). Changing epidemiology of the American population. *Clinics in Geriatric Medicine*, *35*(1), 1–12. https://doi.org/10.1016/j.cger.2018.08.001.

Harris-Kojetin, L., Sengupta, M., Lendon, J. P., Rome, V., Valverde, R., & Caffey, C. (2016). Long-term care providers and services users in the United States: data from the National Study of Long-Term Care Providers, 2013-2014. Vital & health statistics. Series 3. *Analytical and epidemiological studies*(38). x–105.

Heaney, C. A., & Israel, B. A. (2008). Social networks and social support. In K. Glanz, B. K. Rimer, & K. Viswanath (Eds.), *Health behavior and health education: Theory, research, and practice* (4th ed., pp. 189–210). Jossey-Bass.

Helgeson, V. S., Novak, S. A., Lepore, S. J., & Elton, D. T. (2004). Spouse social control efforts: Relations to health behavior and well-being among men with prostate cancer. *Journal of Social & Personal Relationships*, *21*(1), 53–68. https://doi.org/10.1177/0265407504039840.

Heron, M. (2019). National vital statistics reports. In United States Department of Health and Human Services Health Resources and Services Administration (Series Ed.). *National Vital Statistics Reports, Vol. 68*

Hirschman, K. B., & Hodgson, N. A. (2018). Evidence-based interventions for transitions in care for individuals living with dementia. *Gerontologist*, *58*(Suppl. 1), S129–S140. https://doi.org/10.1093/geront/gnx152.

Hogan, K. -A., Burnett, S., & Roberts, S. (2017). Help me get home safely: Preventing medically unnecessary hospitalizations. *Perspectives: Journal of the Gerontological Nursing Association*, *39*(4), 23–25. http://search.ebscohost.com/login.aspx?direct=true&AuthType=ip,uid&db=rzh&AN=129270265&site=ehost-live&scope=site.

Holt-Lunstad, J., Smith, T. B., Baker, M., Harris, T., & Stephenson, D. (2015). Loneliness and social isolation as risk factors for mortality: A meta-analytic review. *Perspectives on Psychological Science*, *10*(2), 227–237. https://doi.org/10.1177/1745691614568352.

Horwitz, L. I., Krumholz, H. M., Green, M. L., & Huot, S. J. (2006). Transfer of patient care between house staff on internal medicine wards: A national survey. *Archives of Internal Medicine*, *166*(11), 1173–1174.

Horvath, S. (2013). DNA methylation age of human tissues and cell types. *Genome Biology*, *14*(10), R115. https://doi.org/10.1186/gb-2013-14-10-r115.

Institute for Healthcare Improvement. (2020). *Triple aim—The best care for the whole population at the lowest cost.* http://www.ihi.org/Engage/Initiatives/TripleAim/Pages/default.aspx

Institute of Medicine Board on Population Health Public Health Practice: Committee on the Recommended Social Behavioral

Domains Measures for Electronic Health Records. (2015). Capturing social and behavioral domains and measures in electronic health records: Phase 2. https://doi.org/10.17226/18951.

Institute of Medicine (US) Committee on Health Literacy. (2004). Introduction. In L. Nielsen-Bohlman, A. M. Panzer, & D. A. Kindig (Eds.), *Health literacy: A prescription to end confusion*. National Academies Press.

Institute of Medicine (US) Committee on Quality of Health Care in America. (2001). *Crossing the quality chasm: A new health system for the 21st century*. National Academies Press (US). https://pubmed.ncbi.nlm.nih.gov/25057539/.

Institute of Medicine (US) Committee on the Robert Wood Johnson Foundation Initiative on the Future of Nursing, at the Institute of Medicine. (2011). *Transforming practice. The future of nursing: Leading change, advancing health*. https://ipec.memberclicks.net/assets/2016-Update.pdf.

Interprofessional Education Collaborative. (2016). *Core competencies for interprofessional collaborative practice*: 2016 update. https://pubmed.ncbi.nlm.nih.gov/24983041/

Interprofessional Education Collaborative Expert Panel. (2011). *Core competencies for interprofessional collaborative practice: Report of an expertpanel*. https://www.aacom.org/docs/default-source/insideome/ccrpt05-10-11.pdf.

Jaffee, E. G., Arora, V. M., Matthiesen, M. I., Hariprasad, S. M., Meltzer, D. O., & Press, V. G. (2016). Postdischarge falls and readmissions: Associations with insufficient vision and low health literacy among hospitalized seniors. *Journal of Health Communication, 21*(Suppl. 2), 135–140. https://doi.org/10.1080/10810730.2016.1179371.

Johnson J.H., Jr., & Appold, S.J. (2017). *U.S. adults: Demographics, living arrangements, and barriers to aging in place*. https://www.kenaninstitute.unc.edu/wp-content/uploads/2017/06/AgingInPlace_06092017.pdf.

Johnston, M. C., Crilly, M., Black, C., Prescott, G. J., & Mercer, S. W. (2019). Defining and measuring multimorbidity: A systematic review of systematic reviews. *European Journal of Public Health, 29*(1), 182–189. https://doi.org/10.1093/eurpub/cky098.

Joint Center for Housing Studies of Harvard University. (2016). *Disabilities among older adults*. https://www.jchs.harvard.edu/sites/default/files/harvard_jchs_housing_growing_population_2016_1_0.pdf

The Joint Commission. (2012). *Hot topics in health care: Transitions of care: The need for a more effective approach to continuing patient care*. http://www.jointcommission.org/assets/1/18/Hot_Topics_Transitions_of_Care.pdf

Kamitani, T., Fukuma, S., Shimizu, S., Akizawa, T., & Fukuhara, S. (2020). Length of hospital stay is associated with a decline in activities of daily living in hemodialysis patients: A prospective cohort study. *BMC Nephrology, 21*(1), 9. https://doi.org/10.1186/s12882-019-1674-6.

Karliner, L. S., Jacobs, E. A., Chen, A. H., & Mutha, S. (2007). Do professional interpreters improve clinical care for patients with limited English proficiency? A systematic review of the literature. *Health Services Research Journal, 42*(2), 727–754. https://doi.org/10.1111/j.1475-6773.2006.00629.x.

Keller, A. O., Gangnon, R., & Witt, W. P. (2014). The impact of patient-provider communication and language spoken on adequacy of depression treatment for U.S. women. *Health Communication, 29*(7), 646–655. https://doi.org/10.1080/10410236.2013.795885.

Kelly, C., Craft Morgan, J., Kemp, C. L., & Deichert, J. (2020). A profile of the assisted living direct care workforce in the United States. *Journal of Applied Gerontology, 39*(1), 16–27. https://doi.org/10.1177/0733464818757000.

Kirkman, M. S., Briscoe, V. J., Clark, N., Florez, H., Haas, L. B., Halter, J. B., & Swift, C. S. (2012). Diabetes in older adults. *Diabetes Care, 35*(12), 2650. https://doi.org/10.2337/dc12-1801.

Ko, H. C., Wang, L. L., & Xu, Y. T. (2013). Understanding the different types of social support offered by audience to A-list diary-like and informative bloggers. *Cyberpsychology, Behavior and Social Networking, 16*(3), 194–199. https://doi.org/10.1089/cyber.2012.0297.

Kovach, K. A., Reid, K., Grandmont, J., Jones, D., Wood, J., & Schoof, B. (2019). How engaged are family physicians in addressing the social determinants of health? A survey supporting the American academy of family physician's health equity environmental scan. *Health Equity, 3*(1), 449–457. https://doi.org/10.1089/heq.2019.0022.

Kranker, K., Barterian, L. M., Sarwar, R., Peterson, G. G., Gilman, B., Blue, L., & Moreno, L. (2018). Rural hospital transitional care program reduces Medicare spending. *The American Journal of Managed Care, 24*(5), 256–260.

Kripalani, S., Chen, G., Ciampa, P., Theobald, C., Cao, A., McBride, M., & Speroff, T. (2019). A transition care coordinator model reduces hospital readmissions and costs. *Contemporary Clinical Trials, 81*, 55–61. https://doi.org/10.1016/j.cct.2019.04.014.

Kukreja, D., Günther, U., & Popp, J. (2015). Delirium in the elderly: Current problems with increasing geriatric age. *The Indian Journal of Medical Research, 142*(6), 655–662. https://doi.org/10.4103/0971-5916.174546.

Kutner, M., Greenberg, E., Jin, Y., & Paulsen, C. (2006). *The health literacy of America's adults: Results from the 2003 national assessment of adult literacy*. https://nces.ed.gov/pubs2006/2006483.pdf.

Lee, A., Lee, K. -W., & Khang, P. (2013). Preventing falls in the geriatric population. *The Permanente Journal, 17*(4), 37–39. https://doi.org/10.7812/TPP/12-119.

Lopez-Otin, C., Blasco, M. A., Partridge, L., Serrano, M., & Kroemer, G. (2013). The hallmarks of aging. *Cell, 153*(6), 1194–1217. https://doi.org/10.1016/j.cell.2013.05.039.

LoPresti, M. A., Dement, F., & Gold, H. T. (2014). End-of-life care for people with cancer from ethnic minority groups: A systematic review. *American Journal of Hospice and Palliative Medicine, 33*(3), 291–305. https://doi.org/10.1177/1049909114565658.

MacLeod, S., Musich, S., Gulyas, S., Cheng, Y., Tkatch, R., Cempellin, D., & Yeh, C. S. (2017). The impact of inadequate health literacy on patient satisfaction, healthcare utilization, and expenditures among older adults. *Geriatric Nursing, 38*(4), 334–341. https://doi.org/10.1016/j.gerinurse.2016.12.003.

MacPherson, A. L., & Parikh, R. B. (2017). Policy and politics to drive change in end-of-life care: Assessing the best and worst places to die in America. *Generations, 41*(1), 94–101. http://search.ebscohost.com/login.aspx?direct=true&AuthType=ip,uid&db=rzh&AN=123060337&site=ehost-live&scope=site.

Mandal, B., & Roe, B. (2008). Job loss, retirement and the mental health of older Americans. *Journal of Mental Health Policy and Economics, 11*(4), 167–176.

Mate, K. S., Berman, A., Laderman, M., Kabcenell, A., & Fulmer, T. (2018). Creating age-friendly health systems—A vision for better care of older adults. *Healthcare (Amsterdam), 6*(1), 4–6. https://doi.org/10.1016/j.hjdsi.2017.05.005.

Maxwell, C. J., Campitelli, M. A., Diong, C., Mondor, L., Hogan, D. B., Amuah, J. E., & Bronskill, S. E. (2018). Variation in the health outcomes associated with frailty among home care clients: Relevance of caregiver distress and client sex. *BMC Geriatrics, 18*(1), 211. https://doi.org/10.1186/s12877-018-0899-8.

May, P., Garrido, M. M., Cassel, J. B., Kelley, A. S., Meier, D. E., Normand, C., & Morrison, R. S. (2016). Palliative care teams' cost-saving effect is larger for cancer patients with higher numbers of comorbidities. *Health Affairs (Millwood), 35*(1), 44–53. https://doi.org/10.1377/hlthaff.2015.0752.

Melrose, S. (2019). Late life depression: Nursing actions that can help. *Perspectives in Psychiatric Care, 55*(3), 453–458. https://doi.org/10.1111/ppc.12341.

Mitchell, S. E., Laurens, V., Weigel, G. M., Hirschman, K. B., Scott, A. M., Nguyen, H. Q., & Li, J. (2018). Care transitions from patient and caregiver perspectives. *Annals of Family Medicine, 16*(3), 225–231. https://doi.org/10.1370/afm.2222.

Moore, C., Wisnivesky, J., Williams, S., & McGinn, T. (2003). Medical errors related to discontinuity of care from an inpatient to an outpatient setting. *Journal of General Internal Medicine, 18*(8), 646–651. https://doi.org/10.1046/j.1525-1497.2003.20722.x.

Morris, N. S., MacLean, C. D., Chew, L. D., & Littenberg, B. (2006). The single item literacy screener: Evaluation of a brief instrument to identify limited reading ability. *BMC Family Practice, 7*, 21. https://doi.org/10.1186/1471-2296-7-21.

Muezzinler, A., Zaineddin, A. K., & Brenner, H. (2014). Body mass index and leukocyte telomere length in adults: A systematic review and meta-analysis. *Obesity Reviews, 15*(3), 192–201. https://doi.org/10.1111/obr.12126.

National Association of Boards of Pharmacy. (2019). 2019 NABP E-profile aggregate data. https://www.aacp.org/node/416

National Association of Social Workers. (n.d.). A*bout social workers*. https://www.socialworkers.org/News/Facts/Social-Workers

National Hospice and Palliative Care Organization. (2018). *NHPCO Factsandfigures*,2018edition.https://www.nhpco.org/hospice-facts-figures/

National Hospice and Palliative Care Organization. (2019). Palliative care or hospice? The right service at the right time for seriously ill individuals.https://www.nhpco.org/wp-content/uploads/2019/04/PalliativeCare_VS_Hospice.pdf

National Institute on Aging. 2017. *Aging in place*: Growing older at home. https://www.nia/nih.gov.health/aging-place-growing-older-home

National League for Nursing. (2014). *A vision for recognition of the role of licensed practical/vocational nurses in advancing the nation's health*. https://www.nln.org/docs/default-source/uploadedfiles/about/nlnvision_7.pdf?sfvrsn=c7e06e45_3

Nemko, M. (2007). Ahead-of-the-curve careers. *U.S. News & World Report*. Retrieved from https://money.usnews.com/money/careers/articles/2007/12/19/ahead-of-the-curve-careers

Newsom, J. T., Rook, K. S., Nishishiba, M., Sorkin, D. H., & Mahan, T. L. (2005). Understanding the relative importance of positive and negative social exchanges: Examining specific domains and appraisals. *The Journals of Gerontology Series B: Psychological Sciences and Social Sciences, 60*(6), P304–P312. https://doi.org/10.1093/geronb/60.6.p304.

NICHE and age-friendly health systems: An interview with Dr. Terry Fulmer, PhD, RN, FAAN President, The John A. Hartford Foundation. (2019). *Geriatric Nursing*, 40(6), 651–652. https://doi.org/10.1016/j.gerinurse.2019.11.005

Noelke, C., & Beckfield, J. (2014). Recessions, job loss, and mortality among older US adults. *American Journal of Public Health, 104*(11), 126. https://doi.org/10.2105/AJPH.2014.302210.

Noordman, J., van der Weijden, T., & van Dulmen, S. (2012). Communication-related behavior change techniques used in face-to-face lifestyle interventions in primary care: A systematic review of the literature. *Patient Education and Counseling, 89*(2), 227–244. https://doi.org/10.1016/j.pec.2012.07.006.

North, B. J., & Sinclair, D. A. (2012). The intersection between aging and cardiovascular disease. *Circulation Research, 110*(8), 1097–1108. https://doi.org/10.1161/circresaha.111.246876.

O'Mahony, D., O'Sullivan, D., Byrne, S., O'Connor, M. N., Ryan, C., & Gallagher, P. (2015). STOPP/START criteria for potentially inappropriate prescribing in older people: Version 2. *Age and Ageing, 44*(2), 213–218. https://doi.org/10.1093/ageing/afu145.

Office of Disease Prevention and Health Promotion. (2020a). *Social determinants of health*. https://health.gov/healthypeople/objectives-and-data/social-determinants-health

Office of Disease Prevention and Health Promotion. (2020b). *Healthy people 2030*. https://health.gov/healthypeople

Okun, M. A., Huff, B. P., August, K. J., & Rook, K. S. (2007). Testing hypotheses distilled from four models of the effects of health-related social control. *Basic and Applied Social Psychology, 29*(2), 185–193.

Ortman, J., & Velkoff, V. (2014). *An aging nation: The older population in the United States*. https://www.census.gov/prod/2014pubs/p25-1140.pdf

Paasche-Orlow, M. K., & Wolf, M. S. (2008). Evidence does not support clinical screening of literacy. *Journal of General Internal Medicine, 23*(1), 100–102. https://doi.org/10.1007/s11606-007-0447-2.

Panagioti, M., Stokes, J., Esmail, A., Coventry, P., Cheraghi-Sohi, S., Alam, R., & Bower, P. (2015). Multimorbidity and patient safety incidents in primary care: A systematic review and meta-analysis. *PloS One, 10*(8), e0135947. https://doi.org/10.1371/journal.pone.0135947.

Park, H., Satoh, H., Miki, A., Urushihara, H., & Sawada, Y. (2015). Medications associated with falls in older people: Systematic review of publications from a recent 5-year period. *European Journal of Clinical Pharmacology, 71*(12), 1429–1440. https://doi.org/10.1007/s00228-015-1955-3.

Patel, K. V., Guralnik, J. M., Phelan, E. A., Gell, N. M., Wallace, R. B., Sullivan, M. D., & Turk, D. C. (2019). Symptom burden among community-dwelling older adults in the United States. *Journal of the American Geriatrics Society, 67*(2), 223–231. https://doi.org/10.1111/jgs.15673.

Pelton, L., Mate, K., Fulmer, T., & Berman, A. M. Y. (2018). Creating age-friendly health systems. *Health Progress, 99*(1), 87–88. http://search.ebscohost.com/login.aspx?direct=true&AuthType=ip,uid&db=rzh&AN=127389390&site=ehost-live&scope=site.

Person-Centered Care: A Definition and Essential Elements. (2016). *Journal of the American Geriatrics Society*, 64(1), 15–18. https://doi.org/10.1111/jgs.13866

Pooler, J., Levin, M., Hoffman, V., Karva, F., & Lewin-Zwerdling, A. (2016). Implementing food security screening and referral for older patients in primary care: A resource guide and toolkit. Web Page. https://sirenetwork.ucsf.edu/tools-resources/resources/implementing-food-security-screening-and-referral-older-patients-primary.

Power, M. C., Mormino, E., Soldan, A., James, B. D., Yu, L., Armstrong, N. M., & Delano-Wood, L. (2018). Combined neuropathological pathways account for age-related risk of dementia. *Annals of Neurology, 84*(1), 10–22. https://doi.org/10.1002/ana.25246.

Prados-Torres, A., Calderon-Larranaga, A., Hancco-Saavedra, J., Poblador-Plou, B., & van den Akker, M. (2014). Multimorbidity patterns: A systematic review. *Journal of Clinical Epidemiology, 67*(3), 254–266. https://doi.org/10.1016/j.jclinepi.2013.09.021.

Reinhard, S.C.,Young, H.M., Levine, C., Kelly, K., Choula, R.B., Accius, J.C. (2019). *Home alone revisited: Family caregivers providing complex care*. AARP. Retrieved September 10, 2022, from https://www.aarp.org/ppi/info-2018/home-alone-family-caregivers-providing-complex-chronic-care.html

Reynolds, K., Pietrzak, R. H., El-Gabalawy, R., Mackenzie, C. S., & Sareen, J. (2015). Prevalence of psychiatric disorders in U.S. older adults: Findings from a nationally representative survey. *World Psychiatry: Official Journal of the World Psychiatric Association (WPA), 14*(1), 74–81. https://doi.org/10.1002/wps.20193.

Riffin, C., Van Ness, P. H., Wolff, J. L., & Fried, T. (2017). Family and other unpaid caregivers and older adults with and without dementia and disability. *Journal of the American Geriatrics Society, 65*(8), 1821–1828. https://doi.org/10.1111/jgs.14910.

Roberts, A. W., Ogunwole, S. U., Blakeslee, L., & Rabe, M. A. (2018). *The population 65 years and older in the United States: 2016.* https://www.census.gov/content/dam/Census/library/publications/2018/acs/ACS-38.pdf

Rocca, W. A., Boyd, C. M., Grossardt, B. R., Bobo, W. V., Finney Rutten, L. J., Roger, V. L., & St Sauver, J. L. (2014). Prevalence of multimorbidity in a geographically defined American population: Patterns by age, sex, and race/ethnicity. *Mayo Clinic Proceedings, 89*(10), 1336–1349. https://doi.org/10.1016/j.mayocp.2014.07.010.

Romera-Liebana, L., Orfila, F., Segura, J. M., Real, J., Fabra, M. L., Möller, M., & Foz, G. (2018). Effects of a primary care-based multifactorial intervention on physical and cognitive function in frail, elderly individuals: A randomized controlled trial. *The Journals of Gerontology Series A: Biological Sciences & Medical Sciences, 73*(12), 1688–1674. https://doi.org/10.1093/gerona/glx259.

Rosland, A. M., Kieffer, E., Spencer, M., Sinco, B., Palmisano, G., Valerio, M., & Heisler, M. (2015). Do pre-existing diabetes social support or depressive symptoms influence the effectiveness of a diabetes I intervention? *Patient Education and Counseling, 98*(11), 1402–1409. https://doi.org/10.1016/j.pec.2015.05.019.

Rosseter, R. (2019). *Nursing fact sheet.* https://www.aacnnursing.org/News-Information/Fact-Sheets/Nursing-Fact-Sheet

Ryan, C. (2013). *Language use in the United States*: 2011. https://www2.census.gov/library/publications/2013/acs/acs-22/acs-22.pdf

Santos-Parker, J. R., LaRocca, T. J., & Seals, D. R. (2014). Aerobic exercise and other healthy lifestyle factors that influence vascular aging. *Advances in Physiology Education, 38*(4), 296–307. https://doi.org/10.1152/advan.00088.2014.

Saracino, R. M., Bai, M., Blatt, L., Solomon, L., & McCorkle, R. (2018). Geriatric palliative care: Meeting the needs of a growing population. *Geriatric Nursing, 39*(2), 225–229. https://doi.org/10.1016/j.gerinurse.2017.09.004.

Sebastiani, P., Gurinovich, A., Bae, H., Andersen, S., Malovini, A., Atzmon, G., & Perls, T. T. (2017). Four genome-wide association studies identify new extreme longevity variants. *The Journals of Gerontology: Series A, Biological Sciences and Medical Sciences, 72*(11), 1453–1464. https://doi.org/10.1093/gerona/glx027.

Severin, R., Berner, P. M., Miller, K. L., & Mey, J. (2019). The crossroads of aging: An intersection of malnutrition, frailty, and sarcopenia. *Topics in Geriatric Rehabilitation, 35*(1), 79–87. https://doi.org/10.1097/TGR.0000000000000218.

Sheikh, F., Gathecha, E., Bellantoni, M., Christmas, C., Lafreniere, J. P., & Arbaje, A. I. (2018). A call to bridge across silos during care transitions. *The Joint Commission Journal on Quality and Patient Safety, 44*(5), 270–278. https://doi.org/10.1016/j.jcjq.2017.10.006.

Shepperd, S., Gonçalves-Bradley, D. C., Straus, S. E., & Wee, B. (2016). Hospital at home: Home-based end-of-life care. *Cochrane Database of Systematic Reviews* Jul 6;(7):CD009231. https://doi.org/10.1002/14651858.CD009231.pub2.

Skinner, J.S., Duke, L., Wilkins, C.H. (2017). Why ethnogeriatrics is important. In Cummings-Vaughn, L., & Cruz-Oliver, D. M. (n.d.). *Home. VDOC.PUB.* Retrieved September 10, 2022, from https://vdoc.pub/documents/ethnogeriatrics-healthcare-needs-of-diverse-populations-136khovh4g5g

Smith, B. J., McCall, T. C., Slaven, E. M., & Smith, N. (2019). PAs are a solution to the growing need for clinicians to treat an aging population. *Journal of the American Academy of PAs, 32*(12), 46–49. https://doi.org/10.1097/01.Jaa.0000604864.79443.79.

Snow, V., Beck, D., Budnitz, T., Miller, D.C., Potter, J., Wears, R.L., … Williams, M.V. (2009). Transitions of care consensus policy statement: American College of Physicians. In Cummings-Vaughn, L., & Cruz-Oliver, D. M. (n.d.). Home. *VDOC.PUB.* Retrieved September 10, 2022, from https://vdoc.pub/documents/ethnogeriatrics-healthcare-needs-of-diverse-populations-136khovh4g5g

St Sauver, J. L., Boyd, C. M., Grossardt, B. R., Bobo, W. V., Finney Rutten, L. J., Roger, V. L., & Rocca, W. A. (2015). Risk of developing multimorbidity across all ages in an historical cohort study: Differences by sex and ethnicity. *BMJ Open, 5*(2). https://doi.org/10.1136/bmjopen-2014-006413. e006413–e006413.

Stephens, M. A., Rook, K. S., Franks, M. M., Khan, C., & Iida, M. (2010). Spouses use of social control to improve diabetic patients' dietary adherence. *Families, Systems and Health, 28*(3), 199–208. https://doi.org/10.1037/a0020513.

Tindale, L. C., Salema, D., & Brooks-Wilson, A. R. (2019). 10-year follow-up of the super-seniors study: Compression of morbidity and genetic factors. *BMC Geriatrics, 19*(1). https://doi.org/10.1186/s12877-019-1080-8. N.PAG-N.PAG.

Tisminetzky, M., Goldberg, R., & Gurwitz, J. H. (2016). Magnitude and impact of multimorbidity on clinical outcomes in older adults with cardiovascular disease: A literature review. *Clinics in Geriatric Medicine, 32*(2), 227–246. https://doi.org/10.1016/j.cger.2016.01.014.

Triplett, D. P., LeBrett, W. G., Bryant, A. K., Bruggeman, A. R., Matsuno, R. K., Hwang, L., & Murphy, J. D. (2017). Effect of palliative care on aggressiveness of end-of-life care among patients with advanced cancer. *Journal of Oncology Practice, 13*(9), e760–e769. https://doi.org/10.1200/jop.2017.020883.

Tucker, J. S. (2002). Health-related social control within older adults' relationships. *The Journals of Gerontology: Series B, 57*(5), P387–P395.

US Department of Health and Human Services Health Resources and Services Administration. (2018). *The national CLAS standards.* https://minorityhealth.hhs.gov/omh/browse.aspx?lvl=2&lvl=2&lvlid=53

US Department of Health and Human Services, Health Resources and Services Administration, Bureau of Health Workforce, National Center for Health Workforce Analysis. (2017). *Long-term services and supports: Direct care worker demand projections* 2015–2030.

US Department of Health and Human Services. (2018). *Physical activity guidelines for Americans* (2nd ed.).https://health.gov/sites/default/files/2019-09/Physical_Activity_Guidelines_2nd_edition.pdf

US Preventive Services Task Force. (2012). *Understanding task force recommendations.* https://www.uspreventiveservicestaskforce.org/Home/GetFileByID/1869

US Preventive Services Task Force. (2013). *Colorectal cancer: Screening.* https://www.uspreventiveservicestaskforce.org/Page/Document/RecommendationStatementFinal/colorectal-cancer-screening

Valtorta, N. K., Kanaan, M., Gilbody, S., & Hanratty, B. (2016). Loneliness, social isolation and social relationships: What are we measuring? A novel framework for classifying and comparing tools. *BMJ Open, 6*(4), e010799. https://doi.org/10.1136/bmjopen-2015-010799.

van der Heide, I., van Rijn, R. M., Robroek, S. J. W., Burdorf, A., & Proper, K. I. (2013). Is retirement good for your health? A systematic review of longitudinal studies. *BMC Public Health, 13*, 1180. https://doi.org/10.1186/1471-2458-13-1180.

Vangelisti, A.L. (2009). Challenges in conceptualizing social support. *Journal of Social and Personal Relationships*, 26(1), 39–51. https://doi.org/10.1177/0265407509105520; 18 10.1177/02654075091 05520

Vespa, J. (2019). *The graying of America: More older adults than kids by 2035*. https://www.census.gov/library/stories/2018/03/graying-america.html

Watson, K. B., Carlson, S. A., Gunn, J. P., Galuska, D. A., O'Connor, A., Greenlund, K. J., & Fulton, J. E. (2016). Physical inactivity among adults aged 50 years and older—United States, 2014. *MMWR Morbidity and Mortality Weekly Report, 65*(36), 954–958. https://doi.org/10.15585/mmwr.mm6536a3.

Weiss, A.J., & Elixhauser, A. (2014). *Statistical brief #180*.https://www.hcup-us.ahrq.gov/reports/statbriefs/sb180-Hospitalizations-United-States-2012.jsp

Wilkinson, R., Arensberg, M. E., Hickson, M., & Dwyer, J. T. (2017). Frailty prevention and treatment: Why registered dietitian nutritionists need to take charge. *Journal of the Academy of Nutrition & Dietetics, 117*(7), 1001–1009. https://doi.org/10.1016/j.jand.2016.06.367.

Wilson, E., Chen, A. H., Grumbach, K., Wang, F., & Fernandez, A. (2005). Effects of limited English proficiency and physician language on health care comprehension. *Journal of General Internal Medici, 20*(9), 800–806. https://doi.org/10.1111/j.1525-1497.2005.0174.x.

Working Group on Health Outcomes for Older Persons with Multiple Chronic Conditions. (2012). Universal health outcome measures for older persons with multiple chronic conditions. *Journal of the American Geriatrics Society, 60*(12), 2333–2341. https://doi.org/10.1111/j.1532-5415.2012.04240.x.

World Health Organization. (2002). *Proposed working definition of an older person in Africa for the MDS project*. https://www.researchgate.net/publication/264534627_Definition_of_an_older_person_Proposed_working_definition_of_an_older_person_in_Africa_for_the_MDS_Project

World Health Organization. (2010). *Framework for action on interprofessional education & collaborative practice*. http://whqlibdoc.who.int/hq/2010/WHO_HRH_HPN_10.3_eng.pdf

World Health Organization. (2013). *WHO definition of palliative care* https://www.who.int/cancer/palliative/definition/en/.

World Health Organization. (2015). World report on ageing and health. https://www.who.int/ageing/events/world-report-2015-launch/en/

World Health Organization. (2017). *Mental health of older adults*. https://www.who.int/news-room/fact-sheets/detail/mental-health-of-older-adults

World Health Organization. (2018, February 5). Ageing and health. https://www.who.int/news-room/fact-sheets/detail/ageing-and-health

World Health Organization. (2019). *Suicide data*. https://www.who.int/mental_health/prevention/suicide/suicideprevent/en/

World Health Organization. (2020). *About social determinants of health*. https://www.who.int/social_determinants/sdh_definition/en/

Yeatts, D. E., Seckin, G., Thompson, M., Auden, D., Cready, , Cynthia, M., & Shen, Y. (2018). Burnout among direct-care workers in nursing homes: Influences of organisational, workplace, interpersonal and personal characteristics. *Journal of Clinical Nursing, 27*(19–20), 3652–3665. https://doi.org/10.1111/jocn.14267.

Yen, I. H., Fandel Floot, J., Thompson, H., Anderson, L. A., & Wong, G. (2014). How design of places promotes or inhibits mobility of older adults: Realist synthesis of 20 years of research. *Journal of Aging Health, 26*(8), 1340–1372. https://doi.org/10.1177/0898264314527610.

Yourman, L. C., Lee, S. J., Schonberg, M. A., Widera, E. W., & Smith, A. K. (2012). Prognostic indices for older adults: A systematic review. *Journal of the American Medical Association, 307*(2), 182–192. https://doi.org/10.1001/jama.2011.1966.

Yusif, S., Soar, J., & Hafeez-Baig, A. (2016). Older people, assistive technologies, and the barriers to adoption: A systematic review. *International Journal of Medical Informatics, 94*, 112–116. https://doi.org/10.1016/j.ijmedinf.2016.07.004.

Zhang, X., Meng, X., Chen, Y., Leng, S. X., & Zhang, H. (2017). The biology of aging and cancer: Frailty, inflammation, and immunity. *Cancer Journal, 23*(4), 201–205. https://doi.org/10.1097/ppo.0000000000000270.

Ziliak, J.P., & Gundersen, C. (2017). *The health consequences of senior hunger in the United States: Evidence from the 1999–2014 NHANES*. https://www.feedingamerica.org/sites/default/files/research/senior-hunger-research/senior-health-consequences-2014.pdf.

Ziliak, J.P., & Gundersen, C. (2019). *The state of senior hunger in America in 2017*. https://www.feedingamerica.org/sites/default/files/2019-06/The%20State%20of%20Senior%20Hunger%20in%202017_F2.pdf.

4

Ethical Issues in Care

FREDDI SEGAL-GIDAN, PHD, PA AND EDEN RUIZ-LOPEZ, MPA

OBJECTIVES

Student Learning Objectives

After completing this chapter, the student should be able to do the following:

1. List the four key principles of medical ethics and how these apply to medical decision making and informed consent for patients.
2. Describe types of elder abuse or mistreatment and common risk factors associated with abuse.
3. Explain how ageism and cultural considerations interplay with ethical considerations in the care of older adults.

Practitioner Objectives

After completing this chapter, the practitioner should be able to do the following:

1. Apply the key principles of medical ethics to medical decision making in the care of older adults.
2. Incorporate patient values and preferences on a routine basis in care decisions for older adults.
3. Identify elder abuse or mistreatment, and know how to intervene and report.
4. Have awareness of the unique ethical issues faced by providers when caring for older adults and when involved in research with older adult subjects.

Introduction

Ethical issues can occur when caring for patients of any age, but they are encountered more frequently with older adults. It is therefore imperative that those caring for older adults are familiar with the principles of medical ethics, how they are applied to the older adult patient population, and common situations medical providers of older adults encounter that may include ethical conflicts. Advance directives and the presentation of personal wishes through the use of documents such as a living will, power of attorney for health care, and orders for life-sustaining care are ways that enable older adults communicate their values and wishes for care options to providers should they not be able to do so themselves. Clinicians need to be aware of the ongoing, often hidden impact of ageism in medical care and how it influences care for older adults is a component of aspects of medical care and decision making involving older adults. The assessment of decisional capacity and its impact on the ability for older adults to provide informed consent is at the heart of many of the ethical issues commonly encountered in the care of older adults. Elder mistreatment is an area of special concern when caring for older adults and one in which ethical conflicts are frequently encountered. Participation of older adults in research is important and to be encouraged, but this is another area where attention must be paid to potential ethical conflicts to ensure that older adults are treated properly.

Interprofessional Collaboration

Ethics committees are a living example of interprofessional collaboration specifically to protect patients and address moral issues that arise when there are conflicts in medical care decisions either among health professionals or among health professionals, patients, and their families. They were established in the latter decades of the 20th century as "a formal mechanism to address some of the value conflicts and uncertainties that arise in contemporary health-care settings" (Auliso & Arnol, 2008, p. 417). These committees are multidisciplinary in composition and usually include a broad spectrum of personnel. In addition to physicians, nurses, and other medical providers, the committee often includes a representative of the institution, often a member of the board, an administrator, a member of the clergy, and in some cases an ethicist, if one is available. Ethics committees have been established in most hospitals and are increasingly being created by long-term care facilities and some large organizations that deliver medical care in order to address ethical conflicts that arise as patients with serious and complex illnesses are being cared for across settings. The role of the ethics committee is to "offer assistance in addressing ethical issues that arise in patient care and facilitate sound decision making that respects participants' values, concerns, and interests" (American Medical Association [AMA], 2020). These committees generally work in an advisory capacity and provide consultation to help patients, families, and health care providers to decide what is the right thing to do in a particular situation involving a specific patient. The committees do not make decisions but provide assistance and facilitate decision making when there is a conflict about what to do or who should make a decision.

CASE STUDY

Mrs. P is a 78-year-old retired teacher, widowed for the past 6 years, who has been living in the home where she raised her three children. Two daughters live within an hour and a son lives out of state. She has type 2 diabetes, a history of breast cancer, which was treated with a left partial mastectomy 12 years ago, and osteoarthritis in her knees. She was recently hospitalized briefly after a fall in the backyard, was treated for a urinary tract infection (UTI) and hyperglycemia, and was found to have two vertebral compression fractures. The daughters noted they were surprised to find the patient's medication bottles in different places throughout the house, a stack of mail including several unpaid bills, and a number of Post-it note reminders on the mirror in the bedroom and on the kitchen cupboards.

The medical team recommended that Mrs. P be discharged to rehabilitation, but she refused and insisted on going home. Both daughters offered for her to stay with them and receive outpatient therapy while they helped her to recover, but again she refused and insisted on going home. She signed the discharge papers and a daughter drove her home from the hospital, stayed for 4 nights, met the home health nurse, and tried to hire an in-home aide for a few hours a day, but the patient refused, insisting that she could manage on her own. The daughter then returned to her home, and she or her sister now phone the patient daily and have arranged for one of them to visit on the weekend.

It has now been 10 days since Mrs. P was discharged to her home, and the home health physical therapist is calling your office and asks to speak with you as the primary care provider. She is concerned about the patient's ability to manage in her home on her own and believes she needs more care. Because the hospital discharged the patient home, it appears that hospital administrators determined she had the capacity to make this decision. Your review of the hospital notes does not show that there was any formal assessment of cognition performed, but the social worker's discharge planner did note that the daughters were concerned about the patient's ability to return to her home without assistance. In your clinic files there is a notation that the patient has a living trust and her two daughters are named jointly as her health care proxy/power of attorney for health care.

The patient has an appointment scheduled with you in 2 days You ask the office receptionist to contact the daughters and request that at least one but preferably both accompany the patient to the appointment. You also note that an assessment of capacity is needed, as well as a depression and mental status screening. Mrs. P has been a patient in the practice where you work for over a decade, so you know her well and have met her family. You know her values, know that she has long ties to the community, and have heard her express her intention is to remain in her own home, care for herself, and "not be a burden" to her children. You are conflicted about respecting Mrs. P's wishes and values and the potential risk and harm that the current situation presents to her health and well-being.

Principles of Medical Ethics

Ethical principles of medical care and practice are shared across health professions. Four basic ethical principles in medicine are used to guide decision making: autonomy, justice, beneficence, and nonmaleficence. Each one of these basic principles is considered when there is conflict or confusion about what is to be done. These principles are broad and nonspecific. They do not tell the clinician what to do but serve as reminders of what should be considered when engaged in medical decision making. Medical providers caring for older adults frequently face the challenge of balancing these competing principles, and due to a patient's advancing age and multiple medical conditions, conflicts between these principles as guidance for clinical decision making occur more frequently.

Respect for the autonomy of the individual acknowledges that every patient has the right to make decisions regarding his or her own medical care. Within this principle is the assumption that all adult patients have free will and the capacity to understand and act in their own best interest without any undue outside influence. Implicit in this principle is the understanding that individual decisions may differ based on one's beliefs, values, and personal history. In the clinical context, *autonomy* is generally understood to refer to an individual patient's authority over decisions affecting his or her own health care and body. As medical providers, physician assistants (PAs) and nurse practitioners (NPs) must respect patients' choices regarding their care and should not influence this choice based on their own values or other motivations. The principle of respect for autonomy is what underlies the concept of "informed consent" that is key to interactions, particularly those involving procedures, between patients and medical providers.

Patient autonomy has been the cornerstone of clinical bioethics for several decades. Traditionally, it has focused on the patients' capacity of to make their own decisions and on the clinician's obligation to provide patients with information that will facilitate their ability to do so adequately. Another approach is relational, where consideration is given to the social, political, and economic conditions that influence the person, process, and decision. Relational autonomy is explicitly concerned with protecting and promoting the autonomy of members of oppressed groups, which some argue should include older adults due to the ageism that is pervasive throughout society and within the medical system.

In the United States, individual choice and freedom are highly valued and closely align with the ethical principle of autonomy. In the care of older adults, the principle of autonomy comes into play when there are questions about an individual patient's decision-making ability and capacity for self-determination. This may involve conflict between patients and their family members when there is disagreement about how to proceed, whether the patient's expressed wishes are well informed or being influenced by others. Another common situation involving the principle of autonomy is when a patient is making a decision that may lead to harm through self-neglect or impaired judgment and reasoning.

Nonmaleficence requires that there is no intention to create harm or injury to the patient, through acts of either commission or omission. This principle dates back to ancient times, when the 4th-century BCE physician-philosopher

Hippocrates is said to have directed physicians "to help and do no harm." There is a fundamental commitment, some would say a duty, of health care professionals to protect patients in their care and shield them from harm. Today, it is deemed negligent if a medical provider places a patient in a position where there is an unreasonable risk of harm.

Nonmaleficence is considered a constant duty, meaning that a health professional should never harm a patient or other individual. The duty to avoid harm is central to the role of all health care providers. As patients advance in age, the risk for potential harm in providing medical care increases, which puts increased attention on this principle in the course of clinical care and decision making. The decreased physiologic reserve treatments that are considered the standard of care for young and middle-aged adults with minimal risk may become associated with more adverse effects in older patients. The presence of multiple coexisting conditions in many older adults and the medications or other treatment interventions also create an environment where the potential for harm increases. In caring for older adults, especially those who are vulnerable or frail, it may not always be possible to "avoid harm," but it is important to consider options that minimize potential harm.

Another aspect of nonmalfeasance is to refrain from providing treatment that is ineffective. This is applicable in the medical care for older adults when there is a lack of scientific information about the use of a specific drug or device in older populations. It also applies to the widespread use of many over-the-counter vitamins, herbals, and supplements that have no proven efficacy but have been shown to not be harmful. These products are sold and marketed to older adults as "safe" or "natural" solutions for a variety of ailments, and many older adults readily purchase and consume them on a regular basis.

The principle of beneficence requires health care providers to act in the best interests of the patient and by doing so to act in a manner that prevents or reduces harm to that individual patient. This is the foundation of the trust between patients and medical providers, and it underlies the core belief that medical providers are motivated to help and to heal. This principle can be applied not only to the individual but to society as a whole where the expectation is that licensed health care providers will work toward the good of all, to the benefit of everyone.

Beneficence requires that the actions health care professionals take benefit others by providing for their good. To do so requires compassion and an understanding of the patient's value system; this includes the determination of "good," which is not an absolute. The determination of "good" varies by individual and depends on a person's expressed preferences. Besides differing between patients, what an individual patient views as beneficial at one time in life may change depending on the person's life experiences and circumstances.

Justice in medical care is defined as fairness, the belief that everyone should be treated fairly. On an individual level the principle of justice translates into treating all patients equally without preferential treatment to any one person or class of individuals. On a societal level it involves the fair and equitable distribution of resources. Issues about the proper distribution of medical care services and resources to meet the needs of the older adult population often involve questions around distributive justice.

Documentation of Individual Values

To support patient autonomy and ensure that an individual's wishes are known, it is highly recommended that clinicians discuss preferences with patients and encourage patients to communicate these in writing. Since the 2010s several different documents have been developed, referred to as advance directives or advance health care directives, to facilitate written communication by patients of their values and wishes to clinicians and others. These include a living will, a health care power of attorney, and a physician/provider order for life-sustaining treatment (POLST).

An advance directive or advance health care directive refers to a legal document on which individuals specify what actions they desire regarding their health should they no longer be able to make decisions for themselves due to illness or loss of cognitive capacity. The completion of an advance directive provides an opportunity for people to think ahead about the kind of care they want or do not want in the future and to discuss this with family members and others. Its focus is solely on health care decisions, and its purpose is to serve as a guide to family members and medical providers. In the United States these documents have legal status, but in other countries they are sometimes only considered to be legally persuasive.

A living will is the broadest form of an advance directive, and the two terms are often used interchangeably. A living will is a written, legal document that focuses on end-of-life care and spells out the medical treatments a person does or does not desire in order to be kept alive. It can also include preferences for specific medical treatments, such as dialysis or use of a feeding tube, pain management, or organ donation. Five Wishes (www.fivewishes.org) is an "easy-to-use legal advance directive document written in everyday language. It helps all adults, regardless of age or health, to consider and document how they want to be cared for at the end of life." It is available in 28 languages, and there are many supportive documents on the website that can help both clinicians and patients.

The health care power of attorney (HCPOA) or power of attorney for health care (POA-HC) is a legal document that names a specific person to speak on behalf of the person executing the document should there be a time or situation when the individual is unable to communicate her or his wishes. The person who is named in the document is considered to be the health care proxy or surrogate proxy. Patients should be encouraged to discuss their preferences with the person they name as their health care proxy and to provide that person with a copy of the document. The document empowers the named person to speak with others and make decisions concerning medical treatment for the person who named him or her, as if he or she were that individual. Depending on where one lives, the terminology for the person who is designated to make medical decisions on behalf of someone may differ and be referred to by a variety of terms:

- Health care agent
- Health care proxy
- Health care surrogate
- Health care representative
- Health care attorney-in-fact
- Patient advocate

Every adult, but especially older adults, should have an HCPOA completed. For older patients it is important that this be done at a time when they are in good health and there is no question of the person's cognitive capacity to complete such a document. In an effort to encourage all adult patients to complete an advance directive, the Patient Self-Determination Act (PSDA) requires hospitals, home health agencies, nursing homes, and hospice providers to offer new patients information about advance directives. It is reported that about a third of adults have completed some type of advance directive (Yadav et al., 2017). This presents lots of opportunity for improvement and for every clinician to encourage older adult patients who have not completed one of these documents to do so. The completion of a HCPOA does not require a lawyer and can be accomplished easily. The rules and forms differ by state, so it is essential that all practicing clinicians know what is required by the state where they work. The HCPOA can be changed or revoked at any time, might require a witness, and in most cases does not need to be notarized.

The physician order for life-sustaining treatment (POLST) was developed as an end-of-life planning tool that patients can use to communicate their wishes. Depending on the state, it is also known by one of the following names:

- Portable order for life-sustaining treatment (POLST)
- Medical order for life-sustaining treatment (MOLST)
- Medical order on scope of treatment (MOST)
- Physician's order on scope of treatment (POST)
- Transportable physician order for patient preferences (TPOPP)

A national POLST form (https://polst.org/national-form/) was created in 2019 to make it easier to "honor patient treatment wishes across the United States" and promote the proper use of the form.

It does not replace an advance directive, is more specific than a durable power of attorney for health care (DPAHC) or living will, and is usually completed at a time when a patient is ill, often hospitalized or on hospice. It is also increasingly being included in forms that are completed upon admission to many long-term care facilities, such as assisted living and skilled nursing homes. The goal is to prevent unwanted to ineffective treatment at the end of life and to ensure that a patient's wishes are respected.

The POLST/MOLST was designed to give seriously ill patients a way to express more specifically their desires for particular forms of end-of-life care. The form contains instructions about medical treatments for specific medical emergencies or conditions, such as use of cardiopulmonary resuscitation (CPR), intubation, defibrillation, or a feeding tube. The form is designed to travel with the patient from one facility to another. It is printed on bright colored paper, often pink or green, so it cannot be missed or overlooked in a printed chart. Once the patient has completed the document, it is signed a physician, NP, or PA. The POLST form is a medical order and as such emergency medical personnel are required to follow its instructions regarding CPR and other emergency care.

A do not resuscitate order (or DNR) is a direction to not engage in CPR if the heart stops or a person stops breathing. It is among the most common requests included as part of an advance directive and can also be verbally requested by patient. Once entered into a person's chart, this order is followed by medical providers in all states as part of standard medical practice.

The American Medical Association (1991) has published guidelines for the appropriate use of CPR. These acknowledge the routine use of CPR in hospitalized patients who experience cardiac or respiratory arrest and that "consent to administer CPR is presumed" (p. 417). The document also recognizes that the two exceptions to this presumption favoring CPR are when a patient or a designated surrogate declines, either verbally or in writing, or when the treating physician judges that it would be futile.

The use of DNR orders varies widely across settings, diseases, and age groups. In the mid-1990s 11% of Medicare beneficiaries were found to have a DNR (Wenger et al., 1996). Two decades later, in a study of older adults' attitudes toward CPR, 44% of participants reported having a DNR (Adams & Snedden, 2008). Survival to discharge rates from CPR in a hospitalized patient are less than 10% (Di Bari et al., 2000), which has led to a growing consensus that CPR may be inappropriate for some patients and actually constitute medical futility in many cases. Although this is not true for all older adults, among those who have multiple complex medical problems, poor function, and are frail, it may be particularly true.

Factors affecting decisions around the use of CPR and DNR orders have been extensively studied, and the role of age remains controversial. Age has been found to increase the use of DNR orders, which some have argued may represent ageism, whereas others point out that it is the outcome of carrying out the wishes of the individual (Cook et al., 2017). If decisions against active resuscitation are based purely on a patient's chronologic age without considering the likelihood of survival, quality of life, or the patient's wishes, this may constitute ageism.

Ageism

The term *ageism* was first used by the gerontologist Robert Butler (2011) to describe discrimination against older people, and today is used more broadly to describe any age-based discrimination. Ageism, defined as "prejudice towards, stereotyping, or discrimination against persons solely on chronological age" is pervasive in modern society but remains hidden and not openly acknowledged or addressed (Williams, 2007, p. 1). In fact, ageism, in the form of pervasive negative attitudes about older persons, is widely accepted and normative for most cultures (Boduroglu, 2006). It is similar to other known forms of discrimination such as gender-based discrimination (sexism) and ethnicity-based discrimination (racism), but it receives far less attention.

Older persons are often overlooked, if not actively excluded, and prejudice with respect to age remains acceptable among young people. In a culture that glorifies youth, negative stereotypes of older adults abound, and aging is often treated with fear and aversion. Three common stereotypes of aging or older adults held by younger people include succession, consumption, and identification (North & Fisk, 2012). Succession refers to the belief that older individuals have "had their turn" and should step aside for younger generations. Consumption refers to the use of resources by older adults and the feeling among younger people that there are limited resources and older adults are using resources that should be available to them. Identification refers to the belief that older people should "act their age," not try to act younger than they are, or not adopt dress and speech of younger people.

Ageism is systemic; can be found in the media, the workplace, and also in health care; and is often implicit. It can be seen in how older adults are portrayed and in the use of language, images, and in attitudes. A report issued by the Institute of Medicine (2008) argued that negative attitudes toward older adults occur in the health care across professional disciplines and across care settings. Health care professionals routinely receive education and training in the care of children (pediatrics), but not in the care of the aging population. Geriatric training is not required and far fewer hours of lecture and clinical training are devoted to the care of older adults, although this population spans 3 to 4 decades and is growing, than to that of children. Older adults are often excluded from clinical trials, even though those in this population are among the largest users of drugs and devices. Screening for common medical conditions and preventive care too often does not occur—or when it does, it is an afterthought—in the provision of medical care to older adults.

There is a considerable body of research that has documented negative attitudes toward older patients by health care providers. More recently, however, there are encouraging indications of a shift in attitudes among medical students, physicians, and nurses (Liu 2012). The concern is that such attitudes produce a negative implicit bias that can influence clinical practice and decision making in the medical care for older adults. For example, studies have shown that older adults with breast cancer and lung cancer were less likely to be offered more aggressive care or some types of follow-up care than younger patients for the same type of tumor (Madan, 2006; Peak, 2003).

Communication and the language used is important factor considering any form of discrimination. Language carries and conveys meaning, which feeds assumptions and judgments that can contribute to the development of stereotypes and discrimination. The use of terms like "little old lady" or "grumpy old man" and words like "sweetie" and "dearie" when speaking with or about older patients overtly expresses a negative bias and has no place in modern medicine. The fast pace of medicine and time demands on clinicians often lead to hurried conversations, rapid speech, and distractions, which may hinder communication and lead older people to perceive that they are not being valued; in addition, the older patient may interpret the behavior as poor bedside manner or disrespect. Using a person's age as a reason or explanation for that patient's complaint is a form of ageism.

Older adult patients may themselves possess ageist attitudes and biases, referred to as self-ageism, and this can negatively impact their health care. For example, the belief that pain is normal and to be expected with increasing age may lead older adults to minimize their pain or be less likely to seek treatment (Makris et al., 2015). Negative age stereotypes held earlier in life have been found to be associated with a later increased risk for Alzheimer brain pathology (Levy et al., 2016). On the flip side, positive aging attitudes and youthful identities have been shown to contribute to better health and increased longevity in later life (Westerhof et al., 2014).

Decisional Capacity

Many ethical questions that arise in the care of older adults have to do with whether the older adult has the mental capability to make a medical decision. This focuses on issues of decisional capacity and requires a clear understanding of *competency* and *capacity*, terms that are often used interchangeably but should not be. Both terms refer to whether a person is considered able, or no longer able, to perform a specific function, in this case to make a decision. Although the two terms overlap, they are not synonymous and clinicians must have a clear understanding of the distinction between the two.

Competency describes the quality or condition of being legally qualified to perform an act. It includes the mental ability to distinguish right from wrong and to manage one's own affairs. It is a legal term, a quality that one either has or does not have, and is solely determined by the judicial system. In the United States all adults, persons over age 18, are presumed to have legal competency unless a court has determined otherwise. There are three basic minimum criteria or standards for competency: (1) the ability to communicate one's preferences or choices, (2), the ability to demonstrate an understanding of the information presented to the individual, and (3) the ability to appreciate the consequences of a decision.

Capacity differs from competency. It is a medical term that describes the ability to do, experience, or understand.

It is situation or context specific, which means that capacity can vary depending on a number of factors. It may wax and wane due to underlying medical conditions, medication affects, and the complexity of the situation and decision that needs to be made. A patient who is determined to lack decision-making capacity due to an acute illness or delirium may regain the ability with appropriate treatment.

Clinicians intuitively assess capacity at every medical encounter. If there is a reason to question a patient's decision-making ability, a more formal evaluation of capacity may be required. The determination is based on an objective assessment of the individual, either through a specific test or observable action. Medical providers, including PAs and NPs, may be asked to provide an assessment of an individual's capacity. Sometimes this may be in the context of a medical procedure or treatment, or it may be to inform a legal question regarding competency.

The standard for determining capacity varies relative to the benefits and harms expected as a consequence of the choice made. As the risk associated with a patient's choice increases, there is an increasing necessity for the clinician to pay attention to capacity and to more strictly assess whether the patient does or does not have capacity for the specific decision. A patient's refusal of recommended treatment does not mean that she or he lacks decision-making capacity (Ganzini et al., 2004). Nor does the presence of a psychiatric diagnosis or cognitive impairment in and of itself mean that the individual lacks decisional capacity.

As clinicians, PAs and NPs are obligated to promote the patient's decision-making capacity and the patient's ability to exercise autonomy. Presenting medical information using language the patient understands, avoiding medical jargon, and using terms appropriate to the patient's educational level are essential elements to enhance decision-making capacity. Asking a patient to express key ideas in his or her own words is a helpful way to evaluate the patient's understanding, especially of complex information. Making certain that patients wear glasses or use hearing aids, as needed, is important to ensure the patient's ability to understand and communicate. Whenever possible, patients should not be interviewed or asked to make a medical decision when they are experiencing pain other distressing symptoms.

Questions about medical decision-making capacity in older adults often arise in the course of caring for older adults, yet research shows that less than half the time physicians identify patients who are found to lack capacity by formal evaluation (American Bar Association, 2008). This reflects the increased prevalence of cognitive impairment that occurs with advanced age along with the interaction of chronic and acute medical conditions, the use of and interaction of multiple medications by older adults, and the complex decisions that are often required regarding evaluation or treatment in the care of older adults. Therefore it is imperative that clinicians caring for older adults be prepared for this, expect it to occur, and know how to proceed.

A patient may elect to involve others in the decision-making process or to delegate decision making to another individual, usually a family member. This can be done by verbally giving permission to another to make a decision or may be implicit by the patient's inclusion of another individual in a visit or meeting. In the latter situation it would be appropriate for a clinician to verbally ask the patient if she or he wishes to include the other individual in the decision-making process. This should be done in private to avoid the potential for undue influence or possible coercion by the other individual.

Informed Consent

Informed consent is at the core of medical decision making. It is a process based on the principle of autonomy that ensures patients are adequately informed to make medical care choices. The requirement for informed consent is considered a basic patient right. It has become an essential component of medical care whenever there is a procedure or other interventions that include any potential risk. The purpose of informed consent is to promote autonomy, to protect patients from undesired treatment, and to help patients make decisions about medical issues that align with their personal values (Ivashkov & Van Norman, 2009). Informed consent is not just a document indicating the patient's authorization; instead, it should be the result of a process that involves discussion between the provider and the patient that indicates the patient's understanding of the need for and the risk and benefit of a specific medical intervention.

The three core elements of informed consent are disclosure, decision-making capacity, and voluntariness (Sessums et al., 2011). Disclosure involves the sharing of medical information about the risks and benefits of a proposed procedure or treatment by a medical provider with a patient. The goal in disclosure is to provide the patient with sufficient information to make a decision. The challenge for the provider is to provide the information in a way that it can be adequately understood, to not provide too much information that it is overwhelming or not understandable, and to not provide too little information. Disclosure for true informed consent also requires that a provider outline the risks associated with doing nothing, such as not having a specific test or declining treatment. Decision-making capacity was discussed previously. Voluntariness means that the older adult is making the decision without coercion from anyone. Sometimes this can be difficult to assess, especially in certain cultures where patients are expected to defer to the medical provider or decisions are traditionally made by a certain family member, such as a spouse or eldest son.

Informed consent involves shared decision making, a process that consists of an *active* exchange between the medical provider and the older adult patient. The medical provider shares with the patient information about the diagnosis, prognosis, and treatment. The older adult communicates her or his values, preferences, expectations, and goals. The result is a decision made by the patient in collaboration with the provider that is the best possible one for that patient given the available options and the patient's wishes. Underlying shared decision making is the ethical principle of autonomy and the right to self-determination. There is also some evidence that shared decision making leads to better outcomes and care (Stacey et al., 2017).

The shared decision-making process requires that the treating medical provider or members of the medical team have a discussion with older adult patients that includes what their understanding is of their medical condition or diagnosis, the severity of their illness, the prognosis, what tests or treatments are being recommended and why, what treatment options are available and the potential risks and benefits of each, and the likely outcome from each test or treatment that is being proposed. For example, is a test being recommended that would change the diagnosis or the treatment, or is a treatment going to cure the problem or merely keep it from getting worse, and how sick is the treatment likely to make the patient? Within the context of this discussion, what are the patient's wishes, what is the patient's desired outcome, and how much discomfort is the older adult patient willing to endure?

Assessment and Evaluation of Capacity

Clinicians who care for older adults may be asked to assess a patient's capacity for decision making. There may be a question regarding the older adult's capacity to provide informed consent for medical care or concern about the ability of some individuals to care for themselves. Family members may want to help an older adult relative and ask for a determination by the provider of the individual's capacity. Risk factors for impaired medical decision making have been identified (Box 4.1), which includes advanced age (over 85 years). A patient who has one or more of these risk factors should never be automatically considered to be impaired or lacking a medical decision-making capacity. Rather, the clinician caring for a patient with one or more of these risk factors needs to be aware that these place the person at higher risk for impaired capacity and should be prepared to try to mitigate the risk whenever possible and, if and when necessary, be prepared to assess capacity if the need arises.

Also, a growing number of older adults have no family or friends to rely on, and in these situations a capacity evaluation may be needed in order to get the courts to appoint a guardian for a person who lacks capacity to make decisions independently. A capacity evaluation is the physician or other provider's opinion, based on objective findings, as to whether a person does or does not retain the ability to make a sound decision, usually about medical care or finances.

• BOX 4.1 Risk Factors for Impaired Medical Decision-Making Capacity

- Age <18 or >85 years
- Chronic neurologic condition
- Chronic psychiatric condition
- Low education level
- Cultural or language barrier
- Fear or discomfort with institutional medical setting

A stepwise approach to capacity assessment with an older adult is recommended. Prior to initiating a formal evaluation, it is essential to make sure that there are no communication barriers that could hinder the older adult's abilities to communicate and understand information. Does the older adult have vision or hearing difficulties, and if so, do they have glasses, hearing aids, or other devices to help compensate for these sensory deficits? What is the older adult's primary language? If the provider does not speak that language, then engagement of an interpreter is required. It is important to present the information in a manner that is consistent with the older adult's level of education and health literacy level. Medical terms should be avoided, but when they have to be used, the clinician should then provide an explanation and have the older adult repeat the information in his or her own words to ensure that the patient understands.

The next step is to evaluate for any reversible conditions that could cause impaired capacity. This requires a complete, current medical evaluation. Conditions that commonly occur in older adults and can cause the person to have impaired capacity at the time, but that may resolve with treatment, include infections, adverse effects of a medication or the interaction of two or more medications, illicit drug use, hypoxia, metabolic abnormalities, acute neurologic (e.g., stroke, subdural hematoma) or psychiatric disorders, delirium, and any acute illness.

At the outset it is important to identify any language or communication barriers that might interfere with a patient's understanding. This would include expressive language preference and access to interpreter services, expressive or receptive speech difficulties, and the presence of vision or hearing loss with correction if feasible. Next, any reversible causes of impaired capacity, such as delirium, medications, or psychiatric illness, should be identified and treated.

A directed clinical interview with the older adult is the most commonly used approach by clinicians to assess capacity regarding a proposed medical procedure or treatment. This is usually done indirectly as part of the patient interview and history taking. If the patient demonstrates basic logic during the conversation, then it is generally assumed the person has the capacity to make medical decisions. To assist clinicians conducting an evaluation of medical decision-making capacity, a series of questions directed around the four key elements of capacity—understanding, appreciation, reasoning, and the ability to communicate clearly—has been proposed (Box 4.2). The mnemonic CURVES (Choose and communicate, Understand, Reason, Value, Emergency, Surrogate) offers a quick and easy way to recall the abilities a patient must possess in order to have decision-making capacity (Chow et al., 2010).

BOX 4.2 Principles of Medical Ethics

- Autonomy
- Nonmaleficence
- Beneficence
- Justice

When there is a question about a patient's capacity for medical decision, making a more formal evaluation of capacity sometimes is necessary. Several assessment tools have been developed that clinicians can utilize to provide a more standardized and objective assessment of capacity. The Aid to Capacity Evaluation (ACE) is widely used and considered the best available online tool. It includes seven items that address each of the four key elements of capacity and has been found to have high interrater reliability when used with hospitalized medically ill patients. The MacArthur Competence Assessment Tool for Treatment (MacCAT-T) and the MacArthur Competence Assessment Tool for Clinical Research (MacCAT-CR) (Grisso & Applebaum, 1997) were designed specifically to assess capacity to consent to treatment and research. The MacCAT-T is a semistructured interview that was developed to assess all four aspects of capacity specifically for decision making about medical treatment. It is relatively quick to administer, requiring approximately 15 to 20 minutes, and has been used in psychiatric patients (those diagnosed with conditions such as schizophrenia, major depressive disorder,or anorexia nervosa), patients with dementia, and hospitalized medically ill patients. The MacCAT-CA is a 22-item structured interview that uses a vignette and scored questions to measure competence-related abilities in understanding, reasoning, and appreciation. Another tool, the Capacity to Consent to Treatment Instrument (CCTI) is a semistructured assessment that involves two hypothetical vignettes and takes about 20 minutes to complete (Marson & Cody, 1995). It assesses the four aspects of capacity, with the addition of another element, reasonableness of the decision, and has shown high interrater reliability when used to assess capacity in patients with Alzheimer dementia and Parkinson disease.

Capacity instruments improve reliability of the clinician's assessment of capacity and should be used as an aid in conducting a clinical assessment of capacity. They can help to structure the evaluation and make sure that all key elements are covered when conducting an assessment of medical decision-making capacity.

Cultural Considerations

Awareness and sensitivity to cultural and ethnic differences is essential to creating a relationship of trust between clinicians and patients. An appreciation for the cultural, religious, and ethnic backgrounds of older adult patients is essential to provide care that is informed by a respect for the patient's values and preferences. Older adults from similar ethnic backgrounds or religious affiliations, even family members, may not share the same beliefs and values, as these are also influenced by life experience. Therefore as part of the medical history, questions should be included that elicit information and insights into an older adult patient's cultural, ethnic, and religious background, beliefs, and values.

Culture connects humans to one another in ways that include shared values, beliefs, and practices concerning illness and health. Understanding different cultural views helps to shape questions to be asked and to understand responses and choices of patients. Knowing the specific content of a patient's health-related values, beliefs, preferences, or behaviors requires a willingness to ask the older adult directly about these. The clinician may or may not personally agree with these views or be able to accommodate them in a health care setting, but the medical professional should be able to recognize what they are and what is important to the patient.

We live and work in a culturally diverse society and must recognize the cultures of our own medical professions and institutions, which may at times contribute to and interfere with understanding a patient's or family's perspective. Cultural competency in medical care requires that clinicians develop respect for diversity and an understanding of how cultural values shape how people think and behave concerning their health and medical care. Students and practicing clinicians must learn to recognize their own cultural influences and to identify their own perceptions and biases that may prevent them from seeing the effects of professional medical culture on their interactions with patients and their families. When the decisions or behaviors of a patient go against our expectations, this provides an ideal opportunity to evaluate what cultural beliefs may be influencing the patient, or the clinician's, behavior. Thinking critically, as a normal part of health care work, about situations in which references to the "culture" of a patient, family, or population may represent the clinician's own uncertainty or distress.

When an older adult becomes seriously ill, the cultural expectations around decision making and family roles may become more important and apparent. In some cultures, there are beliefs that older adults should not be informed about a life-threatening condition but should be shielded from this information, with the family taking on the responsibility of carrying the burden of this information. Or there may be a belief that hearing bad news will worsen the outcome and hasten death, so information is kept from a patient. If a patient verbally asks to not be informed or requests that the clinician speak with the family, then it would be appropriate to respect the patient's wishes and do so. However, acting on the wishes of a family member without the patient's consent would not be appropriate for patients who have the capacity to make their own decision. If a patient has identified a health care proxy and that person requests that the patient not be included or told certain information, the clinician will need to establish whether this is appropriate, or not. Does the patient lack capacity to the extent that the proxy has authority to act for the patient?

Families may invoke cultural differences as the reason for requesting a clinician speak with them first and not the patient, or for excluding an older adult patient from participating in a meeting about diagnosis disclosure or treatment options. Agreeing to such a request would not be ethically appropriate if the patient retains decision-making capacity. Patients have the legal right to receive medical information about their condition or to delegate this right to someone else. Family members do not have the right, regardless of their cultural beliefs and background, to determine if a patient can or cannot participate in her or his care. And it would be wrong to assume that a patient has no preference. The burden falls on the clinician to find out how involved patients wish to be in their own medical care, how much they wish to be told, and who else they wish to include in having this information.

When a family member uses culture as a reason to exclude the patient from the decision-making process, this provides the clinician with an opportunity for further questioning and exploration. Asking questions such as "Could you help me understand what your cultural belief is?" or "I'd like to better understand what you mean. Can you explain this further?" can help to start a conversation and possibly avoid a confrontation. In this situation it may be helpful to identify a health care provider or member of the clergy who shares the same ethnic or religious background to help elucidate the cultural values and beliefs.

Elder Mistreatment (Abuse and Neglect)

Incidence/Prevalence

Elder mistreatment is a multifaceted issue that is vastly underdetected and underreported. Nationally, one in ten Older Americans over the age of 60 have encountered some form of abuse, neglect, or exploitation (Acierno et al., 2010), and this affects one in six older adults globally (Yon et al., 2017). For every case that reaches the attention of authorities, another 23.5 cases go unreported (Lachs & Berman, 2011). A meta-analysis from 2017 asserted that a more up-to-date rate of prevalence was 15.7% (Yon et al., 2017). For older people residing in the community, a 2010 study cited that as many as 11% percent had experienced abuse (Acierno et al., 2010).

The average age of an older person experiencing abuse is in the mid to upper 70s, and two-thirds of the victims are female (Roberto, 2016). People with dementia are twice as likely to experience abuse (Mosqueda et al., 2016) as are people of any age who are dependent on others for activities of daily living (ADLs). Thirty percent of adults with disabilities who used personal assistance services (PAS) for assistance with activities of daily living reported one or more types of mistreatment by their care provider (Oktay & Tompkins, 2004).

Consequences of Elder Mistreatment

The consequences of elder mistreatment are grave. Older persons who are victimized are three times more likely to die as a result of elder abuse and may experience great financial losses or psychological trauma (Storey et al.,1998). Outcomes and consequences spanning physical and mental deterioration, injury, long-term emotional illness, hospitalization, being institutionalized, frailty, and even mortality have all been noted (Podnieks & Thomas, 2017). This issue is also a global threat to public health (Yunus et al., 2019). Additional research has pointed out that sleeping problems (Olofsson et al., 2012), gastrointestinal symptoms (Stöckl & Penhale, 2015), and suicidal ideation (Wu et al., 2013) may be present in victims. Loneliness and a tendency to be socially withdrawn—which occurs when older people socially isolate themselves and choose not to undertake hobbies; visit family members, friends, or neighbors; and participate in social activities within their communities—is another often underrecognized consequence (Wong & Waite, 2017). There is also the social consequence of an increase of expenditures to offset those lost due to exploitation (Anetzberger, 2004).

Definitions of Types of Abuse

The National Center on Elder Abuse defines elder abuse as referring to any known, intentional, or negligent act by a caregiver or any other person that causes harm or a serious risk (of harm) to an older person (National Center on Elder Abuse, 2016b). There are several other accepted definitions of elder abuse, and the most relied on are cited from both the Centers for Disease Control and Prevention (CDC) and the World Health Organization (WHO). The CDC (2021) defines elder abuse as "an intentional act or failure to act that causes or creates a risk of harm to an older adult" (p. 1), and the WHO (2021) refers to it as "a single, or repeated act, or lack of appropriate action, occurring within any relationship where there is an expectation of trust which causes harm or distress to an older person" (p. 1).

The types of elder abuse or elder mistreatment are categorized as physical, emotional, or psychological, and sexual abuse, neglect, and financial exploitation. It is not uncommon to hear of an older person experiencing more than one form of mistreatment at the same or different time, which is called polyvictimization. Polyvictimization is defined as "multiple co-occurring or sequential types of elder abuse by one or more perpetrators, or one type of abuse perpetrated by multiple others with whom the older adult has a personal, professional, or care recipient relationship in which there is a societal expectation of trust" (Ramsey-Klawsnik et al., 2014, p. 5; Ramsey-Klawsnik, 2017).

Physical abuse can manifest in several ways, where an older person is physically injured or impaired and a perpetrator uses physical force, coercion, or constraints. Signs that physical abuse may be occurring are evidence of cuts, bruises, burns, welts (National Center on Elder Abuse, 2018), and signs of the use of restraints to make an older person bed or chair bound. In a study of bruising patterns, bruises located in specific areas of the body may be characteristic of physical abuse (Fig. 4.1). The researchers found that bruises located on the lateral or anterior surface of an older person's arm, back, or face may have been inflicted as

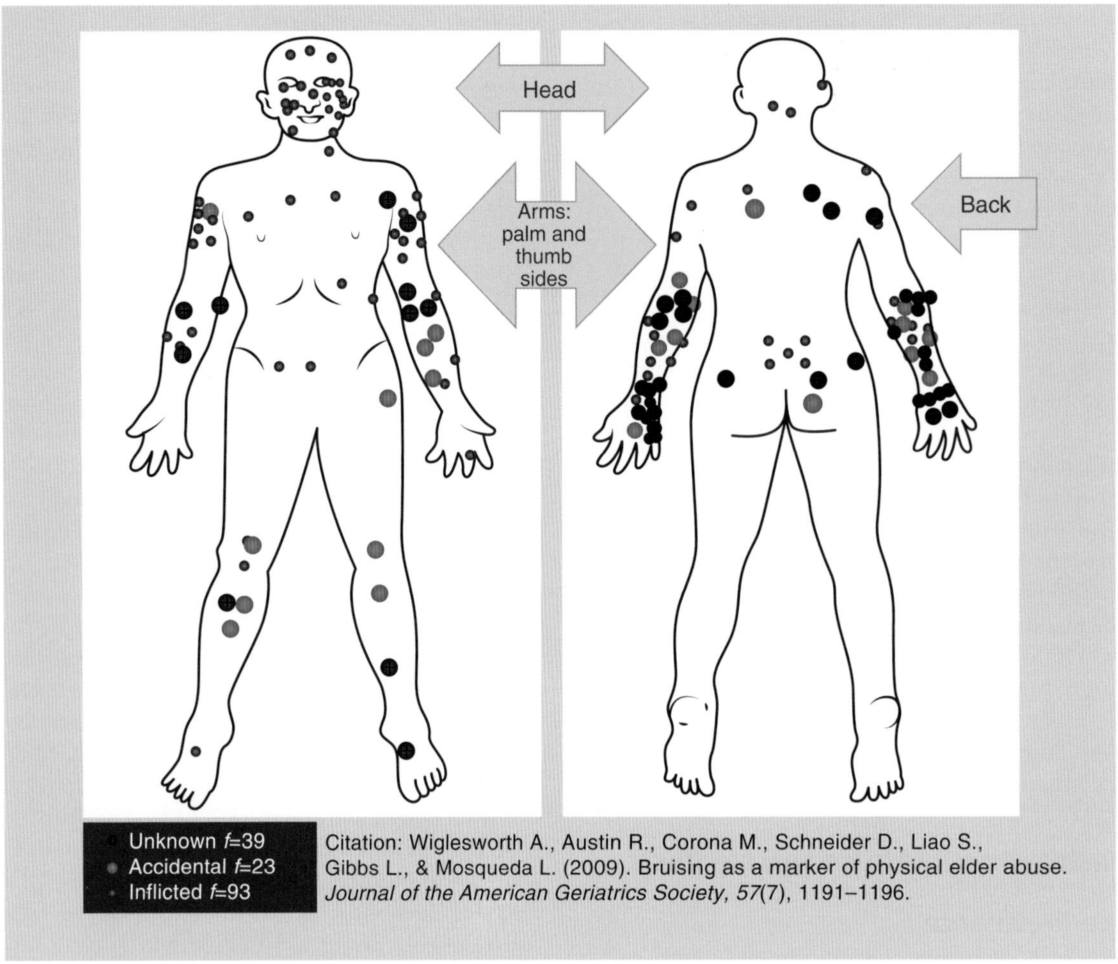

• **Fig. 4.1** Bruising patterns elder abuse. (Adapted from Wiglesworth, A., Austin, R., Corona, M., Schneider, D., Liao, S., Gibbs, L., & Mosqueda, L. [2009]. Bruising as a marker of physical elder abuse. *Journal of the American Geriatrics Society, 57*[7], 1191–1196.)

a result of physical abuse, especially if at least one bruise was 5 centimeters or larger (Mosqueda et al., 2005). Medication misuse as a chemical restraint to excessively or needlessly sedate an older person is also considered a form of physical abuse that can often be overlooked or missed.

Psychological or emotional abuse consists of threats, isolation, belittling, emotional rejection, or verbally attacking an older person. Evidence of this type of abuse may include someone exhibiting anxiety, being fearful, showing signs of depression or psychological distress, being socially withdrawn, showing signs of restlessness or sleeplessness, isolation, or behavioral changes (National Center on Elder Abuse, 2018).

Sexual abuse involves any nonconsensual act that is often forced, tricked, or threatened upon an older person. It may also happen in the form of unwanted touching, being exposed to someone's genitals (National Center on Elder Abuse, 2018), or a person being forced to watch pornography. It is not uncommon to see other forms of abuse grouped with sexual abuse—for example, psychological abuse. Older people who have been sexually abused might show signs of anxiety, avoidance, and apprehension. An older person may have contracted a sexually transmitted infection or may have ripped and soiled clothing.

Neglect is defined as the inability to meet an older person's basic needs, which may jeopardize the person's safety and emotional or physical well-being. Some common symptoms of neglect include bedsores, unattended medical needs, a disheveled appearance, evidence of poor hygiene, and unusual weight loss or evidence of malnutrition (National Center on Elder Abuse, 2018). Evidence of neglect may include an older person (1) lying in his or her own urine and feces for extended periods of time, (2) being malnourished or having pressure sores due to a lack of appropriate care, (3) having a dirty, disheveled appearance, elongated nails, and living in a filthy environment, or (4) existing in hazardous or unsafe living conditions or arrangements (e.g., in domiciles where there is improper wiring, no heat, or no running water).

Not all states recognize the term self-neglect or screen for it in intervention efforts or direct response. Self-neglect may rather be considered a form of neglect because there is a failure or refusal of people in an older adult's life to provide the essentials such as food, water, clothing, shelter, personal hygiene, medicine, comfort, and personal safety based on an implied or agreed-upon responsibility to the older adult. It is in situations of self-neglect where ethical issues of autonomy and self-determination by the patient and the duty of the medical provider to "do good" and "do no harm" come sharply into conflict.

Financial exploitation is thought to be the most prominent form of abuse (some argue that neglect is actually the most prevalent but is underrecognized) because it is often the most reported form. It can be elaborate and committed by either someone known to the older person or a complete stranger who is trying to scam that older person. Financial exploitation is defined as theft or fraud, and it results from the abuse of power by someone who intends to have illegal access to a person's property, possessions, or money. Signs of financial exploitation may include forging signatures on documents, committing theft, unauthorized use of debit or credit cards, liquidating assets, or extorting money through cash, wire transfers, or gift cards (National Center on Elder Abuse, 2018).

Older patients might come into a hospital or clinical setting and tell the clinician that they cannot afford to fill prescriptions because they lent money to a caregiver who needed help with rent and utilities for the month. Patients may tell clinicians that they did not receive an order of sanitizer, gloves, and other household disinfecting supplies, and they do not know what to do. It may also not be uncommon for a caregiver to accompany a patient into the clinic for an appointment and then pull the clinician aside to request capacity assessments or signatures on power of attorney documents. Although this is not always abuse, this common scenario has the potential for ethical conflict, and clinicians need to recognize that the situation may not be as benign as it appears.

Risk Factors of Abuse

Social isolation is the leading risk factor for abuse, and it may lead to a lack of access to supports and resources as well as unmet physical, mental, and emotional needs. In a review of elder abuse and neglect risk factors, Storey (2020) found problems with physical health, mental health, substance abuse, dependency, stress and coping, and attitudes that excuse or justify perpetrator behavior or lead to low worth and value, as well as victimization (meaning that older persons who experienced child abuse or domestic violence face a higher likelihood of experiencing abuse in later life) (Acierno et al., 2010; Fulmer et al., 2005; Lachs & Pillemer, 1995).

Who Are the Perpetrators?

Perpetrators are oftentimes in a known and trusted relationship with the older person; for example, the perpetrator could be a child, grandchild, or caregiver. Although family members are most often the perpetrators of elder abuse (Holtfreter et al., 2014; Lachs & Berman, 2011; Naughton et al., 2012), the characteristics and identity of perpetrators will vary according to the type. Financial exploitation has been found to most often be perpetrated by family members or care workers, followed by partners (Jackson, 2016). Neglect is frequently committed by adult children, paid caregivers, and spouses (Lach & Berman, 2011). Partners or spouses and acquaintances are most frequently the perpetrators of physical abuse (Acierno et al., 2009). Although there are scant data on perpetrators of sexual abuse, a 2009 study reported that sexual abuse was most often perpetrated by partners or spouses, followed by acquaintances and strangers (Acierno et al., 2009). Pertaining to psychological or verbal abuse, partners or spouses are most often the perpetrators, along with acquaintances, followed by other relatives (Acierno et al., 2009; Jackson, 2016).

The average perpetrator is 45 years old (Brownell et al., 1999; Jackson & Hafemeister, 2011), 56% to 62% are Caucasian males (Brownell et al., 1999; Jackson & Hafemeister, 2011), 70% are unmarried (Jackson & Hafemeister, 2011), between one-third and two-thirds are unemployed (Acierno et al., 2009; Brownell et al., 1999; Jackson & Hafemeister, 2011; Naughton et al., 2012), and 25% to 35% have a mental illness (Amstadter et al., 2011; Brownell et al., 1999; Clancy et al., 2011; Jackson & Hafemeister, 2011; Lowenstein et al., 2009).

Assessment Tools

It is not always easy to recognize elder mistreatment or abuse. The American Medical Association (AMA, 2020) recommends that screening for elder abuse should be part of the care for all older adults (Burnett et al., 2014). In busy medical practices, cases can easily get overlooked or signs and symptoms missed or dismissed by clinicians. It takes vigilance and a willingness on the part of clinicians to consider the possibility that intentional harm is being inflicted on an older adult patient in the person's home by a trusted family member or in a facility by a professional paid staff member. Screening has been shown as a way to help prevent and detect elder abuse. There is no gold standard or single accepted universal screening tool. A number of validated tools have been developed to help clinicians identify and assess for elder abuse with the goal of improving identification and decreasing both the number of victims and the severity of abuse. Table 4.1 provides a brief listing of a few commonly used elder abuse screening tools and the setting for which they are designed to be used.

Reporting

An older person's account of being abused should be taken seriously. When questioned directly, a patient may deny the abuse or lack insight about being victimized, whether or not tthe patient has cognitive impairment. It is not the role of a clinician to prove that abuse is occurring but to report suspected abuse to the appropriate authority for further investigation. Licensed health care providers, including PAs and NPs, are considered mandated reporters and have a

TABLE 4.1 Elder Abuse Screening Tools

Tool	Number of Items	Setting
Elder Abuse Suspicion Index (EASI)	6	Family practice and ambulatory care
Hwalek-Sengstock Elder Abuse Screening Test (H-S/EAST)	6	Outpatient or emergency dept
Vulnerability to Abuse Screening Scale (VASS)	12	Emergency medical settings

Adapted from Burnett, J., Achenbaum, W. A., & Murphy, K. P. (2014). Prevention and early identification of elder abuse. *Clinics in Geriatric Medicine, 30*(4), 743–759.

TABLE 4.2 Red Flags for Potential Elder Abuse

Type of Abuse	Signs or Symptoms
Physical	Broken bones, bruises, welts, burns Untreated bed sores Torn, stained blood under clothing Unexplained sexually transmitted disease Dirtiness, poor nutrition, poor hygiene Poor living conditions Lack of medical aids (glasses, dentures, medications)
Emotional and psychological	Unusual changes in behavior or sleep Fear or anxiety Isolated or nonresponsive Depression
Financial	Unusual changes in bank account or money management Unusual changes in will, trust or other financial documents Fraudulent signatures on financial documents Unpaid bills

Adapted from the National Center on Elder Abuse (NCEA). (2018). Signs of elder abuse. Retrieved from https://ncea.acl.gov/NCEA/media/Publication/NCEA_SignsEA.pdf

legal as well as ethical duty to identify and report suspected abuse. Beyond reporting, the ethical duty to care for one's patient requires that clinicians seek help if they hear or see red flags of abuse (Table 4.2) while meeting with a patient. For example, clinicians may turn to a social worker or other professionals who are capable of assisting with filing reports. If someone's life is in imminent danger, it is important to contact 9-1-1.

To report suspicions of abuse for a community-dwelling older person, reports should be filed with both local law enforcement and Adult Protective Services (APS). APS can ensure that the safety and well-being of older persons is upheld and that the organization is able to triage and investigate allegations. Beyond that, APS can provide referrals for local social services, housing, medical or legal service programs, and other supportive services and can monitor and evaluate each case it receives (National Center on Elder Abuse, 2019), among other interventions available in the victim's location.

For people residing in long-term care settings (e.g., nursing home, acute rehabilitation facilities, or assisted living), a combination of reports should be filed with law enforcement and long-term care ombudsmen, otherwise known as resident advocates and the department of public health (the licensing and certification division) or community care licensing depending on the classification of facility. The long-term care ombudsman program is by design a consent-based program, so victims will have to provide consent in order for an ombudsman to investigate complaints. The ombudsman will seek to resolve complaints and provide education, regular facility visits, and promote council involvement to residents and family members (National Center on Elder Abuse, 2019).

Any person who has assumed full or intermittent responsibility for the care or custody of an older person or a person with a disability regardless of age, often referred to as a dependent adult, whether or not that person is paid for the role, is considered a mandated reporter. This is an area where rules vary state by state. Such persons may include administrators, supervisors, and any licensed staff of a public or private facility that provides care or services to people. Also included among mandated reporters are any care custodians, health practitioners, clergy members, and employees of a county adult protective services agency or a local law enforcement agency. Failure of a mandated reporter to report any form of abuse, neglect, or exploitation can result in fines, prison time, or other legal consequences. It also leaves the older adult vulnerable to continued victimization and the likelihood that the situation will get worse. The ethical duty to do good and avoid harm requires that clinicians report suspected elder abuse. Information on mandatory reporting laws and other state-specific laws that focus on filing charges, state statues, and consumer protection statues can be found at the National Center on Elder Abuse (NCEA) website.

Not surprisingly, there are a number of barriers to the detection and reporting of suspected elder mistreatment by clinicians. Five barriers that have been identified are professional orientation, how to conduct an assessment, interpretation of the assessment, the requirement to report a suspected case within the medical institution, and the requirement to alert the external public health or social service system. Lack of knowledge and adequate education for assessing and addressing the abuse and neglect of older adults has been found to be a hindrance across multiple professions. To address these barriers, some health care systems have developed protocols to assist clinicians. Additional strategies include photographically documenting the home environment, additional training, improved direct communication with social workers, a dedicated location on existing forms or new forms to document concerns, a reporting hotline, and a system to provide feedback to emergency medical services and community paramedics (Rosen et al., 2017).

Resources

The NCEA is one of 27 federally funded resource centers administered by Health and Human Services and the Administration for Community Living developed to improve the national response to elder abuse, neglect, and exploitation. The center educates and shares the latest research, publicizes information on national policy, and promotes best practices in the field (National Center on Elder Abuse, 2016a). The NCEA has developed a wealth of resources for both the public and medical providers (Box 4.3) that can be easily accessed from its website. For example, with partners at the National Adult Protective Services Association (NAPSA), the center has created "Adult Protective Services, What You Must Know," which provides a thorough explanation of what APS is and what it does, coupled with a helpful set of frequently asked questions (FAQs). Working with partners at the National Consumer Voice for Quality, Long-Term Care, the organization has published a fact sheet, "Long-Term Care Ombudsman Program, What You Must Know," that explains what the ombudsman program is as well as what ombudsmen do, provides an overview of residents' rights, and walks through some helpful FAQs.

Driving and Older Adults

With one in five drivers over age 65, providers caring for older adults will increasingly encounter issues about when a patient is no longer safe to drive and face ethical conflicts that are inherent in this area of clinical practice. The ethics of clinical decision making about when to report the health-related driving risk of an older driver to state licensing authorities are challenging and not an area of medical practice for which there are easy-to-apply guidelines. At its core is the conflict between patient autonomy and safety. As health care providers, PAs and NPs have responsibility to provide care and maintain confidentiality, but they also have a duty to ensure public health and safety. Additional ethical considerations include confidentiality and trust, which form the basis of the therapeutic relationship between patients and providers. Added to this is the uncertainty about how to determine individual driving risk and safety.

Physiologic changes associated with normal aging and diseases that commonly affect older adults may compromise their ability to drive safely. Older adults are more than twice as likely to have a medical problem that can make driving difficult compared to younger adults. Determining when in the course of aging or a specific disease an individual is no longer safe to drive is not always apparent. Changes in sensory processing, especially vision but also hearing, can impact one's ability to drive. Chronic diseases such as diabetes with peripheral neuropathy, dementia, and other neurologic conditions, as well as medication or drug use that compromises cognitive processing and response time, may increase the risk of crashes while driving. Some states require reporting of specific conditions (i.e., seizures), but few offer exact guidelines while placing the onus on medical providers for determining medical competence to drive.

Driving is a privilege, not a right, that is granted by the state, but it also carries a lot of social value. When the question of competence to operate a motor vehicle arises, the ethical issues of benefit of continued driving for the individual versus potential risk to that individual, others, or society must be considered.

There is a lot of uncertainty when it comes to determining individual driving safety and risk. Providers must employ clinical reasoning and judgment, risk assessment, and knowledge of state reporting laws in determining how to act. Most older adults are safe drivers, but when there is impairment, patients are often reluctant or unable to recognize that they are impaired or to accurately assess the risk for potential harm to themselves or others. This anosognosia (lack of awareness or lack of insight) is in itself an indication that the older adult has an impairment.

Clinicians need to be prepared to address the issue of driving impairment with their older patients. Asking about any recent automobile accidents or driving tickets is a nonthreatening way to raise the topic of driving safety. When there are concerns about a patient's ability to safely operate a motor vehicle, it may be useful to ask family members whether they have noticed any scratches or damage to the person's car or if they have any concerns about their relative's ability to drive. A positive answer to one or more of three

• BOX 4.3 Selected Elder Abuse Resources

Available Through the National Center on Elder Abuse (NCEA; https://ncea.acl.gov)

Elder Abuse Screening Tools for Healthcare Professionals
Mandated Reporting of Abuse of Older Adults and Adults with Disabilities
Taking Care of You—Tips for The Family Caregiver
Archstone Caregiver Brochure—You Are Their Advocate
The Facts of Elder Abuse
Research to Practice Translation: Bruising in Older Adults (2014)

Signs of Elder Abuse Available on Other Websites

Center for Elder Justice: https://eldermistreatment.usc.edu/
Elder Abuse Guide for Law Enforcement: https://eagle.usc.edu/
Training Resources on Elder Abuse: https://trea.usc.edu/

simple questions should alert the clinician to a need for further assessment of driving safety:

1. Do you feel safe riding in the car with this person driving?
2. Would you allow a young child to ride in the car with this person driving?
3. Would you feel safe knowing that a young child was playing on the street where this person was driving?

Research Participation

Ethical issues are frequently encountered in the area of research that involves the participation of human subjects. The ethical issues that arise in the design and conduct of research involving older adults are the same as those related to research on human subjects generally, but they become more evident and potentially problematic when older adults are involved due to some of the unique aspects of this population. PAs and NPs will increasingly be involved in caring for older patients who are engaged in research studies and in facilitating referrals of older adult patients in their care to clinical trials and other research studies. Thus it is imperative that they have a solid understanding of the ethical issues related to the research participation of older adults so they can both support older adult participation in research and know when to advocate for or against the participation in research of an older adult whose care they are involved in.

Until the 1980s those over age 65 were automatically excluded from clinical trials, as well as many research studies. This underrepresentation in clinical trials was found to cause difficulties for clinicians with subsequent disadvantage to older adults (Crome et al., 2011). Although there are problems associated with the inclusion of the older adults in clinical trials, their exclusion altogether poses greater problems. Excuses in protocols have been found to be rooted in ageism, where those of advanced age (sometimes 60, 65, or 70) and above are often excluded based on erroneous concerns that patients over this age are not reliable or fully competent, are unable to follow instructions, and have a higher rate of poor compliance and increased likelihood of dropping out.

Older adults as a group were considered to be in the category of a vulnerable population that required special consideration when included in research. A vulnerable population is defined for purposes of research as a group that requires special consideration due to an inherent increased risk associated with the group's characteristics. Three identified vulnerable populations when conducting research are children, pregnant women, and prisoners. Age by itself does not meet the criteria of vulnerability, and thus most older individuals should be considered eligible to participate in research.

Some groups of older adults, not all, clearly do fall within the definition of a vulnerable population that will require additional safeguards, but members of these groups may still be suitable for research participation. Such subgroups of older adults include those with multiple chronic medical problems, chronic mental health conditions, nursing home residents, home bound patients, those with impaired cognitive capacity, and those who are terminally ill and dying. Research can proceed with individuals from these populations but requires additional measures to assure that those participating are doing so within accepted clinical and ethical practice.

With the growing older adult population, the need for knowledge about the older population based on data that include representation from this population and is not extrapolated from younger persons has become increasingly apparent and necessary. Research involving young and middle-aged persons as subjects of medical investigations may have limited applicability to an older adult and does not necessarily benefit the older population. It is essential that inclusion of older adults in research is promoted based on the principle of distributive justice. The application of an appropriate ethical framework can facilitate the engagement of older persons in all areas of biomedical research. This has required a change in thinking about inclusion and exclusion criteria, how to assess the benefit-burden ratio, and consideration of issues related to the process of informed consent, assessment of competency, and protection of privacy (Sepett et al., 2011).

Realistically there are a number of very real reasons that make involvement of older adults in research challenging. The existence of one or more chronic conditions and daily use of multiple medications may place them at higher risk for adverse events and often excludes older adults from meeting inclusion criteria for studies. Practical difficulties such as the research study location, transportation, and social and cultural barriers also serve to discourage older adults from participation. The older adult population has also been a less attractive potential market for pharmaceutical companies and other product developers, but that is changing with the growth of the older adult population in the United States and worldwide.

Recruitment of older adults into research studies involves a number of potential ethical conflicts, some that are obvious and others that are more subtle. It is well recognized that individuals are more inclined to participate in a study if it is recommended to them by their health care provider, in whom they have an established relationship and trust (Stevens & Pletsch, 2002). Patients may feel unintentionally pressured to agree to participate when approached by their medical provider or an associate. They may want to please the provider by agreeing to participate, or they may believe they will get better care by participating. On the other hand, there may be a concern that they will receive poor care, be considered uncooperative, or be abandoned by their medical provider if they decline participation (Steinke, 2004). Older adults who are socially isolated or lonely may seek to participate in research as a way of social interaction, and those who are poor may view research participation as a way to gain increased access to care.

One area of ethical conflict in clinical research that often goes unrecognized by clinicians is therapeutic misconception. This refers to a situation in which research participants mistakenly believe they are to receive some form of treatment or care (Lidz & Applebaum, 2002). This is most common in clinical trials but can occur in any research that involves a clinical intervention. A related issue is researcher role conflict, which occurs when the researcher is expected to perform two roles with different and sometimes opposing sets of expectations—that of the researcher and that of the health care provider. This can be confusing to the research participant who is unclear when interacting with the health professional whether it is as research participant and researcher or patient and medical provider.

An essential component of research participation, as outlined in the Nuremburg code, is that consent be voluntary. In order to do research, a participant must have the capacity to give informed consent, which requires that the individual possess sufficient knowledge and comprehension of the elements of the research including the purpose, risks and benefits, duration of participation, and any conflicts of interest and institutional affiliations of the researchers. This is where ethical issues can arise with more frequency when older adults are involved. The determination of capacity to give informed consent becomes more of an issue among research participants of advanced age or those at any age who have identified medical conditions (stroke, dementia, psychiatric illness, vision or hearing loss, etc.) that are known to impact memory, comprehension, or judgment, or that may eventually do so if the study requires participation over time. When an older adult is legally incompetent, physically or mentally unable to give consent, or found to lack capacity, informed consent must be obtained from the older adult's legally authorized representatives in accordance with applicable law.

Exclusion of cognitively impaired older adults from research has been justified based on the principle of autonomy. This, however, violates the principle of justice, especially if the research could not otherwise be conducted in a way that would benefit the older population. Thus current thinking among researchers, clinicians, and ethicists is that regardless of age or other circumstances that may make older adults more vulnerable, they should not systematically be excluded from research.

Unique Situations of Ethical Conflict for Physician Assistants and Nurse Practitioners

The working relationship of PAs and NPs with physicians creates a situation that can lead to ethical conflicts. These are not confined to working with older adults and may occur when caring for patients of any age, but they become more complicated when the patient is an older and possibly dependent adult. What are PAs or NPs to do when they disagree with the physician they work with about the plan of care or treatment? If the patient is someone who the PA or NP has an established relationship with and the physician does not, this may become an especially difficult situation. How these situations are avoided or handled requires discussions between clinicians *before* the circumstances arise, starting with the recognition that these are real possibilities in modern-day practice.

Whether employed in a private practice or by a health system, it is important for clinically practicing PAs and NPs to have a possibly difficult but necessary frank and open conversation with the physician or physicians with whom they work about how best to handle situations in which providers disagree about appropriate care. The situation is no different than when such disagreement occurs between two treating physicians. Foremost to keep in mind is patient-centered care and the principle of autonomy. Providing the patient with information and options, as unbiased as possible, would be the preferred course, as well as to follow the patient's expressed wishes, or those of the patient's surrogate if the patient is unable to express her or his wishes at the time.

NPs and PAs often experience ethical conflict associated with their perceived professional obligations to advocate for patients. Clinical providers can find themselves caught between the rules and expectations of the health plan or system in which they work and advocating for their patients' best interests and needs. The increasing role that insurance providers, and in particular managed care companies, play in determining treatment options adds to this dilemma. Similar to studies focusing on physicians, studies on NPs have found that they experience ethical conflicts in providing primary care to patients in managed care settings (Ulrich et al., 2003). With a growing portion of Medicare beneficiaries enrolled in managed care plans (Medicare Advantage), clinicians caring for older adults can expect to experience more challenges to their treatment decisions and increasing conflicts with their role as patient advocates. Many experience, on a daily to weekly basis, third-party decisions by insurance companies that interfere with their ability to provide necessary treatment. The tension between the obligation to the patient and costs of care is an ever-present reality in today's medical system that can create ethical conflict for medical providers. Payers, usually insurance companies, face very real financial pressures to limit services or access to expensive procedure or treatments. Barriers of additional paperwork, such as requests for medical records and completion and submission of prior authorization, require providers to spend time that is often not reimbursable or not considered as part of productivity.

The conflict of interest between pharmaceutical representatives and health care providers has been receiving increased scrutiny. PAs and NPs are not immune from this challenge and need to be aware of research that has documented the influence pharmaceutical marketing can have on providers and the care they provide. Psychological research has shown that the impulse to "return the favor" exists in the recipient of even a small gift. Thus it is not surprising that the receipt of gifts from vendors has been shown to influence provider prescribing behavior (Brennat et al., 2006).

Key Points

- Ethical principles of care are the same for older adults as for individuals of any age.
- Ethical conflicts arise more commonly in the care of older adults and most often are around questions of capacity for decision-making and end-of-life care.
- Older adults can assure their values are honored and potentially reduce ethical conflicts by completing an advance health care directive.
- Elder abuse and driving are two areas where medical providers caring for older adults often encounter ethical issues.
- The inclusion of older adults in research requires attention to ethical considerations unique to this population.

More information about tools and Interprofessional Education Collaborative (IPEC) competencies mentioned in this chapter can be found in Appendix 1: Tools and Appendix 2: IPEC Competencies.

References

Acierno, R., Hernandez, M. A., Amstadter, A. B., Resnick, H. S., Steve, K., Muzzy, W., & Kilpatrick, D. G. (2010). Prevalence and correlates of emotional, physical, sexual, and financial abuse and potential neglect in the United States: The national elder mistreatment study. *American Journal of Public Health, 100*(2), 292–297.

Acierno, R., Hernandez, M. A., Muzzy, W., & Steve, K. (2009). *National elder mistreatment study* (Final report submitted to the National Institute of Justice. Document No. 226456). https://www.ncjrs.gov/pdffiles1/nij/grants/226456.pdf.

Adams, D. H., & Snedden, S. P. (2008). How misconceptions among elderly patients regarding survival outcomes of inpatient cardiopulmonary resuscitation affect do-not-resuscitate orders. *Journal of the American Osteopathic Association, 106*, 402–404.

American Bar Association, American Psychological Association. (2008). *Assessment of older adults with diminished capacity: A handbook for psychologists*. http://www.apa.org/pi/aging/programs/assessment/capacity-psychologist-handbook.pdf.

American Medical Association. (1991). Guidelines for the appropriate use of do-not-resuscitate orders. Council on Ethical and Judicial Affairs, American Medical Association. *Journal of the American Medical Association, 265*(14), 1868–1871.

American Medical Association. (2020). *Ethics committees in health care institutions*. https://www.ama-assn.org/delivering-care/ethics/ethics-committees-health-care-institutions.

Amstadter, A. B., Cisler, J. M., McCauley, J. L., Hernandez, M. A., Muzzy, W., & Acierno, R. (2011). Do incident and perpetrator characteristics of elder mistreatment differ by gender of the victim? Results from the national elder mistreatment study. *Journal of Elder Abuse & Neglect, 23*, 43–57.

Anetzberger, G. (2004). *The clinical management of elder abuse*. Hawthorne Press.

Auliso, M. P., & Arnol, R. M. (2008). Role of the ethics committee: Helping to address value conflicts or uncertainties. *Chest, 134*(20), 417–424.

Barstow, C., Shahan, B., & Roberts, M. (2018). Evaluating medical decision-making capacity in practice. *American Family Physician, 98*(1), 40–46.

Boduroglu, A., Yoon, C., Luo, T., & Park, D. C. (2006). Age-related stereotypes: A comparison of American and Chinese cultures. *Gerontology, 52*, 324–333.

Brownell, P., Berman, J., & Salmone, A. (1999). Mental health and criminal justice issues among perpetrators of elder abuse. *Journal of Elder Abuse & Neglect, 11*(4), 81–94.

Butler, R. (2011). *The longevity prescription*. Avery.

Burnett, J., Achenbaum, W. A., & Murphy, K. P. (2014). Prevention and early identification of elder abuse. *Clinics in Geriatric Medicine, 30*(4), 743–759.

Centers for Disease Control and Prevention. (2021). *Violence prevention: Elder abuse*. https://www.cdc.gov/violenceprevention/elderabuse/index.html.

Chow, G. V., Czarny, M. J., Hughes, M. T., & Carrese, J. A. (2010). CURVES: A mnemonic for determining medical decision-making capacity and providing emergency treatment in the acute setting. *Chest, 137*(2), 421–427.

Clancy, M., McDaid, B., O'Neill, D., & O'Brien, J. G. (2011). National profiling of elder abuse referrals. *Age and Ageing, 40*, 346–352. https://doi.org/10.1093/ageing/afr023.

Cook, I., Kirkup, A. L., Langham, L. J., Malik, M. A., Marlow, G., & Sammy, I. (2017). End of life care and do not resuscitate orders: How much does age influence decision making? A systematic review and meta-analysis. *Gerontology & Geriatric Medicine, 3*. https://doi.org/10.1177/2333721417713422.

Crome, P., Lally, F., Cherubini A., et al. (2011). Exclusion of older people from clinical trials: Professional views from nine European countries participating in the PREDICT study. *Drugs Aging, 28*(8), 667–677. (PMID:21812501)

Di Bari, M., Chiarlone, M., Fumagalli, S., Boncinelli, L., Tarantini, F., Ungar, A., et al. (2000). Cardiopulmonary resuscitation of older, inhospital patients: Immediate efficacy and long-term outcome. *Critical Care Medicine, 28*, 2320–2325.

Fulmer, T., Paveza, G., VandeWeerd, C., Fairchild, S., Guadagno, L., Bolton-Blatt, M., & Norman, R. (2005). Dyadic vulnerability and risk profiling for elder neglect. *The Gerontologist, 45*(4), 525–534. https://doi.org/10.1093/geront/45.4.525.

Ganzini, L., Volicer, L., Nelson, W. A., Fox, E., & Derse, A. (2004). Ten myths about decision-making capacity. *Journal of the American Medical Directors Association, 5*, 263–267.

Grisso, T., Appelbaum, P., & Hill-Fotouhi, C. (1997). The MacCAT-T: A clinical tool to assess patient's capacities to make treatment decisions. *Psychiatric Services, 48*, 1415–1419.

Holtfreter, K., Reisig, M. D., Mears, D. P., & Wolfe, S. E. (2014). *Financial exploitation of the elderly in a consumer context* (Final report submitted to the National Institute of Justice. Document No. 245388). https://www.ncjrs.gov/pdffiles1/nij/grants/245388.pdf.

Institute of Medicine. (2008). *Retooling for an aging America: Building the health care workforce*. National Academies Press.

Ivashkov, Y., & Van Norman, G. A. (2009). Informed consent and the ethical management of the older patient. *Anesthesiology Clinic, 27*(3), 569–580.

Jackson, S. (2016). All elder abuse perpetrators are not alike: The heterogeneity of elder abuse perpetrators and implications for intervention. *International Journal of Offender Therapy and Comparative Criminology, 60*(3), 265–285. https://doi.org/10.1177/0306624X14554063.

Jackson, S. L., & Hafemeister, T. L. (2011). Risk factors associated with elder abuse: The importance of differentiating by type of elder maltreatment. *Violence and Victims, 26*, 738–757.

Lachs, M., & Berman, J. (2011). Under the radar: New York state elder abuse prevalence study, self-reported relevance and documented case surveys. http://www.ocfs.state.ny.us/main/reports/Under%20the%20Radar%2005%2012%2011%20final%20report.pdf.

Lachs, M. S., & Pillemer, K. (1995). Abuse and neglect of elderly persons. *The New England Journal of Medicine, 332*(7), 437–443. https://doi.org/10.1056/NEJM199502163320706.

Levy, B. R., Ferrucci, L., Zonderman, A. B., Slade, M. D., Troncoso, J., & Resnick, S. M. (2016). A culture-brain link: Negative age stereotypes predict Alzheimer's disease biomarkers. *Psychology and Aging, 31*(1), 82–88.

Lidz, C. W., & Applebaum, P. S. (2002). The therapeutic misconception problems and solutions. *Medical Care, 40*(Suppl), V55–V63.

Liu, Y. E., While, A. E., Norman, I. J., & Ye, W. (2012). Health professionals' attitudes toward older people and older patients: A systematic review. *Journal of Interprofessional Care, 26*(5), 397–409.

Lowenstein, A., Eisikovits, Z., Band-Winterstein, T., & Enosh, G. (2009). Is elder abuse and neglect a social phenomenon? Data from the first national prevalence survey in Israel. *Journal of Elder Abuse & Neglect, 21*, 253–277.

Madan, A. K., Cooper, L., Gratzer, A., & Beech, D. J. (2006). Ageism in breast cancer surgical options by medical students. *Tennessee Medicine, 99*(5), 37–38. 41.

Marson, D., Ingram, K., Cody, H., & Harrell, L. E. (1995). Assessing the competency of patients with Alzheimer's disease under different legal standards. *Archives of Neurology, 52*, 949–954.

Mosqueda, L., Burnight, K., & Liao, S. (2005). The life cycle of bruises in older adults. *Journal of the American Geriatrics Society, 53*(8), 1339–1343.

Mosqueda, L., Burnight, K., Gironda, M. W., Moore, A. A., Robinson, J., & Olsen, B. (2016). The abuse intervention model: A pragmatic approach to intervention for elder mistreatment. *Journal of the American Geriatrics Society, 64*(9), 1879–1883.

National Center on Elder Abuse. (2016a). *About us*. https://ncea.acl.gov/About-Us.aspx.

National Center on Elder Abuse. (2016b). *Data and statistics*. https://ncea.acl.gov/About-Us/What-We-Do/Research/Statistics-and-Data.aspx#05.

National Center on Elder Abuse. (2018). *Signs of elder abuse*. https://ncea.acl.gov/NCEA/media/Publication/NCEA_SignsEA.pdf.

National Center on Elder Abuse. (2019). *Frequently asked questions*. https://ncea.acl.gov/FAQ.aspx.

The National POLST Paradigm Taskforce: National POLST Paradigm Webpage [online]. www.polst.org.

Naughton, C., Drennan, J., Lyons, I., Lafferty, A., Treacy, M., Phelan, A., & DeLaney, L. (2012). Elder abuse and neglect in Ireland: Results from a national prevalence survey. *Age and Ageing, 41*, 98–103. https://doi.org/10.1093/ageing/afr107.

North, M. S., & Fiske, S. T. (2012). An inconvenienced youth? Ageism and its potential intergenerational roots. *Psychological Bulletin, 138* (5), 982–997. https://doi.org/10.1037/a0027843.

Oktay, J. S., & Tompkins, C. J. (2004). Personal assistance providers' mistreatment of disabled adults. *Health & Social Work, 29*(3), 177–188.

Olofsson, N., Lindqvist, K., & Danielsson, I. (2012). Fear of crime and psychological and physical abuse associated with ill health in a Swedish population aged 65–84 years. *Public Health, 126*(4), 358–364.

Peake, M. D., Thompson, S., Lowe, D., & Pearson, M. G. (2003). Ageism in the management of lung cancer. *Age and Ageing, 32*(2), 171–177.

Podnieks, E., & Thomas, C. (2017). The consequences of elder abuse: *Elder abuse* (pp. 109–123). Cham: Springer.

Ramsey-Klawsnik, H. (2017). Older adults affected by polyvictimization: A review of early research. *Journal of Elder Abuse & Neglect, 29*(5), 299–312.

Ramsey-Klawsnik, H., Heisler, C., Gregorie, T., Quinn, K., Roberto, K. A., & Teaster, P. B. (2014). Polyvictimization in later life. *Victimization of the Elderly and Disabled, 17*(1), 3–6. http://www.napsa-now.org/wp-content/uploads/2016/08/701-Polyvictimization-in-Later-Life.pdf.

Roberto, K. (2016). The complexities of elder abuse. *The American Psychologist, 71*(4), 302–311.

Seppet, E., Pääsuke, M., Conte, M., Capri, M., & Franceschi, C. (2011). Ethical aspects of aging research. *Biogerontology, 12*(6), 491–502.

Sessums, L. L., Zembrzuska, H., & Jackson, J. L. (2011). Does this patient have medical decision-making capacity? *Journal of the American Medical Association, 306*, 420–427.

Stacey, D., Légaré, F., Lewis, K., Barry, M. J., Bennett, C. L., Eden, K. B., et al. (2017). Decision aids for people facing health treatment or screening decisions. *Cochrane Database of Systematic Reviews,* Issue 4, Art No. NCD001431.

Steinke, E. E. (2004). Research ethics, informed consent, and participant recruitment. *Clinical Nurse Specialist, 18*, 88–95.

Stevens, P. E., & Pletsch, P. K. (2002). Informed consent and the history of inclusion of women in clinical research. *Health Care for Women International, 23*, 809–819.

Stöckl, H., & Penhale, B. (2015). Intimate partner violence and its association with physical and mental health symptoms among older women in Germany. *Journal of Interpersonal Violence, 30*(17), 3089–3111.

Storey, J. E. (2020). Risk factors for elder abuse and neglect: A review of the literature. *Aggression and Violent Behavior, 50*, 101339.

Ulrich, C. M., Soeken, K. L., & Miller, N. (2003). Ethical conflict associated with managed care: Views of nurse practitioners. *Nursing Research, 52*, 168Y175.

Wenger, N. S., Pearson, M. L., Desmon, K. A., Harrison, E. R., Rubenstein, L. V., Rogers, W. H., et al. (1996). Epidemiology of do-not-resuscitate orders: Disparity by age, diagnosis, gender, race, and functional impairment. *Archives of Internal Medicine, 156*, 2497–2498.

Westerhof, G. J., Miche, M., Brothers, A. F., Barrett, A. E., Diehl, M., Montepare, J. M., et al. (2014). The influence of subjective aging on health and longevity: A meta-analysis of longitudinal data. *Psychology and Aging, 29*(4), 793–802.

Williams, M. (2007). Invisible, unequal, and forgotten: Health disparities in the elderly. *Notre Dame Journal of Law, Ethics, and Public Policy, 21*, 442–478.

Wong, J. S., & Waite, L. J. (2017). Elder mistreatment predicts later physical and psychological health: Results from a national longitudinal study. *Journal of Elder Abuse & Neglect, 29*(1), 15–42.

World Health Organization. (2021). *Ageing and the life-course: Elder abuse.* https://www.who.int/ageing/projects/elder_abuse/en/

Wu, L., Shen, M., Chen, H., Zhang, T., Cao, Z., Xiang, H., & Wang, Y. (2013). The relationship between elder mistreatment and suicidal ideation in rural older adults in China. The. *American Journal of Geriatric Psychiatry*, *21*(10), 1020–1028.

Yadav, K. N., Gabler, N. B., Cooney, E., Kent, S., Kim, J., Herbst, N., Mante, A., Halpern, S. D., & Courtright, K. R. (2017). Approximately one in three US adults completes any type of advance directive for end-of-life care. *Health Affairs (Millwood)*, *36*(7), 1244–1251. https://doi.org/10.1377/hlthaff.2017.0175. PMID: 28679811.

Yon, Y., Mikton, C. R., Gassoumis, Z. D., & Wilber, K. H. (2017). Elder abuse prevalence in community settings: A systematic review and meta-analysis. *The Lancet Global Health*, *5*(2), e147–e156.

Yunus, R. M., Hairi, N. N., & Choo, W. Y. (2019). Consequences of elder abuse and neglect: A systematic review of observational studies. *Trauma, Violence, & Abuse*, *20*(2), 197–213.

5

Sexuality in Older Adults

PHYLLIS ATKINSON, RN, GNP-BC

OBJECTIVES

Student Learning Objectives

After completing this chapter, the student should be able to do the following:

1. Identify the myths surrounding sexual practice in older adults.
2. Describe the normal changes of the male and female sexual systems.
3. Describe the pathologic problems of the aging male and female sexual systems.
4. Discuss environmental barriers to older adults' sexual practices and the ways to manipulate these barriers.
5. Conduct an assessment interview related to an older adult's sexuality and intimacy.
6. Identify alternatives to an older adult's sexual practice other than sexual intercourse.

Practitioner Objectives

After completing this chapter, the practitioner should be able to do the following:

1. Generate knowledge from clinical practice to improve practice and patient outcomes related to sexuality and sexual health.
2. Evaluate the ethical consequences of patients' decisions related to sexuality and sexual health.
3. Provide patient-centered care recognizing cultural diversity and the patient or designee as a full partner in decision making about sexual health.
4. Educate professional and lay caregivers to provide culturally and spiritually sensitive appropriate care around issues of sexuality and sexual health.
5. Demonstrate interpersonal and communication skills that result in effective information exchange with patients, patients' families, physicians, professional associates, and other individuals within the health care system about sexuality and sexual health.
6. Demonstrate a high level of responsibility, ethical practice, and sensitivity to sexuality and sexual health among a diverse patient population.
7. Assess, evaluate, and improve patients' care practices surrounding their sexuality.

Overview of Sexuality in Older Adults

The sexual well-being of older adults is a topic that received little attention or scientific study until the 2010s. Much of what was taught or believed to be true was based on folklore, hearsay, and individual experience. With the aging population increasing, not only in the United States but across the world, the importance of sexuality among older adults has been recognized and the research has increased.

The Global Study of Sexual Attitudes and Behaviors (GSSAB) was first published online in 2004. It was the first large, multicountry survey to systematically study the attitudes, beliefs, and health in sexual relationships in middle-aged and older adults. There were 13,888 women and 13,618 men, ages 40 to 80 years, in 29 countries (Laumann et al., 2005). Until 2007, there were no comprehensive, nationally representative, population-based data available to inform health care providers' understanding of the sexual norms and problems of older adults. Lindau et al. (2007) designed the National Social Life, Health, and Aging Project (NSHAP) to provide data on the sexual behaviors and problems of older adults. Their landmark study had a sample of 1550 women and 1435 men, ages 57 to 85, residing in the United States and found sexual activity was an important part of older adults' lives.

DeLamater (2012) completed an extensive review of the literature dating back to 1996 and concluded that men and women remain sexually active into their 70s and 80s. He and Koepsel completed another review of the literature in 2015 and found men reported greater incidence and frequency of sexual activity, including sexual intercourse than women.

Sexuality is a key component of health and functioning that changes with age (Waite et al., 2017). Human sexuality includes various types of intimate activity, as well as the sexual knowledge, beliefs, attitudes, and values of individuals. After retirement, older adults often feel useless and lose self-esteem. Remaining sexually active can improve feelings of self-esteem and usefulness. Sexually active older adults help their partners express love, affection, and loyalty. It can also enhance personal growth, creativity, and communication. Older persons, especially older women, who feel desirable and attractive often report also feel younger (Messinger-Rapport et al., 2003).

Although the need to express sexuality continues as one ages, older adults face several barriers to sexual expression, including problems arising from low desire, aging, disease, and medications; societal beliefs; and changes in social circumstances (Lindau et al., 2007). Nurse practitioners (NPs) and physician assistants (PAs) are in a pivotal position to assess normal aging changes, along with those caused by disabling medical conditions and medications, and to intervene at an early point to enhance sexuality in older adults.

According to the World Health Organization (WHO, 2013), sexual health is defined as a state of physical, mental, and social well-being in the sphere of sexuality. It is not limited by age. Intrinsic to the right to sexual health is a positive and respectful approach to sexuality and sexual relationships, as well as the possibility of having sexual experiences that are pleasurable and safe, free from coercion, discrimination, violence, and disease. Sexuality is influenced by the interaction of biologic, psychological, social, economic, political, cultural, ethical, legal, historical, religious, and spiritual factors (WHO, 2002).

The absence of male partners for older women generates the stereotype that older adults should not participate in sexual relationships. The life span of men in the United States is shorter than that of women. According to "The Population 65 Years and Older in the United States: 2016 American Community Survey Reports," there were more females than males. Among the older population, those ages 65 to 74 had the highest sex ratio (88), while the population 85 and older had the lowest sex ratio (53), representing nearly two females for every male. Although most of the older population had been married at some point in their lives, a majority of older females (72%) were widowed by the age of 85 and older, while more than half of their male counterparts were still married. This often leaves older women without sexual partners. The loss of a partner does not necessarily mean that women do not have continuing sexual needs. Liu et al. (2016) found men were more likely to report being sexually active, having sex more often and more enjoyably than older women. Greater life expectancy and improved health care results in older adults living longer with chronic conditions that impact all aspects of their life, including sexuality. PAs and NPs in all settings need to be able to provide the tools and resources older adults need to cope with sexual health changes that will be impacted by chronic diseases (Traeen et al., 2017).

Flynn and Gow (2015) found frequency of sexual behavior had a significant association with quality of life in the social relationship domain. They also found the importance of sexual behaviors was significantly associated with the psychological domain. This association was independent of the presence of a spouse/partner and self-reported health. In a 2017 study, Wardecker et al. (2018) found that heterosexuals as well as lesbian and gay individuals experienced increases in life satisfaction across adulthood, whereas bisexuals' life satisfaction did not increase. Syme et al. (2013) also found sexuality to be integral to quality of life for older adults.

Santos-Iglesias, Byers, and Moglia (2016) studied the sexual well-being (SWB) of 149 men and 148 women from ages 65 to 75 and found they overall reported a positive SWB. Both men and women reported a positive SWB despite whether they were or were not in a relationship. Those who were in a relationship engaged in frequent genital and no-genital sexual activity. Two-thirds of the participants had experienced at least one sexual difficulty in the previous 3 months, and only 25% were distressed by the difficulty. Similarly, Gillespie (2017) found that older adults with active and satisfying sex lives reported situational, behavioral, and attitudinal synchronicity. Many of the participants reported that good sex was an important part of life.

Waite et al. (2017) studied the effect of those with optimistic personalities and concluded that husbands who were high in positivity showed higher levels of sexual activity. These findings were mediated by individuals thinking about sex and believing sex was an important part of one's quality of life.

Sexuality Process

There are several normal physiologic changes associated with aging that affect sexual function. DeLamater's 2012 and DeLamater and Koepsel's 2015 review of the literature found that these aging-related physical changes do not always lead to a decline in sexual function. In fact, they stated there is little evidence to support the belief that age-related physical changes are associated with reduced sexual activity. DeLamater et al. (2015) summarized that age-related changes can contribute to sexual functioning; however, an individual's sexual satisfaction is dependent upon that individual's response to the age-related changes (Box 5.1).

Women usually do not have difficulty maintaining sexual function in older age unless a medical condition intervenes. The most noticeable changes in women are due to the declining function of the ovaries during climacteric and subsequent hormonal changes with a marked decrease in estrogen. There is vaginal dryness and atrophy associated with this decline in estrogen that occurs after menopause. The atrophic vagina leads to vaginitis and irritation, as well as pain and bleeding during intercourse (DeLamater, 2012). A lack of sexual interest (33.2%) and lubrication difficulties (21.5%) were the most common female sexual problems found in Laumann et al. (2005, 2009) studies. Urinary incontinence from detrusor insufficiency or stress can cause embarrassment during intercourse (Messinger-Rapport et al., 2003). The age-related shortening and narrowing of the vagina may further compromise pleasurable intercourse (Butler and Lewis, 2000). Women may also have increased facial hair from decreased estrogen levels, causing them to feel less attractive (Butler and Lewis, 2000). Decline in the erotic sensitivity of nipple, clitoral, and vulvar tissue during sexual activity is also common among older women (Agronin 2017. Traeen and colleagues' review of the literature in their 2017 article cited the most important predictors of sexual problems and distress among older women was whether they have a partner and whether that partner has sexual problems.

Common physiologic changes associated with aging men is a slow decline in testosterone production, which may lead

• BOX 5.1 Normal Changes of the Aging Male Sexual System

Normal Changes of the Aging Male Sexual System

- The penis may take longer to become firm and may not be as firm as at a younger age; therefore, a longer period of foreplay should be planned.
- Ejaculation may take longer to achieve, may be less expulsive, and may be shorter in duration. The client should conserve strength and not work hard at the beginning of intercourse, which could result in tiring before climax.
- The erection diminishes more quickly after climax, so if condoms are being used, the client should plan to withdraw immediately after climax.
- It takes longer to achieve a second orgasm, so the client should plan to resume foreplay or use this time to touch or talk.
- Rectal sphincter contractions may be experienced, but these do not interfere with orgasm.

Normal Changes of the Aging Female Sexual System

- Vaginal secretions diminish; the use of an artificial water-based lubricant helps decrease discomfort.
- The vagina becomes shorter and does not expand as well to accommodate the penis. Some discomfort may be experienced, so alternative positions for intercourse (see Fig. 13.1) may help decrease discomfort.
- Orgasmic contractions are fewer and may be accompanied by painful uterine contractions. However, these generally do not indicate pathologic problems.
- Vaginal irritation and clitoral pain are common and do not signify illness.
- The breasts lose tone, and the areolar area does not enlarge as considerably.
- Infrequent rectal sphincter contractions that do not interfere with orgasm and the postcoital need to void may be experienced.

to slower erections, less firm erections, and decreased likelihood of orgasms (DeLamater, 2012). Men also experience less preejactulatory fluid, and semen that is less forceful at ejaculation (Butler & Lewis, 2000; Messinger-Rapport et al., 2003). The refractory period between ejaculations is long. Andropause (male menopause) has several physical, sexual, and emotional symptoms. There is disagreement about which term should be used to accurately describe the phenomenon. Most endocrinologists now use the term *ADAM*, an acronym for Androgen Decline in the Aging Male (Blackwell, 2006). Serum sex hormone-binding globulin (SHBG) concentrations gradually increase as a function of age, resulting in less free testosterone. Testosterone levels diminish with age from a reduction in both testosterone production and metabolic clearance. These hormonal changes lead to a loss of libido, decreased muscle mass and strength, alterations in memory, diminished energy and well-being, an increase in sleep disturbance, and possibly osteoporosis secondary to a decrease in bone mass. Testosterone appears to influence the frequency of nocturnal erections; however, low testosterone levels do not affect erections produced by erotic stimuli (Kaiser, 2000; Messinger-Rapport et al., 2003). Despite these physiologic changes, aging men can still experience orgasmic pleasure (Messinger-Rapport et al., 2003). Early ejaculation (26.2%) and erectile dysfunction (22.5%) were the most common male sexual problems reported in the Laumann et al. (2009) study.

Libido appears to be testosterone dependent in both men and women. Women experience a decline in both ovarian hormones and adrenal androgens in the years preceding menopause. In both genders, the reduced availability of sex hormones in older adults results in less rapid and less extreme vascular responses to sexual arousal (Wise & Crone, 2006). Although some older adults view this gradual slowing as a decline in function, others do not consider it an impairment, as it merely results in taking more time to achieve orgasm (Butler and Lewis, 2000).

Erectile dysfunction (ED) (impotence), the inability to develop and sustain an erection for satisfactory sexual intercourse in 50% or more attempts at intercourse, can occur at any age but does increase with age. For example, over their 9-year study period, sexual intercourse or activity frequency decreased by less than once per month, two times per month, and three times per month in men in their 40s, 50s, and 60s, respectively. The number of erections per month declined by 3, 9, and 13 in men in their 40s, 50s, and 60s, respectively (Araujo et al., 2004). Waite et al. (2017) found few health factors were associated with differences in frequency of sex. Erectile dysfunction revealed the strongest negative association with frequency of sex. Erectile disorder affects 20% to 40% of men in their 60s and 50% to 70% of men in their 70s to 80s (Agronin, 2017). Causes of erectile dysfunction include structural abnormalities of the penis; the adverse effects of drugs; psychologic disorders; and vascular, neurologic, and endocrine disorders. In addition to age, the best predictors of ED are diabetes mellitus, hypertension, obesity, dyslipidemia, cardiovascular disease, smoking, and medication use (Agronin, 2017). The frequency of ED in men with diabetes increases with age. In one report, the prevalence increased from 6% in men ages 20 to 24 years to 52% in those ages 55 to 59 years (Agronin, 2017). It is most common to have more than one cause of erectile dysfunction in older men (Wise & Crone, 2006).

To assist older adults in fulfilling their sexual desires most effectively, NPs and PAs need to understand the normal changes of the aging sexual system. Knowledge about these normal changes enable providers to work more confidently with individuals to compensate for these changes, to assist them in understanding these changes, and to become aware of possible pathologic problems within the aging sexual system. In 1966, Masters and Johnson developed the sexual response cycle, which encompassed four phases that included excitement, plateau, orgasm, and resolution. More current models have attempted to demedicalize the cycle and added stages to include psychological and physiologic changes: desire, arousal or excitement, plateau, orgasm, and resolution. The 2019 Geriatrics at Your Fingertips chapter on the sexuality of older adults (Ruben et al., 2019) noted that older men have a delay in erection, decreased tensing of the scrotal sac, and loss of testicular elevation in the excitement phase. Older women's clitorises require longer direct stimulation, and they experience reduced and delayed vaginal lubrication. Older males may be able to stay in the plateau phase longer before they climax, in comparison to when they were younger, which may or may not enhance the overall pleasure. Older men have reduced preejaculatory secretion, and older women have less expansion and congestion of the vagina. For older men and women, orgasm is reduced in intensity and duration. Older men experience a prolonged refractory period between erections. Older women experience a more rapidly loss of vascular congestion during the resolution phase.

Conditions Affecting Older Adults' Sexual Response

There are many illnesses, surgeries, and medications as well as environmental and psychological barriers that affect sexual function in an older adult. Sexual function is a process that depends on the interaction of the neurologic, endocrine, and vascular systems. These organ systems are increasingly involved with diseases as one ages that can contribute directly or in combination to changes in sexual function (see Table 5.1). A thorough laboratory assessment is also needed to rule out conditions contributing to sexual dysfunction. Refer to Box 5.2.

Sexual function is also influenced by several psychosocial factors, including family and religious beliefs, the sexual partner, and the individual's self-esteem (Wise & Crone, 2006). Previous levels of sexual interest and function are strongly correlated with sexual activity later in life (Dhingra et al., 2016).

Syme et al. (2013) used data from the Wisconsin Longitudinal Study to perform a case-control study on the risk factors for sexual unwellness in older adults ages 63 to 67. They concluded there was a higher risk for lack of such a sexual satisfaction associated with poor spousal health, a history of diabetes, and fatigue symptoms. In addition, being of male gender, being satisfied with martial support, and having better spousal health reduced the risk of being sexually unsatisfied. Higher risk for being unable to maintain the sexual relationship was independently associated with higher education level, poorer self-related health, better spousal health, a history of diabetes, prostate cancer, fatigue, sexual pain, and a history of depression. They found a greater number of partnership factors, more than individual health factors, were related to lack of sexual satisfaction. Individual health factors were prominent when predicting whether an older adult is decreasing or stopping sexual activity. Their review of the literature concluded sexual well-being probably plays a significant role in successful aging. Similarly, DeLamater (2012) and DeLamater and Koepsel (2015) found a positive relationship between good physical and mental health and frequency of sexual activity in both men and women. Through a review of the literature, DeLamater and Koepsel (2015) found positive attitudes about the importance of sexual expression are associated with increased sexual activity. Men are more likely to rate sex as important to themselves. As individuals age, married couples as well as lesbian couples desire emotional intimacy, stability and continuity

TABLE 5.1 Organ System and Impact on Sexual Function

Common Diseases for Each Organ System	Impact of Sexual Function
Chronic renal disease	Fatigue, malaise, lower testosterone
Cardiovascular disease	Erectile and ejaculatory dysfunction, desire, arousal, and orgasm
Diabetes mellitus	Erectile dysfunction, hypogonadism, loss of lubrication, hypogonadism, dyspareunia, and reduced orgasm
Chronic pulmonary disease	Testosterone depression, inability to participate, secondary shortness of breath
Cancer	Dysphoria, decreased orgasmic ability, decreased libido, dyspareunia, vaginal dryness
Genitourinary	Erectile dysfunction, ejaculatory dysfunction, and hypoactive sexual desire, avoidance of sexual activities due to psychological distress, arousal disorders, painful sexual intercourse, orgasmic phase difficulties, and reduced sexual satisfaction
Muscular skeletal	Impaired sexual activity due to pain and stiffness
Sensory deficits	Loss of sexual excitement due to loss of familiar stimuli
Neuropsychiatric	Depression and anxiety: decreased sexual desire and arousal Chronic pain: reduced libido Dementia: inappropriate sexual behaviors, reduced sexual interest, aggressive or insensitive sexual behaviour Parkinson disease: sexual disorders due to incoordination Schizophrenia: lower rates of coital orgasm Personality disorders: erectile dysfunction

From Wise, T. N., & Crone, C. (2006). Sexual function in the geriatric patient. *Clinical Geriatrics*, *14*(12), 17–26. https://searchebscohostcom.ezproxy.libraries.wright.edu/login.aspx?direct=true&db=rzh&AN=106272806&site=eds-live; Dhingra I, DeSousa A, Sonavance S. (2016). Sexuality in older adults: Clinical and psychological dilemmas. *Journal of Geriatric Mental Health* 3, 131–139; Agronin, M. (2017). *Sexual dysfunction in older adults*. https://www.uptodate.com/contents/sexual-dysfunction-in-older-adults

• BOX 5.2 Laboratory Tests to Guide Sexual Assessment

- Total serum testosterone
- Dihydrotestosterone
- Estradiol
- Mean gonadotropin-releasing hormone
- Serum luteinizing hormone
- Serum prolactin
- Prostate-specific antigen
- Complete blood count
- Complete metabolic panel
- Thyroid-stimulating hormone

instead of penetrative sex (DeLamater & Koepsel 2015). Depressive symptoms were broadly associated with worse sexual health, more so than physical function, anxiety or stress, or age itself (Wang et al., 2015).

High frequency of sex is positively related to later risk of cardiovascular events for men but not women, and good sexual quality seems to protect women but not men from cardiovascular risk in later life (Liu et al., 2016.) Liu et al. also found no evidence that poor cardiovascular health interferes with later sexuality for either gender.

Surgeries can also affect an older adult's sexual responses. Some of these surgeries include coronary artery bypass surgery, hysterectomy, mastectomy, prostatectomy, orchiectomy, and removal of anus and rectum.

HIV

According to the Centers for Disease Control (CDC) and Prevention HIV Surveillance Report (2017), nearly half of people in the United States living with diagnosed HIV are ages 50 and older. Though new HIV diagnoses are declining among people ages 50 and older, around one in six HIV diagnoses in 2016 were in this group. People ages 50 and older accounted for 17% (6812) of the 39,782 new HIV diagnoses in 2016 in the United States. People ages 50 to 54 accounted for 43% (2959) of the new diagnoses among people ages 50 and older. Among people ages 55 and older who received an HIV diagnosis in 2015, 50% had HIV 4.5 years before diagnosis, the longest diagnosis delay for any age group.

A study by Lovejoy et al. (2008) revealed that sexual activity was more prevalent among HIV-positive older adults who were not cognitively impaired, were younger, and considered themselves to be in good health. According to their study, most of those having sex were male, took Viagra, and were in a relationship.

Per the CDC (2022) people may have many of the same HIV risk factors as their younger counterparts, but they also face unique issues placing them at higher risk. Social capital as defined by the Organization for Economic Co-operation and Development (OECD) are "networks together with shared norms, values and understandings that facilitate co-operation within or among groups." Amin (2016, p. 983) used the General Social Survey (GSS) from 2012 and found social capital was positively associated with other human immunodeficiency virus/sexually transmitted disease risk behaviors such as sex with strangers, having multiple sex partners, injecting drugs, and having male-to-male sex. Older women are no longer worried about becoming pregnant so are less likely to use a condom to practice safer sex. Age-related thinning and dryness of vaginal tissue may raise older women's risk for HIV infection. Although older adults visit their health care providers more frequently, they are less likely than younger people to discuss their sexual or drug use behaviors with them and health care providers are less likely to ask their older patients about these issues. Stigma and isolation due to illness or loss of family and friends may prevent older adults from seeking HIV care and disclosing their HIV status. HIV increases the risk for cardiovascular disease, bone loss, and certain cancers, which makes aging with HIV infection present special challenges to older adults and their medical providers. Older HIV patients need to be careful about interactions between the medications used to treat HIV, cholesterol, and obesity. According to the CDC, older adults also see sexually transmitted infections (STIs) as something that happens to somebody else. Women outnumber men, giving men many partners to choose from; older women may try to please their male partners by agreeing to unprotected sex. Today's older adults grew up when men made most of the decisions in a relationship, and if a man does not want to use a condom, then it is not used. Favors are also known to occur in community settings such as retirement homes, assisted living facilities, and even long-term care facilities, including women performing sex acts in trade for cigarettes.

Malignancies

One of the most common and distressing consequences of cancer treatment is sexual dysfunction. Altered gonadal function and surgical disfigurement can be long-term results affecting sexuality in cancer survivors among older adults. Bober and Varela (2012) reviewed the most common sexual problems found among cancer survivors and highlighted the most promising evidence-based practices for assessment and interventions. Bober and Varela list low desire, arousal, pain, and lubrication problems as being the most common difficulties with sexuality among female cancer survivors. Male cancer survivors typically have issues with erectile dysfunction, loss of libido, and loss orgasmic satisfaction. Other issues men may face are hot flashes, fatigue, gynecomastia, and emotional lability (Bober & Varela, 2012). Bober and Varela's review of the literature revealed most women over the age of 65 are more likely to stop sexual activity after surgery for gynecologic cancer. Older women also report lower sexual functioning and quality of life after treatment for vulvar malignancy. Older men take twice as long to recover their sexual function compared to their younger counterparts after undergoing a radical prostatectomy (Table 5.2).

TABLE 5.2 Cancer Type and Impact on Sexual Function

Type of Cancer	Effect on Sexuality
Breast	Decreased desire, problems with lubrication, arousal, lubrication, and orgasm, dyspareunia, body image concerns, poor nipple sensation, fatigue, decreased libido
Prostate	Erectile dysfunction: may take 2–3 years to recover, retrograde ejaculation
Colorectal	Erectile and ejaculatory disorder, dyspareunia decreased libido, changes in orgasm
Bladder	Erectile dysfunction
Vaginal	Pain
Bone marrow	Orgasm problems, pain, vaginal dryness
Female genitourinary	Lower desire, dyspareunia, vaginal atrophy

Data from Bober, S., & Varela, V. (2012). Sexuality in adult cancer survivors: Challenges and interventions. *Journal of Clinical Oncology, 30*(30). 3712–3719; and Wise, T. N., & Crone, C. (2006). Sexual function in the geriatric patient. *Clinical Geriatrics*, *14*(12), 17–26. https://searchebscohostcom.ezproxy.libraries.wright.edu/login.aspx?direct=true&db=rzh&AN=106272806&site=eds-live.

Breast cancer, one of the leading cancers affecting older women, has clear implications for self-esteem and sexual functioning. Dysphoria from the disease, fears of death, and disfigurement may diminish sexual desire before treatment begins (Wise & Crone, 2006). The presence of medical illnesses, as well as myths about sexuality and the benefit of treatment to older adults, often prevents clinicians from aggressively treating older women with breast cancer. Tamoxifen induces premature menopause and accelerates sexual difficulties. Alternative sexual positions and vaginal lubrication decrease problems.

Prostate cancer is the most common cancer in men and the second leading cause of death from cancer in men in the United States. The risk of developing prostate cancer increases with age. Radical prostatectomy, a curative treatment, involves massive disturbance of hormone-producing glands, surrounding nerves, and urinary structures. This often results in temporary urinary incontinence and impotence, both affecting a male's sexuality. The introduction of nerve-sparing techniques has greatly decreased sexual dysfunction; however, men may need to wait 2 to 3 years for maximum function to return. Phosphodiesterase inhibitors and prosthetic devices can be useful to modify postradiation treatment dysfunctions that have occurred in 50% of those receiving treatment (Wise & Crone, 2006).

Colon cancer may result in the need for an ostomy, which can result in fear of fecal spillage and odor, inhibiting sexual pleasure. Women with ostomies can develop dyspareunia secondary to fistula formation (Wise & Crone, 2006).

Dementia

Lindau and colleagues (2018) sampled 3196 home-dwelling older adults with a mean Montreal Cognitive Assessment (MoCA 0–30 points) of 22.7. Their findings revealed that 59% men and 51% women were sexually active, including 41% of those ages 80 to 91. Seventy-seven percent reported having sexual function problems.

Dementia in older adults can lead to various sexual disturbances. Factors associated with dementia that can affect sexual functioning include failure to recognize a partner, misidentification of a partner, delusions, hallucinations, personality changes, and disinhibition (Lesser, Hughes & Kumar, 2005). One behavior common among individuals with dementia is hypersexuality, also referred to as inappropriate sexual behavior (ISB) and sexual disinhibition (Srinivasan & Weinberg, 2006; Wallace & Safer, 2009). ISB has been reported to occur in 7% to 25% of dementia patients, with higher prevalence in residents of skilled nursing facilities and in patients with more severe cognitive impairments (De Giorgi & Series, 2016). Older adults with dementia may masturbate in public, strip themselves of clothing, expose themselves, or make overt gestures to others. Sexual impulsivity and inappropriate behavior can occur during the course of many different dementing illnesses but occurs early on in the course of a form of frontotemporal dementia (FTD). These behaviors are disturbing to others and often difficult to address. Although there may be no apparent explanation for such behavior, family and caregivers should consider the possibility that these behaviors are triggered by unmet intimacy needs or may also indicate pain, hyperthermia, or trying to be freed from a restrained situation (Messinger-Rapport et al., 2003; Wallace & Safer, 2009).

The research division of the Hebrew Home for the Aged, under a state-sponsored grant, completed a training video titled "Freedom of Sexual Expression: Dementia and Resident Rights in Long-Term Care Facilities." More information on the video can be found at https://terranova.org/film-catalog/freedom-of-sexual-expression-dementia-and-resident-rights-in-long-term-care-facilities/.

Medications

Many medications affect the sexuality of older adults. Sexual dysfunction is a common, unwanted side effect of many types of drug therapy. NPs and PAs need to consider all prescribed medications as well as any over-the-counter medications including herbals and oils (Table 5.3).

Drugs that affect libido act centrally and reduce desire by causing sedation or hormonal disturbance. Drugs that interfere with the autonomic system will have negative effects on erectile function, ejaculation, and orgasm. Drugs interfering with hormones, such as tamoxifen, will also affect vaginal response (Smith, 2007). Antihypertensives

TABLE 5.3 Medications and Sexual Function

Classification of Medications	Effect on Sexuality
Benzodiazepines	Reduction in desire, disinhibiting, can increase libido
Antihypertensives	Beta-blockers, angiotensin-converting enzyme inhibitor, thiazide diuretics and calcium channel blockers: erectile dysfunction
Antidepressants	Tricyclic antidepressants: erectile failure in men and anorgasmia in women Selective serotonin reuptake inhibitors (SSRIs): loss of sexual interest, erectile dysfunction, ejaculatory delay or failure, anorgasmia Monoamine oxidase inhibitors: orgasm failure, erectile dysfunction Venlafaxine: less dysfunction that SSRIs Mirtazapine: Low incidence of sexual dysfunction Trazodone: Associated with priapism and is used to treat erectile dysfunction
Antiepileptics	Hyposexuality
Antipsychotics	Marked sexual dysfunction: disturbances of erection and ejaculation, changes in libido, and priapism in men and decreased libido, orgasmic dysfunction in women
Prostate medications	Alpha-blockers: ejaculatory problems Finasteride: reduces sexual desire Antiandrogens and gonadotrophin-releasing hormone analogues: impair testosterone, reduce libido and erectile dysfunction
Anti-Parkinsonian medications	Levodopa may cause hypersexuality
Recreational medications	Alcohol: increased sexual desire, erectile failure with intoxication; reduced testosterone with long-term use Tobacco: erectile dysfunction

Data from Smith, S. (2007). Drugs that cause sexual dysfunction. *Psychiatry, 6*(3), 111–114. https://doi-org.ezproxy.libraries.wright.edu/10.1016/j.mppsy.2006.12.004; Thornhill, T. (2007). Aging and sexuality. *U.S. Pharmacist, 32*(6), HS5–HS18.

(especially beta-blockers and diuretics), antiandrogens, and many psychotropic medications can affect sexual function. The autonomic effect of beta-blockers increases risk of erectile dysfunction. Vasodilators and angiotension-2 receptor antagonists are free of side effects for sexual dysfunction.

Older adults on antidepressants, especially selective serotonin-reuptake inhibitors (SSRIs) or venlafaxine, suffered sexual dysfunction, with higher rates in men. This is through the activation of 5-HT2 receptors, which inhibits both noradrenergic and dopaminergic transmission. It is important to determine what the patient's sexual functioning was prior to starting an antidepressant, as depressions alone can cause sexual dysfunction. Erection is triggered by both parasympathetic and sympathetic neuronal stimulation and is adversely affected by anticholinergic agents, such as tricyclic antidepressants (TCAs), that block this neurotransmitter.

Trazodone has moderate to high affinity for alpha-1 and alpha-2 receptors, which can account for its positive effect on libido and erectile function. Duloxetine has less sexual dysfunction than SSRIs but more than placebo.

Antiepileptics cause hyposexuality through hormonal effects on the hypothalamic-pituitary-adrenal axis. This is seen more with the hepatic-enzyme-inducing antiepileptic drugs, such as carbamazepine, phenytoin, and Depakote. Lamotrigine does not affect sexual function Benzodiazepines cause drowsiness and reduce sexual desire. This appears to be dose related.

Antipsychotic medications are associated with marked sexual dysfunction. They can cause disturbances of erection and ejaculation, changes in libido, and priapism in men and decreased libido, orgasmic dysfunction in women. Sexual dysfunction is estimated to occur in 30% to 60% of patients taking antipsychotic medications and often leads to nonadherence. The sexual dysfunction side effect is secondary to autonomic and hormonal mechanisms. Thioridazine, aliphatic phenothiazines (chlorpromazine), sulpiride, and risperidone result in the greatest sexual dysfunction. Prolactin-raising antipsychotics are associated with greater sexual dysfunction. Medications such as quetiapine, aripiprazole, and olanzapine have been associated with less sexual dysfunction. The adrenergic mechanism of clozapine, a prolactin-sparing medication, causes sexual dysfunction.

Medications used to treat benign prostatic hypertrophy reduce sexual desire as a known direct effect of these medications. Alpha-blockers may cause ejaculatory problems. Finasteride, a 5-apha-reductasse inhibitor, reduces sexual desire. Medications used to treat prostate cancer include antiandrogens such as cyproterone acetate and flutamide as well as gonadotrophin-releasing hormone analogues such as goserelin and leuprorelin; these impair testosterone, reduce libido, and may cause erectile dysfunction.

Levodopa, a key ingredient in the commonly prescribed Parkinson medication carbidopa/levodopa (Sinemet), may cause hypersexuality. Alcohol may increase sexual desire. Intoxication may result in erectile failure. Long-term use of alcohol interferes with the hypothalamic-pituitary-adrenal axis, resulting in reduced testosterone, which in turn reduces sex drive and performance.

Tobacco can cause erectile dysfunction by damaging the lining of blood vessels in the genital region and causing erectile dysfunction. Many recreational drugs have also been reported to be associated with impaired sexual performance and dysfunction including cannabis and opiates (Smith,

2007). Before initiating medication that may affect sexual function, it is prudent of health care providers to have open discussions with patients about the potential adverse side effects of sexual dysfunction and to not assume that because the patient is an older adult he or she will not care.

Environmental and Psychological Barriers to Sexual Practice

Older adults may be reluctant to begin dating, feeling unfamiliar with dating practices. How to date and make new relationships can be challenging at any age but presents unique challenges with the older adult population (Butler & Lewis, 2000). Alternatively, masturbation is a method in which both men and women can be sexually fulfilled in the absence of partners. Lindau et al. found that the prevalence of masturbation was lower at older ages and high among men (2007).

In Wang et al.'s Successful Aging Evaluation (SAGE) population-based study, older men and women (606) who had a partner reported frequent engagement in and satisfaction with sexual activity. The mean age of the sample was 75.2 years. Over 80% of those who responded had engaged in sexual activity the previous year. Over 70% had engaged in sexual activity weekly or more than once a week, and over 60% were somewhat or very satisfied with their sex lives Depressive symptoms were broadly associated with worse sexual health, more so than physical function, anxiety or stress, or age itself.

Satisfaction with a marriage was a mediating variable that led to continued sexual activity (Waite et al., 2017). Martial conflict reported by the husband led to decreased sexual activity and martial conflict reported by the wife led to increased sexual activity. Laumann and Waite (2008) reported sexual problems among older adults were responses to the presence of stressors in multiple life domains. They found older women's sexual health was more sensitive to their physical health than men. Their study found the link of life stress with sexual problems was more likely secondary to poor mental health and relationship dissatisfaction.

One of the most difficult problems encountered when intervening to assist older adults with meeting sexual needs is overcoming environmental barriers. In the community setting, older couples may be hindered by a lack of assistive equipment needed to safely fulfill their sexual desires. In long-term and acute care settings as well as in assisted living settings, lack of privacy often prevents older individuals from pursuing sexual relationships. Due to a fear of becoming the topic of conversation among staff members as well as their peers, older adult, become hesitant to seek advice from staff or pursue opportunities for sexual fulfillment. The issue of privacy of information becomes a reality for older adults desiring sexual relations (Rheaume & Mitty, 2008). There is a lack of guidelines on how to assess and accommodate nursing home residents' preferences for intimate sexual activity (Metzger, 2017). Sexuality assessment is needed to effectively determine older adults' sexual needs in long-term care facilities (Lichtenberg, 2014). Nurse practitioners and physician assistants need to assist in creating an environment that is respectful of patient autonomy and preferences. Long-term care facilities should create staff policies that address the sexuality of their residents (Lichtenberg, 2014). There should be plans that include how to accommodate sexual intimacy. Providers should determine statutes and case law on sexual consent for the provider's practicing state. Metzger (2017) has proposed that facilities have a resident sexuality consultation team, similar to a wound care team. He also suggested that "intimacy rooms" be created to provide privacy with appropriate signage. Providers should furnish educational material for staff and families and hold staff training sessions. Aids such as lubricants should be provided.

Sexual dysfunction may be a signal of other psychosocial disorders, such as depression, delirium, and dementia. Sexuality can also be affected by anxiety concerning partner availability and lifestyle issues. Many older individuals may be self-medicating with alcohol and drugs as a way of managing depression or anxiety symptoms, coping with loneliness or loss, or dealing with pain, which can impact sexual function (Lesser et al., 2005). Completing a thorough assessment for medications, depression, delirium, and an older adult's sexuality will assist NPs and PAs in determining the root cause of sexual dysfunction.

Clients with dementia should be given special attention to ensure their safety when they decide to engage in sexual relationships. Health care professionals working with cognitively impaired older adults need to determine if the individual is actually consenting to a sexual activity. Metzger (2017) has suggested that the standard for sexual consent capacity might be influenced but the nature of the sexual activity in question. For example, consent to kiss or hold hands would be different than consent for sexual penetration. If the person is unable to consent to participation in a sexual activity and has a surrogate decision maker, that person should be involved with judgments regarding the benefits or potential harm associated with that person's sexual expression (Rheaume & Mitty, 2008). In long-term care settings, including assisted living facilities, a resident's attempt at sexual expression is often viewed as a "problem" behavior (Rheaume & Mitty, 2008). In fact, more literature about the sexuality of older adults pertains to the inappropriateness of the behavior than literature about the need for sexual expression among older adults.

Assessment of Sexuality

Health care providers should be cognizant of indications of sexual interest in older adults. Overt gestures of sexuality in public areas or hints of sexual interest during conversations with older adults should not be ignored or punished; they should be viewed as an indication of sexual interest between older adults.

Older adults should not thoughtlessly enter into sexual relationships. Among older adults, there is the added risk factor of potential cognitive impairments, which may hinder clients' decision-making ability. Before a sexual relationship commences, it may be appropriate for providers to meet with both older adults individually and together to discuss their intentions and expectations regarding the sexual relationship. In so doing, their fears and apprehensions may be expressed and their questions answered. In addition, such a discussion may reveal whether one of them is being coerced into the relationship or is not mentally competent to decide to enter into such a relationship.

A cognitive assessment such as the Montreal Cognitive Assessment (MoCA) should be performed as part of the assessment of older adult's capacity for decision making, including the decision to become involved in a sexual relationship. The information gained from this assessment is useful if the family or the provider suspects the older adult is cognitively impaired and unable to make decisions to participate in sexual relationships. If the cognitive assessment does not provide sufficiently clear information regarding decision-making abilities, a more thorough assessment by a psychological team may be necessary to prevent anyone from taking advantage of an older adult.

Sexual health may have a direct impact on the well-being of an individual with chronic illnesses (Nusbaum et al., 2003). Therefore, it is essential to obtain a sexual history, but one of the greatest obstacles in assessing the sexuality of older adults occurs at the beginning of the assessment. Getting started with the sexual history becomes easier with experience. One challenge providers face is to help older adults develop and sustain the intimate relationship they desire. This involves active assessment, including actively reviewing health concerns and conditions that affect sexual functioning (Szwabo, 2003). Although discomfort in this area is understandable, increased proficiency comes with experience. According to the National Social Life, Health and Aging Project (NSHAP), a total of 38% of men and 22% of women reported having discussed sex with a physician since the age of 50 years (2007). Healthy sexuality depends on good communication between the health professional and the patient. NPs and PAs are in a pivotal position to begin this communication.

The PLISSIT model has been used to assess and manage the sexuality of adults since 1976 (Annon, 1976). PLISSIT is an acronym for Permission, Limited Information, Specific Suggestions, and Intensive Therapy (Rheaume & Mitty (2008). The model offers suggestions for initiating and maintaining the discussion of sexuality of older adults. It was first used with young adults but has been used successfully with older adults as well. The PLISSIT model is applicable for minority populations, such as LGBTQ+ people, sex workers, and nonmonogamous individuals, who have their own unique sexual health considerations that need to be included in the assessment of an older adult's sexuality. The PLISSIT model is optimal when providers reflect on their own biases and seek to provide safe spaces for all populations, using additional resources like conferences, books, and webinars that focus on various communities' specific needs. The model consists of four steps:

1. The provider creates the space for a patient to bring up sexual health concerns, usually through open-ended questions such as "Is there anything about your sexual health you'd like to discuss?"
2. Once the patient has identified a concern, the provider can offer targeted information, including potential causes of the symptoms.
3. A differential diagnosis is offered, with specific suggestions for how to begin addressing the problem. The provider can let the patient know that this is just the first attempt at addressing the issue and that there are other treatment options if this suggestion does not solve the patient's problem.
4. If necessary, a referral can be made to a sexual health specialist, such as a sex therapist, pelvic floor specialist, or sex educator, to provide more comprehensive support and guidance.

A detailed sexual history should be completed by the primary care practitioner as part of a complete history or when appropriate given the presenting complaint. The goal of the assessment, regardless of the model used, is to gather information that allows older adults to express sexuality safely and to feel uninhibited by normal or pathologic problems. A quiet, private meeting place should be provided and interruptions during the discussion should be avoided. Providers should sit at eye level with the patient and ask questions in a manner that is not threatening. Providers should avoid using terms that may suggest they are making assumptions about sexual behavior or orientation. For example, when asking about an older adult's sexual orientation, they should avoid using the term *husband* or *wife*, instead using the term *partner*. They also need to avoid medical terminology and the use of slang words (Nusbaum & Hamilton, 2002).

Other components of the sexual history taking include reviewing medications and medical conditions that may contribute to sexual dysfunction. The review of medications is often an opportunity to discuss sexual function by using an opening comment such as "I see you are taking [name of medication]. [Name of medication] can be associated with sexual problems. Are you having any difficulty?" Tactics like this often puts the older adult at ease and opens the lines of communication. In addition, providers should review the older adult's early experiences, if he or she is willing to share. The patient may have a history of sexual abuse or rape that is now affecting the individual's sexual function and emotional well-being. A physical assessment of the breasts and genital tissue is an essential part of the assessment of sexuality. Laboratory tests may be useful in determining reductions in hormone levels that may contribute to decreased libido or erectile dysfunction. (See Box 5.3.)

Providers should also obtain information on sexual preferences. An assessment of the environments in which patients

• BOX 5.3 Questions on Sexuality

- Are you currently sexually active? If so, with one or more than one partner?
- Do you have a male or female partner?
- Are your sexual desires being met?
- Do you have any questions or concerns about your sexual function? About your partner's sexual function?
- What kind of information would you like?

live should follow. Providers should determine where the older adult plans to participate in sexual activity. In acute, long-term care, and assisted living settings, the environment should be assessed for privacy and safety. This enables older adults to proceed with sexual activity safely and comfortably. In the community setting, the environment should be assessed for safety and the availability of adaptive equipment such as side rails, trapezes, and specialized beds, which may be needed to allow older adults to practice sexual activity safely within the home.

Sexuality and sexual expression were not formally or informally taught during the developmental years of today's cohort of older adults. In fact, sexuality was hidden behind closed doors during many older adults' lives. Therefore, the sexuality assessment of an older adult may be the first opportunity he or she has to openly discuss sexuality. Embarrassment, shyness, and apprehension in this area are common. In addition, older adults may view the normal changes of aging as embarrassing or indicative of illness and may be reluctant to discuss these matters with health care providers.

Laumann et al. (2008) looked at data from the Global Study of Sexual Attitudes and Behaviors (GSSAB), which was a population survey of 27,500 men and women, ages 40 to 80 in 29 countries. They extracted data from the United States and found of the 1491 individuals surveyed, less than 25% of those with sexual problems actually reported the sexual problem. They also found a correlation between erectile dysfunction and depression; however, it was not clear if the depression and consequently the medications to treat the depression were the cause of erectile dysfunction or if erectile dysfunction caused the depression. They did suggest that when someone is reporting sexual dysfunction, assessing for depression cannot be overlooked. The findings also indicated that feeling that the problem was sensitive or that they were not been bothered by the problem may keep older adults from raising the subject and other sexual difficulties with their health care provider. The researchers also found that health care providers in the United States rarely ask patients about their sexual health during a routine consultation. Lindau and colleagues (2008) had similar findings when they looked at the curriculum in medical schools across the country. They found medical schools were not educating students on how to perform a sexual history. When sexual history taking was included in the curriculum, students performed a sexual history 98% of the time in the obvious-relevance cases compared to 86% being completed by students who had not had sexual history taking as part of their curriculum. In the least-obvious relevance cases, no students initiated a sexual history.

Lindau et al. (2018) found that individuals with dementia who were having sex were less likely to discuss their problems with a provider. Discussing sexual history in a sensitive manner should improve the provider-patient relationship and offer greater professional satisfaction as well as improved functioning for the older adult.

Instruments such as the ADAM Questionnaire, created by Morley (2000), is a helpful screening tool to assess sexual function of older men. It should prompt further work-up, including a testosterone level and a prostate-specific antigen (Blackwell, 2006).

In a 2015 editorial by Kob and Sewell, the researchers commented that one area in need of research is how to best assist health care providers of all types to become more comfortable and more adept at asking older individuals about their sexuality. Neglecting to ask older adults about their sex lives may be a missed opportunity to help older individuals avoid sexually transmitted diseases and to improve their quality of life (Kob & Sewell, 2015).

Since the 2007 Lindau et al. study, other researchers have found that older women had a similar number of sexual concerns as younger women but were less likely to have the topic of sexual health raised during health care visits. Health care providers working with older adults need to be open to discussing sexuality and assess the sexual health concerns of all those they serve (Syme et al., 2013).

As advanced practice providers assess the sexuality of older adults, they need to be mindful that many of the studies done to date include surveys of older adults. There may be a bias with underreporting of sexual problems, as older adults answering the surveys are usually those who are very satisfied or very dissatisfied.

Gillespie (2017) found two characteristics pertaining to older adult sexuality. These characteristics, sexual synchronicity and open sexual communication, are major influences to self-reported sex frequency and satisfaction. Health care providers should also have open communication about individuals' sexuality, assessing their open communication with their partners about their individual needs.

Bauer and coworkers (2013) found that although knowledge may be increased through education, unless the formal caregiver changes her or his personal biases toward older adult sexuality, change would not occur. Bauer et al. (2013) suggested that education needs to focus on how to conduct a sexual health and sexual needs assessment. Furthermore, they recommended that these assessments need to be supported by guidelines and policy.

Granville and Pregler (2018) suggested routine screening questions for older women's sexual health to include questions such as the following:

- Do you have any concerns about keeping yourself sexually healthy and safe?
- Have you been satisfied with the frequency and nature of your sexual activities?
- Do you have the difficulty becoming aroused?

- Are you able to become adequately lubricated for vaginal sex?
- Have you had difficulty having an orgasm?
- Within the past year have you had sex with another person?
- How many partners in the past year?
- Have your sexual partners been men, women, or both?
- Have you ever had a sexually transmitted infection?
- What are you doing to prevent sexually transmitted infections?
- What specific sexual activities have you engaged in?
- Has anyone ever of coerced or forced you to have sex?
- Have you ever been touched in a sexual way that was unwanted?

In acute care settings, providers are in a key position to address newly developed or potential sexual dysfunctions before a patient is discharged to a community setting or long-term care environment. However, because of discomfort, myths, and lack of training in the area of sexuality, these problems are often ignored. The result is that older adults are discharged home or to another setting with a newly developed or chronic condition that prevents them from functioning sexually.

In the community setting, providers have access to the older adult's entire family unit in his or her natural surroundings. The information needed to make a sexual assessment is therefore readily accessible. Yet providers may feel intimidated or uncomfortable questioning older adults about their sexual desires and needs. Consequently, the information needed for proper intervention is not obtained.

Providers are reluctant to venture into such uncharted territory. The result is that sexually interested older adults are in a situation in which they may have multiple disabilities, no privacy, no support, and no appropriate way in which to express their sexual feelings (Wallace, 2003).

Alternative Sexual Practice Among Older Adults

Amin (2016) used the General Social Survey (GSS) from 2012 to further examine the sexual behaviors of older adults. He found that in adults ages 55 years and older, 87% of the 547 who responded did not use a condom, and 15% reported engaging in sexually risky behaviors such as causal sex, paid sex, male-to-male sex, and drug use.

Waite et al. (2017) found the husband's comorbidity burden was associated with differences in the frequency of sex. They found that those individuals still achieved sexual satisfaction with different kinds of sexual activity.

The literature has established that in addition to older adults' ongoing need to express their sexuality through traditional sexual methods, older adults also must fulfill the human need to touch and to be touched. A person's need for intimacy and closeness to another does not end at any age (Kaiser, 2000). There is little information about the role of touch as a substitute or addition to the sexual practices of older adults. It is known that touch is an overt expression of closeness, intimacy, and sexuality and is an integral part of sexuality.

The importance of touch is often undervalued by society. In fact, touch is often thought of as the invasion of a person's space, and caregivers should not assume that a person likes or wants to be touched (Rheaume & Mitty, 2008). Non-task-related "affective" touching, such as simply stroking a person's check or holding one's hand, may be viewed as assaultive, erotic, comforting, or presumptuous, depending on a person's culture, personal comfort level, and relationship with the one doing the touching (Rheaume & Mitty, 2008). For legal as well as privacy reasons, many people have shied away from touching. To older adults experiencing touch deprivation, the social rules that govern touch may be devastating. It is important to remember that touch is a way in which older adults may fulfill their sexuality with each other. Touch may be both a welcome addition to traditional sexual methods and an alternative means of sexual expression when intercourse is not desired or possible.

When sexual intercourse is not the preferred method of intimacy or is not possible for an older couple, the couple may be taught alternative methods of intimacy in the form of touch. Touch is a means of expressing intimacy and closeness that may fulfill older clients' sexual needs and desires. Touch can best be fulfilled by finding a comfortable environment in which an older adult couple can expose parts of their bodies to each other as they feel comfortable. A shower or bath may be enjoyable. The couple should be taught to move their fingertips slowly or lightly over each other's skin while enjoying the closeness of the other person. Massage therapy, books, and videos may provide older adults with a way to touch that results in the fulfillment of sexual desires. Soft music may add to the conducive environment for older couples.

In addition to the burden caused by society's lack of understanding of the sexuality of older adults, aging homosexuals have the additional burden of society's lack of understanding of homosexuality. According to the 2006 MetLife study of LGBTQ+ seniors, they are twice as likely to live alone, half as likely to have a life partner or significant other, half as likely to have close relatives to call on for help, and four times less likely to have children to help them. Gays and lesbians who have "come out" to others often need to go into hiding when they need health care services. Aging networks' attitudes and practices toward gay and lesbian older adults have gone unchallenged, resulting in a senior health care system that is even more homophobic than other health care systems (MetLife, 2006). Despite prevailing stereotypes, it is important for NPs and PAs to recognize that same-sex companionship is an acceptable expression of sexuality for both men and women.

Providers need to be sure that their own personal beliefs about alternative sexual practices do not prevent older homosexual clients from fulfilling their sexual desires. Examination of his or her own feelings toward this alternative sexual practice may allow providers to recognize the meaning of the homosexual lifestyle to the older adult. Homosexual partners should be encouraged to participate in the sexual assessment and planning when appropriate. Providers should also remember that no information about the sexual orientation of their patients should be shared with the family unless permission has been given.

Cultural Beliefs and Differences/Cultural Competency

Fredriksen-Goldsen and colleagues created 10 core competencies to promote the well-being of the lesbian, gay, bisexual, and transgender (LGBT) older adults. It is predicted that by 2030 the LGBT community will double and comprise between 3% to 4% of the general US adult population. See Box 5.4 for the list of the competencies.

NPs and PAs have ethical mandates to be knowledgeable and competent when working with diverse populations. Although the competencies discussed in this section are for the LGBT population, they can also be applied to all older adults.

There are culturally based differences in sexual activity, including what different cultures think about kissing, foreplay, oral sex, masturbation, abstinence, homosexuality and same-sex relationships, and marriage. These beliefs are established early in an individual's life, depending on where one was raised and what religious beliefs one has had from a young age. It is important for NPs and PAs to be cognizant of these rooted beliefs. Orel and Watson (2012) uses the acronym ADDRESSING to illustrate 10 cultural factors and personal attributes that impact sexuality (refer to Table 5.4).

• BOX 5.4 Core Competencies for LGBT Older Adults

1. Critically analyze personal and professional attitudes toward sexual orientation, gender identity, and age, and understand how factors such as culture religion, media, and health and human service systems influence attitudes and ethical decision making
2. Understand and articulate the ways that larger social and cultural contexts may have negatively impacted LGBT older adults as a historically disadvantaged population
3. Distinguish similarities and differences within the subgroups of LGBT older adults, as well as their intersecting identities (such as age, gender, race, and health status) to develop tailored and responsive health strategies
4. Apply theories of aging and social and health perspectives and the most up-to-date knowledge available to engage in culturally competent practice with LGBT older adults
5. When conducting a comprehensive biopsychosocial assessment, attend to the ways that the larger social context and structural and environmental risks and resources may impact LGBT older adults
6. When using empathy and sensitive interviewing skills during assessment and intervention, ensure the use of language is appropriate for working with LGBT older adults to establish and build rapport
7. Understand and articulate the ways in which agency, program, and service policies do or do not marginalize and discriminate against LGBT older adults
8. Understand and articulate the ways that local, state, and federal laws negatively and positively impact LGBT older adults, to advocate on their behalf
9. Provide sensitive and appropriate outreach to LGBT older adults, their families, caregivers, and other supports to identify and address service gaps, fragmentation, and barriers that impact LGBT older adults
10. Enhance the capacity of LGBT older adults and their families, caregivers, and other supports to navigate aging, social, and health services

From Fredriksen-Goldsen, K. I., Hoy-Ellis, C. P., Goldsen, J., Emlet, C. A., & Hooyman, N. R. (2014). Creating a vision for the future: Key competencies and strategies for culturally competent practice with lesbian, gay, bisexual, and transgender (LGBT) older adults in the health and human services. *Journal of Gerontological Social Work, 57*(2–4), 80–107. https://doi.org/10.1080/01634372.2014.890690

Strategies to Enhance Sexual Function in Older Adults

Even though the literature supports the existence of sexual interest and practice in older adults, health care professionals carry out few interventions to facilitate older adults' expression of sexuality. One reason for this is that society continually equates sexuality with sexual intercourse. There are special considerations NPs and PAs can implement to improve the older adults' sexuality. Some of these include ways to reduce fatigue and pain, which may include taking analgesics prior to sexual activity, performing muscle stretches, or using nasal oxygen or inhalers prior to sex. NPs and PAs should educate older adults about different sexual positions, such as side-by-side lying or rear entry braced by pillows to reduce physical exertion or stress on other body parts. Educating older adults about over-the-counter lubricants will also reduce the sexual dysfunction of vaginal dryness many older women experience. Educating older adults about the changes that occur with aging in relation to sexual activity, such as the fact that extra time for foreplay is needed to provide sufficient arousal to achieve orgasm, will alleviate anxiety and improve overall sexuality. NPs and PAs may want to recommend psychotherapy for a couple. Other interventions might include increasing socialization for older women to assist them with finding new partners.

Medications to enhance men's sexual function were discussed previously. There are other tools men can use, which include penile rings, that can help men maintain an erection. A penile pump can help men achieve erections. The American Urological Association ED guidelines approve vacuum erection devices with a vacuum limiter for the safe treatment of ED (Burraro et al., 2014).

Even though the Food and Drug Administration does not approve supplements, patients will ask about them, and

TABLE 5.4 ADDRESSING Cultural Factors

Cultural Factors	Explanation
Age and cohort effects	Society assumes older adults are asexual
Degree of physical ability	Effect of chronic diseases; ability to perform activities of daily living
Degree of cognitive ability	Mental health issues, attitude toward self as a sexual being, level of sexual knowledge and comfort with intimacy
Religion	Must be included in a sexual health history
Ethnicity and race	Avoid generalizations
Socioeconomic status	Level of education, economic class, style of life, occupation, and living conditions need to be considered
Sexual orientation	
Individualistic life experiences	Most significant is past history of sexual experiences and activities, past history of abuse, violence, trauma, natural disasters history of sexually transmitted infections (STIs), HIV, AIDs
Natural origin	One's country of origin
Gender	

From Orel, N., & Watson, W. (2012, Spring). Addressing diversity in sexuality and aging: Key considerations for healthcare providers. *Journal of Aging and Life Care*.https://www.aginglifecarejournal.org/addressing-diversity-in-sexuality-and-aging-key-considerations-for-healthcare-providers/

NPs and PAs need to be cognizant of what is on the market. Yohimbine is an herbal used by men to treat ED, and it is used by men and women for sexual stimulation. It should not be used in older adults with renal or hepatic impairment. Potential side effects include arrhythmias, anxiety, irritability, bronchospasm, and death (Burraro et al., 2014).

Butea gel is a product from Thailand and available on the Internet. It stimulates erections and can also be used as a sexual stimulant for women. The main ingredient in Butea gel is Butea superb, an herb commonly used in Thailand as an aphrodisiac. Other ingredients include Elephanttopus scabar linn, Betula aionoides Buch Ham, and Tinospora Tuberculata Beumee (Burraro et al., 2014).

The amino acid L-argingine, ArginMax, an herbal available for both men and women that can be taken prior to intercourse. It is a naturally occurring amnio acid that increases the production of nitric oxide, a chemical released by the genital nerves during arousal, delivering increased blood flow to the area (Burraro et al., 2014).

Osphena, a selective estrogenreceptor modulator (SERM), is being used to treat dyspareunia and vaginal dryness. It has a black box warning for increased endometrial cancer and cardiovascular risk including thromboembolic stroke, hemorrhagic stroke, and DVT.

Refer to Box 5.5 for further strategies to enhance sexual function. Further interventions are discussed in the Interprofessional Collaboration in the Management of Sexuality in Older Adults section, presented next.

BOX 5.5 Strategies to Enhance Sexual Function in Older Adults

Dietary Strategies

- Avoid alcohol or tobacco.
- Discuss well-balanced meals with a registered dietitian.

Medication Strategies

- Take pain medications before sexual activity if needed.
- Discuss with primary care provider (medical doctor or nurse practitioner) discontinuing medications that may impair sexual function.

Environmental Adaptations

- Plan for sexual activity when most rested.
- Allow conjugal visits or home visits.
- Live pets provide sensory stimulation.
- Offer objects to touch, fondle, and hold such as dolls or stuffed animals for demented older adult.

Psychologic Strategies

- Communicate desires to partner.
- Discuss fears and concerns with primary care provider.
- Encourage routine visits to hairdresser to promote self-esteem and well-being.
- Join a support group.
- Use relaxation techniques.

Physical Strategies

- Improve exercise tolerance by participating in supervised exercise program.
- Use touch, kissing, and hugging.
- Use pillows under painful joints.
- Take a warm shower before activity.
- Get regular check-ups.

Modified from Arena, J, & Wallace, M. (2008). Sexuality issues in aging. Nursing standard of practice protocol: Sexuality in older adults. In C. Rheaume & E. Mitty, (2008). Sexuality and intimacy in older adults. *Geriatric Nursing, 29*(5), 342–349.

Interprofessional Collaboration in the Management of Sexuality in Older Adults

Since the 1990s, the World Health Organization (WHO) has encouraged integrated care. Working in multidisciplinary teams is crucial for ensuring high-quality care for older adults across the world (Asakawa et al., 2017). In dealing with the sexuality of older adults, team members need to include the primary care provider, physical therapist, occupational therapist, social worker, and pharmacist. Depending on the location of the older adult, other team members may include nursing aides, nurses, and the activities director if the older adult resides in a nursing facility, including an assisted living facility.

The occupational therapists and nursing aids are often around older adults during acts of intimate care such as toileting, bathing, and dressing. This lends more opportunities for them to approach the topic of intimacy and sexuality goals and desires (Lichtenburg 2014).

Pelvic physical therapy can help not only with myofascial pelvic pain but it may also reduce symptoms of other conditions caused by pelvic floor problems, such as urinary and fecal incontinence, painful intercourse, and sexual dysfunction. Pelvic physical therapy is performed by physical therapists who go through specialized training (Harvard Health Publishing, 2018). Physical therapists play a vital role on the interprofessional team by assisting older adults to relieve pain from arthritis, as well as educating them on alternative positions to achieve their sexual goals.

Pharmacists are often the first health care provider older adults approach with questions about their medications affecting their sexuality (Thornhill, 2007). Pharmacists serve a valuable role on the interprofessional team by providing insight into medications already being taken that may be contributing to sexual dysfunction. Medication profiles should be screened for medications that can case sexual dysfunction. Pharmacists can serve as an educational resource for older adults as well as for health care providers. Consultant pharmacists in long-term care facilities can serve on committees to help draft facility policies and provide education to residents, staff, and families (Thornhill, 2007). Pharmacists also serve as a resource for pharmacotherapy for the treatment of sexual dysfunction in older adults. Pharmacists can discuss nonpharmacologic treatment strategies such as weight loss, smoking cessation, and alcohol reduction as well as pharmacologic treatments of sexual dysfunction. Medication classifications, including intracavernosal alprostadil and the phosphodiesterase type-5 inhibitors such as sildenafil, vardenafil, and tadalafil, can be discussed with the older adult and the interprofessional team. The pharmacist can also screen for potential drug or concomitant disease interactions (Thornhill).

Social workers are unique partners on the interprofessional team, as they infuse the notion of "personhood" into interventions largely predicated on a biomedical model of aging that reduces older adults (including patients and caregivers) to the medical functioning of the body and mind. In a survey completed by Salisu (2017), older adults indicated they preferred that social workers initiate the conversation about sexuality and that they would rather discus their sexual activities privately, without family members.

There is documented lack of knowledge among nursing home staff of late-life sexuality (DiNapoli et al., 2013; Monteiro et al., 2017). DiNapoli et al. utilized focus groups to conclude a lack of knowledge among formal caregivers in relation to the perception of older adult sexuality. DiNaploi et al. stated there is a need for effective interventions to balance resident safety and autonomy. Providing education to the staff and families is a role of NPs and PAs, who are to educate professional and lay caregivers to provide culturally and spiritually sensitive, appropriate care. This education needs to include the nursing staff's ability to examine their personal biases (Bauer et al., 2013).

Santos-Iglesias et al. (2016) has encouraged health care providers to become active in the education of the public, formal caregivers and clinicians in the beliefs surrounding the sexuality of older adults. They also encourage providers to become active in public policy changes that recognize the needs and rights of older adults regarding their sexuality. Policies need to be written to support sexual needs assessments and sexual health assessments (Bauer et al., 2013).

Becoming more prevalent are policies that incorporate the sexual needs of older adults in care plans (Messinger-Rapport et al., 2003). Acute and long-term care facilities should make proper arrangements for privacy to allow for older adults' sexual experiences. The physical facilities within each setting vary. The ideal situation is to set up a pleasant room that can be used for a variety of activities but may also be reserved by older adults for private visits with a spouse or partner. In most settings this may not be possible, and client rooms may be used while the nursing staff gains permission from and plans alternate activities for their roommates.

In any setting, older adults' safety should be maintained. The call lights should be easily accessible. Side rails on the bed should be used if necessary, and the room should be situated so that the nursing staff is aware of when it is in use.

Staff education about the sexuality and intimacy of older adults should include recognition of cues, desires, and interest in sexual activity, and intimacy. It should also include the use of and access to pornographic material, especially through the Internet, which many older adults now access. Education of nursing staff needs to also address eliminating stereotypes, such as "the dirty old man" (Rheaume & Mitty, 2008). Open discussion of attitudes and sexual issues among staff can increase comfort with sexual issues. Case studies and games such as trivia games can be an effective means of education. Education should also be available to the family. The training should begin by discussing and dispelling the myths surrounding older adults' sexual desires and activity. The training should include normal changes associated with older men and women, and how to compensate for specific physical disabilities. A more positive attitude toward the sexual expression of older adults may develop with increased knowledge and may allow such expression to become a natural part of the aging process.

Training should conclude with discussion groups to allow staff and family to examine their own feelings about sexuality and its role in the life of older adults. Role-playing may be an effective technique to gain understanding of the effect of the staff and family's personal values on older adults.

CASE STUDY

Case 1

LA is an 84-year-old woman who comes to your office for a wellness check. She is active with no significant health problems. She reports she just started a sexual relationship with her next-door neighbor in the retirement community. After listening to her friends, she doubts he is monogamous.

Case 2

PH is a 77-year-old woman who has lived with BP for 25 years. She seeks your advice on the lack of intimacy since he started treatments for prostate cancer. BP has been more distant, and not only does PH feel her sexual needs are not being met, she feels her emotional intimacy has also suffered.

Case 3

SB is a 93-year-old woman residing in a retirement community. She has vascular dementia but has been able to remain functional within the routine of the retirement community. She calls her son and daughter-in-law (DIL) to report she has a boyfriend and they are having sex. After further questioning, the son and DIL feel the couple are not having intercourse but are probably engaging in foreplay. They call you seeking advice.

Case 4

BC is a 78-year-old woman who resides in a memory care unit. She is still married, and her husband visits often. Other than her dementia, she is in good physical health. She is frequently seen ambulating the hallways with 86-year-old PS, who suffers from vascular dementia as well as congestive heart failure (CHF), chronic kidney disease (CKD), and peripheral artery disease (PAD). PS is also married, and his wife visits frequently. The manager of the building contacts you to report they found both of them in bed together unclothed. The manager is asking for your advice.

Summary

In all of these cases the approach is the same. NPs and PAs must educate the older adult, family members, and caregivers about the importance of sexuality throughout the life span, including older age. Myths and biases need to be eliminated.

In case 1, the risk of unprotected sex needs to be discussed. A thorough sexual history needs to be done, and LA needs to feel comfortable discussing her involvement with her neighbor.

In case 2, a thorough sexual history needs to occur. PH needs to be empowered to discuss her concerns with BP. Alternatives to intercourse need to be discussed. If BP is also your patient, a thorough sexual history may reveal his issues and concerns.

In case 3, whether or not SB is capable of making her own decisions about her sexuality needs to be determined. If she is not capable, her son needs to decide if he is going to allow her to continue to engage in an intimate relationship. The family needs to be educated about older adult sexuality. Meeting with the director of wellness as well as the family of the partner should be encouraged. SB needs to be protected from potential financial exploitation.

In case 4, both individuals need to be examined for their capacity to make decisions about their sexual health. A meeting privately with each family and then as a group to discuss the management of the memory care should occur with documentation of the outcome.

Key Points

- Sexual desire and interest persist throughout the life span of older adults.
- NPs and PAs are often subject to myths surrounding the sexual practices of older adults and often lack the knowledge and training on how to assist older adults in fulfilling their sexual desires.
- Older adults may experience normal, age-related changes in their sexual systems, which may hinder their sexual response but not eliminate their ability to achieve sexual fulfillment.
- Pathologic problems with the aging sexual response are often related to illnesses and medication.
- Older adults with dementia may display inappropriate sexual behavior and may not be competent to participate in sexual relationships.
- Environmental barriers in the home, as well as in acute and long-term care settings, may prevent older adults from fulfilling their sexual desires.
- It is imperative that all older adults receive a sexual assessment so that normal and pathologic changes can be identified.
- Normal changes of aging can be compensated for by teaching older adults about the changes.
- Interventions used to assist older adults in adapting to age-related changes include manipulation of the environment and procurement of assistive equipment and devices needed to continue to function sexually.
- Touch can be an alternative to sexual intercourse and can provide the intimacy some older adults need.

More information about tools and Interprofessional Education Collaborative (IPEC) competencies mentioned in this chapter can be found in Appendix 1: Tools and Appendix 2: IPEC Competencies.

References

Agronin, M. (2017). *Sexual dysfunction in older adults*. https://www.uptodate.com/contents/sexual-dysfunction-in-older-adults

Amin, I. (2016). Social capital and sexual risk-taking behaviors among older adults in the United States. *Journal of Applied Gerontology, 35*(9), 982–999. https://doi.org/10.1177/073346481454704.

Annon, J. (1976). The PLISSIT model: A proposed conceptual scheme for behavioral treatment of Sexual Problems. *Journal of Sex Education and Therapy, 2*, 1–15.

Araujo, A., Mohr, B., & Mckinlay, J. (2004). Changes in sexual function in middle-aged and older men: Longitudinal data from the Massachusetts male aging study. *Journal of American Geriatrics Society, 52*(9), 1502–1509.

Arena, J., & Wallace, M. (2008). *Sexuality issues in aging. Nursing standard of practice protocol: Sexuality in older adults*. https://www.guidelinecentral.com/summaries/sexuality-in-the-older-adult-in-evidence-based-geriatric-nursing-protocols-for-best-practice/

Asakawa, T., Kawabata, H., Kisa, K., Terashita, T., Murakami, M., & Otaki, J. (2017). Establishing community-based integrated care for elderly patients through interprofessional teamwork: A qualitative analysis. *Journal of Multidisciplinary Healthcare, 10*, 399–407. https://doi.org/10.2147/JMDH.S144526. https://www.health.harvard.edu/womens-health/pelvic-physical-therapy-another-potential-treatment-option.

Bauer, M., McAuliffe, L., Nay, R., & Chenco, C. (2013). Sexuality in older adults: Effect of an education intervention on attitudes and beliefs of residential aged care staff. *Educational Gerontology, 39*(2), 82–91. https://doi-org.ezproxy.libraries.wright.edu/10.1080/03601277.2012.682953.

Blackwell, J. (2006, June). Androgen and the aging man. *Advance for Nurse Practitioners, 14*(6), 39–42.

Bober, S., & Varela, V. (2012). Sexuality in adult cancer survivors: Challenges and interventions. *Journal of Clinical Oncology, 30*(30), 3712–3719.

Burraro, T., Koeniger-Donohue, R., & Hawkins, J. (2014). Sexuality and quality of life in aging: Implications for practice. *Journal for Nurse Practitioners, 10*(7), 480–485.

Butler, R., & Lewis, M. (2000). Sexuality. In M. Beers & R. Berkow, R (Eds.), *The Merck manual of geriatrics*. Merck.

Centers for Disease Control and Prevention. (2017, November). *HIV surveillance report, 2016*, vol. 28. http://www.cdc.gov/hiv/library/reports/hiv-surveillance.html.

Centers for Disease Control and Prevention. (2022, June 28). HIV by age. Centers for Disease Control and Prevention. Retrieved September 11, 2022, from https://www.cdc.gov/hiv/group/age/index.html?CDC_AA_refVal=https%3A%2F%2Fwww.cdc.gov%2Fhiv%2Fgroup%2Fage%2Folderamericans%2Findex.html.

De Giorgi, R., & Series, H. (2016). Treatment of inappropriate sexual behavior in dementia. *Current Treatment Options in Neurology, 18*(9), 41. https://doi.org/10.1007/s11940-016-0425-2. https://terranova.org/film-catalog/freedom-of-sexual-expression-dementia-and-resident-rights-in-long-term-care-facilities/.

DeLamater, J. (2012). Sexual expression in later life: A review and synthesis. *Journal of Sex Research, 49*(2–3), 125–141.

DeLamater, J., & Koepsel, E. (2015). Relationships and sexual expression in later life: Biopyychosocial perspective. *Sexual and Relationship Therapy, 30*(1), 37–59.

Dhingra, I., DeSousa, A., & Sonavance, S. (2016). Sexuality in older adults: Clinical and psychological dilemmas. *Journal of Geriatric Mental Health, 3*, 131–139.

Di Napoli, E. A., Breland, G. L., & Allen, R. S. (2013). Staff knowledge and perceptions of sexuality and dementia of older adults in nursing homes. *Journal of Aging and Health, 25*(7), 1087–1105. https://doi.org/10.1177/0898264313494802.

Flynn, T., & Gow, A. J. (2015). Examining associations between sexual behaviours and quality of life in older adults. *Age and Ageing, 44*(5), 823–828. https://doi.org/10.1093/AGEING/AFV083.

Fredriksen-Goldsen, K., Hoy-Ellis, P., Goldsen, J., Emlet, C., & Hooyman, N. (2014). Creating a vision for the future: Key competencies and strategies for culturally competent practice with lesbian, gay, bisexual, and transgender (LGBT) older adults in the health and human services. *Journal Gerontological Social Work, 57*(2–4), 80–107. https://doi.org/10.1080/01634372.2014.890690.

Gillespie, J. (2017). Sexual synchronicity and communication among partnered older adults. *Journal of Sex & Martial Therapy, 43*(5), 441–455.

Granville, L., & Pregler, J. (2018). Women's sexual health and aging. *Journal of American Geriatrics Society, 66*, 595–601.

Kaiser, F. (2000). Sexual dysfunction in men. In M. Beers & R. Berkow (Eds.), *The Merck manual of geriatrics*. Merck.

Kob, S., & Sewell, D. D. (2015). Sexual functions in older adults. *The American Journal of Geriatric Psychiatry, 23*(3), 223–226. https://doi.org/10.1016/J.JAGP.2014.12.002.

Laumann, E., Glasser, D., Neves, R., & Moreia, E. (2009). A population-based survey of sexual activity, sexual problems and associated help-seeking behavior patterns in mature adults in the United States of America. *International Journal of Impotence Research, 21*(3), 171–178. https://doi.org/10.1038/ijir.2009.7.

Laumann, E., Nicolosi, A., Glasser, D., Paik, A., Gingell, C., Moira, E., & Wang, T. (2005). Sexual problems among women and men aged 40–80y: Prevalence and correlates identified in the global study of sexual attitudes and behaviors. *Internal Journal of Impotence Research, 17*, 39–57.

Laumann, E., & Waite, L. (2008). Sexual dysfunction among older adults: Prevalence and risk factors from a nationally representative U.S. probability sample of men and women 57–85 years of age. *Journal of Sexual Medicine, 10*, 2300–2311.

Lesser, J., Hughes, S., & Kumar, S. (2005). Sexual dysfunction in the older woman: Complex medical, psychiatric illnesses should be considered in evaluation and management. *Geriatrics, 60*(8), 18–21.

Lichtenberg, P. A. (2014). Sexuality and physical intimacy in long-term care. *Occupational Therapy in Health Care, 28*(1), 42–50. https://doi.org/10.3109/07380577.2013.865858. PMID: 24354331; PMCID: PMC4550102.

Lindau, S., Dale, W., Feldmeth, G., Gavrilova, N., Langa, K., Makelarski, J., & Wroblewski, K. (2018). Sexuality and cognitive status: A U.S. nationally representative study of home- dwelling older adults. *Journal of American Geriatrics Society, 66*, 1902–1910.

Lindau, S., Goodrich, K., Leitsch, S., & Cook, S. (2008). Sex in the curriculum: The effect of a multi-modal sexual history-taking module on medical student skills. *Sex Education, 8*(1), 1–9. https://doi-org.ezproxy.libraries.wright.edu/10.1080/14681810701811753.

Lindau, S. T., Schumm, L. P., Laumann, E. O., Levinson, W., O'Muircheartaigh, C. A., & Waite, L. J. (2007). A study of sexuality and health among older adults in the United States. *The New England Journal of Medicine, 357*(8), 762–774. https://doi.org/10.1056/NEJMoa067423.

Liu, H., Waite, L., Shen, S., & Wang, D. (2016). Is sex good for your health? A national study on partnered sexuality and cardiovascular risk among older men and women. *Journal of Health and Social Behavior, 57*(3), 276–296.

Lovejoy, T., Heckman, T., Sikkema, K., Hansen, N., Kochman, A., Suhr, J., Garske, J., & Johnson, C. (2008). Patterns and correlates of sexual activity and condom use behavior in persons 50-plus years of age living with HIV/aids. *Aids and Behavior, 12*(6), 943–956.

Masters, W. H., & Johnson, V. E. (1966). *Human sexual response.* Little, Brown & Company.

Messinger-Rapport, B., Sandhu, S., & Hujer, M. (2003). Sex and sexuality: Is it over after 60? *Clinical Geriatrics, 11*(10), 45.

MetLife. (2006). *Out and aging: The MetLife study of lesbians and gay baby boomers.* www.asaging.org/networks/LGAIN/OutandAging.pdf.

Metzger, E. (2017). Ethics and intimate sexual activity in long-term care. *AMA Journal of Ethics, 19*(7), 640–648. https://journalofethics.ama-assn.org/article/ethics-and-intimate-sexual-activity-long-term-care/2017-07.

Monteiro, A., Von Humboldt, S., & Leal, I. (2017). How do formal caregivers experience the sexuality of older adults? Beliefs and attitudes towards older adults' sexuality. *Psychology, Community & Health, 6*(1), 77–92.

Morley, J. (2000). Validation of a screening questionnaire for androgen deficiency in aging males. *Metabolism, 49*(9), 1239–1242.

Nusbaum, M., & Hamilton, C. (2002). The proactive sexual health history. *American Family Physician, 66*(9), 1705.

Nusbaum, M., Hamilton, C., & Lenahan, P. (2003). Chronic illness and sexual functioning. *American Family Physician, 67*, 347.

Orel, N., & Watson, W. (Spring 2012). Addressing diversity in sexuality and aging: Key considerations for healthcare providers. *Journal of Aging and Life Care, 22*(1). https://www.aginglifecare.org/ALCA_Web_Docs/journal/GCM_journal_april2012.pdf.

Rheaume, C., & Mitty, E. (2008). Sexuality and intimacy in older adults. *Geriatric Nursing, 29*(5), 342–349.

Ruben, D., Herr, K., Pacala, J., Pellock, B., Potter, J., & Semla, T. (2019). Sexuality: *Geriatrics at your fingertips.* American Geriatrics Society.

Salisu, M. (2017). *Older adults' sexuality: Role of social workers-can they talk to us?.* [Poster presentation]. Society for Social Work and Research Bissonet (New Orleans Marriott).

Santos-Iglesias, P., Byers, E. S., & Moglia, R. (2016). Sexual well-being of older men and women. *Canadian Journal of Human Sexuality, 25*(2), 86–98. https://doi-org.ezproxy.libraries.wright.edu/10.3138/cjhs.252-A4.

Smith, S. (2007). Drugs that cause sexual dysfunction. *Psychiatry, 6*(3), 111–114. https://doi-org.ezproxy.libraries.wright.edu/10.1016/j.mppsy.2006.12.004.

Srinivasan, S., & Weinberg, A. (2006). Pharmacologic treatment of sexual inappropriateness in long-term care residents with dementia. *Annals of Long-Term Care, 14*(10), 20–28.

Syme, M. L., Klonoff, E. A., Macera, C. A., & Brodine, S. K. (2013). Predicting sexual decline and dissatisfaction among older adults: The role of partnered and individual physical and mental health factors. *The Journals of Gerontology: Series B: Psychological Sciences and Social Services, 68*(3), 323–332. https://doi-org.ezproxy.libraries.wright.edu/10.1093/geronb/gbs087.

Szwabo, P. (2003). Counseling about sexuality in the older person. *Clinical Geriatric Medicine, 19*(3), 595.

Thornhill, T. (2007). Aging and sexuality. *U.S. Pharmacist, 32*(6), HS5–HS18.

Træen, B., Hald, G. M., Graham, C. A., Enzlin, P., Janssen, E., Kvalem, I., Arvalheira, A., & Štulhofer, A. (2017). Sexuality in older adults (65+): An overview of the literature, Part1: Sexual function and its difficulties. *International Journal of Sexual Health, 29*(1), 11–18. https://doiorg.ezproxy.libraries.wright.edu/10.1080/19317611.2016.1224286.

Waite, L., Iveniuk, J., Laumann, E., & McClintock, M. (2017). Sexuality in older couples: Individual and dyadic characteristics. *Archives of Sexual Behavior, 46*, 605–618.

Wallace, M. (2003). Best practices in nursing care to old adults: Sexuality. *Dermatology Nursing, 15*(6). https://www.medscape.com/viewarticle/466153.

Wallace, M., & Safer, M. (2009). Hypersexuality among cognitively impaired older adults. *Geriatric Nursing, 30*(4), 230–237.

Wang, V., Depp, C. A., Ceglowski, J., Thompson, W. K., Rock, D., & Jeste, D. V. (2015). Sexual health and function in later life: A population-based study of 606 older adults with a partner. *The American Journal of Geriatric Psychiatry: Official Journal of the American Association for Geriatric Psychiatry, 23*(3), 227–233. https://doi-org.ezproxy.libraries.wright.edu/10.1016/j.jagp.2014.03.006.

Wardecker, B., Matisck, J., Graham-Engeland, J., & Almeida, D. (2018). Life satisfaction across adulthood in bisexual men and women: Findings from midlife in the United States (MIDUS) study. *Archives of Sexual Behavior, 48*(1), 291–303. https://doi.org/10.1007/s10508-018-1151-5.

Wise, T. N., & Crone, C. (2006). Sexual function in the geriatric patient. *Clinical Geriatrics, 14*(12), 17–26. https://searchebscohostcom.ezproxy.libraries.wright.edu/login.aspx?direct=true&db=rzh&AN=106272806&site=eds-live.

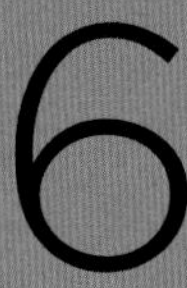

6 Preventive Screenings and Immunizations

VALERIE GRUSS, PHD, APRN, GNP-BC, FAAN, LAUREN DIEGEL-VACEK, DNP, FNP-BC, CNE, AND MARIPAT KING, DNP, RN, ACNP

OBJECTIVES

Student Learning Objectives

After completing this chapter, the student should be able to do the following:

1. Identify the current screening and immunization guidelines for older adults.
2. Discuss concepts related to health promotion and disease prevention to enhance the health of older adults.
3. Recognize the impact of preventive care on enhancing the well-being of older adults.
4. Describe screening tools and immunizations appropriate for older adults.

Practitioner Objectives

After completing this chapter, the practitioner should be able to do the following:

1. Use appropriate geriatric screening tools and immunizations to create preventive patient care plans.
2. Develop proficiency in geriatric screening to evaluate medical, social, and environmental factors that influence overall well-being and identify risks.
3. Develop clinical skills to provide geriatric preventive care using screening tools, immunizations, and the Medicare Annual Wellness Visit to develop patient-centered prevention plans.
4. Improve health outcomes of older adult patients by identifying their modifiable health risks and providing interventions while addressing patients' preferences and values in shared decision making.

Overview

A principal goal of geriatric care is to prevent disease or detect it early so that treatment will be efficacious. Preventive screenings administered to healthy older adults expand the traditional clinic sick visit into a comprehensive wellness visit. Immunizations and screening tools are available for many common diseases and enable the clinician to evaluate older adults for medical and psychosocial problems, as well as cognitive and functional abilities, and to identify those at high risk for common geriatric problems and impairments.

To overcome time-management challenges, clinicians may complete geriatric screenings over multiple visits or use the Medicare Annual Wellness Visit as an opportunity to conduct geriatric screenings and immunizations in a single office visit. This chapter reviews the basic principles of geriatric preventive screening and immunizations in the primary care setting. See Box 6.1 for a list of abbreviations used throughout this chapter.

Interprofessional Collaboration

We focus on collaboration in the management of preventive screenings and immunizations. This chapter is based in the interprofessional collaboration required for geriatric preventive care. Nurse practitioners and physician assistants are defined as "clinicians" because they serve as primary care clinical providers along with other members of the interprofessional team. Information on interprofessional collaboration competencies can be found here:

Core Competencies for Interprofessional Collaborative Practice (IPEC): https://www.ipecollaborative.org/resources.html

Team-Based Competencies: https://nebula.wsimg.com/191adb6df3208c643f339a83d47a3f28?AccessKeyId=DC06780E69ED19E2B3A5&disposition=0&alloworigin=1

Routine Screenings by Age

Functional Status

Necessity

Assessment of functional status identifies the patient's baseline function and provides information about strengths and

HEALTHY PEOPLE 2030 BOX 6.1

Key Overarching Goals

- Increase the proportion of adults who get recommended evidence-based preventative health care—AHS-08

Data from US Department of Health and Human Services. (2020). *Healthy People 2030*. https://health.gov/healthypeople/objectives-and-data/browse-objectives/preventive-care

• BOX 6.1 Top 5 Crash Types for Older Adults

Turning left at an intersection with a stop sign
Turning left at an intersection on a green light without a dedicated green turn arrow
Turning right at a yield sign to merge with traffic at speeds of 40–45 mph
Merging onto a highway from a ramp that has a yield sign
Changing lanes on a road that has four or more lanes

From National Highway Traffic Safety Administration, 2013.

challenges in self-care, which assists in care planning. Early identification of functional change can lead to interventions that provide support and resources to help the patient maintain independence and promote patient safety.

Assessment of functional status includes assessing for activities of daily living (ADLs) and instrumental ADLs (IADLs). ADLs include self-care tasks such as bathing, eating, dressing, ambulating, and toileting. IADLs require executive function and include tasks such as making meals, grocery shopping, using the phone, taking medications, doing laundry, and managing finances (Table 6.1). Typically, impairments of IADLs occur first, but clinicians should screen for both to identify any challenges the patient may be experiencing.

Screening Tools

The clinician may choose to ask brief screening questions or use standard screening tools. For highly functional patients, open-ended questions about their typical day provide a good review of daily function. Global screening questions used to identify potential impairments with ADLs/IADLS may include the following: "Do you need assistance with shopping or finances?" for IADLs and "Do you need assistance with bathing or taking a shower?" for ADLs (Sehgal et al., 2019). Screening for functional status may include patient self-report, caregiver reports, and performance-based measures of ADL functioning; these can be clinically useful, particularly in interdisciplinary settings (Mlinac & Feng, 2016). Standard functional assessment screening tools include tools that measure ADLs alone, IADLs alone, or

CASE STUDY

Scenario

Mr. Brown is a 68-year-old African American man in good health presenting to the primary care clinic for his subsequent Medicare Annual Wellness Visit (AWV). The subsequent AWV is offered every 12 months after the initial examination and first AWV. The primary care provider (PCP) is aware the focus of the visit is on prevention, screening, and coordination of care, and there is no copayment or deductible. The AWV does not provide treatment of chronic care conditions.

Problem

The patient completed the health assessment was completed before the visit. Elements of the health assessment include demographics, self-assessment, psychosocial risks, behavioral risks, activities of daily living (ADLs), and instrumental activities of daily living (IADLs). Mr. Brown's existing medical record was validated by the registered nurse (RN) with elements of the AWV, including the following information: histories (medical, surgical, family); providers (medical, suppliers, durable medical equipment, pharmacy); current medications (HCTZ 25 mg QD, Ramipril 5 mg BID), nonsmoker, exercises three times per week, low-salt diet. Colonoscopy 2018: normal findings, repeat in 5 years; EKG 10 months ago, normal. Psychosocial: widower; active in church, community, and family. Immunizations completed: influenza current year; pneumonia (Pneumovax); tetanus 2017; shingrix two doses (2/6/2018 and 8/7/2018).

The PCP conducted a patient assessment with the following findings: 5'10" (178 cm) 188 lbs. (85.3 kilograms), BMI = 27. Blood Pressure right: 126/78 and left 124/76. Oral screening (SMILE): normal.

The PCP conducted the following screenings:

Screening Tools	Tool/ # Items	Time to Administer	Mr. Brown Findings
Depression screening	GDS short form with 15 items	5–7 minutes	Score 5 = Normal
Alcohol screening	CAGE Screening TAPS tool		Negative
Cognitive screening	Mini-Cog	3 minutes	Score 4 = (Negative)
Fall risk screening	2 questions (neg) Timed up and Go (TUG)	5 minutes	TUG 20 seconds (Neg for fall risk)
Medication risk/review	3 steps to reviewing meds	Previsit review	All meds reconciled
Advance care planning	Power of attorney (POA) Physician orders for life saving treatment (POLST)	10 minutes	Had POA (son) Requested POLST form and will review

Discussion

Findings were discussed with the patient, and the primary care physician (PCP) created a preventive care plan in collaboration with the patient. The PCP completed the annual wellness visit (AWV).

TABLE 6.1 Physical and Instrumental Activities of Daily Living

Activities of Daily Living (Katz ADLs)	Instrumental Activities of Daily Living (Lawton)
Feeding	Using the telephone
Continence	Shopping
Transferring	Preparing food
Toileting	Housekeeping
Dressing	Doing laundry
Bathing	Using transportation
	Managing medications
	Managing finances

ADLs, Activities of daily living.

both. The Katz Index of Independence in Activities of Daily Living (Katz, 1983) is one of the most commonly used tools to measure ADLs. The instrument measures skills of bathing, dressing, transferring, using the toilet, continence, and eating. Clinicians rate individuals as either fully independent (no supervision, direction, or personal assistance needed) or dependent (needing supervision, direction, personal assistance, or total care) across the six skills, with a maximum score of 6 points indicating fully independent, 4 points moderately impaired, and 2 points severely impaired.

The instrument that best addresses IADL activities common to retired older adults is the Instrumental Activities of Daily Living Scale (Lawton & Brody, 1969). This tool is widely used; however, it does not consider more complex social behaviors common among older adults. The IADL takes 10 to 15 minutes to administer and contains eight items (categories of activities), with a summary score from 0 = *low function* to 8 = *high function*. Scoring is determined as follows: Each category item is assigned a score value of 0 or 1. The highest possible score for each category is 1, and the lowest possible score is 0. Category scores are summed for an overall score as follows: 7–8 = *high level of independence*; 5–6 = *moderate level of independence*; 3–4 = *moderate level of independence*; and 1–2 = *dependent*. Although the overall score gives a general assessment of level of independence, category (activity) scores provide a more specific identification of strengths and limitations to guide care plans. The scale can be administered with a written questionnaire or by interview. The patient or a caregiver may provide answers. The scale is generally not useful for older adults in long-term care facilities, where residents perform few IADLs without assistance.

The Older Americans Resources and Services (OARS) Multidimensional Functional Assessment Questionnaire (OMFAQ) is available online (http://www.geri/duke/edu/services/oars.htm). The tool is a 45-minute interview and was designed to determine the impact of services on the functional status of patients. The first part of the tool measures five dimensions of function: social resources, economic resources, mental health, physical health, and ability to carry out ADLs. For each dimension, the information is summarized on a 6-point scale on which the values range from 1 = *excellent functioning* to 6 = *totally impaired functioning*. The second part of the tool is a services assessment with inquiries about the extent of past and current use of services, type of provider, and perceived need for each of 24 services. A summary of the ratings for each of the five dimensions provides an overall impairment score. Individual areas may also be scored to determine level of impairment with specific details.

General health and functional status of an older individual may be captured with the Comprehensive Geriatric Assessment (CGA) tool (Bernabei et al., 2000). This is a well-validated multidimensional evaluation tool that identifies functional status. The time required to administer the CGA is substantial. The CGA includes a cumulative illness rating scale (CIRS), ADLs, IADLs, and short portable mental status questionnaire (SPMSQ). Functional disability is identified by a score of ≥ 3 or a grade 3 or 4 on the CIRS comorbidity index (obtained by dividing the total score by the number of affected organs and systems), or a score ≤ 5 for ADLs or IADLs, or ≥ 5 for the SPMSQ.

Outcomes and Recommendations

A fully independent older adult is a person with no restrictions who requires no assistance or guidance in the 10 areas of ADLs and IADLs (Pfeffer et al., 1982). An older adult with "questionably affected function" remains independent but has greater difficulty than formerly or less skill in the 10 areas of ADLs or IADLs (Pfeffer et al., 1982). A mildly affected person has definite but mild restriction in normal activities or independence and requires supervision or assistance in two or more of the 10 ADLs/IADLs (Pfeffer et al., 1982). A moderately affected person requires assistance with IADLs but performs a portion of the function (i.e., writes own checks or pays at supermarket but someone else balances checkbook, drives, or accompanies the person to appointments; Pfeffer et al., 1982). A moderately severely affected person requires assistance with half or more IADLs and requires three-times-weekly assistance with ADLs (Pfeffer et al., 1982). A severely affected person requires daily assistance in ADLs and total assistance in IADLs (Pfeffer et al., 1982).

It is recommended that the clinician screen the patient and the family/caregiver because the answers may be different. If the screen is positive, the patient should be referred to physical therapy/occupational therapy (PT/OT).

Recommendations

The clinician should also keep in mind that culture, gender, and socioeconomic factors may influence outcomes.

Resources

Katz ADL tool: https://consultgeri.org/try-this/general-assessment/issue-2.pdf

Lawton Instrumental Activities of Daily Living Scale: https://consultgeri.org/try-this/general-assessment/issue-23.pdf

Watch a video demonstrating the use and interpretation of the Lawton Instrumental Activities of Daily Living Scale at http://links.lww.com/A246

The Older Americans Resources and Services (OARS) Multidimensional Functional Assessment Questionnaire (OMFAQ): at http://www.geri/duke/edu/services/oars.htm

HEALTHY PEOPLE 2030 BOX 6.2

Key Overarching Goals

- Increase the proportion of adults who have had a hearing exam in the past 5 years—HOSCD-06

Data from US Department of Health and Human Services. (2020). *Healthy People 2030*. https://health.gov/healthypeople/objectives-and-data/browse-objectives/sensory-or-communication-disorders

Hearing

Necessity

Hearing loss is a decrease in how well one hears. Age-related hearing loss (presbycusis) is one of the most common conditions among older adults. One in three persons ages 65 to 74 years and nearly half of persons older than 75 have hearing loss (National Institute on Deafness and Other Communication Disorders, 2018). Hearing loss typically begins in the sixth decade and is symmetrical, beginning in the high-frequency range. Hearing loss is strongly correlated with depression, decreased quality of life, social isolation, and poorer memory and executive dysfunction.

The American Academy of Family Physicians and the US Preventive Services Task Force (Chou et al., 2011) clinical preventive service recommendations found insufficient evidence to screen for hearing loss in asymptomatic adults ages 50 years or older. However, the Medicare Annual Wellness Visit includes a recommendation to screen adults for hearing impairments.

Screening Tools

Various screening tests are used to detect hearing loss, including a single-item screening question asking, “Do you have difficulty with your hearing?” A yes response should prompt further examination (check for cerumen in ear canal and remove) to rule out a medical etiology. A more comprehensive questionnaire, the 10-item self-administered *Hearing Handicap Inventory for the Elderly*, assesses social and emotional factors associated with hearing loss and requires 2 minutes to complete (Ventry & Weinstein, 1982). If findings indicate a hearing loss is present, a referral to audiology is warranted. The audiologist would identify and measure the type and degree of hearing loss and recommend treatment.

Most hearing problems result from peripheral disease (involvement of the eighth nerve or inner ear). In a quiet room, simple peripheral testing involves asking the patient to compare the sound of rustling fingers (finger rub test) or a ticking watch (watch tick test) bilaterally to test for hearing acuity. With eyes closed, the patient should be instructed to acknowledge hearing the gentle rubbing of the clinician’s fingers approximately 3 to 4 inches away from the patient’s right and left ear. Next a watch is placed at the patient’s ear, and the clinician asks the patient to note when the watch sound disappears as the clinician moves the watch away from the ear. When a man’s watch of average size is used, the tick will be heard by the normal ear of a young adult at a distance of 40 to 50 inches. As people age, the hearing distance for the watch tick diminishes.

Clinical tests used in a primary care setting include the whisper test, in which the clinician stands behind the patient at arm’s length from the ear, covers the untested ear, then whispers a combination of three numbers and letters (e.g., 5-K–2) and asks patient to repeat the set. If the patient is unable to repeat all three, the clinician whispers a second set of three numbers and letters. An inability to repeat at least three of six is positive for impairment.

The physical examination generally includes otoscopy, in addition to the whisper ear test and tuning forks for the assessment of hearing loss. The Weber and Rinne tests, using tuning forks, help distinguish conductive or sensorineural hearing loss and identify asymmetrical hearing loss.

An audiometry test is the most widely used for diagnostic testing for hearing loss. Audiometry checks one’s ability to hear sounds based on loudness (intensity) and tone (speed of sound wave vibrations). Audiometry tests are a simple clinical procedure conducted in a quiet environment with calibrated audiometric equipment by a trained clinician. To test air conduction, the patient wears earphones attached to the audiometer. Pure-tone testing is presented in controlled intensity to one ear at a time. The patient is asked to raise a hand, press a button, or otherwise indicate when she or he hears the sound. Tones are presented across the speech spectrum (500 to 4000 Hz) to determine where the patient’s hearing level falls. The minimum intensity (volume) required to hear each tone is then drawn on a graph, and an attachment called a bone oscillator is placed against the bone behind each ear (mastoid bone) to test bone conduction (Walker et al., 2013). A detailed audiometry test may take 30 to 60 minutes. Patients should ask for the audiogram results because it will serve as a prescription for treatment and hearing aid choice.

Pure-tone screening (PTS) is the gold standard for hearing screening programs in school-age children. Mobile devices, such as mobile phones, are being used for audiometric testing, and findings indicate a high concordance with conventional testing (Chu et al., 2019).

Outcomes and Recommendations

The audiogram results indicate total hearing loss (asymmetrical or symmetrical hearing loss) and high- or low-frequency hearing loss. Normal hearing ranges are 0 to

20 dB in all frequencies. A perfect hearing score is 0 dB at all frequencies. Anything below 20 dB is significantly worse than normal. A 100-dB loss at all frequencies means the patient can hear nothing. Audiometry results indicating a unilateral or asymmetrical hearing loss may indicate a central nervous system lesion and require referral.

The recommended gold standard treatment for hearing loss is a hearing aid. Hearing aids are recommended to improve hearing, communication, and social functioning for some adults with age-related hearing loss. Amplification with hearing aids (any type), personal assistive listening devices, and personal sound amplification devices, with or without additional education or counseling, are helpful. Yet only 10% to 20% of older adults with hearing loss have used hearing aids (Chou et al., 2011). Clinicians need to inform patients that today's hearing aids can be customized to their specific hearing needs, amplify for sounds they have difficulty hearing, and minimize those they do not. There are many types of hearing aids. Some are worn behind the ear or may be worn in the ear and are nearly invisible.

There are many assistive hearing devices to improve a patient's quality of life. These include amplified or captioned phones, FM systems, TV hearing devises, smartphone apps, and hearing loops that connect with hearing aid telecoils. Cochlear implantation may be indicated for patients with severe presbycusis, for which hearing aids are not effective. Cochlear implantation has become a routine procedure. It involves the placement of an electrode array within the inner ear to bypass the damaged cochlea and electronically stimulate the remaining cochlear neurons directly (Blevins, 2020). Cochlear implant outcomes in presbycusis patients may be limited by the age-related reduction in the ability to process sound information, as well as age-related cognitive deficits (Blevins, 2020).

HEALTHY PEOPLE 2030 BOX 6.3

Key Overarching Goals

- Increase the proportion of adults who have had a hearing exam in the past 5 years—HOSCD-06
- Increase the proportion of adults who have had a comprehensive eye exam in the past 2 years—V-02
- Increase access to vision services in community health centers—V-R01
- Reduce vision loss from cataract—V-06
- Reduce vision loss from glaucoma—V-05
- Reduce vision loss from age-related macular degeneration—V-07

Data from US Department of Health and Human Services. (2020). *Healthy People 2030*. https://health.gov/healthypeople/objectives-and-data/browse-objectives/sensory-or-communication-disorders

Vision

Necessity

Several common eye problems occur as people age. Presbyopia is the loss of one's ability to see close objects or small print. Patients report the need to hold reading materials at arm's length or complain of tired eyes while reading. Vision changes related to presbyopia are more noticeable after age 40. Dry eyes are common because the tear glands do not make enough tears. Patients may complain of burning or itching.

Vision loss is common among older adults in the United States, affecting 12% of those 65 to 74 years of age and 15% of those 75 years and older (American Academy of Family Physicians [AAFP], 2016). Common causes of visual impairment include macular degeneration, cataracts, glaucoma, refractive errors, diabetic retinopathy, and temporal arteritis (Siu et al., 2009). Decreased visual acuity and visual impairments increase the risk of falls, fractures, social isolation, and depression and should be treated.

The American Academy of Family Physicians and the US Preventive Services Task Force (USPSTF, 2016, AAFP, 2016) recommendations found insufficient evidence to assess the balance of benefits and harms of screening for impaired visual acuity in older adults (AAFP, 2016; Chou et al., 2016). The Medicare Annual Wellness Visit recommendation is to screen adults annually for visual acuity because visual testing offers little harm and can be accomplished by office staff using a Snellen chart (Snellen, 1868).

Screening Tools

Vision screening tests are used to detect vision changes, including a single-item screening question, "Do you have trouble seeing, reading, or watching TV (with glasses, if used)?" A yes response should prompt further examination to determine visual impairment.

Yearly visual acuity screening may be completed by a Snellen chart testing eye examination. The Snellen test uses a chart with various sized letters arranged in eleven rows. The first line has one very large letter, and subsequent rows have letters that decrease in size. This chart helps determine how well the patient can see letters. Patients are asked to remove their glasses or contacts (it may be repeated with glasses or contacts). The chart is viewed from 20 feet away; the patient covers one eye and reads the letters/symbols out loud. The process is repeated with the other eye. The clinician asks the patient to read smaller and smaller letters until the patient can no longer accurately distinguish letters. The smallest row that can be read accurately is the visual acuity in that eye.

"Normal" vision is referred to as 20/20 vision, indicating one can read a letter at 20 feet that most people *should* be able to read at 20 feet. Usually, the 20/20 line of letters is the fourth from the bottom on the Snellen chart, with 20/15, 20/10, and 20/05 below that. The first row is 20/40 indicating one needs to be 20 feet away to see an object that most people can normally see from 40 feet away. To get a driver's license in the United States, your best-corrected visual acuity must be at least 20/40.

Many ophthalmologists are now using an improved chart, the LogMAR or Bailey-Lovie chart, to test for visual acuity (Bailey & Lovie-Kitchin, 2013). This chart was developed at the National Vision Research Institute of Australia in 1976 and is designed to enable a more accurate estimate of acuity than do other charts such as the Snellen.

Outcomes and Recommendations

Presbyopia is typically corrected with reading glasses. Dry eyes may be treated with eye drops that stimulate real tears; a home humidifier may also help. If visual acuity is not 20/20, the patient may need corrective eyeglasses, contact lenses, or surgery. A referral to ophthalmology would be recommended to screen further for visual acuity, test color, peripheral vision, and depth perception.

Pain

Necessity

Pain is common among older adults. The prevalence of pain ("bothersome pain in the last month") was 52.9% among older adults, as reported in the US National Health and Aging Trends Study (Patel et al., 2013), afflicting 18.7 million older adults. Pain prevalence was higher in women and in older adults with obesity, musculoskeletal conditions, and depressive symptoms ($p < 0.001$). Most older adults with pain (74.9%) reported multiple sites of pain, which further complicates effective pain assessment and management (Patel et al., 2013).

Although the prevalence of pain is high, pain among older adults is underdiagnosed and undertreated. An accurate pain assessment is the foundation for treating pain; yet regular and thorough pain assessments are often neglected (Herr, 2011). Pain is underdiagnosed because many older adults live with chronic pain and underreport their pain, and clinicians are not routinely screening older adult patients for pain (Herr, 2011). Pain is undertreated because clinicians may have concerns about the risks of using certain pain medications in older adult patients.

Screening Tools

The presence of pain and its impact should be determined by questioning patients about their pain. Patient self-report is the most reliable and accurate measure for the presence of pain, even for patients with impaired cognition (Pautex et al., 2006). The clinician may begin to assess pain using simple screening questions such as "Do you hurt anywhere?" or "What is stopping you from doing what you want to do?" A positive response indicating the presence of pain and its impact should prompt a thorough assessment using a validated tool appropriate for use among older adults.

Screening tools include unidimensional tools, which measure pain intensity, and multidimensional tools, which are more comprehensive (Karcioglu et al., 2018). The following unidimensional tools have all been used and validated in older adults.

Numeric Rating Scale

The Numeric Rating Scale (NRS) is a single 11-point (0 to 10) scale that can be administered verbally or in writing. It is a unidimensional tool only measuring pain intensity. The NRS tool asks patients to rate their pain on a scale from 0 = *no pain* to 10 = *worst possible pain*. The NRS should not be conducted as a scale from 1 to 10, which does not allow an option of reporting no pain. The pain scores are interpreted as 0 = *no pain*, 1–3 = *mild pain*, 4–6 = *moderate pain*, and 7–10 = *severe pain*.

Verbal Rating Scale

The Verbal Rating Scale (VRS) is a valid unidimensional ordinal scale easily administered with minimal clinical training. The VRS consists of a list of pain intensity descriptors used to represent various levels of pain: no pain, mild pain, moderate pain, and severe pain. Patients are instructed to select the one descriptor that best describes their current pain. The descriptor result is assigned a number and recorded.

Visual Analogue Scale

The Visual Analogue Scale (VAS) is a unidimensional tool widely used to estimate the severity of pain and to determine the extent of pain relief. The VAS is a continuous scale comprised of a horizontal or vertical line, usually 10 cm long, anchored by two verbal/written descriptors, 0 being "no pain" and 10 being "the wort pain imaginable." Patients are asked to rate their current pain by selecting a point on the scale line.

Faces Pain Scale-Revised

The Faces Pain Scale-Revised (FPS-R) is a unidimensional self-report measure of pain intensity. It was adapted from the original Faces Pain Scale to score the sensation of pain on a widely accepted 0-to-10 metric. It is easy to administer and requires no equipment except for the photocopied faces. The clinician instructs the patient as follows: "These faces show how much something can hurt. This face *[point to left-most face]* shows no pain. The faces show more and more pain *[point to each from left to right]* up to *this* one *[point to right-most face]*. It shows very much pain. Point to the face that shows how much you hurt *[right now]*." The clinician scores the chosen face 0, 2, 4, 6, 8, or 10, counting left to right, so 0 = *no pain* and 10 = *very much pain* (Hicks et al., 2001). Like the VAS, minimal language translation difficulties support the use of FPS-R across cultures and languages.

Other Screening Tools

An important component of geriatric pain assessment is an evaluation of its effect on the patient's function and quality of life (Herr, 2011). The Brief Pain Inventory (BPI) is a self-report or interview tool that assesses the intensity of pain and its impact on functioning for persons with chronic pain. The BPI is available in a short form and long form (with additional descriptors). The short form takes 5 minutes to complete, and the long form takes 10 minutes. The BPI assesses pain severity, impact on daily function, location of pain, pain medications, and amount of pain relief in the past 24 hours or past week. There is no scoring algorithm, but the rating mean of the four severity items can measure severity, and the mean of the seven interference items can measure the impact of pain on function. The BPI has been translated into dozens of languages and used for cancer patients and patients with chronic pain (Cleeland & Ryan, 1991).

Pain is a multidimensional experience that should be evaluated beyond intensity. The Geriatric Pain Measure (GPM) Short Form (Blozik et al., 2007) is a 12-item self-report or interview questionnaire that captures the multidimensional nature of pain. The GPM-12 covers three of the five subscales of the original GPM (pain intensity, pain with ambulation, and disengagement because of pain). The GPM-12 has two questions that ask about pain intensity and 10 items related to pain impact. Calculation of the GPM-12 (12-item version) score is as follows: items 11 and 12 (pain intensity) are scored 0–10; all other items are scored *yes* = 2 and *no* = 0; total score 5 sum of all items (0–40); transformation to a 0–100 scale is determined by multiplying the raw total score by 2.5. The GPM-12 has demonstrated good validity and reliability in European and US populations of older adults. Despite its short form, the GPM-12 captures the multidimensional nature of pain in older adults.

Outcomes and Recommendations

Pain screening should be comprehensive and include an assessment for pain intensity, pain's impact on function, and quality of life. Pain screening and assessment is key to developing a comprehensive pain management plan. Pain management approaches for older adults should include a multimodal approach that includes pharmacologic and nonpharmacologic therapies.

The Joint Commission on Accreditation in Healthcare Organizations (2001) identified pain as the fifth vital sign and mandated that pain assessment be evaluated as part of accreditation. Guidelines and protocols for pain assessment and management for older adults are available from the American Geriatrics Society (Rospand, 2002), American Academy of Pain Medicine (2020), and Gerontological Society of America (2015).

Resources

Faces Pain Scale–Revised, 2001, International Association for the Study of Pain [www.iasp-pain.org/FPSR]

Mobility

A fall is an event in which an individual unexpectedly comes to rest on the ground or another lower level without loss of consciousness (World Health Organization [WHO], 2018). Falls are common among older adults and are the leading cause of fatal and nonfatal injuries in persons older than 65 years (Centers for Disease Control and Prevention [CDC], 2018), and falls are associated with morbidity and mortality among older adults. One-third of community-dwelling older adults (over 65 years) fall every year (Bergen et al., 2016). The causes of falls are multifactorial and include poor balance, weakness, chronic illness, visual or cognitive impairment, polypharmacy, and environmental factors such as poor lighting, obstacles, and loose carpets.

The American Academy of Family Physicians (AAFP) does not recommend an automatic comprehensive fall assessment for each older patient; however, the American Geriatric Society (AGS) and British Geriatric Society (BGS) recommend that all adults older than 65 years be screened annually for a history of falls or balance impairment (American Academy of Family Physicians [AAFP], 2012). The CDC developed the Stopping Elderly Accidents, Deaths, and Injuries (STEADI) tool kit for clinicians based on the AGS/BGS guidelines (CDC, 2015). The tool kit includes resources such as an algorithm for fall risk assessment and interventions and the Stages of Change Model. Fall prevention is now reimbursed as part of the medicare Annual Wellness Visit.

Screening for falls and risk for falling is targeted at reducing the risk for falling and preventing falls. Effective fall prevention can reduce serious fall injuries, functional decline, emergency visits, hospitalizations, and nursing home placements.

Screening Tools

Falls often are not reported to clinicians. It is incumbent upon the clinician to ask patients about falls and their fear of falling. There are three key questions:

Have you fallen in the past year?

Do you feel unsteady when standing or walking?

Are you worried about falling?

If the patient responds yes to any question, it indicates the patient may be at increased (high) risk of falling and warrants further assessment. A positive response to question 1 was found to be associated with a 2.8 times higher likelihood of falling in the next year (Ganz et al., 2007). Fall risk screening is an important first step in fall prevention, but it must be followed by a thorough assessment and the development of a fall prevention plan.

Assess: Gait and Mobility

Gait and Balance

Gait and balance should be evaluated as a screen in older individuals reporting a single fall. The clinician should directly assess the gait as a patient enters the examination room. Reduced gait speed has been associated with reduced survival, and patients with slow gait are more likely to fall. Balance may be assessed by semi-tandem stance and full-tandem stance, the Functional Reach test, the Berg Balance Scale, and the Short Physical Performance Battery (SPPB).

Get Up and Go and Timed Up and Go

The Get Up and Go Test measures a patient's ability to rise from a chair, walk 3 m (10 ft), turn, walk back, and sit down again. Evaluation by the clinician may be a simple qualitative assessment of *normal* or *impaired*, but if staff are assessing, then a timed score with the Timed Up and Go Test may be preferable. A patient who takes longer than 12 seconds on the Timed Up and Go Test or a clinician assessment that gait is mildly abnormal or worse should be evaluated further.

Multifactorial Assessment

A multifactorial fall risk assessment can identify the factors that put an older adult at risk of falling. The multifactorial fall risk assessment should be followed by interventions to mitigate the identified risk factors to reduce the risk of falling. The multifactorial assessment includes orthostatic vital signs, visual acuity testing and cataract screening, examination of feet and footwear, gait and balance testing, and medication review. Medication review is for medications associated with falls using the Beers Criteria for potential inappropriate medication use in older adults (American Geriatrics Society 2015 Beers Criteria Update Expert Panel, 2015). An assessment of environmental hazards in the home should be conducted by OT, with recommendations for home modifications, adaptive equipment, and mobility aids.

Outcomes and Recommendations

Report of a single fall in the past 12 months may indicate difficulties or unsteadiness in walking or standing and signify the need for a comprehensive fall risk assessment. Effective multifactorial interventions such as regular exercise and balance training in an evidence-based structure program, minimizing polypharmacy, treating visual impairment, managing hypotension, and using proper footwear can reduce the frequency of falling and may help maintain functional status.

Few studies recommend exercise to prevent falls. Unstructured exercise programs should be initiated with caution because studies indicate it may increase the rate of falls in persons with limited mobility (Panel on Prevention of Falls in Older Persons, American Geriatrics Society and British Geriatrics Society, 2011). Structured, evidence-based fall prevention training programs such as Matter of Balance (National Council on Aging [NCOA], 2008) have shown a significant reduction in falls and improvements in balance and gait. The National Council on Aging is an excellent resource, offering multiple options for other evidence-based programs to present falls.

Shoes with low heel height and high surface contact area are recommended because they reduce the risk for falling. A cane can be used to improve balance. When a patient is being fitted for a cane, the top of the cane should be at the top of the greater trochanter or at the break of the wrist when the patient stands with arms at the side; when the patient holds the cane, there should be, approximately, a 15-degree bend at the elbow.

A walker is recommended when a cane provides insufficient stability. The patient must be fitted for a walker. Front-wheeled walkers allow a more natural gait and are easier for cognitively impaired patients to use. Four-wheeled rolling walkers (i.e., Rollators) have the advantage of a smoother, faster gait but require more coordination because of the brakes. They are practical for outside walking.

Resources

National Council on Aging, Evidence-Based Falls Prevention Programs: https://www.ncoa.org/healthy-aging/falls-prevention/falls-prevention-programs-for-older-adults-2/

HEALTHY PEOPLE 2030 BOX 6.4

Key Overarching Goals

- Increase the proportion of older adults with dementia or their caregivers who know they have it—DIA-01
- Increase the proportion of adults with subjective cognitive decline who have discussed their symptoms with a provider—DIA-03

Data from US Department of Health and Human Services. (2020). *Healthy People 2030.* https://health.gov/healthypeople/tools-action/browse-evidence-based-resources/final-recommendation-statement-cognitive-impairment-older-adults-screening

Mentation: Cognitive Screen

The US Preventive Services Task Force (USPSTF, 2020) reports there is insufficient evidence to support or refute whether screening for cognitive impairment in nonsymptomatic older adults is beneficial. Yet the benefits of screening for mild cognitive impairment seem clear. Key benefits include safety issues related to whether independent living is safe and concerns about driving safely.

The Medicare Annual Wellness Visit and 4M screening recommendations include screening older adults for mentation. Early identification of cognitive impairment provides an opportunity for the patient and family to be involved in shared decision making and to make future plans based on their personal preferences.

The American Academy of Neurology suggests cognitive screening when cognitive impairment is suspected (Petersen et al., 2001), with reported warning signs or symptoms. If warning signs appear, screening should be conducted, and, if positive, clinical assessment should be conducted to determine if there is a medical etiology to symptoms that may be reversible, such as polypharmacy or depression.

Screening Tools

The presence of cognitive changes and their impact may be determined by questioning the patient about changes in mentation, "Do you or any family/friends think you have a problem with your memory?" (Kane et al., 2018). A positive response would warrant cognitive screening with a validated instrument. The following are common cognitive screening tests. Cognitive screening tests do not substitute for a complete diagnostic workup. A positive screening test indicates a person may have cognitive impairment and should confirm this with a diagnostic assessment and workup.

The Mini-Cog cognitive screening tool is a three-item word recall and clock drawing test to detect cognitive impairment in older adults. The Mini-Cog is free, takes 2 to 4 minutes to administer, and has less ethnic/language bias and similar sensitivity and specificity as the Mini-Mental State Exam. The Mini-Cog can be used effectively after brief training in both health care and community settings. Studies conducted in primary care settings have shown that nonprofessionals, including medical assistants, can administer the Mini-Cog with high reliability after minimal training and practice. The Mini-Cog website (https://mini-cog.com/) provides the free tool and information on administering and scoring the Mini-Cog.

The Mini-Mental State Exam (MMSE) or Folstein test (Folstein et al., 1975) is a 30-point questionnaire published in 1975. The MMSE was widely and freely distributed for decades. It was one of the most commonly used cognitive screening tools; however, several limitations exist. The length of administering the test (7–8 minutes) may be prohibitive. Other tool limitations include age bias, education bias, and that the tool is not sensitive for mild dementia. Further, in 2010 it was determined that Psychological Assessment Resources (PAR) has exclusive rights to publish and license the MMSE. PAR (https://www.parinc.com/Products/Pkey/237) sells an officially licensed version of the MMSE for $1.23 per test and enforces its exclusive rights to distribute the MMSE. As a result, use of this tool has diminished.

The Montreal Cognitive Assessment (MoCA) is a 30-item questionnaire that takes longer (10–12 minutes) to administer. The MoCA evaluates orientation, short-term memory/delayed recall, executive function/visuospatial ability, language ability, and abstraction. It also includes the clock drawing test. It is more sensitive than the MMSE in predicting mild cognitive impairment. The MoCA became proprietary in September 2019. Each user must be trained and certified for a fee of $125 and recertify every 2 years to administer the tool. Ziad Nasreddine, the MoCA's author and copyright holder (Nasreddine et al., 2005) has created a company (MoCA Test Inc.; www.mocatest.org) to manage certification, licensing, administration, scoring, and communication. Under the new requirements and subject to uncertain future iterations, users must register a unique profile, obtain consent, and enter selected patient data and test responses through an online portal for centralized scoring.

The Saint Louis University Mental Status (SLUMS) screening tool consists of 11 items, takes 7 minutes to administer, and has better sensitivity than the MMSE for mild dementia. The 11 items measure orientation, short-term memory, calculations, naming of animals, the clock drawing test, and recognition of geometric figures. Scores range from 0 to 30. Scores of 27 to 30 are considered normal in a person with a high school education. Scores between 21 and 26 suggest mild neurocognitive disorder, and scores between 0 and 20 indicate dementia. The SLUMS Test is available for free (http://aging.slu.edu/pdfsurveys/mentalstatus.pdf).

Outcomes and Recommendations

If cognitive screening outcomes suggest cognitive impairment, further diagnostic assessment and testing is warranted. First, a medical etiology for cognitive changes should be ruled out. If there is no medical etiology related to the cognitive changes, a comprehensive neuropsychological assessment should be conducted by a trained and licensed neuropsychologist. Neuropsychological assessment includes a lengthy battery of tests assessing memory, executive functioning, language skills, math skills, visual and spatial skills, mood, and other abilities related to cognitive functioning to help diagnose an individual's condition accurately. Neuropsychological assessment can determine the impact of the cognitive changes on the individual's functioning and identify areas of impairment that may need assistance; it also ascertains areas of strength.

Recommendations

Useful websites to which to refer patients and families include the following:

National Institute on Aging (the Alzheimer's Disease Education and Referral Center) https://www.nia.nih.gov/health/about-adear-center
Alzheimer's Association https://act.alz.org/
National Alliance for Caregiving https://www.caregiver.org/

HEALTHY PEOPLE 2030 BOX 6.5

Key Overarching Goals

- Improve cardiovascular health in adults—HDS-01
- Reduce the proportion of adults with high blood pressure—HDS-04
- Reduce cholesterol in adults—HDS-06

Data from US Department of Health and Human Services. (2020). *Healthy People 2030*. https://health.gov/healthypeople/objectives-and-data/browse-objectives/heart-disease-and-stroke/improve-cardiovascular-health-adults-hds-01

Disease-Specific Screenings

Cardiovascular

Necessity

The American Heart Association (AHA) and the American College of Cardiology (ACC) formed a task force that reviews and modifies the guidelines for hypertension based on published standards from organizations such as the Institute of Medicine (Arnett et al., 2019). The overall goal is to improve cardiovascular health, which for many people has its basis in hypertension. To ensure that guidelines and recommendations remain current, revisions are coordinated on 6-year cycles. Historically, between 1934 and 1954, almost 5 million insured adults demonstrated a direct relationship between level of blood pressure (BP) and risk of clinical complications and death (Aprahamian et al., 2018). Currently, rates of hypertension increase dramatically as the age of the person goes up. They are higher in men than in women and higher in African Americans than in Caucasians, Hispanic Americans, and Asian Americans (Savji et al., 2013). Control of hypertension is considerably lower for those > 75 years of age (46%) and only 39.8% for adults > 80 years of age. Age modifies the association between high BP and health risks. In adults age 50 years or older who participated in the first National Health and Nutrition Examination Survey (NHANES) and had their

BP measured, systolic blood pressure (SBP) of 140 mm Hg or greater was associated with increased mortality, regardless of diastolic blood pressure (DBP; Aronow, 2020).

Despite the proven benefits of BP reduction in older individuals, there is considerable disagreement between major guidelines surrounding the optimal levels of BP treatment and control to be achieved. In the FRAIL study (fatigue, resistance, ambulation, illnesses, and loss of weight) conducted in 2019, hypertension, physical activity, number of prescribed drugs, and cognitive performance were significantly associated with frailty status (Aronow, 2020). Untreated hypertension was more prevalent in frail older patients and was significantly associated with frailty. Intensive control of hypertension could influence the trajectory of frailty, and this hypothesis should be explored in future prospective clinical trials. Given the high prevalence of older adults with hypertension, nurse practitioners should critically examine the overall benefit of treatment, use of antihypertensive therapies, and BP targets to provide high-quality care to this patient population.

Screening Tools

Office measurement of blood pressure should be performed with a manual or automated sphygmomanometer. Proper protocol is to use the mean of two measurements taken while the patient is seated. The patient should be allowed to sit comfortably for at least 5 minutes upon entry to the office. It is important to use the appropriate-sized cuff and to place the patient's arm at the approximate level of the right atrium. Multiple measurements over time have a better positive predictive value than a single measurement. Certainly the "white coat syndrome" should be evaluated, and patients should be encouraged to have their blood pressure taken in different environments to ensure adequate evaluation.

According to the AHA/ACC (Arnett et al., 2019) and the JNC-9 screening guidelines, it is recommended that all persons over the age of 60 have hypertension screening at least yearly (Arnett et al., 2019). For patients who have known hypertension, the recommendation is to be checked at least twice a year so that BP goals are met. Patients should be carefully educated to report dizziness or other signs and symptoms of overmedication, as well as to refrain from stopping an antihypertensive medication precipitously as this may cause rebound hypertension.

Outcomes and Recommendations

The treatment of hypertension in patients older than 65 years has been demonstrated to reduce mortality by 26% and cardiovascular mortality by 43% (Arnett et al., 2019). The 2017 ACC/AHA hypertension guidelines recommend treatment of noninstitutionalized ambulatory community-dwelling adults ages 65 years and older with an average SBP of 130 mm Hg or higher with lifestyle measures plus an antihypertensive drug to lower the BP to less than 130/80 mm Hg (Benenson et al., 2020). For older adults with hypertension and a high burden of comorbidities and limited life expectancy, clinical judgment, patient preference, and a team-based approach to assess risk/benefit are reasonable for decisions about the intensity of SBP lowering and the choice of antihypertensive drugs to use for treatment.

The initial antihypertensive drug for older persons with primary hypertension is a thiazide diuretic (preferably chlorthalidone) or a calcium channel blocker. If three antihypertensive drugs are needed, they should be a thiazide diuretic plus a calcium channel blocker plus an angiotensin-converting enzyme inhibitor or angiotensin receptor blocker. If a fourth antihypertensive drug is needed to treat resistant hypertension, a mineralocorticoid antagonist should be added. The choice of antihypertensive drug therapy would be modified depending on the comorbidities present.

Coronary Artery Disease (Cad)

Necessity

To date in the older adult age group, the only effective therapy with lipid-lowering medication proven to reduce cardiovascular risk is to lower the concentration of cholesterol containing atherogenic particles via lipid-altering therapies (Bibbins-Domingo et al., 2016). From the standpoint of lipid lowering, older adult patients can be stratified into two groups:

1. Patients ages 65 to 74 years, in whom there is strong evidence of the benefit of cholesterol lowering. In these patients, the decision-making process depends solely on the evaluation of cardiovascular risk in patients without known cardiovascular disease and the risk versus benefit in patients with significant noncardiovascular comorbidity.
2. Patients older than 75 years in whom there is no direct evidence of benefit or lack of cholesterol lowering. For these patients, the practitioner makes a recommendation to the patient based on the risk of atherosclerotic cardiovascular disease, comorbidity burden, lifestyle/socioeconomic status, and presence of frailty. Treatment in this age group is based on the assessment of risk versus benefit and patient preference.

The safety of lipid-lowering drugs is of interest in older adults because the likelihood of an adverse event increases with age and the evidence for clinical benefit decreases with age (Bibbins-Domingo et al., 2016). Disorders resulting in a higher likelihood of drug-related adverse events include impairments of major organs, such as chronic kidney disease, liver disease, heart failure, or diabetes/hypothyroid endocrine disorders. Drug-related toxicity in older adults is attributed to drug accumulation to toxic concentrations. The risk of occurrence of this accumulation increases with age through a series of mechanisms:

- There is an age-related decrease in the glomerular filtration rate.
- There is an age-related decrease in hepatic blood flow and a decrease in drug clearance.
- Aging may be associated with changes in induction and inhibition of different Cyp-450 enzymes.

- Aging might be associated with an increased expression of P-glycoproteins, resulting in alterations in the rate of drug transport across cellular membranes.
- Frailty (but not aging per se) has been associated with diminished drug esterase and conjugation activity.

Screening Tools

There is good evidence that high levels of total cholesterol and low-density lipoprotein (LDL) cholesterol, and low levels of high-density lipoprotein (HDL) cholesterol, are important risk factors for coronary heart disease (CHD; Bibbins-Domingo et al., 2016). However, abnormalities of lipoprotein metabolism include elevations of total cholesterol, LDL cholesterol, or triglycerides, or deficiencies of HDL cholesterol. An age to stop screening has not been established. Screening may be appropriate in older persons who have never been screened; repeated screening is less important in older persons because lipid levels are less likely to increase after 65 years of age. However, because older adults have an increased baseline risk of CHD, they stand to gain greater absolute benefit from the treatment of dyslipidemia, compared with younger adults (USPSTF, 2018).

Outcomes and Recommendations

Treatment decisions should take into account a person's overall risk of heart disease rather than lipid levels alone. Overall risk assessment should include the following factors: age, sex, diabetes, elevated blood pressure, family history (in younger adults), and smoking. Risk calculators that incorporate specific information on multiple risk factors provide a more accurate estimation of cardiovascular risk than tools that count numbers of risk factors.

In patients 40 to 75 years of age with diabetes mellitus and an LDL-C level of ≥ 70 mg/dL (≥ 1.8 mmol/L), moderate-intensity statins can be initiated without calculating the patient's 10-year atherosclerotic cardiovascular disease (ASCVD) risk. In patients with diabetes mellitus at higher risk, especially those with multiple risk factors or those 50 to 75 years of age, it is reasonable to use a high-intensity statin to reduce the LDL-C level by ≥50%.

In adults 40 to 75 years of age evaluated for primary ASCVD prevention, a clinician-patient risk discussion should take place before starting statin therapy. The risk discussion should include a review of major risk factors (e.g., cigarette smoking, elevated blood pressure, LDL-C, hemoglobin A1C [if indicated], and calculated 10-year risk of ASCVD), the presence of risk-enhancing factors, the potential benefits of lifestyle and statin therapies, the potential for adverse effects and drug-drug interactions, consideration of costs of statin therapy, and patient preferences and values in shared decision making.

In adults 40 to 75 years of age without diabetes mellitus and with LDL-C levels ≥ 70 mg/dL (≥ 1.8 mmol/L) at a 10-year ASCVD risk of ≥ 7.5%, use of a moderate-intensity statin should begin if a discussion of treatment options favors statin therapy, such as risk-enhancing factors. If risk status is uncertain, use of coronary artery calcium (CAC) to improve specificity should be considered. If statins are indicated, LDL-C levels can be reduced by ≥ 30%, and if 10-year risk is ≥ 20%, LDL-C levels can be reduced by ≥ 50%.

In adults 40 to 75 years of age without diabetes mellitus and a 10-year risk of 5% to 19.9%, risk-enhancing factors favor the initiation of statin therapy. Risk-enhancing factors include a family history of premature ASCVD; persistently elevated LDL-C levels ≥ 160 mg/dL (≥ 4.1 mmol/L); metabolic syndrome, chronic kidney disease, and a history of preeclampsia or premature menopause (55 years of age). For any patient, if the CAC score is ≥ 100 Agatston units or ≥ the 75th percentile, statin therapy is indicated unless otherwise deferred by the outcome of the clinician-patient risk discussion.

Adherence and percentage response to LDL-C-lowering medications and lifestyle changes can be assessed with repeat lipid measurement 4 to 12 weeks after statin initiation or dose adjustment, repeated every 3 to 12 months as needed. Responses to lifestyle and statin therapy are defined by percentage reductions in LDL-C levels compared with baseline. In ASCVD patients at very high risk, triggers for adding nonstatin drugs are defined by threshold LDL-C levels ≥ 70 mg/dL (≥ 1.8 mmol/L) on maximal statin therapy.

Once patients begin a therapy, practitioners should reassess in 4 to 12 weeks with a fasting cholesterol, and once tolerance has been established, patients should be retested every 3 to 12 months as needed.

In older adults with an LDL-C level of 70 to 189 mg/dL (1.7–4.8 mmol/L), the clinician may initiate a moderate-intensity statin. However, statin therapy may be stopped when the patient's physical or cognitive functional decline, multimorbidity, frailty, or reduced life expectancy limit the potential benefits. In adults 76 to 80 years of age with an LDL-C level of 70 to 189 mg/dL (1.7–4.8 mmol/L), the clinician can measure CAC to reclassify those with a CAC score of zero to avoid statin therapy.

Hyperlipidemia

Necessity

To date in the older adult age group, the only effective therapy with lipid-lowering medication to reduce cardiovascular risk is to lower the concentration of cholesterol containing atherogenic particles via lipid-altering therapies (Arnett et al., 2019). From the standpoint of lipid lowering, older adult patients can be stratified into two groups:

1. Patients ages 65 to 74 years, in whom there is strong evidence of the benefit of cholesterol lowering. In these patients, the decision-making process depends solely on the evaluation of cardiovascular risk in patients without known cardiovascular disease and the risk versus benefit in patients with significant noncardiovascular comorbidity.
2. Patients older than 75 years in whom there is no direct evidence of benefit or lack of benefit for cholesterol lowering. For these patients, the practitioner makes a recommendation to the patient based on the risk of

atherosclerotic cardiovascular disease, comorbidity burden, lifestyle/socioeconomic status, and presence of frailty. Treatment in this age group is based on the assessment of risk versus benefit and patient preference. The safety of lipid-lowering drugs is of interest in older adults because the likelihood of an adverse event increases with age and the evidence for clinical benefit decreases with age. Disorders resulting in a higher likelihood of drug-related adverse events include impairments of major organs such as chronic kidney disease, liver disease, heart failure, or diabetes/hypothyroid endocrine disorders. Drug-related toxicity in older adults is attributed to drug accumulation to toxic concentrations. The risk of occurrence of this accumulation increases with age through a series of mechanisms:

- There is an age-related decrease in the glomerular filtration rate.
- There is an age-related decrease in hepatic blood flow and a decrease in drug clearance.
- Aging may be associated with changes in induction and inhibition of different Cyp-450 enzymes.
- Aging might be associated with an increased expression of P-glycoproteins, resulting in alterations in the rate of drug transport across cellular membranes.
- Frailty (but not aging per se) has been associated with diminished drug esterase and conjugation activity.

Screening Tools

There is good evidence that high levels of total cholesterol and LDL cholesterol, and low levels of HDL cholesterol, are important risk factors for CHD. However, abnormalities of lipoprotein metabolism include elevations of total cholesterol, LDL cholesterol, or triglycerides, or deficiencies of HDL cholesterol (USPSTF, 2018). An age to stop screening has not been established. Screening may be appropriate in older persons who have never been screened; repeated screening is less important in older persons because lipid levels are less likely to increase after 65 years of age. However, because older adults have an increased baseline risk of CHD, they stand to gain greater absolute benefit from the treatment of dyslipidemia, compared with younger adults.

Outcomes and Recommendations

Treatment decisions should consider a person's overall risk of heart disease rather than lipid levels alone. Overall risk assessment should include the following factors: age, sex, diabetes, elevated blood pressure, family history (in younger adults), and smoking. Risk calculators that incorporate specific information on multiple risk factors provide a more accurate estimation of cardiovascular risk than tools that count numbers of risk factors.

In patients 40 to 75 years of age with diabetes mellitus and an LDL-C level of ≥ 70 mg/dL (≥ 1.8 mmol/L), moderate-intensity statins can be initiated without calculating 10-year ASCVD risk. In patients with diabetes mellitus at higher risk, especially those with multiple risk factors or those 50 to 75 years of age, it is reasonable to use a high-intensity statin to reduce the LDL-C level by ≥ 50%.

In adults 40 to 75 years of age evaluated for primary ASCVD prevention, a clinician-patient risk discussion should take place before starting statin therapy. The risk discussion should include a review of major risk factors (e.g., cigarette smoking, elevated blood pressure, LDL-C, hemoglobin A1C [if indicated], and calculated 10-year risk of ASCVD), the presence of risk-enhancing factors, the potential benefits of lifestyle and statin therapies, the potential for adverse effects and drug-drug interactions, consideration of costs of statin therapy, and patient preferences and values in shared decision making.

In adults 40 to 75 years of age without diabetes mellitus and with LDL-C levels ≥ 70 mg/dL (≥ 1.8 mmol/L) at a 10-year ASCVD risk of ≥ 7.5%, use of a moderate-intensity statin should begin if a discussion of treatment options favors statin therapy, such as risk-enhancing factors. If risk status is uncertain, use of CAC to improve specificity should be considered. If statins are indicated, LDL-C levels can be reduced by ≥ 30%, and if 10-year risk is ≥ 20%, reduced LDL-C levels can be reduced by ≥ 50%.

In adults 40 to 75 years of age without diabetes mellitus and a 10-year risk of 5% to 19.9%, risk-enhancing factors favor the initiation of statin therapy. Risk-enhancing factors include a family history of premature ASCVD, persistently elevated LDL-C levels ≥ 160 mg/dL (≥ 4.1 mmol/L), metabolic syndrome, chronic kidney disease, a history of preeclampsia, and premature menopause (55 years of age). For any patient, if the CAC score is ≥ 100 Agatston units or ≥ the 75th percentile, statin therapy is indicated unless otherwise deferred by the outcome of the clinician-patient risk discussion.

Adherence and percentage response to LDL-C-lowering medications and lifestyle changes can be assessed with repeat lipid measurement 4 to 12 weeks after statin initiation or dose adjustment, repeated every 3 to 12 months as needed. Responses to lifestyle and statin therapy are defined by percentage reductions in LDL-C levels compared with baseline. In ASCVD patients at very high risk, triggers for adding nonstatin drugs are defined by threshold LDL-C levels ≥ 70 mg/dL (≥ 1.8 mmol/L) on maximal statin therapy.

Once patients begin a therapy, practitioners should reassess in 4 to 12 weeks with a fasting cholesterol and, once tolerance has been established, patients should be retested every 3 to 12 months as needed.

In older adults with an LDL-C level of 70 to 189 mg/dL (1.7–4.8 mmol/L), the clinician may initiate a moderate-intensity statin. However, statin therapy may be stopped when the patient's physical or cognitive functional decline, multimorbidity, frailty, or reduced life expectancy limit the potential benefits. In adults 76 to 80 years of age with an LDL-C level of 70 to 189 mg/dL (1.7–4.8 mmol/L), the clinician can measure CAC to reclassify those with a CAC score of zero to avoid statin therapy.

Stroke

Necessity

Stroke (or cerebral vascular accident) is the fourth leading cause of death in the United States. Additionally, it causes more long-term disability than any other disease (CDC, 2017; Go et al., 2001). Older persons are at higher risk of having a stroke. One major risk factor for stroke is hypertension, which older people naturally develop. Additionally, the rate of atrial fibrillation in the older population is much higher than that in younger adults (Wolf et al., 1991). Atrial fibrillation is the most common type of cardiac arrhythmia (irregular heartbeat), and its prevalence increases with age, affecting about 3% of men and 2% of women ages 65 to 69 years and about 10% of adults 85 years and older (Go et al., 2001). Atrial fibrillation is a major risk factor for ischemic stroke, increasing risk of stroke by as much as fivefold (Wolf et al., 1991). Approximately 20% of patients who have a stroke associated with atrial fibrillation are first diagnosed with atrial fibrillation at the time of the stroke or shortly thereafter. Clots traveling from the left atrium through the carotid arteries may occlude the cerebral circulation, thereby causing an ischemic stroke. The USPSTF (Bibbins-Domingo et al., 2016) found adequate evidence that treatment with anticoagulant therapy reduces the incidence of stroke in patients with symptomatic atrial fibrillation. Without treatment with anticoagulant therapy, patients with atrial fibrillation have an approximately fivefold increased risk of stroke, and strokes associated with atrial fibrillation tend to be more severe than strokes attributed to other causes (Curry et al., 2018). Approximately one-third of patients with atrial fibrillation who have a stroke die within the year, and up to 30% of survivors have some type of permanent disability (Curry et al., 2018). Atrial fibrillation does not always cause noticeable symptoms, and some persons may not be aware that they have it. For approximately 20% of patients who have a stroke associated with atrial fibrillation, stroke is the first sign that they have the condition. If persons with undiagnosed atrial fibrillation could be detected earlier and start preventive therapy earlier, some of these strokes might be avoided.

Screening Tools

- Electrocardiogram to monitor patients for atrial fibrillation, atrial flutter, or other dysrhythmias, which place patients at higher risk of stroke; patients in atrial fibrillation need to be evaluated for anticoagulation therapy
- Blood pressure management: Over 67% of patients who experience a stroke have a BP in excess of 140/90 mm Hg
- Carotid artery auscultation and ultrasound of carotid arteries
- Diabetes: Fasting blood glucose < 120 mg/dl and A1C < 7%
- Fat and cholesterol level measurement.

Current Guidelines

- Triglycerides < 150 mg/dl
- LDL < 100 mg/dl
- HDL > 50 mg/dl
- Total cholesterol < 200 mg/dl

Outcomes and Recommendations

Older persons who have multiple comorbidities putting them at high risk for strokes are advised to do the following:

- Have a biannual screening for heart rate and rhythm; electrocardiogram.
- Have their carotid arteries assessed, followed by ultrasound if bruit is auscultated.
- Monitor and maintain control of BP.
- Cease smoking.
- Control and monitor cholesterol.
- Control and monitor diabetes, if appropriate.
- Maintain a healthy diet.
- Maintain regular exercise and activity.

Abdominal Aortic Aneurysm

An aneurysm is a bulge in an artery due to a weakening of the wall. The ballooning of the artery may grow larger and tear if not diagnosed and repaired. A ruptured abdominal aortic aneurysm (AAA) is a life-threatening emergency, and 15,000 people die as a result of a ruptured AAA each year in the United States (Owens et al., 2019).

Necessity

The older a patient is, the higher the risk of AAAs. Men are more likely to have an AAA than women. Smoking increases your risk of developing an AAA eightfold. Risk factors for developing an AAA include the following:

- Age over 60 years
- Tobacco use
- Family history of AAA
- History of peripheral artery disease
- History of heart disease
- History of poorly controlled hypertension

Screening Tools

Current recommendations are to screen all patients who have smoked > 40 years or who are currently smoking by annual radiograph, ultrasound, or computed tomography, depending on the patient's body habitus. AAA is typically an asymptomatic disorder, but occasionally it is picked up incidentally on a radiograph of the abdomen. Occasionally, a patient may notice a pulsatile area in the abdomen. If a patient does feel anything, it may be lower abdominal pain or back pain. Tests to diagnose a AAA include an ultrasound, radiograph, and an abdominal CT.

Outcomes and Recommendations

Treatment prior to rupture is critical in terms of survival. AAAs that are < 4 cm should be carefully and closely monitored so that, if they grow, they can be repaired. Those AAAs that are 5 cm or greater need to be repaired. There are two standard methods of treatment:

- Since the early 1970s, the standard method of AAA repair has been the placement of a synthetic graft over the tear in the operating room under general anesthesia. Typically, the patient is in the hospital for 8 to 10 days following surgery and makes a full recovery.
- More recently, an endovascular graft can be placed via small incisions in the femoral artery of the groin. Fluoroscopic guidance is used to place the graft accurately inside the AAA. The graft is then expanded and held in place with metallic hooks. Patients go home in 1 or 2 days and can resume work in 1 week in most cases. Endovascular grafts are scanned on a regular basis to ensure the status of the repair.

The endovascular graft is a much-desired approach, especially in the older adult population, because the risk of complications decreases exponentially with a less invasive approach.

HEALTHY PEOPLE 2030 BOX 6.6

Key Overarching Goals

- Reduce the number of diabetes cases diagnosed yearly—D-01
- Increase the number of people with diabetes who get formal diabetes education—D-06
- Reduce the rate of death from any cause in adults with diabetes—D-09

Data from US Department of Health and Human Services. (2020). *Healthy People 2030*. https//health.gov/healthypeople/objectives-and-data/browse-objectives/diabetes

Diabetes

Necessity

The percentage of adults with type 2 diabetes increases with age (CDC, 2017). About 25% of Americans over age 65 have type 2 diabetes, 50% have prediabetes, and approximately 2 million older adults have undiagnosed diabetes (CDC, 2017).

Screening Tools

Fasting plasma glucose (FPG) or hemoglobin A1C blood tests (United States Preventive Services Task Force [USPSTF], 2015) are used to screen for type 2 diabetes.

Outcomes and Recommendations

Adults ages 40 to 70 should be screened every 1 to 3 years for abnormal glucose if they have the following risk factors: overweight, obesity, family history, personal history of gestational diabetes, or if they are members of certain racial/ethnic groups who may be at risk at an earlier age (African American, Asian American, Hispanic, American Indian, Alaskan Indian, Native Hawaiian, Pacific Islander; USPTF, 2015). The American Diabetes Association recommends screening at 3-year levels for older adults with a body mass index $\geq 25\,kg/m^2$ (ADA, n.d.). Both groups recommend an FPG or A1C test for all individuals older than age 45 at 3-year intervals to detect prediabetes or diabetes, particularly those with a body mass index (BMI) $\geq 25\,kg/m^2$ (Lee & Halter, 2017). For older adults, a person-centered approach is used to evaluate individuals and their risk factors.

HEALTHY PEOPLE 2030 BOX 6.7

Key Overarching Goals

- Reduce the rate of acute hepatitis C—IID-12

Data from US Department of Health and Human Services. (2020). *Healthy People 2030*. https://health.gov/healthypeople/objectives-and-data/browse-objectives/infectious-disease/reduce-rate-acute-hepatitis-c-iid-12

Hepatitis C Screen

Necessity

Older adults are more likely to have the hepatitis C virus (HCV) due to several risk factors that include receiving a blood transfusion prior to 1992 (before universal HCV screening of blood and blood products) and a history of other exposure factors including sexual transmission and injection drug use (USPTF, 2013). Additionally, alcoholic liver disease and chronic hepatitis are the most common causes of end-stage liver disease in older adults (Kelly et al., 2017).

Screening Tools

The Hepatitis C Virus Rapid Antibody Test (CDC, 2013) is used to screen for hepatitis C.

Outcomes and Recommendations

Adults born between 1945 and 1965 should be tested once, regardless of HCV risk factors. Individuals with additional risk factors such as use of intranasal or injection drug use, incarcerations, unregulated tattoos, or long-term hemodialysis should be tested periodically (USPTF, 2013).

HEALTHY PEOPLE 2030 BOX 6.8

Key Overarching Goals

- Reduce the overall cancer death rate—C-01
- Reduce the female breast cancer death rate—C-04
- Reduce the colorectal cancer death rate—C-06
- Reduce the prostate cancer death rate—C-08
- Increase the proportion of cancer survivors who are living 5 years or longer after diagnosis—C-11

Data from US Department of Health and Human Services. (2020). *Healthy People 2030*. https://health.gov/healthypeople/objectives-and-data/browse-objectives/cancer

Cancer

Colorectal Cancer

Necessity

Colorectal cancer has a high incidence, and approximately 60% of colorectal cancer patients are older than 70, with this incidence likely increasing in the near future (García-Albéniz et al., 2017). Older adult patients (> 70–75 years of age) are a heterogeneous group, ranging from the very fit to the very frail (Millan et al., 2015). Studies suggest that fit older adult patients can be treated the same way as their younger counterparts (García-Albéniz et al., 2017). The treatment of frail older patients should be discussed carefully with the patient and family, taking into account fitness for treatment, wishes of the patient and family, and quality of life.

Screening Tools

The guidelines recommend screening for colorectal cancer using fecal occult blood testing, sigmoidoscopy, or colonoscopy in adults, beginning at age 50 years and continuing until age 75. The guidelines recommend against routine screening for colorectal cancer in adults ages 76 to 85 years. According to the US Preventive Service Task Force, some types of screening (fecal occult blood testing [FOBT], sigmoidoscopy, or total colonoscopy) are recommended for persons 50 to 75 years of age; however, the decision to screen patients 76 to 85 years of age is based on individual judgment. Furthermore, screening is not recommended for persons ≥ 85 years of age (Bibbins-Domingo et al., 2016).

Outcomes and Recommendations

Colonoscopy for colorectal cancer screening is currently thought to be unnecessary in the oldest populations, who are considered to be in generally poor physical condition and whose remaining life spans are presumed to be short (Ko & Sonnenberg, 2005). However, older adult patients who are in good health and can be expected to have longer remaining life spans, but are not being screened, should benefit from screening colonoscopy (Ko & Sonnenberg, 2005). Although colonoscopy is not an easily tolerated test for older adults, the early detection of colorectal cancer is considered to be just as beneficial for older adults as it is for younger patients (Kudo & Kudo, 2017). It is therefore not ideal to avoid colonoscopy just because a person is older; instead, this procedure should be conducted as much as possible if colorectal cancer is suspected, with due consideration of the patient's general physical condition. It is essential that the treatment of older adult patients is performed cautiously, accounting for potential risks and benefits on an individual basis. The report by García-Albéniz et al. is extremely valuable in this sense and suggests the need for further discussion on the significance of screening tests in older adults.

Lung Cancer

Since the 1960s, there has been a concerted effort to reduce the uptake of cigarette smoking and to help smokers quit, and to determine if screening could reduce the burden of disease among those at high risk of lung cancer due to prolonged cigarette smoking. On November 4, 2010, the director of the National Cancer Institute (NCI) announced that an ongoing evaluation of the National Lung Screening Trial (NLST) data had shown a statistically significant 20% reduction in lung cancer mortality in a group of adults at high risk of lung cancer who were screened using low-dose computed tomography (National Lung Screening Trial Research, 2011).

Necessity

In the United States, lung cancer is the leading cause of death from cancer. This has been observed for men since the mid-1950s and for women since the mid-1980s. Although lung cancer is the third most common cancer diagnosed among men and women, the annual burden of disease is larger than that of any other cancer (Smith et al., 2009). In 2012, the American Cancer Society determined that lung cancer accounted for 160,340 deaths, which was approximately 28% of all deaths from cancer in the United States. Average 5-year lung cancer survival is among the poorest of all cancers (16.8%), and, although 5-year survival is considerably better when the disease is diagnosed while still localized (52.2%), the majority of patients with lung cancer are diagnosed with regional and distant disease (Marcus et al., 2000).

The estimated direct medical cost of lung cancer was $12.1 billion in the United States in 2010, accounting for approximately 10% of the total medical expenditure on cancer (Wender et al., 2013). Findings from the National Cancer Institute's National Lung Screening Trial established that lung cancer mortality in specific high-risk groups can be reduced by annual screening with low-dose computed tomography (Field et al., 2012; Jaklitsch et al., 2012; National Lung Screening Trial Research, 2011). These findings indicate that the adoption of lung cancer screening could save lives.

Guidelines

The National Cancer Institute's National Lung Screening Trial recommended that clinicians with access to high-volume, high-quality lung cancer screening and treatment centers should initiate a discussion about screening with apparently healthy patients ages 55 to 74 years who have at least a 30-pack-year smoking history and who currently smoke or have quit within the previous 15 years (National Lung Screening Trial Research, 2011).

Screening Tools

The screening tool used annually is low-dose computed tomography.

Outcomes and Recommendations

Clinicians should ascertain the smoking status and smoking history of their patients ages 55 to 74 years (Table 6.2). Clinicians with access to high-volume, high-quality lung cancer screening and treatment centers should initiate a discussion about lung cancer screening with patients ages 55 to 74 years who have at least a 30-pack-year smoking history, currently smoke or have quit within the past 15 years, and

TABLE 6.2 Eligibility Criteria for the National Lung Screening Trial

Criteria	Definition
Age	Ages 55–74 years, with no signs or symptoms of lung cancer.
Smoking history	Active or former smoker with a 30–pack-year history (a pack-year is the equivalent of 1 pack of cigarettes per day per year; 1 pack per day for 30 years or 2 packs per day for 15 years would both be 30 pack-years).
Active smoker	If active smoker, should also be vigorously urged to enter a smoking cessation program.
Former smoker	If former smoker, must have quit within the past 15 years.
General health exclusions	Life-limiting comorbid conditions. Metallic implants or devices in the chest or back. Requirement for home oxygen supplementation.

who are in relatively good health. Core elements of this discussion should include the following benefits, uncertainties, and harms of screening.

The American Lung Association recommends annual lung cancer screening with low-dose computed tomography (LDCT) based on the NLST entry criteria (American Lung Association [ALA], n.d.). The National Comprehensive Cancer Network (NCCN) guidelines recommend annual LDCT for adults who meet the NLST entry criteria and for individuals age 50 years or older with a smoking history of 20 or more pack-years who have one other known risk factor for lung cancer (family history, significant exposure to radon, etc.). The American Association for Thoracic Surgery guidelines (Marcus et al., 2009) recommend annual lung cancer screening with LDCT for adults ages 55 to 79 years with a 30-pack-year history of smoking, and annual screening beginning at age 50 for adults with a 20-pack-year history who have an additional cumulative risk of developing lung cancer of 5% or greater over the following 5 years. The recommendations from these organizations are conservative and mostly restricted to the NLST study protocol because there are many questions inherent in a lung cancer screening guideline that cannot fully be answered at this time.

Now that rigorous evidence supports the value of screening for lung cancer with LDCT, it is important that the implementation of lung cancer screening proceeds in a manner that focuses on maximizing benefits and minimizing harms (Gohagan et al., 2005). At this time, there is sufficient evidence to support screening, provided that the patient has undergone a thorough discussion of the benefits, limitations, and risks and can be screened in a setting where the clinicians have experience in lung cancer screening (Bach et al., 2012).

HEALTHY PEOPLE 2030 BOX 6.9

Key Overarching Goals

- Increase the proportion of adults with depression who get treatment—MHMD-05

Data from US Department of Health and Human Services. (2020). *Healthy People 2030*. https://health.gov/healthypeople/objectives-and-data/browse-objectives/mental-health-and-mental-disorders/increase-proportion-adults-depression-who-get-treatment-mhmd-05

Psychosocial and Substance Use

Mood: Depression

Necessity

Since the 1920s the number of Americans over the age of 65 years increased from 3 million to nearly 45 million in 2013, accounting for 13% of the population. Meanwhile, the population over age 85 grew from 100,000 in 1900 to nearly 6 million in 2013 (US Census Bureau, 2019). A report from the National Institute on Aging and the US State Department points out that, by 2030, the number of adults over age 65 will likely reach 72 million, or just over 20% of the total population. Ten million of those people will be over age 85 (National Institute on Aging, 2016).

Depression in the population over 65 is common, both for those with comorbidities and those without. Depression is recognized as the most common psychiatric disorder in this age group, leading to poor quality of life, limited activities of daily living, and an increased risk of medical comorbidity and suicide. The incidence and prevalence of depression has been consistently high in residential aged care homes (i.e., nursing homes), ranging from 6% to 24% for major depression and 25% to 40% for depressive symptoms or minor depression. Approximately 54% of all permanent aged care residents in the United States are reported to have mild, moderate, or major depressive symptoms over the first year of stay (Manetti et al., 2014). The treatment and management of depression among older adults remains a challenge (Park & Unützer, 2011). The presence of comorbid illness and grief often confound the presentation of depression. As a result, it can remain undetected despite its significant adverse impact on quality of life, morbidity, and mortality. Suicide rates are almost twice as high among older persons when compared with the general population, with the rate highest for white men over 85 years of age. Detecting late-life depression in the primary setting helps with the many comorbidities that are associated with depression (Manetti et al., 2014). There are a variety of validated screening tools that are useful in screening for depression in the geriatric population.

Screening Tools

The Geriatric Depression Scale (GDS; Yesavage & Sheikh, 1986) and Patient Health Questionnaire (PHQ-9; Kroenke & Spitzer, 2002) are useful depression screening tools in the ambulatory setting. Any positive screening test result should initiate a full diagnostic interview. When screening for depression in older adults, it is particularly important to have systems in place to provide feedback of screening results, a readily accessible means of making an accurate diagnosis, and a mechanism for providing treatment and careful follow-up. Research indicates that the addition of therapeutic counseling to pharmacologic therapy provides additional benefit for older, frail patients with depression.

The Geriatric Depression Scale (GDS) is 15 items long, and the Montgomery–Asberg Depression Rating Scale (MADRS; Fantino & Moore, 2009) is 10 items long. These multiple-question scales require a trained professional to administer them. The St. Louis University (SLU) Appetite, Mood, Sleep, Activity, and thoughts of Death (AM SAD) questionnaire (Chakkamparambil et al., 2015) was developed with five items and was psychometrically tested. This test can be administered by health care professionals not specifically trained in depression screening and can be used as a first-line test when depression is suspected. Referrals can then be made to a trained professional.

Outcomes and Recommendations

All geriatric patients who are displaying symptoms of depression, including changes in appetite, mood, sleep, activity level, thoughts of death, changes in weight, withdrawal or crying, displays of anger, and the like, should be screened for depression. Treatment measures among practitioners should follow evidence-based depression care management. Medicare and home health care agencies must ensure compliance to depression care management, including a depression care plan, therapeutic counseling, antidepressant medication, and cognitive therapy. Practitioners should follow up regularly with patients who had positive screens in their depression assessments.

Resources

Geriatric Depression Scale: https://consultgeri.org/try-this/general-assessment/issue-4.pdf

Sexually Transmitted Infections

Necessity

Typically, sexually transmitted infections (STIs) are associated with adolescents and young adults, yet sexually active older adults are also at risk of infection (CDC, 2018). Data regarding epidemiology, clinical presentation, and diagnosis of STIs in older adults are still lacking, although a number of studies show that the incidence of STIs, including human immunodeficiency virus (HIV) infection, is significant and has been increasing over the years, as older adults may live and maintain health and fitness into their eighth and ninth decades (Griffiths & David, 2013).

HEALTHY PEOPLE 2030 BOX 6.10

Key Overarching Goals

- Reduce sexually transmitted infections and their complications, and improve access to quality STI care
- Reduce the rate of new HIV diagnoses

Data from US Department of Health and Human Services. (2020). *Healthy People 2030*. https://health.gov/healthypeople/objectives-and-data/browse-objectives/sexually-transmitted-infections

Screening Tools

STI screening prevents complications and is cost effective. Screening of adults for STIs should occur regardless of age, based on guidelines such as those from the CDC (2019) and US Preventive Services Task Force (Parekh et al., 2018; USPSTF, 2019). Annual screening is recommended in sexually active women and older women at increased risk (CDC, 2019). Cervical cancer (CC) screening guideline changes in 2009 and 2012 recommended less frequent screening; however, in patients who are sexually active, annual cervical screening in women and serum bloodwork screening in men are recommended to assess for and appropriately treat STIs in this age group (USPSTF, 2018).

Outcomes and Recommendations

There are many opportunities for health care providers to take an active role in primary and secondary prevention of STIs. First, clinicians and patients alike must overcome ageist assumptions that STIs are not an important health consideration for mature adults. Health care providers can improve the diagnosis and treatment of STIs for older adults in the primary care setting through screening, comprehensive history taking (including sexual histories), physical examination, and prevention tailored for this age group (Nunes et al., 2016).

HIV

Necessity

Older adults are the fastest growing segment of society of people living with HIV (Ellman et al., 2014; Sankar et al., 2011). Many of these adults are not aware of their positive status. Practitioners and health care providers are often reluctant to ask older patients about their sexual histories and current status to evaluate their risk factors for HIV. Additionally, older adults may have incorrect perceptions related to their risk for acquiring HIV. According to the *Journal of Gerontological Social Work* (Oraka et al., 2018), older adults account for 17% of new HIV diagnoses in the United States and are more likely to be diagnosed with HIV later in the course of the disease compared to younger people. An estimated 16.3% of sexually active older adults have tested for HIV, and 15.9% were at increased risk for HIV infection (reported injection of drugs or crack-cocaine use, paying money for sex, more than three sex partners in the past year, or men who reported having sex with another man; Ford et al., 2015). In the adjusted model, adults ages 65 to 75, not married, self-identified as gay/bisexual, and at increased risk for HIV infection were more likely to have tested for HIV

(Ford et al., 2015). An estimated 83.7% of sexually active older adults have never tested for HIV (Ford et al., 2015).

Screening Tools

In the past, HIV screening required pretest counseling and often written patient consent. However, the most recent CDC recommendations are for routine, voluntary, opt-out screening (Adekeye et al., 2018; CDC, 2018). For this approach, an HIV test is ordered after the patient is informed that the test will be performed, and the patient may elect to decline or defer testing. Consent is inferred unless the patient declines testing. Formal pretest counseling and written consent are no longer required. The rationale for this approach is that including HIV testing as a routine part of medical practice will increase the number of individuals screened and thus the number of those with HIV infection who will be identified and referred for treatment. It is also possible that routine HIV testing will improve patient-provider communication about uncomfortable subjects such as sexual practices and drug use. As a baseline, persons of all ages should have a lifetime HIV test, in accordance with both the CDC and USPSTF recommendations for routine HIV testing (Ford et al., 2015). After that lifetime test, the frequency of testing should be determined by the patient's risk behaviors and the underlying HIV prevalence in the patient's community. Providers who treat older adults in primary care and inpatient settings should consider both individual-level (risk, age) and community-level (prevalence) factors when determining the appropriate HIV testing strategy. Older patients with routine engagement in risk behaviors should receive HIV testing and HIV prevention education on a regular basis. However, some patients may have an infrequent prompt for a subsequent HIV test, such as the initiation of a new sexual partnership, whereas others have no change in risk behavior and therefore no indication for a subsequent HIV test. To attain this level of customized HIV testing for each patient, providers must engage their patients in honest and open discussions of risk behaviors and revisit this risk assessment at regular intervals to determine changes in risk behavior. As Ford et al. recommended, providers must "talk directly with their older patients during their clinical visits to promote HIV prevention, assess risk, and provide HIV screening" (Ford et al., 2015).

Outcomes and Recommendations

According to the CDC, older adults underestimate their risk for acquiring HIV infection, underreport symptoms that could be related to HIV infection, and receive less attention from public health outreach and HIV prevention programs (Adekeye et al., 2018; Lindau et al., 2007). There are many opportunities for health care providers to take an active role in primary and secondary prevention of this disease. First, clinicians and patients alike must overcome ageist assumptions that sexually transmitted infections (STIs, including HIV) are not an important health consideration for mature adults. Health care providers can improve HIV-related outcomes for older adults in the primary care setting through screening, comprehensive history-taking (including sexual histories), physical examination, and prevention tailored for this age group. It is imperative that practices and policies are developed and implemented to increase HIV awareness and screening in the older adult population. Increased health care provider awareness of the importance of HIV screening, especially for those 65 and older, is critical. Health policies and clinical guidelines should be revised to promote and support HIV screening of all adults (Sanders et al., 2008).

HEALTHY PEOPLE 2030 BOX 6.11

Key Overarching Goals

- Reduce the proportion of people who had alcohol use disorder in the past year—SU-13
- Reduce the proportion of people who had drug use disorder in the past year—SU-15
- Increase the rate of people with opioid use disorder getting medications for addiction treatment—SU-D03

Data from US Department of Health and Human Services. (2020). *Healthy People 2030*. https://health.gov/healthypeople/objectives-and-data/browse-objectives/drug-and-alcohol-use

Substance Use/Misuse

Although rates of substance abuse generally decrease after early adulthood, according to the most recent data available, more than 1 million older adults had a substance use disorder (SUD) in 2014 (Center for Behavioral Health Statistics and Quality, [CBHSQ]; Lipari & Van Horn, 2017). Abused substances included alcohol, marijuana, cocaine, and prescription drugs such as narcotic pain relievers and benzodiazepines (Lipari & Van Horn, 2017). Older adults who abuse opioids and benzodiazepines are at increased risk for suicidal thoughts (National Institute on Drug Abuse, 2019) and should be screened (Substance Abuse and Mental Health Services Administration [SAMHSA], 2020).

Alcohol Use

Necessity

A moderate level of alcohol use (two 8-oz. drinks/day) has some benefits associated with decreased risk of cardiovascular disease (Halter et al., 2017). Drinking above that recommendation can have detrimental effects on all organ systems and increases the risk of hypertension, cancer, cognitive function, seizures, insomnia, and depression (Lei & Louise, 2017).

Screening Tool

The CAGE screening tool has four questions (Williams, 2014).

- Have you ever felt you needed to **C**ut down on your drinking?
- Have people **A**nnoyed you by criticizing your drinking?
- Have you ever felt **G**uilty about drinking?
- Have you ever felt you needed a drink first thing in the morning? (**E**ye-opener)

Interpretation. A yes response to two of the questions should prompt further questioning about an individual's alcohol use.

Outcomes and Recommendations

Screen at least once or whenever a drinking problem is suspected (Lee & Walter, 2017).

Resources

CAGE screening tool: https://www.mirecc.va.gov/visn22/CAGE.pdf

HEALTHY PEOPLE 2030 BOX 6.12

Key Overarching Goals

- Reduce current use of tobacco use in adults—TU-01
- Increase Medicaid coverage of evidence-based treatment to help people quit using tobacco—TU-16

Data from US Department of Health and Human Services. (2020). *Healthy People 2030*. https://health.gov/healthypeople/objectives-and-data/browse-objectives/tobacco-use/reduce-current-tobacco-use-adults-tu-01

Tobacco Use

Necessity

Statistics show that 8.5% of adults in the United States ages 65 and older are smokers (CDC, 2019). Smoking has adverse effects on every organ of the body, and tobacco use is responsible for one in five deaths in the United States annually (CDC, 2020). Smoking cessation is the major modifiable risk factor to decrease the risk of lung cancer in all age groups, and the risk for developing it increases with pack-years (Presley et al., 2017).

Screening Tools

Ask all adults about tobacco use and offer behavioral and approved Food and Drug Administration pharmacotherapeutic interventions (USPTF, 2015).

Outcomes and Recommendations

Screening for tobacco use should be done once and, for patients dependent on tobacco, intervention options offered at each visit (USPTF, 2015).

Drug Misuse and Abuse

Necessity

As the baby boomer generation ages, the prevalence of recreational and illicit drug use in older adults is increasing and resulting in drug-related emergency department visits (Lipari & Van Horn, 2017). Tobacco, alcohol, illicit drugs, and nonmedical prescription use contribute to morbidity and mortality.

Recreational Drugs

Older adults should be screened for use of recreational drugs such as marijuana, heroin, and cocaine (Lee & Walter, 2017).

Prescription Drugs

Older adults should be screened for the misuse or abuse of prescription drugs, including prescription and nonprescription pain relievers and benzodiazepines.

Screening Tools

The Tobacco, Alcohol, Prescription Medication, and Other Substance Use (TAPS) tool is a validated tool that screens for tobacco, alcohol, and drug use in primary care settings and identifies unhealthy substance use in primary care patients (Gryczynski et al., 2017). The TAPS tool is made up of two parts: a rapid screen (TAPS-1) consisting of four items that ask about the patient's use, during the past 12-months, of substances in four categories, with response options of never, less than monthly, monthly, weekly, and daily or almost daily, and a brief assessment section (TAPS-2) for those who screen positive on TAPS-1.

Outcomes and Recommendations

The identification of patients who have problem use can inform the clinician of the need for a more detailed clinical assessment.

Resources

The Tobacco, Alcohol, Prescription Medication, and Other Substance Use tool: https://www.drugabuse.gov/taps/#/

Routine Screenings by Gender

Gender-Specific: Female

Breast Cancer

Necessity

Guidelines for breast cancer screening in the older female vary by organization and are intended for women who are asymptomatic, do not have a history of breast cancer, and are at average risk for the disease. Mammography screening is covered by Medicare without an age limit (Chang et al., 2016).

Screening Tools

Mammography is an x-ray image of the breasts used to screen for breast cancer. This type of mammogram is ordered as a *screening* mammogram. It usually involves two or more images of each breast. A *diagnostic* mammogram takes longer, and the total dose of radiation is higher because more images are needed to obtain views of the breasts from several angles. For women with a history of breast cancer, diagnostic mammograms should be ordered for a more comprehensive screening.

Outcomes and Recommendations

United States Preventive Task Force (USPTF) Guidelines. Biennial mammography screening is recommended for women age 50 to 75. The USPTF guideline is based on a calculated risk versus benefit of screening and determined that there is insufficient evidence to recommend screening mammography after age 75 years for women without symptoms (USPTF, 2013).

American Cancer Society (ACS) Guidelines. Annual mammography is recommended beginning at age 40, with no specific age recommended to discontinue screening. Instead, clinicians should use individualized assessments of a woman's health status for guiding the decision to discontinue (Walter & Schonberg, 2014).

Cervical Cancer

Necessity

ThePap smear screens for cervical cancer and precancers. A human papilloma virus (HPV) test sample is taken at the same time to evaluate for HPV strains linked to a high risk for the development of cervical cancer (Halter et al., 2017).

Screening Tools

Pap smear
HPV test

Outcomes and Recommendations

Women are recommended to have these screenings every 5 years, beginning at around age 21 (Halter et al., 2017). There is consensus among USPTF, ACS, and the American College of Gynecology (ACOG) that screening for cervical cancer should be discontinued at age 65 if there is a documented history of adequate prior screening with normal results (Lee & Walter, 2017).

HEALTHY PEOPLE 2030 BOX 6.13

Key Overarching Goals

- Reduce the proportion of adults with osteoporosis—O-01
- Increase the proportion of older adults who get screened for osteoporosis—O-D01
- Increase the proportion of older adults who get treated for osteoporosis after a fracture—O-D02
- Reduce hip fractures among older adults—O-02

Data from US Department of Health and Human Services. (2020). *Healthy People 2030*. https://health.gov/healthypeople/objectives-and-data/browse-objectives/osteoporosis

Osteoporosis

Necessity

Half of American women over age 50 will have a fracture secondary to osteoporosis (National Osteoporosis Foundation, 2020). The risk of primary osteoporosis increases with age and varies by race and ethnicity (USPTF, 2018). Early detection of osteopenia or osteoporosis identifies women who may benefit from therapies to improve bone density. Evidence-based treatments include pharmacologic, nutritional, and lifestyle recommendations to lower the risk of fractures in older women (Rothmann et al., 2017).

Screening Tools

Dual-energy X-ray absorptiometry (DEXA) scan measures bone density.

Fracture Risk Assessment Tool (FRAX) calculates the 10-year risk of fracture and guides the clinical approach for prevention: https://www.sheffield.ac.uk/FRAX/

Outcomes and Recommendations

All women ages 65 years and older should be screened for osteoporosis (USPTF, 2018).

Other Screens

Frailty

Necessity

Physical frailty in older adults is a medical syndrome resulting from age-associated declines across multiple physiologic systems (Johns Hopkins, n.d.). Frailty is highly prevalent among older adults and increases older adults' vulnerability to adverse outcomes such as falls, disability, immobility, dementia, delirium, poor surgical outcomes, hospitalizations, and death. After exposure to a stressful event (such as a hospitalization), frail older adults may not return to their functional baseline.

A standardized gold definition has not been established; however, a phenotype of frailty in older adults has been developed from data from the Cardiovascular Health Study (CHS; Fried et al., 2001). The CHS phenotype model characterizes frailty around five indicators.

1. Unintentional weight loss (as evidenced by > 4–5 kg or > 5%/y)
2. Exhaustion/fatigue (as indicated by inability to walk several hundred yards or > 3–4 d/week feeling exhausted)
3. Low activity (as evidenced by < 383 kcal/week in men and < 270 kcal/week in women)
4. Weakness (demonstrated with low grip strength)
5. Slowness (demonstrated as slow gait speed)

Screening Tools

Other models and frailty screening tools (e.g., Frailty Index, Frailty Index for Elders, Vulnerable Elderly Survey [VES-13]) combine elements of functional and biologic indicators to identify frailty.

The Frailty Index (FI; Rockwood et al., 2005) is a cumulative deficit model that identifies frailty by the presence of 25 or more clinical deficits, conditions, symptoms, or laboratory values, scored as the proportion of total indicators present. These 70 clinical deficits include cognition, mood, and social resources, along with physiologic components to define frailty (Rockwood et al., 2005). The original FI requires a large number of variables, making clinical sensitivity difficult to interpret and the FI less practical in a clinical setting.

The Frailty Index for Elders (FIFE; Tocchi et al., 2014) was developed to assess for frailty risk in older adults. FIFE is a 10-item validated assessment instrument with scores ranging from 0 o 10. A score of 0 indicates no frailty; a score of 1 to 3 indicates frailty risk; and a score of 4 or greater indicates frailty. For clinicians, the FIFE may be useful as an assessment instrument to determine frailty using all items and to determine risk for frailty using individual items.

The Vulnerable Elder Survey-13 (VES-13) is a self-administered 13-item tool that evaluates functional and physical performance. The VES-13 identifies community-dwelling older adults at risk for death or functional decline. A score of 3 or higher on the 13-item scale indicates a four-fold increase risk of adverse outcomes and identified the one-third of older adults who were most at risk for functional decline or death (Saliba et al., 2001). The VES-13 provides clinicians with additional information that can be used in postoperative optimization of treatment in high-risk groups of patients and can be a useful prescreening tool to avoid more extensive and time consuming comprehensive geriatric evaluations.

Outcomes and Recommendations

Care of identified frail older patients is challenging for clinicians due to their complex needs and fragile health status. At the same time, the interprofessional geriatric team is poised to provide the type of comprehensive patient-centered care needed to stabilize these patients. The recommended first step is to screen and identify those older adults who are frail or at risk for frailty. Clinicians then may address how recognizing frailty helps us in managing older adults who are frail to develop a comprehensive care plan to address their complex needs.

HEALTHY PEOPLE 2030 BOX 6.14

Key Overarching Goals

- Increase the use of oral health care systems—OH-08

Data from US Department of Health and Human Services. (2020). *Healthy People 2030*. https://health.gov/healthypeople/objectives-and-data/browse-objectives/health-care/increase-use-oral-health-care-system-oh-08

Oral Health

Necessity

Poor oral health can impact patients' ability to chew, smile, interact with others, and communicate. Older Americans with the poorest oral health tend to be those who are economically disadvantaged, lack insurance, and are members of racial and ethnic minorities. Being disabled, homebound, or institutionalized (e.g., seniors who live in nursing homes) also increases the risk of poor oral health (https://www.cdc.gov/oralhealth/basics/adult-oral-health/adult_older.htm). Currently, Medicare does not cover oral health unless the patient is in the hospital and it is a required procedure. Dental care is among the top five costs that older adults incur. Due to the high cost of dental care, many older adults go without dental care. Options for receiving dental care at a reduced cost may include federally qualified health centers, public health clinics, and dental schools.

Cancers of the mouth (oral and pharyngeal cancers) primarily occur in older adults; median age at diagnosis is 62 years (National Cancer Institute. Surveillance, Epidemiology, and End Results Program [SEER], n.d.), and the incidence of oral cancer increases with age. Oral cancers represent approximately 3% of all cancers diagnosed in the United States (Fedele et al., 1991). Oral squamous cell carcinoma accounts for 90% of all oral cancers (https://oralcancerfoundation.org/facts/). Early carcinomas often go undetected because pain usually is not a factor until the lesion is large.

Early diagnosis is the most important consideration for improving patient survival. Yet oral cancer screenings are often omitted during physical assessments, although older adults visit their primary care providers 5 to 7 times more often than they visit their dentists. Older adults consult about oral lesions more with their medical providers than their dental professionals because Medicare does not cover dental visits.

Screening Tools

Oral screening includes inspection of lips, tongue, gums and tissues, saliva, natural teeth (dentures), oral cleanliness, and dental pain. The Kayser-Jones Brief Oral Health Status Examination (BOHSE) designed for nursing home residents (both cognitively intact and cognitively impaired) may be used in primary care settings (https://oralcancerfoundation.org/facts/; Kayser-Jones et al., 1995). The oral screening includes examination of lips, tongue, tissue inside cheek, floor and roof of mouth, gums between teeth or under artificial teeth, saliva, condition of natural teeth, condition of artificial teeth, pairs of teeth in the chewing position (natural or artificial), and oral cleanliness. Each item is scored 0, 1, or 2, with 0 being normal. Although the cumulative score is helpful, individuals who score 2 on items should be referred for a dental evaluation, examination, and follow-up immediately.

Oral cancer screening includes comprehensive head, neck, and oral examinations that include direct extraoral observation, palpation, and intraoral measurements of ulcerations, lumps, swellings, or growths. These screenings are easy to perform, take 5 minutes to complete, and can be done bedside or chairside.

Smile Tool

Screen for oral cancer beginning with history and the extraoral examination by palpating the head and neck.

Mention abnormalities to the patient to solicit further information. (Any lesion lasting more than 2 weeks should be suspicious for oral cancer.)

Inspect the intraoral area for raised lesions and red or white patches.

Localize abnormalities by inspecting and palpating the lips, mucosa, palate, tonsillar area, floor of the mouth, and tongue. (The most common locations of oral cancer are the tongue and the floor of the mouth.)

Evaluation, measurement, description, documentation, and referral when indicated (referral to an ear, nose, and throat [ENT] specialist).

Outcomes and Recommendations

Much research has demonstrated the impact of oral health on quality of life and general health, particularly among older adults (Petersen & Yamamoto, 2005). Poor oral health and poor general health are interrelated, primarily because of their common risk factors, including aging and chronic diseases. Education and continuous training of clinicians must ensure that health care providers have skills in and a profound understanding of the importance of oral health (Petersen & Yamamoto, 2005).

The World Health Organization (WHO) recommends that countries adopt certain strategies for improving the oral health of older adults (Petersen & Yamamoto, 2005). US public health programs should incorporate oral health promotion and disease prevention based on the common risk factors approach. Control of oral disease and illness in older adults should be strengthened through organization of affordable oral health services that meet their needs.

The American Cancer Society (ACS) recommends that primary care providers examine patients at risk for oral cancer as part of a routine checkup because this would give providers the opportunity to detect oral cancer at an early stage (https://www.cancer.org/cancer/oral-cavity-and-oropharyngeal-cancer.html). This is important because the 5-year survival rate is 83% for patients diagnosed with localized lesions, compared to a 63% survival rate for all stages combined (https://www.cancer.net/cancer-types/oral-and-oropharyngeal-cancer/statistics).

HEALTHY PEOPLE 2030 BOX 6.15

Key Overarching Goals

- Reduce food insecurity and hunger—NWS-01
- Reduce the proportion of adults with obesity—NWS-03

Data from US Department of Health and Human Services. (2020). *Healthy People 2030*. https://health.gov/healthypeople/objectives-and-data/browse-objectives/nutrition-and-healthy-eating/reduce-household-food-insecurity-and-hunger-nws-01

https://health.gov/healthypeople/objectives-and-data/browse-objectives/health-care/increase-use-oral-health-care-system-oh-08. https://health.gov/healthypeople/objectives-and-data/browse-objectives/overweight-and-obesity/reduce-proportion-adults-obesity-nws-03

Nutrition

Necessity

Good nutrition is critical to overall health and well-being, yet many older adults are at risk of inadequate nutrition. Undernutrition is associated with an increased need for health care services and increased mortality. Among older adults receiving home health care, 12% were malnourished, and 51% were at risk of malnourishment (Yang et al., 2011). Thus, it is important to screen all older adults' nutritional status.

Medicare defines normal body mass index (BMI) in older adults as 23 to 30 kg/m^2; a BMI of less than 23 kg/m^2 is associated with increased health service utilization and mortality (Yang et al., 2011). It is not enough to assess anthropometrics alone among older adults because BMI 18.5 kg/m^2 is consistently found to be an unreliable indicator of malnutrition in older populations.

Screening Tools

Screening for nutritional impairment in older adults can be accomplished by asking a single question (e.g., "Have you lost weight in the past 6 months?"), monitoring weight, or asking patients or caregivers to complete the Mini Nutritional Assessment (MNA-SF). The MNA-SF is a screening tool used to identify older adults (> 65 years) who are malnourished or at risk of malnutrition. The MNA-SF is based on the full MNA, the original 18-item questionnaire published in 1994 by Guigoz and colleagues (Guigoz et al., 2006). The most recent version of the MNA-SF was developed in 2009 (Kaiser et al., 2009) and consists of six questions on food intake, weight loss, mobility, psychological stress or acute disease, the presence of dementia or depression, and BMI. When height or weight cannot be assessed, then an alternate scoring for BMI includes the measurement of calf circumference. Scores of 12 to 14 are considered normal nutritional status, 8 to 11 indicate risk of malnutrition, and 0 to 7 indicate malnutrition (https://consultgeri.org/try-this/general-assessment/issue-9.pdf).

An advantage of the tool is that no laboratory data are needed. An in-depth assessment and physical examination should be performed when patients are identified as malnourished or at nutritional risk. Symptoms and objective clinical findings should be assessed in addition to the patient's cultural factors, preferences, and social needs/desires surrounding meals. A 72-hour food diary recording the patent's consumption is another important supplement to the MNA-SF. The Malnutrition Screening Tool (MST; https://www.ncoa.org/center-for-healthy-aging/resource-hub/community-orgs-and-professionals/professional-resources/malnutrition-screening-tools/) is a quick and easy validated tool to screen patients for risk of malnutrition. The tool is suitable for a residential aged care facility or for adults in the inpatient or outpatient hospital setting. Nutrition screening parameters include weight loss or appetite. This brief tool asks the following questions:

1. Have you recently lost weight without trying? If yes, how much weight have you lost?
2. Have you been eating poorly because of a decrease appetite?

The two questions are then scored: 0 or 1 = *no risk* and 2 or more = *risk*. A positive screen recommends rapid implementation of nutrition interventions and ordering a nutrition consult within 24 to 72 hours, depending on risk.

Outcomes and Recommendations

Clinicians should regularly screen older adult patients for nutritional status, address risk factors of malnutrition, treat underlying conditions causing malnutrition, change a restricted diet, recommend vitamin and mineral supplements, and refer to registered dietician for guidance. The clinician should educate patient and family to monitor the patient's weight at home and keep a record. Caregivers should spend mealtimes together at home to observe eating habits, help with meal plans, use local services that provide at-home delivered meals, and if needed access a food pantry or other nutrition services. The local Area Agency on Aging or county social workers can provide information on local available services (https://www.ncoa.org/center-for-healthy-aging/resourcehub/community-orgs-and-professionals/professional-resources/malnutrition-screening-tools/). Practitioners should encourage physical activity because this may stimulate appetite.

Recommendations

Older adults who unintentionally lose 5% or more of their body weight in 6 months or have a low BMI require further evaluation for poor nutrition. Through the Choosing Wisely Campaign, the American Geriatrics Society (https://www.choosingwisely.org/societies/american-geriatrics-society/) recommends against the use of appetite stimulants or high-calorie supplements because of the lack of proven effectiveness in long-term survival or improvement in quality of life. Instead, it recommends discontinuing medications that contribute to weight loss and diminish appetite, providing appealing foods, ensuring social support, and offering feeding assistance.

Driving Safety

Necessity

There are approximately 46 million people age 65 or older, projected to more than double to more than 98 million by 2060 (Insurance Institute for Highway Safety [IIHS], 2018). A total of 4973 people ages 70 and older died in motor vehicle crashes in 2018 (IIHS, 2018). The high fatality rates are attributed in part to older adults' increased comorbidities and frailty, which make it more difficult for an older adult to survive a crash (Box 6.2).

The number of older adults is increasing, and normal aging may include declines in sensory systems such as vision, hearing, motor skills, and cognition. However, not all changes that occur with age indicate an individual is not able to drive.

When determining ability to drive, consider the person's functional abilities rather than age. When assessing a patient's driving safety, it is important to consider dementia as a factor. Although cognitively intact older drivers made considerably fewer driving errors than those with dementia, they did make errors across all driving situations, such as turn position errors, positioning errors, and overcautiousness (Barco et al., 2015).

The clinician may notice changes that may indicate a potential driving concern, or the patient may bring a notice from the state indicating the need for a medical release to continue driving due to a recent accident or citation. The clinician will need to address the medical concerns and determine fitness to drive for the older adult. Additionally, the clinician may need to help the older adult and significant other connect with resources to assist in the determination or to access driving retirement resources.

• BOX 6.2 Abbreviations

ACIP = Advisory Committee on Immunization Practices
ACOG = American College of Gynecologists
ACS = American Cancer Society
ADA = American Diabetes Association
ADLs = Activities of daily living
ASCVD = Atherosclerotic cardiovascular disease
AWV = Medicare Annual Wellness Visit
BMI = Body mass index
BP = Blood pressure
CAC = Coronary artery calcium
CAD = Coronary artery disease
CC = Cervical cancer
CDC = Centers for Disease Control and Prevention
CHD = Coronary heart disease
DBP = Diastolic blood pressure
FPG = Fasting plasma glucose
HDL = High-density lipoprotein cholesterol
HPV = Human papilloma virus
IADLs = Instrumental ADLs
LDL = Low-density lipoprotein cholesterol
SBP = Systolic blood pressure
STIs = Sexually transmitted infections
USPTF = United States Preventive Task Force

Many older adults may restrict or self-impose limitations on their driving to improve safety, such as not driving at night, driving during less busy times of day, and avoiding driving in bad weather. But older drivers with cognitive impairment may have limited insight into any changes they may be experiencing and will not likely self-impose driving limitations willingly (Andrew et al., 2015).

Screening Tools

A simple screening tool to assess at-risk drivers is "The 4 Cs." Older drivers are rated on a scale of 1 to 4 in each of the four areas below. Total scores range from 4 to 16. Higher scores indicate a high risk of unsafe driving. A score of 9 or above was able to identify 84% of unsafe drivers from a road test (O'Connor et al., 2010).

- Crashes/citations
- Concern (family report)
- Clinical status (medical history, medications)
- Cognition

Evidence-based screening and assessments can identify impairments that might put older adults at risk for unsafe driving. Clinicians should screen for chronic medical conditions and conduct a medication history and a driving history. The driving history should include obtaining information from the older person, family, friends, and caregivers. The clinician should inquire about history of crashes, traffic citations; reduced driving mileage; aggressive or impulsive personality; and family' or friends' reports of driving ability as marginal or unsafe.

Screening for chronic medical conditions that may contribute to unsafe driving include the following:

- Neurocognitive disorders: Alzheimer disease and related dementias
- Visual impairment: Macular degeneration, glaucoma, retinopathy, cataracts
- Hearing impairment: Hearing loss
- Behavioral/mental health conditions: Depression, psychosis
- Mobility conditions: Arthritis, Parkinson disease, falls, poor range of motions
- Other: Chronic obstructive pulmonary disease (COPD), asthma, sleep disturbance, diabetes, fatigue, cardiovascular disease, epilepsy
- Acute medical conditions: Dizziness/syncope, hypotension, hypoglycemia, seizures, recent injury or surgery

The clinician should obtain a thorough medication history, examine the list of medications, and look for any medications that may impair driving, such as antipsychotics, decongestants/antihistamines, hypnotics, narcotics, tranquilizers, muscle relaxants, and some antidepressants. Roadwise RX is a free online tool developed by the American Automobile Association Foundation for Traffic Safety. It allows anyone to enter the names of medications and check if the medication can affect driving: http://www.roadwiserx.com

Driving is a complicated activity that involves many areas of cognition, perception, sensory, and motor systems. It is important to screen for cognitive impairment (see the section on screenings).

The most comprehensive approach to assess for unsafe driving is to refer the patient to a certified driver rehabilitation specialist (CDRS) or an occupational therapist who is specially trained to assess driving safety (specialty certification in driving and community mobility [SCDCM]). This specialist will evaluate competency by having the patient perform tasks under simulated real-life conditions. This requires a battery of tests that will predict the patient's ability to perform well on a road test. This battery of tests may include the following elements:

- Assessment of Driving Related Skills (ADReS) available at https://www.nhtsa.gov/sites/nhtsa.dot.gov/files/documents/811113.pdf
- DriveABLE http://driveable.com/
- Rockwood Driving Battery https://www.pearsonclinical.co.uk/Psychology/AdultCognitionNeuropsychologyandLanguage/AdultGeneralAbilities/RookwoodDrivingBattery(RDB)/Resources/Rookwood-overview.pdf

Studies predicting road test performance in drivers with dementia have used the following battery of tests: Trail Making Test A (TMT-A), Clock Drawing Test, and Alzheimer's Detection 8 (AD8). This screening battery can be performed in less than 10 minutes and predicted with good results the failure rate for the on-road driving test (Carr et al., 2011). Driving evaluations include an assessment of motor skills, with specific tests of reaction time and brake reaction tests, which can be performed on special equipment or simulators.

Outcomes and Recommendations

To keep older adults safe in their communities as long as possible, we must consider ways to enhance driving safety. The clinician should do the following:

- Encourage older drivers to see their primary care provider regularly if there are concerns.
- Recommend that older drivers drive cars with automatic transmission, power steering, back-up mirrors, large mirrors.
- Recommend routine vision checks.
- If the patient reports trouble seeing in the dark, recommend no nighttime driving.
- Review safe driving tips (e.g., avoid high traffic areas, leave more space between cars, drive in the right-hand lane on highways, avoid driving in bad weather).
- Warn about medications that may impact driving, and encourage patients to always read labels.
- Encourage refresher courses in driving.
- Encourage older drivers to stay physically active and exercise.

Decision to Stop Driving

The decision to stop driving can happen in a variety of ways: as the result of a family decision, a provider decision, or a law enforcement decision; an older driver may make the decision; or it may result from a combination of factors.

To ease the transition to driving retirement, the clinician should develop a Mobility Action Plan. The goal of the Mobility Action Plan is to keep the "retired driver" busy and active in community activities. Clinicians can create a schedule and involve the retired driver by asking what are the important activities that he or she wants to go to and how will he or she get there? It may also help to assign a chauffeur among family, friends, and neighbors, and then ask the drivers to rotate. Clinicians should consider involving volunteer drivers from senior organizations or churches and can rehearse with the patient how to use public transportation, the senior bus service, and or senior cab passes/discounts.

Outcomes and Recommendations

State laws have key provisions pertaining to older driver licensing requirements. These provisions may include mandated vision and driving tests at certain ages, such as every 2 years for drivers ages 81 years to 86 years and every year for drivers > 87 years. State provisions may require an examination (vision test, written drivers test) and an actual demonstration of the ability to exercise ordinary and reasonable control of the motor vehicle for drivers ages 75 years and older. Laws for individual states can be found at https://www.nhtsa.gov/sites/nhtsa.dot.gov/files/keyprovisionsolderdrivers.pdf.

Resources

Vision requirements for individual states: https://lowvision.preventblindness.org/2003/06/06/state-vision-screening-and-standards-for-license-to-drive/

AAA: Evaluate Your Driving Ability: http://www.seniordriving.aaa.com/evaluate-your-driving-ability

AARP Driving Resource Center: interactive tools, games, traffic laws in your state, exercise programs: https://www.aarp.org/auto/driver-safety/driving-tips/

CMA Driver's Guide: http://ammac.org/Residents/CMA-Drivers-Guide-8th-edition-e.pdf

Exercise Safety Behind the Wheel video: http://www.aarp.org/home-family/getting-around/driving-resource-center/info-08-2013/exercise-for-safety.html

Acknowledgment

Peggy Barco, OTD, OTR/L, SCDCM CDRS, https://engageil.com/wp-content/uploads/2018/04/Driving-Safety-of-the-Older-Adult-One-Slide-per-Page.pdf

Elder Abuse

Necessity

Elder abuse includes physical, sexual, or psychological abuse, as well as neglect, abandonment, and financial exploitation of an older person by another entity. Elder abuse may occur in any setting (e.g., at home, in a facility, or in the community; Table 6.3). Abuse occurs in a relationship where there is an expectation of trust or when the older person is specifically targeted based on age or disability. There are no definitive statistics on the occurrence of elder abuse or self-neglect; however, 1 in 10 persons over age 60 and living at home experience abuse or neglect (CDC, 2015). Multiple forms of abuse may occur at the same time.

Self-neglect is an adult's inability, due to physical or mental impairment or diminished capacity, to perform essential self-care duties, including obtaining essential food, clothing, shelter, and medical care; to obtain goods and services necessary to maintain physical health, mental health, and emotional well-being; and to ensure general safety because of impairment in the ability to manage one's own financial affairs. Self-neglectors are vulnerable persons who have multiple deficits in a variety of social, functional, and physical domains. It is the most commonly reported form of mistreatment and an independent risk factor for death. Note that lifestyle choices or living arrangements alone do not prove self-neglect, and self-neglect may occur simultaneously with other forms of elder abuse and may precede or follow elder abuse victimization.

Many older adults do not report abuse because of fear of retaliation, lack of physical or cognitive ability to report, or an unwillingness to get the abuser in trouble (Tatara et al., 1998). However, financial exploitation is self-reported at a rate considerably higher than self-reported rates of emotional, physical, and sexual abuse or neglect. Professionals who lack proper training to detect abuse often miss it (NCEA, n.d.). It is imperative that clinicians develop skills to identify elder abuse.

Screening Tools

When screening an older adult for abuse, the clinician should follow these guidelines (US Preventive Services Task Force, 2013):

- Ensure privacy and address confidentiality.
- Separate survivors from caregivers.
- Allow adequate time for responses.
- Recognize cultural differences.
- Progress from general to more specific/direct questions.
- Do not blame the older adult who may be victimized.
- Do not blame or confront the perpetrator.
- Acknowledge that this process may require multiple interviews.
- Be attentive to the impact of the screening on the provider-patient relationship.

Initially, screening may include asking the patient some general screening questions such as "Are there any problems with family or household members that you would like to tell me about?" A positive response requires more direct questions to determine specifics.

- Abandonment: Is there anyone you can call to come and take care of you?

TABLE 6.3 Types of Elder Abuse

Type of Elder Abuse	Prevalence	Definition
Neglect	49%	Refusal or failure to fulfill any part of a person's obligations or duties to an older person
Emotional/psychological abuse	35%	Inflicting mental pain, anguish, or distress on an older person through verbal or nonverbal acts
Physical abuse	30%	Use or threat of the use of physical force that may result in bodily injury, physical pain, or impairment
Financial exploitation	26%	The illegal or improper use of a vulnerable adult's funds, property, or assets
Abandonment	4%	Desertion of an older adult by an individual who had assumed responsibility for providing care for the adult, or by a person with physical custody of the adult
Sexual abuse	1%	Nonconsensual sexual contact of any kind

- Physical abuse: Has anyone at home every hit you or hurt you?
- Exploitation: Has anyone taken your things?
- Neglect: Are you receiving enough care at home?
- Psychological abuse: Has anyone ever scolded or threatened you? Has anyone made fun of you?

There are multiple validated tools for elder abuse screening.

- The Elder Abuse Suspicion Index (EASI; Yaffe et al., 2008) was developed to raise a clinician's suspicion about elder abuse to a level at which it might be reasonable to propose a referral for further evaluation by social services, Adult Protective Services, or equivalents. Although all six questions should be asked, a response of yes on one or more of questions 2 through 6 may establish concern (https://medicine.uiowa.edu/familymedicine/sites/medicine.uiowa.edu.familymedicine/files/wysiwyg_uploads/EASI.pdf).
- The Elder Assessment Instrument (EAI; Fulmer, 2003) should be used as a comprehensive approach for screening suspected elder abuse victims in the clinical setting. The instrument evaluates evidence of five domains: general assessment (4 items), possible abuse indicators (6 items), possible neglect indicators (13 items), possible exploitation indicators (5 items), and possible abandonment indicators (3 items). There is no score for the instrument. A patient should be referred to social services (1) if there is any positive evidence without sufficient clinical explanation, (2) whenever there is a subjective complaint by the older adult of elder mistreatment, or (3) whenever the clinician deems there is evidence of abuse, neglect, exploitation, or abandonment (https://medicine.uiowa.edu/familymedicine/sites/medicine.uiowa.edu.familymedicine/files/wysiwyg_uploads/EAI.pdf)
- The Hwalek-Sengstock Elder Abuse Screening Test (H-S/EAST; Neale et al., 1991) is a 15-item screening tool used to identify people at high risk for the need of protective services. A response of no to items 1, 6, 12, and 14; a response of "someone else" to item 4; and a response of yes to all others is scored in the abused direction (https://medicine.uiowa.edu/familymedicine/sites/medicine.uiowa.edu.familymedicine/files/wysiwyg_uploads/HS_EAST.pdf).
- The Self-Neglect Severity Scale (SSS) (Dyer et al., 2007) assesses three domains of self-neglect (hygiene, functioning, and environment) and can detect the severity of neglect within each domain. The tool relies on observational ratings and interview responses and assesses subjects' physical appearance and environment. It is administered in the home to include an environmental assessment. There are 37 items, and most are scored on a 0-to-4 scale with 0 = *no problem* to 4 = *among the worst I've ever seen*. Most items are completed using direct observation, except for items in the impaired function domain. These items are scored with inputs from the Wolf-Klein Clock Test (Wolf-Klein et al., 1989) the Adult Protective Services (APS) data extraction sheet (a comprehensive social history form), and a physical examination of the subject. One item requires a verbal response from the subject. A global 0-to-10 scale "overall risk assessment" item is also included. The three individual domain summation scores and a composite summation score are calculated and recorded on the SSS (http://www.ncbi.nlm.nih.gov/pubmed/17972656).

Outcomes and Recommendations

When elder abuse or self-neglect is suspected, many states have mandated reporting laws for health professionals. These laws vary by state and change periodically. Mandated reporting promotes safety for older adults who otherwise might not seek services and provides an opportunity for the older adult to seek help that may not be available without competent reporters. Prior to making a report, the clinician should advise the older adult about confidentiality and its limits. Be sure that the older adult understands what may happen if she or he discloses abuse or neglect. The older adult should be made aware that any clinician who determines there is abuse or neglect is mandated to report it. The clinician who suspects abuse or neglect must inform the older adult that she or he has some concerns and will be making a report; the clinician can then discuss with the older adult the possible reactions and consequences to the patient and the patient's caregivers or perpetrators. The clinician must document that the report has been made and devise a safety plan. When making a report, the clinician should contact the appropriate agency and call police at 9-1-1 if the older adult is in immediate, life-threatening danger. If there is no immediate life-threatening danger, the clinician should call to the state Adult Protective Services (APS) agency at http://www.napsa-now.org/get-help/help-in-your-area/. The clinician does not need to prove the abuse is occurring.

When reporting to APS, the clinician should be prepared to provide the name, address, and contact information for the older adult, as well as details about the concern. The person making the report will be asked his or her name and contact information, but this information will not be released to the alleged abuser or to the older adult.

The goal of APS is to promote safety, independence, and quality of life for older persons and persons with disabilities who are being mistreated or in danger of being mistreated and who are unable to protect themselves. The APS will investigate, assess the victim's risk, assess the victim's capacity to understand his or her risk and ability to give informed consent, and develop a case plan with necessary services. These services may include arranging for emergency shelter, medical care, legal care, counseling services, and supportive services as needed. APS creates an intervention plan and provides ongoing monitoring for up to 15 months. In cases of self-neglect, older adults often can continue to live in the community with interventions designed to ameliorate some or all gaps in the performance of self-care and self-protection domains.

Resources

The National Adult Protective Services Association (NAPSA) has helpful resources: http://www.napsa-now.org/wp-content/uploads/2014/11/Mandatory-Reporting-Chart-Updated-FINAL.pdf; NCEA, state resources: https://ncea.acl.gov/resources/state.htm.

HEALTHY PEOPLE 2030 BOX 6.16

Key Overarching Goals

- Increase the proportion of people who get the flu vaccine every year—IID-09

Data from US Department of Health and Human Services. (2020). *Healthy People 2030*. https://health.gov/healthypeople/objectives-and-data/browse-objectives/vaccination/increase-proportion-people-who-get-flu-vaccine-every-year-iid-09

Immunizations

Influenza Vaccine

Necessity

All adults are recommended to receive an influenza vaccination annually to prevent seasonal flu (CDC, 2020). Immunization of older adults has been shown to reduce rates of respiratory illness, hospitalization, and death (CDC, 2020). Approximately 70% to 85% of deaths due to flu are in adults over 65 years of age (CDC, 2019). The high-dose vaccine has demonstrated a reduction in the incidence of influenza-like illness in older adults; however, there is not sufficient evidence for changing the recommendation from the standard-dose vaccine (Doyle et al., 2020).

Screening Tools

History of annual immunization.

Outcomes and Recommendations

Annual immunization of influenza vaccine prior to beginning of flu season is recommended. All older adults are at a higher risk of complications from flu, especially those with chronic diseases such as chronic obstructive pulmonary disease, asthma, cancer, cardiovascular disease, diabetes, HIV, and immunosuppression (CDC, 2020).

Pneumococcal Vaccine

Necessity

Over one-third of adults 65 years and older do not report having received a pneumococcal vaccine (CDC, 2018).

Screening Tools

History of pneumococcal immunization.

Outcomes and Recommendations

All adults 65 years or older should receive one dose of the pneumococcal conjugate vaccine (PCV13) followed in 6 to 12 months by one dose of the pneumococcal polysaccharide vaccine PPSV23 (CDC, 2020).

Tetanus-Diphtheria-Pertussis (Td/Tdap)

Necessity

The CDC reports that four out of five adults ages 65 and older did not report receiving a TD vaccine (CDC, 2018). Older adults, especially women over 65, are at the highest risk of developing tetanus due to lack of booster vaccinations (CDC, 2018). Adults ages 65 and older should also be immunized for pertussis because epidemiologic studies show that older adults may not have adequate immunity and may be a cause of the spread of pertussis (CDC/MMWR, 2012). Tdap would provide necessary protection (CDC/MMWR, 2012).

Screening Tools

History of Td vaccination in past 10 years.

Outcomes and Recommendations

A Td booster vaccination every 10 years or after a moderate traumatic skin injury such as a burn, puncture, or soft tissue wound is recommended (CDC, 2018). At least one of the Td boosters after age 65 should be a Tdap to include the pertussis component, either Boostrix or Adacel (MMWR, 2012). Patients with an unknown Td immunization history should have the complete series (CDC, 2018).

Herpes Zoster Vaccine

Necessity

Herpes zoster is more common in older adults, who also have a higher incidence of postherpetic neuralgia (PHN; CDC, 2019). PHN pain can be debilitating and chronic, lasting for weeks, months, and sometimes years after resolution of the rash. Other complications of zoster include ophthalmic involvement with risk of vision loss, encephalitis, and bacterial infection of the skin lesions (CDC, 2019). Older adults with compromised immune systems are more likely to have complications and a higher incidence of PHN (CDC, 2019). According to the CDC, only one-third of older adults have received a zoster vaccination, identifying an opportunity for primary care providers to assess and advise patients to be appropriately vaccinated (CDC, 2018).

Screening Tool

Screening for a history of varicella infection (chicken pox) and previous shingrix vaccination is recommended.

Outcomes and Recommendations

The Advisory Committee on Immunization Practices recommends two doses of shingrix, 2 to 6 months apart, for adults over age 50. This is regardless of whether patients have had shingles or received the Zostavax vaccine (CDC, 2019). shingrix is the preferred vaccination because it is 90% effective in protecting against herpes zoster and PHN (CDC, 2019).

Key Points

- Older adults are at increased risk of multiple chronic conditions, functional impairments, and changes in well-being.
- Preventive interventions including screenings and immunizations, can limit disease and disability among older adult patients.
- Age-based screening and immunization guidelines provide strategies for clinicians to use when developing preventive care plans to enhance the health and well-being of their older adult patients.

More information about tools and Interprofessional Education Collaborative (IPEC) competencies mentioned in this chapter can be found in Appendix 1: Tools and Appendix 2: IPEC Competencies.

References

Adekeye, O. A., Heiman, H. J., Onycabor, O. S., & Hyacinth, H. I. (2018). The new invincibles: HIV screening among older adults in the US. *PLoS One, 7*(8), E43618. https://doi.org/10.1371/journal.pone.0043618.

American Academy of Family Physicians. (2012). *Clinical preventive service recommendation. Fall prevention in older adults.* https://www.aafp.org/patient-care/clinical-recommendations/all/fall-prevention.html.

American Academy of Family Physicians. (2016). *Clinical preventive service recommendation. Visual difficulties and impairment.* https://www.aafp.org/patient-care/clinical-recommendations/all/visual.html.

American Academy of Pain Medicine. (2020). AAPM pain treatment guidelines. *AAPM, April 2020.* https://painmed.org/clinician-resources/clinical-guidelines.

American Diabetic Association. (n.d.). *Overview.* https://www.diabetes.org/diabetes.

American Geriatrics Society. (n.d.). *Choosing wisely.* https://www.choosingwisely.org/societies/american-geriatrics-society/

American Geriatrics Society 2015 Beers Criteria Update Expert Panel, Fick, D. M., Semla, T. P., Beizer, J., Brandt, N., Dombrowski, R., & Giovannetti, E. (2015). American Geriatrics Society 2015 updated beers criteria for potentially inappropriate medication use in older adults. *Journal of the American Geriatrics Society, 63*(11), 2227–2246. https://doi.org/10.1111/jgs.13702.

American Lung Association. (n.d.). *Guidance on lung cancer screening.* https://www.lung.org/lung-health-diseases/lung-disease-lookup/lung-cancer/saved-by-the-scan/resources.

Andrew, C., Traynor, V., & Iverson, D. (2015). An integrative review: Understanding driving retirement decisions for individuals living with a dementia. *Journal of Advanced Nursing, 71*(12), 2728–2740. https://doi.org/10.1111/jan.12727.

Aprahamian, I., Sassaki, E., dos Santos, M. F., Izbicki, R., Pulgrossi, R., Biella, M., Borges, C., Sassaki, M., Torres, L., Fernandez, I., Piao, O., Castro, P., Fontenele, P., & Yassuda, M. (2018). Hypertension and frailty in older adults. *Journal of Clinical Hypertension, 20*(1), 186–192. https://doi.org/10.1111/jch.13135.

Arnett, D. K., Blumenthal, R. S., Albert, M. A., Buroker, A. B., Goldberger, Z. D., Hahn, E. J., & Michos, E. D. (2019). 2019 ACC/AHA guideline on the primary prevention of cardiovascular disease: Executive summary: A report of the American College of Cardiology/American Heart Association Task Force on Clinical Practice Guidelines. *Journal of the American College of Cardiology, 74*(10), 1376–1414. https://doi.org/10.1016/j.jacc.2019.03.009.

Aronow, W. S. (2020). Managing the elderly patient with hypertension: Current strategies, challenges, and considerations. *Expert Review of Cardiovascular Therapy, 18*(2), 117–125. https://doi.org/10.1080/14779072.2020.1732206.

Bach, P. B., Mirkin, J. N., Oliver, T. K., Azzoli, C. G., Berry, D. A., Brawley, O. W., Byers, T., Colditz, G., Gould, M., Jett, J., Sabichi, A. L., Smith-Bindman, R., Wood, D. E., Qaseem, A., & Deterbeck, F. C. (2012). Benefits and harms of CT screening for lung cancer: A systematic review. *Journal of the American Medical Association, 307*(22), 2418–2429. https://doi.org/10.1001/jama.2012.5521.

Bailey, I. L., & Lovie-Kitchin, J. E. (2013). Visual acuity testing. From the laboratory to the clinic. *Vision Research, 90,* 2–9. https://doi.org/10.1016/j.visres.2013.05.004.

Barco, P. P., Baum, C. M., Ott, B. R., Ice, S., Johnson, A., Wallendorf, M., & Carr, D. B. (2015). Driving errors in persons with dementia. *Journal of the American Geriatrics Society, 63*(7), 1373–1380. https://doi.org/10.1111/jgs.13508.

Benenson, I., Waldron, F. A., & Bradshaw, M. J. (2020). Treating hypertension in older adults: Beyond the guidelines. *Journal of the American Association of Nurse Practitioners, 32*(3), 193–199. https://doi.org/10.1097/JXX.0000000000000220.

Bergen, G., Stevens, M. R., & Burns, E. R. (2016). Falls and fall injuries among adults aged ≥65 years—United States, 2014. *Morbidity and Mortality Weekly Report, 65*(37), 993–998.

Bernabei, R., Venturiero, V., Tarsitani, P., & Gambassi, G. (2000). The comprehensive geriatric assessment: When, where, how. *Critical Reviews in Oncology/Hematology, 33*(1), 45–56. https://doi.org/10.1016/S1040-8428(99)00048-7.

Bibbins-Domingo, K., Grossman, D. C., Curry, S. J., Davidson, K. W., Epling, J. W. J., & Garcia, F. A. (2016). US preventive services task force, statin use for the primary prevention of cardiovascular disease in adults. US preventive services task force recommendation statement. *Journal of the American Medical Association, 316*(19), 1997–2007. https://doi.org/10.1001/jama.2016.15450.

Blevins, N. (2020). *Presbycusis. UpToDate.* Retrieved March 12, 2020, from https://www.uptodate.com/content/presbycusis.

Blozik, E., Stuck, A. E., Niemann, S., Ferrell, B. A., Harari, D., Renteln-Kruse, W. V., Gillman, G., Beck, J., & Clough-Gorr, K. M. (2007). Geriatric pain measure short form: Development and initial evaluation. *Journal of the American Geriatrics Society, 55*(12), 2045–2050. https://doi.org/10.1111/j.1532-5415.2007.01474.x.

Cancer Net. (n.d.). *Oral cancer statistics.* https://www.cancer.net/cancer-types/oral-and-oropharyngeal-cancer/statistics.

Carr, D. B., Barco, P. P., Wallendorf, M. J., Snellgrove, C. A., & Ott, B. R. (2011). Predicting road test performance in drivers with dementia. *Journal of the American Geriatrics Society, 59*(11), 2112–2117. https://doi.org/10.1111/j.1532-5415.2011.03657.x.

Centers for Disease Control and Prevention (CDC). (2013). *HCV rapid antibody test (Assay) CDC 2013 guideline*. https://www.cdc.gov/mmwr/pdf/wk/mm62e0507a2.pdf

Centers for Disease Control and Prevention (CDC). (2015) *Algorithm for fall risk assessment and interventions*. http://www.cdc.gov/steadi/pdf/algorithm_2015-04-a.pdf.

Centers for Disease Control and Prevention (CDC). (2015). *Elder abuse prevention*. http://www.cdc.gov/features/elderabuse/

Centers for Disease Control and Prevention (CDC). (2017). *Atrial fibrillation* [fact sheet]. https://www.cdc.gov.proxy.cc.uic.edu/dhdsp/data_statistics/fact_sheets/fs_atrial_fibrillation.htm.

Centers for Disease Control and Prevention (CDC). (2018). National Center for Injury Prevention and Control (WISQARS). http://www.cdc.gov/injury/wisqars/

Centers for Disease Control and Prevention (CDC). (2018). *Vaccines 2018*. https://www.cdc.gov/vaccines/imz-managers/coverage/adult vaxview/pubs-resources/NHIS-2016.html.

Centers for Disease Control and Prevention (CDC). (2019). *Flu deaths*. https://www.cdc.gov/flu/highrisk/65over htm#anchor_1554994347538.

Centers for Disease Control and Prevention (CDC). (2019). *Flu risk*. https://www.cdc.gov/flu/highrisk/65over.htm#anchor_1554994347538.

Centers for Disease Control and Prevention (CDC). (2019). *Oral health*. https://www.cdc.gov/oralhealth/basics/adult-oral-health/adult_older.htm.

Centers for Disease Control and Prevention (CDC). (2019). *Sexually transmitted disease surveillance 2018*. Atlanta, GA: US Department of Health and Human Services. https://www.cdc.gov/std/stats18/default.htm.

Centers for Disease Control and Prevention (CDC). (2019). *Shingles* [fact sheet]. https://www.cdc.gov/shingles/hcp/clinicaloverview.html#complications.

Centers for Disease Control and Prevention (CDC). (2020). *Recommended adult immunization schedule for ages 19 years or older, United States, 2020, Age 65 years and older*. https://www.cdc.gov/vaccines/schedules/hcp/imz/adult.html#table-age.

Centers for Disease Control and Prevention (CDC). (2020). *Smoking and tobacco use: Fast facts*. https://www.cdc.gov/tobacco/data_statistics/fact_sheets/fast_facts/index.htm.

Centers for Disease Control and Prevention (CDC). (2020). *Tobacco campaign*. https://www.cdc.gov/tobacco/campaign/tips/resources/data/cigarette-smoking-in-united-states.html#age_group.

Chakkamparambil, B., Chibnall, J. T., Graypel, E. A., Manepalli, J. N., Bhutto, A., & Grossberg, G. T. (2015). Development of a brief validated geriatric depression screening tool: The SLU "AM SAD." *American Journal of Geriatric Psychiatry, 23*(8), 780–783. https://doi.org/10.1016/j.jagp.2014.10.003.

Chang, C. H., Bynum, J. P., Onega, T., Colla, C. H., Lurie, J. D., & Tosteson, A. N. (2016). Screening mammography use among older women before and after the 2009 US Preventive Services Task Force Recommendations. *Journal of Women's Health, 25*(10), 1030–1037. https://doi.org/10.1089/jwh.2015.5701.

Chou, R., Dana, T., Bougatsos, C., Fleming, C., & Beil, T. (2011). Screening adults aged 50 years or older for hearing loss: A review of the evidence for the US preventive services task force. *Annals of Internal Medicine, 154*(5), 347–355.

Chu, Y. C., Cheng, Y. F., Lai, Y. H., Tsao, Y., Tu, T. Y., Young, S. T., Chen, T. S., Chung, Y. F., Lau, F., & Liao, W. H. (2019). A mobile phone–based approach for hearing screening of school-age children: Cross-sectional validation study. *JMIR mHealth and uHealth, 7*(4), e12033. https://doi.org/10.2196/12033.

Cleeland, C. S., & Ryan, K. M. (1991). The brief pain inventory. *Pain Research Group*, 143–147. https://www.mdanderson.org/research/departments-labs-institutes/departments-divisions/symptom-research/symptom-assessment-tools/brief-pain-inventory.html.

Curry, S. J., Krist, A. H., Owens, D. K., Barry, M. J., Caughey, A. B., Davidson, K. W., Doubeni, A. A., Eping, J. A., Kemper, A. R., Kubik, M., & Laundefeld, C. S. (2018). Screening for atrial fibrillation with electrocardiography: US Preventive Services Task Force recommendation statement. *Journal of the American Medical Association, 320*(5), 478–484. https://doi.org/10.1001/jama.2018.10321.

Doyle, J. D., Beacham, L., Martin, E. T., Talbot, H. K., Monto, A., Gaglani, M., Middleton, D. B., Silveriera, F. P., Zimmerman, R. K., Alyanak, E., & Smith, E. R. (2020). Relative and absolute effectiveness of high-dose and standard-dose influenza vaccine against influenza-related hospitalization among older adults—United States, 2015–2017. *Clinical Infectious Diseases, ciaa160*. https://doi.org/10.1093/cid/ciaa160.

Dyer, C. B., Kelly, P. A., Pavlik, V. N., Lee, J., Doody, R. S., Regev, T., Pickens, S., Burnett, J., & Smith, S. M. (2007). The making of a self-neglect severity scale. *Journal of Elder Abuse & Neglect, 18*(4), 13–23. https://doi.org/10.1300/j084v18n04_03.

Ellman, T. M., Sexton, M. E., Warshafsky, D., Sobieszczyk, M. E., & Morrison, E. A. (2014). A forgotten population: Older adults with newly diagnosed HIV. *AIDS Patient Care and STDS, 28*(10), 530–536. https://doi.org/10.1089/apc.2014.0152.

Fantino, B., & Moore, N. (2009). The self-reported Montgomery-Åsberg depression rating scale is a useful evaluative tool in major depressive disorder. *BMC Psychiatry, 9*(1), 26. https://doi.org/10.1186/1471-244X-9-26.

Fedele, D. J., Jones, J. A., & Niessen, L. C. (1991). Oral cancer screening in the elderly. *Journal of the American Geriatrics Society, 39*(9), 920–925. https://doi.org/10.1111/j.1532-5415.1991.tb04461.x.

Field, J. K., Smith, R. A., Aberle, D. R., Oudkerk, M., Baldwin, D. R., Yankelevitz, D., Pedersen, J. H., Swanson, S. J., Travis, W. D., Wisbuba, I. I., & Noguchi, M. (2012). International Association for the Study of Lung Cancer Computed Tomography Screening Workshop 2011 report. *Journal of Thoracic Oncology, 7*(1), 10–19. https://doi.org/10.1097/jTO.0b013e31823c58ab.

Folstein, M. F., Folstein, S. E., & McHugh, P. R. (1975). Mini-mental state: A practical method for grading the cognitive state of patients for the clinician. *Journal of Psychiatric Research., 12*(3), 189–198.

Ford, C. L., Godette, D. C., Mulatu, M. S., & Gaines, T. L. (2015). Recent HIV testing prevalence, determinants, and disparities among US older adult respondents to the behavioral risk factor surveillance system. *Sexually Transmitted Diseases, 42*(8), 405. https://doi.org/10.1097/OLQ.0000000000000305.

Fried, L. P., Tangen, C. M., Walston, J., Newman, A. B., Hirsch, C., Gottdiener, J., Seeman, T., Tracy, R., Kop, W. J., Burke, G., & McBurnie, M. W. (2001). Frailty in older adults: Evidence for a phenotype. *The Journals of Gerontology Series A: Biological Sciences and Medical Sciences, 56*(3), M146–M157. https://doi.org/10.1093/gerona/56.3.M146.

Fulmer, T. (2003). Elder abuse and neglect assessment. *Journal of Gerontological Nursing, 29*(6), 4–5. https://doi.org/10.3928/0098-9134-20030601-04.

Ganz, D. A., Bao, Y., Shekelle, P. G., & Rubenstein, L. Z. (2007). Will my patient fall? *Journal of the American Medical Association, 297*(1), 77–78. https://doi.org/10.1001/jama.297.1.77.

García-Albéniz, X., Hsu, J., Bretthauer, M., & Hernan, M. A. (2017). Effectiveness of screening colonoscopy to prevent colorectal cancer among Medicare beneficiaries aged 70 to 79 years: A prospective observational study. *Annals of Internal Medicine, 166*(1), 18–26. https://doi.org/10.7326/M16-0758.

Gerontological Society of America. (2015). National pain strategy (NPS) by the Interagency Pain Research Coordinating Committee (IPRCC). https://www.geron.org/images/gsa/May2015_Statement.pdf.

Go, A. S., Hylek, E. M., Phillips, K. A., Change, Y., Henault, L. E., Selby, J. V., & Singer, D. E. (2001). Prevalence of diagnosed atrial fibrillation in adults: National implications for rhythm management and stroke prevention: The anticoagulation and risk factors in atrial fibrillation (ATRIA) study. *Journal of the American Medical Association, 285*(18), 2370–2375. https://doi.org/10.1001/jama.285.18.2370.

Gohagan, J. K., Marcus, P. M., Fagerstrom, R. M., Pinsky, P. F., Kramer, B. S., Prorok, P. C., Ascher, S., Bailey, W., Brewer, B., Church, T., & Engelhard, D. (2005). Final results of the lung screening study, a randomized feasibility study of spiral CT versus chest x-ray screening for lung cancer. *Lung Cancer, 47*(1), 9–15. https://doi.org/10.1016/j.lungcan.2004.06.007.

Griffiths, M., & David, N. (2013). Sexually transmitted infections in older people. *International Journal of STD & AIDS, 24*, 756–757. https://doi.org/10.1177/0956462488768.

Gryczynski, J., McNeely, J., Wu, L. T., Subramaniam, G. A., Svikis, D. S., Cathers, L. A., Sharma, G., King, J., Jelstrom, E., Nordeck, C. D., & Sharma, A. (2017). Validation of the TAPS-1: A four-item screening tool to identify unhealthy substance use in primary care. *Journal of General Internal Medicine, 32*(9), 990–996. https://doi.org/10.1007/s11606-017-4079-x.

Guigoz, Y. (2006). The Mini Nutritional Assessment (MNA®) review of the literature-What does it tell us? *Journal of Nutrition Health and Aging., 10*(6), 466.

Halter, J. B., Ouslander, J. G., Studenski, S., High, K. P., Asthana, S., Supiano, M. A., & Ritchie, C. (Eds.). (2017). *Hazzard's geriatric medicine and gerontology* (7th ed.). McGraw-Hill.

Herr, K. (2011). Pain assessment strategies in older patients. *Journal of Pain, 12*(3), S3–S13. https://doi.org/10.1016/j.j.pain.2010.11.011.

Hicks, C. L., von Baeyer, C. L., Spafford, P., van Korlaar, I., & Goodenough, B. (2001). The Faces Pain Scale—Revised: Toward a common metric in pediatric pain measurement. *Pain, 93*(2), 173–183. https://doi.org/10.1016/S0304-3959(01)00314-1.

Insurance Institute for Highway Safety. (2018). *Fatality statistics older people*. https://iihs.org/topics/fatality-statistics/detail/older-people.

Jaklitsch, M. T., Jacobson, F. L., Austin, J. H., Field, J. K., Jett, J. R., Keshavjee, S., MacMahon, H., Mulshine, J. L., Munden, R. F., Salgia, R., & Strauss, G. M. (2012). The American Association for Thoracic Surgery guidelines for lung cancer screening using low-dose computed tomography scans for lung cancer survivors and other high-risk groups. *Journal of Thoracic and Cardiovascular Surgery, 144*(1), 33–38. https://doi.org/10.1016/j.jtcvs.2012.05.060.

Johns Hopkins Medicine. (n.d.). *Frailty assessment calculator*. https://www.johnshopkinssolutions.com/solution/frailty/

Joint Commission on the Accreditation of Healthcare Organizations. (2001). *Accreditation guide for hospitals*. https://www.jointcommission.org/-/media/deprecated-unorganized/imported-assets/tjc/system-folders/topics-library/171110_accreditation_guide_hospitals_final.pdf.

Kaiser, M. J., Bauer, J. M., Ramsch, C., Uter, W., Guigoz, Y., Cederholm, T., Thomas, D. R., Anthony, P., Charlton, K. E., Maggio, M., & Tsai, A. C. (2009). Validation of the mini nutritional assessment short-form (MNA®-SF): A practical tool for identification of nutritional status. *Journal of Nutrition, Health and Aging, 13*(9), 782. https://doi.org/10.1007/s12603-009-0214-7.

Kane, R. L., Ousland, J. G., Resnick, B., & Malone, M. L. (2018). *Essential of clinical geriatrics* (pp. 35–70) (8th ed.). McGraw-Hill.

Karcioglu, O., Topacoglu, H., Dikme, O., & Dikme, O. (2018). A systematic review of the pain scales in adults: Which to use? *American Journal of Emergency Medicine, 36*(4), 707–714. https://doi.org/10.1016/j.ajem.2018.01.008.

Katz, S. (1983). Assessing self-maintenance: Activities of daily living, mobility, and instrumental activities of daily living. *Journal of the American Geriatrics Society, 31*(12), 721–727. https://doi.org/10.1111/j.1532-5415.1983.tb03391.x.

Kayser-Jones, J., Bird, W. F., Paul, S. M., Long, L., & Schell, E. S. (1995). An instrument to assess the oral health status of nursing home residents. *The Gerontologist, 35*(6), 814–824. https://doi.org/10.1093/geront/35.6.814.

Kelly, S. G., Barancin, C., & Lucey, M. R. (2017). Hepatic disease. In J. B. Halter, J. G. Ouslander, S. Studenski, K. P. High, S. Asthana, M. A. Supiano, & C. Ritchie (Eds.), *Hazzard's geriatric medicine and gerontology* (7th ed.). McGraw-Hill. http://accessmedicine.mhmedical.com.proxy.cc.uic.edu/content.aspx?bookid=1923§ionid=144526298.

Ko, C. W., & Sonnenberg, A. (2005). Comparing risks and benefits of colorectal cancer screening in elderly patients. *Gastroenterology, 129*(4), 1163–1170. https://doi.org/10.1053/j.gastro.2005.07.027.

Kroenke, K., & Spitzer, R. L. (2002). The PHQ-9: A new depression diagnostic and severity measure. *Psychiatric Annals, 32*(9), 509–515. https://doi.org/10.3928/0048-5713-20020901-06.

Kudo, S., & Kudo, T. (2017). The necessity of colorectal cancer screening for elderly patients. *Translational Gastroenterology and Hepatology, 2*. https://doi.org/10.21037/tgh.2017.03.03.

Lawton, M. P., & Brody, E. M. (1969). Assessment of older people: Self-maintaining and instrumental activities of daily living. *Gerontologist., 9*(3 Part 1), 179–186.

Lee, P. G., & Halter, J. B. (2017). Diabetes mellitus. In J. B. Halter, J. G. Ouslander, S. Studenski, K. P. High, S. Asthana, M. A. Supiano, & C. Ritchie (Eds.), *Hazzard's geriatric medicine and gerontology* (7th ed). McGraw-Hill. http://accessmedicine.mhmedical.com.proxy.cc.uic.edu/content.aspx?bookid=1923§ionid=144561220.

Lee, S. J., & Walter, L. (2017). Prevention and screening. In J. B. Halter, J. G. Ouslander, S. Studenski, K. P. High, S. Asthana, M. A. Supiano, & C. Ritchie (Eds.), *Hazzard's geriatric medicine and gerontology* (7th ed). McGraw-Hill. http://accessmedicine.mhmedical.com.proxy.cc.uic.edu/content.aspx?bookid=1923§ionid=144518165.

Lindau, S. T., Schumm, L. P., Laumann, E. O., Levinson, W., O'Muircheartaigh, C. A., & Waite, L. J. (2007). A study of sexuality and health among older adults in the United States. *New England Journal of Medicine, 357*(8), 762–774.

Lipari, R.N., & Van Horn, S.L. (2017). Trends in substance use disorders among adults aged 18 or older. The CBHSQ Report. Center for Behavioral Health Statistics and Quality (CBHSQ), SAMHSA, and by RTI International in Research Triangle Park, North Carolina. https://www.samhsa.gov/data/sites/default/files/report_2790/ShortReport-2790.html.

Manetti, A., Hoertel, N., Le Strat, Y., Schuster, J. P., Lemogne, C., & Limosin, F. (2014). Comorbidity of late-life depression in the United States: A population-based study. *American Journal of Geriatric Psychiatry, 22*(11), 1292–1306. https://doi.org/10.1016/j/japg.2013.05.001.

Marcus, P. M., Bergstralh, E. J., Fagerstrom, R. M., Williams, D. E., Fontana, R., Taylor, W. F., & Prorok, P. C. (2000). Lung cancer mortality in the Mayo Lung Project: Impact of extended follow-up. *Journal of the National Cancer Institute, 92*(16), 1308–1316. https://doi.org/10.1093/jnci/92.16.1308.

Millan, M., Merino, S., Caro, A., Feliu, F., Escuder, J., & Francesch, T. (2015). Treatment of colorectal cancer in the elderly. *World Journal of Gastrointestinal Oncology, 7*(10), 204. https://doi.org/10.4251/wjgo.v7.i10.204.

Mini-Cog. (n.d.). Mini-Cog screening for dognitive impairment in older adults. https://mini-cog.com/

Mlinac, M. E., & Feng, M. C. (2016). Assessment of activities of daily living, self-care, and independence. *Archives of Clinical Neuropsychology, 31*(6), 506–516. https://doi.org/10.1093/arclin/acw049.

Morbidity and Mortality Weekly Report (MMWR). Centers for Disease Control and Prevention. (2012). Updated recommendations for use of tetanus toxoid, reduced diphtheria toxoid, and acellular pertussis (Tdap) vaccine in adults aged 65 years and older—Advisory Committee on Immunization Practices (ACIP). https://www.cdc.gov/mmwr/preview/mmwrhtml/mm6125a4.htm.

Nasreddine, Z. S., Phillips, N. A., Bédirian, V., Charbonneau, S., Whitehead, V., Collin, I., Cummings, J. L., & Chertkow, H. (2005). The Montreal Cognitive Assessment, MoCA: A brief screening tool for mild cognitive impairment. *Journal of the American Geriatrics Society, 53*(4), 695–699. https://doi.org/10.1111/j.1532-5415.2005.53221.x.

National Cancer Institute. Surveillance, Epidemiology, and End Results (SEER) Program. (n.d.). *Oral cavity and pharynx cancer [fact sheet].* http://seer.cancer.gov/statfacts/html/oralcav.htmlexternalicon.

National Center on Elder Abuse. (n.d.). https://ncea.acl.gov/

National Council on Aging. (2008). *Matter of balance: Falls prevention program.* https://www.ncoa.org/resources/program-summary-a-matter-of-balance/

National Council on Aging (n.d.). *Malnutrition screening tools.* https://www.ncoa.org/center-for-healthy-aging/resourcehub/community-orgs-and-professionals/professional-resources/malnutrition-screening-tools/

National Institute on Aging. (2016). *World's older population grows dramatically.* https://www.nih.gov/news-events/news-releases/worlds-older-population-grows-dramatically.

National Institute on Deafness and other Communication Disorders (NIDCD). (2018). *Hearing loss and older adults.* https://www.nidcd.nih.gov/health/hearing-loss-older-adults.

National Institute on Drug Abuse. (2019). *Drug use and its consequences increase among middle-aged and older adults.* https://www.drugabuse.gov/news-events/nida-notes/2019/07/drug-use-its-consequences-increase-among-middle-aged-older-adults.

National Lung Screening Trial Research Team. (2011). Reduced lung-cancer mortality with low-dose computed tomographic screening. *New England Journal of Medicine, 365*(5), 395–409.

National Osteoporosis Foundation. (2020). *What women need to know.* https://www.nof.org/preventing-fractures/general-facts/what-women-need-to-know/.

National Highway Traffic Safety Administration. (2013). TRAFC Safety Acts - Transportation. (n.d.). Retrieved September 12, 2022, from https://crashstats.nhtsa.dot.gov/Api/Public/Publication/812199.

Neale, A. V., Hwalek, M. A., Scott, R. O., & Stahl, C. (1991). Validation of the Hwalek-Sengstock elder abuse screening test. *Journal of Applied Gerontology, 10*(4), 406–418. https://doi.org/10.1177/073346489101000403.

Nunes, S., Azevedo, F., & Lisboa, C. (2016). Sexually transmitted infections in older adults–raising awareness for better screening and prevention strategies. *Journal of the European Academy of Dermatology and Venereology, 30*(7), 1202–1204. https://doi.org/10.1111/jdv.13124.

O'Connor, M., Kapust, L., Lin, B., Hollis, A., & Jones, R. (2010). The 4Cs (crash history, family concerns, clinical condition, and cognitive functions): A screening tool for the evaluation of the at-risk driver. *Journal of the American Geriatrics Society, 58*(6), 1104–1108. https://doi.org/10.1111/j.1532-5415.2010.02855.

Oraka, E., Mason, S., & Xia, M. (2018). Too old to test? Prevalence and correlates of HIV testing among sexually active older adults. *Journal of Gerontological Social Work, 61*(4), 460–470. https://doi.org/10.1080/01634372.2018.1454565.

Oral Cancer Foundation. (n.d.). *Oral cancer facts: Rates of occurrence in the United States.* https://oralcancerfoundation.org/facts/

Owens, D. K., Davidson, K. W., Krist, A. H., Barry, M. J., Cabana, M., Caughey, A. B., Doubeni, C. A., Epling, J. W., Kubik, M., Landefeld, C. S., & Mangione, C. M. (2019). Screening for abdominal aortic aneurysm: US Preventive Services Task Force Recommendation Statement. *Journal of the American Medical Association, 322*(22), 2211–2218. https://doi.org/10.1001/jama.2019.18928.

Panel on Prevention of Falls in Older Persons, & American Geriatrics Society and British Geriatrics Society. (2011). Summary of the updated American Geriatrics Society/British Geriatrics Society clinical practice guideline for prevention of falls in older persons. *Journal of the American Geriatrics Society, 59*(1), 148–157. https://doi.org/10.1111/j.1532-5415.2010.03234.x.

Parekh, N., Donohue, J. M., Corbelli, J., Men, A., Kelley, D., & Jarlenski, M. (2018). Screening for sexually transmitted infections after cervical cancer screening guideline and Medicaid policy changes. *Medical Care, 56*(7), 561–568. https://doi.org/10.1097/MLR.0000000000000925.

Park, M., & Unützer, J. (2011). Geriatric depression in primary care. *Psychiatric Clinics, 34*(2), 469–487. https://doi.org/10.1016/j.psc.2011.02.009.

Patel, K. V., Guralnik, J. M., Dansie, E. J., & Turk, D. C. (2013). Prevalence and impact of pain among older adults in the United States: Findings from the 2011 National Health and Aging Trends Study. *Pain, 154*(12), 2649–2657. https://doi.org/10.1016/j.pain.2013.07.029.

Pautex, S., Michon, A., Guedira, M., Emond, H., Lous, P. L., Samaras, D., Michel, J. P., Herrmann, F., Giannakopoulos, P., & Gold, G. (2006). Pain in severe dementia: Self-assessment or observational scales? *Journal of the American Geriatrics Society, 54*(7), 1040–1045. https://doi.org/10.1111/j.1532-5415.2006.00766.x.

Petersen, P. E., & Yamamoto, T. (2005). Improving the oral health of older people: The approach of the WHO Global Oral Health Programme. *Community Dentistry and Oral Epidemiology, 33*(2), 81–92. https://doi.org/10.1111/j.1600-0528.2004.00219.x.

Petersen, R. C., Stevens, J. C., Ganguli, M., Tangalos, E. G., Cummings, J. L., & DeKosky, S. T. (2001). Practice parameter: Early detection of dementia: mild cognitive impairment (an evidence-based review). Report of the Quality Standards Subcommittee of the American Academy of Neurology. *Neurology, 56*(9), 1133–1142. https://doi.org/10.1212/WNL.56.9.1133.

Pfeffer, R. I., Kurosaki, T. T., Harrah, C. H., Jr., Chance, J. M., & Filos, S. (1982). Measurement of functional activities in older adults in the community. *Journal of Gerontology, 37*(3), 323–329. https://doi.org/10.1093/geronj/37.3.323.

Presley, C., Maggiore, R., & Gajra, A. (2017). Lung cancer. In J. B. Halter, J. G. Ouslander, S. Studenski, K. P. High, S. Asthana, M. A. Supiano, & C. Ritchie (Eds.), *Hazzard's geriatric medicine and gerontology* (7th ed). McGraw-Hill. http://accessmedicine.mhmedical.com.proxy.cc.uic.edu/content.aspx?bookid=1923§ionid=144527301.

Rockwood, K., Song, X., MacKnight, C., Bergman, H., Hogan, D. B., McDowell, I., & Mitnitski, A. (2005). A global clinical measure of fitness and frailty in elderly people. *Canadian Medical Association Journal, 173*(5), 489–495. https://doi.org/10.1503/cmaj.050051.

Rospand, M. R. (2002). AGS panel on persistent pain in older person: The management of persistent pain in older person. *Journal of American Geriatrics Society, 50*(6), 205–224. https://doi.org/10.1046/j.1532-415.50.6s.1.x.

Rothmann, M. J., Möller, S., Holmberg, T., Højberg, M., Gram, J., Bech, M., Brixen, K., Hermann, A. P., Gluer, C. C., Barkmann, R., & Rubin, K. H. (2017). Non-participation in systematic screening for osteoporosis—The ROSE trial. *Osteoporosis International, 28*(12), 3389–3399. https://doi.org/10.1007/s00198-017-4205-y.

Saliba, D., Elliott, M., Rubenstein, L. Z., Solomon, D. H., Young, R. T., Kamberg, C. J., Carol-Roth, R. N., MacLean, C. H., Shekelle, P. G., Sloss, E. M., & Wenger, N. W. (2001). The Vulnerable Elders Survey: A tool for identifying vulnerable older people in the community. *Journal of the American Geriatrics Society, 49*(12), 1691–1699. https://doi.org/10.1046/j.1532-5415.2001.49281.x.

Sanders, G. D., Bayoumi, A. M., Holodniy, M., & Owens, D. K. (2008). Cost-effectiveness of HIV screening in patients older than 55 years of age. *Annals of Internal Medicine, 148*(12), 889–903.

Sankar, A., Nevedal, A., Neufeld, S., Berry, R., & Luborsky, M. (2011). What do we know about older adults and HIV? A review of social and behavioral literature. *AIDS Care, 23*(10), 1187–1207. https://doi.org/10.1080/09540121.564115.

Savji, N., Rockman, C. B., Skolnick, A. H., Guo, Y., Adelman, M. A., Riles, T., & Berger, J. S. (2013). Association between advanced age and vascular disease in different arterial territories: A population database of over 3. 6 million subjects. *Journal of the American College of Cardiology, 61*(16), 1736–1743. https://doi.org/10.1016/j.jacc.2013.01.054.

Sehgal, M., Hidlebaugh, E., Checketts, M. G., & Reyes, B. (2019). Geriatrics screening and assessment. *Primary Care: Clinics in Office Practice, 46*(1), 85–96.

Siu, A. L., Bibbins-Domingo, K., Grossman, D. C., Baumann, L. C., Davidson, K. W., Ebell, M., Garcia, F. A., Gillman, M., Herzstein, J., Kemper, A. R., & Krist, A. H. (2009). Screening for impaired visual acuity in older adults: US Preventive Services Task Force recommendation statement. *Journal of the American Medical Association, 315*(9), 908–914. https://doi.org/10.1001/jama.2016.0763.

Smith, B. D., Smith, G. L., Hurria, A., Hortobagyi, G. N., & Buchholz, T. A. (2009). Future of cancer incidence in the United States: Burdens upon an aging, changing nation. *Journal of Clinical Oncology, 27*(17), 2758–2765. https://doi.org/10.1200/JCO.2008.20.8983.

Snellen, H. (1868). Probebuchstaben zur Bestimmung der Sehschärfe. Peters.

Substance Abuse and Mental Health Services Administration. (2020). *National Survey on Drug Use and Health 2017–2018. State level data.* https://www.samhsa.gov/data/report/2017-2018-nsduh-other-sources-state-level-data.

Tatara, D. C., Kuzmeskus, L. B., Duckhorn, E., Bievens, L., Thomas, C., & Gertiz, J. (1998). *The national elder abuse incidence study: Final report.* National Center on Elder Abuse. http://aoa.gov/AoA_Programs/Elder_Rights/Elder_Abuse/docs/ABuseReport_Full.pdf.

Tocchi, C., Dixon, J., Naylor, M., Jeon, S., & McCorkle, R. (2014). Development of a frailty measure for older adults: The frailty index for elders. *Journal of Nursing Measurement, 22*(2), 223–240. https://doi.org/10.1891/1061-3749.22.2.223.

US Census Bureau. (2019) *Quick facts: United States.* https://www.census.gov/quickfacts/fact/table/US/PST045219

US Department of Health and Human Services, Office of Disease Prevention and Health Promotion. (2020). In *Health People 2030.* (n.d.). Retrieved from https://health.gov/healthypeople.

US Preventive Services Task Force, United States (USPSTF). Office of Disease Prevention & Health Promotion. (2015). *Abnormal blood glucose and type II diabetes mellitus: Screening, final recommendation statement.* US Department of Health and Human Services, Office of Public Health and Science, Office of Disease Prevention and Health Promotion. https://www.uspreventiveservicestaskforce.org/Page/Document/UpdateSummaryFinal/screening-for-abnormal-blood-glucose-and-type-2-diabetes.

US Preventive Services Task Force, United States (USPSTF). Office of Disease Prevention & Health Promotion. (2015). *Tobacco smoking cessation in adults, including pregnant women: Behavioral and pharmacotherapy interventions.* US Department of Health and Human Services, Office of Public Health and Science, Office of Disease Prevention and Health Promotion. https://www.uspreventiveservicestaskforce.org/Page/Document/UpdateSummaryFinal/tobacco-use-in-adults-and-pregnant-women-counseling-and-interventions1.

US Preventive Services Task Force, United States (USPSTF). Office of Disease Prevention & Health Promotion. (2016). *Breast cancer: Screening. Final recommendation statement.* US Department of Health and Human Services, Office of Public Health and Science, Office of Disease Prevention and Health Promotion. https://www.uspreventiveservicestaskforce.org/Page/Document/UpdateSummaryFinal/breastcancer-screening1.

US Preventive Services Task Force, United States (USPSTF). Office of Disease Prevention & Health Promotion. (2018). *Cervical cancer: Screening. adolescent, adult, senior.* US Department of Health and Human Services, Office of Public Health and Science, Office of Disease Prevention and Health Promotion. https://www.uspreventiveservicestaskforce.org/uspstf/recommendation/cervical-cancer-screening.

US Preventive Services Task Force, United States. Office of Disease Prevention & Health Promotion. (2018). *Hepatitis: Screening.* US Department of Health and Human Services, Office of Public Health and Science, Office of Disease Prevention and Health Promotion. https://www.uspreventiveservicestaskforce.org/Page/Document/ClinicalSummaryFinal/hepatitis-c-screening.

US Preventive Services Task Force, United States (USPSTF). Office of Disease Prevention & Health Promotion. (2018). *Intimate partner violence and abuse of elderly and vulnerable adults: Screening.* US Department of Health and Human Services, Office of Public Health and Science, Office of Disease Prevention and Health Promotion. http://www.uspreventiveservicestaskforce.org/Page/Document/RecommendationStatementFinal/intimate-partner-violence-and-abuse-o-elderly-and-vulnerable-adults-screening.

US Preventive Services Task Force, United States (USPSTF). Office of Disease Prevention & Health Promotion. (2018). *Osteoporosis to prevent fractures: Screening. Adult, senior.* US Department of Health and Human Services, Office of Public Health and

Science, Office of Disease Prevention and Health Promotion. https://www.uspreventiveservicestaskforce.org/Page/Document/RecommendationStatementFinal/osteoporosis-screening1.

US Preventive Services Task Force, United States (USPSTF). Office of Disease Prevention & Health Promotion. (2020). *Cognitive impairment in older adults: Screening*. US Department of Health and Human Services, Office of Public Health and Science, Office of Disease Prevention and Health Promotion. https://www.uspreventiveservicestaskforce.org/uspstf/recommendation/cognitive-impairment-in-older-adults-screening?mod=article_inline.

Ventry, I. M., & Weinstein, B. E. (1982). The hearing handicap inventory for the elderly: A new tool. *Ear and Hearing*, *3*(3), 128–134. https://doi.org/10.1097/00003446-198205000-00006.

Walker, J. J., Cleveland, L. M., Davis, J. L., & Seales, J. S. (2013). Audiometry screening and interpretation. *American Family Physician.*, *87*(1), 41–47.

Walter, L. C., & Schonberg, M. A. (2014). Screening mammography in older women: A review. *Journal of American Medical Association*, *311*(13), 1336–1347. https://doi.org/10.1001/jama.2014.2834.

Wender, R., Fontham, E. T., Barrera, E., Colditz, G. A., Church, T. R., Ettinger, D. S., Etzioni, R., Flowers, C. R., Scott-Gazelle, G., Kelsey, D. K., & LaMonte, S. J. (2013). American Cancer Society lung cancer screening guidelines. *CA: A Cancer Journal for Clinicians*, *63*(2), 106–117. https://doi.org/10.3322/caac.21172.

Williams, N. (2014). The CAGE questionnaire. *Occupational Medicine*, *64*(6), 473–474. https://doi.org/10.1093/occmed/kqu058.

Wolf, P. A., Abbott, R. D., & Kannel, W. B. (1991). Atrial fibrillation as an independent risk factor for stroke: The Framingham Study. *Stroke*, *22*(8), 983–988. https://doi.org/10.1161/01.STR.22.8.983.

Wolf-Klein, G. P., Silverstone, F. A., Levy, A. P., Brod, M. S., & Breuer, J. (1989). Screening for Alzheimer's disease by clock drawing. *Journal of the American Geriatrics Society*, *37*(8), 730–734. https://doi.org/10.1111/j.1532-5415.1989.tb02234.x.

World Health Organization. (2018). Falls. [Fact sheet]. https://www.who.int/news-room/fact-sheets/detail/falls.

Yaffe, M. J., Wolfson, C., Lithwick, M., & Weiss, D. (2008). Development and validation of a tool to improve physician identification of elder abuse: The Elder Abuse Suspicion Index (EASI)©. *Journal of Elder Abuse and Neglect*, *20*(3), 276–300. https://doi.org/10.1080/08946560801973168.

Yang, Y., Brown, C. J., Burgio, K. L., Kilgore, M. L., Ritchie, C. S., Roth, D. L., West, D. S., & Locher, J. L. (2011). Undernutrition at baseline and health services utilization and mortality over a 1-year period in older adults receiving Medicare home health services. *Journal of the American Medical Directors Association*, *12*(4), 287–294. https://doi.org/10.1016/j.hamda.2010.08.017.

Yesavage, J. A., & Sheikh, J. I. (1986). 9/Geriatric Depression Scale (GDS) recent evidence and development of as shorter version. *Clinical Gerontologist*, *5*(1–2), 165–173. https://doi.org/10.1300/j018v05n01_09.

7

Promotion of Healthy Aging

C. KIM STOKES, DMSC, MHS, PA-C

OBJECTIVES

Student Learning Objectives

After completing this chapter, the student should be able to do the following:

1. Describe wellness as it pertains to the older adult.
2. Summarize the approach to promoting health in the aging adult.
3. Appraise the unique aspects of physical as well as psychosocial dynamics and how they affect the health and well-being of the older adult.

Practitioner Objectives

After completing this chapter, the practitioner should be able to do the following:

1. Use best available evidence to advocate for patients and continuously improve the quality of clinical practice for the aging patient.
2. Understand, evaluate, and apply interventions for the prevention of disease and health promotion/maintenance.
3. Utilize interpersonal skills to create and sustain a therapeutic and ethically sound relationship with aging patients and families to thereby promote health.
4. Develop practice approaches based on patient information, psychosocial conditions, living environment, current scientific evidence, and informed clinical judgment and integrate research, theory, and practice knowledge for the aging adult.

Overview of Promoting Healthy Aging

Definition of Healthy Aging in the Older Adult

Health, by definition, is the state of being free from illness or injury. Promoting healthy aging involves preventing injury and illness, as well as fostering overall well-being. There are as many as nine dimensions of wellness described in the literature, including physical, emotional, creative, environmental, financial, occupational, intellectual, social, and spiritual (Melynk & Neale, 2018). As people age, each of these dimensions should be considered. Additionally, to promote healthy aging, one must understand the social determinants of health and how they impact health and health care (Office of Disease Prevention and Health Promotion [ODPHP], 2014; World Health Organization [WHO], 2008). (See Fig. 7.1.) The dimensions of wellness and their relationship to healthy aging are further discussed later in this chapter.

The Burden of Unhealthy Practices and Environments in the Older Adult Population

The burden of unhealthy aging ultimately results in a myriad of problems for the patient as well as for the patient's caregivers, formal and informal. Perhaps the most striking example of the multifactorial nature of "healthy aging" can be observed through examining falls and fall risk. Many factors contribute to falls in the aging population, ranging from overall health to hearing/vision problems to the home environment.

To go a step farther, consider the economic impact of falls in the aging population. A person falls, enters the hospital environment, and possibly requires admission with or without surgical intervention, followed by potential deconditioning from immobilization for recovery. This one event could result in multiple weeks of missed wages and potentially a change in the quality of life for the remainder of the individual's lifetime. A fall also increases the risk of nosocomial infection, deep vein thrombosis, delirium, and hospital readmission.

Stevens and Lee (2018) reported implementing a single intervention (of seven studied in their research) that could prevent between 9500 and 45,000 medically treated falls, at a savings of $94 million to $442 million in direct medical costs annually. They noted the highest yield change was home modification delivered by the services of occupational therapists ($38.2 million, as noted in Table 7.1). This is noteworthy for understanding the value of interprofessional care for the aging population.

Direct medical costs include fees for hospital and nursing home care, doctors and other professional services, rehabilitation, community-based services, use of medical equipment, prescription drugs, and insurance processing. Direct costs do not account for the indirect long-term effects of these injuries, such as disability, dependence on others, lost time from work and household duties, and reduced quality of life. Additional information regarding the direct costs of falls can be found from

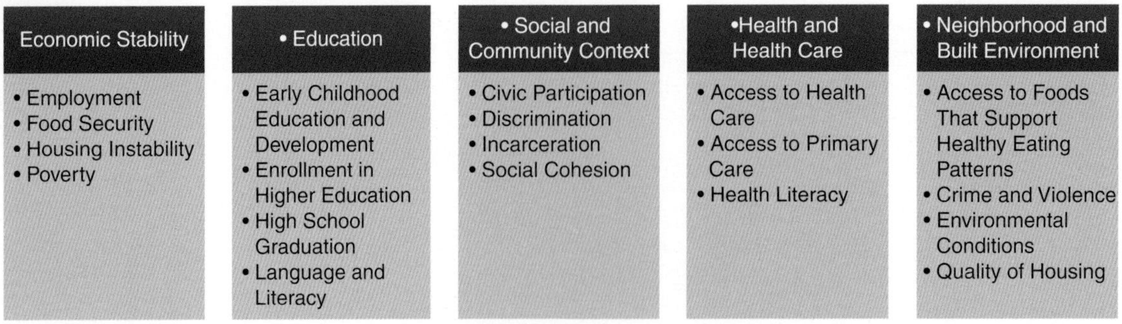

Economic Stability	• Education	• Social and Community Context	•Health and Health Care	• Neighborhood and Built Environment
• Employment • Food Security • Housing Instability • Poverty	• Early Childhood Education and Development • Enrollment in Higher Education • High School Graduation • Language and Literacy	• Civic Participation • Discrimination • Incarceration • Social Cohesion	• Access to Health Care • Access to Primary Care • Health Literacy	• Access to Foods That Support Healthy Eating Patterns • Crime and Violence • Environmental Conditions • Quality of Housing

• **Fig. 7.1** Overview of Social Determinants of Health. (Adapted from Healthy People. [2020]. WHO Healthy People 2020 framework. https://www.healthypeople.gov/2020/topics-objectives/topic/social-determinants-of-health.)

TABLE 7.1 **Estimating Medical Costs Averted by Conducting Clinical Fall Prevention Interventions in the United States**

A. Risk of contributing factor (prevalence)[b]	B. No. of older adults with risk factor (millions)	C. Interventions (effectiveness)[b]	D. Type of older adults eligible for intervention	E. % of older adults potentially eligible for intervention
Poor balance associated with neurologic gait disorders (24.0)[20]	11.5	Tai chi (29)[9]	No history of falls	65.1[1]
		Otago Program by physical therapist (32)[10]	History of falls	34.9[1]
Mobility problems (27.4)[21]	13.1	Tai chi (29)[9]	Excellent to good health	78.8[5]
		Otago Program by physical therapist (32)[10]	Fair or poor health	21.2[5]
Taking a medication potentially linked to falls (21.3)[22]	10.2	Medication review and modification (39)[8]	All people aged ≥ 65 years	100.0
Vitamin D insufficiency (<50 ng/mL) (35.0)[23]	16.7	Vitamin D supplementation (14)[7]	All people aged ≥ 65 years	100.0
Visual impairment: cataract (24.7)[24]	11.8	Expedited first eye cataract surgery (34[c])[12]	Poor vision	100.0
Poor depth perception from multifocal eyewear (32.4)[25,26]	15.5	Single vision distance lenses for outdoor activities (40)[11]	Active older adults	36.4[5]
Home hazards (80.0)[27]	38.2	Home modifications delivered by occupational therapist (31)[13]	Some functional decline	35.4[5]

[a]Calculations should be done from left to right to avoid rounding errors.
[b]Values in parentheses are percentages.
[c]The intervention was only tested among women, yet we assume there would be similar effectiveness among both men and women.
From Stevens, J. A., & Lee, R. (2018). The potential to reduce falls and avert costs by clinically managing fall risk. *American Journal of Preventive Medicine 55*(3), 290–297. https://doi.org/10.1016/j.amepre.2018.04.035
Note: Column B (number of older adults with the risk factor) = Column A (prevalence of the risk factor) × (47.8 million older adults); Column F (total eligible population) = Column B (number of older adults with the risk factor) × Column E (% of older adults eligible for the intervention); Column G (number of older adults likely to adopt intervention) = Column F (total eligible population) × 10% (estimated adoption rate); Column H (expected number of falls) = Column G (number eligible and likely to adopt the intervention) × (28.7% [the estimated incidence of falls in the U.S. 3[6]]) × (1,000,000); Column I (number of falls prevented) = Column H (expected number of falls) × Column C (intervention effectiveness); Column J (number of medically treated falls prevented) = Column I (number of falls prevented with intervention) × (37.5% [the estimated proportion of medically treated falls[36]]); Column K (direct medical costs averted) = Column J (number of medically treated falls prevented)x ($9,780 [the average cost of a medically treated fall[3']])/1,000,000.
No., number.

the US Centers for Disease Control and Prevention (CDC, "Physical activity for healthy weight," 2015). Publications from the *Journal of Public Health Management and Practice* (Haddad et al., 2019) as well as *the Journal of the American Geriatrics Society* (Florence et al., 2018) have also addressed the economic burden of falls.

For the informal caregiver, the burden of a fall equates to lost time at work as well as changed quality of life that is difficult to quantify. It is known that approximately 75% of all caregivers are women, with 50% being spouses, 25% being formal caregivers (part of the health care workforce), and another 25% being other informal caregivers—sisters, daughters, daughters-in-law, and granddaughters. Many times, these informal caregivers give up their occupation to care for loved ones or are forced to take paid or unpaid leave from work, which has even more financial repercussions on the economy, not to mention the caregiver's overall well-being.

Prevention of Unhealthy Practices and Environments for Older Adults

Unhealthy practices and environments increase the physical, emotional, and financial burden of the aging population. Common unhealthy practices in any age group might include exacerbating medical conditions or poor wound

F. Total eligible population (millions)	G. No. of eligible adults likely to adopt to intervention (millions)	H. Expected no. of falls among eligible adopters	I. No. of falls prevented with intervention	J. No. of medically treated falls prevented	K. Direct medical costs averted, $ (millions)
7.5	0.7	214,339	62,158	23,309	228
4.0	0.4	114,907	36,770	13,789	135
10.3	1.0	296,201	85,898	32,212	315
2.8	0.3	79,689	25,500	9,563	94
10.2	1.0	292,206	113,960	42,735	418
16.7	1.7	480,151	67,221	25,208	247
11.8	1.2	338,849	115,209	43,203	423
5.6	0.6	161,792	64,717	24,269	237
13.5	1.4	388,511	120,438	45,164	442

healing as a result of smoking, dietary indiscretion, or failure to wear a seatbelt. However, in the aging population, it is worth mentioning a few more, such as avoidance of mental health interventions, substance use/abuse, unsafe sexual practices, overmedication or medications that may increase the risk for falls, being unprepared for medical urgencies and emergencies, being financially unprepared for personal needs, or the loss of a spouse/significant other.

Given the multidimensional definition of *health*, it is evident that a medical provider (physician, nurse practitioner [NP], or physician assistant [PA]) cannot address the needs of the aging population alone. An interprofessional team-based care model (WHO, 2010) is imperative to ensuring needs are met and healthy practices can be implemented (Gilbert et al., 2010).

Interprofessional Collaboration in Healthy Aging

Nurse Practitioner and Physician Assistant Roles

The role of the NP and PA in promoting healthy aging is to truly listen to the patient; to review medical records for accuracy in the documentation of past medical history, family history, social and occupational history, and screening history; and to coordinate care from a patient-centered perspective. Additional dimensions of wellness and social determinants of health should also be considered and may require additional team members to get a fuller picture of the patient.

From here, a plan of evaluation should be initiated, which may include a geriatric comprehensive assessment (Ramani et al., 2014), with screening for cognition and mental health (specifically depression and substance abuse), as well as a review of activities of daily living (ADLs) and instrumental activities of daily living (IADLs). Diagnostic screening, a plan of vaccination and/or additional tests may be indicated. The NP or PA should remain up to date on screening guidelines set forth by the US Preventive Services Task Force (USPSTF) and the CDC, as well as Beers criteria (Fick et al., 2019), which provide medication management suggestions to prevent adverse outcomes in those over the age of 65. It is imperative for the provider to speak openly and honestly regarding prognostication and to advocate both for the patient and for advanced care planning.

Roles of Other Members of the Interprofessional Team

The nature of multiple comorbidities makes evaluation of the aging patient more complex. Thus, evaluations related to cognition, mood, finances, social wellness, and spiritual well-being may require more than one office visit, more than one type of health care provider, and the need to evaluate the patient in more than one environment. Every vital aspect of the aging patient's health cannot be visualized in the clinic alone. A patient-centered medical home with access to a variety of health professionals is ideal (Gilbert et al., 2010; WHO, 2010).

Behavioral health professionals (e.g., psychiatrists, health psychologists, marriage and family therapists, social workers, or other licensed counselors) integrated into clinical settings may assist with screenings related to mood and cognition, as well as offer advice to the provider or counseling for the patient and family. Additionally, these professionals are a valuable lifeline to community resources the aging patient may desperately need, from access to food to access to respite care. Social workers, home health nurses, nursing assistants, occupational therapists, and physical therapists have a valuable role in promoting healthy aging. These health professionals commonly have access to the patient's home environment and may provide additional pieces of vital information, including details about home safety and a better understanding of social supports and the home dynamic.

Physical therapists may also assist in the treatment of deconditioning to decrease fall risk. The role of a clinical pharmacist (PharmD) cannot be overstated. These professionals can review medication lists to ensure best practices are adhered to and work with patients to find affordable alternatives, both of which are keys to patient compliance. Audiology or ophthalmology referrals may be necessary to ensure patients can see and hear, as visual and auditory impairment can be confused with cognitive impairment. Besides the obvious diabetes education that a trained nutritionist may provide, the quality of life in patients with heart failure and chronic kidney disease may also be improved by a family referral to a nutritionist, especially when the person responsible for cooking and shopping is included in these appointments.

What is the value of good quality food if you cannot eat it? A dentist should also be part of the team of health professionals that cares for an aging patient to ensure the patient has proper dentition to allow for the best nutritional outcomes. Poor dentition can cause pain and be a source of systemic infection and systemic inflammation that can worsen health outcomes. In addition, dentition matters can affect wound healing after surgery because healing tissues depend on adequate blood flow and require the patient have enough dietary protein for healing. A patient with poor dentition may avoid many proteins due to difficulty with chewing or swallowing or may be unaware of how to get protein from plant sources. This person would be at a higher risk of postoperative wound infections or nonhealing (Brown et al., 2018; Whitson, 2019).

Promoting Healthy Aging

Promoting Healthy Diet and Lifestyle

Approach to a Healthy Diet and Lifestyle in the Aging Patient

Possibly the most profound promotion of healthy aging can be obtained through diet and lifestyle changes. Maintaining a

CASE STUDY

Scenario

Mary Smith is a 65-year-old woman who has been a factory worker since she turned 16. She assembles parts for electrical devices. She goes into work at 11 p.m. and gets off at 7 a.m. Once, she had planned to retire at 65, but due to her 83-year-old mother's chronic kidney disease, frequent falls, and heart failure and her spouse's severe chronic obstructive pulmonary disease (COPD), Mary has been the sole provider for the household for the past few years and needs the additional income. Overall, she feels she is in fair health. She takes an aspirin each day and "a pill" for her blood pressure. She sleeps about 4 hours a night and eats regularly because she makes all the meals in the house. Her kids live a couple of hours away. She has one grandchild who lives in town, attends the local college, and stays at the house while Mary works at night. Upon physical exam, Mary's blood pressure is found to be elevated at 180/94 and she has lost 5 lbs. She indicates she has trouble sleeping and feels tired during the day. She has a bruise on her left hip that she states came from tripping over the oxygen tubing at her home. She is up to date on screening exams and immunizations.

Problem

Mary has not been in to see you for over a year, noting she "just hasn't had time because someone has to be at the house all the time." She is here today because she is just so tired and is hoping you can give her something for rest. Even on her days off Mary lacks energy and has trouble falling asleep.

Discussion

Mary represents many people in the United States today. Older patients are living longer, working longer, and dealing with more medical conditions and stress than in previous decades. Mary's fatigue could be related to several possible diagnoses, including exhaustion, heart failure, chronic kidney disease, depression, sleep apnea, thyroid disease, caregiver burnout, and even cancer. When caring for patients like Mary, it is important for the practitioner to keep an open mind in order to think critically and to consider the overall wellness of the patient. The easy answer for Mary is for her provider to write a prescription for something to help her sleep. However, these medications increase fall risk and the risk of cognitive impairment in the aging population. By reviewing Mary's situation with a more critical eye, the practitioner may identify an underlying cause and help eliminate or alleviate it.

healthy weight (body mass index [BMI], hip-to-waist ratio) through middle age and older slows the aging process in vasculature and the brain, as well as reduces the physiologic load on weight-bearing joints and the spine. If genes, nutrition, lifestyle, environment, and chance together make up the human aging process, 40% of the process can potentially be altered through modifications of diet (nutrition) and lifestyle alone, with an additional benefit resulting from promoting an environment with access to care and safety (Shamsuddin, 2018).

In addition to physical activity, lifestyle intervention should include smoking cessation, reducing alcohol intake, preventing polypharmacy, maintaining optimal nutritional intake, and encouraging adequate sleep hygiene. A thorough history should include diet consumed, who is responsible for cooking and shopping, access to fresh foods and produce, as well as what the patient enjoys eating and doing. As for lifestyle, asking about smoking, drugs, and alcohol is valuable. In a thorough history, the NP or PA may discover the patient is struggling with sleep and using alcohol or other over-the-counter medications to assist with sleep. Regular exercise, adequate nutrition, stimulus control, and access to mental health resources may help older adults regulate sleep patterns without medications or substances that increase fall risk (Reid et al., 2010). Stimulus control for insomnia should include a recommendation to remove all nonsleep activities out of the bed, including television or technology (iPads, tablets, e-readers, etc.) (Martin et al., 2017). Regarding exercise, it is reasonable for the provider to inquire about what resources are available and affordable as well as the types of activity the patient enjoys.

Steps to Diagnosing Healthy Diet and Lifestyle Concerns

Low BMI (<20), rapid weight loss (more than 10 lb. or 4.5 kg in 6 months) and rapid weight gain (more than 4 lb. or 1.8 kg in a single day for heart failure patients) warrant further evaluation. Listening to the patient/family, taking a history of what is being consumed, asking who purchases the groceries and with what funds are all worthwhile and relevant questions. Asking such questions may seem intrusive, but the answers will provide key information for the care of your patient. Also, close collaboration with nutrition professionals can be essential to preventing hospitalization due to dietary indiscretion.

Factors to Consider in Healthy Diet and Lifestyle Education

The same social determinants of health that affect health care access may limit access to nutrition and lifestyle resources, from the ability to afford nutritious food to the safety of the potential environment for cardiovascular exercise. Encouraging a healthy diet rich in all food groups should include ensuring food can be obtained, ingested, and processed correctly. As noted earlier, an adequate oral exam for dentition is crucial, so patients should be referred to a dentist when needed. Poststroke patients or those with abnormal muscle tone (such as those affected by Parkinson disease) may need to be referred to a speech therapist or occupational therapist for a swallowing evaluation to help prevent aspiration and associated sequelae.

Many patients require specialty diets as they age, from sodium restriction in the hypertensive or heart failure patient to multiple restrictions (sodium, potassium, magnesium, etc.) in the patient with chronic kidney disease. Patient and family education is imperative and may have to be revisited multiple times with patience.

Cardiovascular and overall health must be considered before implementing lifestyle change. Traditionally, the screening for exercise tolerance has been established with the use of exercise stress tests. However, the US Physical Activity Guidelines for Americans (Department of Health and Human Services [DHHS], 2008) recommend against this practice for low-risk, asymptomatic persons. Currently, several approaches have been noted in the literature that are appropriate for use with older adults. "Exercise Assessment and Screening for You" (Chodzko-Zaiko et al., 2012) is one example. This tool may also allow for directed goal setting or other advice. Note the focus on falls and fall risk that should be addressed in the aging population to avoid exercise-related injury. This type of questionnaire may also allow for better advice on exercises to begin with or allow more patient choice, which improves adherence.

Advising Aging Patients on Healthy Diet and Lifestyle

Current dietary advice for all adults includes a healthy balanced diet, avoidance of tobacco and recreational drugs, and limited alcohol intake. The US Department of Health and Human Resources and the US Department of Agriculture (2012) develop dietary guidelines for Americans every 5 years; the current recommendations are summarized in Box 7.1 (DeSalvo et al., 2016).

Although many adults could benefit from caloric restriction (Stevens & Lee, 2018), recent understanding of optimal nutrition for those over 65 includes balancing macronutrients (protein, carbohydrates, and fat; Levine et al., 2014) and maintaining a BMI between normal and overweight (25–35). Optimizing calcium and vitamin D is highly encouraged, but the utilization of other supplements is not routinely recommended (Fick et al., 2019; Friedman et al., 2019).

• BOX 7.1 Summary of Dietary Guidelines for Americans 2015–2020

Guidelines

1. Follow a healthy eating pattern[a] across the life span.
2. Focus on variety, nutrient density, and volume.
3. Limit calories from added sugars and saturated fats, and limit sodium[b] intake.
4. Shift to healthier food and beverage choices.
5. Support healthy eating patterns for all.

Further Clarification

[a]*Healthy eating pattern* includes a variety of vegetables from all the subgroups (all colors, legumes, starchy, etc.); fruits, especially whole fruits; grains, at least half of which are whole grains; fat-free or low-fat dairy products; a variety of protein foods including seafood, lean meats and poultry, eggs, legumes, nuts, seeds, and soy products; oils.

[b]*Sodium intake* should be limited to less than 2300 mg/day. (See also Institute of Medicine. [2013]. *Sodium intake in populations: Assessment of evidence*. National Academies Press.)

Persons should also meet the *Physical Activity Guidelines for Americans*.

Adapted from US Department of Health and Human Services: US Department of Agriculture. (2015, December). *2015–2020 dietary guidelines for Americans* (8th ed.). US Dept of Health and Human Services.

For physical activity, the National Institutes of Health (NIH) recommends a focus on the need in older adults for a combination of endurance (aerobic activity), strength (muscle-strengthening exercise), balance training, and flexibility through the Go4Life campaign (NIH, n.d.).

The US Department of Health and Human Services (DHHS, 2008) further clarifies aerobic activity for older adults as 150 minutes of moderate intensity aerobic activity per week as their abilities and conditions allow. Balance training may be obtained in a variety of ways. A list of evidence-based fall preventions programs can be found on the National Council on Aging website (NCOA, n.d.). Patients should also be educated on whether and how their medical conditions affect exercise to better prepare and ensure safe environments for physical activity. Additionally, the American Geriatrics Society recommends osteoarthritis and osteoporosis management as the primary prevention (see Table 7.3) strategy for these conditions (Friedman et al., 2019), to include maintenance of a healthy weight and an adequate dietary intake of calcium and nutrients to reduce bone loss. Currently, management of osteoarthritis additionally includes the use of acetaminophen for chronic pain control.

Promoting Emotional, Social, and Spiritual Wellness

Approach to Emotional, Social, and Spiritual Wellness in the Aging Patient

Addressing the physical health of the aging population without considering overall wellness is a disservice. A variety of sources discuss the value of "wellness" or "well-being" as it pertains to healthy aging in terms of both health and cognitive benefits (Melynk & Neale, 2018; Strout & Howard, 2012, 2015; Strout et al., 2016). Dimensions of wellness include emotional, financial, social, spiritual, occupational, physical, intellectual, and environmental factors. Primary prevention strategies recommended in the American Geriatrics Society (AGS) White Paper on Healthy Aging (Friedman et al., 2019) includes a focus beyond the physical, noting several dimensions of wellness across a variety of domains (Table 7.2). Without adequate emotional, social, and spiritual wellness, chronic illness or chronic pain could be exacerbated (Swarbrick, 2006). An integrated approach to behavioral health can aid in identifying and addressing these concerns but do not substitute for a provider who seeks to understand the needs of the patient.

Steps to Discover Disruptions in Emotional, Social, or Spiritual Concerns in the Aging Patient

In the busy day-to-day activities of any clinical environment, it can be easy for a health care provider to go from room to room and chart to chart without meaningfully interacting with the patient, which would involve direct eye contact, appropriate open body language, a reassuring tone, and a genuine reassuring demeanor. But these interactions are essential to understanding the aging patient. Likewise, for

TABLE 7.2 Correlating American Geriatrics Society (AGS) Primary Prevention Recommendations to the Dimensions of Wellness

AGS Domain	AGS Primary Prevention Recommendation	Dimension of Wellness
Promoting health, preventing injury, and managing chronic conditions	Maintain healthful balanced nutrition	Physical wellness
	Avoid tobacco	
	Avoid recreational drugs or excess alcohol	
	Maintain sleep hygiene	
	Maintain ideal body weight	
	Practice oral hygiene	
	Manage stress	
	Regular physical activity	
	Manage stress	Emotional wellness
Optimizing cognitive health	Lifelong learning	Intellectual wellness
	Lifelong intellectual engagement	
Optimizing mental health	Engaging in meaningful work	Occupational/career wellness
Optimizing mental health	Finding life purpose	Spiritual wellness
Optimizing mental health	Participating in enriching social activities	Social wellness and emotional wellness
Facilitating social engagement	Forming meaningful relationship with people who share interests	
	Engaging in civic activities	
Facilitating social engagement	Meeting safety, financial, and housing needs	Environmental wellness
Facilitating social engagement	Meeting safety, financial, and housing needs	Financial wellness

Adapted from Friedman, S. M., Mulhausen, P., Cleveland, M. L., Coll, P. P., Daniel, K. M., Hayward, A. D., . . . White, H. K. (2019). Healthy aging: American geriatrics society white paper executive summary: AGS White Paper on Healthy Aging. *Journal of the American Geriatrics Society, 67*(1), 17–20. https://doi.org/10.1111/jgs.15644; Melnyk, B. M., & Neale, S. (2018). 9 dimensions of wellness: Your health and well-being isn't just about nutrition and exercise. *American Nurse Today, 13*(1), 10; Swarbrick, M. (2006). A wellness approach. *Psychiatric Rehabilitation Journal, 29*(4), 311–314. https://store.samhsa.gov/system/files/sma16–4958.pdf

emotional concerns, collaborating with behavioral health professionals or completing questionnaires (such as those that screen for depression, anxiety, or burnout) can identify problems for appropriate referral ad enhance the focus on well-being when caring for an older adult. Burnout, typically associated with work environments, is commonly seen in patients who are acting as caregivers at home, especially in older adults who are caring for persons in the home with neurocognitive disorders. Up to half of informal caregivers have been shown to experience burnout that can progress to depression and anxiety (Kim et al., 2014). A variety of screening tools exist that have been used in older adults, including the Pines Burnout Measure (Takai et al., 2008).

A medical evaluation may reveal something through a lab test or diagnostic study that was missed in the history of present illness (HPI) assessment and may trigger additional questions. With emotional, social, and spiritual concerns, the provider who does not ask will likely never know. The NP and PA cannot rely on ancillary staff to ask all these questions. Asking directly and with compassion is most likely to strengthen the patient-provider relationship and establishes trust.

Factors to Consider in Screening for Emotional, Social, and Spiritual Wellness

It is important not to press your own beliefs on the patient; rather explore the patient's needs from the standpoint of cultural humility. Additionally, some patients withdraw socially without even realizing it. This could be the result of psychological disorders (such as depression) or neurologic conditions (such as altered mental status) as well as caregiver burnout. Our scenario tells the tale of Mary Smith who has left her social network (ceased self-care activities) to care for both her spouse and an aging parent with multiple comorbidities. This describes the burden of many aging patients who are not only patients themselves but are also informal caregivers to other older adults. This points out the need, when caring for an older adult, to ask whether that individual is caring for anyone else, such as an aging parent, dependent spouse/partner, sibling, adult child, or in some cases, even a young grandchild.

Asking aging patients about emotional health/well-being, time for self-care or respite, access to additional resources or support (siblings, family members, home health, other community resources), and social activities or spiritual care is pivotal for improving the quality of life and reducing stress levels of informal caregivers. Statistically, the key to keeping the caregiver's patient healthy is to keep the caregiver healthy (Erlingsson et al., 2012). This quality of life and personal well-being also decreases the risk of elder abuse and neglect.

Fear and anxiety regarding the health of a loved one or personal health or outcomes may affect health. Generating a conversation with your patients and caregivers regarding advance care directives or a durable health care power of attorney (HCPOA) to ensure the patient has the support to make his or her wishes known may alleviate worry and fear, in both the patient and the caregivers (Dingfield & Kayser, 2017).

Resources for Emotional, Social, or Spiritual Concerns in the Aging Patient

Resources available to address emotional, social, and spiritual concerns are largely regionally/locally dependent. As a start, the NP or PA can reach out to the local Council on Aging (https://www.ncoa.org/) and inquire as to if or when caregiver support groups meet. These agencies also commonly have a "respite" service for caregivers, which provides a few hours of rest time for family caregivers weekly. The National Council on Aging also has a listing of "senior centers" or special populations groups offered by city parks and recreation departments. Knowing a local chaplain or common houses of worship in the area may also help the NP or PA care for aging patients by informing them about a place of worship, a connection to like-minded persons, or programs offered through outreach ministries.

Promoting Safe Environments

Approach to Discussing Safe Living and Work Environments With the Aging Patient

Simply speaking, a safe living and work environment would include a space that is free of fall risk and environmentally controlled (heating, air, etc.). For example, when a patient has experienced a fall, asking about throw rugs, stairs coming into the home, and the like could be telling. However, some of the most awkward conversations can also arise when discussing safe living and work environments. It feels so personal to ask, "Do you feel safe at home?" or "Do you feel safe at work?" However, asking these questions can save lives, especially in the case of elder abuse. Finding a way to ask these questions without a caregiver present is imperative. And there are more comfortable ways to ask than by using these direct questions. For example, one might say, "How are things going at work?" or "This must be stressful for you. How are things at home?" Then the practitioner can watch for body language (breaking eye contact, withdrawing) that may indicate there is a concern.

Additionally, asking simply about "safety" at home is not clear enough to cover all that really needs to be addressed. Questions such as "Do you feel safe in your home physically?" or "Do you fear a break in or theft of your possessions or money?" better address concerns about physical and psychological safety. The following questions better address concerns about abuse and neglect:

- Do you feel safe with your caregiver?
- Does your caregiver ever make you feel small or use words that make you feel bad about yourself?
- Does your caregiver ever leave you alone when you really need something?
- What are the sleeping arrangements in your home?

Questions such as "Does your home have stairs with rails, running water, or throw rugs?" better address concerns regarding hazards.

Steps for Recognizing Unsafe Living and Work Environments for the Aging Patient

It can be difficult to recognize when a patient is in an unsafe living or work environment. Many patients are private and feel these matters should remain private. Others may or may not realize they are being taken advantage of or that they are at a disadvantage (e.g., an aging patient who is not digitally literate allows a younger family member to do online banking on the patient's behalf and money goes missing). Medical providers may not recognize the need to focus on these areas as part of routine medical care, may not feel comfortable asking these questions, or may discount the need to do so because they seem less important and of a low priority given the time pressures in many medical settings.

As with emotional, social, and spiritual well-being, the practitioner who does not ask these questions may never know whether or not the patient is in a safe environment. Also, there are some observable signs that may signal a bigger problem and, at minimum, should trigger inquiry, such as fractures or injuries that do not correlate to the mechanism of injury, falls with a long downtime before being discovered, a prolonged length of time between injury and treatment, pressure ulcers, controlled substance prescriptions that need refill before expected date, and multiple falls at home.

Factors to Consider in Living and Work Environments for the Aging Patient

If there are legitimate concerns about patient well-being related to the patient's living environment or other safety issues, a call to adult protective services (APS) through the local Department of Social Services (DSS) is warranted. Placing a call and discussing the situation with a caseworker could save a life or greatly improve the quality of life for the patient. Each situation is considered closely and investigated. In an inpatient or emergency room setting, the caregiver may need to be removed for the safety of the patient. Health care professionals should follow the guidelines set forth in their facility.

It is important not to jump to conclusions and assume the person with falls and fractures is being abused or neglected. Rather, a kind, considerate approach with an open door of communication is ideal. Family dynamics are more than the medical provider can handle alone and she or he will require assistance. Reporting concerns to DSS may cause a rift between the provider and the patient or unsettle the provider-patient-family relationship. However, this should not delay a referral if there are significant concerns.

Resources to Promote Safe Living and Work Environments for the Aging Patient

One of the best ways to get a better idea of your patient's home environment is to order an occupational therapy (OT) evaluation with a home assessment (Stevens & Lee, 2018). This study has also been shown to reduce fall risk, improve the ability to age in place, and ultimately decrease the economic burden of aging. The occupational therapist may recommend a ramp into the home, removal of throw rugs, reorganization of cabinets to make commonly used items more accessible (and to decrease the need for step stools), or the addition of rails in the bathroom to aid in standing after toileting, among other modifications. In some situations, OT cannot be ordered as a stand-alone service. In this case, the PA or NP can consider other needs of the patient. In the case study, for example, the patient, Mary, also has high blood pressure that is not well controlled. A nurse visit to check Mary for hypertension along with an OT home evaluation may be appropriate to augment or reduce the need for more frequent office visits and ultimately provide better access to care and influence over outcomes.

In addition to considering a patient's home environment, referrals to a social worker or behavioral health specialist may prove beneficial. The social worker may be able to assist the patient in finding access to services that will improve health and aging. The behavioral health practitioner may be able to assist the patient with alcohol reduction/cessation and address underlying mental health concerns.

Work environments may prove difficult to assess. One exception is that of farmers and agricultural laborers. NPs and PAs who work in areas with many farmers, fishers, or loggers may consider making a referral to the local agromedicine team. This team can evaluate the working environment, give advice for safety and wellness in the agricultural environment, and help to decrease the risk of occupational injury related to falls, equipment accidents, exposure to harmful chemicals, musculoskeletal injury, and similar hazards (Morera et al., 2014; Rudolphi & Donham, 2015).

Promoting Financial Wellness

Approach to Discussing Financial Wellness With the Aging Patient

Financial wellness may seem an odd topic to include in a medical text. However, it is relevant to the care of older adults. Many aging patients are ill prepared for the financial burden of their disease and the potential costs of short or long-term care, so they may be disillusioned in terms of understanding what is and is not covered by Medicare or Medicaid. Additionally, elder abuse includes financial abuse—the use of the patient's assets for personal gain, thus making the situation even worse. Older adults are also prone to financial scams, which may be furthered by the use of technology (Gorney et al., 2020). Cybercrime is also a problem in the older adult population (Munanga, 2019).

Steps for Recognizing Financial Concerns in the Aging Patient

Some patients will never bring up financial insecurities with their providers, but many will, especially when it comes to the cost of prescriptions or the cost of long-term care. It is worthwhile to start the conversation with the patient by saying, "You're taking several medications. Do you have any trouble paying for them? Maybe I can help." Then the clinician can look through the list to see what medications might be discontinued. Financial concerns may also lead to food insecurity or lack of psychological/physical safety in the home due to disrepair or infestation. Again, humble inquiry is key: "It's been a cold winter; how is your home heated? Do you have enough oil/wood?" "I noticed you're losing weight. You been eating okay? What have you been eating? How do you get your groceries?" Symptoms as "routine" in the aging patient as constipation can be related to hunger, food insecurity, or financial concerns. Identifying an older adult who may be caught in a scam or cyberscam can be difficult and, for the clinician, may only be discovered in retrospect.

Factors to Consider When Addressing Financial Concerns in the Aging Patient

It is not the role of the medical provider to advise patients and their families regarding financial matters. However, it is important to recognize the impact of finances on a patient's care and to vigilantly advocate for the patient if need be. It is helpful to advise patients to consider the value of a durable HCPOA as well as an estate manager or other financial adviser, as medical care expenses may mount, long-term care may be considered, or the patient may be left cognitively unable to manage a household. This is also an excellent opportunity to discuss or complete an advance directive in a controlled environment versus taking this step during a time of high stress and pressure, such as after a significant illness or injury has occurred.

Having honest, straight-forward conversations with the patient and their family regarding illness and prognostication best allows patients to prepare for the future. One of the most urgent situations during which these conversations should be at the forefront involves irreversible neurocognitive impairment related to Alzheimer disease, Parkinson disease, vascular dementia, and frontotemporal dementia. These conditions are not curable and follow a progression. Early recognition and conversations allow time for important communication between the patient, the family/community, and the provider. These decisions can ultimately ease the burden of caregivers by providing peace and guidance from the patient. Patients should share their decisions with family/decision makers.

No one enjoys discovering they have been party to deceit. Thus, older adults who have fallen prey to cybercrime or some other financial scam may not report the crime. To avoid financial scams and cybercrimes, the Federal Bureau of Investigation (FBI) has provided a list of basics for computer and Internet security (Box 7.2). Additionally, if someone in the household has a neurocognitive disorder, the clinician should inform the caregivers to closely monitor financial statements and consider changes in monetary management as appropriate, which may include canceling credit cards, for example.

Resources to Promote Financial Wellness

The local Council on Aging should have information regarding how to understand Medicare and Medicaid and dates for

• BOX 7.2 Risk Reduction of Cybercrime in Older Adults

- Avoid shopping online.
- Do not give away financial information over the telephone or Internet.
- Have computers and Internet checked for malware and protected frequently.
- Visit known and trustworthy websites and avoid unfamiliar websites, which may have programs that take personal information even without consent.
- Be suspicious and click with care.
- Avoid opening e-mails from unknown senders.
- Use telephones with caller identification, and talk to only known individuals.
- Avoid making charitable contributions over the telephone.

Adapted from the Federal Bureau of Investigation (FBI), (2018). *Elder fraud.* https://www.fbi.gov/scams-and-safety/common-fraud-schemes/seniors

enrollment. If a clinician suspects financial abuse, the best approach is to contact Adult Protective Services through the local department of social services. Additionally, local hospitals, law offices, and the Internet have templates that can be used to guide discussions. Some states have also simplified the advance care directive to streamline the discussion (e.g., NC Medical Orders for Scope of Treatment (MOST) form). Additionally, the local Council on Aging and public libraries commonly have basic computer and technology courses to help anyone become computer literate and aware of issues related to cybersafety.

Special Consideration

Driving

Approach to Driving in Relation to Older Adults

Discussions with older adults related to driving can prove difficult because of the independence that comes with driving. However, the NP or PA has a role in these discussions, especially when older patients could be impaired due to vision loss, physical changes, or neurocognitive changes. Older drivers are also more likely to have slowed motor reflexes, impaired hearing, or a reduction in strength or coordination, which can make driving a matter of public safety. Although it may be tempting to punt these topics to another clinician, having an open and honest conversation with patients and their families is the best place to start.

Steps to Diagnosing Problems With Driving

Inquiries about driving-related accidents or getting lost offer the simplest way to find out if there are big problems. These questions should be asked of both the older adult and people who have been passengers in the vehicle. Sometimes, the first indicator of neurocognitive impairment is getting lost in a vehicle, even driving hundreds of miles. The passengers of older adults may be able to give insight as to the older adult's quality of driving. For instance, does the car stay on the correct side of the road? Does the driver adequately signal or miss turns, and so forth?

Resources for Patient and Clinicians

The CDC recommends the use of "MyMobilityPlan" to make a plan to stay mobile and independent. Additionally, an occupational therapist may be utilized for a "car fit" test to ensure patients can adequately sit in a vehicle, reach the equipment, and see over the dashboard, among other things. The National Institute on Aging (NIA, 2018) also has a guide for patients to understand when it may be time to stop driving. After there has been an honest and open conversation with the older adult regarding the health and safety of the patient and others, the local Department of Motor Vehicles (DMV) may prove to be the best resource. The NP or PA could request a senior driving evaluation or anonymously report a problem to the DMV.

If a conversation with the older adult is not successful, reporting is always an option. Advice to families may include using memory loss to their advantage by "losing" keys, "taking the car for repairs," or having a friend "borrow" the car. Disabling the car or selling the car is also an option, but this may cause undesired distress. The family member should be advised to keep her or his own car keys close or hidden, especially if memory loss is a consideration.

Key Points

- Promoting healthy aging goes beyond physical health to include multiple dimensions of wellness.
- Overlooking the other dimensions of wellness and social determinants of health can be detrimental to the health of the older adult.
- The most reasonable approach to the multiple comorbidities associated with aging includes an interprofessional approach to care, with an integrated behavioral health practitioner if possible.
- Home evaluations through OT may offer the largest benefit in reducing falls and fall risk.
- Before an older patient begins a new physical activity, the primary provider should complete a screening.
- The National Council on Aging, National Institutes of Aging, and American Geriatrics Society have invaluable resources to promote healthy aging.

More information about tools and Interprofessional Education Collaborative (IPEC) competencies mentioned in this chapter can be found in Appendix 1: Tools and Appendix 2: IPEC Competencies.

References

Brown, T. A., Brown, J. E., Britton, B., & Caldon, T. L. (2018). Effects of early recovery after surgery protocol on clinical outcomes after Whipple surgery. *Journal of the American College of Surgeons, 227*(4), e172–e172. https://doi.org/10.1016/j.jamcollsurg.2018.08.468.

Center for Disease Control and Prevention (CDC). (2015). *Physical activity for healthy weight.* https://www.cdc.gov/healthyweight/physical_activity/index.html

Center for Disease Control and Prevention (CDC). (2016). *Cost of falls among older adults.* https://www.cdc.gov/homeandrecreationalsafety/falls/fallcost.html

Center for Disease Control and Prevention (CDC). (2020). *Older adult drivers.* https://www.cdc.gov/motorvehiclesafety/older_adult_drivers/index.html

Chodzko-Zajko, W. J., Resnick, B., & Ory, M. G. (2012). Beyond screening: Tailoring physical activity options with the EASY tool. *Translational Behavioral Medicine, 2*(2), 244–248. https://doi.org/10.1007/s13142-012-0134-7.

DeSalvo, K. B., Olson, R., & Casavale, K. O. (2016). Dietary guidelines for Americans. *Journal of the American Medical Association, 315*(5), 457–458. https://doi.org/10.1001/jama.2015.18396.

Dingfield, L. E., & Kayser, J. B. (2017). Integrating advance care planning into practice. *Chest, 151*(6), 1387–1393. https://doi.org/10.1016/j.chest.2017.02.024.

Erlingsson, C. L., Magnusson, L., Hanson, E., Linnéuniversitetet, Institutionen för hälso- och vårdvetenskap, H. V., & Fakultetsnämnden för hälsa, socialt arbete och beteendevetenskap. (2012). Family caregivers' health in connection with providing care. *Qualitative Health Research, 22*(5), 640–655. https://doi.org/10.1177/1049732311431247.

Fick, D. M., Semla, T. P., Steinman, M., Beizer, J., Brandt, N., Dombrowski, R., … By the 2019 American Geriatrics Society Beers Criteria® Update Expert Panel. (2019). American geriatrics society 2019 updated AGS Beers criteria® for potentially inappropriate medication use in older adults. *Journal of the American Geriatrics Society, 67*(4), 674–694. https://doi.org/10.1111/jgs.15767.

Florence, C. S., Bergen, G., Atherly, A., Burns, E. R., Stevens, J. A., & Drake, C. (2018). Medical costs of fatal and nonfatal falls in older adults. *Journal of the American Geriatrics Society, 66*(4), 693–698. https://doi.org/10.1111/jgs.15304.

Friedman, S. M., Mulhausen, P., Cleveland, M. L., Coll, P. P., Daniel, K. M., Hayward, A. D., … White, H. K. (2019). Healthy aging: American geriatrics society white paper executive summary: AGS white paper on healthy aging. *Journal of the American Geriatrics Society, 67*(1), 17–20. https://doi.org/10.1111/jgs.15644.

Gilbert, J. H. V., Yan, J., & Hoffman, S. J. (2010). A WHO report: Framework for action on interprofessional education and collaborative practice. *Journal of Allied Health, 39*(1), 196–197.

Gorney, R., Cassidy-Eagle, E., & Smith, K. (2020). Easy money: Financial scams and older adults. *The American Journal of Geriatric Psychiatry, 28*(4), S6–S6. https://doi.org/10.1016/j.jagp.2020.01.020.

Haddad, Y. K., Bergen, G., & Florence, C. S. (2019). Estimating the economic burden related to older adult falls by state. *Journal of Public Health Management and Practice, 25*(2), E17–E24. https://doi.org/10.1097/PHH.0000000000000816.

Institute of Medicine. (2013). *Sodium intake in populations: Assessment of evidence.* National Academies Press.

Kim, Y., Shaffer, K. M., Carver, C. S., & Cannady, R. S. (2014). Prevalence and predictors of depressive symptoms among cancer caregivers 5 years after the relative's cancer diagnosis. *Journal of Consulting and Clinical Psychology, 82*, 1–8.

Levine, M. E., Suarez, J. A., Brandhorst, S., Balasubramanian, P., Cheng, C. W., Madia, F., Fontana, L., Mirisola, M. G., Guevara-Aguirre, J., Wan, J., Passarino, G., Kennedy, B. K., Wei, M., Cohen, P., Crimmins, E. M., & Longo, V. D. (2019). Low protein intake is associated with a major reduction in IGF-1, cancer, and overall mortality in the 65 and younger but not older population. *Cell Metabolism, 19*, 407–417.

Munanga, A. (2019). Cybercrime: A new and growing problem for older adults. *Journal of Gerontological Nursing, 45*(2), 3–5. https://doi.org/10.3928/00989134-20190111-01.

Martin, J. L., Song, Y., Hughes, J., Jouldjian, S., Dzierzewski, J. M., Fung, C. H., & Alessi, C. A. (2017). A four-session sleep intervention program improves sleep for older adult day health care participants: Results of a randomized controlled trial. *Sleep, 40*(8), zsx079. https://doi.org/10.1093/sleep/zsx079.

Melnyk, B. M., & Neale, S. (2018). 9 dimensions of wellness: Your health and well-being isn't just about nutrition and exercise. *American Nurse Today, 13*(1), 10.

Morera, M. C., Monaghan, P. F., Tovar-Aguilar, J. A., Galindo-Gonzalez, S., Roka, F. M., & Asuaje, C. (2014). Improving health and safety conditions in agriculture through professional training of Florida farm labor supervisors. *Journal of Agromedicine, 19*(2), 117–122. https://doi.org/10.1080/1059924X.2014.886318.

National Council on Aging (NCOA). (n.d.). *Evidence-based falls prevention programs.* https://www.ncoa.org/healthy-aging/falls-prevention/falls-prevention-programs-for-older-adults-2/

National Institute of Health (NIH): National Institute of Aging. (n.d.). *Exercise and physical activity: Getting fit for life.* https://www.nia.nih.gov/health/exercise-and-physical-activity-getting-fit-life

National Institute of Health (NIH): National Institute of Aging. *Go4Life® from the National Institute on Aging at NIH.* https://go4life.nia.nih.gov/

National Institute of Health (NIH): National Institute of Aging. (2018). *Older drivers.* https://www.nia.nih.gov/health/older-drivers

Office of Disease Prevention and Health Promotion (ODPHP). (2014). *Healthy people 2020: Social determinants of health.* https://www.healthypeople.gov/2020/topics-objectives/topic/social-determinants-of-health.

Ramani, L., Furmedge, D. S., & Reddy, S. P. (2014). Comprehensive geriatric assessment. *British Journal of Hospital Medicine, 75* (Suppl. 8), C122–C125. https://doi.org/10.12968/hmed.2014.75.Sup8.C122.

Reid, K. J., Baron, K. G., Lu, B., Naylor, E., Wolfe, L., & Zee, P. C. (2010). Aerobic exercise improves self-reported sleep and quality of life in older adults with insomnia. *Sleep Medicine, 11*(9), 934–940. https://doi.org/10.1016/j.sleep.2010.04.014.

Rudolphi, J. M., & Donham, K. J. (2015). Toward a national core course in agricultural medicine and curriculum in agricultural safety and health: The "building capacity" consensus process. *Journal of Agromedicine*, *20*(1), 77–83. https://doi.org/10.1080/1059924X.2014.977503.

Simpson, S. J., Couteur, D. G. L., Raubenheimer, D., Solon-Biet, S. M., Cooney, G. J., Cogger, V. C., & Fontana, L. (2017). Dietary protein, aging and nutritional geometry. *Ageing Research Reviews*, *39*, 78–86. https://doi.org/10.1016/j.arr.2017.03.001.

Shamsuddin, A. (2018). Diseases of aging. In R. Hines (Ed.), *Stoelting's Anesthesia and co-existing disease* (7th ed., pp. 327–343m). Elsevier.

Stevens, J. A., & Lee, R. (2018). The potential to reduce falls and avert costs by clinically managing fall risk. *American Journal of Preventive Medicine*, *55*(3), 290–297. https://doi.org/10.1016/j.amepre.2018.04.035.

Strout, K. A., David, D. J., Dyer, E. J., Gray, R. C., Robnett, R. H., & Howard, E. P. (2016). Behavioral interventions in six dimensions of wellness that protect the cognitive health of community-dwelling older adults: A systematic review. *Journal of the American Geriatrics Society*, *64*(5), 944–958. https://doi.org/10.1111/jgs.14129.

Strout, K. A., & Howard, E. P. (2012). The six dimensions of wellness and cognition in aging adults. *Journal of Holistic Nursing*, *30*, 195–204.

Strout, K. A., & Howard, E. P. (2015). Five dimensions of wellness and predictors of cognitive health protection in community-dwelling older adults: A historical COLLAGE cohort study. *Journal of Holistic Nursing*, *33*, 6–18.

Swarbrick, M. (2006). A wellness approach. *Psychiatric Rehabilitation Journal*, *29*(4), 311–314. https://store.samhsa.gov/system/files/sma16-4958.pdf.

Takai, M., Takahashi, M., Iwamitsu, Y., Ando, N., Okazaki, S., Nakajima, K., … Miyaoka, H. (2008, 2009). The experience of burnout among home caregivers of patients with dementia: Relations to depression and quality of life. *Archives of Gerontology and Geriatrics*, *49*(1), e1–e5. https://doi.org/10.1016/j.archger.2008.07.002.

US Department of Health and Human Services. (2008). *2008 Physical activity guidelines for Americans*. US Dept of Health and Human Services. Office of Disease Prevention and Health Promotion (ODPHP) publication U0036.

US Department of Health and Human Services: US Department of Agriculture. (2015, December). *2015–2020 Dietary guidelines for Americans* (8th ed.). US Dept of Health and Human Services. http://www.health.gov/DietaryGuidelines.

Whitson, B. A. (2019). Early to extubate, early to discharge—Providing further evidence in favor of fast tracking and early recovery after surgery pathways. *Journal of Thoracic and Cardiovascular Surgery*, *159*(1), P191. https://doi.org/10.1016/j.jtcvs.2019.03.117.

World Health Organization (WHO). (2008). Commission on social determinants of health. closing the gap in a generation: Health equity through action on the social determinants of health. http://www.who.int/social_determinants/en

World Health Organization (WHO). (2010). *Framework for action on interprofessional education and collaborative practice*. https://www.who.int/hrh/resources/framework_action/en/

8

Medication Use in Older Adults

TATYANA GURVICH, PHARMD, BCGP, YUEN NG, PHARMD, AND JANET CHO, PHARMD, BCGP

OBJECTIVES

Student Learning Objectives

After completing this chapter, the student should be able to do the following:

1. Identify concerns of medication use in the older adults.
2. Identify polypharmacy and medication cascades.
3. Identify and discuss differences in drug response in older patients.
4. Describe a practical approach to prescribing in older patients.
5. Explain how to dose and titrate medications safely in older patients.
6. Utilize the Beers Criteria to identify potentially harmful medications in older adults.
7. Describe a practical and safe approach to the use of pain medications in older patients.
8. Describe a practical approach to older patients' use of over-the-counter medications, supplements, and cannabis.
9. Describe various methods of coordinating care with a clinical pharmacist to improve medication use in older adults.
10. Discuss the value of medication reconciliation for older patients during transitions of care.

Practitioner Objectives

After completing this chapter, the practitioner should be able to do the following:

1. Identify concerns of medication use in older adults, and implement a tracking system in one's clinical practice to minimize occurrence of misuse.
2. Implement strategies into your clinical practice to avoid polypharmacy and medication cascades in older patients.
3. Utilize differences in the drug response of older patients in the selection of prescribed medications.
4. Utilize dosing guidelines and titration schedules that have been established for older patients.
5. Utilize Beers criteria in the management of medical problems and decisions regarding the discontinuation of medications.
6. Develop clinical strategies to use pain medications safely in older patients.
7. Develop clinical strategies to help older patients use over-the-counter medications, supplements, and cannabis safely.
8. Integrate the expertise of a clinical pharmacist into the geriatric clinical practice.
9. Develop effective strategies to implement medication review during older adults' transitions of care.

Introduction

Older adults constitute 10% to 15% of the total adult population in the United States, yet they consume a disproportionally large number of prescription and over-the-counter medications and supplements. Most patients are medically complicated because they have accumulated multiple chronic diseases over the years. Each chronic disease often requires multiple drugs for treatment. It is not uncommon for older adults to take 10 to 20 medications daily. Long medication lists produce adverse events, polypharmacy, and confusion due to complicated medication regimens, all of which increase overall health care costs. The total estimated health care expenditure related to potentially inappropriate medications is $7.2 billion (American Geriatrics Society, 2012; Fu et al., 2007). Older adults account for 49.8% of hospital admissions due to adverse drug events (Budnitz et al., 2006). The rate is the greatest for ages 85+. Adverse events happen in all health care settings. This chapter discusses the basic principles of geriatric pharmacology and geriatric prescribing. Concepts such as polypharmacy, prescribing cascades, and deprescribing, as well as commonly utilized tools to improve patient outcomes and quality of life will be discussed.

Overview of Medication Use in the Older Adult

Epidemiology

Although older adults are living longer, the burden of multiple chronic conditions in this population, defined as having two or more, will increase (Barnett et al., 2012). Approximately 80% of older adults will have at least one chronic health condition, and more than 60% will have multiple chronic conditions (Ralph et al., 2013). Of those multiple chronic conditions, the most common chronic conditions in older adults are hypertension, hyperlipidemia, and diabetes (US Centers for Medicare & Medicaid Services, 2017). (See Table 8.1.)

The most common chronic conditions require medications for treatment, and older adults may accumulate numerous prescribing providers. Thus it is not surprising

CASE STUDY

A patient is newly diagnosed with dementia due to Alzheimer disease, and his neurologist starts him on a regimen of donepezil at 5 mg daily. He tolerates this dose well. A month later, he is asked to increase the dose to 10 mg daily. During the next appointment with his primary care provider, the patient reports he has been experiencing new-onset diarrhea and increased frequency of urination that has resulted in incontinence, plus watery eyes and rhinorrhea that he attributes to seasonal allergies. His pulse has also been lower than usual (50–55 beats per minute). To treat some of these symptoms, his wife has been giving him an over-the-counter (OTC) medication, 25 mg of diphenhydramine, several times per day for "allergies." With regard to his memory, he seems to be a little more confused than before.

Donepezil is a cholinesterase inhibitor that increases levels of acetylcholine. It is essentially a cholinergic drug. Therefore, common adverse reactions are cholinergic in nature: diarrhea, urinary frequency, watery eyes, runny nose, and low pulse. The new symptoms the patient is describing are consistent with the side effects of donepezil. Although the patient tolerated the lower dose of donepezil without issue, side effects emerged at the increased dose that are now requiring more medication.

A troubling outcome of this scenario is the patient's use of diphenhydramine, a medication that should not be used routinely in older adults given its anticholinergic profile and its potential for causing both confusion and cognitive decline. Although it may be treating some of the side effects of donepezil, its mechanism of action is also essentially counteracting that of donepezil. Although other dementia medications may be trialed instead of donepezil to avoid the side effects the patient is experiencing, it is also appropriate to reevaluate the dose of donepezil. The patient may be best served by the lower dose of donepezil, as he appeared to have tolerated it well.

that 40% of older adults take 5 to 9 medications, and 18% take 10 or more (Kaufman et al., 2002).

Medication use increases with age. According to the 2015–2016 National Health and Nutrition Examination Survey, only 18% of children under age 12 years used prescription drugs compared to 85% of adults ages 60 and over in the past 30 days (Martin et al., 2019). There were no significant differences between males and females in the older age group. However, there were differences in race: the highest prescription drug use was among non-Hispanic white persons and the lowest prescription drug use among non-Hispanic Asian and Hispanic persons.

In 2017, Medicare part D estimated as many as 1.5 billion prescription drug events, which account for as much as $100 billion in prescription expenditures for 40.5 million beneficiaries (US Centers for Medicare & Medicaid Services, 2019). The top five prescriptions dispensed were atorvastatin, gabapentin, lisinopril, hydrocodone-acetaminophen, and amlodipine—medications used to treat high cholesterol, hypertension, and pain. Due to the high usage and cost of medications required to treated chronic conditions in older adults, it is imperative to evaluate the appropriate use of medications.

TABLE 8.1 Medications That May Be Affected by Changes in Absorption With Age

Example	Possible Mechanism Affected	Possible Adverse Effect
Cefpodoxime[a]	↓ Gastric motility, intestinal surface area, and splanchnic blood flow	Subtherapeutic dose absorbed
Calcium carbonate[b]	↓ Active transport	↑ Risk for constipation
Enteric-coated formulations[c]	↓ Gastric acid production	↑ Risk for gastrointestinal adverse effects

Data from [a]Giarratano, A., Green, S. E., & Nicolau, D. P. (2018). Review of antimicrobial use and considerations in the elderly population. *Clinical Interventions in Aging, 13*, 657–667. https://doi.org/10.2147/cia.s133640; [b]Veldurthy, V., Wei, R., Oz, L., Dhawan, P., Jeon, Y. H., & Christakos, S. (2016). Vitamin D, calcium homeostasis and aging. *Bone Research, 4*(1). https://doi.org/10.1038/boneres.2016.41; [c]Ruscin, J. M., Linnebur, S. A., Porter, R. S., & Kaplan, J. L. (2018). Drug categories of concern in older adults. *Merck Manual*. https://www.merckmanuals.com/professional/geriatrics/drug-therapy-in-older-adults/drug-categories-of-concern-in-older-adults

Polypharmacy

Polypharmacy is the concomitant use of several drugs by a single person (Morin et al., 2018). It is the use of unnecessary medications regardless of the number of medications being taken. In other words, it is taking more medications than is clinically necessary. Given that more than half of older adults have at least two chronic conditions, polypharmacy is a common issue in the older population (Gujjarlamudi, 2016; Maher, Hanlon, & Hajjar, 2014; National Institute on Aging [NIA], 2017). Polypharmacy can lead to adverse drug reactions, drug-drug interactions, and nonadherence, which can increase the risk for hospitalization, morbidity, and mortality (Gujjarlamudi, 2016). For example, compare patient A and patient B, both 70-year-old female patients who take seven different medications for five different indications. (See Table 8.2.)

Based on the numeric polypharmacy definition, both patient A and patient B can be categorized with polypharmacy. However, take a closer look at the medications, the indication for use, and the medical necessity. When evaluating for medication appropriateness, the provider may find that patient B is taking an additional medication to tackle another medication's side effect (an over-the-counter medication that was recommended by the patient's friend because it helps with sleep), and that medications within the same class and used to treat the same chronic condition have been prescribed by two different doctors. Without interviewing the patients for medication adherence and side effects, it would appear in this scenario that patient B is taking several inappropriate medications, whereas all of patient A's medications appear to be medically necessary. The shift in defining polypharmacy using a descriptive approach enhances the medication review process to better assess for clinical appropriateness and safety of medications.

Clinical Application

A common guideline that can easily be applied to any clinical practice is that for any patient who is taking five or more medications daily (prescription, over-the-counter, or herbal medicines), the clinician should review the list carefully for necessity. The number "five" is a trigger for putting the patient at risk for polypharmacy.

Health care providers can minimize the consequences of polypharmacy by assessing the patient's medications at each visit, identifying prescription and OTC medication use that can be concerning for older adults, discussing with the patients as well as their family members and caregivers the risks and benefits of each medication, and eliminating any unnecessary medications from the list.

TABLE 8.2 Examples of Medications That Are Affected by Distribution Changes

Example	Possible Mechanism Affected	Possible Effect
Lithium[a]	↓ Total body water	↑ Risk for toxicity
Amiodarone[a]	↑ Total body fat	↑ Drug half-life
Phenytoin[a,b]	↓ Serum albumin	↑ Risk for toxicity
Macrolides[c]	↑ Serum α_1-glycoprotein	↓ Free concentration of drug

Data from [a]Turnheim, K. (2003). When drug therapy gets old: Pharmacokinetics and pharmacodynamics in the elderly. *Experimental Gerontology, 38*(8), 843–853. https://doi.org/10.1016/s0531-5565(03)00133-5; [b]Ruscin, J. M., Linnebur, S. A., Porter, R. S., & Kaplan, J. L. (2018). Drug categories of concern in older adults. *Merck Manual.* https://www.merckmanuals.com/professional/geriatrics/drug-therapy-in-older-adults/drug-categories-of-concern-in-older-adults; [c]Giarratano, A., Green, S. E., & Nicolau, D. P. (2018). Review of antimicrobial use and considerations in the elderly population. *Clinical Interventions in Aging, 13*, 657–667. https://doi.org/10.2147/cia.s133640

Prescribing Cascades

Any symptom in an elderly patient should be considered a drug side effect until proven otherwise.

Jerry Gurwitz, MD

A prescribing cascade is a phenomenon leading to *polypharmacy*, triggered by an initial drug-induced adverse event that mimics symptoms of disease, which are then treated with one or more additional medications (Fig. 8.1). If a cascade is unrecognized, the vicious chain reaction can self-propagate, with devastating consequences for the patient. Prescribing cascades occur either when patients initiate the cycle by self-medicating with over-the-counter (OTC) treatments without the knowledge and input of their health care provider or when a provider fails to carefully review a patient's medication list prior to initiating a new prescription. Most commonly, a patient will present with a new "symptom" that is in fact a medication side effect. This "symptom" is ascribed to a new medical problem and an additional medication is prescribed to treat it. The preferred approach would begin with a thorough review of the current medication list, allowing the provider to determine if the new symptom is in fact an adverse reaction to a new medication for this patient. If the provider determines that the symptom is actually a medication side effect, there are two potential options: continue the current medication and treat the side effect or stop

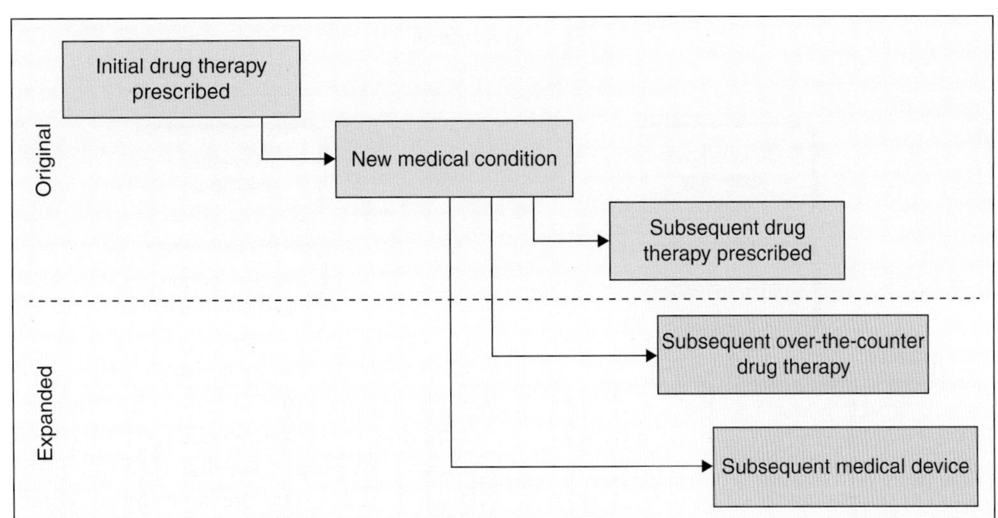

• **Fig. 8.1** Example of a prescribing cascade. (From Rochon, P. A., & Gurwitz, J. H. [2017]. The prescribing cascade revisited. *The Lancet, 389*, 1778–1780.)

the offending medication and try another with a different side effect profile? Ultimately, the provider is responsible for determining which option is safest for a given patient.

Clinical Application

Figs. 8.2 and 8.3 are examples of prescribing cascades one might see in clinical practice. An activating antidepressant can lead to a patient developing activating types of symptoms, such as anxiety or insomnia, which may result in more prescriptions for those new symptoms. A class of antihypertensives, called Ca channel blockers, may cause peripheral edema and gastroesophageal reflux disease (GERD) as side effects, which then may cause the provider to prescribe medications to treat those symptoms.

Any time a health care provider decides to prescribe a new medication, she or he should review potential side effects with the patient and go through a risk and benefit analysis for using this medication. If side effects emerge and require treatment, the provider should reassess the need to continue the medication that caused the side effect. Alternatives may be available that will prevent the need to add more medications to the list.

Medication Burden in the Older Adult

The consequences of polypharmacy and potentially inappropriate medications are numerous and significant. They include adverse drug events, drug interactions, medication nonadherence, worsening of a variety of geriatric syndromes, and greater health care costs (Maher et al., 2014). (See Box 8.1.)

Polypharmacy has been cited as a major risk factor for adverse drug events and drug interactions, including drug-drug, drug-disease, and drug-food interactions (Nguyen et al., 2006). These have the potential to cause

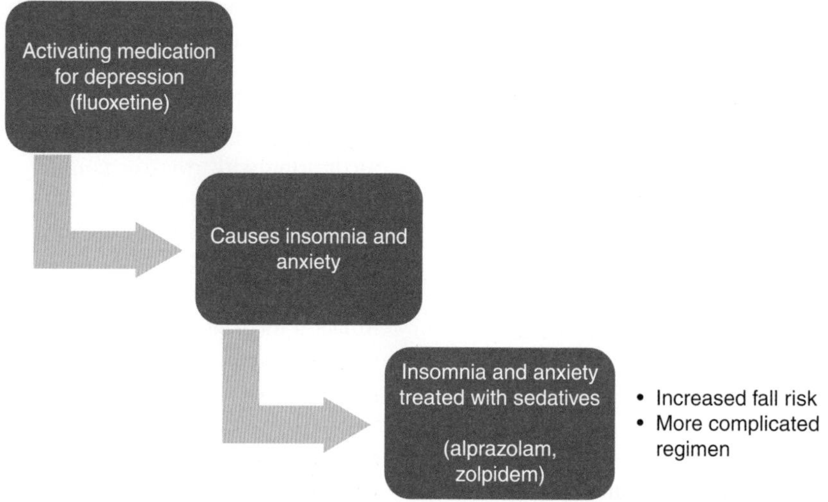

• **Fig. 8.2** Medication cascade with fluoxetine. (Developed by Tatyana Gurvich, PharmD, BCGP)

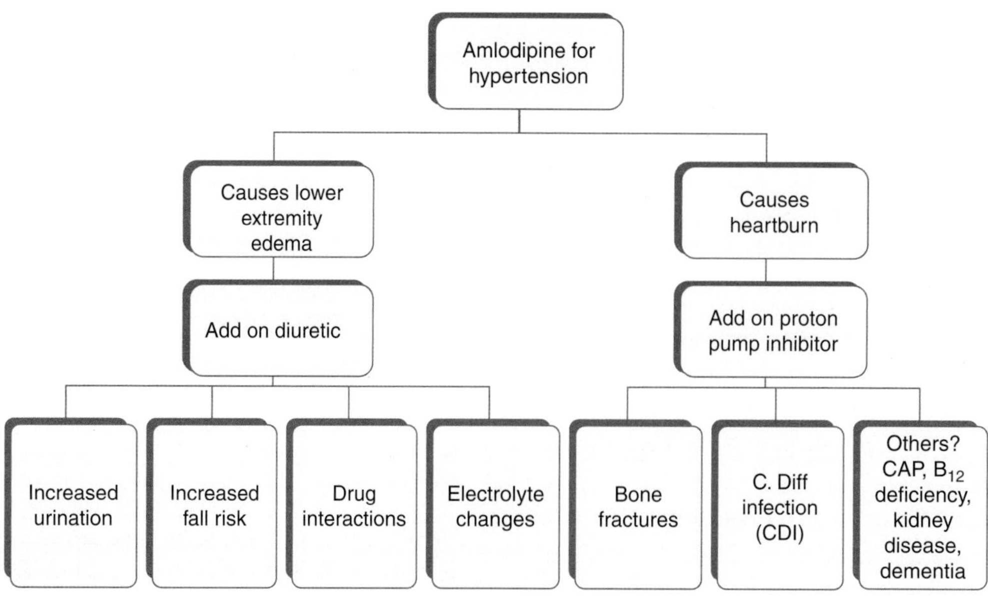

• **Fig. 8.3** Prescribing cascade with amlodipine. (Developed by Tatyana Gurvich, PharmD, BCGP)

• BOX 8.1 Risks of Polypharmacy

- Adverse drug events
- Medication cascades
- Worsening of existing medical problems and emergence of new diagnoses
- Increased risk of falls
- Increased risk for confusion and cognitive decline
- Increased risk of health care costs

• BOX 8.2 Drugs That Increase the Risk of Hospitalizations

- 50% drug related hospitalizations:
    - Antiplatelet drugs, NSAID, diuretics, anticoagulants
- 21% of preventable hospital admissions:
    - Beta-blockers, ACEIs ARBs, digoxin, opioids, insulin, and oral diabetic agents

medication-related hospitalizations and emergency room visits, especially in older adults. Medication nonadherence due to complex medication regimens may produce negative outcomes, including treatment failure and the progression of disease and disease-related complications.

Geriatric syndromes are worsened as a result of polypharmacy. It has been associated with a decline in function status, a decreased ability to perform instrumental activities of daily living (IADLs), and diminished physical functioning. Polypharmacy is also a risk factor for cognitive impairment, seen with delirium and dementia in older adults. Older adults in particular have a higher risk of falling and increased urinary incontinence. Certain medications may precipitate or exacerbate falls or urinary incontinence and should be reevaluated for appropriateness and safety in use. Additionally, an older adult's nutritional status may be negatively affected by polypharmacy, as evidenced by reports of higher malnutrition in those taking 10 or more medications. Overall, the negative health outcomes due to polypharmacy may augment health care costs to both patients and the health care system due to an increase in outpatient visits, hospitalizations, and prescription drug expenditures.

Older adults are especially vulnerable to adverse drug events and seven times more likely to require a hospitalization compared to younger adults (Budnitz et al., 2006). More than 99,000 emergency hospitalizations occur each year in the older adult population due to adverse drug events (Budnitz et al., 2011). The predominant drugs implicated in these hospitalizations are warfarin, insulin, oral antiplatelet agents, and oral hypoglycemic agents (Budnitz et al., 2011). (See Box 8.2.)

As the population ages, the incidence of emergency department visits due to adverse drug events increases. For adults 65 years or older, the number of emergency department visits rose nearly 9% in less than one decade: 25.6% in 2005–2006 to 34.5% in 2013–2014 (Shehab et al., 2016). The growing problem of using more medications than medically necessary poses serious negative health risks in the older adult population, as well as increased health care costs in the United States (Charlesworth et al., 2015). Safety measures need to be applied to require close attention on polypharmacy and potentially inappropriate medications.

Quality Measures for Medication Use

Quality measures are tools used to ensure safe, effective, patient-centered, and high-quality health care (US Centers for Medicare & Medicaid Services, 2019). The National Committee for Quality Assurance (NCQA) developed the Healthcare Effectiveness Data and Information Set (HEDIS), a widely used performance improvement tool for physicians and organizations. Medication management and care coordination measures pertinent to the older adult population include annual monitoring for patients on persistent medications, medication reconciliation post discharge, transitions of care, and follow-up after emergency department visits for people with multiple high-risk chronic conditions.

Persistent medications use is defined as an outpatient medication used at least 180 days per year. Annual monitoring for patients on select persistent medications may reduce the occurrence of preventable adverse drug events. Medication reconciliation post discharge requires a patient's medications to be reconciled within 30 days from an inpatient facility discharge, such as the hospital or emergency department. This is particularly important for patients who take multiple medications to ensure the safe and appropriate use of medications following discharge. Transitions of care include four reported rates after discharge from an inpatient facility. These are notification of inpatient admission, receipt of discharge information, patient engagement after inpatient discharge (such as a primary care appointment), and medication reconciliation postdischarge. For people with multiple high-risk chronic conditions, follow-up with one's primary care provider within 7 days of an emergency department visit is important in order to minimize emergency department readmission, hospitalization, and negative health outcomes.

Additionally, measures of overuse/appropriateness include medication management that focuses on identifying potentially harmful drug-disease interactions in older adults, as well as the use of high-risk medications in the older population. These quality measures aid in addressing negative health outcomes related to polypharmacy and potentially inappropriate medications, and they facilitate monitoring high-risk medications associated with increased hospitalization rates.

Age-Related Changes That Alter Drug Response in Older Adults

Pharmacokinetic Changes

Pharmacokinetics refers to the process by which drugs are disposed of in the body or, more simply, what the body does to the drug. The four basic pharmacokinetic parameters are *absorption*, *distribution*, *metabolism*, and *excretion*.

Each of these parameters is affected by age and thus may significantly alter clinical practice. Some changes are mainly theoretic and of limited clinical utility. Others are significantly more important and impact drug selection, dosing, and the everyday clinical decisions a health care provider might make when treating older patients.

Absorption

Of all the pharmacokinetic parameters, this is the one least affected by age. The absorption of a medication is altered by any changes in intestinal epithelial surface area, splanchnic blood flow, gastric motility, gastric acid production, or active transport. The overall surface area of the intestinal epithelium and splanchnic blood flow decreases with age, as do the rate of gastric emptying and intestinal motility, both of which delay the movement of drugs through the gastrointestinal tract. Gastric acid secretion also decreases, causing a subsequent increase in gastric pH.

So how do these changes collectively affect drug absorption in geriatric patients? Not only may it take longer for medications to get primarily absorbed across the gastrointestinal epithelium, but it also takes longer for the medication to pass through the gastrointestinal tract. Furthermore, drugs that require a more acidic environment for optimal absorption may not be absorbed as well given the higher pH. These processes are slow, naturally occurring changes that take place in all older adults, but some of these changes do not begin until age 80 (Klotz, 2009). What can safely be said about drug absorption in older adults is that although medications may be absorbed at slower rates and with a possibly delayed onset of the drug's effect, the final extent of absorption is largely unchanged. Table 8.1 lists examples of medications that may be affected by changes in absorption with age.

Clinical Application

An older patient decides to take a single dose of ibuprofen for a headache. For this acute, one-time event, the onset of pain relief may be slightly delayed relative to the onset in a younger patient due to slower absorption. If the same patient is chronically taking the same dose of ibuprofen for osteoarthritis pain multiple times per day, and thus has established a normal steady-state concentration, it is likely that the cumulative effect of ibuprofen will be identical for this older patient as compared to a younger counterpart.

Another issue to consider in older adults, in addition to age-related absorptive changes, is the effect of certain medications on the overall absorption of all medications. In this setting, the clinical implications of changes in absorption become much more substantial. For example, it is common for older adults to take one or more acid blockers, including a proton pump inhibitor, a histamine-2 receptor antagonist, or an antacid. Any of these medications alone or in combination can further alkalinize the already less acidic gastric environment, further impairing normal drug absorption. As an additional example, opioids or medications with anticholinergic activity may further slow down gastric emptying. When they are taken on a daily basis, the cumulative effect of reduced gastric emptying may further delay the onset of the effect of other medications being given concurrently.

Distribution

Drug distribution is defined as the movement of a drug to and from the blood and various tissues of the body (e.g., fat and muscle) and the organs of the body (e.g., brain, liver, kidney). There are two important parameters related to distribution to consider: volume of distribution (Vd) and protein binding. Volume of distribution is a theoretic calculation that is used to determine how easily a drug distributes in the body's tissues. To be precise, the Vd is the volume that would be needed to create an equivalent concentration of drug in the body tissues as in the blood plasma. For example, if the Vd for a drug is high, that drug easily distributes through the body tissues and is thus present at a high concentration relative to the concentration in the blood; as such, a large theoretic volume of "tissue" would be needed to make the concentrations in the tissue and blood equal. Protein binding determines the free fraction of a drug, which is the fraction that exerts a medication's pharmacologic effect. Protein binding is typically listed as a percentage. A drug that is >90% protein bound is considered to be a highly protein-bound drug. This means that 90% of the available drug is bound to protein, either albumin or alpha-1-acid glycoprotein, and only 10% of the drug is free to enter the body tissues and be pharmacologically active.

The volume of distribution is a pharmacokinetic parameter that is significantly altered by age and is associated with important clinical implications. Aging causes significant body composition and plasma protein level changes. As we age, total body fat increases and total body water decreases. This happens in both men and women and is not necessarily related to changes in total weight. Even when an older adult's weight remains constant throughout life, the relative percentage of fat and water still changes. According the National Health and Nutrition Examination Survey taken by the Centers for Disease Control and Prevention (CDC), the average percentage of body fat increases by 35% for men and by 21% for women, when comparing those ages 16 to 19 to those ages 60 to 79. The percentage of body water decreases by the same amount. These changes will affect the distribution of both fat-soluble (lipophilic) drugs and water-soluble (hydrophilic) drugs. The Vd for lipophilic drugs tends to increase with age because of the increase in body fat, resulting in an increased distribution of the drug into the body's fat tissue, along with an increase in the elimination half-life due to rediffusion of the drug from fatty tissue (Mahabadi, n.d.). This leads to an accumulation of the drug that, with continued use, can result in prolonged clinical activity and more adverse events (Mahabadi, n.d.). Conversely, hydrophilic drugs tend to have a smaller Vd in older patients and will have higher serum concentrations for any given dose. Change in Vd is one of the primary contributing factors that necessitates careful dosing of medications in older patients. Table 8.2 lists some examples of drugs that may be impacted by changes in distribution as described earlier.

Clinical Application

All benzodiazepines are highly lipophilic medications, and most have a prolonged effect in older adults. They tend to sit on the adipose tissues, and continued use will usually result in adverse effects such as oversedation, confusion, or falls. This is one of the reasons benzodiazepines appear in all references that discuss inappropriate prescribing in older adults.

Drug protein binding is also significantly affected by age. Medications that are highly protein bound are more affected, given the changes in protein levels that occur with aging. With age, plasma albumin levels decrease, resulting in an increased free fraction of some medications. This can lead to an exaggerated medication effect and even toxicity. Concentrations of alpha-1-acid glycoprotein are typically increased, leading to a decrease in the free fraction of some drugs, particularly alkaline medications, and a reduced effect.

Clinical Application

When reviewing a pharmacokinetic parameter of a new drug, the health care provider must always pay particular attention to the percentage of protein binding in drugs that also have a narrow therapeutic window. Warfarin is a common example usually used in this case. It is 97% protein bound. That means that only 3% constitutes the free fraction (i.e., the amount of drug that is exerting the anticoagulant effect). If albumin levels drop and the free fraction increases as a result, the patient could be prescribed a dose that is too high and might lead to a dangerous bleeding event.

Metabolism

When we talk about drug metabolism, we must look at the Cytochrome P 450 pathways and what effect age has on this set of enzymes. Box 8.3 lists the specific CYP pathways that may be impacted by age alone. We also must look at patient-specific parameters that can impact drug metabolism, such as preexisting liver disease, the individual patient's lifestyle choices, and genetic predisposition, which determines the level of activity of some of the individual CYP450 enzymes. Table 8.3 lists selected lifestyle and health issue and their impact on metabolism of drugs. Hepatic metabolism of medications can decrease with advancing age due to reductions in liver mass, cytochrome P_{450} (CYP) enzyme activity, hepatic blood flow, and first-pass metabolism. Alterations in all of these factors can increase the risk of adverse effects (Kinirons & O'Mahony, 2004; Mangoni & Jackson, 2004; Rivera & Antognini, 2009; Turnheim, 2003). First-pass metabolism is defined as the process that breaks down some of the orally administered medications before they reach systemic circulation. It has been shown to decline by approximately 1% per year beginning at age 40 (Ruscin et al., 2018a). Additionally, some medications that are metabolized by the liver may have a 30% to 40% reduction in metabolic clearance (Ruscin et al., 2018a; Turnheim, 2003). Table 8.4 lists selected medications and various metabolic mechanisms that may impact the therapeutic effects of those drugs.

• BOX 8.3 Aging and the Effect on the Cytochrome P450 Enzymes

Decreased	Decreased or Unchanged	Unchanged
CYP 1A2 CYP 2C19	CYP 2A CYP 2C9 CYP 3A4	CYP 2D6

From Cusack, B. J. (2004). Pharmacokinetics in older persons. *American Journal of Geriatric Pharmacotherapy, 2*(4):274–302.

TABLE 8.3 Factors That Impact Liver Metabolism in Older Adults

Factor	Result
Smoking	Induction
Alcohol chronic use Binge drinking	Induction Inhibition
Drugs	Induction/inhibition
Diet	Variable
Malnutrition	Inhibition, if severe
Frailty	Inhibition

Data from O'Mahoney, M. S, & Woodhouse, K. W. (1994). Age, environmental factors and drug metabolism. *Pharmacology & Therapeutics, 61*(1–2), 279–287.

Clinical Application

Whenever possible, it is important for the health care professional to choose medications that are less affected by the CYP 450 metabolism. Within pharmacologic classes of medications, there may be those that are affected less. Medications like citalopram, escitalopram, pravastatin, and rosuvastatin are less dependent on the P450 pathway compared to other medications in their respective classes.

Excretion

Excretion is the most affected pharmacokinetic parameter in older adults. Most geriatric patients will develop some degree of renal insufficiency as they get older. When assessing renal function in any patient, clinicians usually look at the serum creatinine and the glomerular filtration rate (GFR). Creatinine is a by-product of muscle breakdown. Older adults have less muscle mass, and therefore just looking at the serum creatinine alone is not enough and can be misleading because it can overestimate renal function. Urinary excretion of medications declines with advancing age due to decreased glomerular filtration and tubular secretory function (Lau & Abernethy, 2012; Turnheim, 2003).

TABLE 8.4 Examples of Medications That Are Impacted by Changes in Metabolism and Old Age

Example	Possible Mechanism Affected	Possible Effect
Fluoroquinolones[a]	↓ CYP enzyme activity	↑ Drug half-life
Propranolol[b]	↓ First-pass metabolism	↑ Risk for cardiovascular adverse effects
Morphine[c]	↓ Hepatic blood flow	↑ Risk for central nervous system (CNS) depression adverse effects

Data from [a]Giarratano, A., Green, S. E., & Nicolau, D. P. (2018). Review of antimicrobial use and considerations in the elderly population. *Clinical Interventions in Aging, 13,* 657–667. https://doi.org/10.2147/cia.s133640; [b]Mangoni, A. A., & Jackson, S. H. (2004). Age-related changes in pharmacokinetics and pharmacodynamics: Basic principles and practical applications. *British Journal of Clinical Pharmacology, 57*(1), 6–14. doi.org/10.1046/j.1365-2125.2003.02007; [c]Johnny Lau, S. W., & Abernethy, D. R. (2012). Chapter 26: Drug therapy in the elderly. In A. J. Atkinson, S. M. Huang, J. J. Lertora, & S. P. Markey (Eds.), *Principles of Clinical Pharmacology* (3rd ed., pp. 437–453). Academic Press. https://www.sciencedirect.com/science/article/pii/B978012385471100026X

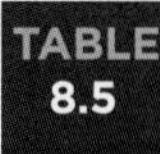

TABLE 8.5 Examples of Medications That Are Affected by Changes in Renal Excretion

Example	Possible Mechanism Affected	Possible Effect
Digoxin[a]	↓ Glomerular filtration	↑ Risk for toxicity
Cimetidine[b]	↓ Tubular secretory function	↑ Risk for central nervous system (CNS) adverse effects

Data from [a]Johnny Lau, S. W., & Abernethy, D. R. (2012). Chapter 26: Drug therapy in the elderly. In A. J. Atkinson, S. M. Huang, J. J. Lertora, & S. P. Markey (Eds.), *Principles of clinical pharmacology* (3rd ed., pp. 437–453). Academic Press; Turnheim, K. (2003). When drug therapy gets old: Pharmacokinetics and pharmacodynamics in the elderly. *Experimental Gerontology, 38*(8), 843–853. https://doi.org/10.1016/s0531-5565(03)00133-5; The 2019 American Geriatrics Society Beers Criteria® Update Expert Panel. (2019). American Geriatrics Society 2019 Updated AGS Beers Criteria® for potentially inappropriate medication use in older adults. *Journal of the American Geriatrics Society, 67*(4), 674–694. https://doi.org/10.1111/jgs.15767; Johnny Lau, S. W., & Abernethy, D. R. (2012). Chapter 26: Drug therapy in the elderly. In A. J. Atkinson, S. M. Huang, J. J. Lertora, & S. P. Markey (Eds.), *Principles of Clinical Pharmacology* (3rd ed., pp. 437–453). Academic Press. https://www.sciencedirect.com/science/article/pii/B978012385471100026X

Even though serum creatinine levels may stay within normal limits in many older adults, creatinine clearance is reduced on average by 8 mL/min/1.73 m^2 per decade after age 40, and the glomerular filtration rate is reduced by 25% to 50% in people ages 20 to 90 (Ruscin et al., 2018b; Turnheim, 2003). Table 8.5 provides examples of medications that are affected by changes in excretion.

Most labs now provide eGFR as a standard measure for all patients getting a chemistry panel. Levels 60 and above are considered normal. Creatinine clearance can also be calculated and provides an accurate estimate of the patient's renal function. Most drug information resources refer to creatinine clearance when they discuss dosing adjustments for renally cleared drugs in patients with renal insufficiency. The Cockroft and Gault equation is the most common calculation used to estimate renal function in older patients because it incorporates age as one its parameters:

$$\text{Clcr} = (140 \times \text{Age})\ \text{wt(kg)Scr} \times 72$$

For women the number is further multiplied by 85%. Table 8.6 provides some clinical benchmarks of how to evaluate reduced clearance in older patients.

Which value to use for weight becomes an issue for older patients. Using total body weight, especially in overweight patients, can cause one to overestimate renal function, because the bulk of that extra weight comes from fat not muscle mass in an older adult. The only time when it may be appropriate to use total body weight may be in a frail geriatric patient who is underweight. In an overweight patient, an adjusted body weight provides a more clinically relevant number. To get the most conservative value for renal function, ideal body weight (IBW) should be used in this calculation. Box 8.4 show the formulas that are used to determine ideal or adjusted body weight.

Clinical Application

Because most older patients will have some degree of renal insufficiency, it is helpful to review the medication list in order to screen for drugs that are renally cleared. The provider should choose those that do not have to be renally adjusted. If an anticoagulant is necessary and renal function prohibits the use of newer anticoagulants, coumadin may be an option. Insulin is usually reserved for patients who cannot handle renally cleared oral medications. Linagliptin is one DPP4 inhibitor that does not have to be renally adjusted. Amlodipine can be used safely in renally impaired patients. Table 8.7 lists commonly used medications that are renally cleared. These medications may not be safe to use in patients with renal insufficiency or may require dosage adjustments to accommodate declining renal function.

Pharmacodynamic Changes

Pharmacodynamics can explain the actions of a drug on the body through biochemical, physiologic, and molecular mechanisms (Farinde et al., 2019). In other words, pharmacodynamics describes what a drug does to the body (Farinde

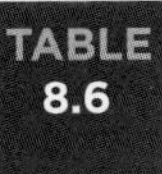

TABLE 8.6 How to Clinically Evaluate a Creatinine Clearance Calculation

Cl_{cr}	Action
50 ml/min or greater	Renal function is good. No dosage adjustment necessary.
30–50 ml/min	Some renal impairment: Dose adjustment may be necessary. Clinical judgment comes into play.
Less than 30 ml/min	Significant renal impairment. Some mediations should not be used. Others may be used at a significantly reduced dose.

TABLE 8.7 Selected Medications That Require Dosing Adjustments or Should Not Be Used With Reduced Kidney Function

Drug Names/Drug Class	Drug Names/Class
Beta-blockers: Acebutolol, atenolol, bisoprolol, nadolol, sotalol	Gout medications: Allopurinol colchicine
Metformin	Bisphosphonates
H2 blockers: Famotidine	Nonsteroidal antiinflammatory drugs (NSAIDs)
Antibiotics: Fluroquinolones, Bactrim, nitrofurantoin	New anticoagulants
ACE: Lisinopril, Enalapril	DPP4 inhibitors: Alogliptin, saxagliptin, sitagliptin
Thiazides and K sparing diuretics	SGLT2 inhibitors
Valacyclovir, acyclovir	Lithium
Narcotics: Codeine, morphine, tramadol, oxycodone	Duloxetine, paroxetine
Gabapentin, pregabalin, topiramate	Memantine

• BOX 8.4 Ideal and Adjusted Body Weight Equations

Estimate Ideal Body Weight in Kilograms[a]

Males: IBW = 50 kg + 2.3 kg for each inch over 5 feet
Females: IBW = 45.5 kg + 2.3 kg for each inch over 5 feet

Adjusted Body Weight[b, c]

AjBW = IBW + 0.4(ABW − IBW)

AjBW, Adjusted body weight; *IBW*, ideal body weight.

Data from [a]Devine, B. J. (1974). Gentamicin therapy. *Drug Intelligence & Clinical Pharmacy, 8*, 650–655; [b]Bauer, L. A. (2001). *Applied clinical pharmacokinetics* (pp. 93–179). McGraw Hill; [c]Winter, M. E. (2004). *Basic pharmacokinetics*. Lippincott Williams and Williams.

et al., 2019; Le et al., 2019). In addition to pharmacokinetic changes, older adults may experience age-related changes in pharmacodynamics due to altered receptor properties and homeostatic mechanisms (Farinde et al., 2019; Turnheim, 2003). Some receptors may be downregulated in older adults, decreasing the therapeutic effect of the medication. Conversely, reductions in homeostatic mechanisms and counterregulatory measures may lengthen the time needed to return to the original steady-state, which may in turn increase the risk for adverse effects (Turnheim, 2003).

Clinical Application

Older patients are simply more sensitive to the therapeutic and side effects of medications. Adverse reactions are more common and more severe in this patient population. Sometimes clinicians see rare side effects in older adults that they just do not see in younger patients. Older patients will sometimes have medication side effects that occur in only 1% to 2% in the general population. Timolol eye drops, which are considered to be topical agents, have been known to produce bradycardia or depression in older patients. Beta agonist inhalers will cause tachycardia anxiety and agitation in frail older patients. Pseudoephedrine is more likely to cause hypertension and activation in this patient population. Table 8.8 lists medications that may produce an altered response in older adults due to age-related pharmacodynamic changes.

Prescribing Challenges in Older Adults

An older adult's medication list should be critically reviewed frequently and with extra care. Any changes that have been made as a result of either prescribing or deprescribing must be done in a rational manner, utilizing a risk-benefit analysis. Equally careful attention must be paid to OTC medications, herbal supplements, and vitamins. Simply taking a medication history is not enough. A provider must spend time evaluating the appropriateness of each medication and its respective dose, while looking for potential drug cascades and drug-disease and drug-drug interactions. Duplicative medications must be discontinued. Issues related to medication adherence and medication administration must be discussed thoroughly to ensure patient safety. If this evaluation is not completed during each visit, medication lists will typically grow, with polypharmacy as the likely outcome.

Dosing of Medications in an Older Adult

There are no official dosing parameters for older patients. Package inserts for drugs published by pharmaceutical companies only provide dosing guidelines and titrations for average adults. Dosing adjustment guidelines are provided for patients with renal or hepatic insufficiency, but

TABLE 8.8 **List of Medications That May Be Affected by Changes in Pharmacodynamics**

Example	Possible Mechanism Affected	Possible Effect
Beta-blockers[a]	↓ β-adrenoreceptors	↓ Antihypertensive effect
Sulfonylureas[a]	↓ Glucose counter-regulation	↑ Risk of hypoglycemia
Drugs with anticholinergic profile[b]	↓ Acetylcholine	↑ Likelihood/severity of anticholinergic side effects including central anticholinergic effects: Confusion
Anti-psychotics[c]	↓ Decline in dopamine levels	↑ Sensitivity to EPS side effects and tardive dyskinesia
Blood-brain barrier[d]	↑ Permeability	More likely to have CNS adverse effects

Data from [a]Turnheim, K. (2003). When drug therapy gets old: Pharmacokinetics and pharmacodynamics in the elderly. *Experimental Gerontology, 38(8)*, 843–853. https://doi.org/10.1016/s0531-5565(03)00133-5; [b]Feinberg 1993; [c]Berry 2016; [d]Daneman 2015.

no information is officially provided for how to dose medications in older adults who do not have renal or hepatic disease.

Clinical Application

Start low, go slow, but do go!
A common dosing mantra in geriatric pharmacology

When treating geriatric patients, the starting dose of most drugs should be lower than for average patients. Sometimes this means starting at a dose 50% lower than the standard recommended dose. The titration schedule for most drugs is also slower, sometimes at half the speed normally used with average patients. Despite "starting low" and "going slow," a maximum dose may still be necessary for some patients to achieve a full therapeutic response. In other words, a slow, deliberate titration schedule should not dissuade a provider from increasing a dose as needed to achieve the desired therapeutic effect. This strategy should be utilized with most chronic medications, including those for hypertension, diabetes mellitus, and hyperlipidemia, as well as for psychoactive medications. Older adults are more sensitive to each drug's therapeutic and adverse effects, so a lower starting dose and a slower titration schedule ensures that a patient will better tolerate a new medication and increases the chance of treatment success. When dosing medications for an acute problem, such as infection, careful attention must be paid to recent renal and hepatic function, with dosing determined only after evaluating these parameters.

Deprescribing is a common practice in geriatric medicine, defined as stopping a medication that is either inappropriate or no longer necessary. It also includes reducing the dose of a medication that is causing a side effect or contributing to a drug-drug interaction. A provider may deprescribe to correct polypharmacy or to avoid an unintended medication cascade. The whole process of deprescribing is somewhat counterintuitive for providers because they are primarily trained to diagnose and treat new medical problems. Reducing treatment, when appropriate, is something that should be considered constantly in geriatrics in order to reduce the risk of polypharmacy and inappropriate prescribing. Deprescribing is always done with the prescriber's guidance and in agreement with the patient. Patient self-deprescribing is never recommended and can be a dangerous practice, depending on the drugs involved.

Five steps for deprescribing have been identified:

- Identify potentially inappropriate medications.
- Determine if a medication can be stopped or a dosage can be reduced
- Develop a tapering plan.
- Monitor the patient carefully for adverse events.
- Document outcomes.

What are priorities for deprescribing in older patients (Farrell et al., 2015)? Box 8.5 provides a list of drugs that are considered the most likely to be deprescribed:

When looking at published literature on deprescribing, it becomes apparent that prescribers often require evidence-based guidance on how to do it. *A risk-versus-benefit analysis for using each drug must be done. When medications are stopped, patients must be carefully monitored to ensure a positive outcome.*

• BOX 8.5 Drugs Most Likely to Be Deprescribed

- Benzodiazepines
- Atypical antipsychotics
- Statins
- Tricyclic antidepressants
- Proton pump inhibitors
- Urinary anticholinergics
- Typical antipsychotics
- Cholinesterase inhibitors
- Opioids
- Selective serotonin-reuptake inhibitors (SSRIs)
- Bisphosphonates
- Anticonvulsants
- Beta-blockers
- Antiplatelets

Beers Criteria

Although certain medications can be safely or reasonably used in younger adults, they may pose additional risks when used in older adults (Ruscin et al., 2018b). In 1991, Dr. Mark Beers developed criteria to identify the types of medications that are not appropriate for use in older adults residing in nursing homes (Beers et al., 1991; Marcum & Hanlon, 2012). Although the Beers list was initially developed primarily to address medication mismanagement in long-term care settings, it is now applied in all areas of health care: ambulatory care settings, hospitals, transitional care units, and long-term care facilities. The American Geriatrics Society has been updating the Beers Criteria every couple of years since 2011, with the most recent version appearing in 2019 (AGS, 2019). The selected medications from the Beers criteria table are an abbreviated list of commonly used medications that should be avoided in older adults. However, it is important to note that the Beers Criteria should be referred to as a guideline for treatment decision making, as some of the listed medications may still be used in clinically appropriate situations. Table 8.9 lists selected medications discussed in the Beers Criteria.

HEALTHY PEOPLE 2030 BOX 8.1

- Reduce the rate of hospital admissions for diabetes among older adults
- Reduce the number of high-risk medication uses in older adults
- Reduce the risk of polypharmacy in older adults
- Use safe methods of de-prescribing when appropriate in older adults

A Practical Approach to Prescribing Medications to Older Patients

Clinical Application

The following issues must be considered each time providers review the medication list:

- Each medication on the list must have a current indication that is appropriate given the patient's age, disease progression, and outcome measures.
- The safest drug in its therapeutic class must be selected to minimize risks of more adverse events, side effects, and drug-drug interactions, reducing the possibility of prescribing cascades.
- Dosing considerations and a reasonable administration schedule are critical in order to maintain good therapeutic outcomes and compliance.
- Careful monitoring for therapeutic and adverse effects is crucial after drugs are started or stopped.
- Monitoring for medication compliance should be ongoing as long as medications are being prescribed. Reasons for nonadherence must be addressed with patients and caregivers.
- Patient and caregiver education about each drug is critical. A clear understanding of what to expect from each medication and when to seek additional help is necessary for good therapeutic outcomes.
- The cost of medications may be prohibitive for some patients. An annual review of a patient's medication drug plan during Medicare open enrollment can help to address this issue.

Approach to Newly Approved Drugs

On average, the Food and Drug Administration (FDA) approves 25 to 50 new drugs each year. When a new drug is FDA approved and becomes available to the public, relatively little information is available to determine whether it will be safe or well tolerated in older patients. The older patient population is poorly represented in clinical trials, with up to 35% of published trials excluding older people. There are many reasons why older adults are underrepresented in clinical studies (Box 8.6), but there are also benefits to be gained by including older adults in drug trials (Table 8.10). When older patients are used in premarketing trials, they are divided into two age groups: 65 to 75 and over 75. On average 10% to 20% of patients in clinical trials will be 65 years old and over, whereas only 10% of that population will be over the age of 75. If a new drug is tested in 4000 patients, that means 400 to 800 patients may be over the age of 65 and 40 to 80 patients will be over the age of 75. Because most pharmacokinetic and dynamic changes happen after age 75, it is impossible to predict efficacy and safety in the very old when new drugs are released on the market. Standard package inserts may include the following statement in the geriatric section: "No overall differences in safety or effectiveness were observed between geriatric and younger subjects, and other reported clinical experience has not identified differences in responses between the older and younger patients, but greater sensitivity of some older adults cannot be ruled out." Although the FDA encourages pharmaceutical companies to include older patients in trials to measure safety and efficacy, while also allowing for comparisons with counterparts who are not older adults, the inclusion of older adults in studies adds a layer of complexity that may ultimately affect outcomes. Multiple comorbid conditions and long medication lists can contribute to drug-disease and drug-drug interactions not seen in younger patients. Older adults may also have issues with mobility or cognition, which may make it more difficult for them to follow complicated study instructions or follow protocols. They may also need more supportive care, which may limit their participation in clinical trials.

Clinical Application

As a general rule, do not use medications newly added to the market, if it can be avoided, as they are poorly studied in older adults. Drug-drug interaction information is typically limited to single-dose studies, and the full impact of drug-drug interaction potential is unknown. Drug side effects are typically more pronounced and more common in older adults. When

TABLE 8.9 Selected Medications From the Beers Criteria

Medication Category With Examples	Recommendation	Rationale
First-generation antihistamines[a,b] Brompheniramine Chlorpheniramine Dimenhydrinate Diphenhydramine Doxylamine Hydroxyzine Meclizine Promethazine	Avoid	↑ Risk for confusion, falls, and anticholinergic effects (e.g., dry mouth, constipation)
Peripheral α1 blockers[a,c] Doxazosin Prazosin Terazosin	Avoid use for treatment of hypertension	↑ Risk for orthostatic hypotension and related issues (e.g., falls)
Antidepressants[a,d,e] Amitriptyline Doxepin >6 mg/day Nortriptyline Paroxetine	Avoid	↑ Risk for orthostatic hypotension, falls, and anticholinergic effects (e.g., dry mouth, constipation)
Antipsychotics (APs)[a] First-generation APs Second-generation APs	Avoid, except when clinically indicated (e.g., schizophrenia, bipolar disorder)	↑ Risk of mortality in older adults with dementia
Benzodiazepines[a] Alprazolam Clonazepam Lorazepam Temazepam	Avoid	↑ Risk for falls, delirium, and motor vehicle accidents
Nonbenzodiazepine hypnotics[a] Eszopiclone Zaleplon Zolpidem	Avoid	↑ Risk for falls, delirium, and motor vehicle accidents
Sulfonylureas[a] Glimepiride Glyburide	Avoid	↑ Risk for hypoglycemia
Proton-pump inhibitors (PPIs)[a,f] Esomeprazole Lansoprazole Omeprazole Pantoprazole	Avoid routine use for >8 weeks, except when clinically indicated (e.g., oral corticosteroid use, erosive esophagitis)	↑ Risk for clostridium difficile infection, osteoporosis, and fractures
Nonselective nonsteroidal antiinflammatory drugs (NSAIDs)[a] Aspirin >325 mg/day Diclofenac Ibuprofen Meloxicam Naproxen	Avoid chronic use, except when alternative treatments are ineffective and used with gastroprotective agent	↑ Risk for gastrointestinal bleeding, peptic ulcer disease, elevated blood pressure, and kidney injury

Data from [a]American Geriatrics Society Beers Criteria® Update Expert Panel. (2019). American Geriatrics Society 2019. Updated AGS Beers Criteria® for potentially inappropriate medication use in older adults. *Journal of the American Geriatrics Society, 67*(4), 674–694. https://doi.org/10.1111/jgs.15767; [b]Cho, H., Myung, J., Suh, H., & Kang, H. Y. (2018). Antihistamine use and the risk of injurious falls or fracture in elderly patients: A systematic review and meta-analysis. *Osteoporosis International, 29*(10), 2163–2170. https://doi.org/10.1007/s00198-018-4564-z; [c]Mol, A., Bui Hoang, P. T. S., Sharman, S., Reijinierse, E. M., Van Wezel, R. J. A., Meskers, C. G. M., & Maier, A. B. (2019). Orthostatic hypotension and falls in older adults: A systematic review and meta-analysis. *Journal of the American Medical Directors Association, 20*(5), 589–597. https://doi.org/10.1016/j.jamda.2018.11.003; [d]Hegeman, J., van den Bemt, B., Weerdesteyn, V., Nienhuis, B., van Limbeek, J., & Duysens, J. (2011). Unraveling the association between SSRI use and falls: an experimental study of risk factors for accidental falls in long-term paroxetine users. *Clinical Neuropharmacology, 34*(6), 210–215. https://doi.org/10.1097/WNF.0b013e31823337d1;
[e]Marcum, Z. A., Perera, S., Thorpe, J. M., Switzer, G. E., Castle, N. G., Strotmeyer, E. S., et al. (2016). Antidepressant use and recurrent falls in community-dwelling older adults: Findings from the Health ABC Study. *Annals of Pharmacotherapy, 50*(7), 525–533. https://doi.org/10.1177/1060028016644466;
[f]Ito, T., & Jensen, R. T. (2010). Association of long-term proton pump inhibitor therapy with bone fractures and effects on absorption of calcium, vitamin B_{12}, iron, and magnesium. *Current Gastroenterology Reports, 12*(6), 448–457. https://doi.org/10.1007/s11894-010-0141-0

• BOX 8.6 Reasons for the Underrepresentation of Older Adult Patients in Clinical Studies

- Challenges in gaining informed consent
- Multiple comorbid conditions may pose challenges in outcomes assessment
- Polypharmacy may lead to drug-drug interactions
- Challenges in complying with clinical study procedures
- May necessitate age-relevant formulations and packing
- Fear or failure due to confounding behavior of the drug in older adults
- Sponsors may incur higher cost for medical management and compensation
- Institutional and logistic problems
- May need supportive care
- Investigator's preferences and perceived difficulties in screening
- Protocol restrictions with exclusion criteria on age

TABLE 8.10 Benefits of Older Adult Patients' Participation in Clinical Studies

Problem Statement	Benefits of Participation
Underrepresentation in clinical trials	Researchers can learn more about the new drugs, therapies, medical devices, surgical procedures, or tests
Special health needs in elderly	Special health needs that are different from those of younger population could be established during clinical development
Different dosage requirements	Different dosages of a drug to have the right results and appropriate in elderly could be established
Inadequate evidence and knowledge about responses	Adverse drug reactions specific to older adults could be established
Majority users of many medicines	Risk associated with exposure to large population could be predicted
Generalizability of clinical trial findings	Would form representative population, particularly if the study drug will be used in elderly patients
Discrimination	Demonstrated fairness and equity in research participation

From Premnath Shenoy, P., & Harugeri, A. (2015). Elderly patients' participation in clinical trials. *Perspectives in Clinical Research, 6*(4), 184–189. https://www.ncbi.nlm.nih.gov/pmc/articles/PMC4640010/

reviewing lists of adverse reactions of a new drug, the provider must pay attention to all of them, including the side effects that occur in less than 2% of average adult patients, as they may occur more commonly in older patients.

If possible, it is important to wait 1 to 2 years before prescribing new medications in older patients. Postmarketing surveillance occurs after the drug is released in order to track adverse reactions and drug-drug interactions not seen in premarketing trials. This can add valuable clinical information that may help the provider when deciding whether to use this medication in older patients.

In most clinical situations, it may be safer to start with an older, established drug. The side effect profile and drug-drug and drug-disease interaction potential will have already been well established. As such, the response of an older patient to this medication will be much more predictable and easier to manage.

Areas That Call for Special Attention

Over-the-Counter (OTC) Medications

In the United States, adults who are at least 65 years of age account for 30% of the use of nonprescription medications, even though they constitute only 13% of the population (Centers for Disease Control and Prevention [CDC], 2004). Although OTC medications are convenient and easily accessible, they can increase the risk of drug-drug interactions and adverse drug reactions (CDC, 2019; World Health Organization [WHO], 2005). OTC medications can be confusing for both patients and health care providers, especially those that come in different formulations and with different active added ingredients. Therefore, it is important for providers to be familiar with the properties of each medication and all active ingredients, and it is essential to assess each patient's use of OTC medications.

Each year, 30 million older adults experience at least one fall, with 20% of the falls causing serious injury (CDC, 2019). Some OTC medications contain active ingredients that may increase the risk for confusion and falls, such as those with strong anticholinergic properties (AGS, 2019). First-generation antihistamines (e.g., brompheniramine, diphenhydramine, meclizine) are widely available and can be used for a variety of indications, including allergic rhinitis, insomnia, motion sickness, and nausea. OTC medications with anticholinergic properties can increase the risk for falls and can cause central (e.g., confusion, memory impairment, paradoxical excitation) and peripheral adverse effects (e.g., dry mouth, constipation, urinary retention), especially if taken in combination with other medications that have anticholinergic properties (Lieberman, 2004; Scolaro, 2017). Central nervous system (CNS) depressants (e.g.,

HEALTHY PEOPLE 2030 BOX 8.2

- Reduce fall-related deaths among older adults
- Reduce the proportion of older adults who use inappropriate medications
- Reduce the rate of emergency department visits due to falls among older adults
- Reduce the proportion of preventable hospitalizations in older adults with dementia

alcohol, sedatives, opioids) can also increase the risk for falls and central adverse effects (Welch, 2017). Safer alternatives include less-sedating medications (e.g., second-generation antihistamines, intranasal medications) and nonpharmacologic methods (e.g., lifestyle modification, sleep hygiene) (Melton & Kirkwood, 2017; Scolaro, 2017; Welch, 2017).

Studies have shown that the risk of gastrointestinal bleeding may be quadrupled in older adults who use nonsteroidal antiinflammatory drugs (NSAIDs) (Wongrakpanich et al., 2018). NSAIDs work by inhibiting cyclooxygenase enzyme (COX-1 and COX-2) activity, which in turn inhibits prostaglandin and thromboxane synthesis. Although COX-2 inhibition is largely responsible for the desired effects of NSAIDs, COX-1 inhibition contributes to many of the adverse effects of NSAIDs, including decreased renal perfusion, increased blood pressure, and weakening of the protective gastrointestinal mucosal barrier (Wongrakpanich et al., 2018). The risk of gastrointestinal bleeding increases further in patients with a history of peptic ulcer disease or bleeding dyscrasias. Bleeding is also increased when NSAIDs are used in combination with other prescription medications or supplements that can potentiate bleeding (e.g., anticoagulants, antiplatelets, corticosteroids, other NSAIDs) (Wilkinson & Tromp, 2017; Wongrakpanich et al., 2018).

Despite these concerns, oral OTC NSAIDs (e.g., aspirin, ibuprofen, naproxen) are commonly used for treating headache and musculoskeletal pain (National Institute on Aging [NIA], 2019; Wilkinson & Tromp, 2017). Safer alternatives include non-NSAID oral analgesics (e.g., acetaminophen), topical analgesics (e.g., counterirritants, salicylates, anesthetics), and pharmacologic methods (e.g., physical therapy) (Olenak, 2017). If chronic oral NSAID therapy is needed, gastrointestinal protective agents (e.g., proton pump inhibitors, histamine-2 receptor antagonists) should be considered (Olenak, 2017; Wongrakpanich et al., 2018). Although acetaminophen use in in an older adult should not exceed 3 grams per day, a lower daily limit may be needed for older patients at an increased risk of acetaminophen-associated liver toxicity, such as those with liver disease, concomitant hepatotoxic medication use, poor nutrition, or those who consume at least three alcoholic drinks daily (Wilkinson & Tromp, 2017). Counterirritants are topical agents that stimulate sensory nerves with a less severe pain to distract from the more intense underlying pain, whereas anesthetic agents inhibit nerve impulse conduction (Olenak, 2017). To prevent medication-overuse headaches, OTC analgesic use should not exceed 3 days per week for treatment of chronic headaches (Wilkinson & Tromp, 2017).

Although proton pump inhibitors (PPIs) can be helpful for symptoms of acid reflux and to prevent gastrointestinal bleeding from chronic NSAID use, long-term use of PPIs has been associated with an increased risk for community-acquired pneumonia, *Clostridium difficile* infection, bone fractures, and vitamin B_{12} deficiency (Olenak, 2017; Whetsel & Zweber, 2017; Wongrakpanich et al., 2018). According to the 2019 Beers Criteria, PPIs should not be used for more than 8 weeks, except in high-risk patients (Lieberman, 2004). Safer alternatives for symptoms of heartburn include antacids (e.g., calcium carbonate), histamine-2 receptor antagonists (H2RAs; e.g., famotidine, ranitidine), and nonpharmacologic methods (e.g., avoiding trigger foods, eating smaller meals) (Whetsel & Zweber, 2017). Antacids containing calcium and aluminum are associated with constipation, whereas those containing magnesium are associated with diarrhea. Magnesium- and aluminum-containing antacids should be used with caution in patients with impaired renal function, and sodium-containing antacids should be avoided in patients with cardiovascular conditions (Whetsel & Zweber, 2017). Antacids can be taken at symptom onset and can provide relief within 5 minutes but have a limited duration of 20 to 30 minutes and may impair the absorption of certain medications when taken concomitantly (e.g., antibiotics, levothyroxine) (Maton & Burton, 1999; Whetsel & Zweber, 2017).

HEALTHY PEOPLE 2030 BOX 8.3

- Reduce the rate of hospital admissions for pneumonia among older adults
- Reduce hip fractures among older adults

H2RAs have a longer duration of relief of 4 to 10 hours and can be taken at symptom onset or 30 to 60 minutes before symptoms are expected. Lower doses of H2RAs may be needed in patients with decreased renal function. Cimetidine is generally not recommended because it has a higher risk for adverse drug reactions and drug-drug interactions compared to other H2RAs (Whetsel & Zweber, 2017). Table 8.11 lists selected OTC items that may be problematic in older patients and safer alternatives if available.

HEALTHY PEOPLE 2030 BOX 8.4

- Reduce the rate of hospital admissions for pneumonia among older adults
- Reduce hip fractures among older adults

Complementary and Alternative Medications and Integrative Health

Surveys conducted in the United States have shown that more than half of older adults have used complementary and alternative medicine (CAM), defined as a nonmainstream practice that is used to add to or replace conventional medicine (Jamshed et al., 2014; National Cancer Institute [NCI], 2020; National Center for Complementary and Integrative Health [NCCIH], 2019c). Integrative health (IH) combines conventional and complementary medicine in a coordinated manner (NCCIH, 2019c). These practices may include dietary supplements, naturopathy, homeopathy, traditional Chinese medicine (TCM), and Ayurveda (Tsourounis & Dennehy, 2018; Ulbricht & Ko, 2018).

TABLE 8.11 **Selected Over-the-Counter (OTC) Medications That Can Pose Problems in Older Patients**

Type of OTC Medication	Concerns With Older Adults	Safer Nonprescription Alternatives
First-generation antihistamines[a,b,c,d] Brompheniramine Chlorpheniramine Dimenhydrinate Diphenhydramine Doxylamine Meclizine	Increase risk for Falls Central anticholinergic effects (e.g., confusion, memory impairment) Peripheral anticholinergic effects (e.g., dry mouth, constipation, urinary retention, blurry vision)	**Allergic Rhinitis** Second-generation antihistamines Loratadine Fexofenadine Levocetirizine Cetirizine* Intranasal products Corticosteroids Cromolyn Nonpharmacologic methods Avoid allergen triggers Nasal saline solutions Insomnia Nonpharmacologic methods Sleep hygiene **Motion Sickness/Nausea** Antacids Calcium carbonate Aluminum hydroxide Magnesium hydroxide Sodium bicarbonate Histamine-2 receptor antagonist (H2RA) Famotidine Ranitidine Nonpharmacologic methods Acupressure wristband Avoid overeating Avoid trigger foods, beverages, and scents
Oral nonsteroidal antiinflammatory drugs (NSAIDs)[a,d,e,f,g] Aspirin >325 mg/day Ibuprofen Naproxen	Increase risk for Bleeding Renal toxicity Cardiovascular toxicity	Oral analgesics Acetaminophen Topical analgesics Anesthetics Lidocaine Counterirritants Methyl salicylate Camphor Menthol Methyl nicotinate Capsaicin Salicylate Trolamine salicylate Gastrointestinal protection Proton pump inhibitor (PPI) Omeprazole Esomeprazole Lansoprazole Histamine-2 receptor antagonist (H2RA) Famotidine Ranitidine Nonpharmacologic methods Headache Stress management Avoid trigger substances and situations Musculoskeletal pain Rest injured area Ice therapy for swelling Heat therapy for stiffness Compress injured area Elevate injured body part Osteoarthritis Weight loss if overweight Physical exercise Heat or ice therapy

(Continued)

TABLE 8.11 Selected Over-the-Counter (OTC) Medications That Can Pose Problems in Older Patients—cont'd

Type of OTC Medication	Concerns With Older Adults	Safer Nonprescription Alternatives
Proton pump inhibitors (PPIs)[a,h] Omeprazole Esomeprazole Lansoprazole	Increase risk for Community-acquired pneumonia Clostridium difficile infection Bone fractures Vitamin B_{12} deficiency	Antacids Calcium carbonate Aluminum hydroxide Magnesium hydroxide Sodium bicarbonate Histamine-2 receptor antagonists (H2RAs) Famotidine Ranitidine Nonpharmacologic methods Avoid trigger foods and beverages Eat smaller meals Stop or reduce smoking Wear loose-fitting clothes Avoid eating within 3 hours of lying down Elevate the head of the bed or use a foam pillow wedge

Data from [*]Causes sedation in approximately 10% of patients.[c] [a]American Geriatrics Society Beers Criteria® Update Expert Panel. (2019). American Geriatrics Society 2019. Updated AGS Beers Criteria® for potentially inappropriate medication use in older adults. *Journal of the American Geriatrics Society, 67*(4), 674–694. https://doi.org/10.1111/jgs.15767; [b]Melton, S. T., & Kirkwood, C. K. (2017). Chapter 46: Insomnia, drowsiness, and fatigue. In D. L. Krinsky (Ed.), *Handbook of nonprescription drugs: An interactive approach to self-care* (19th ed.). American Pharmacists Association. doi-org.libproxy1.usc.edu/10.21019/9781582122656.ch46; [c]Scolaro, K. L. (2017). Chapter 11: Colds and allergy. In D. L. Krinsky (Ed.), *Handbook of nonprescription drugs: An interactive approach to self-care* (19th ed.). American Pharmacists Association. doi-org.libproxy1.usc.edu/10.21019/9781582122656.ch11; [d]Welch, A. C. (2017). Chapter 19: Nausea and vomiting. In D. L. Krinsky (Ed.), *Handbook of nonprescription drugs: An interactive approach to self-care* (19th ed.). American Pharmacists Association. doi-org.libproxy1.usc.edu/10.21019/9781582122656.ch19; [e]Olenak, J. L. (2017). Chapter 7: Musculoskeletal injuries and disorders. In D. L. Krinsky (Ed.), *Handbook of nonprescription drugs: An interactive approach to self-care* (19th ed.). American Pharmacists Association. doi-org.libproxy1.usc.edu/10.21019/9781582122656.ch7; [f]Wilkinson, J. J., & Tromp, K. (2017). Chapter 5: Headache. In D. L. Krinsky (Ed.), *Handbook of nonprescription drugs: An interactive approach to self-care* (19th ed.). American Pharmacists Association. doi-org.libproxy1.usc.edu/10.21019/9781582122656.ch5; [g]Wongrakpanich, S., Wongrakpanich, A., Melhado, K., & Rangaswami, J. (2018). A comprehensive review of non-steroidal anti-inflammatory drug use in the elderly. *Aging and Disease, 9*(1), 143–150. doi.org/10.14336/AD.2017.0306; [h]Whetsel, T., & Zweber, A. (2017). Chapter 13: Heartburn and dyspepsia. In D. L. Krinsky (Ed.), *Handbook of nonprescription drugs: An interactive approach to self-care* (19th ed.). American Pharmacists Association. doi-org.libproxy1.usc.edu/10.21019/9781582122656.ch13

CAM and IH may provide potential treatment options to address conditions for which conventional medicine has been ineffective and can improve patient empowerment. Some of these therapies have been scientifically and clinically tested (Ulbricht & Ko, 2018). However, it is a common misconception that all CAM and IH therapies are safe due to their natural origins. In fact, many of these treatments lack strong scientific and clinical evidence of effectiveness and may even cause adverse effects or dangerous interactions with prescription medications (Jamshed et al., 2014; NCCIH, 2019c; Ulbricht & Ko, 2018). Therefore, it is important to determine if patients use CAM and IH and to discuss the risks and benefits of their use.

Many patients commonly take dietary supplements that may contain vitamins, minerals, herbs, amino acids, or other substances (US Food and Drug Administration [FDA], 2019b). Under the Dietary Supplement Health and Education Act (DSHEA) of 1994, the Food and Drug Administration (FDA) performs postmarketing surveillance of dietary supplements, but the manufacturers are responsible for adhering to current good manufacturing practice standards for the labeling, safety, and efficacy of their products (Bridgeman & Rollins, 2018; Tsourounis & Dennehy, 2018; US Food and Drug Administration [FDA], 2019a, 2019b). Despite these regulations, there have been concerns that some dietary supplements may be contaminated with substances other than the labeled active ingredients, may be marketed with false or misleading health claims, and may increase the risk for adverse effects and drug interactions (Bridgeman & Rollins, 2018; US Food and Drug Administration [FDA], 2007). Table 8.12 includes a list of common dietary supplements, their uses, and their potential adverse effects and drug interactions.

Homeopathy is a medical system based on two theories: "like cures like" and "the law of minimum dose" (NCCIH, 2019d). In other words, the same substance that can produce symptoms if used in large doses can also treat the symptoms if used in small doses (Ulbricht & Ko, 2018). Additionally, the potency of a homeopathic medicine can be increased with further dilution (NCCIH, 2019d; Ulbricht & Ko, 2018). Homeopathic medicines are derived from various substances, including botanical sources and toxic materials, but they are often diluted to contain a minute or even undetectable amount of active ingredient (NCCIH, 2019d; Ulbricht & Ko, 2018). There is limited evidence supporting the use of homeopathy, and some have proposed that homeopathic medicine may be similar to placebo (Shurtleff, 2019; Ulbricht & Ko, 2018). Although homeopathic formulations are regulated under the Federal Food, Drug, and Cosmetic Act (FDCA), the FDA does not perform safety

TABLE 8.12 Commonly Used Supplements in Older Adults

Dietary Supplement	Common Uses[a,b]	Possible Adverse Effects[b,c]	Possible Drug Interactions[a,b]
Black cohosh	Menopause support	Stomach upset, weight gain, hepatotoxicity	↑ Adverse effects with tamoxifen
Cinnamon	Glucose metabolism	Rash, hepatotoxicity	↑ Hypoglycemic risk with antihyperglycemic agents
Chondroitin	Bone health	Nausea, stomach upset, allergic reactions	↑ Bleed risk with warfarin
Coenzyme Q10	Cardiac health	Nausea, stomach upset	↓ Anticoagulant effect of warfarin
Cranberry	Urinary tract health	Kidney stones, diarrhea	↑ Bleed risk with warfarin
Fish oil	Cardiac health	Stomach upset, "fish burp"	↑ Bleed risk at doses >4 g/day
Garlic	Cardiac and immune health	Nausea, heartburn, garlic breath	↑ Bleed risk with warfarin
Ginger	Digestive health and anti-emesis	Heartburn, belching	↑ Bleed risk with warfarin
Ginkgo	Brain health	Stomach upset, headache, allergic skin reactions	↓ Clearance of atorvastatin
Ginseng (Panax)	Performance enhancement and immune health	Insomnia, headache, rash	↑ Hypoglycemic risk with antihyperglycemic agents
Glucosamine	Bone health	Nausea, stomach upset, drowsiness	↑ Bleed risk with warfarin
Green tea	Cardiac health and performance enhancement	Stomach upset, cardiac stimulation	↓ Anticoagulant effect of warfarin
Melatonin	Sleep aid	Nausea, morning grogginess, headache	↓ Antihypertensive effects of nifedipine
Red yeast rice	Cardiac health	Stomach upset, ↑ liver function enzymes, rhabdomyolysis	↑ Adverse effects with gemfibrozil
Saw palmetto	Prostate health	Stomach upset, fatigue, headache	↑ Bleed risk with warfarin
St. John's wort	Mood support	Nausea, fatigue, skin reactions	↓ Levels of CYP3A4 substrates
Turmeric	Healthy inflammatory response	Stomach upset, nausea	↑ Levels of sulfasalazine
Valerian	Sleep aid	Headache, excitability	↑ Sedative effect with alcohol
Vitamin K	Bone health	Nausea, diarrhea, stomach upset	↓ Anticoagulant effect of warfarin

[a]Data from Bridgeman, M. M., & Rollins, C. J. (2018). Chapter 23: Essential and conditionally essential nutrients. In D. L. Krinsky (Ed.), *Handbook of nonprescription drugs: An interactive approach to self-care* (19th ed.). American Pharmacists Association. doi-org.libproxy1.usc.edu/10.21019/9781582122656.ch23; [b]McQueen, C. E., & Orr, K. K. (2018). Chapter 51: Natural products. In D. L. Krinsky (Ed.), *Handbook of nonprescription drugs: An interactive approach to self-care* (19th ed.). American Pharmacists Association. doi-org.libproxy1.usc.edu/10.21019/9781582122656.ch51; [c]Therapeutic Research Center Natural Medicines. (2020). *Vitamin K*. https://naturalmedicines-therapeuticresearch-com/databases/food,-herbs-supplements/professional.aspx?productid=983

and efficacy evaluations of homeopathic products. Despite having a low risk for adverse effects due to the extensive dilution process, one example of an unintended adverse effect was a zinc nasal spray that was commonly used for colds but was withdrawn from the US market due to numerous reports of loss of smell (Ulbricht & Ko, 2018). Some homeopathic products have also been reported to contain excessive amounts of active ingredients that could lead to adverse effects and drug interactions (NCCIH, 2019d; Ulbricht & Ko, 2018).

Traditional Chinese medicine (TCM) uses a variety of modalities to address health problems, including acupuncture, tai chi, and herbal medicine (Ulbricht & Ko, 2018). Some research has shown that acupuncture may be helpful for osteoarthritis and nausea and that Tai Chi may improve balance in older adults. TCM can also be seen in Western medicine, such as naturally made lovastatin from red yeast rice. However, more rigorous testing is needed to support the efficacy and safety of TCM (Ulbricht & Ko, 2018). In 2004, the FDA prohibited the sale of ephedra-containing products, which were commonly used for weight loss and athletic performance enhancement, due to an alarming number of reported serious adverse effects (National Institutes of Health [NIH] Office of Dietary Supplements, 2020; *Traditional Chinese Medicine: What you need to know*, 2013). Given its similarity to ephedrine, ephedra has been shown to share drug interactions that are similar to those for ephedrine (NIH, 2004). In addition, some TCM products have been found to be contaminated with toxins, heavy metals, and prescription medications (Ulbricht & Ko, 2018).

Ayurveda is an ancient Indian medical system that uses a holistic approach with natural products and lifestyle methods to optimize physical, psychological, and spiritual health (Chen et al., 2015; Ulbricht & Ko, 2018). Some small studies have shown that some Ayurvedic medicine may have an effectiveness that is similar to that for certain conventional treatments for pain and rheumatoid arthritis (Chen et al., 2015). However, there are few robust clinical and scientific studies that support the efficacy and safety of Ayurvedic medicine. There have been concerns that some Ayurvedic preparations may contain toxic amounts of heavy metals and can possibly interact with medications, foods, and other herbs (Chen et al., 2015; Ulbricht & Ko, 2018). For example, using garlic or ginger with anticoagulants can increase the risk of bleeding (NCCIH, 2019e).

Naturopathy is a medical system that uses a holistic approach with natural treatment and preventive therapies, including dietary counseling, acupuncture, homeopathy, and dietary supplements (Ajanal et al., 2013; Ulbricht & Ko, 2018). Although some naturopathic regimens, such as preventing cardiovascular disease with a healthy diet, have been shown to be effective and are integrated in conventional medicine, other naturopathic treatments, as previously mentioned, may need further studies to assess their safety and efficacy (Ulbricht & Ko, 2018).

Given the increasing prevalence of CAM and IH use among older adults, health care providers are more likely to encounter patients who are utilizing CAM and IH therapies (Jamshed et al., 2014). Therefore, it is important for providers of conventional, complementary, and integrative medicine to work collaboratively to treat patients. In general, patients should be advised to take caution when using CAM or IH therapies and to purchase CAM and IH products from trustworthy sources (Ulbricht & Ko, 2018). Table 8.12 lists some of the supplements commonly used by older adults.

Pain Management and Geriatrics

There are reports suggesting that approximately 25% to 85% of older adults worldwide experience chronic pain (Stompór et al., 2019). A Medicare part D analysis using data from 2016 showed that more than 500,000 beneficiaries received high doses of opioids that were, on average, greater than recommended by the manufacturer. With the aging baby boomer generation and the expected increase of the older adult population in the United States, the Administration on Aging (AOA) and the Substance Abuse and Mental Health Services Administration (SAMHSA) predict that the misuse of opioids among older adults will increase twofold from 2004 to 2020 (Minnesota Prevention Resource Center, 2017). This can become problematic, as opioids are associated with concerns related to misuse and polypharmacy (e.g., confusion, falls, respiratory depression) and undertreated pain can lead to disturbances to quality of life (e.g., depression, social isolation, cognitive impairment) (American Geriatrics Society, 2019; Cavalieri, 2007; Dowell et al., 2016). As a result, health care providers have the difficult responsibility of balancing appropriate pain management while minimizing adverse effects.

According to the 2016 Guideline for Prescribing Opioids for Chronic Pain from the Centers for Disease Control and Prevention (CDC), nonpharmacologic therapy and nonopioid medication are preferred for chronic pain management, excluding active cancer, palliative, and end-of-life indications. Chronic pain is defined as pain that lasts for more than 3 months or the amount of time that is normally needed for tissue healing (Dowell et al., 2016). There are many treatment options depending on the type or cause of pain. For example, studies have shown that physical therapy (e.g., hip/knee osteoarthritis, low back pain, fibromyalgia), weight loss (e.g., knee osteoarthritis), and psychological therapy are effective nonpharmacologic methods. If pharmacologic therapy is needed, providers can consider topical (e.g., NSAIDs, lidocaine) or injectable (e.g., intraarticular or subacromial corticosteroid) formulations for localized pain. Systemic medications may be necessary for nonlocalized nociceptive pain (e.g., acetaminophen, NSAIDs) and neuropathic pain (e.g., select antidepressants, anticonvulsants). If pharmacologic therapy is used, it is important to weigh the risks and benefits, including potential adverse effects (e.g., fall risk with antidepressants and anticonvulsants, bleed risk with nonselective NSAIDs) (American Geriatrics Society, 2019; Dowell et al., 2016).

However, health care providers may need to consider opioid therapy, especially if there is inadequate pain control with nonpharmacologic and nonopioid medication therapy. In general, it is recommended that providers start with an immediate-release formulation, use the lowest effective dose, limit duration of treatment to what is medically necessary (e.g., typically ≤3 days for acute pain), titrate cautiously, and avoid high opioid doses (e.g., ≥90 morphine milligram equivalents [MME]/day), especially when managing older adults (Dowell et al., 2016). Some analgesics may have unique properties that can lead to additional drug interactions or adverse effects (e.g., serotonergic effects of tramadol and methadone, psychoactive properties of cannabis) (Baldo & Rose, 2020; Elikottil et al., 2009). Providers should perform regular evaluations to ensure that the expected benefits outweigh the risks of opioid use and consider incorporating nonopioid methods for optimal chronic pain management. There are different steps that providers can take to minimize serious adverse events and opioid misuse, such as assessing prescription drug monitoring program (PDMP) reports, utilizing treatment agreements, counseling patients on common adverse effects (e.g., constipation, central nervous system depression, tolerance), addressing risks factors for overdose (e.g., identifying red flags, minimizing drug interactions, performing urine drug tests, prescribing naloxone), and taking caution when tapering opioid therapy (e.g., monitoring for withdrawal symptoms, tapering as slow as necessary) (Dowell et al., 2016). Although controversial, providers may want to assess for pseudoaddiction—a concept that explains how patients may exhibit behaviors associated with addiction when pain is undertreated (Greene & Chambers, 2015). Given the multifaceted aspects of chronic pain management, utilizing multimodal and multidisciplinary approaches can help address patient-specific concerns as well as improve pain and function (Dowell et al., 2016).

HEALTHY PEOPLE 2030 BOX 8.5

- Reduce the proportion of adults with chronic pain that frequently limits life or work activities
- Increase self-management of chronic pain that frequently limits life or work activities
- Reduce the impact on loved ones of chronic pain that frequently limits life or work activities
- Reduce the proportion of adults with arthritis who have moderate or severe joint pain
- Reduce the proportion of people who misused prescription opioids in the past year
- Reduce the proportion of people who started misusing prescription opioids in the past year

The Use of Cannabis

Although historical evidence suggests that cannabis has been used medicinally for more than 5000 years, its use has been associated with social stigma, ethical controversies, and legal implications. However, the perception of cannabis use in the United States has been evolving as numerous states and territories have legalized its use (Bridgeman & Abazia, 2017). This is reflected in studies showing that 2.9% of adults 65 years and older had used cannabis in the past year in 2015–2016 compared to 0.4% in 2006–2007 (Han & Palamar, 2020). With its increasing prevalence, health care providers can expect to encounter cannabis use more frequently in patient-care settings.

Although there are ≥60 active compounds found in cannabis, two major cannabinoids that are commonly used for therapeutic purposes are tetrahydrocannabinol (THC) and cannabidiol (CBD) (Bridgeman & Abazia, 2017; Elikkottil & Gupta, 2009). THC is known to have psychoactive properties, as it has partial agonistic effects on endogenous cannabinoid receptors that are located throughout the human body, such as the brain and immune cells. However, CBD is nonpsychoactive, as it has low affinity for these receptors (Bruni et al., 2018). As cannabinoids can also exert their effects through noncannabinoid receptors (e.g., opioid, serotonin, nicotinic) and ion channels (e.g., calcium, potassium, sodium), studies have suggested that cannabis may potentially offer a variety of therapeutic benefits given its ability to affect different systems in the body (Bridgeman & Abazia, 2017).

Cannabinoid-containing products are available in various formulations and routes of administration (e.g., oral, inhalation, intranasal, topical) (Bruni et al., 2018). Inhaled formulations have a rapid onset of effect that peaks within 30 minutes and lasts from 6 to 24 hours, whereas oral formulations have a slower onset of effect that peaks within 4 hours and lasts up to 12 to 24 hours (Canadian Centre on Substance Use and Addiction, 2019). There are currently four pharmaceutical-grade formulations, but only three are available in the United States: dronabinol, nabilone, and a CBD-based oral solution. Although these medications only have a few FDA-approved indications (e.g., chemotherapy-induced nausea and vomiting, AIDS-associated anorexia, seizure disorders), some studies have shown that medicinal cannabinoids may also have therapeutic use in many other conditions (e.g., chronic pain, multiple sclerosis, Parksinon disease, Alzheimer disease, glaucoma) (Bridgeman & Abazia, 2017; Bruni et al., 2018). Given the variability of botanicals and the potential for impurities in non-FDA-approved formulations, patients should be advised to take caution and to purchase cannabis-containing products from trustworthy sources (National Institute on Drug Abuse [NIDA], 2019; NCCIH, 2019b).

Although more studies are needed to evaluate the long-term effects of medicinal cannabis use, patients and their caregivers should be counseled to monitor for potential adverse effects (e.g., falls, gastrointestinal issues, changes in mood and behavior), including psychoactive effects (e.g., euphoria) if using THC-containing products (Abuhasira et al., 2019; Bridgeman & Abazia, 2017). Therefore, it is important to reconcile medication lists at each visit as well as to identify medications, herbals, and supplements that can interact with cannabinoid-containing products (e.g., inhibitors/inducers of cytochrome P450 isoenzyme 2C9 and 3A4 for THC and 2C19 and 3A4 for CBD) (Bridgeman & Abazia, 2017). As more scientific and clinical information on cannabis use and its effects become available, health care providers will be able to make more guided clinical decisions with their patients.

HEALTHY PEOPLE 2030 BOX 8.6

- Increase the proportion of adults whose health care providers checked their understanding
- Increase the proportion of adults whose health care providers involved them in decisions as much as they wanted

Clinical Application

If older patients decide the try cannabis products, the recommendation should be to use the lowest effective dose,

• BOX 8.7 Summary of Guidelines on Cannabis Use

1. Use the lowest effective dose.
2. Start with half the average adult dose and titrate up slowly.
3. Be aware that THC-dominant products are more likely to cause psychoactive side effects.
4. Monitor for new onset symptoms or side effects, such as dizziness, confusion, falls, or cognitive decline.
5. Treat using cannabis just like you would any other prescription medication
6. Screen patients for side effects and drug-drug interactions with cannabis.

Data from Abuhasira, R., Ron, A., Sikorin, I., & Novack, V. (2019). Medical cannabis for older patients—treatment protocol and initial results. *Journal of Clinical Medicine, 8*(11), 1819. https://doi.org/10.3390/jcm8111819; Bridgeman, M. B., & Abazia, D. T. (2017). Medical cannabis: History, pharmacology, and implications for the acute care setting. *Pharmacy and Therapeutics: A Peer-Reviewed Journal for Formulary Management, 42*(3), 180–188.

use products that are CBD dominant, and carefully monitor for side effects: dizziness, increased falls, and any kind of confusion or cognitive decline. Patients with preexisting respiratory disease are at risk for exacerbations if they are using the inhaled route of administration. Topical formulations are tolerated better than others. Box 8.7 provides a summary of guidelines for product selection and dosing for older patients if they choose to try cannabis for their various medical problems.

Coordination of Care With the Pharmacy: An Interdisciplinary Approach

- Geriatrics is a team sport. Older patients are medically, pharmacologically, and psychosocially complicated. A single provider cannot adequately address all needs of older adults.
- Numerous published literatures support a variety of direct patient care roles that can be provided by pharmacists, including patient counseling, medication management, chronic disease management (Santschi et al., 2011), and health care professional education (Nkansah et al., 2010).
- Patient counseling entails medication education on new and existing therapies. Pharmacist-delivered education would include the medication's name, indication, expected effects and benefits, expected onset of action, medication route, dosage form, dosage, administration, how to prepare and administer medication, how to respond to a missed dose, common and severe side effects, potential interactions (including drug-drug, drug-food, drug-disease interactions), contraindications, proper storage and disposal, as well as how to access the pharmacist and the refill process (American Society of Health-System Pharmacists, 2013). It is essential that patients understand their medications and can manage their own care.
- Medication management is the process of addressing medication safety issues. This may include medication contraindication, drug interactions, overprescribing, underprescribing, duplications, prescribing errors, and patient medication adherence (Agency for Healthcare Research and Quality. 2018). To effectively manage medications, medication reconciliation is required to ensure there is a complete and accurate medication list, including over-the-counter medications, herbals, and supplements. Medication reconciliation entails comparing the current medication list to what the patient is currently taking, including the dose, route, frequency, and adherence.
- Chronic disease management can be provided through pharmacist-driven clinics. They may provide management of chronic disease states such as hypertension, dyslipidemia, diabetes, heart failure, asthma, chronic obstructive pulmonary disease, and smoking cessation. Additionally, pharmacists can manage high-risk medications with a narrow therapeutic index, such as warfarin for anticoagulation. Chronic disease management by pharmacists includes education on disease state, expected effects of chronic disease on the patient's life, recognition of possible disease complications (American Society of Health-System Pharmacists, 2013), and therapeutic regimens to treat. Depending on the pharmacy clinic protocol and collaborative practice agreements, pharmacists may be able to start, stop, and adjust medication dosages.
- Pharmacists can deliver high-quality health care professional education. The type of education may vary based on the health care setting but can range from answering specific medication questions (i.e., correct administration, alternative dosage forms, drug-drug interactions, etc.) to providing drug monographs, detailed drug information consults, in-service presentations on new therapies, and clinical guidelines updates.
- In geriatric care, pharmacists may be more involved in various roles ranging from polypharmacy and adherence management, chronic disease management, interprofessional team care, and medication error prevention during transition points (Lee et al., 2015).
- See Box 8.8.
- Polypharmacy and adherence management can be provided by pharmacists through medication reconciliation and medication management. Inventions used in older adult populations may include simplifying complex medication regimens; utilizing medication adherence tools such as medication charts, pill boxes, or medication reminder systems; and providing education on medication to address medication misunderstandings. Pharmacists may also implement these techniques while managing chronic diseases. Hypertension, diabetes, heart failure, chronic obstructive pulmonary disease (COPD), anticoagulation, and osteoporosis are some of the chronic conditions in older adults that have shown positive outcomes by pharmacist-driven management (Lee et al., 2015).

• BOX 8.8 Role of a Clinical Pharmacist in the Care of a Geriatric Patient

- Perform accurate medication reconciliations with recommendations for pharmacotherapeutic changes.
- Provide general pharmacotherapy assessments or chronic disease-targeted interventions.
- Serve as a drug information resource to providers and patients.
- Assist in navigating Medicare part D plans and reducing medication costs.
- Be aware that pharmacists are available at every health care setting, including the community, hospital, clinic, and long-term care settings.

- Medication errors during transition points are prevalent, and these errors have the potential to cause great harm to older adults who are vulnerable to transition-related medication misadventures. Pharmacists should perform medication reconciliation during transition points—including home to hospital, or hospital to home, rehabilitation facility, or nursing home (Lee et al., 2015)—to decrease readmission rates and provide health care cost savings.
- Because they are the medication experts on the interprofessional care team, most studies favor the practice of having pharmacists offer medication and therapeutic management, provider education to improve prescribing patterns, and patient education to improve clinical outcomes (Lee et al., 2015). Geriatric pharmacists integrated into multidisciplinary geriatric care teams have provided a range of services and interventions, leading to a reduction in hospitalizations, emergency department visits, and overall positive clinical outcomes (Campbell et al., 2018). Additionally, for geriatric fall risk assessments, pharmacists can evaluate medication regimens for drugs and drug classes associated with falls, such as anticholinergic medications, central nervous system depressants, and cardiovascular medications (Fritsch & Shelton, 2019).

Transitions of Care

Older adults are especially susceptible to medication therapy problems during transitions of care to other facilities or when returning to the community. During hospital admission or discharge, up to 70% of patients are left with medication discrepancies, about 30% of which have the potential to cause patients harm (Mueller et al., 2012). Particularly, older adults with multiple chronic conditions and polypharmacy are at a higher risk for medication misadventures (Surbhi et al., 2003). In an effort to reduce hospital readmissions and medication-related problems, pharmacists have been utilized to perform medication reconciliation or comprehensive medication review during hospital admission and discharge (Berquist et al., 2019). Berquist studied pharmacists who were board certified in geriatrics to examine the interventions that took place after hospital discharge for 365 patients of a geriatric primary clinic. During the 14-month study, pharmacists identified more than 600 medication discrepancies and proposed greater than 1000 recommendations to the primary provider. Pharmacists can offer a positive impact by delivering direct patient care in the older adult population, particularly during the precarious time when a patient is transitioning from one care setting to another.

Summary of Basic Recommendations

As this chapter has shown, geriatric pharmacotherapy is both complex and nuanced. Older adults tend to accumulate medical problems with age. Often those medical problems require pharmacotherapy, with more than one drug necessary to treat each disease state. Therefore, it is not uncommon for health care providers to see long medication lists when taking care of an older adult. To avoid additional complications, medication lists must be reviewed frequently. The medication list must be rational and free from unnecessary medications, as well as medications that might cause drug-drug interactions or adverse effects. Medications that are poorly tolerated by older patients should be avoided. Choosing the right medication at the right dose is imperative.

Key Points

- Review all lists of five or more medications on a regular basis to avoid polypharmacy.
- Pay attention to vitamins, supplements, and over-the counter medications.
- Ensure that each medication on the list has an appropriate indication.
- Avoid duplications.
- Assume any new symptom is a drug side effect until that possibility has been ruled out.
- Screen for medications highlighted on the Beers list and other geriatric criteria.
- When making changes to the medication list, try to work with one drug at a time.
- When starting a new medication, *start low, go slow, but do go.*
- Avoid new drugs on the market.
- Create a medication list that is practical and affordable for the patient.

More information about tools and Interprofessional Education Collaborative (IPEC) competencies mentioned in this chapter can be found in Appendix 1: Tools and Appendix 2: IPEC Competencies.

References

Abuhasira, R., Ron, A., Sikorin, I., & Novack, V. (2019). Medical cannabis for older patients- treatment protocol and initial results. *Journal of Clinical Medicine*, *8*(11), 1819. https://doi.org/10.3390/jcm8111819.

Agency for Healthcare Research and Quality. (2018). Topic: Medical errors. AHRQ. (2018.). Retrieved from https://www.ahrq.gov/topics/medical-errors.html.

Ajanal, M., Nayak, S., Prasad, B. S., & Kadam, A. (2013). Adverse drug reaction and concepts of drug safety in Ayurveda: An overview. *Journal of Young Pharmacists*, *5*(4), 116–120. https://doi.org/10.1016/j.jyp.2013.10.001.

American Geriatrics Society. (2019). For older people, medications are common; updated AGS Beers Criteria® aims to make sure they're appropriate, too. https://www.americangeriatrics.org/media-center/news/older-people-medications-are-common-updated-ags-beers-criteriar-aims-make-sure.

American Geriatrics Society 2012 Beers Criteria Update Expert Panel. (2012). American Geriatrics Society updated Beers Criteria for potentially inappropriate medication use in older adults. *Journal of the American Geriatric Society*, *60*(4):616–631. https://doi.org/10.1111/j.1532–5415.2012.03923.x.

American Society of Health-System Pharmacists. (2013). ASHP's comments on Chronic Care Options. ASHP. (n.d.). Retrieved September 12, 2022, from https://www.ashp.org/advocacy-and-issues/key-issues/other-issues/additional-advocacy-efforts/ashps-comments-on-chronic-care-options?loginreturnUrl=SSOCheckOnly.

Baldo, B. A., & Rose, M. A. (2020). The anaesthetist, opioid analgesic drugs, and serotonin toxicity: A mechanistic and clinical review. *British Journal of Anaesthesia*, *124*(1), 44–62. https://doi.org/10.1016/j.bja.2019.08.010.

Barnett, K., Mercer, S. W., Norbury, M., Watt, G., Wyke, S., & Guthrie, B. (2012). Epidemiology of multimorbidity and implications for health care, research, and medical education: a cross-sectional study. *Lancet (London, England)*, *380*(9836), 37–43. https://doi.org/10.1016/S0140-6736(12)60240-2.

Beers, M. H., Ouslander, J. G., Rollingher, I., Reuben, D. B., Brooks, J., & Beck, J. C. (1991). Explicit criteria for determining inappropriate medication use in nursing home residents. *Archives of Internal Medicine*, *151*(9), 1825–1832. https://doi.org/10.1001/archinte.151.9.1825.

Berquist, K., Linnebur, S. A., & Fixen, D. R. (2019). Incorporation of Clinical Pharmacy Into a Geriatric Transitional Care Management Program. *Journal of pharmacy practice.*, *33*(5), 661–665.

Berry, S. D., Placide, S. G., Mostofsky, E., Zhang, Y., Lipsitz, L. A., Mittleman, M. A., & Kiel, D. P. (2016). Antipsychotic and Benzodiazepine Drug Changes Affect Acute Falls Risk Differently in the Nursing Home. *The journals of gerontology. Series A, Biological sciences and medical sciences*, *71*(2), 273–278. https://doi.org/10.1093/gerona/glv091.

Bridgeman, M. B., & Abazia, D. T. (2017). Medical cannabis: History, pharmacology, and implications for the acute care setting. *P & T: A Peer-Reviewed Journal for Formulary Management.*, *42*(3), 180–188.

Bridgeman, M. M., & Rollins, C. J. (2018). Chapter 23: Essential and conditionally essential nutrients. In D. L. Krinsky (Ed.), *Handbook of nonprescription drugs: An interactive approach to self-care* (19th ed.). American Pharmacists Association https://doi.org.libproxy1.usc.edu/10.21019/9781582122656.ch23.

Bruni, N., Della Pepa, C., Oliaro-Bosso, S., Pessione, E., Gastaldi, D., & Dosio, F. (2018). Cannabinoid delivery systems for pain and inflammation treatment. *Molecules*, *23*(10), 2478. https://doi.org/10.3390/molecules23102478.

Budnitz, D. S., Lovegrove, M. C., Shehab, N., & Richards, C. L. (2011). Emergency hospitalizations for adverse drug events in older Americans. *New England Journal of Medicine*, *365*(21), 2002–2012. https://doi.org/10.1056/nejmsa1103053.

Budnitz, D. S., Pollock, D. A., Weidenbach, K. N., Mendelsohn, A. B., Schroeder, T. J., & Annest, J. L. (2006). National surveillance of emergency department visits for outpatient adverse drug events. *Journal of the American Medical Association*, *296*(15), 1858–1866. https://doi.org/10.1001/jama.296.15.1858.

Campbell, B. K., Le, T., Gubner, N. R., & Guydish, J. (2018). Health risk perceptions and reasons for use of tobacco products among clients in addictions treatment. *Addictive behaviors.*, *91*, 149–155.

Canadian Centre on Substance Use and Addiction. (2019). Cannabis: *Inhaling vs ingesting*. https://www.ccsa.ca/sites/default/files/2019-06/CCSA-Cannabis-Inhaling-Ingesting-Risks-Infographic-2019-en_1.pdf.

Cavalieri, T. A. (2007). Managing pain in geriatric patients. *Journal of the American Osteopathic Association.*, *107*(Suppl. 4), ES10–ES16.

Centers for Disease Control and Prevention. (2004). *The state of aging and health in America*. https://www.cdc.gov/aging/pdf/State_of_Aging_and_Health_in_America_2004.pdf.

Centers for Disease Control and Prevention. (2019). *Keep on your feet—Preventing older adult falls*. https://www.cdc.gov/injury/features/older-adult-falls/index.html.

Charlesworth, C. J., Smit, E., Lee, D. S., Alramadhan, F., & Odden, M. C. (2015). Polypharmacy Among Adults Aged 65 Years and Older in the United States: 1988-2010. *The journals of gerontology. Series A, Biological sciences and medical sciences*, *70*(8), 989–995. https://doi.org/10.1093/gerona/glv013.

Chen, K. C., Lu, R., Iqbal, U., Hsu, K. C., Chen, B. L., Nguyen, P. A., et al. (2015). Interactions between traditional Chinese medicine and western drugs in Taiwan: A population-based study. *Computer Methods and Programs in Biomedicine*, *122*(3), 462–470. https://doi.org/10.1016/j.cmpb.2015.09.006.

Cho, H., Myung, J., Suh, H., & Kang, H. Y. (2018). Antihistamine use and the risk of injurious falls or fracture in elderly patients: a systematic review and meta-analysis. *Osteoporosis International*, *29*(10), 2163–2170. https://doi.org/10.1007/s00198-018-4564-z.

Daneman, R., & Prat, A. (2015 Jan 5). The blood-brain barrier. *Cold Spring Harb Perspect Biol*, *7*(1), a020412. https://doi.org/10.1101/cshperspect.a020412. PMID: 25561720; PMCID: PMC4292164.

Dowell, D., Haegerich, T. M., & Chou, R. (2016). CDC guideline for prescribing opioids for chronic pain—United States. *2016. Morbidity and Mortality Weekly Report*, *65*(1), 1–49.

Elikottil, J., Gupta, P., & Gupta, K. (2009). The analgesic potential of cannabinoids. *Journal of Opioid Management*, *5*(6), 341–357.

Farinde, A., Porter, R. S., & Kaplan, J. L. (2019). Overview of pharmacodynamics—Clinical pharmacology. *Merck Manual*. https://www.merckmanuals.com/professional/clinicalpharmacology/pharmacodynamics/overview-of-pharmacodynamics.

Farrell, B., Tsang, C., Raman-Wilms, L., Irving, H., Conklin, J., & Pottie, K. (2015). What are priorities for deprescribing for elderly patients? Capturing the voice of practitioners: A modified delphi process. *PLoS One*, *10*(4), e0122246.

Feinberg, M. (1993). The problems of anticholinergic adverse effects in older patients. *Drugs & aging*, *3*(4), 335–348. https://doi.org/10.2165/00002512-199303040-00004.

Fritsch, M. A., & Shelton, P. S. (2019). Geriatric Polypharmacy: Pharmacist as Key Facilitator in Assessing for Falls Risk: 2019 Update. *Clinics in geriatric medicine*, *35*(2), 185–204. https://doi.org/10.1016/j.cger.2019.01.010.

Fu, A. Z., Jiang, J. Z., Reeves, J. H., Fincham, J. E., Liu, G. G., & Perri, M., 3rd. (2007). Potentially inappropriate medication use and healthcare expenditures in the US community-dwelling elderly. *Medical Care*, *45*(5), 472–476. https://doi.org/10.1097/01.mlr.0000254571.05722.34.

Giarratano, A., Green, S. E., & Nicolau, D. P. (2018). Review of antimicrobial use and considerations in the elderly population. *Clinical Interventions in Aging*, *13*, 657–667. https://doi.org/10.2147/cia.s133640.

Greene, M. S., & Chambers, R. A. (2015). Pseudoaddiction: Fact or fiction? An investigation of the medical literature. *Current Addiction Reports*, *2*(4), 310–317. https://doi.org/10.1007/s40429-015-0074-7.

Gujjarlamudi, H. B. (2016). Polytherapy and drug interactions in elderly. *Journal of Mid-life Health*, *7*(3), 105–107. https://doi.org/10.4103/0976-7800.191021.

Han, B. H., & Palamar, J. J. (2020). Trends in cannabis use among older adults in the United States, 2015–2018. *JAMA Internal Medicine*, E1–E3. 2020 Apr 1;180(4):609-611. doi: 10.1001/jamainternmed.2019.7517. PMID: 32091531; PMCID: PMC7042817.

Hegeman, J., van den Bemt, B., Weerdesteyn, V., Nienhuis, B., van Limbeek, J., & Duysens, J. (2011). Unraveling the association between SSRI use and falls: an experimental study of risk factors for accidental falls in long-term paroxetine users. *Clinical Neuropharmacology*, *34*(6), 210–215. https://doi.org/10.1097/WNF.0b013e31823337d1.

Ito, T., & Jensen, R. T. (2010). Association of long-term proton pump inhibitor therapy with bone fractures and effects on absorption of calcium, vitamin B12, iron, and magnesium. *Current Gastroenterology Reports*, *12*(6), 448–457. https://doi.org/10.1007/s11894-010-0141-0.

Jamshed, S. Q., Min, C. S., Siddiqui, M. J., & Verma, R. K. (2014). Role of complementary and alternative medicine in geriatric care: A mini review. *Pharmacognosy Reviews*, *8*(16), 81–87. https://doi.org/10.4103/0973-7847.134230.

Johnny Lau, S. W., & Abernethy, D. R. (2012). Chapter 26: Drug therapy in the elderly. In A. J. Atkinson, S. M. Huang, J. J. Lertora, & S. P. Markey (Eds.), *Principles of Clinical Pharmacology* (3rd ed., pp. 437–453). Academic Press. https://www.sciencedirect.com/science/article/pii/B978012385471100026X.

Kaufman, D. W., Kelly, J. P., Rosenberg, L., Anderson, T. E., & Mitchell, A. A. (2002). Recent patterns of medication use in the ambulatory adult population of the United States: the Slone survey. *JAMA*, *287*(3), 337–344. https://doi.org/10.1001/jama.287.3.337.

Kinirons, M. T., & O'Mahony, M. S. (2004). Drug metabolism and ageing. *British Journal of Clinical Pharmacology*, *57*(5), 540–544. https://doi.org/10.1111/j.1365-2125.2004.02096.x.

Klotz, U. (2009). Pharmacokinetics and drug metabolism in the elderly. *Drug Metabolism Reviews.*, *41*(2), 67–76.

Le, J., Porter, R. S., & Kaplan, J. L. (2019). Overview of pharmacokinetics—Clinical pharmacology. *Merck Manual*. https://www.merckmanuals.com/professional/clinical%20pharmacology/pharmacokinetics/overview-of-pharmacokinetics.

Lieberman, J. A., 3rd (2004). Managing anticholinergic side effects. *Primary care companion to the Journal of Clinical Psychiatry.*, *6*(Suppl. 2), 20–23.

Mahabadi, N. (n.d.). Volume of distribution - StatPearls - NCBI Bookshelf. StatPearls. https://www.ncbi.nlm.nih.gov/books/NBK545280/

Maher, R. L., Hanlon, J., & Hajjar, E. R. (2014). Clinical consequences of polypharmacy in elderly. *Expert Opinion on Drug Safety*, *13*(1), 57–65. https://doi.org/10.1517/14740338.2013.827660.

Mangoni, A. A., & Jackson, S. H. (2004). Age-related changes in pharmacokinetics and pharmacodynamics: basic principles and practical applications. *British Journal of Clinical Pharmacology*, *57*(1), 6–14. https://doi.org/10.1046/j.1365-2125.2003.02007.x.

Marcum, Z. A., & Hanlon, J. T. (2012). Commentary on the new American Geriatric Society Beers Criteria for potentially inappropriate medication use in older adults. *American Journal of Geriatric Pharmacotherapy*, *10*(2), 151–159. https://doi.org/10.1016/j.amjopharm.2012.03.002.

Marcum, Z. A., Perera, S., Thorpe, J. M., Switzer, G. E., Castle, N. G., Strotmeyer, E. S., et al. (2016). Antidepressant use and Recurrent falls in community-dwelling older adults: Findings from the Health ABC Study. *Annals of Pharmacotherapy*, *50*(7), 525–533. https://doi.org/10.1177/1060028016644466.

Martin, C. B., Hales, C. M., Gu, Q., & Ogden, C. L. (2019). Prescription Drug Use in the United States, 2015-2016. *NCHS data brief*.(334), 1–8.

Maton, P. N., & Burton, M. E. (1999). Antacids revisited: A review of their clinical pharmacology and recommended therapeutic use. *Drugs*, *57*(6), 855–770. https://doi.org/10.2165/00003495-199957060-00003.

McQueen, C. E., & Orr, K. K. (2018). Chapter 51: Natural products. In D. L. Krinsky (Ed.), *Handbook of nonprescription drugs: An interactive approach to self-care* (19th ed.). American Pharmacists Association doi-org.libproxy1.usc.edu/10.21019/9781582122656.ch51.

Melton, S. T., & Kirkwood, C. K. (2017). Chapter 46: Insomnia, drowsiness, and fatigue. In D. L. Krinsky (Ed.), *Handbook of nonprescription drugs: An interactive approach to self-care* (19th ed.). American Pharmacists Association doi-org.libproxy1.usc.edu/10.21019/9781582122656.ch46.

Minnesota Prevention Resource Center. (2017). Resources list: Opioid use in the older adult population. *SAMHSA's State Technical Assistance Contract*, *1*(1), 1–6. https://mnprc.org/wp-content/uploads/2019/01/resources-opiod-use-older-adult-pop.pdf.

Mol, A., Bui Hoang, P. T. S., Sharman, S., Reijinierse, E. M., Van Wezel, R. J. A., Meskers, C. G. M., & Maier, A. B. (2019). Orthostatic hypotension and falls in older adults: A systematic review and meta-analysis. *Journal of the American Medical Directors Association*, *20*(5), 589–597. https://doi.org/10.1016/j.jamda.2018.11.003.

Morin, L., Johnell, K., Laroche, M. L., Fastbom, J., & Wastesson, J. W. (2018). The epidemiology of polypharmacy in older adults: Register-based prospective cohort study. *Clinical Epidemiology*, *10*, 289–298. https://doi.org/10.2147/CLEP.S153458.

Mueller, S. K., Sponsler, K. C., Kripalani, S., & Schnipper, J. L. (2012). Hospital-based medication reconciliation practices: a systematic review. *Archives of internal medicine*, *172*(14), 1057–1069. https://doi.org/10.1001/archinternmed.2012.2246.

National Cancer Institute. (2020). Complementary and alternative medicine (CAM). National Cancer Institute. (n.d.). https://www.cancer.gov/about-cancer/treatment/cam

National Center for Complementary and Integrative Health. (2013). *Traditional Chinese medicine: What you need to know*. https://nccih.nih.gov/health/whatiscam/chinesemed.htm#hed2

National Center for Complementary and Integrative Health. (2019b). *Cannabis (marijuana) and cannabinoids: What you need to know.* https://www.nccih.nih.gov/health/cannabis-marijuana-and-cannabinoids-what-you-need-to-know

National Center for Complementary and Integrative Health. (2019c). *Complementary, alternative, or integrative health: What's in a name?* https://nccih.nih.gov/health/integrative-health

National Center for Complementary and Integrative Health. (2019d). *Homeopathy.* https://nccih.nih.gov/health/homeopathy#hed2

National Center for Complementary and Integrative Health. (2019e). *Using dietary supplements wisely.* https://nccih.nih.gov/health/supplements/wiseuse.htm#hed8

National Institute on Aging. (2019). *Safe use of medicines for older adults.* https://www.nia.nih.gov/health/safe-use-medicines-older-adults

National Institute on Drug Abuse. (2019). *Marijuana.* https://www.drugabuse.gov/publications/research-reports/marijuana/marijuana-safe-effective-medicine

National Institutes of Health Office of Dietary Supplements. (n.d.). *Ephedra.* https://ods.od.nih.gov/Health_Information/Ephedra.aspx

National Institutes of Health Office of Dietary Supplements. (2004). *Ephedra and ephedrine alkaloids for weight loss and athletic performance.* https://ods.od.nih.gov/factsheets/ephedraandephedrine-HealthProfessional

Nguyen, J. K., Fouts, M. M., Kotabe, S. E., & Lo, E. (2006). Polypharmacy as a risk factor for adverse drug reactions in geriatric nursing home residents. *The American journal of geriatric pharmacotherapy, 4*(1), 36–41. https://doi.org/10.1016/j.amjopharm.2006.03.002.

Nkansah, N., Mostovetsky, O., Yu, C., Chheng, T., Beney, J., Bond, C. M., & Bero, L. (2010). Effect of outpatient pharmacists' non-dispensing roles on patient outcomes and prescribing patterns. *The Cochrane database of systematic reviews, 2010*(7), CD000336. https://doi.org/10.1002/14651858.CD000336.pub2.

Olenak, J. L. (2017). Chapter 7: Musculoskeletal injuries and disorders. In D. L. Krinsky (Ed.), *Handbook of nonprescription drugs: An interactive approach to self-care* (19th ed.). American Pharmacists Association doi-org.libproxy1.usc.edu/10.21019/9781582122656.ch7.

Ralph, N. L., Mielenz, T. J., Parton, H., Flatley, A. -M., & Thorpe, L. E. (2013). Multiple Chronic Conditions and Limitations in Activities of Daily Living in a Community-Based Sample of Older Adults in New York City, 2009. *CUNY Graduate School of Public Health & Health Policy., 100,* 1–10.

Rivera, R., & Antognini, J. F. (2009). Perioperative drug therapy in elderly patients. *Anesthesiology, 110*(5), 1176–1181. https://doi.org/10.1097/aln.0b013e3181a10207.

Ruscin, J., Porter, R. S., & Kaplan, J. L. (2018a). Pharmacokinetics in older adults—Geriatrics. *Merck Manual.* https://www.merckmanuals.com/professional/geriatrics/drug-therapy-in-older-adults/pharmacokinetics-in-older-adults.

Ruscin, J. M., Linnebur, S. A., Porter, R. S., & Kaplan, J. L. (2018b). Drug categories of concern in older adults. *Merck Manual.* https://www.merckmanuals.com/professional/geriatrics/drug-therapy-in-older-adults/drug-categories-of-concern-in-older-adults.

Santschi, V., Chiolero, A., Burnand, B., Colosimo, A. L., & Paradis, G. (2011). Impact of pharmacist care in the management of cardiovascular disease risk factors: a systematic review and meta-analysis of randomized trials. *Archives of internal medicine, 171*(16), 1441–1453. https://doi.org/10.1001/archinternmed.2011.399.

Scolaro, K. L. (2017). Chapter 11: Colds and allergy. In D. L. Krinsky (Ed.), *Handbook of nonprescription drugs: An interactive approach to self-care* (19th ed.). American Pharmacists Association doi-org.libproxy1.usc.edu/10.21019/9781582122656.ch11.

Shehab, N., Lovegrove, M. C., Geller, A. I., Rose, K. O., Weidle, N. J., & Budnitz, D. S. (2016). US Emergency Department Visits for Outpatient Adverse Drug Events, 2013–2014. *JAMA, 316*(20), 2115–2125. https://doi.org/10.1001/jama.2016.16201.

Shenoy, P., & Harugeri, A. (2015). Elderly patients' participation in clinical trials. *Perspectives in Clinical Research., 6*(4), 184–189.

Shurtleff, D. (2019). Workshop summary outlines current landscape and future prospects for cannabis research. *National Center for Complementary and Integrative Health.* https://www.nccih.nih.gov/research/blog/workshop-summary-outlines-current-landscape-and-future-prospects-for-cannabis-research.

Stompór, M., Grodzicki, T., Stompór, T., Wordliczek, J., Dubiel, M., & Kurowska, I. (2019). Prevalence of chronic pain, particularly with neuropathic component, and its effect on overall functioning of elderly patients. *Medical Science Monitor, 25,* 2695–2701. https://doi.org/10.12659/msm.911260.

Therapeutic Research Center Natural Medicines. Vitamin K. (2020). https://naturalmedicines-therapeuticresearch-com/databases/food,-herbs-supplements/professional.aspx?productid=983

Tsourounis, C., & Dennehy, C. (2018). Chapter 50: Introduction to dietary supplements. In D. L. Krinsky (Ed.), *Handbook of nonprescription drugs: An interactive approach to self-care* (19th ed.). American Pharmacists Association doi-org.libproxy1.usc.edu/10.21019/9781582122656.ch50.

Turnheim, K. (2003). When drug therapy gets old: Pharmacokinetics and pharmacodynamics in the elderly. *Experimental Gerontology, 38*(8), 843–853. https://doi.org/10.1016/s0531-5565(03)00133-5.

The 2019 American Geriatrics Society Beers Criteria® Update Expert Panel. (2019). American Geriatrics Society 2019 Updated AGS Beers Criteria® for potentially inappropriate medication use in older adults. *Journal of the American Geriatrics Society, 67*(4), 674–694. https://doi.org/10.1111/jgs.15767.

Ulbricht, C., & Ko, E. M. (2018). Chapter 52: Common complementary and integrative medicine health systems. In D. L. Krinsky (Ed.), *Handbook of nonprescription drugs: An interactive approach to self-care* (19th ed.). American Pharmacists Association doi-org.libproxy1.usc.edu/10.21019/9781582122656.ch52.

U.S. Centers for Medicare & Medicaid Services. (2017). Chronic conditions. CMS. (2017). https://www.cms.gov/Research-Statistics-Data-and-Systems/Statistics-Trends-and-Reports/Chronic-Conditions/CC_Main

U.S. Food and Drug Administration (FDA). (2007). *Backgrounder on the final rule for current good manufacturing practices (CGMPs) for dietary supplements.* https://www.fda.gov/food/current-good-manufacturing-practices-cgmps-food-and-dietary-supplements/backgrounder-final-rule-current-good-manufacturing-practices-cgmps-dietary-supplements

U.S. Food and Drug Administration (FDA). (2019a). *Dietary supplements.* https://www.fda.gov/food/dietary-supplements

U.S. Food and Drug Administration (FDA). (2019b). *Questions and answers on dietary supplements.* https://www.fda.gov/food/information-consumers-using-dietary-supplements/questions-and-answers-dietary-supplements

Veldurthy, V., Wei, R., Oz, L., Dhawan, P., Jeon, Y. H., & Christakos, S. (2016). Vitamin D, calcium homeostasis and aging. *Bone Research, 4*(1). https://doi.org/10.1038/boneres.2016.41.

Welch, A. C. (2017). Chapter 19: Nausea and vomiting. In D. L. Krinsky (Ed.), *Handbook of nonprescription drugs: An interactive approach to self-care* (19th ed.). American Pharmacists Association doi-org.libproxy1.usc.edu/10.21019/9781582122656.ch19.

Whetsel, T., & Zweber, A. (2017). Chapter 13: Heartburn and dyspepsia. In D. L. Krinsky (Ed.), *Handbook of nonprescription drugs: An interactive approach to self-care* (19th ed.). American Pharmacists Association doi-org.libproxy1.usc.edu/10.21019/9781582122656.ch13.

Wilkinson, J. J., & Tromp, K. (2017). Chapter 5: Headache. In D. L. Krinsky (Ed.), *Handbook of nonprescription drugs: An interactive approach to self-care* (19th ed.). American Pharmacists Association doi-org.libproxy1.usc.edu/10.21019/9781582122656.ch5.

Wongrakpanich, S., Wongrakpanich, A., Melhado, K., & Rangaswami, J. (2018). A comprehensive review of non-steroidal anti-inflammatory drug use in the elderly. *Aging and Disease*, *9*(1), 143–150. https://doi.org/10.14336/AD.2017.0306.

World Health Organization (WHO). (2005). NSAIDs—Black box warning for both prescription and OTC products *WHO Pharmaceuticals Newsletter* (3, pp. 4–5) https://apps.who.int/medicinedocs/pdf/s8118e/s8118e.pdf.

9

Complementary and Integrative Therapies for Older Adults

KERRY S. FANKHAUSER, DNP, RN, AHN-BC, UZIT

OBJECTIVES

Student Learning Objectives

After completing this chapter, the student should be able to do the following:

1. Describe the history and evolution of complementary and alternative therapies into Western medicine practice for the older adult.
2. Identify the five broad complementary and alternative therapy categories as defined by the National Center for Complementary and Integrative Health.
3. List common complementary and alternative therapies and rationale of therapies used by the older adult.

Practitioner Objectives

After completing this chapter, the practitioner should be able to do the following:

1. Demonstrate and critically analyze complementary and integrative health data and evidence in clinical situations to improve advanced practice.
2. Apply clinical science regarding complementary and integrative health to diagnose health conditions using advanced decision making, clinical problem solving, and evidence-based practices.
3. Acknowledge the individual's environmental, social, and cultural influences, and assess the patient's and caregiver's educational needs to provide personalized health care.
4. Collaborate with other professionals to integrate complementary and integrative health care with other health interventions.

Definition and History of Complementary and Alternative Therapies in the Older Adult

In about the early 1800s, biomedicine, the concept that the mind and body are separate, was created from the *reductionist approach* founded by René Descartes (1596–1650) (Fontaine, 2015). Prior to this view, many cultures over thousands of years throughout the world had used traditional healing practices that incorporated holistic healing of the whole person (mind, body, and spirit) and one's belonging and balance within nature and the world (Ross, 2009). Even Hippocrates (circa 460 BC), the father of medicine, believed in a holistic approach to create harmony between an individual and nature to promote wellness (Dossey & Keegan, 2016).

There have been many names to describe therapeutic practices that cover a broad range of concepts, approaches, and modalities; these have amalgamated with Western allopathic medicine, which is a medical system that focuses on treating symptoms and diseases. Alternative therapies are modalities or practices that are used in place of or instead of mainstream or biomedical modalities, and complementary therapies are practices used in conjunction with allopathic therapies (Koithan, 2009). Integrative medicine refers to therapies that integrate the practitioner and patient relationship, the whole person along with one's preferences, culture and community, and care that is informed by evidence; it also utilizes a combination of appropriate therapies to promote optimal health of the individual (Koithan, 2009).

Understanding the healing modalities and their effects on a person's well-being is a concept that continues to evolve worldwide. In the United States, the National Center for Complementary and Alternative Medicine (NCCAM), as part of the National Institute of Health (NIH), was founded in 1998 by Congress and coined the term *complementary and alternative medicine (CAM)* (NIH, 2005). Within the NCCAM, five categories were identified regarding healing modalities: (1) mind-body therapies, (2) biology-based therapies, (3) manipulative and body-based methods, (4) energy therapies, and (5) whole medical and alternative systems (Koithan, 2009; Ness et al., 2005). Because CAM includes various worldviews, philosophies, principles, modalities, products, and types of practices, a more encompassing nomenclature was needed to reflect these modalities fully. In 2014, Congress changed the name of the NCCAM to the National Center for Complementary and Integrative Health (NCCIH) to reflect the center's research commitment more accurately, which was to study inclusive health approaches being used by the American public (NIH, 2015). NCCIH has condensed the five categories into three categories: (1) natural

CASE STUDY

A 65-year-old white female presents to her community clinic and is seen by the nurse practitioner (NP). Her chief complaint is that after her fall 2 days ago (for which no fractures were noted by the emergency department health care provider), she feels pain and stiffness in her joints, more than the usual arthritic "aches and pains" generalized in her joints, and is also worried that she will fall again. The patient also states that she is feeling anxious over the possibility that her children in another state will "make" her move out of her home and into a long-term care facility, as she now lives alone because her husband passed away 9 months ago. She displays sadness when talking about her husband. The patient wants to nonpharmacologically reduce her overall stiffness by improving her circulation. She also wants to have better balance to prevent the likelihood of another fall, which might reduce her independence. She's worried that adding more oral medications might make her lightheaded and dizzy. She states she is open to trying something new.

History

- Hypertension for 10 years

List of Medications

1. Hydrochlorothiazide (HCTZ) 25 mg PO, once in the morning
2. Potassium supplement (K-tab) 20 milliequivalents (mEq) PO once in the morning
3. Acetaminophen 650 mg PO daily as needed for arthritis pain

Assessment

- 5′4″, 132 lbs (60 kgs)
- Vital statistics: Blood pressure (B/P): 140/82, pulse (P): 71 (resting), R: 16, temperature (T): 98.2
- Arthritic pain level: 3

Problem

The NP is generally aware of complementary and integrative practices. She asks the patient if she is aware of therapies such as yoga, aromatherapy, tai chi, meditation, and the extent of the support system in her community.

Discussion

1. The NP expresses her rationale for suggesting that the patient use a community resource in her neighborhood—for instance, a senior citizen center (SCC) that offers simple classes such as chair yoga or tai chi classes. The NP suggests that the patient attend these classes two to three times per week. The NP knows that the evidence supports the use of yoga and tai chi to reduce arthritis pain and, with regular practice, improve one's sense of balance. Also, the SCC offers an inexpensive way to promote exercise that can increase the patient's overall circulation.
2. The NP also knows that utilization of the SCC will help the patient feel less isolated and may improve her outlook on life since losing her husband. If the SCC is in close proximity to the patient's home, she might know some of the individuals at the SCC, some of whom may be her neighbors.
3. The NP also suggests that the patient consider using aromatherapy, such as one that would incorporate lavender for its antiinflammatory and analgesic properties. The NP states that the patient can try to use an essential oil in a diffuser first and then apply the diluted oil topically to her feet in the evening prior to sleep. The NP knows that evidence supports the use of lavender for sleep, which might benefit the patient's overall mood and help her to avoid depression as she works through the loss of her husband and the changes this has brought to her life.
4. The NP wants the patient to continue her regular medications and to be seen again in the clinic in 6 months to check her vital statistics, potassium (K+) level, arthritis pain, and balance issues (additional falls), and to gauge patient's use and any benefits gained from the SCC, yoga or tai chi, and aromatherapy.

products, (2) mind and body practices (Fig. 9.1), and (3) other complementary health approaches. Because the three new categories are nondescriptive, for the purposes of this chapter the original five categories will be delineated to provide a more in-depth understanding of modalities.

The need for more holistic approaches is especially important in the older adult community, as there is an emphasis on quality of life, pain management, and maintaining health as opposed to mainly curing treatments. First one must understand the concept of holism and its effect in health care. Holism, from the Greek word *holos* meaning "whole," as termed in the early 1900s by Jan Smuts from Cambridge University (as cited in Erickson, 2007), is the natural tendency for groups of units to be organized together. Although often in health care "whole" has been defined as the sum of its parts, many holistic practitioners view this concept differently; these parts regarding a human should not be broken down into detached subcategories of systems, as reflected in the reductionist model, or made separate from one's environment (Erickson, 2007). The concept of holism includes wholeness of the person, focused on wellness and the ever-present interconnection to others and the environment (Hani & Ahmad, 2016).

The National Center for Health Statistics (NCHS) conducts interviews approximately every 5 years regarding the use of complementary and alternative therapies by different age groups. The NCHS noted that yoga, meditation, and chiropractic usage all increased among US adults from 2012 to 2017 (Clarke et al., 2018). Many older adults use complementary, alternative, and integrative modalities specifically for chronic conditions such as arthritis, hypertension, cardiovascular and circulatory ailments, pain management, psychosocial conditions, and orthopedic impairments (Eliopoulos, 2015).

Evidence Supporting Complementary and Alternative Therapies in the Older Adult

The health care community continues to promote care that is based on evidence and drives how care needs to be implemented or how holistic care can be combined with allopathic care. The NIH-NCCIH conducts and

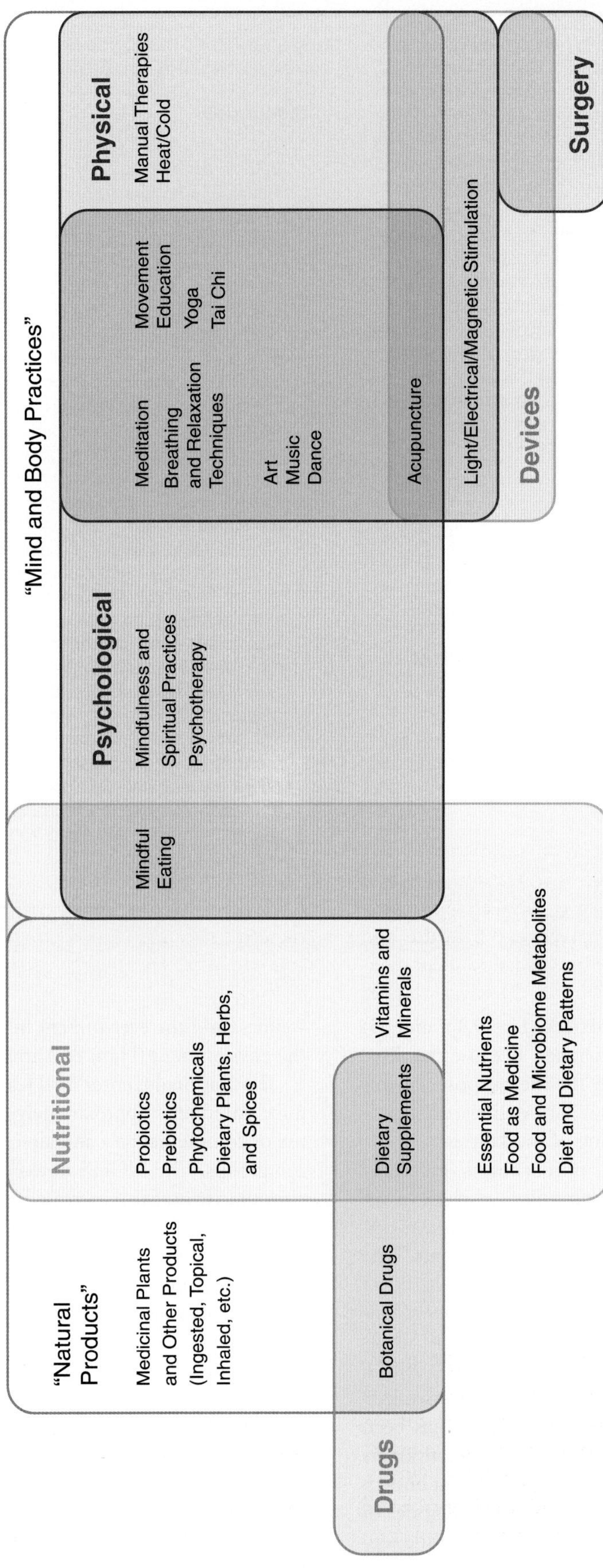

• **Fig 9.1** Example of complementary health approaches that fall within the categories: Psychological, Physical, and Nutritional. (From https://www.nccih.nih.gov/health/complementary-alternative-or-integrative-health-whats-in-a-name.)

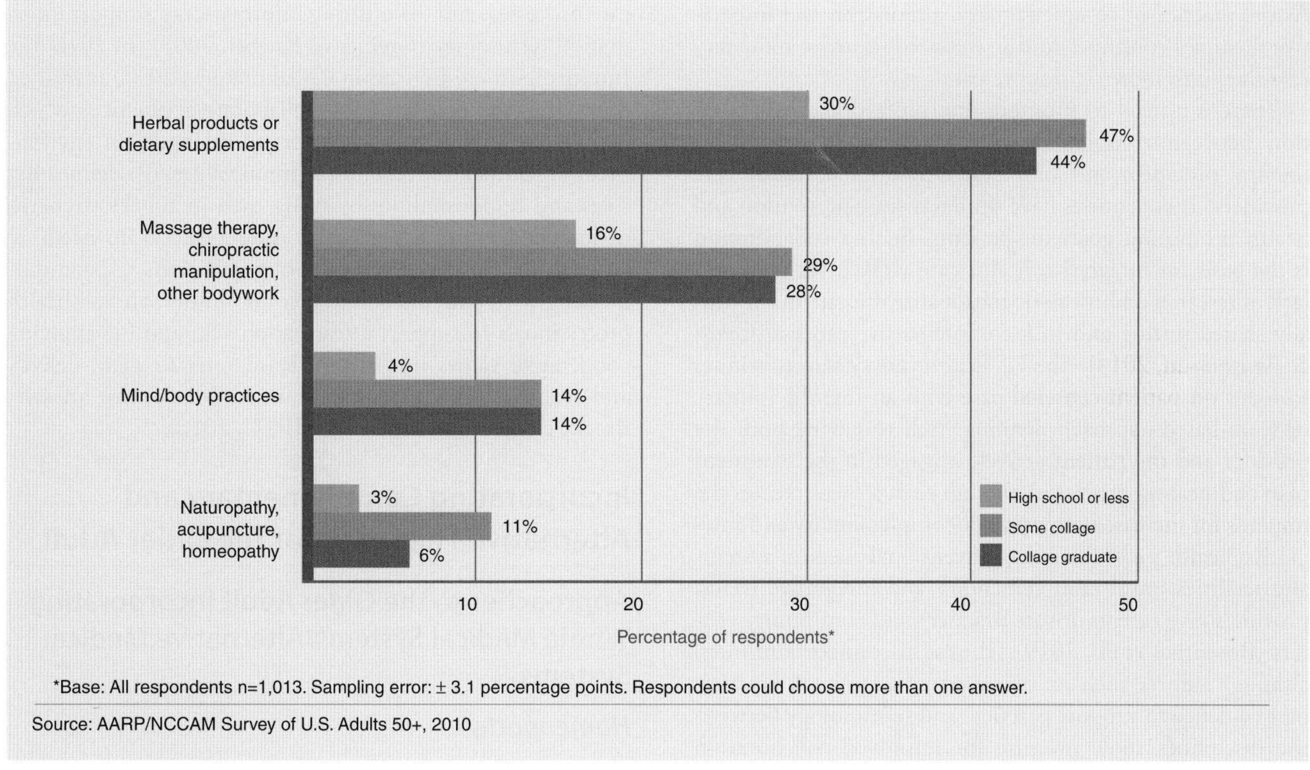

• **Fig. 9.2** Education level and type of CAM used in the past 12 months (From AARP and National Center for Complementary and Alternative Medicine Survey Report. [2011, April]. https://files.nccih.nih.gov/s3fs-public/news/camstats/2010/NCCAM_aarp_survey.pdf.

supports complementary, alternative, and integrative therapies research while providing evidential information. The Institute of Medicine (IOM) endorses education for health care professionals that emphasizes a proactive comprehensive approach that integrates best practices for health and wellness (Alperson, 2017). Due to the older adult population's growing chronic conditions, the IOM advises higher learning institutions to include integrative healing or integrative holistic health care (IHHC) into their curricula. It is crucial that NPs and physician assistants (PAs) have education regarding the benefits and risks of complementary, alternative, and integrative therapies to patients not only to know how to use them but also to provide evidence regarding these therapies to their patients.

The 2010 NCCAM survey report (Fig. 9.2) showed that individuals age 50 and older most often learned of complementary, alternative, and integrative practices from family or friends (26%) and the Internet (14%), whereas only than a third of these older adults learned about these practices from their physicians or health care providers (NIH, 2011). One reason for the lack of discussion is that health care providers do not bring up or initiate the topic for discussion. Additionally, if not asked, patients do not know or feel comfortable elaborating on the subject (NIH, 2011). The National Institute on Aging provides evidence-based resources regarding complementary, alternative, and integrative therapies for older adults. Additionally, the Natural Standard research collaboration provides peer-reviewed and evidence-based practices regarding complementary, alternative, and integrative therapies (Kreitzer & Koithan, 2014).

The American Holistic Nurses Association (AHNA) also is an excellent complementary, alternative, and integrative therapies resource and was founded in 1981 in the United States by Charlotte McGuire and 75 other members (Dossey & Keegan, 2016). The AHNA supports the use of evidence-based practice in healing modalities. The AHNA recognizes the categories of CAM therapies and the trends within holistic nursing and health care reform in the *Patient Protection and Affordable Healthcare Act (HR 3590)* authorized in the United States. NPs and PAs determined to identify the most recent and current research regarding complementary, alternative, and integrative therapies are encouraged to view these findings at http://www.nlm.nih.gov/medlineplus/complementaryandalternativemedicine.html.

Preventive Care and Holistic Approach of Complementary and Alternative Therapies

When health care providers are assessing the gerontologic population, it is crucial to identify all elements of healing a patient is using to promote the health and well-being. Because so many older adults are living with chronic conditions and have limited financial resources, seniors are seeking complementary, alternative, and integrative therapies to supplement the use of expensive pharmaceuticals, which often have high risks of side effects and adverse reactions (Eliopoulos, 2015).

As the practice of complementary, alternative, and integrative therapies continues to rise, the need to invest monetary resources into more rigorous research exists.

There is a need to promote interprofessional collaboration between complementary and alternative/integrative therapy providers and biomedical/traditional health care providers. These entities have similar disease prevention and health promotion goals for patients. Such a collaboration is the basis for integrative health care (IHC), yet there is a lack of research on how to operationalize the care in a mutually shared setting and in a comprehensive process (Grant & Bensoussan, 2014). The US health care system continues to focus on patient-centered care with an interdisciplinary or team-based approach, lending itself to having both the provider and the patient actively engaged in the treatment plan and healing process. Although such a focus creates the impetus for increased inclusion of complementary and integrative health providers into conventional medical systems and facilities, most complementary and integrative health providers give care in private practices and community centers (Rosenthal et al., 2019). Thus a disconnect continues, although efforts such as increased education of practice, best evidence to support practice, and terminology between the disciplines show promise for improved collaboration (Grant et al., 2014; Rosenthal et al., 2019).

Nurse Practitioner and Physician Assistant Roles

For the older adult population, it is important for NPs and PAs to consider all aspects of a patient's life when assessing health needs. A holistic gerontologic assessment is useful when obtaining health information. One approach would be to use the Shuler NP Practice Model to guide the health care provider when conducting an assessment and developing a treatment plan focused on wellness, natural, alternative, and complementary therapies (NAC), and pharmacologic therapies (Shuler et al., 2001). This model emphasizes an individual's personal level of functioning, psychological responses when not in balance, physical capacities, beliefs, and cultural and spiritual influences and beliefs regarding health and treatment (Shuler et al., 2001). The Shuler model promotes a holistic approach to health care and is patient centered. It incorporates both the complementary and integrative therapies with allopathic health care as needed for patients' healing processes.

Roles of Other Members of the Interprofessional Team

When team members are collaborating in treatment plans and care for patients, it is important for all members of the team to be competent in their areas of expertise. The IOM delineated five core competencies for all health care professionals to follow, which include (1) providing patient-centered care, (2) working in interdisciplinary teams, (3) employing evidence-based practice, (4) applying quality improvements to care processes, and (5) utilizing informatics to support information technology (Greiner & Knebel, 2003). In 2016, the Interprofessional Education Collaborative (IPEC) identified four core competencies for collaborative practice, which included (1) working with others to maintain an environment of mutual respect and common values, (2) delineating roles and responsibilities by using each member's strengths of knowledge and expertise to assess health care needs of patients and promote the health of populations, (3) communicating with patients/families, communities, and all health professionals to support a team approach, and (4) applying cooperative values in different team roles to plan, deliver, and evaluate health care programs and policies that are safe, timely, efficient, and equitable (IPEC, 2016).

Incorporating Complementary and Alternative Therapies for the Older Adult

Approaches to the Older Adult Incorporating Whole Medical Systems/Alternative Medical Systems

Homeopathy

A German physician and chemist, Samuel Hahnemann, developed the therapeutic system known as *homeopathy* in the late 1700s (Fontaine, 2015). Homeopathy, from the Greek words *omiois* ("similar") and *pathos* ("feeling"), is based on the "principles of similars," meaning "like cures like." The technique is based on using repeatedly diluted ingredients to heal an ill person that, if they were nondiluted, would normally cause illness in a healthy person (Teut et al., 2010). The premise is that the symptoms reflect the body's effort to heal, and using minute dosages of the substance that in high dosages would create sickness in a healthy person will have a curative effect on an ill person (Dossey & Keegan, 2016). These repeated dilutions are vigorously shaken (succession) to increase the vibration of the remedy, enhancing the magnetic fields of the resonance frequencies (Dossey & Keegan, 2016). Although this system is not scientifically based, it is widely used throughout the world, with rates in the United States ranging from 1.7% to 4.4% of the population (Relton et al., 2017). Homeopathic ingredients include substances from plants, animals, minerals, and chemicals and are so vastly diluted that no molecules of the original substance are noted (Dossey & Keegan, 2016).

Teut et al. (2010) found that older people frequently used homeopathic remedies for hypertension, sleep hygiene, diabetes, sciatica and low back pain, osteoarthritis, and depression. Regarding the older adult population using homeopathy, general questions from NPs and PAs include asking specifically about the patient's use and knowledge of complementary and integrative therapies. Although no gold-standard type of history assessment is noted in the literature, questions need to be nonjudgmental yet thorough. These questions should allow the practitioner to determine what types of therapies are being used, what they are being used for, how much (dosage) or how often they are being used, and if the therapies are being prescribed by a health care provider. Resources that NPs and PAs can use with their patients are available from the American Institute of Homeopathy and the National Center for Homeopathy.

Evidence for Homeopathy

According to the NIH's National Center for Complementary and Integrative Health, the evidence to support the efficacy of homeopathy is minimal. Additionally, homeopathy is used for various conditions, and there is little research regarding the safety of homeopathy products.

Naturopathy

Naturopathy is a medicinal system that relies on the healing power within nature to promote health, prevent disease, and support the responsibility of the patient to be educated regarding one's health (McCabe, 2000). In the 19th century, Dr. John Scheel from New York City was the originator of the term *naturopathy*, although Benedict Lust is credited with validating naturopathy as a medicinal system (Fontaine, 2015). Its focus is on health versus disease and, similar to the nursing practice, has a holistic perspective of health with an emphasis on patient education. Naturopathy was practiced in ancient Greece and is now supported by research for nutritional guidance, herbal applications, and the promotion of holistic health. Hippocrates once stated: "*It is more important to know what sort of person has a disease than to know what sort of disease a person has*" (cited by Fontaine, 2015). Naturopathic medicine emphasizes clinical counseling for self-care and preventive practices (Oberg et al., 2014). Naturopathic physicians are utilized as primary care practitioners, thus they do not provide emergency or surgical care (Fontaine, 2015).

The basic principles of a naturopathic medicine include (1) first do no harm, (2) use therapies that are harmonious with restorative powers found in nature, (3) identify causative factor(s) diminishing a patient's health state, (4) treat the whole person in her or his contextual environment, (5) reestablish one's vitality and optimal healthy balance, (6) use preventive medicine, and (7) educate the patient (McCabe, 2000). Harmonious therapies noted in nature include sunshine, clean air and water, good sleep hygiene, suitable food, and herbals, along with physical movement, proper elimination, and having purpose in life (McCabe, 2000). Deficiencies in any of these categories may be a cause for imbalance or disease. Florence Nightingale also understood the importance of one's environment to promote optimal conditions for healing (Huisman et al., 2012). Nightingale felt that the patient needed to be supported by the best conditions for nature to assist in the healing process (McCabe, 2000).

In the older adult population, it is important for NPs and PAs to have a cursory understanding of naturopathy and to identify what naturopathy remedies patients are using and why they are using them. Oberg et al. (2014) noted that the older adult primarily used naturopathic medicines for fatigue, anxiety, diabetes, diarrhea, upper respiratory infections (URIs), depression, insomnia, limb pain, GERD, and hypertension. Examples of naturopathy remedies for anxiety and depression may include vitamins, minerals, nutritional supplements, pharmaceuticals, herbals, acupuncture, and even some homeopathic treatments (Breed & Bereznay, 2017). Resources available to NPs and PAs include those provided by the American Botanical Council, the American Herbalist Guild, the Herb Research Foundation, the Herb Society of America, the American Association of Naturopathic Physicians, the International Listening Association, and the National Center for Complementary and Integrative Health (NIH-NCCIH).

Evidence for Naturopathy

The evidence for using naturopathy, which supports health maintenance, illness prevention, patient education, and patient responsibility, is growing. An example is the use of herbs and herbals, which are an element of naturopathy. Older adults frequently use herbs and herbals such as ginkgo biloba for maintenance of memory, echinacea to strengthen the immune system, St. John's Wort to ward off depression, and garlic to reduce cholesterol in the body (Altizer et al., 2013). The use of naturopathic medicines has been shown to result in statistically significant improvements in patients treated for depression and anxiety (Breed & Bereznay, 2017). When naturopathic medicine has been used in clinical settings with older adults, the patients exhibited improved self-care behaviors (Oberg et al., 2014).

Ayurveda

Another major medical system is Ayurveda, which originated in India more than 5000 years ago and accentuates the science of life and longevity (Fontaine, 2015). *Ayurveda* in the Sanskrit language derives from *ayur* ("life") and *veda* ("knowledge") and recognizes the interdependence of an individual's health and the quality of one's life within one's natural world and the cosmos (Fontaine, 2015). The World Health Organization (WHO) recognizes Ayurveda as a medical science in which holistic principles include primary, secondary, and tertiary preventive practices, along with patient empowerment and self-efficacy (Kessler et al., 2013). This ancient system integrates modern science and technology with biomedical science and quantum physics using the principles of the five elements: earth, water, fire, air, and space containing both matter and energy. In Ayurvedic medicine, all individuals have properties of all these elements that combine to regulate one's mind, body, and spirit. These individual combinations contribute to a person's body as *doshas* (three vital energies: *Vata*, *Pitta*, and *Kapha*), *dhatus* (seven tissues: plasma, blood, muscle, fat, bone, marrow/nerve, and reproductive tissue), and *malas* (three excretions: urine, stool, and sweat). Being healthy in Ayurvedic tradition means having a balance of the doshas as is needed for an individual (Fontaine, 2015).

Ayurveda views geriatrics (*vārdhakya*) as the aging process (*jarā*) of change in physical, psychological, emotional, and

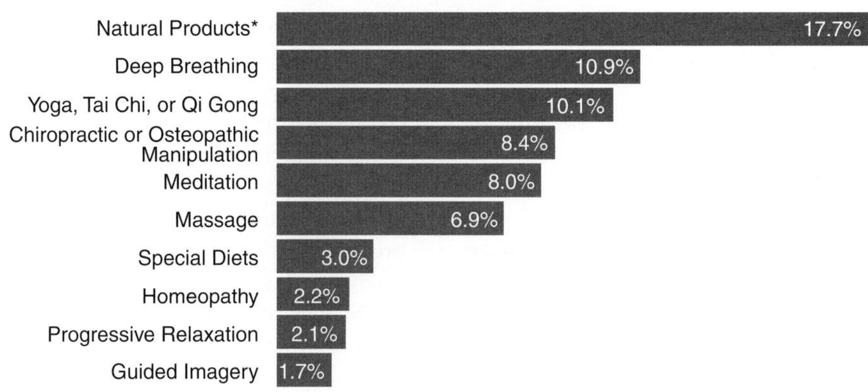

• **Fig. 9.3** 10 Most common complementary health approaches among adults—2012 (From https://www.nccih.nih.gov/health/complementary-alternative-or-integrative-health-whats-in-a-name.)

social aspects (Burdak & Gupta, 2015). Ayurvedic diagnoses involve a holistic approach, which uses a history assessment that includes a medical and family assessment, along with lifestyle questions, and identifies patterns in behavior. The physical exam includes an examination of the skin and tongue, along with osculation of the heart, lungs, and intestines (Narayanasami & Narayanasami, 2006). In Ayurveda, a preventive approach is to be initiated long before an individual reaches old age, thus discipline to one's adherence to diet, lifestyle, and social activities is crucial for longevity (Shukla, 2015). There is also an emphasis on the "tripods of life" (*trayopastambha*), which include food (*ahara*), sleep (*nidra*), and controlled sex (*brahmacarya*) (Burdak & Gupta, 2015). Ayurvedic treatments are focused on prevention and an individualistic approach using treatments such as nutrition, herbs, exercise, yoga, breathing techniques, meditation, massage, aromatherapy, music, and purification (Fontaine, 2015) (Fig. 9.3). Thus it is important for NPs and PAs to include these elements in their history assessments for patients that practice Ayurvedic medicine. Ayurvedic resources for NPs and PAs include those provided by the Alliance of International Aromatherapists, the American Herbalist Guild, the American Meditation Institute, the Herb Society of America, the Institute of Integrative Aromatherapy, the Yoga Alliance, Yoga Research Foundation, the American Holistic Nurses Association, the American Massage Therapy Association, the American Yoga Association, the International Association of Yoga Therapists, the National Association for Holistic Aromatherapy, the National Ayurvedic Medical Association, and the National Center for Complementary and Integrative Health (NIH-NCCIH).

Traditional Chinese Medicine/Acupuncture

Traditional Chinese medicine (TCM) encompasses many traditional practices, techniques, and medicines originating in China and then spreading into East Asian countries (Takayama & Iwasaki, 2017). TCM is more than 2500 years old, is practiced worldwide, and includes treatments such as acupuncture and acupressure, moxibustion and cupping, oriental massage, herbals, and oriental dietetics (Figueira et al., 2010). The goal of TCM is to promote health and quality of life by focusing on the person, not on the sickness or disease (Dossey & Keegan, 2016). There are three pillars in Chinese medicine theory: (1) the theory of yin-yang, (2) the theory of the five elements, and (3) the theory of Qi (Maciocia, 2015). Its philosophy, as noted in the Chinese textbook *Yellow Emperor's Classic of Internal Medicine* (*Huangdi Neijing*), stresses the exploration for harmony and balance within a constantly changing environment utilizing the union of opposites in yin (passive female principle of the universe) and yang (active male principle of the universe); the five phases or elements, which are (1) wood: liver/gallbladder, (2) fire: heart/small intestine, (3) earth: spleen/stomach, (4) metal: lungs/large intestine, and (5) water: kidneys/bladder); seasonal effects (spring, summer, late summer, autumn, and winter); the principles of qi (炁) (circulating energy); and treatment regimens (Fontaine, 2015).

Qi is distributed throughout all organisms via meridians (*Jingmai*) or networks that connect all parts to create wholeness of itself and interconnectedness to the universe (Dossey & Keegan, 2016). There are 12 paired primary meridians (6 yang and 6 yin symmetrical pairs) that correspond to the 12 major functions of the body, and there are also 8 secondary meridians (Wagner, 2015). In some texts, 14 meridians are noted because the 2 single midmeridians (the Governing Vessel flowing into the Conception Vessel) are important (Fontaine, 2015). When qi is blocked, an imbalance of matter and energy occur, and illness and disease can follow (Wagner, 2015). Along these meridians are 361 acupuncture points that, if activated, can unblock and reregulate the flow of qi (Covington, 2001).

Many people turn to TCM due to untoward side effects they may have experienced with allopathic medicine, along with the fact that allopathic medicine usually has no curative attributes for chronic conditions. Also, many older adults who are on fixed incomes cannot afford the high costs of commercial pharmaceuticals or have a microbial resistance to some medications (Figueira et al., 2010). Incorporating TCM into health care can be useful for older adult patients with issues such as chronic pain, stroke, bowel function, sleep hygiene, appetite stimulation, and quality-of-life improvement (Barad et al., 2008). Many local community health centers and senior citizen facilities offer seniors a variety of Chinese modalities such as tai chi, qigong, acupressure, and educational seminars either free as part of membership or at nominal fees. Resources that NPs and PAs can suggest to their older patients include those provided by seniorliving.org along with local senior citizen centers as well as those offered by the NCOA's National Institute of Senior Centers (NISC), Silver Sneakers, the Taoist Tai Chi Society, the American Association of Acupuncture and Oriental Medicine, the American Tai Chi and Qigong Association, the NIH-NCCIH, and the Therapeutic Massage & Bodywork Resource Center.

Native American Traditions

Prior to the establishment of European communities, there were approximately 5 million to 10 million people from different communities, with unique languages, cultures, and governance structures, living in America (Braun & LaCounte, 2015). Currently there are 573 recognized tribal nations (National Congress of American Indians, 2019). Although there is variation among nations, most have high respect for older adults because of their accrued wisdom, and older adults usually serve as community leaders (Dossey & Keegan, 2016). Family structure for Native Americans is unique from the Anglo-Saxon concept of "family." Native American family systems are extended kin and nonkin networks that form one's culture, socialization, and sense of selfhood shaping one's values and care concepts of physical, emotional, cultural, spiritual, and communal needs (Red Horse, 1980).

Customarily in Native American traditions there is an emphasis on harmony with nature, an orientation to the present moment (versus the past or the future), and an integration of rituals and ceremony being incorporated into daily life (Dossey & Keegan, 2016). Due to colonization, many indigenous communities suffered from subjugation, a loss of land and culture, and a loss of traditional lifestyles and power, all of which can be linked to health and social issues (Braun et al., 2015). In spite of the losses, many native American folk healing traditions are still practiced and have valued acceptance for healing by honoring the four constructs: (1) spirituality (Creator, Mother Earth, Great Father), (2) society (family, clan, tribe/nation), (3) milieu (daily life, nature, balance), and (4) self (inner desires and peace, beliefs, and principles) (Portman & Garrett, 2006). Many Native Americans do not differential religion from spirituality. They believe "spirituality means 'walking the path of Good Medicine' (living a good way of life) 'in harmony and balance' (through the harmonious interaction of mind, body spirit, and natural environment) 'with all our relations' (with all living beings in the Circle of Life)" (Portman & Garrett, 2006, p. 457).

Healing practices can include ceremonies, dancing, smudging (a ritual that utilizes smoke from ignited herbs to cleanse surrounding negative energies), and prayers for special occasions such as funerals and youth events. Although practices differ among specific nations, other traditional medicinal remedies for balance, harmony, and health are herbs, teas, tobacco, salves or poultices for physical infirmities, along with massage, therapeutic touch, and bodywork practices (Broome & Broome, 2007). Of great importance is the relationship and connection that one has with one's inner self, others, nature, the world, and the cosmos.

There are several culturally appropriate considerations NPs and PAs can use to bridge the cultural gap. Such actions include avoiding forceful eye contact, asking if the patient wants others to be part of the conversation, using a light touch handshake, and conveying information in a calm, straightforward, and tranquil voice tone (Broome & Broome, 2007). It is important for NPs and PAs to ask about the use of native plants for healing. Resources regarding these plants/herbs and their usage can be located through reputable websites such as NIH's Traditional Healing–American Indian and Alaska Native Health. NPs and PAs need to remember that regardless of the nation affiliation of the older Native American, three cultural principles remain paramount for optimum health: family connectedness, the need for physical activity, and access to healthy foods. Thus having a holistic approach that encompasses a bio-psycho-socio-spiritual perspective will help to build trust in the healing relationship with the patient. NPs and PAs can utilize relevant resources such as those provided by the American Society on Aging; Indian Health Services; the National Indigenous Women's Resource Center; the National Resource Center for American Indian, Alaska Native and Native Hawaiian Elders; the National Resource Center for Native Hawaiian Elders; the National Resource Center on Native American Aging; and the Office of Minority Health.

An important aspect for NPs and PAs to recognize is that all of these systems—homeopathy, naturopathy, Ayurveda, TCM, and Native American traditions—share common themes. First, they stress oneness with nature, environment, and a body-mind-culture premise. Second, these systems are meant to keep an individual in balance and optimal health. Curing diseases or illnesses is not the main emphasis as it is for the Western allopathic health system.

Additionally, many of these systems share similar healing modalities such as herbal remedies, aromatherapy, and massage. Although the types of herbals or aromatherapy plants or varieties of massage slightly differ, the intent for balance and wellness is comparable.

Evidence for Native American Traditions

The evidence indicates that Native Americans have a higher propensity for illnesses, chronic conditions, and death than Caucasian Americans (Braun & LaCounte, 2015; Broome & Broome, 2007). This includes twice as high rate of diabetes mellitus, stomach and liver cancers, and infant mortality, along with higher rates of unintentional injuries and suicide. Additionally, indigenous Americans' life expectancies are lower than that of the general population rates

(Braun et al., 2014). Although there are variations in different indigenous cultures, Hopkins and colleagues (2007) indicated that the inclusion of family, a focus on physical activity, and the concern for a healthy diet were important elements for healthy aging for native elders. Community-based approaches to improving the health of older Native Americans have been shown to be highly effective in engaging this vulnerable population, assessing needed care, and promoting intergenerational relationships, which is crucial to native elders' cultural identity (Browne et al., 2015).

Approaches to the Older Adult Incorporating Manipulative and Body-Based Methods

Massage/Acupressure

The use of massage, acupressure, and bodyworks can be found in many of the traditional healing practices such as in Ayurveda, TCM, and Native American traditions. Healing through touch is an ancient practice, as described in the Chinese *Huang Ti Nei Ching* over 5000 years ago when discussing internal medicine in relation to acupuncture points and energy pathways (Dossey & Keegan, 2016). In the Indian Vedic scriptures and part of Ayurvedic medicine, massage is regarded as a necessary part of healing. Gentle, rhythmic Ayurvedic massage has been shown to be effective in decreasing chronic pain conditions, such as low back pain, and improving fatigue, which is a quality-of-life factor (Kumar et al., 2017). During ancient Greek civilization, Hippocrates noted the benefits of massage and manipulation regarding whole-body therapies that involved touch (Dossey & Keegan, 2016). In the Bible there are two New Testament passages (New Revised Standard Version: Mark 5:25–34; Luke 6:18–19) regarding Jesus' healing touch and energy fields.

The theory of how touch is therapeutic varies from Eastern to Western worldviews. In Eastern cultures, healing occurs due to energy that flows in the body through a practitioner to a person in a fashion similar to magnetic flow patterns on earth and in the universe (Dossey & Keegan, 2016). In Western worldviews, healing happens due to a physical effect of cellular changes with the touch manipulation. The concept of touch and its therapeutic value has changed over time as cultures have changed. In the 1600s, during the European Puritan culture, touch became synonymous with sin and was discouraged as a healing modality. Although this attitude has evolved, health care practitioners need to be mindful of appropriate and culturally sensitive approaches to using touch and massage. In the United States "massage" is regulated and licensed as a practice used specifically by massage therapists and nurse massage therapists (Harris & Richards, 2010). Nurses and PAs have a license to "touch" and can use therapeutic touch in the form of back rubs and hand massages as a treatment therapy (Sparber, 2001).

Ever since the time of Florence Nightingale, nurses have been trained in the art of massage as a nursing skill, and it has been an essential part of patient care plans (Westman & Blaisdell, 2016). Massage has been shown to decrease stress levels and feelings of fatigue, decrease pain perception, positively affect the inflammatory process, promote postburn healing, and improve a sense of well-being (Fellowes et al., 2004; Khaledifar et al., 2017; Metin & Ozdemir, 2016; Westman & Blaisdell, 2016). Massage also promotes the therapeutic relationship between nurses and patients by empowering patients to be more engaged in their healing processes (Westman & Blaisdell, 2016).

As a rule, older adults in the United States are deprived of touch more than other populations and can benefit greatly, both physically and psychologically, from back rubs and hand massages with few contraindications (Harris & Richards, 2010). Therapeutic touch and massage have been shown to increase muscle balance, decrease spasms, improve gait and movement, and increase circulation in older persons (Sefton et al., 2012). When slow-stroke massage (neck to waist on back) was used on patients with Alzheimer disease, pacing, wandering, and resisting decreased significantly (Rowe & Alfred, 1999).

Chiropractic/Osteopathy Manipulation

Chiropractic services and osteopathy manipulations are growing in demand, especially in the older population. Approximately 15% of adults 65 years or older seek chiropractic care (Hawk et al., 2017). Although many people may equate chiropractic care with only the osteopathic manipulations, there are several other treatment modalities that doctors of chiropractic (DCs) use. These include spinal manipulative therapy (SMT), acupuncture and acupressure, physical exercises, nutritional evaluation, and counseling, along with fall prevention (Dougherty et al., 2012). Chiropractic care is often considered a complementary or integrative therapy used in conjunction with other allopathic medicine such as pharmaceuticals, surgical and medical procedures, and prescribed physical therapy. The DC, however, can serve more of a primary management role depending on the chronicity of an individual's pain or the accessibility to a DC in the region where an older adult lives. Additionally, the scope of a DC's practice can vary depending on state laws (NIH, 2019). Regardless of the DC's role, NPs and PAs should verify that the DC is providing care that is evidence based and is patient centered (Hawk et al., 2017).

Due to the diversity of chiropractic modalities, many of these therapies can be noted in the different traditional health care systems. In the homeopathy and naturopathy systems, several compounds and treatments are used for the relief of chronic pain. Therefore DCs may combine some of these treatments to augment chiropractic services and enhance the pain management process (Owen, 2003). NPs and PAs need to determine if the DC is combining any homeopathic or naturopathic medicine into the treatment. Chiropractic-type services can be noted in the Ayurvedic system. TCM uses acupuncture and acupressure that often aligns with treatment plans in chiropractic services.

In the older population, chiropractic services are most often used for musculoskeletal symptoms (Dougherty et al.,

2012). Because these services are diverse, they also can be utilized for overall wellness and illness prevention, improvement of energy, and maintenance of immune function (Evans et al., 2010). Regardless of the reason for chiropractic needs, NPs and PAs should engage in interdisciplinary communication with a person's DC due to the neurologic and musculoskeletal age-related changes and verify that physical examinations are being routinely performed so that chiropractic services are being adapted to meet these changing needs (Hawk et al., 2017). Although severe adverse incidents are rare, minor side effects such as muscle soreness or stiffness may occur after chiropractic services. NPs and PAs need to be cognizant of these side effects and advise the older adult appropriately. Additionally, NPs and PAs should work with the DC so that information is flowing in both directions, thereby optimizing the patient's well-being. Resources NPs and PAs can utilize if the patient is seeking chiropractic services or wants additional information include those provided by the American Association of Acupuncture and Oriental Medicine, the American Board of Physician Specialties, the American Chiropractic Association, the American Chronic Pain Association, the American Counseling Association, and the Therapeutic Massage & Bodywork Resource Center.

Reflexology

Reflexology is considered a manipulative and energy-based therapy that is like massage but utilizes specific hand/finger techniques, applying pressure to stimulate the endocrine system (Wang et al., 2008, 2016, as cited in Metin & Ozdemir, 2016). The use of reflexology for the stimulation of toxin flushing is usually limited to acupressure points, or reflexes, most notably on the feet, hands, and ears (Fontaine, 2015). Reflexology has been found to be effective for headaches, musculoskeletal pain, muscle strength, and tone improvement (Metin & Ozdemir, 2016). Naseri-Salahshour et al. (2019) found that reflexology on hemodialysis patients reduced the severity of nausea. Other uses include treatment of "addictions, allergies, bronchitis, cerebral palsy, depression, diabetes, hemorrhoids, hepatitis, herpes, infertility, irritable bowel syndrome, nausea, premenstrual syndrome, stroke, and ulcers" (Fontaine, 2015, p. 209). Both massage and auricular therapy (reflexology/acupressure to the ears) have been shown to be effective for treating sleep disturbances in older adults (Gooneratne, 2008).

Approaches to the Older Adult Incorporating Mind-Body Interventions

Yoga

Yoga has been in existence in Eastern countries for thousands of years, originating in India (Diamond, 2012). Yoga practices in the traditional Patanjali sutras, from an ancient Indian sage, have eight limbs, which include (1) the yamas (abstinences) in which there are five subgroups: ahimsa (nonviolence), satya (truthfulness), asteya (nonstealing), brahmacharya (nonlust), and aparigraha (nongreed); (2) the niyamas (personal disciplines), which have five subgroups: soucha (purity), santosha (contentment), tapas (self-discipline), svadyaya (self-study), and ishvarapranidhana (surrendering to a greater force than oneself); (3) the asanas (poses); (4) pranayama (breathing techniques); (5) pratyahara (withdrawal of senses); (6) dharana (intense focus); (7) dhyana (state of meditation); and (8) samadhi (state of oneness) (Fontaine, 2015). Be mindful that spelling may differ in various texts, yet the intent and meaning are the same. Yoga has been used to maintain a balance of mental, emotional, and physical health and well-being for individuals. Patients who are often "out of balance" are in vulnerable situations as they deal with diagnoses, unfamiliar environments, and pain/discomfort whether it be acute or chronic. Such situations can cause hyperarousal of the nervous system, which can negatively influence breathing patterns and energy levels and can exacerbate the perception of pain (Vallath, 2010). The practice of yoga has the potential to decrease metabolism by slowing one's breathing, reducing muscle tension, and minimizing the sensation of fatigue (Vallath, 2010).

Yoga has been shown to be beneficial for pain management, which can positively influence patients' healing processes and may reduce in-patient stays, thereby improving patient satisfaction scores (Greene, 2010; Hayes & Chase, 2010). Yoga has also been shown to be effective for different painful conditions such as acute injury, arthritis, and chronic low back pain (Wren et al., 2011, as cited in Villemure et al., 2014). Niedzialek et al. (2019) noted that the practice of yoga improved control of tinnitus, sleep hygiene, and quality of life in patients with chronic tinnitus. Kusnick et al. (2012) postulated that health care providers should be educated in the use of modalities such as yoga and use them as part of allopathic medicine treatment, especially for pain management.

Spirituality/Prayer

Within the process of health care and healing, health care providers are cognizant that the healing environment is a crucial factor that will allow the health care provider to care for the whole person. In healing environments, all elements of physical, mental, emotional, and spiritual caring are necessary for holistic healing (Fontaine, 2015). It is important to note the difference between spirituality, which is the essence of one's being, purpose, relationships, and outward expression of living, versus religion, which is an organized system within a group of people regarding mutual beliefs, values, and practices (Dossey & Keegan, 2016). Both religiousness and spirituality affect human health by providing buffers to life's demands and stressors (Harrington, 2016). Puchalski (2010), as cited in Harrington (2016), found that older adults want their physicians to recognize their spiritual aspects and integrate them into treatment. The Joint Commission requires health care organizations who service older adults to do spiritual assessments (Hodge et al., 2012). Unfortunately, patients' spiritual needs are not always addressed adequately in health care settings either because spirituality is confused with religion or because the practitioner is unfamiliar or uncomfortable with assessing the

TABLE 9.1 Types of Complementary and Alternative Medicine

CAM	How It Helps
Relaxation and meditation	"[H]elpful tools for coping with stress and promoting long-term health by slowing down the body and quieting the mind. Such techniques generally entail: refocusing attention (for example, noticing areas of tension), increasing body awareness, and exercises (such as meditation) to connect the body and mind together. Used daily, these practices can lead to a healthier perspective on stressful circumstances." https://www.stlukes-stl.com/health-content/medicine/33/000359.htm
Guided imagery	"[G]uided imagery involves listening to a trained therapist or a guided imagery CD to move into a state of deep relaxation. Once in a relaxed state, the images that come up in your mind can help you uncover important realizations about your emotional, spiritual, and physical health." https://www.stlukes-stl.com/health-content/medicine/33/000359.htm
Hypnosis	"Hypnotherapists use exercises that bring about deep relaxation and an altered state of consciousness... During hypnosis, your body relaxes and your thoughts become more focused. Like other relaxation techniques, hypnosis lowers blood pressure and heart rate, and changes certain types of brain wave activity. In this relaxed state, you will feel at ease physically yet fully awake mentally, and you may be highly responsive to suggestion. Your conscious mind becomes less alert and your subconscious mind becomes more focused. Some people respond better to hypnotic suggestion than others." https://www.stlukes-stl.com/health-content/medicine/33/000353.htm
Biofeedback	"Biofeedback is a technique that trains people to improve their health by controlling certain bodily processes that normally happen involuntarily, such as heart rate, blood pressure, muscle tension, and skin temperature... Researchers are not sure exactly how or why biofeedback works." https://www.stlukes-stl.com/health-content/medicine/33/000349.htm

patients' spirituality, even though it is linked to improved client satisfaction (Hodge et al., 2012). In the older adult, often the shift from longevity of life to quality of life is done in the context of one's sense of belonging and life satisfaction, both of which are directly linked to one's spiritual practices (Guerrero-Castañeda & Flores, 2017).

Relaxation/Meditation/Guided Imagery/Hypnosis/Biofeedback/Cognitive-Behavioral Therapy

Relaxation and meditation are woven into many complementary and alternative therapies (Table 9.1). These therapies can have benefits in physical, emotional, mental, spiritual, and even biologic processes such as antiinflammation (Bower & Irwin, 2016). Inflammatory processes, which are the body's response to injury, are at the root of many diseases such as different types of cancers, infectious diseases, and some autoimmune disorders (Hunter, 2012). In the 1960s, cardiologist Dr. Herbert Benson noted the mind-body connection to health and identified a physiologic relaxation response in which there is "decreases in oxygen consumption, respiratory rate, and blood pressure, along with an increased state of well-being" (Dusek & Benson, 2009, p. 47). Normally, when a person experiences stress and responds to it, vital signs increase and the sympatho-adreno-medullary axis and the hypthothalamus-pituitary-adreno axis are activated, causing the release of adrenocorticotropic hormone (ACTH), which stimulates the release of catecholamines, epinephrine, and norepinephrine (Dusek & Benson, 2009). When the body is constantly overstimulated this way, chronic inflammation can occur, causing damage to the body. Reversing this process through relaxation and meditation encourages biologic changes to occur at the cellular level that positively change stress-induced alterations.

Guided imagery is a technique that uses one's imagination, evoking all five senses to enrich health, creative abilities, or overall performance (Wood & Patricolo, 2013). Clinically, guided imagery can be used in three ways: (1) diagnostically to identify basic issues or problems, (2) mentally to help prepare patients for upcoming medical events, and (3) physiologically to produce an intended effect such as relaxation (Wood & Patricolo, 2013). The American College of Critical Care Medicine advocates for nonpharmacologic interventions, and guided imagery has been noted for helping patients to relax and has even been useful for weaning patients from mechanical ventilators (Hadjibalassi et al., 2018). Case et al. (2018) noted improved physical and mental well-being in patients with multiple sclerosis who participated in guided imagery.

Forms of mental images or hypnotic trances used by traditional healers have been in existence for thousands of years throughout the world (Fontaine, 2015). In the 18th century, *hypnotherapy* was termed by Dr. Franz Anton Mesmer, for which the word *mesmerize* was coined (Fontaine, 2015). The definition of hypnosis is therapy that creates an altered state of consciousness (Tabish, 2008). For the older adult, hypnosis can be a helpful nonpharmacologic tool used to reduce the perception of pain, especially in the management of chronic or arthritic pain (Ardigo et al., 2016). Ashton et al. (1997, as cited in Ardigo et al., 2016) studied patients undergoing coronary artery bypass surgery who were taught self-hypnosis; these patients used less postoperative narcotics and reported less anxiety and tension after surgeries.

Biofeedback and cognitive behavioral therapy (CBT) are therapeutic approaches that influence involuntary body responses such as vital signs along with thoughts, feelings, and behaviors (Dossey & Keegan, 2016; Tamish, 2008). Biofeedback is often utilized for pain control, sleep hygiene, and stress management (Kreitzer & Koithan, 2014). Alhasan et al. (2017) showed that visual biofeedback, which is a type of virtual reality, or exergaming such as using a Wii product can improve balance for older individuals. CBT, which most often is used to address anxiety and depression, focuses on the premise that stress and suffering distort emotions and behaviors and can be changed to prevent negative consequences affecting health and wellness (Dossey & Keegan, 2016). CBT can be an effective tool for older adults to use as they cope with the many changes in their health and lifestyles and end-of-life decisions.

Contemplative Listening

Contemplative listening, contemplative or compassionate silence, and mindful listening are all indicative of a type of nonjudgmental awareness that can occur when one is present with another person. It is a method of discussion for the listener that facilitates a patient's internal dialogue (Perelman & Olbrechts-Tyteca, 1969, as cited in Evers, 2017). Health care practitioners using contemplative listening allow time for the patient to speak without the practitioner setting the agenda, trying to fix a problem, or finding a solution (Back et al., 2009). Contemplative training is a behavioral technique for which the practitioner acquires mental pliancy that focuses on the "in-the-moment" awareness or "presence," giving complete attention on the patient so as to promote a setting of compassion with respect and understanding (Back et al., 2009). Contemplative listening motivates the patient to "tell the story" and "own" the process for healing (Evers, 2017). This technique empowers the patient to be an integral part of the healing process. Contemplative listening by a practitioner is patient centered and contains an unconditional, supportive regard for "allowing space" for patient discussion (de Groot & van Hoek, 2017).

Music/Art/Dance/Animal-Assisted Therapies

"Little as we know about the way in which we are affected by form, by colour, and by light, we do know this, that they have an actual physical effect...People say the effect is only on the mind. It is no such thing. The effect is on the body, too...Variety of form and brilliancy of color in the objects presented to patients are actual means of recovery" (Nightingale, as cited in Dossey & Keegan, 2016 p. 59). Art therapy has many forms and mediums depending on one's preference to foster creativity, cultivate resilience, and promote healing. In the older adult, art therapy is used to meet psychological needs; improve motivation, self-esteem, and self-confidence; and help maintain cognitive functions (Stallings & Thompson, 2012). Examples of art therapy include coloring books for adults, pottery, paper crafts, watercolor arts, jewelry making, and sculpture. When art therapy is done in groups, it also fosters connectedness and social interactions that promote the older adults' psychosocial well-being (Fave et al., 2018). Art therapy has been shown in studies to be an effective intervention for anxiety and depression (Kreitzer & Koithan, 2014).

Dance is also a form of expression and creativity for which older adults can connect with others socially. Not only is dance physiologically beneficial, it is an opportunity to reminisce to the music of the older adults' generation while integrating psychological and sociologic components (Vankova et al., 2014). Dance activity, if only once a week for an hour, even for wheelchair-bound persons, has been shown to reduce depressive symptoms in the older adult (Vankova et al., 2014).

Approaches to the Older Adult Incorporating Biology-Based Approaches

Diets/Food Fermentation/Nutrition

In Chinese tradition, diet is important for maintaining health and combating illness (Covington, 2001). Also, diet plays a crucial role in Ayurvedic medicine. Food fermentation was a method for preserving foods before the invention of refrigerators and freezers. Overall nutrition has always played a role in health. Let food be your medicine and medicine be your food.

Herbs/Botanicals/Extracts/Essential Oils-Aromatherapy

Aromatherapy includes several techniques, such as inhalation, diffusion, application, and ingestion (in countries other than the United States), that use essential oils to address various ailments and preventive self-care (Kreitzer & Koithan, 2014). Essential oils derived from plants (roots, leaves, blooms), trees (sap and bark), and flowers have been utilized for more than 5000 years in many places around the world, such as countries in the Middle East as well as India and Egypt. Benefits are derived from essential oils that are used in aromatherapy for their antiinflammatory, antibacterial, antiviral, and antifungal chemical compounds (Allard & Katseres, 2016). Lavender has been shown to improve sleep hygiene in patients (Cho et al., 2017; Fismer & Pilkington, 2012). Essential oils such as lavender, Roman chamomile, mandarin, neroli, sandalwood, geranium, and palmarosa have been shown to have analgesic properties for pain management in perioperative and critical care settings (Buckle, 1999). Sweet marjoram, lavender, peppermint, ginger, and mandarin have been noted for reducing patient-reported pain, anxiety, and nausea in an acute care setting (Johnson et al., 2016). Citrus essential oils such as lime, wild orange, grapefruit, tangerine, and lemon have been used to reduce perceived stress levels in surgical patients (Reynolds et al., 2018). Massage is often used in conjunction with aromatherapy due to the improved absorption of the essential oils into the skin with massage, and this is one of the most used CIT applications worldwide (Fellowes et al., 2004; Metin & Ozdemir, 2016).

Supplements/Vitamins/Prebiotics/Probiotics

This is an important part of the history taking to explore with the older adult what supplements, vitamins, prebiotics, or probiotics the patient takes on a regular and even occasional basis.

Approaches to the Older Adult Incorporating Energy Therapies

Biofield Therapies

- *Tai Chi* and *Qi Gong* are ancient practices from Eastern Asian cultures.
- *Reiki* is an energy modality that incorporates a holistic approach to healing and balance.
- *Healing Touch* is an energy therapy.
- *Therapeutic Touch* was developed.
- *Bioelectromagnetic-based therapies* refer to a newer adjunct therapy.

Safety Concerns

There are several safety concerns that NPs and PAs need to keep in mind when assessing, planning, and treating older adults using complementary and alternative/integrative therapies. First, determine if the patient is confiding all of the pertinent information. Second, identify the evidence that supports the CIT modality. Third, ascertain if there are overlaps, conflicts, or other issues when combining the CIT and traditional therapies, especially pharmaceuticals. The NP or PA should also inquire not only about what is being digested but also about what is being absorbed (via the skin) or inhaled/diffused in the air. In addition, the health care provider should ask if CIT is being used in the environment (i.e., cleaning supplies).

Nonjudgmental, Culturally Sensitive, Holistic Approach With the Use of Complementary and Alternative Therapies in the Older Adult

Each health care provider enters a patient–health care provider relationship with her or his own bias, whether or not one recognizes it. It behooves the health care provider to explore her or his own values, beliefs, and opinions regarding CIT before treating the patient.

Key Points

- Terminology
  - Balance
  - CAM
  - CIT
  - Holism
  - TCM
  - Traditional healing practices
- Evidence to Support Complementary and Alternative Therapies
  - Resources
  - Academy for Guided Imagery
  - Academy of Nutrition and Dietetics
  - Alliance of International Aromatherapists
  - Alliance of Therapies Dogs
  - American Board of Hypnotherapy (ABH-NLP)
  - American Board of Physician Specialties
  - American Botanical Council
  - American Geriatric Society
  - American Herbalist Guild
  - American Institute of Homeopathy
  - American Meditation Institute
  - American Society of Clinical Hypnosis
  - Bioelectromagnetics Society
  - Commodity Supplemental Food Program (CSFP)
  - Community Innovations for Aging in Place Initiative (CIAIP)
  - Emergency Food Assistance Program (TEFAP)
  - Herb Research Foundation
  - Herb Society of America
  - Imagery International
  - Indian Health Service
  - Institute of Integrative Aromatherapy
  - International Society for the Studies of Subtle Energies and Energy Medicine
  - Medline Plus
  - National Council on Aging (NCOA)
  - National Council on Aging's National Institute of Senior Centers (NISC)
  - National Indian Council on Aging
  - National Institute on Aging
  - North American Society of Homeopaths (NASH)
  - Office of Minority Health
  - Pet Partners.org
  - Senior Farmers' Market Nutrition Program (SFMNP)
  - Seniorliving.org
  - Silver Sneakers
  - Taoist Tai Chi Society
  - Supplemental Nutrition Assistance Program (SNAP)
  - World Health Organization (WHO)
  - Yoga Alliance
  - Yoga Research Foundation

2. Associations
- American Art Therapy Association
- American Association of Acupuncture and Oriental Medicine
- American Association of Naturopathic Physicians
- American Association of Retired Persons (AARP)
- American Chiropractic Association
- American Chronic Pain Association
- American Counseling Association
- American Dance Therapy Association
- American Holistic Nurses Association
- American Massage Therapy Association
- American Music Therapy Association
- American Tai Chi and Qigong Association (ATCQA)
- American Yoga Association
- Association for Applied Psychophysiology and Biofeedback
- Association for Behavioral and Cognitive Therapies
- Healing Touch International Association
- Healing Touch Professional Association
- Institute for Music and Neurological Function
- International Association of Yoga Therapists (IAYT)
- International Listening Association
- International Scientific Association for Probiotics and Prebiotics (ISAPP)
- National Acupuncture Detoxification Association (NADA)
- National Alaska Native American Indian Nurses Association (NANAINA)
- National Association for Holistic Aromatherapy
- National Ayurvedic Medical Association
- National Coalition of Creative Arts Therapies Associations, Inc.
- Reflexology Association of America
- Spiritual Care Association
- Therapeutic Touch International Association

3. Centers
- Center for Contemplative Mind in Society
- Center for Mind-Body Medicine
- International Center for Reiki Training
- Local senior citizen centers
- National Center for Complementary and Integrative Health (NIH-NCCIH)
- National Center for Homeopathy
- National Center for Health Statistics (NCHS)
- National Indigenous Women's Resource Center
- National Resource Center for American Indian, Alaska Native & Native Hawaiian Elders
- National Resource Center for Native Hawaiian Elders
- National Resource Center on Native American Aging
- Therapeutic Massage & Bodywork Resource Center

More information about tools and the Interprofessional Education Collaborative (IPEC) competencies mentioned in this chapter can be found in Appendix 1: Tools and Appendix 2: IPEC Competencies.

References

Alhasan, H., Hood, V., & Mainwaring, F. (2017). The effect of visual feedback on balance in elderly population: A systematic review. *Clinical Interventions in Aging, 12*, 487–497. https://doi.org/10.2147/CIA.S127023.

Allard, M. E., & Katseres, J. (2016). Using essential oils to enhance nursing practice and for self-care. *American Journal of Nursing, 116*(2), 42–49. https://doi.org/10.1097/01.NAJ.0000480495.18104.db.

Alperson, S. Y. (2017). Integrative healing health care: Brief experiential education for octor of nursing practice students. *Nursing & Primary Care, 1*(6), 1–17. https://doi.org/10.33425/2639-9474.1037.

Altizer, K., Quandt, S. A., Grzywacz, J. G., Bell, R. A., Sandberg, J., & Arcury, T. A. (2013). Traditional and commercial herb use in health self-management among rural multiethnic older adults. *Journal of Applied Gerontology, 32*(4), 387–407. https://doi.org/10.1177/0733464811424152.

American Holistic Nurses Association. (2018). *Holistic geriatric care resource center*. https://www.ahna.org/Home/Resources/Geriatric-Care

Ardigo, S., Herrmann, F. R., Moret, V., Dérame, L., Giannelli, S., Gold, G., & Pautex, S. (2016). Hypnosis can reduce pain in hospitalized older patients: A randomized controlled study. *BMC Geriatrics, 16*(1), 1–8. https://doi.org/10.1186/s12877-016-0180-y.

Back, A. L., Bauer-Wu, S. M., Rushton, C. , H., & Halifax, J. (2009). Compassionate silence in the patient-clinician encounter: A contemplative approach. *Journal of Palliative Medicine, 12*(12), 1113–1117. https://doi.org/10.1089/jpm.2009.0175.

Barad, A., Maimon, Y., Miller, E., Merdler, S., Goldray, D., Lerman, Y., & Lev-ari, S. (2008). Acupuncture treatment in geriatric rehabilitation: A retrospective study. *Journal of Acupuncture and Meridian Studies, 1*(1), 54–57. https://doi.org/10.1016/S2005-2901(09)60008-X.

Bower, J. E., & Irwin, M. R. (2016). Mind-body therapies and control of inflammatory biology: A descriptive review. *Brain, Behavior, and Immunity, 51*, 1–11. https://doi.org/10.1016/j.bbi.2015.06.012.

Braun, K. L., Browne, C. V., Ká opua, L. S., Kim, B. J., & Mokuau, N. (2014). Special issue: Remembering our roots. *The Gerontologist, 54*(1), 117–126. https://doi.org/10.1093/geront/gnt067.

Braun, K. L., Kim, B. J., Ká opua, L. S., Mokuau, N., & Browne, C. V. (2015). Native Hawaiian and Pacific Islander elders: What gerontologists should know. *Gerontological Society of America, 55*(6), 912–919. https://doi.org/10.1093/geront/gnu072.

Braun, K. L., & LaCounte, C. (2015). The historic and ongoing issue of health disparities among native elders. *American Society on Aging: Generations, 38*(4), 60–69. https://www.researchgate.net/publication/274391737_The_historic_and_ongoing_issue_of_health_disparities_among_native_elders.

Breed, C., & Bereznay, C. (2017). Treatment of depression and anxiety by naturopathic physicians: An observational study of naturopathic medicine within an integrated multidisciplinary community health center. *Journal of Alternative and Complementary Medicine, 23*(5), 348–354. https://doi.org/10.1089/acm.2016.0232.

Broome, B., & Broome, R. (2007). Native Americans: Traditional healing. *Urologic Nursing, 27*(2), 161–163. 173.

Browne, C. V., Carter, P., & Gray, J. S. (2015). National resource centers focus on indigenous communities. *Generations: Journal of the American Society on Aging, 38*(4), 70–73.

Buckle, J. (1999). Aromatherapy in perianesthesia nursing. *Journal of PeriAnesthesia Nursing, 14*(6), 336–344. https://www.ncbi.nlm.nih.gov/pubmed/10839071.

Burdak, S. L., & Gupta, N. (2015). A review of preventative health care in geriatrics through Ayurveda. *International Journal of Ayurvedic Medicine, 6*(2), 100–112. https://www.ijam.co.in/index.php/ijam/article/view/06122015.

Case, L. K., Jackson, P., Kinkel, R., & Mills, P. J. (2018). Guided imagery improves mood, fatigue, and quality of life in individuals with multiple sclerosis: An exploratory efficacy trial of healing light guided imagery. *Journal of Evidence-Based Integrative Medicine, 23*, 1–8. https://doi.org/10.1177/2515690X17748744. 2515690X17748744.

Cho, E. H., Lee, M. -Y., & Hur, M. -H. (2017). The effects of aromatherapy on intensive care unit patients' stress and sleep quality: A nonrandomized controlled trial. *Evidence-Based Complementary and Alternative Medicine, 2017*, 1–10. https://doi.org/10.1155/2017/2856592. 2856592.

Clarke, T. C., Barnes, P. M., Black, L. I., Stussman, B. J., & Nahin, R. L. (2018). Use of yoga, meditation, and chiropractors among U.S. adults aged 18 and over. *National Center for Health Statistics Data Brief, 325*, 1–8. https://www.ncbi.nlm.nih.gov/pubmed/30475686.

Covington, M. B. (2001). Traditional Chinese medicine in the treatment of diabetes. *Diabetes Spectrum, 14*(3), 154–159. https://doi.org/10.2337/diaspect.14.3.154.

De Groot, J., & van Hoek, M. E. C. (2017). Contemplative listening in moral issues: Moral counseling redefined in principles and method. *Journal of Pastoral Care &Counseling, 71*(2), 106–113. https://doi.org/10.1177/1542305017708155.

Diamond, L. (2012). The benefits of yoga in improving health. *Primary Health Care: Clinics in Office Practice, 22*(2), 16–19. https://doi.org/10.7748/phc2012.03.22.2.16.c8961.

Dossey, B. M., & Keegan, L. (2016). *Holistic nursing: A handbook for practice* (7th ed.). Jones & Bartlett Learning.

Dougherty, P. E., Hawk, C., Weiner, D. K., Gleberzon, B., Andrew, K., & Killinger, L. (2012). The role of chiropractic care in older adults. *Chiropractic & Manual Therapies, 20*(3), 1–9. https://doi.org/10.1186/2045-709X-20-3.

Dusek, J. A., & Benson, H. (2009). Mind-body medicine: A model of the comparative clinical impact of the acute stress and relaxation responses. *Minnesota Medicine, 92*(5), 47–50.

Eliopoulos, C. (2015). Safe integration of complementary and alternative therapies in geriatric care. *American Holistic Nurses Association: Nurse Competence in Aging CNE*, 1–18. https://www.ahna.org/.

Erickson, H. L. (2007). Philosophy and theory of holism. *Nursing Clinics of North America, 42*(2), 139–163. https://doi.org/10.1016/j.cnur.2007.03.001.

Evans, M. W., Ndetan, H., & Hawk, C. (2010). Use of chiropractic or osteopathic manipulation by adults aged 50 and older: An analysis of data from the 2007 national health interview survey. *Topics in Integrative Health Care, 1*(2). ID: 1.2005.

Evers, H. (2017). Contemplative listening: A rhetorical-critical approach to facilitate internal dialog. *Journal of Pastoral Care & Counseling, 71*(2), 114–121. https://doi.org/10.1177/1542305017708154.

Fave, A. D., Bassi, M., Boccaletti, E. S., Roncaglione, C., Bernardelli, G., & Mari, D. (2018). Promoting well-being in old age: The psychological benefits of two training programs of adapted physical activity. *Frontiers in Psychology, 9*(828), 1–13. https://doi.org/10.3389/fpsyg.2018.00828.

Fellowes, D., Barnes, K., & Wilkinson, S. S. M. (2004). Aromatherapy and massage for symptom relief in patients with cancer (review). *Cochrane Database of Systematic Reviews, 3(CD002287).* https://doi.org/10.1002/14651858.CD002287.pub2.

Figueira, H. A., Figueira, O. A., Figueira, A. A., Figueira, J. A., Giani, T. S., & Dantas, E. H. M. (2010). Elderly quality of life impacted by traditional Chinese medicine techniques. *Clinical Interventions in Aging, 5*, 301–305. https://doi.org/10.2147/CIA.S10615.

Fismer, K. L., & Pilkington, K. (2012). Lavender and sleep: A systematic review of the evidence. *European Journal of Integrative Medicine, 2012*, e436–e447. https://doi.org/10.1016/j.eujim.2012.08.001.

Fontaine, K. (2015). *Complementary & alternative therapies for nursing practice* (4th ed.). Pearson Education.

Gooneratne, N. S. (2008). Complementary and alternative medicine for sleep disturbances in older adults. *Clinics in Geriatric Medicine, 24*(1), 121–138. https://doi.org/10.1016/j.cger.2007.08.002.

Grant, S. J., & Bensoussan, A. (2014). The process of care in integrative health care settings: A qualitative study of US practices. *BMC Complementary and Alternative Medicine, 14*(1), 1–13. https://doi.org/10.1186/1472-6882-14-410.

Green, M. A. (2010). Paying for nursing orientation. *Journal for Nurses in Staff Development, 26*(6), E3–E7. https://doi.org/10.1097/NND.0b013e3181fc0459.

Greiner, A. C., & Knebel, E. (2003). The core competencies needed for health care professionals. In A. C. Greiner & E. Knebel (Eds.), *Health professions education: A bridge to quality*. National Academies Press (US).

Guerrero-Castañeda, R. F., & Flores, T. C. (2017). Spiritual care in old age: nursing reflection. *MOJ Gerontology & Geriatrics, 2*(4), 259–261. https://doi.org/10.15406/mojgg.2017.02.00055.

Hadjibalassi, M., Lambrinou, E., Papastavrou, E., & Papathanassoglou, E. (2018). The effect of guided imagery on physiological and psychological outcomes of adult ICU patients: A systematic literature review and methodological implications. *Australian Critical Care, 31*(2), 73–86. https://doi.org/10.1016/j.aucc.2017.03.001.

Hani, M. B., & Ahmad, M. (2016). Refinement of the concept of holism in nursing care. *Persian Journal of Medical Sciences, 3*, 1–12. https://www.researchgate.net/publication/310805599_Evaluation_of_the_concept_of_holism_in_nursing_care.

Harrington, A. (2016). The importance of spiritual assessment when caring for older adults. *Ageing & Society, 36*(1), 1–16. https://doi.org/10.1017/S0144686X14001007.

Harris, M., & Richards, K. C. (2010). The physiological and psychological effects of slow-stroke back massage and hand massage on relaxation in older people. *Journal of Clinical Nursing, 19*(7–8), 917–926. https://doi.org/10.1111/j.1365-2702.2009.03165.x.

Hawk, C., Schneider, M. J., Haas, M., Katz, P., Dougherty, P., Gleberzon, B., & Weeks, J. (2017). Best practices for chiropractic care for older adults: A systematic review and consensus update. *Journal of Manipulative and Physiological Therapeutics, 40*(4), 217–229. https://doi.org/10.1016/j.jmpt.2017.02.001.

Hayes, M., & Chase, S. (2010). Prescribing yoga. *Primary Care, 37*(1), 31–47. https://doi.org/10.1016/j.pop.2009.09.009.

Hodge, D. R., Horvath, V. E., Larkin, H., & Curl, A. L. (2012). Older adults' spiritual needs in health care settings: A qualitative meta-synthesis. *Research on Aging, 34*(2), 131–155. https://doi.org/10.1177/0164027511411308.

Hopkins, S. E., Kwachka, P., Lardon, C., & Mohatt, G. V. (2007). Keeping busy: A yup'ik/cup'ik perspective on health and aging.

International Journal of Circumpolar Health, 66(1), 42–50. https://doi.org/10.3402/ijch.v66i1.18224.

Huisman, E. R. C. M., Morales, E., van Hoof, J., & Kort, H. S. M. (2012). Healing environment: A review of the impact of physical environment factors on users. *Building and Environment, 58,* 70–80. https://doi.org/10.1016/j.buildenv.2012.06.016.

Hunter, P. (2012). The inflammatory theory of disease. *EMBO (European Molecular Biology Organization) Reports, 13*(11), 968–970. https://doi.org/10.1038/embor.2012.142.

Interprofessional Education Collaborative (IPEC), (2016). *IPEC core competencies for interprofessional collaborative practice: 2016 update.* Interprofessional Education Collaborative. https://hsc.unm.edu/ipe/resources/ipec-2016-core-competencies.pdf.

Johnson, J. R., Rivard, R. L., Griffin, K. H., Kolste, A. K., Joswiak, D., Kinney, M. E., & Dusek, J. A. (2016). The effectiveness of nurse-delivered aromatherapy in an acute care setting. *Complementary Therapies in Medicine, 25,* 164–169. https://doi.org/10.1016/j.ctim.2016.03.006.

Kessler, C., Wischnewsky, M., Michalsen, A., Eisenmann, C., & Melzer, J. (2013). Ayurveda: Between religion, spirituality, and medicine. *Evidence-Based Complementary and Alternative Medicine,* 1–11. https://doi.org/10.1155/2013/952432. 952432.

Khaledifar, A., Nasiri, M., Khaledifar, B., Khaledifar, A., & Mokhtari, A. (2017). The effect of reflexology and massage therapy on vital signs and stress before coronary angiography: An open-label clinical trial. *ARYA Atherosclerosis, 13*(2), 50–55. https://www.ncbi.nlm.nih.gov/pmc/articles/PMC5628851/.

Koithan, M. (2009). Introducing complementary and alternative therapies. *Journal for Nurse Practitioners, 5*(1), 18–20. https://doi.org/10.1016/jnurpra.2008.10.012.

Kreitzer, M. J., & Koithan, M. (2014). *Integrative nursing.* Oxford University Press.

Kumar, S., Rampp, T., Kessler, C., Jeitler, M., Dobos, G. J., Lüdtke, R., & Michalsen, A. (2017). Effectiveness of Ayurvedic massage (sahacharadi taila) in patients with chronic low back pain: A randomized controlled trial. *Journal of Alternative and Complementary Medicine, 23*(2), 109–115. https://doi.org/10.1089/acm.2015.0272.

Kusnick, C., Kraftsow, G., & Hilliker, M. (2012). Building bridges for yoga therapy research: The Aetna, Inc., mind-body pilot study on chronic and high stress. *International Journal of Yoga Therapy, 22*(1), 91–92. http://tinyurl.com/hl75cg9.

Maciocia, G. (2015). *The foundations of Chinese medicine: A comprehensive text* (3rd ed.). Elsevier.

McCabe, P. (2000). Naturopathy, Nightingale, and nature cure: A convergence of interests. *Complementary Therapies in Nursing & Midwifery, 6*(1), 4–8. https://doi.org/10.1054/ctnm.1999.0401.

Metin, Z. G., & Ozdemir, L. (2016). The effects of aromatherapy massage and reflexology on pain and fatigue in patients with rheumatoid arthritis: A randomized controlled trial. *Pain Management Nursing, 17*(2), 140–149. https://doi.org/10.1016/j.pmn.2016.01.004.

Narayanasami, A., & Narayanasami, M. (2006). Ayurvedic medicine: An introduction for nurses. *British Journal of Nursing, 15*(21), 1185–1190. https://doi.org/10.12968/bjon.2006.15.21.22378.

Naseri-Salahshour, V., Sajadi, M., Abedi, A., Fournier, A., & Saeidi, N. (2019). Reflexology as an adjunctive nursing intervention for management of nausea in hemodialysis patients: A randomized clinical trial. *Complementary Therapies in Clinical Practice, 36*(2019), 29–33. https://doi.org/10.1016/j.ctcp.2019.04.006.

National Centers for Complementary and Integrative Health (NCCIH). (2015). Complementary and integrative health for older adults. *U.S. Department of Health and Human Services: National Institutes of Health.* https://nccih.nih.gov/health/providers/digest/age

National Congress of American Indians. (2019, May). *Tribal nations & the United States: An introduction.* http://www.ncai.org/tribalnations/introduction/Tribal_Nations_and_the_United_States_An_Introduction-web-.pdf

National Institutes of Health (NIH). (2011, April). Complementary and alternative medicine: What people aged 50 and older discuss with their health care providers. *AARP and National Center for Complementary and Alternative Medicine Survey Report: U.S. Department of Health and Human Services.* https://www.nccih.nih.gov/sites/nccam.nih.gov/files/news/camstats/2010/NCCAM_aarp_survey.pdf

National Institutes of Health (NIH). (2005). *National center for complementary and alternative medicine: A resource guide.* https://www.aamc.org/research/adhocgp/pdfs/nccam.pdf

National Institutes of Health (NIH). (2015). NIH complementary and integrative health agency gets new name. *National Center for Complementary and Integrative Health (NCCIH).* https://nccih.nih.gov/news/press/12172014

National Institutes of Health (NIH). (2018, July). Complementary, alternative, or integrative health: What's in a name? *National Center for Complementary and Integrative Health (NCCIH).* https://nccih.nih.gov/health/integrative-health

National Institutes of Health (NIH). (2019, April). *Chiropractic.* https://nccih.nih.gov/health/chiropractic

Ness, J., Cirillo, D. J., Weir, D. R., Nisly, N. L., & Wallace, R. B. (2005). Use of complementary medicine in older Americans: Results from the health and retirement study. *The Gerontologist, 45*(4), 516–524. https://www.ncbi.nlm.nih.gov/pmc/articles/PMC1557639/https://www.ncbi.nlm.nih.gov/pmc/articles/PMC1557639/.

Niedzialek, I., Raj-Koziak, D., Milner, R., Wolak, T., Ganc, M., Wójcik, J., & Skarżyński, P. H. (2019). Effect of yoga training on the tinnitus induced distress. *Complementary Therapies in Clinical Practice, 36*(2019), 7–11. https://doi.org/10.1016/j.ctcp.2019.04.003.

Oberg, E. B., Thomas, M. -S., McCarty, M., Berg, J., Burlingham, B., & Bradley, R. (2014). Older adults' perspectives on naturopathic medicine's impact on healthy aging. *Explore, 10*(1), 34–43. https://doi.org/10.1016/j.explore.2013.10.003.

Owen, J. (2003). The use of homeopathic remedies by the chiropractic physician. *Dynamic Chiropractic, 21*(2). https://www.dynamic-chiropractic.com/mpacms/dc/article.php?id=8985.

Portman, T. A. A., & Garrett, M. T. (2006). Native American healing traditions. *International Journal of Disability, Development and Education, 53*(4), 453–469. https://doi.org/10.1080/10349120601008647.

Red Horse, J. G. (1980). Family structure and value orientation in American Indians. *Social Casework: The Journal of Contemporary Social Work, 61*(8), 462–467. https://doi.org/10.1177/104438948006100803.

Relton, C., Cooper, K., Viksveen, P., Fibert, P., & Thomas, K. (2017). Prevalence of homeopathy use by the general population worldwide: A systematic review. *Homeopathy, 106*(2), 69–78. https://doi.org/10.1016/j.homp.2017.03.002.

Reynolds, J., Parker, B., Wells, N., & Card, E. (2018). Using aromatherapy in the clinical setting: Making sense of scents. *American Nurse Today, 13*(6). https://www.americannursetoday.com/aromatherapy-clinical-setting/.

Rosenthal, B., Gravrand, H., & Lisi, A. J. (2019). Interprofessional collaboration among complementary and integrative health providers in private practice and community health centers. *Journal of*

Interprofessional Education & Practice, 15(1), 70–74. https://doi.org/10.1016/j.xjep.2019.02.007.

Ross, C. L. (2009). Integral healthcare: The benefits and challenges of integrating complementary and alternative medicine with a conventional healthcare practice. *Integrative Medicine Insights, 4*, 13–20. https://doi.org/10.4137/IMI.S2239.

Rowe, M., & Alfred, D. (1999). The effectiveness of slow-stroke massage in diffusing agitated behaviors in individuals with Alzheimer's disease. *Journal of Gerontological Nursing, 25*(6), 22–34. https://doi.org/10.3928/0098-9134-19990601-07.

Sefton, J. M., Yarar, C., & Berry, J. W. (2012). Six weeks of massage therapy produces changes in balance, neurological and cardiovascular measures in older people. *International Journal of Therapeutic Massage and Bodywork, 5*(3), 28–40. https://doi.org/10.3822/ijtmb.v5i3.181.

Shukla, R. (2015). Geriatric care in Ayurved: Evidence based review. *HSOA Journal of Alternative, Complementary & Integrative Medicine, 1*(1), 1–4. https://doi.org/10.24966/ACIM-7562/100005.

Shuler, P. A., Huebscher, R., & Hallock, J. (2001). Providing wholistic health care for the elderly: Utilization of the Shuler nurse practitioner practice model. *Journal of the American Academy of Nurse Practitioners, 13*(7), 297–303. https://doi.org/10.1111/j.1745-7599.2001.tb00039.x.

Sparber, A. (2001). State boards of nursing and scope of practice of registered nurses performing complementary therapies. *Online Journal of Issues in Nursing, 6*(3). www.nursingworld.org/MainMenuCategories/ANAMarketplace/ANAPeriodicals/OJIN/TableofContents/Volume62001/No3Sept01/ArticlePreviousTopic/CmplementaryTherapiesReport.aspx.

Stallings, J. W., & Thompson, S. K. (2012). Use of art therapy in geriatric populations. *Annals of Long-Term Care: Clinical Care and Aging, 20*(6), 28–32. https://www.managedhealthcareconnect.com/articles/use-art-therapy-geriatric-populations.

Tabish, S. A. (2008). Complementary and alternative healthcare: Is it evidence-based? *International Journal of Health Sciences, 2*(1), 5–9. https://www.ncbi.nlm.nih.gov/pmc/articles/PMC3068720/.

Takayama, S., & Iwasaki, K. (2017). Systematic review of traditional Chinese medicine for geriatrics. *Geriatrics & Gerontology International, 17*(5), 679–688. https://doi.org/10.1111/ggi.12803.

Teut, M., Lüdtke, R., Schnabel, K., Willich, S. N., & Witt, C. M. (2010). Homeopathic treatment of elderly patients – A prospective observational study with follow-up over a two year period. *BMC Geriatrics, 10*, 10. https://doi.org/10.1186/1471-2318-10-10.

Vallath, N. (2010). Perspectives on yoga inputs in the management of chronic pain. *Indian Journal of Palliative Care, 16*(1), 1–7. https://doi.org/10.4103/0973-1075.63127.

Vankova, H., Holmerova, I., Machacova, K., Volicer, L., Veleta, P., & Celko, A. M. (2014). The effect of dance on depressive symptoms in nursing home residents. *Journal of American Medical Directors Association (JAMDA), 15*(8), 582–587. https://doi.org/10.1016/j.jamda.2014.04.013.

Villemure, C., Ceko, M., Cotton, V. A., & Bushnell, M. C. (2014). Insular cortex mediates increased pain tolerance in yoga practitioners. *Cerebral Cortex, 24*(10), 2732–2740. https://doi.org/10.1093/cercor/bht124.

Wagner, J. (2015). Incorporating acupressure into nursing practice. *American Journal of Nursing, 115*(12), 40–45. https://doi.org/10.1097/01.NAJ.0000475290.20362.77.

Westman, K. F., & Blaisdell, C. (2016). Many benefits, little risks: The use of massage in nursing practice. *American Journal of Nursing, 116*(1), 34–39. https://doi.org/10.1097/01.NAJ.0000476164.97929.f2.

Wood, D., & Patricolo, G. E. (2013). Using guided imagery in a hospital setting. *Alternative and Complementary Therapies, 19*(6), 301–305. https://doi.org/10.1089/act.2013.19604.

Zhao, H., & Luo, Y. (2017). Traditional Chinese medicine and aging intervention. *Aging and Disease, 8*(6), 688–690. https://doi.org/10.14336/AD.2017.1002.

10 Clinical Assessment: Cognitive, Psychological, Social, Functional, and Medications

LESLIE CHANG EVERTSON, DNP, RN, GNP-BC AND KEMI IYABO REEVES, MSN, RN, GNP-BC

OBJECTIVES

Student Learning Objectives

After completing this chapter, the student should be able to do the following:

1. Describe the process of completing a geriatrics-focused history.
2. Understand normal age-related changes in order to identify abnormal findings.
3. Demonstrate a comprehensive geriatric-focused clinical examination.

Practitioner Objectives

After completing this chapter, the practitioner should be able to do the following:

1. Identify culturally competent factors when developing a patient-centered treatment plan.
   a. *Competencies for the nurse practitioner profession:* Independent practice and ethics
   b. *Competencies for the physician assistant profession:* Systems-based practice
2. Distinguish the purpose and appropriate use of geriatrics-focused screening tools to address health promotion and patient safety.
   a. *Competencies for the nurse practitioner profession:* Independent practice
   b. *Competencies for the physician assistant profession:* Medical knowledge
3. Describe the professional role of the nurse practitioner and physician assistant in a clinical setting and the methods they can use to work effectively with an interdisciplinary team.
   a. *Competencies for the nurse practitioner profession:* Health delivery system
   b. *Competencies for the physician assistant profession:* Interpersonal and communication skills

Introduction

The clinical assessment of a patient is the foundation for making an accurate medical diagnosis. To correctly identify acute and chronic diseases, a clinician needs to gather data through many means. Medical record review, including interpreting laboratory results and imaging, is often necessary. Arguably the most important step is meeting with the patient and completing a thorough and thoughtful assessment to help arrive at differential diagnoses and eventually the diagnosis(es) and treatment plan. Getting beyond the chief complaint and finding out enough information to make the visit and the medical recommendations successful takes astute observational and interviewing skills, an approachable demeanor, and the ability to communicate clearly and compassionately. A complete physical such as in a preventive visit or a Medicare Annual Wellness Exam (Medicare.gov, n.d.) is detailed and comprehensive and is not done at every appointment, but the screening and assessment tools employed in a comprehensive exam can be used in problem-focused visits as well. Knowing which ones to use and when comes with experience and practice.

Interprofessional Collaboration

The role of the geriatric assessment team (GAT) is a model that relies on a multidisciplinary diagnostic and treatment process to address physical health, psychosocial conditions, functional limitations, and socioenvironmental circumstances. GATs offer a unique opportunity for an in-depth patient-focused assessment to improve collaboration and communication among practitioners from a variety of disciplines, including a medical provider (physician, nurse practitioner [NP], and physician assistant [PA]), nurse, social worker, pharmacist, physical therapist, occupational therapist, nutritionist, and psychologist. A PA or NP can serve as the primary medical provider or can collaborate with one or more physicians on a GAT. PAs and NPs are ideally suited to serve as GAT leaders, where they can use their skills and training to facilitate communication and collaboration with the goal of improved outcomes for older adults, especially those with complex medical problems.

CASE STUDY SAFETY

A 78-year-old man is scheduled to see you for the first time. He is a referral from the emergency department physician at the local hospital. The discharge summary from his last emergency department visit a couple of weeks ago describes several previous visits for altered mental status and falls with incomplete medical histories and a vague mention of possible prior alcohol abuse. He has left the emergency department against medical advice on more than one occasion. The office staff explain that he arrived 15 minutes late and alone.

Upon entering the room, you notice that he appears disheveled. His clothes are unwashed and he needs a shave and a haircut. He looks up at you when you enter the room. You introduce yourself and ask how he is doing today. He leans in closer to you and asks for your name again. You repeat it, noting that he seems to be straining to hear you. He is unable to tell you what medications he is taking but says he has bottles at home that he did not bring with him today. He says he used to drink but not anymore and says it has been "years." When you ask about where he lives and if he has any friends or family nearby, he becomes upset and wants to know why any of that is your business anyway. His vital signs are normal although you notice that he is thin, and unfortunately the last emergency department discharge summary does not have a weight. He looks like he wants to leave. He says that he only came because he needs help getting his driver's license back after someone took it away.

He says he sleeps fine but that he gets up at night a few times to go to the bathroom. He does not use a walker or a cane. When asked about his falls, he cannot recall the details. You ask if he has fallen at night when going to the bathroom, and he mentions that he uses the bathroom in the hallway. You ask if there is a bathroom connected to the bedroom that would be closer, and he tells you that his wife uses that bathroom. You ask if his wife came with him today, and he mutters that she died a year ago. He looks tearful, and you tell him you are sorry for his loss. You ask how he has been getting along since she passed, and you learn that she passed suddenly and that the doctors were of no help. He tells you that he does not speak to his children who live out of state, and then he asks if can he leave. When he gets up to leave, you notice that he is unsteady and needs to lean on the furniture to get up and walk. You ask if he would please stay and say that you want to help. He agrees.

Based on your interaction with the patient so far, you would like more information about his alcohol consumption, his nutritional status, his cognition, possible depression, and gait and balance concerns.

Greeting the Patient

One of the most difficult skills to learn as a new clinician is how to remember all the components of a comprehensive clinical assessment. You can have a checklist, flash cards or a detailed template and still miss key information that can be learned in the first few minutes when you meet a patient for the first time. When you knock on the door, walk in, introduce yourself and smile, then start taking mental notes:

- Did your patient look up at you when you walked in?
  - If not consider hearing loss, cognitive impairment, or physical debility.
- Did the patient smile or look upset?
  - If your patient appears happy, do not be remiss and assume that this is the case. Always inquire about mood and screen for depression as needed.
  - If your patient appears upset or has a flat affect, be sure to ask how he or she is currently feeling and check the medical record for a history of depression or other conditions such as Parkinson disease, which could possibly present as masked faces.
- Consider the patient's ability to pay attention during a conversation. Inattention can be attributed to anxiety, cognitive impairment, or another neurologic disorder.
- Does your patient appear thinner than you remember? Heavier than you remember?
- How was the patient dressed?
  - If your patient is well groomed, take note so that you will be aware of changes in the future. If you notice changes in hygiene or indifference regarding appearance, try to find the reason for the change. This could indicate an unstable living condition or lack of access to laundry facilities. Additionally, patients with cognitive impairment may not notice that their clothes are soiled or that they need to shower.
- Are the patient's clothes clean but mismatched to the weather?
  - For example, if the patient is wearing a winter coat and hat in the middle of summer, is it because the patient feels cold despite the heat or because the patient does not realize that he or she is dressed inappropriately.
- When you introduce yourself, you might shake hands and you may note your patient's ability to reciprocate, grip strength, and social cues.
  - Is the patient able to keep up social graces? If not (e.g., disinhibited behavior, anger, agitation), is this a change from the last visit (which may indicate a mood disorder or a dementia-related behavior)?
- If you've seen the patient before, does the patient remember you? Does the patient remember the purpose of the visit?
  - If your patient does not remember meeting you and cannot recall the reason for the visit, this could be cause for concern.
- If the patient stands to greet you or to walk from a chair to an exam table, note whether the patient needs to use the arms of the chair to stand? Does the patient use a walking aid? Should the patient have been using a walking aid because of unsteady gait?
  - Although formal gait and balance assessments are important, a lot of information can be garnered within the first few minutes of your interaction with your patient.
- What is your patient's ability to communicate? Is your patient able to participate in a conversation and provide his or her own history?
  - Does the patient have word-finding difficulty? Is the patient aphasic or dysarthric? Was this always the case, or is this a change? Has the patient had a stroke in the

past? Is the patient seeing a neurologist? Should she or he be seeing a speech therapist?

- Did the patient come alone, or was she or he accompanied by somebody? Did the patient look to a family member for answers to questions about the history of present illness?
  - Is this new? Does the patient get upset if the family member offers information? If your patient has dementia, is this family member a legal decision maker?
- Always explain what you plan to accomplish during your visit.
  - Is it a physical? Is it a problem-focused visit? Is it a follow-up visit regarding an ongoing problem?
  - Was there an interval hospitalization or emergency room visit?
- Remember to ask about other providers involved in the patient's care. Again, note whether the patient can remember which specialists are involved and for what reason.

Eye Contact

Consider how you look to the patient and family—communication goes both ways. When you walk into the room, look up at your patient, not down at the chart. Make eye contact, and take inventory of what you see. Be mindful that patients are coming to see you for a reason. If you use an electric medical record and are charting while seeing the patient, try not to turn your back to the patient for most of the visit. Many clinicians are pressured to see a certain number of patients in a day. This can make anyone feel rushed and become task oriented. Consider for a moment how good it feels when someone acknowledges you and your concerns in any situation, but most certainly when you do not feel well and may be nervous and possibly frightened. Those first few minutes when you walk into a patient's exam room can set the mood for the rest of the visit, provide valuable assessment information, and build rapport between clinician and patient.

Room Configuration

When seeing older adult patients, make sure that you can conduct your assessment in a safe and as stress-free environment as possible. Here are a few considerations:

- Try to schedule the appointment in a room large enough to accommodate a walker or wheelchair in addition to your patient and possibly a family member. Patients are offered and can accept the presence of a medical chaperone as well.
- It is important to have low exam table to make getting on and off easier and safer for your older adult patient. Many of these tables can convert into a chair position with a pullout step for patients to rest their feet on.
- Include chairs for sitting comfortably if the exam table is not needed and, if possible, extra chairs for family members.
- Privacy is important. The door must close, because maintaining privacy for the physical exam as well as during discussions of health-related issues is professional and required. If the room has windows, make sure there are blinds that can block any view into the room from the outside.
- Consider the temperature of the room. A separate thermostat is preferred as an older adult may want the exam room warmer than a typical office temperature. This is important if you are asking patients to disrobe and wait for your exam. Having extra blankets in the room can also be helpful.
- If you have a computer in the room, try to position it so that you do not have your back to the patient and family during the visit.

History

When taking a patient history, there are unique considerations in the care of older adults:

- The patient may have multiple complaints rather than a single chief complaint.
- Multiple chronic diseases and a past history of medical and surgical problems could contribute to or cause new problems.
- Remember to ask about pain, both acute and chronic. Document location, quality, what makes it feel better, and what makes it feel worse. Consider using a number scale, having your patient rate the pain on a scale of 0 to 10.
- Inquire about the patient's advance directives, physician's/provider order for life-sustaining treatment (POLST) forms, and, if possible, document all goals-of-care discussions.
- There may be a need for corroboration or involvement of the family or others. As a clinician you need to consider the Health Insurance Portability and Accountability Act (HIPAA), patient privacy, and the need for independence.

For older adults, the importance of psychosocial factors such as living situation, social support, and finances is essential in understanding the problem in addition to the impact of these factors on management and treatment decisions.

Medication Review

Medication reconciliation is a critical component of serving as a primary care provider to the older adult population. Aging is associated with an increase in chronic medical conditions, an increase in the number of specialists involved, and an increase in the number of medications used to treat comorbidities. This combination sets the stage for disjointed care resulting in delays, medication errors, and poor health outcomes, and it is a significant public health problem. Between 2013 and 2014 in the United States, 41% of all emergency department visits for individuals 65 to 79 years of age resulting in a hospitalization stemmed from adverse drug events and increased to 47% for individuals 80 years of age or older (Shehab et al., 2016). This is a systemic problem that begins in primary care offices, and for a provider focusing on the older adult population, mitigating risk is should be a primary focus.

Medication review should be a routine activity that is a significant component of each patient encounter. This is even more important when managing patients with multiple comorbidities and advanced age. An in-depth medication reconciliation should be completed (1) when patients are establishing care, (2) during annual wellness visits, (3) during any transition of care (hospital to home, hospital to skilled nursing facility, or skilled nursing facility to home), and (4) when changes in a patient's condition are identified. Changes in a patient's condition can be both physiologic (e.g., changes in gait pattern, dizziness, falls) or changes in mental status (e.g., disorientation, poor regulation of emotions), but they should always lead to a review of medication as a part of the evaluation and differential diagnostic workup.

SAFETY ALERT

Transitions of care are a time during which frequent medication changes occur, and often patients and families are not clear on what medications should be discontinued or continued for ongoing long-term management. Conducting an extended follow-up visit allows for in-depth medication reconciliation, health education, and health promotion counseling.

A *brown bag medication review* is used in geriatric practices and begins at the time of scheduling the visit. Patients should be advised to bring all their medications with them to the appointment. They are instructed to bring any medication used in the past 12 months, including prescription medications, over-the-counter medications, vitamins, herbal supplements, nutritional supplements, and topical creams. When patients arrive, they should be prompted to set out all the medications so they can be recorded accurately. At the start of the encounter, providers should begin their brown bag medication review by assessing for and recording medication allergies and intolerances. Then the provider should review and record each medication that is brought. The record should include the medication's name, dosage, frequency, and route of administration. While taking an inventory of medications, it is important for the provider to ask about substance use (alcohol, tobacco, caffeine, marijuana/cannabis, and recreational drugs) for a more complete assessment. As each medication is recorded, it is important to engage patients and caregivers in the review process and acknowledge the purpose of the medication while reinforcing instructions and assessing for understanding. Medication reconciliation is a complex process of documenting, counseling, and evaluating the appropriateness of each medication with special attention paid looking for polypharmacy, medication nonadherence, and suspect medications (see Chapter 8). Once the brown bag medication review is complete, an updated medication list identifying medications to be continued, with clear administration instruction, and medications to be discontinued should be provided to patients. Communication between patients and providers as discussed previously is very important; however, it is key to involve the other members of the health care team, with special attention paid to other prescribing providers. Preventing disjointed care will greatly improve the quality of care the practitioner is able to provide and optimize outcomes.

Special consideration: There should be special attention paid when patients indicate they use marijuana. Many states have passed laws legalizing the medicinal use of marijuana, and more states are passing subsequent regulations regarding the recreational use of marijuana. The provider should take special care to note the following:

- *Type of use:* Medicinal verses recreational
- *Type of marijuana product:* Hemp or cannabidiol/CBD (marginal concentrations of tetrahydrocannabinol or THC) versus marijuana
- *Content:* Refers to both tetrahydrocannabinol (the psychoactive component of cannabis) and cannabidiol content
- *Form taken:* Topical preparation, edible, inhalant, and so on

SAFETY ALERT

Medication reconciliation provides an opportune time to begin an assessment of patients' and caregivers' health literacy by asking why each medication is being taken and what provider prescribed the medication. Health literacy is essential for patients to successfully navigate their health care and make informed health decisions. Medication counseling and health promotion behaviors can occur simultaneously to reinforce good health behaviors.

SAFETY ALERT

The Food and Drug Administration (FDA), the Drug Enforcement Administration, and the Environmental Protection Agency have provided guiding principles for the proper disposal of expired, unused, and unwanted medications (both prescription and over the counter). Water treatment plants are not designed to remove pharmaceuticals from water; therefore, medications flushed down the toilet or disposed of down a drain eventually end up in drinking water, rivers, and streams. Concentrations of pharmaceutical pollutants are escalating and are found to have a negative impact on aquatic and terrestrial ecosystems. It is important to counsel patients about local resources and programs for proper medication disposal. Many pharmacies have options for proper medication disposal including drug collection units, drop-off kiosks, or mail-back programs. These often exclude disposal of sharps or injectable medication, as special safety measures are provided for this class of medication. It is also important to note that the FDA has compiled a list of medications approved for toilet or drain disposal. Medications included on the "flush list" are listed due to their hazardous nature and potential danger posed to children, pets, and other individuals if accidentally ingested, touched, or misused. Table 10.1 is the approved flush list, most recently revised by the FDA in 2018.

TABLE 10.1 FDA-Approved "Flush List" of Medications

Active Ingredients	Found in Brand Names
Benzhydrocodon/acetaminophen	Apadaz
Buprenorphine	Belbuca, Bunavail, Butrans, Suboxone, Subutex, Zubsolv
Diazepam	Diastat/ Diastat AcuDial rectal gel
Fentanyl	Abstral, Actiq, Duragesic, Fentora, Onsolis
Hydrocodone	Anexsia, Hysingla ER, Lortab, Norco, Reprexain, Vicodin,Vicoprofen, Zohydro ER
Hydromorphone	Dilaudid, Exalgo
Meperidine	Demerol
Methadone	Dolophine, Methadose
Methylphenidate	Daytrana transdermal patch system
Morphine	Arymo ER, Embeda, Kadian, Morphabond ER, MS Contin, Avinza
Oxycodone	Combunox, Oxaydo (formerly Oxecta), OxyContin, Percocet,Percodan, Roxicet, Roxicodone, Targiniq ER, Xartemis XR,Xtampza ER, Roxybond
Oxymorphone	Opana, Opana ER
Sodium oxybate	Xyrem oral solution
Tapentadol	Nucynta, Nucynta ER

FDA, Food and Drug Administration.
From https://www.fda.gov/drugs/disposal-unused-medicines-what-you-should-know/drug-disposal-fdas-flush-list-certain-medicines

Polypharmacy refers to the presence of multiple medications prescribed for chronic use in a patient. Polypharmacy is commonly recognized when five or more medications are present. As patients age and develop comorbidities, prescribing multiple medication may not be clinically inappropriate; however, it is necessary to continuously monitor for adverse events, minimal or no therapeutic effect, nonadherence, and poor health outcomes as a result of aggressive medication management. Adverse drug events can arise due to a variety of reasons such as drug-drug interactions, cognitive changes, physiologic age-related changes, visual impairments, and gait and balance disorders. For this reason, providers must recognize opportunities to discontinue medications and actively de-prescribe medications, if appropriate, during patient encounters. Providers must actively engage and educate patients as to why a medication is being discontinued and provide an updated medication list for patients to reference at home with instructions as to what medications are to be continued and what medications should be stopped.

Medication nonadherence is another identifiable obstacle affecting patient outcomes and should be consider when performing medication reconciliation. If medication nonadherence is identified during medication reconciliation, the discrepancy in medication administration should be documented and the barrier hindering compliance investigated. There are a variety of barriers that can result in medication nonadherence. Common barriers include medication cost, transportation issues, medication intolerance or adverse effects, changes in cognition, and poor health literacy. Interventions can vary and are most successful when a patient-centered approach is used. It is vital for the provider to fully understand the complexity of each patient's situation and involve patients when developing an intervention to improve medication adherence. Limited access to transportation is a prevalent issue in the older adult population and a frequent barrier to maintaining medication adherence; this situation can be improved with options like prescribing a 90-day supply of medications or providing information for mail-order pharmacies. When diminishing cognitive performance is the identifiable barrier to medication adherence, providers can engage and support caregivers to take a more active role in medication administration. Cost is an unfortunate but common barrier to medication adherence, and it has been identified that approximately 4% of individuals 65 years of age and older delay or do not receive medical treatment or prescriptions drugs due to cost (Centers for Disease Control and Prevention, 2017). There are a variety of options providers can use to assist patients with accessing care. Referencing the medication formulary of patients' insurance provider, discontinuing inessential medications, or referring patients to prescription assistance programs can offer the most affordable management options and improve medication adherence.

The older adult population is very susceptible to adverse reactions to medication due to age-related changes in pharmacokinetics and pharmacodynamics. The Beers Criteria for Potentially Inappropriate Medication Use in Older Adults, also known as the Beers criteria, refer to a set of guiding principles that health care professionals can use to improve the safety of prescribing medications for older adults. The Beers criteria were initially developed in 1991 by a geriatrician, Dr. Mark Beers, who worked with colleagues to identify a list of medications that posed additional health risk to the aged (Reuben et al., 2019). Since Beers' death in 2009 the Beers criteria have been updated and maintained by the American Geriatrics Society; these criteria are best used to guide prescribing and de-prescribing practices when assessing for potentially inappropriate medications in the geriatric population and have been proven to have predictive ability regarding a patient's risk for adverse drug events, emergency room visits, and hospitalizations.

E	1	20/200
F P	2	20/100
T O Z	3	20/70
L P E D	4	20/50
P E C F D	5	20/40
E D F C Z P	6	20/30
F E L O P Z D	7	20/25
D E F P O T E C	8	20/20
L E F O D P C T	9	
F D P L T C E O	10	
P D Z O L O F T D	11	

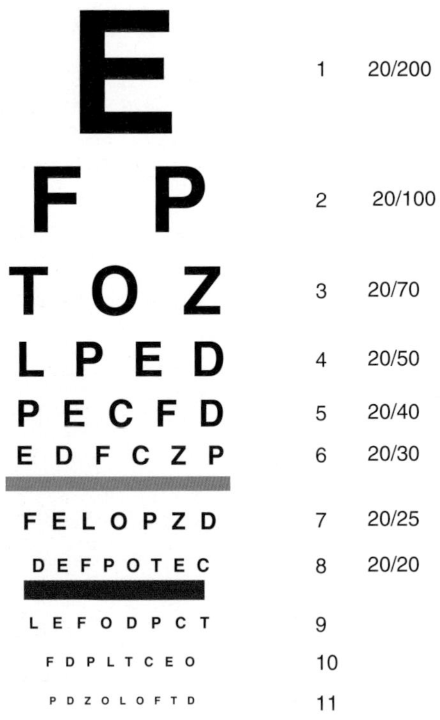

• **Fig. 10.1** Snellen Eye Chart (From Azzam, D., & Ronquillo, Y. [2021]. Snellen chart. In *StatPearls*. StatPearls Publishing. PMID: 32644387.)

Physical Assessment

A geriatrics-focused physical assessment should concentrate on aspects that affect function, including vision, hearing, urinary incontinence, gait, and balance.

Visual impairment is prevalent among the aged, but it is often underreported. The National Center for Health Statistics (2017) found that 13.4% of individuals 65 to 74 years of age have vision impairment, and that increases to 18.9% for individuals 75 years of age or older (US Department of Health and Human Services, Centers for Disease Control and Prevention, 2017). Screening for visual impairments in acuity, peripheral vision, contrast sensitivity, and depth perception is important to identify older people at risk for difficulty with driving, instrumental activities of daily living dysfunctions, or falls and fractures.

The most common visual screening test performed is use of the Snellen chart (Fig. 10.1) or a random E chart, which evaluates visual acuity. Visual acuity is patients' ability to discern the shapes and details of the things they see. It is expressed as a fraction (e.g., 20/20), which means a patient's visual acuity at 20 feet away from an object is normal. Patients who score 20/40 need to be 20 feet away to see an object that people can normally see from 40 feet away. Severe visual impairment or legal blindness is identified at a visual acuity of 20/200 or worse in the better eye. Driving laws vary state to state; however, a visual acuity of 20/40 is the most common standard used when a person is seeking to qualify for a driver's license. Providers caring for older adults need to be aware of driving laws in their state regarding vision and requirements for advising or reporting patients who have significant visual impairment (National Institute on Aging, 2018; Reuben et al., 2019).

Assessment of visual fields is another common vision screening used in primary geriatric care to assess for losses in a patient's central and peripheral vision, most commonly due to glaucoma. Glaucoma is the second leading cause of blindness and a major source of morbidity and disability in older Americans (Gupta et al., 2016). Unfortunately, there are no symptoms in the early stages of glaucoma, thus many persons affected are unaware until considerable damage to their vision is done. It is estimated that 2.3 million people 60 years of age and older have a glaucoma diagnosis, with the prevalence highest in non-Hispanic blacks, followed by non-Hispanic whites, and Mexican Americans (Gupta et al., 2016). Glaucoma has characteristic optic cupping and nerve damage resulting in loss of peripheral vision fields, requiring ophthalmologist management every 6 to 12 months. There are a variety of approaches to assess visual fields, but most commonly primary care providers use confrontation visual field testing (Fig. 10.2).

The provider faces the patient and asks the patient to look straight ahead at a fixed item. The provider will present an object, often two fingers, slowly moving in the patient's peripheral visual field while the patient's gaze remains straight ahead. Patients are instructed to alert the provider when they detect the peripheral object. This helps identify where patients' peripheral vision begins and ends. For earlier glaucoma detection, primary care providers can rely on the assistance of an ophthalmologist to perform a dilated eye exam for direct evaluation of the optic nerve and to measure the intraocular pressure of the eye.

In addition to general vision screenings, there are diagnosis-specific considerations that require attention when managing the older adult population. A biennial full examination by an ophthalmologist is recommended for patients greater than 65 years old and annually for those with glaucoma, macular degeneration, diabetes, retinopathy, or being treated with hydroxychloroquine (Plaquenil). In most cases vision can be corrected; therefore it is the role of the provider to identify those at risk for visual impairments and complete routine visual screenings to identify the visual impairment and make appropriate referrals to ophthalmologists or optometrists.

Hearing impairment is the most common sensory impairment in the aged. The National Center for Health Statistics found that 27.3% of individuals 65 to 74 years of age have hearing impairment, and that increases to 45.1% for individuals 75 years of age or older (US Department of Health and Human Services, Centers for Disease Control and Prevention, 2017). Hearing impairment can negatively affect a patient's ability to communicate clearly and socialize, and it can impact cognitive performance. The correlation between hearing loss and dementia is well documented in research; however, it is not clear if hearing impairment is a risk factor or early sign of dementia (Golub et al., 2017).

Hearing screening should be a routine assessment completed for all patients. Screening begins by asking these questions: Do you feel you have hearing loss? Do others complain that you don't hear them or they have to repeat themselves? Do others complain that you have the television or radio too loud? If the patient answers yes, the first step is to examine the ear and ear canal and rule out cerumen impaction; this step is essential prior to performing any additional screening. Once clear, providers can proceed with the whisper test or use an AudioScope to determine the pattern of loss and if the loss is unilateral or bilateral. It is important to document the intensity of the test tone (i.e., dB level) and what losses are present at the different frequencies (e.g., 500, 1000, 2000, 4000 Hz). The whisper test is an exercise whereby the provider stands behind the patient an arm's length away from the ear being tested. The provider asks the patient to occlude the untested ear. Next the provider fully exhales, whispers a combination of three numbers and a letter (e.g., 7 K 4), and then asks the patient to repeat the combination. If the patient is unable to repeat all three characters, the provider whispers a second set. If the patient is unable to repeat at least three of the six characters, he or she is positive for hearing impairment. Once it is established that a hearing impairment is present, a referral should be placed to an audiologist to provide a more specific classification of the hearing disorder—sensorineural hearing loss, conductive hearing loss, central auditory processing disorders, for example—and discuss corrective treatments. Not all patients are interested in corrective treatments for their hearing loss; however, there are still strategies that can be used to improve communication during patient encounters. In clinical practice when evaluating a patient with an identified or known hearing loss who does not use hearing amplification, it is useful for the medical provider to have available a portable assistive hearing device, such as a Pocketalker or earphones that connect to a mobile phone with an amplification application that can be used to augment hearing. These are relatively inexpensive, portable, and often demonstrate to patients who are reluctant to acknowledge hearing loss how much conversation they are missing.

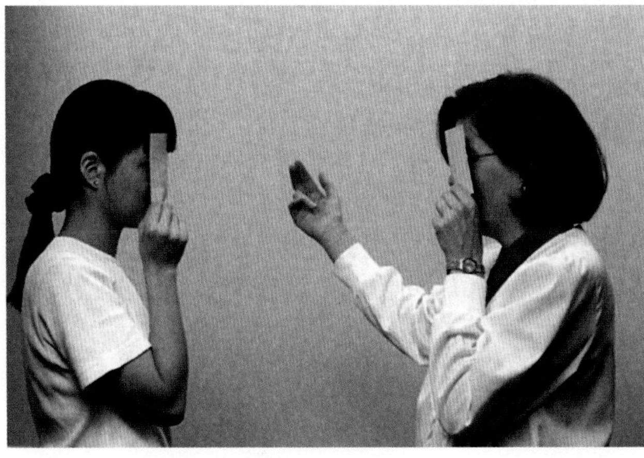

• **Fig. 10.2** Visual Field Assessment. (From Wilson, S. F., & Giddens, J. F. [2013]. *Health assessment for nursing practice* (5th ed.). Mosby.)

Fall incidents can be the result of multiple factors: intrinsic factors (poor balance, visual impairment, generalized weakness, and cognitive decline), extrinsic factors (medication adverse effects), and environmental factors (stairs, poor lighting, and throw rugs). "Falls are the leading cause of injury-related morbidity and mortality among older adults in the United States. In 2014, 28.7% of community-dwelling adults 65 years or older reported falling, resulting in 29 million falls (37.5% of which needed medical treatment or restricted activity for a day or longer) and an estimated 33,000 deaths in 2015" (Force, 2018, p. 1699). The role of the geriatric provider is to identify patients with an increased risk for falling and to implement an intervention to decrease fall incidents. Falls risk should be assessed upon establishing care, at annual wellness visits, during transitions of care, with changes in condition (including fall incidents), and after starting a medication or adjusting medication dosages.

There are a variety of screening tools used to assess gait and balance, typically by evaluating quadricep strength, static balance, dynamic balance, gait speed, and gait quality:

- *Orthostatic hypotension:* To evaluate for postural hypotension, the blood pressure and pulse are measured in lying, sitting, and standing positions. Initially, the patient is assisted into a lying position and requested to remain lying for 5 minutes. After 5 minutes, the blood pressure and pulse rate are measured. Next, the patient is assisted into a standing position, and after 3 minutes the blood pressure and pulse rate are measured. A test is considered abnormal if the systolic blood pressure drops 20 or more points, if the diastolic blood pressure drops 10 or more points, or if the patient reports syncope, lightheadedness, dizziness, blurred vision, diaphoresis, head or neck pain, or decreased hearing.
- *Timed up and go:* All you need for this screening is a standard armchair and measured distance of 10 feet. Once set up, you ask the patient to take a seat in a standard armchair and provide the following instructions: "When

I say go, I would like you to (1) stand up from the chair. (2) Walk to the line on the floor at your normal pace. (3) Turn. (4) Walk back to the chair at your normal pace. (5) Sit down again." It is acceptable for patients to use an assistive device if needed. On the word *go*, you will begin timing the patient and monitoring for abnormalities: slow gait speed, loss of balance, short strides, shuffling gait, little or no arm swing, steadying self on walls or furniture, a discontinuous turn, or inappropriate use of an assistive device. This screening tool evaluates both static and dynamic balance, but patients are noted to have an elevated risk for falls if the time is greater than or equal to 12 seconds.

- *Tandem stance:* For this test you will be evaluating a patient's static balance. You will inform patients that they will be demonstrating four standing positions and should maintain the stance for 10 seconds prior to moving to the next position. If they are able to maintain the position without moving their feet or needing to steady themselves for 10 seconds, they will move on to the next position for a total of four positions: (1) feet side by side, (2) feet semitandem, (3) feet full tandem, and (4) standing on one foot (Fig. 10.3). Patients should not use assistive devices during this screening, but you should stand next to the patients, hold their arm, and help them assume the correct position to ensure safety. When patients are steady, let go, and time how long they can maintain the position, but remain ready to assist patients if they should lose their balance.

Falls are a prevalent occurrence within the older population and result in serious injury, functional decline, decreased quality of life, fear of falling, and poor health outcomes. In addition to using the screening tool discussed earlier to assess gait pattern and balance, contributing factors must be considered when assessing fall risk and recommending patient-specific interventions.

Special consideration: Osteoporosis is a skeletal disorder characterized by loss of bone mass resulting in a bone fragility and increased risk of fractures. Osteoporosis is usually asymptomatic until a fracture occurs. The USPSTF recommends routine screening of at-risk populations for osteoporosis with a goal of preventing osteoporotic fractures. Routine screening is recommended for the following patients:

- Women 65 years of age and older
- Postmenopausal women younger than 65 years of age but at increased risk of osteoporosis
- Men at increased risk of osteoporosis (U.S. Preventative Services Task Force: Final Recommendation Statement Osteoporosis to Prevent Fractures: Screening, n.d.).

SAFETY ALERT

The following systems may contribute to fall risk:

- *Neurologic:* Hemiparesis, changes in gait pattern, ataxia, tremor
- *Neuropathy:* Altered sensation and proprioception of the lower extremities
- *Ophthalmologic conditions:* Poor depth perception, impaired peripheral and central vision
- *Cardiovascular disease:* Orthostatic hypotension, distress on exertion
- *Pulmonary disease:* Poor oxygenation
- *Musculoskeletal conditions:* Structural changes, decreased range of motion

Once fall risk is identified and patients have been classified as having a low, moderate, or high fall risk, an intervention, if necessary, can be implemented.

Instructions to the patient:

- I'm going to show you four positions.
- Try to stand in each position for 10 seconds.
- You can hold your arms out, or move your body to help keep your balance, but don't move your feet.
- For each position I will say, **"Ready, begin."** Then, I will start timing. After 10 seconds, I will say, "Stop."

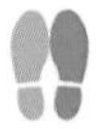	**① Stand with your feet side-by-side.**	Time: ________ seconds
	② Place the instep of one foot so it is touching the big toe of the other foot.	Time: ________ seconds
	③ Tandem stand: Place one foot in front of the other, heel touching toe.	Time: ________ seconds
	④ Stand on one foot.	Time: ________ seconds

• **Fig. 10.3** Tandem Stance Balance Test Lateral (A) and back view (B) of an individual performing the tandem stance balance test with visual feedback in real time (yellow dot, center of pressure; red dot, target point). (From the Centers for Disease Control and Prevention: National Center for Injury Prevention and Control.)

Functional Assessment

During a physical exam, a clinician can discover a great deal about a patient using assessment techniques and observational skills. But what patients can do in their day-to-day life outside of the clinic is not as easy to ascertain. To live independently in the community, a person must be able to perform certain tasks. Changes in health, hospitalizations, and even normal aging can change functional ability. Several scales have been developed to help determine a patient's functional status. These can be helpful in determining a patient's current state as well as the progression of disease states. Some of the most commonly used scales are the Lawton-Brody instrumental activities of daily living scale and the Katz index of independence in activities of daily living scale.

The Lawton–Brody instrumental activities of daily living (IADL) scale assesses skills such as one's ability to use the telephone, shop, prepare food, clean the house, do laundry, handle transportation, manage medications, and handle finances (Lawton & Brody, 1969).

The Katz index of independence in activities of daily living (ADL) scale assesses a person's ability to satisfactorily perform her or his own personal care, ambulate, and eat independently (Katz et al., 1963).

A commonly used performance status test is the Karnofsky scale, which can be helpful in determining disability status (Karnofsky, 1949).

Elder Abuse

According to the National Council on Aging, approximately 10% of Americans age 60 and older have been the victim of some type of elder abuse (National Council on Aging [NCOA], n.d.). Elder abuse can include physical, sexual, financial, and emotional abuse, as well as neglect and self-neglect (National Center on Elder Abuse [NCEA], n.d.). If elder abuse is suspected, the Elder Abuse Suspicion Index (EASI) can be used for cognitively intact patients to assess the need to refer a patient to social services or adult protective services (Yaffe et al., 2008).

Lower Urinary Tract Symptoms (LUTS)

When completing the review of systems, it is important to ask patients if they have had any new or ongoing urinary symptoms such as urine leakage or incontinence, nocturia, or frequency. Consider the onset of any symptoms, recent or long-standing, and other associated problems such as mobility, cognition, or recent medication changes that may help determine the cause and perhaps treatment and potentially help improve the patient's quality of life.

If the patient complains of incontinence, it is important to ask how long it has been a problem and to what degree. For example, was it a one-time occurrence that could be explained, or has it happened on several occasions? Does it only happen under certain circumstances or during a certain time of day? Bear in mind the different types of incontinence: stress, overflow, urge, functional, and mixed.

If the patient complains of nocturia, it is important again to find out how long it has been occurring and how frequently the patient has to get up at night. Is the patient taking diuretic medications? How much caffeine or alcohol is the patient drinking? Did you notice lower extremity edema during the physical exam?

Is the patient complaining of urinary frequency? How often does the patient have to urinate? Is the patient able to completely empty his or her bladder? For male patients, ask about difficulty starting or stopping a stream of urine and if there is any dribbling, which may indicate an enlarged prostate. Is there any pain with urination?

Nutritional Assessment

Changes that occur with aging increase nutritional risk for older adults, resulting in 1 in 10 older persons experiencing malnutrition (Veronese et al., 2019). Malnutrition is a "deficiency, excess or imbalance in a person's intake of energy and/or nutrients" (World Health Organization [WHO] https://www.who.int/news-room/fact-sheets/detail/malnutrition; Veronese et al., 2019). There is a strong correlation between malnutrition and diminished physical performance, mobility limitations, and frailty (Lelli et al., 2019). Nutritional needs are attributable to several factors including health conditions, caloric requirements, activity level, energy expenditures, food preferences, and the ability to access, ingest, and digest food. Body mass index (BMI) is a measure of a person's weight in relation to his or her height. Body mass index serves as an easily assessable method clinicians use to estimate body fat, as there is a strong correlation between body mass index and other direct measures of body fat. Body mass index is classified as follows:

- Underweight: Less than 18.5
- Normal weight: 18.5 to 24.9
- Overweight: 25.0 to 29.9
- Obese: Greater than or equal to 30.0

The World Health Organization explains undernutrition as a broad concept encompassing malnutrition, overweight conditions, and obesity. There is evidence indicating no increased mortality risk for adults 65 years of age or older that are overweight (Ard et al., 2016). However, there is some benefit to weight loss in persons with obesity who have osteoarthritis, diabetes mellitus, coronary heart disease, and activity intolerance (Ard et al., 2016). Therefore, weight loss interventions are targeted at persons with a BMI greater than 30, with the greatest benefits seen in physical function, blood sugar levels, lipids, and quality of life (Ard et al., 2016).

Nutritional assessment in older adults focuses on weight loss, undernutrition, and nutrient deficiencies. Screening for nutritional status is an elemental component of geriatrics-focused primary care and needs to be assessed on annual wellness visits and with any significant changes in weight. Clinically significant weight loss is defined as follows:

- Greater than or equal to 2% weight loss in 1 month
- Greater than or equal to 5% weight loss in 3 months

- Greater than or equal to 10% weight loss in 6 months

Unintentional weight loss, especially in those with a body mass index less than 30, poses a negative impact on morbidity and mortality. Unintentional weight loss is a complicated occurrence and may be the result of a variety of factors, including the following:

- Social factors (e.g., social isolation, food insecurity)
- Medical factors (e.g., malignancy, chronic obstructive pulmonary disease [COPD], dysphagia)
- Pharmacologic factors (e.g., selective serotonin-reuptake inhibitors [SSRIs], digoxin)
- Psychological factors (e.g., depression, dementia, alcoholism)
- Physiologic factors (e.g., diminished taste, early satiety, delayed gastric emptying, and smell sensitivity)

Routine weight monitoring and body mass index tracking offer a simple screen of nutritional health. However, using validated screening tools allows for a targeted approach to identifying at-risk patients so that clinicians can initiate nutritional support when indicated. Validated nutritional screening tools are designed to detect undernutrition and patients at risk of becoming undernourished. Here is a list of widely used validated nutritional screening tools and their targeted risk group:

- *Malnutrition Universal Screening Tool (MUST):* Targeted to detect undernutrition based on the correlation between impaired nutritional status and impaired function (Jensen et al., 2019)
- *Mini Nutritional Assessment-Short Form (MNA):* Targeted to detect undernutrition and older patients at risk receiving care in their home, in a skilled nursing facility, or in the hospital setting (Jensen et al., 2019)
- *Nutritional Risk Screening-2002 (NRS-2002):* Targeted to detect undernutrition in hospitalized older patients (Jensen et al., 2019)

In 2016, leaders from several global nutritional societies met at the American Society for Parenteral and Enteral Nutrition Conference to develop an approach to diagnosing malnutrition. Consensus was agreed upon for the use of any validated nutritional screening tool, providing a diagnostic structure for malnutrition, and finally grading the severity of malnutrition. Leaders identified three phenotype or sign criteria: unintentional weight loss, low body mass index, and reduced muscle mass; and two etiologic criteria: reduced food intake and disease burden/inflammation (Jensen et al., 2019). A diagnosis of malnutrition occurs when a patient exhibits at least one phenotype criterion and one etiologic criterion (Jensen et al., 2019).

When patients present with a complaint of decreased appetite or weight loss, an evaluation of nutritional history is needed, including questions about appetite, dietary changes, and percentage of meal intake. It is important that a medication review be included in a nutritional assessment, with particular attention paid to medications with a recent dose change or that have been recently initiated. An evaluation of contributing, comorbid conditions should be assessed for progression or acute exacerbation as an underlying contributor to malnutrition. The negative impact chronic diseases, such as chronic obstructive pulmonary disease, congestive heart failure, and diabetes mellitus, have on appetite and nutrition absorption heavily impact an individual's ability to keep up with nutritional needs. Therefore identifying what comorbid conditions are present provides a physiologic etiology for a generalized symptom of appetite loss.

Prealbumin is a precursor to albumin, a vital protein used to restore and repair tissue. Testing prealbumin levels is another objective way to assist clinicians and support a diagnosis of malnutrition when assessing nutritional health. In addition to more apparent consequences of malnutrition, the depletion of micronutrients (e.g., vitamin B_{12}, calcium, vitamin D) is a common consequence, so testing vitamin levels is standard as supplementation may be indicated.

Psychological

Depression

A comprehensive physical assessment would not be complete without including a psychological assessment. Clinicians and patients need to remember that depression is not a normal consequence of aging. For some patients, their health care professional may be the only person who ever asks them how they are feeling. Understanding what screening and diagnostic tools to use can make your questions pertinent and actionable. The Patient Health Questionnaire (PHQ-9) is self-administered (although it can be interviewer-administered) and is not only a diagnostic tool for depression but can also assess its severity (Kroenke et al., 2001).

The PHQ-2 is the shortened screening version of the PHQ-9. In a busy primary care practice where efficiency is desired, the patient may be asked to complete the PHQ-2, which consists of the first two questions of the PHQ-9: *Over the last two weeks, how often have you had little interest or pleasure in doing things? Over the last two weeks, have you felt down, depressed, or hopeless?* Then a clinician can determine whether or not the patient should complete the entire PHQ-9 (Arroll et al., 2010). If the patient confirms feeling "little interest or pleasure in doing things" or "feeling down, depressed, or hopeless," the clinician should ask the remaining questions. The PHQ-9 can be used to monitor the severity of depression over time. When treating a patient who is on antidepressants, initial follow-up should occur within 2 to 4 weeks with the goal of three visits in 12 weeks, and the PHQ-9 should be used to monitor progress (DeJesus et al., 2007).

The Geriatric Depression Scale (GDS) is a 30-question depression screening tool designed for the older adult population (Yesavage et al., 1982). A shorter 15-question form is often used for patients who are medically frail or have mild dementia (Marc et al., 2008). The tool can be self-administered or interviewer administered, although studies have shown that the scores tend to be higher when self-administered (de Waal et al., 2012). As with the PHQ-9, the GDS can be used to monitor the severity of depression over time.

Anxiety

Although many patients have both depression and anxiety, it is possible for a patient to have high anxiety symptoms and not have high depression symptoms (Spitzer et al., 2006). Examples of anxiety symptoms include overwhelming worry, sleep disturbance, trouble concentrating, and muscle tension (Hoge et al., 2012). The Generalized Anxiety Disorder (GAD-7) is a seven-question anxiety scale (Spitzer et al., 2006). The GAD-7 can be used to screen for anxiety and to monitor severity. It can be both self-administered and interviewer administered. The GAD-7 can be used in the older adult population; however, some studies suggest that the cut point may need to be lowered (Wild et al., 2014).

Sleep Hygiene

Insomnia

As providers, we understand the importance of asking our patients about their diet and exercise, but equally important is to inquire about their quality of sleep. Older adult patients will more than likely have trouble staying asleep versus falling asleep (McCall, 2004). Insomnia is characterized by one or more of the following: difficulty falling asleep, difficulty staying asleep, or early morning wakening with an inability to fall back asleep. The patient must report that the symptoms have been present for at least 3 months (Glasheen et al., 2016).

Sleep Apnea

When assessing a patient's quality of sleep, a clinician may become suspicious that obstructive sleep apnea (OSA) may be the culprit, especially if the patient or patient's partner complains of snoring. A simple screening tool is the STOP-Bang questionnaire, which takes just a few minutes and has been found to have the highest sensitivity for detecting moderate-severe sleep apnea when compared to other screening tools (Chung et al., 2016).

Periodic Limb Movement Disorder/Restless Leg Syndrome

When asking patients about their sleep, especially if they report poor-quality sleep, pay attention to symptoms such as "tossing and turning" or a compelling urge to move a limb. Periodic limb movement disorder (PLMD) is defined as intermittent leg movements >15/hour together with sleep disturbance and daytime fatigue (Scofield et al., 2008). Restless leg syndrome (RLS) is described as unpleasant feelings in the legs that causes an uncontrollable need to move, symptoms that are worse at rest, and symptoms that can often be relieved by moving or pacing (Allen et al., 2005). If sleep apnea has been suspected in the past, the patient may have a polysomnographic monitoring, which, along with an electrogram, can detect the presence of limb movement while sleeping (Walters, 2001). If periodic limb movement disorder or restless leg syndrome is suspected, a sleep study may be needed for further evaluation.

Substance Use Disorder

Substance use disorder is a chronic relapsing brain disorder characterized by an impaired ability to stop or control substance use despite unfavorable social, occupational, or health consequences. The most commonly misused substances are marijuana, alcohol, opioids, and illicit drugs and cost the United States an estimated $64 billion annually in health care costs (National Institute on Drug Abuse [NIDA], n.d.[b]). Substance use has been shown to cause poor health outcomes and increased mortality (National Institutes of Health, n.d.). Mental health problems and substance use disorders share underlying causes, including changes in brain composition, genetic vulnerabilities, and early exposure to stress or trauma (US Department of Health & Human Services, n.d.). More than one in four adults living with serious mental health problems have a concurrent substance use disorder (US Department of Health & Human Services, n.d.). Symptoms of substance use disorder may include behavior, physical, or social changes with symptoms defined by the *Diagnostic and Statistical Manual of Mental Disorders*, fifth edition *(DSM-5)* criteria, including the following:

- Continuing to use a substance despite adverse consequences
- Repeated inability to carry out roles at work or home as a result of use
- Recurrent use in physically hazardous situations
- Continued use despite persistent social and interpersonal problems during use
- Tolerance, needing an increased dose to achieve some effect, or a diminished effect with the use of the same dose
- Withdrawal syndrome or use of the substance to avoid withdrawal
- Using more substance or using for a more extended period than intended
- Persistent desire to cut down use or unsuccessful attempts to control use
- Spending a significant amount of time obtaining, using, or recovering from use
- Stopping or reducing important occupational, social, or recreational activities due to use
- Craving or strong desire to use

Alcohol misuse can occur at any age but is the primary substance misused in the older adult population, which poses a unique set of complications (Reuben et al., 2019). Alcohol misuse is often unrecognized because of the reduced social and occupational responsibilities of retirees, but it accounts for 20% of alcohol-related deaths in persons 65 years of age and older (National Institutes of Health, n.d.). "Alcohol is a factor in 30 percent of suicides, 40 percent of crashes and burns, 50 percent of drownings and homicides, and 60 percent of falls" (National Institute on Drug Abuse [NIDA], n.d.[a]). The National Institute on Alcohol Abuse and Alcoholism defines at-risk drinking for anyone age 65 years or older as having more than seven drinks a week or three drinks on one occasion (Reuben et al., 2019).

• BOX 10.1 Medication Classes That Interact With Alcohol

- Tylenol
- Anesthetics
- Antihypertensives
- Antihistamines
- Antipsychotics
- Narcotic analgesics
- Nonsteroidal antiinflammatory drugs (NSAIDs)
- Sedatives
- Antidepressants
- Anticonvulsants
- Nitrates
- Beta-blockers
- Oral hypoglycemic agents
- Anticoagulants

Alcohol tolerance changes with age due to decreased lean body mass and total body water resulting in higher blood concentrations per amount of alcohol consumed. Often the consequences of alcohol misuse can be mistaken for other age-related conditions—for example, memory changes or gait and balance changes. Alcohol misuse can also worsen comorbid health conditions like diabetes, osteoporosis, hypertension, memory loss, and mood disorders, as well as can lead to malignancy. Many drugs interact with alcohol; therefore, a medication review becomes an elemental component of assessment when suspecting alcohol misuse. The provider must also be mindful of the concurrent use of alcohol with certain medications (Box 10.1).

In addition, clinicians need to be mindful not only to screen for illicit and recreational substances but also to assess for the misuse of prescribed medications. According to the National Institute on Drug Abuse, the most common prescription drugs abused are pain medications (opioids), anxiety or insomnia medications (benzodiazepines and sedatives), and medications for attention deficit hyperactivity disorder and narcolepsy (stimulants) (Reuben et al., 2019). The misuse of prescription medications comes with significant complications, the most notable of which are dizziness, somnolence, falls, fractures, mobility impairments, cognitive impairments, pressure ulcers, urinary incontinence, anxiety, depression, hallucinations, and delirium (Reuben et al., 2019).

Cannabis is the most commonly used drug among adults, with a steady increase in use in the United States since 2007, with more prevalent use among particular groups such as baby boomers and military veterans (Mauro et al., 2018). With the legalization of medicinal and recreational marijuana across many American states, older adults are hearing beneficial accounts of marijuana use and experimenting with marijuana, oftentimes without medical supervision. In 2014, the University of Colorado Movement Disorders Center clinic reported about 5% of its Parkinson disease study participants, with an average age of 69, reported using marijuana. In the same clinic, 30% of the general patient population with Parkinson disease inquired about marijuana use over a 6-month period (University of Colorado, Denver, 2019). With such significant increases in the recreational use and medical applications of cannabis, increased attention has been focused on the short- and long-term health effects associated with cannabis use; however, the majority of research is on adolescent cannabis use. It is important to note that researchers have identified changes in executive functions, memory, learning, and impulse control with cannabis use, with a more substantial effect and negative correlation with age (National Institute on Drug Abuse [NIDA], n.d.[c]). Cannabis is an effective treatment for chronic pain, nausea, muscle spasticity, and insomnia. However, patients should be counseled of the washout period and recommended not to drive for 6 hours after inhalation or 9 hours after ingestion. Medication review remains a signification component of assessment. Cannabis has an additive effect when combined with other central nervous system active medications and interacts with warfarin, anticholinergics, alcohol, glipizide, loop diuretics, and statin medications (Reuben et al., 2019).

Opioid use in older persons is associated with the development of geriatric syndromes, specifically cognitive impairment, delirium, falls, reduced appetite, urinary incontinence, and depression (Saraf et al., 2016). It is estimated that prescription misuse and abuse in older people may be as high as 11%, and risk factors include female sex, social isolation, depression, and mental health problems (Reuben et al., 2019). In addition to screening for opioid use, concurrent use of opioids with either benzodiazepines or gabapentinoids increases risk of overdose, severe sedation, respiratory distress, and death (American Geriatrics Society, 2019).

There is a strong correlation of substance use among persons with significant psychological distress; therefore, screening becomes a useful practice to identify patients in need of substance use interventions as well as treatment for comorbid mental health conditions. Thorough questioning about substance use and historical substance use is the standard of care; however, the use of screening tools can increase the feasibility of screening for substance use disorders in a more systematic fashion and assists with identifying at-risk patients. Here is a list of validated tools that can assist clinicians in primary care:

- *The Tobacco, Alcohol, Prescription medication, and other Substance use (TAPS) tool:* This two-step assessment consists of a screening component (TAPS-1) followed by a brief assessment (TAPS-2) for those who screen positive. It can be self-administered or used as an interview tool by a health professional (McNeely et al., 2016).
- *The Cannabis Use Disorder Identification Test-Short Form (CUDIT-R):* This eight-item screening tool assesses for cannabis consumption, problems associated with abuse, dependence, and the psychological consequences for those who are at risk for cannabis misuse (Bonn-Miller et al., 2016).
- *The CAGE questionnaire:* This alcohol screening tool has been validated for use in the older population. A positive response to any of the questions suggests misuse of alcohol and the need for intervention (Reuben et al., 2019).

- *The Alcohol Use Disorder Identification Test-Consumption questionnaire (AUDIT-C):* This questionnaire identifies patients with problem use as well as those with more severe alcohol use disorder. It can be self-administered or used in conjunction with a patient interview (Reuben et al., 2019).
- *The Opioid Risk Tool (ORT):* This self-administered screening tool is used for primary care patients undergoing opioid treatment for chronic pain. It is recommended that the questionnaire be administered when patients establish care or before the initiation of opioid medication to better identify those patients with an elevated risk for misuse (Webster, n.d.).

Clinicians have an opportunity to be extraordinarily impactful when engaging patients about health behaviors and health risks. They are encouraged to foster an open dialogue about substance use to reinforce healthy behaviors, identify patients at risk, and identify patients in need of treatment for substance use disorder.

Cognitive

When assessing cognition, the health care provider will want to consider factors that can influence a patient's performance, such as hearing, vision, hypoxia, medications, substance use, language, and education. If a patient suffers from hearing loss, ensuring that testing is completed while using hearing aids or other amplification is important. For patients with low vision, the provider should consider magnification, prescription eyewear, or a screening test that relies on verbal questions. If during the assessment the provider notes that the older adult patient is hypoxic, correcting the hypoxia should take precedence, as cognition can be affected from low levels of oxygen. Certain medications and substance use can cause sedation or confusion and should be taken into consideration whether or not testing is appropriate at the time. If English is not the patient's primary language, the provider should consider using an interpreter. As a clinician, you should know if your patient has lower education levels or low literacy, as you need to take this into consideration when performing cognitive testing and when providing patient education. A common screening tool for cognitive impairment is the Mini-Cog, which includes a three-item recall and a clock drawing (Borson, n.d.). In an older adult population, compared with longer screening tools, the Mini-Cog is as effective (Borson et al., 2003).

Healthy People Initiatives

Healthy People is a United States initiative centered on improving the health of all people living in the United States of America with a framework focused on health promotion, disease prevention, health information technology, health communication, and addressing all hazards and preparedness for public health issues (e.g., natural disasters, influenza pandemic) (Healthy People 2020: Framework, n.d.). Led by an advisory committee composed of US federal agencies, subject matter experts, and public stakeholders, Healthy People provides a decade-long national objective and structure for policy makers, health systems, and clinicians (Healthy People 2020: Framework, n.d.).

Healthy People 2020's mission focuses on increasing awareness and understanding of social determinants of health. Social determinants of health are social, environmental, and economic conditions that impact health outcomes. "Globally, an estimated 24% of the burden of disease and 23% of all deaths can be attributed to environmental factors" (World Health Organization, n.d.). There is well-founded research comparing the United States to other countries with similar wealth, and the United States has worse life expectancy, mortality, and disease burden rates, which may be due in part to the quality of care provided; however, social determinants likely contribute to some of the cross-national differences (Kamal, 2017). "Fifty percent of inequalities in the distribution within populations of the more important noncommunicable diseases, especially cardiovascular disease and lung cancer, can be accounted for by social inequalities in risk factors" (World Health Organization, n.d.). It is essential when developing plans of care to consider social determinants of health that patients have to navigate in order to provide the necessary support. There are significant associations between the patients' health status and their communities' economic characteristics, including income and inequality in income distribution, wealth, poverty, and the geographic concentration of poverty (Centers for Disease Control and Prevention, n.d.). Healthy People 2020 defined the social determinants of health as follows:

- *Economic stability:* Income/retirement benefits, food insecurity, housing stability, poverty
- *Education:* Early childhood education and development, high school graduation, enrollment in higher education, language, and literacy
- *Social and community context:* Civic participation, community engagement, discrimination, incarceration, social cohesion, social integration, and support systems
- *Health and health care:* Access to health care, access to primary care, health literacy, provider linguistic, cultural competency, and quality of care
- *Neighborhood and built environment:* Access to foods that support healthy eating patterns, crime and violence, transportation, environmental conditions, and quality of housing (Healthy People 2020: Social Determinants of Health, n.d.)

Even when patients are fully engaged in care, there can be circumstances that lead to poor health outcomes; therefore, it is vital to identify patients with elevated risk for individual barriers to care when developing a plan of care keeping social determinants in mind.

Healthy People is in its fifth edition and developing its initiatives for Healthy People 2030. The advisory committee is in the process of developing mission and vision statements, framework, organizational structure, and selection criteria for developing measurable and nationally representative objectives; however, essential concepts that are being considered include the following:

- *Closing gaps:* Health disparities, health equity, and health literacy
- *Cultivating healthier environments:* Physical environments, social environments, and economic environments
- *Increasing knowledge and action:* Shared responsibility across sectors; public health successes; evidence-based laws, policies, and practices; and objectives and data
- *Maintaining health and well-being across the life span*: Physical, mental, and social dimensions, access to quality public health and clinical care (Implementation of Healthy People 2030, n.d.)

Conclusion

This chapter offers tools to assist providers with the detection of conditions prevalent in older adults and to supplement clinical judgment. Medication review is paramount in providing care for the older adult, whether conducting a wellness visit or managing an acute medical issue. As providers caring for an increasingly globalized society, we must contemplate what circumstances are present that lead to poor health outcomes, identify patients with elevated risks, and consider individual barriers to care when developing a treatment plan. Providing age-friendly care through the use of an interprofessional geriatric team is the most effective for the care of frail older adults with multiple comorbid conditions. It is essential for clinicians to provide culturally sensitive, goal-oriented care that prioritizes clinical needs aligned with the patient's goals.

Key Points

- PAs and NPs are ideally suited to serve as geriatric assessment team leaders where they can use their skills and training to facilitate communication and collaboration with the goal of improving outcomes for older adults, especially those with complex medical problems.
- The clinical assessment of a patient starts upon walking into the exam room and greeting the patient. The clinician must observe closely, listen carefully, and communicate clearly in order to gather as much information as possible.
- Obtaining the patient history and completing a medication review will give the clinician a clearer picture of what is actually going on.
- Including a visual, hearing, and gait assessment along with a physical exam allows a clinician to identify potential barriers to understanding the plan of care. Additionally, reviewing the patient's nutritional and functional status will identify potential access to care issues.
- Identifying depression or cognitive impairment in a patient is necessary in order to make appropriate clinical recommendations and to identify when it is necessary to include a family member in their execution.

More information about tools and the Interprofessional Education Collaborative (IPEC) competencies mentioned in this chapter can be found in Appendix 1: Tools and Appendix 2: IPEC Competencies.

References

Allen, R. P., Walters, A. S., Montplaisir, J., Hening, W., Myers, A., Bell, T. J., & Ferini-Strambi, L. (2005). Restless legs syndrome prevalence and impact: REST General Population Study. *Archives of Internal Medicine*, *165*(11), 1286–1292. https://doi.org/10.1001/archinte.165.11.1286.

American Geriatrics Society. (2019). *2019 AGS Beers Criteria Pocketcard.*

Ard, J. D., Gower, B., Hunter, G., Ritchie, C. S., Roth, D. L., Goss, A., ... Locher, J. L. (2016). Effects of calorie restriction in obese older adults: The CROSSROADS Randomized Controlled Trial. *The Journals of Gerontology: Series A*, *73*(1), 73–80. https://doi.org/10.1093/gerona/glw237.

Arroll, B., Goodyear-Smith, F., Crengle, S., Gunn, J., Kerse, N., Fishman, T., ... Hatcher, S. (2010). Validation of PHQ-2 and PHQ-9 to screen for major depression in the primary care population. *Annals of Family Medicine*, *8*(4), 348–353. https://doi.org/10.1370/afm.1139.

Bonn-Miller, M. O., Heinz, A. J., Smith, E. V., Bruno, R., & Adamson, S. (2016). Preliminary development of a brief cannabis use disorder screening tool: The Cannabis Use Disorder Identification Test Short-Form. *Cannabis and Cannabinoid Research*, *1*(1), 252–261. https://doi.org/10.1089/can.2016.0022.

Borson, S. (n.d.). *Mini-Cog: Screening for cognitive impairment in older adults.* https://mini-cog.com/.

Borson, S., Scanlan, J.M., Chen, P., & Ganguli, M. (2003). The Mini-Cog as a screen for dementia: Validation in a population-based sample. *Journal of the American Geriatrics Society*, 51(10), 1451–1454. https://doi.org/10.1046/j.1532-5415.2003.51465.x

Centers for Disease Control and Prevention. (n.d.). *Health Impact in 5 Years.* Retrieved from https://www.cdc.gov/policy/hst/hi5/docs/hi5-overview-v7.pdf.

Centers for Disease Control and Prevention. (2017). *Delay or nonreceipt of needed medical care, nonreceipt of needed prescription drugs, or nonreceipt of needed dental care during the past 12 months due to cost, by selected characteristics: United States, selected years 1997–2016.* https://www.cdc.gov/nchs/data/hus/2017/063.pdf.

Chung, F., Abdullah, H. R., & Liao, P. (2016). STOP-Bang Questionnaire: A practical approach to screen for obstructive sleep apnea. *Chest, 149*(3), 631–638. https://doi.org/10.1378/chest.15-0903.

DeJesus, R. S., Vickers, K. S., Melin, G. J., & Williams, M. D. (2007). A system-based approach to depression management in primary care using the Patient Health Questionnaire-9. *Mayo Clinic Proceedings, 82*(11), 1395–1402. https://doi.org/10.4065/82.11.1395.

de Waal, M. W. M., van der Weele, G. M., van der Mast, R. C., Assendelft, W. J. J., & Gussekloo, J. (2012). The influence of the administration method on scores of the 15-item Geriatric Depression Scale in old age. *Psychiatry Research, 197*(3), 280–284. https://doi.org/10.1016/j.psychres.2011.08.019.

Drug disposal: Flush potentially dangerous medicine. (2018). https://www.fda.gov/drugs/disposal-unused-medicines-what-you-should-know/drug-disposal-flush-potentially-dangerous-medicine#FlushList.

Glasheen, C., Batts, K., Karg, R., Bose, J., Hedden, S., Piscopo, K., Hunter, D., & Tice, P. (2016). *Impact of the DSM-IV to DSM-5 changes on the National Survey on Drug Use and Health.* CBHSQ Methodology Report website, http://www.ncbi.nlm.nih.gov/pubmed/30199183.

Golub, J. S., Luchsinger, J. A., Manly, J. J., Stern, Y., Mayeux, R., & Schupf, N. (2017). Observed hearing loss and incident dementia in a multiethnic cohort. *Journal of the American Geriatrics Society, 65*(8), 1691–1697. https://doi.org/10.1111/jgs.14848.

Gupta, P., Zhao, D., Guallar, E., Ko, F., Boland, M. V., & Friedman, D. S. (2016). Prevalence of glaucoma in the United States: The 2005–2008 National Health and Nutrition Examination Survey. *Investigative Ophthalmology & Visual Science, 57*(6), 2905–2913. https://doi.org/10.1167/iovs.15-18469.

Healthy People 2020: Framework. (n.d.). https://www.healthypeople.gov/sites/default/files/HP2020Framework.pdf

Healthy People 2020: Social Determinants of Health. (n.d.). https://www.healthypeople.gov/2020/topics-objectives/topic/social-determinants-of-health.

Hoge, E. A., Ivkovic, A., & Fricchione, G. L. (2012). Generalized anxiety disorder: Diagnosis and treatment. *BMJ: British Medical Journal, 345*, e7500. https://doi.org/10.1136/bmj.e7500.

Implementation of Healthy People 2030: Recommendations for Implementation and the Framework Graphic for Healthy People 2030. (n.d.). https://www.healthypeople.gov/sites/default/files/Report 8_Implementation and Graphic_Formatted_ EO_508c-final_0.pdf

Jensen, G. L., Cederholm, T., Correia, M. I. T. D., Gonzalez, M. C., Fukushima, R., Higashiguchi, T., & Gossum, A. (2019). GLIM criteria for the diagnosis of malnutrition: A consensus report from the Global Clinical Nutrition Community. *Journal of Parenteral and Enteral Nutrition, 43*(1), 32–40. https://doi.org/10.1002/jpen.1440.

Kamal, R. (2017). *What do we know about social determinants of health in the U.S. and comparable countries? Peterson-Kaiser Health System Tracker*. Peterson-Kaiser Health System Tracker website: https://www.healthsystemtracker.org/chart-collection/know-social-determinants-health-u-s-comparable-countries/?_sf_s=social#item-u-s-obesity-prevalent-among-lower-income-groups-higher-incomes

Karnofsky, D. A. (1949). The clinical evaluation of chemotherapeutic agents in cancer. *Evaluation of Chemotherapeutic Agents*, 191–205.

Katz, S., Ford, A., Moskowitz, R., Jackson, B., & Jaffe, M. (1963). Studies of illness in the aged. *Journal of the American Medical Association, 185*(12), 914. https://doi.org/10.1001/jama.1963.03060120024016.

Kroenke, K., Spitzer, R. L., & Williams, J. B. W. (2001). Validity of a brief depression severity measure. *Journal of General Internal Medicine, 16*(9), 606–613.

Lawton, M. P., & Brody, E. M. (1969). Assessment of older people: Self-maintaining and instrumental activities of daily living. *The Gerontologist, 9*(3 Part 1), 179–186.

Lelli, D., Calle, A., Pérez, L. M., Onder, G., Morandi, A., Ortolani, E., & Inzitari, M. (2019). Nutritional status and functional outcomes in older adults admitted to geriatric rehabilitations: The SAFARI Study. *Journal of the American College of Nutrition, 38*(5), 441–446. https://doi.org/10.1080/07315724.2018.1541427.

Marc, L. G., Raue, P. J., & Bruce, M. L. (2008). Screening performance of the 15-item geriatric depression scale in a diverse elderly home care population. *American Journal of Geriatric Psychiatry: Official Journal of the American Association for Geriatric Psychiatry, 16*(11), 914–921. https://doi.org/10.1097/JGP.0b013e318186bd67.

Mauro, P. M., Carliner, H., Brown, Q. L., Hasin, D. S., Shmulewitz, D., Rahim-Juwel, R., & Martins, S. S. (2018). Age differences in daily and nondaily cannabis use in the United States, 2002-2014. *Journal of Studies on Alcohol and Drugs, 79*(3), 423–431. https://doi.org/10.15288/jsad.2018.79.423.

McCall, W. V. (2004). Sleep in the elderly: Burden, diagnosis, and treatment. *Primary Care Companion to the Journal of Clinical Psychiatry, 6*(1), 9–20. https://doi.org/10.4088/pcc.v06n0104.

McNeely, J., Wu, L. -T., Subramaniam, G., Sharma, G., Cathers, L. A., Svikis, D., & Schwartz, R. P. (2016). Performance of the Tobacco, Alcohol, Prescription Medication, and Other Substance Use (TAPS) tool for substance use screening in primary care patients. *Annals of Internal Medicine, 165*(10), 690–699. https://doi.org/10.7326/M16-0317.

Medicare.gov. (n.d.). *Yearly "wellness" visits.* https://www.medicare.gov/coverage/yearly-wellness-visits.

National Center for Health Statistics. (2017). *Summary health statistics: National Health Interview Survey*, 2017. https://ftp.cdc.gov/pub/Health_Statistics/NCHS/NHIS/SHS/2017_SHS_Table_A-6.pdf.

National Center on Elder Abuse (NCEA). (n.d.). https://ncea.acl.gov/FAQ.aspx.

National Council on Aging (NCOA): Elder Abuse Facts. (n.d.). *Get the facts on elder abuse.* https://www.ncoa.org/public-policy-action/elder-justice/elder-abuse-facts/

National Institute on Aging. (2018). *Older drivers.* https://www.nia.nih.gov/health/older-drivers

National Institute on Drug Abuse. (NIDA). (n.d.[a]). *Comorbidity: Substance use and other mental disorders.* https://www.drugabuse.gov/related-topics/trends-statistics/infographics/comorbidity-substance-use-other-mental-disorders.

National Institute on Drug Abuse. (NIDA). (n.d.[b]). *Trends & statistics.* https://www.drugabuse.gov/related-topics/trends-statistics

National Institute on Drug Abuse. (NIDA). (n.d.[c]). *What are marijuana's long-term effects on the brain?* https://www.drugabuse.gov/publications/research-reports/marijuana/what-are-marijuanas-long-term-effects-brain.

National Institutes of Health. (n.d.). From TAPS website: https://www.drugabuse.gov/taps/#/.

Reuben, D. B., Herr, K. A., Pacala, J. T., Pollock, B. G., Potter, J. F., & Semla, T. (2019). *Geriatrics at your fingertips* (21st ed.). The American Geriatrics Society.

Saraf, A. A., Petersen, A. W., Simmons, S. F., Schnelle, J. F., Bell, S. P., Kripalani, S., & Vasilevskis, E. E. (2016). Medications associated with geriatric syndromes and their prevalence in older hospitalized adults discharged to skilled nursing facilities. *Journal of Hospital Medicine, 11*(10), 694–700. https://doi.org/10.1002/jhm.2614.

Scofield, H., Roth, T., & Drake, C. (2008). Periodic limb movements during sleep: population prevalence, clinical correlates, and racial differences. *Sleep, 31*(9), 1221–1227. https://www.ncbi.nlm.nih.gov/pubmed/18788647.

Shehab, N., Lovegrove, M. C., Geller, A. I., Rose, K. O., Weidle, N. J., & Budnitz, D. S. (2016). US emergency department visits for outpatient adverse drug events, 2013–2014. *Journal of the American Medical Association, 316*(20), 2115–2125. https://doi.org/10.1001/jama.2016.16201.

Spitzer, R. l, Kroenke, K., Williams, J. B. W., & Löwe, B. (2006). A brief measure for assessing generalized anxiety disorder: The GAD-7. *Archives of Internal Medicine, 166*(10), 1092–1097. https://doi.org/10.1001/archinte.166.10.1092.

University of Colorado, Denver. (2019). *A study of tolerability and efficacy of cannabidiol on tremor in Parkinson's disease.* https://clinicaltrials.gov/ct2/show/NCT02818777.

US Department of Health & Human Services. (n.d.). From Mental Health and Substance Use Disorders website: https://www.mentalhealth.gov/what-to-look-for/mental-health-substance-use-disorders.

US Department of Health and Human Services, Centers for Disease Control and Prevention, N.

Veronese, N., Stubbs, B., Punzi, L., Soysal, P., Incalzi, R. A., Saller, A., & Maggi, S. (2019). Effect of nutritional supplementations on physical performance and muscle strength parameters in older people: A systematic review and meta-analysis. *Ageing Research Reviews, 51*, 48–54. https://doi.org/10.1016/j.arr.2019.02.005.

Walters, A. S. (2001). Assessment of periodic leg movements is an essential component of an overnight sleep study. *American Journal of Respiratory and Critical Care Medicine, 164*(8), 1339–1340. https://doi.org/10.1164/ajrccm.164.8.2107127a.

Webster, L.R. (n.d.). *Opioid risk tool.* https://www.drugabuse.gov/sites/default/files/files/OpioidRiskTool.pdf

Wild, B., Eckl, A., Herzog, W., Niehoff, D., Lechner, S., Maatouk, I., & Löwe, B. (2014). Assessing generalized anxiety disorder in elderly people using the GAD-7 and GAD-2 Scales: Results of a validation study. *American Journal of Geriatric Psychiatry, 22*(10), 1029–1038. https://doi.org/10.1016/j.jagp.2013.01.076.

World Health Organization: Department of Public Health, Environmental and Social Determinants of Health. (n.d.). https://www.who.int/phe/about_us/en/.

Yaffe, M. J., Wolfson, C., Lithwick, M., & Weiss, D. (2008). Development and validation of a tool to improve physician identification of elder abuse: The Elder Abuse Suspicion Index (EASI). *Journal of Elder Abuse & Neglect, 20*(3), 276–300. https://doi.org/10.1080/08946560801973168.

Yesavage, J. A., Brink, T. L., Rose, T. L., Lum, O., Huang, V., Adey, M., & Leirer, V. O. (1982). Development and validation of a geriatric depression screening scale: A preliminary report. *Journal of Psychiatric Research, 17*(1), 37–49.

11

Common Geriatric Syndromes

FREDDI SEGAL-GIDAN, PA, PHD

OBJECTIVES

Student Learning Objectives

After completing this chapter, the student should be able to do the following:

1. List common geriatric syndromes and their presentations in the older adult.
2. Describe the approach to diagnosis of common geriatric syndromes in the older adult.
3. Identify the unique aspects of the presentation and management of common geriatric syndromes in the older adult.

Practitioner Objectives

After completing this chapter, the practitioner should be able to do the following:

1. Provide an appropriate clinical evaluation for an older adult presenting with memory problems or confusion, falls, urinary incontinence, or frailty.
2. Develop and execute a management plan for the treatment of an older adult who presents with one of the common geriatric syndromes (confusion, falls, urinary incontinence).
3. Work collaboratively with other team members, as appropriate, to maximize outcomes for an older adult who presents with one of the common geriatric syndromes.

Introduction

Geriatric syndromes are common clinical conditions encountered in older adults that are multifactorial, have shared risk factors, and do not fit into discrete disease categories. They are typical of, but not specific to, aging, interfere with a person's daily life, and are associated with reduced life expectancy. These include many of the most common conditions seen in older adults across medical settings. Conditions most commonly considered geriatric syndromes are cognitive impairment (including delirium), incontinence, falls, and frailty. Sleeping problems, dizziness and syncope, malnutrition and feeding problems leading to unintended weight loss, and self-neglect have also been classified as geriatric syndromes.

The prevalence of geriatric syndromes varies greatly across the older adult population. Among community-dwelling adults over age 65, the prevalence is lower with rates increasing among hospitalized and those living in facilities such as assisted living or nursing homes. The frequency of individual geriatric syndromes varies greatly, with in excess of 80% of the population over age 80 having at least one identifiable geriatric syndrome (Tabue-Teguo, et al., 2017). Multiple co-morbidities are common among older adults as is the co-occurrence of geriatric syndromes, especially among the population over age 80.

Geriatric syndromes significantly impact function, are associated with increased mortality and disability, and can diminish quality of life. These conditions usually have more than one cause and involve multiple organ systems and the shared risk factors of older age, cognitive impairment, functional impairment, and impaired mobility (Inouye et al., 2007). Despite their prevalence, geriatric syndromes often go undiagnosed (Piccoliori et al., 2008). The signs and symptoms associated with geriatric symptoms are what frequently lead older adults to seek medical care. These conditions, especially when not recognized or properly evaluated, can consume large amounts of resources, including multiple providers and recurrent hospitalizations, leading to frustration for patients, caregivers, and health care providers.

Interprofessional Collaboration

Caring for an older adult who has one or more of the common geriatric syndromes requires a team of health professionals in order to provide optimal care and outcome. Geriatric syndromes are primary examples of conditions for which an interprofessional team care approach is preferred. Regardless of setting, physician assistants (PAs) and nurse practitioners (NPs) caring for older adults with one or more of the common geriatric syndromes will need to know how to interface with a wide variety of medical and social service colleagues. The PA or NP working in an emergency department or urgent care takes on the role of initial assessment, data gathering through the history and physical exam, and ordering of appropriate laboratory and radiologic examinations. Consultation with or referral to specialty care may be required and provided either onsite at the time of evaluation or as part of a further evaluation. PAs and NPs in the acute hospital setting might find themselves performing a variety of roles, including serving as a hospitalist or specialty consultant, working with nursing, social service, and therapy staff in the evaluation, management, and discharge plan of a

CASE STUDY

An 82-year-old woman lives with her husband in an independent apartment in a senior living complex. She falls while getting up from the toilet. She is unable to get herself up, so she pulls the emergency cord. Staff arrive and call the paramedics. When the ambulance arrives, the paramedics find her to be alert, able to answer simple questions, and able to move all four extremities. She is bleeding from a laceration on her scalp where her head hit the grab bar but denies any pain. She has history of mild dementia with memory loss for 3 to 4 years, for which she is followed by a community neurologist. She used a cane to assist with ambulation for 5 years until 1 year ago when she began to use a front-wheeled walker. She has a history of polymyalgia rheumatica (PMR) and occasional urinary incontinence for which she wears a pad, but she has no hypertension, diabetes, heart disease, or other chronic illnesses. Her medications are donepezil 10 mg once daily, vitamin D 2000 units daily, and calcium carbonate 800 mg twice daily. Her vital signs are within normal limits, and she is transported to the emergency department for further evaluation.

In the emergency department, her husband reports that this is the third fall she has had in the past month. One occurred when she was getting out of bed a few days before. Staff were present and able to help her up. The other occurred several weeks prior when he was out one evening and he was informed about it by the staff. The patient does not recall either of these prior falls. On physical exam she is found to be an obese older woman. There is a 5-cm laceration along the right temporal region, above her ear. No other evidence of trauma is observed, and the exam is otherwise nonremarkable. Laboratory test results include normal complete blood count (CBC), serum chemistry with mildly elevated blood urea nitrogen (BUN) 32, and urinalysis positive for nitrites. A urine culture and sensitivity test is ordered. The electrocardiogram shows a normal sinus rhythm of 72 beats/min. A CT of the head is ordered, which shows ventricular enlargement with rounding, minimal cerebral atrophy, moderate periventricular white matter changes, and no infarct or mass. The radiologist summary says to "consider normal pressure hydrocephalus (NPH)."

She is admitted to the hospital for overnight observation with mild dehydration and a suspected urinary tract infection (UTI). Intravenous fluids are started, and she is treated empirically with Macrodantin pending the urine culture. The next morning, she is very confused and lethargic, which persists over the next 48 hours and then resolves. A neurologic consult is requested, speech is fluent, the MoCA (Montreal Cognitive Assessment) test is 21/30, and the cranial nerves, motor, and sensory exam is unremarkable. She requires one person to help her to stand with a walker; she has a wide-based gait with slow stride. An MRI is ordered, and quantitative analysis is consistent with possible NPH. The patient declines neurosurgical consultation for a possible shunt placement, and her husband and children support this decision stating it is consistent with her expressed prior wishes. She is discharged home with home health physical therapy and occupational therapy.

patient who is admitted with a geriatric syndrome diagnosis or a patient who develops one of these conditions during admission.

Having a multidisciplinary team that includes, at minimum, a pharmacist and social worker along with a medical provider (physician, NP, PA) has been shown to be ideal for the assessment of geriatric syndromes. Medical specialists (neurologist, cardiologist, urologist, etc.) will frequently need to be part of the evaluation team or available for consultation regarding many of these conditions. Because polypharmacy is so common among older adults and involved in both the underlying cause and management of most geriatric syndromes, the role of the pharmacist is key.

Falls and Gait Instability

Falls occur in one-third of the older population each year and have a significant impact on medical costs, disability, quality of life, and mortality. The frequency of falls and prevalence of fall-related injuries increases with age and are a major factor that impacts the independence of older adults. When asked, 2% of adults over age 65 report a fall-related injury in the prior 6 months (Verma et al., 2016). However, falls often go unreported, especially when there is no associated injury. Routine inquiry about falls, assessment of fall risk, and attention to modifiable risk factors should be part of routine care for older adults.

HEALTHY PEOPLE 2030 BOX 11.1

Reduce the rate of emergency department visits due to falls among older adults—OA-03

The World Health Organization (WHO) defines a fall as "an event which results in a person coming to rest inadvertently on the ground or floor or other lower level" (World Health Organization, 2012). A fall is most often due to a combination of physiologic and environmental factors. Postural stability is maintained by the integration of somatosensory, visual, and vestibular inputs to the central nervous system, followed by outputs to the musculoskeletal system (Fig. 11.1). Function of all the components deteriorates with advancing age, which contributes to the increased fall risk seen in the older adult population.

Age itself is a risk factor for falls, with a 90-year-old being up to four times more likely to fall than a 60-year-old (Stenghagen et al., 2013). Other risk factors include a history of falls, specific medical conditions, and medications that cause sedation or affect gait and balance (Box 11.1). Falls with injury in older adults can have devastating consequences. Up to 20% of patients with a hip fracture die within the first year, and many survivors do not return to their previous level of functioning (McGilton et al., 2009).

HEALTHY PEOPLE 2030 BOX 11.2

Reduce fatal injuries—IVP-01
Reduce unintentional injury deaths—IVP-03
Reduce fall-related deaths among older adults—IVP-08

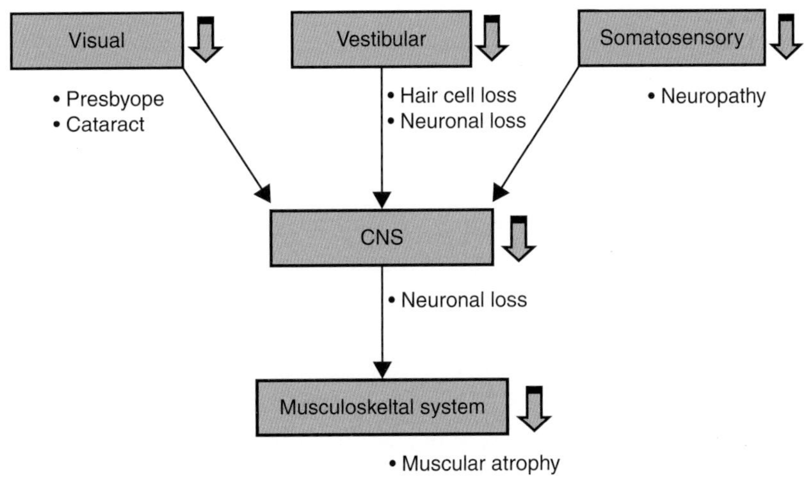

• **Fig. 11.1** Postural Stability (From Iwasaki, S., & Yamasoba, T. [2015]. Dizziness and imbalance in the elderly: Age-related decline in the vestibular system *Aging and Disease* 6[1], 38–47.)

• BOX 11.1 Risk Factors for Falls

- Age
- Prior fall
- Medical conditions
  - Lower extremity osteoarthritis
  - Depression
  - Heart disease
  - Nocturia
- Medications with fall risk

Screening

Many falls can be prevented if risk is identified and appropriate interventions put in place. The Centers for Disease Control and Prevention (CDC) recommends the use of three questions as part of the routine examination of patients over age 65. A positive answer to one or more of these questions should lead to a more in-depth assessment for falls risk and identification of areas for intervention for prevention:

1. Have you fallen in the past 12 months?
2. Have you ever felt unsteady with standing or walking?
3. Are you worried about falling?

A multifactorial assessment of fall risk in community-dwelling older adults based on guidelines developed by the American Geriatrics Society, the British Geriatrics Society, and the National Institute for Health and Care Excellence (NICE) outlines 12 key areas the clinical examination should focus on (Panel on Prevention of Falls 2011, National Institute for Health and Care Excellence, 2013) (Box 11.2). Two tests that are commonly used in clinical practice to assess for fall risk are the Timed Up and Go (TUG) Test and the Functional Reach Test (Table 11.1).

• BOX 11.2 Multifactorial Fall Risk Assessment Areas

- Comprehensive fall history
- Medication list review
- Gait and balance assessment and functional mobility
- Orthostatic vitals
- Heart rate and rhythm
- Neurologic function
- Muscle strength
- Feet and footwear examination
- Visual acuity
- Home safety assessment
- Osteoporosis screening
- Urinary incontinence screening

Assessment

A focused history and physical examination are essential when an older adult presents with a fall. The patient, and often a family member or caregiver who has witnessed the fall, should be interviewed. Questions should be directed to the circumstances surrounding the current fall, as well as previous falls and any injuries from previous falls. Symptoms such as dizziness and palpitations might provide clues to an underlying contributing cause or causes, such as low blood pressure, low blood sugar, or arrhythmia. It is also important to understand the environment and circumstances under which a fall occurs. The primary mechanisms of falling are slipping, tripping, and stumbling. Most falls in older adults occur in the bathroom, followed by the bedroom, kitchen, and living room, and they often involve wet carpets or rugs, the transition areas between carpets and rugs or noncarpeted sections and rugs, and the rush that occurs when a person is hurrying to the bathroom (Rosen et al., 2013).

For community-dwelling older adults, hazards that contribute to fall injuries include stairs, bathtubs without handlebars, electrical cords, clutter, inappropriate lighting, and loose rugs. Nursing home residents are at risk of falls secondary to wet floors, restraints, bedrails, or ties such as tubing or catheters. Even older patients in an inpatient hospital

TABLE 11.1 **Functional Reach Test**

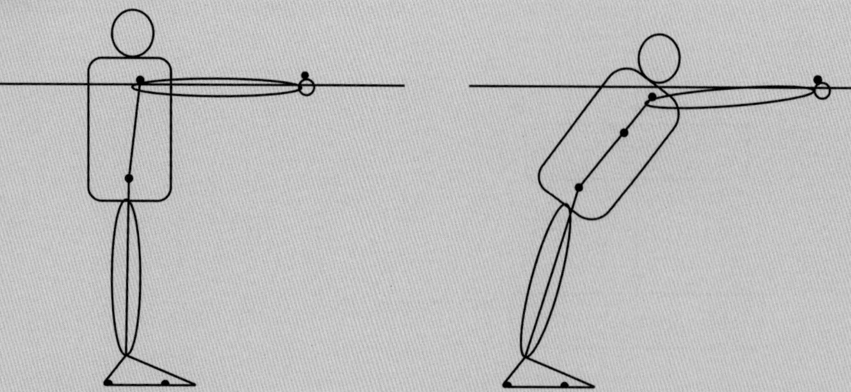

Functional Reach Test

Functional Reach Norms

Age	Men	Women
20–40	42.49 cm	37.19 cm
41–69	38.05 cm	35.08 cm
70–87	33.43 cm	26.59 cm

From Costarella, M., Monteleone, L., Steindler, R., & Zuccaro, S. A. (2010). Decline of physical and cognitive conditions in the elderly measured through the functional reach test and the mini-mental state examination. *Archives of Gerontology and Geriatrics, 50*(3), 332–337.

SAFETY ALERT

Environmental factors contribute to falls in all settings: the home, the hospital, and long-term care. Fall prevention requires attention to these factors, and actions must be taken to remove or reduce hazards that are known to increase fall risk.

setting are at risk of falling. There is little evidence that the addition of rails and the use of restraints, fall-alert bracelets, and bed alarms reduce the risk of falls, although a meta-analysis did suggest that these measures may decrease recurrent falls (Vlaeyen et al., 2015).

The medical history can provide additional information about fall risk factors. Cognitive impairment, sensory impairment (especially vision), Parkinson disease, arthritis of the knees, and any comorbidities that impair gait or balance (e.g., stroke) have been found to be associated with increased fall risk (Ganz et al., 2007). A thorough medication history should be elicited, with attention to drugs that are known to affect gait and balance (Box 11.3).

HEALTHY PEOPLE 2030 BOX 11.3

Reduce the proportion of older adults who use inappropriate medications—OA-02

BOX 11.3 Drug Classes Associated With Fall Risk

- Sedative/hypnotics
- Neuroleptics
- Benzodiazepines
- Antidepressants
- Antihypertensives
- Diuretics
  - Beta-blockers
  - Nonsteroidal antiinflammatory drugs
- Cholinesterase inhibitors

From Woolcott, J. C., Richardson, K. J., Wiens, M. O., Patel, B., Marin, J., Khan, K. M., & Marra, C. A. (2009). Meta-analysis of the impact of 9 medication classes on falls in elderly persons. *Archives of Internal Medicine, 169*, 1952–1960.

Social history should address the patient's support system and living situation, including environmental factors such as rugs, lighting, bath rails, clutter, footwear, and the use of assistive devices. Assessment of functional status should include both basic activities of daily living (ADLs) (e.g., bathing, toileting, feeding, dressing, grooming, and ambulation) and instrumental ADLs (IADLs) (e.g., use of the telephone, shopping, food preparation, managing one's own finances, housekeeping, laundry, and transportation). Any difficulty with IADLs or ADLs has been shown to be associated with an increased risk of falling (Bloch et al., 2010).

The physical examination of an older adult who has experienced a fall should focus on the initial assessment for any injuries. Cardiac, musculoskeletal, and neurologic systems are the three main areas of a fall-focused physical examination. Orthostatic blood pressure, defined as a drop in systolic blood pressure of 20 mm Hg or in diastolic blood pressure of 10 mm Hg at 1 to 3 minutes after the patient repositions from supine to standing, and pulse should be checked. Hypotension when there was a pulse rate that was less than an increase of 6 beats/min measured 30 seconds after standing up has been shown to predict falls (Ganz et al., 2007). A full neurologic examination, including mental status, with a focus on strength, reflexes, sensory, and gait should be done.

Older patients who present to the emergency department (ED) following a fall have a different bodily injury pattern than younger adults, a higher injury severity score, worse outcomes, and higher mortality (Rau et al., 2014). A major difference in the older adult population is skeletal fragility (osteopenia and osteoporosis), which occurs as bones age and become more susceptible to the mechanical forces of trauma. Consequently, older adults sustain more severe injuries from falls with lower force mechanisms than their younger counterparts, who have greater bone density.

Several tools to assess the risk of falls, including the Tinetti Balance and Gait Assessment Tool, the Berg Balance Scale, the Timed Up and Go Test, and the one-legged and tandem stance assessments, can be useful in the clinical assessment of an older adult who has experienced a fall (Gates et al., 2008). The Tinetti Gait and Balance Assessment includes nine measures of balance with a maximum score of 16 and eight measures of gait with a maximum score of 12 (Tinetti et al., 1986). There is a maximum total score of 28 with a score of 18 or less indicating a high risk of fall. The Berg Balance Scale was designed to assess balance in older adults who have had a stroke, but over time this scale has become more generalized for assessing balance in the general older adult population (Berg et al., 1992). The Berg Balance Scale uses a set of 14 items to assess balance, with each item consisting of a 5-point ordinal scale ranging from 0 to 4, with 0 indicating the lowest level of function and 4 the highest level of function. It takes about 20 minutes to complete. The Timed Up and Go Test (TUG) is a simple test easily used by clinicians in a variety of settings. It assesses the time a person takes to rise from a chair, walk three meters, turn around, walk back to the chair, and sit down. An older adult who takes ≥12 seconds to complete the TUG is considered to be at risk for falling.

The Morse Fall Scale (MFS) is another tool used to identify and score fall risk factors. The MFS takes into consideration whether or not the patient has a history of falls, secondary diagnoses, intravenous (IV) access, any use or type of ambulatory aid, as well as the patient's gait type and mental status (Baek et al., 2014). The St. Thomas Risk Assessment Tool in Falling Elderly (STRATIFY) fall score has also been used to assess the risk of falls in older patients and was revalidated in a study of hospital inpatients and nursing home residents (Aranda-Gallardo et al., 2015). This tool comprises five risk factors: past history of falling, patient agitation, visual impairment, incontinence, and transfer and mobility; scores range from 0 to 5 points, and the predictive cutoff of risk of falling is a score ≥ 2 points (Oliver et al., 1997).

Treatment/Management

About 30% to 50% of falls in older adults result in minor injuries, including bruises, abrasions, and lacerations. An estimated 10% of all falls cause major injuries, such as fracture or intracranial injury. One percent of falls in this population result in hip fractures, which lead to a significant risk for post-fall morbidity and mortality (Bradley, 2011). An estimated 75% of all vertebral and nonvertebral fractures occur in those age 65 years or older, and more than 75% of hip fractures affect seniors age 75 years or older.

HEALTHY PEOPLE 2030 BOX 11.4

Reduce hip fractures among older adults—O-02

Treatment should initially focus on any injuries resulting from a fall, and it too often does not include investigation of the cause of the fall. A thorough assessment, as outlined previously, of the underlying causes that contributed to the fall, identification of risk factors, and a program to reduce risk factors and avoid a subsequent fall is essential. A multifactorial intervention program is based on an individualized risk assessment for the patient who reports a fall, has unsteady gait, or is identified as at risk for a fall or experiences a fall with injury. Components of a fall prevention or treatment program are similar and should include exercise, particularly balance, strength and gait training; assessment and modification of the home environment; medication review with goal of minimizing medications; identification and management of postural hypotension; and management of foot problems and footwear. Medication adjustment with dosage adjustments or discontinuation of medications is often necessary. Medication adjustment requires a carefully developed plan that follows good deprescribing practices. Any medication that was started or increased in the time period preceding a fall should be considered as a potential cause or contributing factor. Referral to a physical therapist for evaluation and treatment, and sometimes to an occupational therapist, are an important part of most fall treatment and prevention plans. Referral to a podiatrist should also be considered for those individuals identified with foot problems or where specialized footwear might be appropriate.

A variety of interventions have been studied that apply to both older adults identified at risk for falling and those who have experienced a fall. These have included walking groups, strength and resistance training, and various exercise regimens. Tai chi and physiotherapy have been shown to be moderately effective in preventing falls (Gillespie et al., 2012).

Vitamin D supplementation has received attention as a factor in fall prevention. The US Preventive Services Task Force (2011) draft statement recommends vitamin D supplementation to prevent falls in older adults at increased fall risk. Vitamin D supplementation of at least 800 IU per day is recommended for older persons with proven vitamin D deficiency (American Geriatrics Society [AGS], British Geriatrics Society [BGS], 2010).

Vitamin D supplementation, with or without calcium, has been shown to decrease the number of persons who fell and the number of falls in men and women living in the community with lower baseline vitamin D levels (less than 24 ng per mL [59.90 nmol per L]) (Gillespie et al., 2012).

Once an older adult experiences a fall, especially one with an associated injury, anxiety and fear about falling can occur. Fear of falling ("fallophobia") often leads patients to self-limit their activities, which then leads to further debility and increased risk for falls. The Falls Efficacy Scale and the Activities-Specific Balance Confidence (ABC) scale are two established tools that focus on the impact of balance on daily activities and thus can be used to indirectly assess a patient's fear of falling (Powell & Myers, 1995; Tinetti et al., 1990).

Confusion and Memory Loss

Differentiating normal cognitive changes with aging from those that herald the beginning of a more serious condition can be challenging. The ability to recall and learn new information continues even into advanced age, although with age it may take more repetitions and a longer time to do so. Memory loss, for new information, is not a part of normal aging. There is a continuum of cognitive function recognized from normal, or expected, age-related change to mild cognitive impairment (MCI) and dementia.

MCI involves problems with memory, language, thinking, and judgment that are greater than normal age-related changes but do not interfere with normal functioning. Individuals with MCI have measurable changes in thinking abilities that are noticeable to the person affected and to family members and friends but that do not affect the individual's ability to carry out everyday activities. Fifty percent of individuals with MCI progress to dementia over 5 years, but others do not.

Dementia is the decline in cognitive performance in one or more cognitive domains (memory, language, executive function, attention, visuospatial abilities) that interferes with daily functioning. Dementing illnesses affects more than 6 million people in the United States and increase in prevalence with age. An estimated 10% of the population age 65 years and older has dementia, as do up to 50% in those age 85 years and older (Alzheimer's Association, 2019).

Dementias are the clinical manifestation of underlying neurodegenerative diseases that typically have an insidious onset and are gradually progressive. Delirium, in contrast, has an acute onset with fluctuations in attention and cognitive abilities over hours or days.

The *Diagnostic and Statistical Manual of Mental Disorders* (DSM-5) of the American Psychiatric Association in 2013 incorporated dementia into the diagnostic categories of major and mild neurocognitive disorders, but the term *dementia* is still in common usage as a clinical term (American Psychiatric Association, 2013). To meet DSM-5 criteria for major neurocognitive disorder, an individual must have evidence of significant cognitive decline (e.g., decline in memory, language, learning, calculation, visuospatial ability), and the cognitive decline must interfere with independence in everyday activities (e.g., assistance may be needed with complex activities such as paying bills or managing medications). Deficits do not have to include memory, as was previously required, and in addition may include problems in the following areas:

- Aphasia (language disturbance)
- Apraxia (inability to perform complex movements)
- Agnosia (failure to recognize or identify objects)
- Executive function (judgment and reasoning, problem solving)

Evaluation

When a patient presents with a complaint of memory loss, or more commonly a family member raises concerns about memory and thinking problems, these complaints should be taken seriously and a systematic evaluation undertaken.

HEALTHY PEOPLE 2030 BOX 11.5

Increase the proportion of adults with subjective cognitive decline who have discussed their symptoms with a provider—DIA-03

The history should be obtained from both the patient and a reliable informant, usually a family member, who can confirm and provide additional information. It is not uncommon for a person with a memory disorder to have limited insight or frankly deny the problem. Special attention to the onset and rate of cognitive and functional decline is key to the history in a person with a memory complaint or other cognitive deficit. Changes in personality and behavior, which often occur with these conditions, are also important to document.

Questions about function and ability to perform instrumental activities of daily living (IADLs) and basic activities of daily living (ADLs) should be obtained with a focus on changes that have occurred and over what time period. A thorough medication history, including both prescribed and over-the-counter medications taken on a regular basis, is essential. It is important to pay attention to those classes of medications that can affect memory and cognitive performance (Table 11.2).

An essential component of the evaluation of any person with a memory complaint is bedside mental status testing.

TABLE 11.2 Medications That Cause Cognitive Dysfunction

Category	Medication
Analgesics	Narcotics (fentanyl, meperidine, morphine, propoxyphene)
Antidepressants	Tricyclics (amitriptyline, doxepin)
Antidiarrheals	Atropine, diphenoxylate
Antiepileptics	Long-acting barbiturates
Antihypertensives	Clonidine
Antihistamines	Diphenhydramine
Antipsychotics	Thioridazine, chlorpromazine, haloperidol
Antispasmodics	GI; belladonna, dicyclomineGU; oxybutynin
Benzodiazepines	Diazepam, chlordiazepoxide,
Corticosteroids	Prednisolone
Histamine 2 receptor antagonist	Cimetidine
Muscle relaxants	Cyclobenzaprine, methocarbamol
Sedative-hypnotics	Barbiturates, zolpidem, zaleplon, propofol
Other	Gabapentin, pregabalin, metoclopramide, promethazine

GI, Gastrointestinal; *GU*, genitourinary.
Adapted from multiple sources.

• BOX 11.4 Commonly Used Bedside Mental Status Screening Tools

Folstein Mini Mental State Examination (MMSE)[a]
Modified Mini-Mental State Examination (3MS)
Montreal Cognitive Assessment (MoCA)+
Mini-Cog Screening
St. Louis University Mental Status (SLUMS)

[a]Proprietary + one-time training required to use as of September 2020.

The use of a validated screening instrument in the patient's primary language can provide useful information to serve as a baseline or comparison for the future. Box 11.4 provides a sampling of the more common validated mental status screening tools currently used. Screening for depression using a validated screening instrument such as the Geriatric Depression Scale is also part of the evaluation. The physical examination should include complete cardiovascular and neurologic examinations.

Laboratory testing focuses on identification of underlying conditions that might cause or contribute to cognitive changes. This should at minimum include a complete blood cell count (CBC) with a differential to assess for anemia or underlying infection with an elevated white blood cell count or a left shift; serum chemistry to assess electrolyte imbalance, glucose, renal and liver function, and thyroid-stimulating hormone (TSH) to evaluate for possible underlying hypo- or hyperthyroid disease, a Venereal Disease Research Laboratory [VDRL]) or Rapid Plasma Reagin (RPR) test for syphilis, and vitamin B_{12}

Brain imaging studies (magnetic resonance imaging [MRI] or computed tomography [CT]) are considered part of the basic dementia workup not only to rule out intracranial pathology, but as aids in the diagnostic etiology. An MRI is preferable but cannot be done in patients with a pacemaker, who are claustrophobic, or who cannot lie flat or still for a prolonged period of time. A brain scan should be considered in patients if the following conditions apply:

- Dementia onset occurs at an age younger than 65 years.
- The condition is postacute (symptoms have occurred for < 2 years).
- Focal neurologic deficits are present on physical examination.
- The clinical picture suggests normal-pressure hydrocephalus (triad of onset within 1 year, gait disorder, and unexplained incontinence)

Biomarkers in cerebrospinal fluid and in special positron emission tomography (PET) scans are used in research projects to identify the presence of β-amyloid and tau that can help confirm the diagnosis of Alzheimer's dementia . These biomarkers are not currently used in routine clinical assessments but have been suggested as possible future components when disease specific or modifying treatments have been identified.

Differential Diagnosis

The first step is to determine by history, mental status testing, and examination whether there is evidence of cognitive decline that is beyond what is expected with normal aging.

If there is evidence of cognitive decline, the next step is to evaluate whether this meets the criteria for mild cognitive impairment (MCI), dementia, or delirium. Recognition of dementia may be further complicated by the presence of depression and the need to be aware of treatable conditions that can mimic dementia by their clinical presentation. Medication review, laboratory test results, and brain imaging are useful to identify potentially treatable underlying causes, which should be addressed and treated.

Alzheimer disease (AD) accounts for an estimated 60% to 80% of all dementia cases in older adults (Alzheimer's Association, 2019). Physiologically, there is progressive accumulation of the protein fragment β-amyloid (plaques) outside neurons in the brain and twisted strands of the tau proteins that accumulate inside neurons (tangles) with damage to neuronal function and ultimately the death of neurons. These "tangles and plaques," which were first described by Dr. Alois Alzheimer, begin in the hippocampus and temporal and parietal lobes. Family members, patients, and others often misinterpret initial symptoms of AD (e.g., memory loss) as normal age-related changes. The two greatest risk factors for AD are age and family history, so heightened attention should be paid to patients who report a history of dementia or Alzheimer disease in their parents, grandparents, or siblings.

Known genetic mutations on chromosomes 1, 14, and 21 are responsible for the rare forms of familial AD that typically begin before age 60 years (presenile or early-onset AD). The apolipoprotein E gene *(APOE)* on chromosome 19 is the only currently identified genetic risk factor for the more commonly occurring late-onset AD. Genetic testing is not recommended as part of routine dementia evaluation and should only be considered in very unique circumstances in consultation with a neurologist and genetics counselor.

Gradual onset and progressive decline in cognitive functioning characterize AD. Motor and sensory functions are usually spared until late stages. Seizures, falls, or abnormal findings on the neurologic examination do not occur until very late in the disease process. Memory impairment for new material is a core symptom of dementia (except frontotemporal dementia [FTD]), seen even in the earliest stages of AD. Typical cognitive symptoms evident through the history and mental status testing of AD include the following:

- Difficulty learning and retaining new information
- Disorientation, first to time and then to place
- Language difficulty particularly expressive word finding
- Visuospatial dysfunction (getting lost)
- Impaired judgment and reasoning

Vascular dementia is characterized by multiple infarcts in the cortical and subcortical gray matter or white matter demyelination in the cerebral cortex seen on brain imaging. Typically, the patient with vascular dementia has multiple underlying vascular risk factors such as hypertension, diabetes, coronary heart disease, and hyperlipidemia. Vascular dementia is sometimes referred to as a subcortical dementia with a clinical presentation of slowed thinking and short-term memory problems that respond to cuing. In its pure form this affects approximately 10% of individuals with dementia. However, about 50% of older adults with pathologic evidence of vascular dementia (infarcts) also have Alzheimer pathology, which is referred to as *mixed dementia*.

Other types of dementias have been increasingly recognized over the past several decades. These include *dementia with Lewy bodies (DLB)*, which includes dementia plus Parkinsonian signs (tremor, rigidity, gait disturbance), visual hallucinations rapid eye movement (REM) sleep disorder, and alterations of alertness or attention. In DLB the underling pathology is deposition of synuclein proteins, similar to Parkinson disease, within neurons, called Lewy bodies. *Frontotemporal lobar degeneration (FTD)* is a neurodegenerative disorder that affects the frontal and temporal lobes of the brain. In the early stages, FTD is typically characterized by marked changes in personality and behavior that may be mistaken as late-life psychosis and the patient may be referred to psychiatry or psychology. There are also forms of FTD that present with difficulty producing or comprehending language. In FTD, unlike AD, memory is typically spared until later stages. When the evaluation suggests one of these atypical dementias, patients should be referred to neurology for further evaluation.

The cognitive loss that occurs in dementia is gradual, initially affects ADLs, then basic ADLS become impaired and over many years the patient becomes increasingly dependent on others. Patients with dementia commonly experience symptoms of depression, and depressed patients frequently present with cognitive complaints. Behavioral disturbances are common in dementing illnesses and should be expected in the course of the disease. These disturbances often include anxiety, irritability and agitation, delusional thinking, apathy, and sleep (circadian rhythm) disturbances

Disclosing a diagnosis of Alzheimer disease or one of the other neurodegenerative dementias can be uncomfortable. A separate appointment with the patient and spouse, child, or multiple family members is recommended so that findings and the diagnosis can be presented, questions answered, and the beginning of a treatment plan discussed. It is important to include the patient, even if he or she may not be able to recall being told the diagnosis or fully comprehend the information, as the patient is the one with the experience.

HEALTHY PEOPLE 2030 BOX 11.6

Increase the proportion of older adults with dementia, or their caregivers, who know they have it—DIA-01

Treatment

Primary treatment goals for patients with dementia are to enhance and preserve their quality of life and to optimize functional performance by managing cognition, mood, and behavior (Segal-Gidan, 2011). Currently two classes of medications have been approved by the Food and Drug Administration (FDA) for the symptomatic treatment of dementia: acetylcholinesterase inhibitors and *N*-methyl-D - aspartate (NMDA) agonists. Recommendations are for pharmacologic therapy to be started early in the disease process, beginning with an acetylcholinesterase inhibitor. Three acetylcholinesterase inhibitors are currently available: donepezil (Aricept), rivastigmine (Exelon), and galantamine (Reminyl). These medications can cause gastrointestinal disturbances, ranging from mild nausea and decreased appetite to frank vomiting and diarrhea, and vivid nighttime dreams in some individuals. Close monitoring upon initiation of the medication during the first several months should occur. Memantine (Namenda) is the only NMDA glutamate agonist approved for use in patients with dementia and is usually started after an acetylcholinesterase inhibitor or if a patient cannot tolerate this drug class. It is generally well tolerated, does not interfere with other medications, and dizziness and lethargy are the most frequent side effects. These medications can produce small benefits with a delay in cognitive decline for 12 to 18 months; they do not change the underlying disease process. An open and honest discussion of expected outcomes from treatment and monitoring for common side effects is essential.

Nonpharmacologic treatments, such as physical and cognitive stimulation and reminiscence therapy, are even more important components of a dementia treatment plan. It is of critical importance that clinicians initiate a discussion about long-term health and financial care plans while the patient is still in the early stages of dementia when he or she can participate in these crucial decisions. Caregivers are often subject to enormous stresses and should be encouraged to make sure their medical provider is informed that they are a caregiver for a person with dementia. Referral to sources for caregiver education and attendance at support groups have been shown to be effective in alleviating stress and preserving caregiver health. Respite care and other community resources such as adult day care for dementia patients offer caregivers relief and help postpone patient institutionalization. Familiarity with community resources and referral to social work care management or organizations such as the Alzheimer's Association are essential components of care for patients with dementia and their families.

Delirium

Delirium, an "acute confusional state," is a common geriatric syndrome that is often overlooked and underdiagnosed. Defined in DSM-5, criteria must include acute disturbance in cognition, fluctuating attention, and alteration of the sleep-wake cycle with changes that are primarily related to an underlying medical cause and not better explained by an evolving dementia (American Psychiatric Association, 2013).

Delirium is more common in older adults than younger or middle-aged adults, and the prevalence increases with increasing age among the older adult population. In the very old population, over age 85, living in the community delirium occurs in up to 14%. Up to one-third of all hospitalized elderly patients exhibit some level of delirium, and delirium is the leading complication of hospitalization among older adults (Inouye et al., 2014). Delirium complicates 17% to 61% of major surgical procedures, and as the number of patients of increasing age undergo surgery, the risk for postoperative delirium and prolonged postoperative confusion is increasing. This requires special attention to the risk for delirium in older adults in the preoperative and postoperative settings. Patients with cognitive impairment or a dementia diagnosis are at significantly increased risk for developing delirium. Despite the prevalence of delirium, it frequently goes undetected, with health care professionals identifying only 20% to 50% of cases (Kean & Ryan, 2008).

SAFETY ALERT

Delirium in hospitalized patients in intensive care units is associated with longer hospital stays and a higher rate of death. It is also connected with a greater likelihood of long-term care (nursing home) placement. Early recognition and identification of the underlying cause is essential.

HEALTHY PEOPLE 2030 BOX 11.7

Reduce the proportion of preventable hospitalizations in older adults with dementia—DIA-02

Delirium has been identified as a quality-of-care indicator for older adults and is an independent risk factor for poor medical outcomes in this population. Advanced age, a history of MCI or dementia, poor functional status, and sensory impairment are known predisposing factors for delirium. Beyond age, for hospitalized older adults risk factors for development of delirium are the use of physical restraints, malnutrition, polypharmacy, the use of a urinary catheter, and any iatrogenic event (Inouye & Charpentier, 1996).

The underlying pathophysiology of delirium is not well understood. Inflammatory cytokine response and neurotransmitter disruption are two mechanisms that have been postulated to independently or in conjunction lead to homeostatic disruption that produces clinical delirium. Proinflammatory cytokines released in the peripheral circulation enter the central nervous system, altering endothelial function, diminishing perfusion, activating microglia, and causing neuronal apoptosis and neurotoxicity (van Gool et al., 2010). This process is self-propelling and can last from weeks to months. Cholinergic deficiency is another proposed underlying theory. Anticholinergic medications that can induce or worsen delirium bind to nicotinic and muscarinic receptors in the brain, which modulate cognition and arousal (Hshiehm et al., 2008).

Patients present with either hyperactive delirium, the more common and easily recognized form, or hypoactive delirium, which is less common, frequently overlooked, and associated with a poorer prognosis (Inouye et al., 2014). Hyperactive delirium is associated with agitation, restlessness, excessive wakefulness or inability to sleep, and sometimes hallucinations or other psychotic features. Hypoactive delirium is associated with drowsiness, lethargy, and apathy. It is not uncommon for patients to have both forms at various times during the course of the same illness. It is particularly easy to miss a patient with hypoactive delirium, as they do not call attention to themselves.

The diagnosis of delirium requires a patient interview, a physical examination, cognitive testing, and a review of the medical chart and any collateral information. The Confusion Assessment Method is a practical and useful tool for detecting delirium; it has been validated in a variety of settings and is particularly useful among hospitalized or institutionalized older adults (Inouye et al., 1990). The tool is based on a simple set of questions that can be easily and quickly administered at the patient's bedside by a member of the nursing or medical staff.

A multitude of underlying causes may be involved in delirium, requiring a broad diagnostic approach and an open mind about the possibility of more than one contributing medical problem. The workup should focus on a detailed assessment to search for the precipitant, whether it is an acute medical illness, a change a chronic condition, or medication. Causes of physical discomfort such as constipation and urinary retention are common precipitants that are often overlooked. Acute infection, postoperative state, acute myocardial infarction, and alcohol withdrawal are common precipitating factors. A thorough physical examination to look for evidence of occult infection, volume depletion, abdominal pathology, deep vein thrombosis, and a neurologic cause is a basic part of any delirium evaluation. The patient's medications should be reviewed, with particular attention paid to drugs with anticholinergic effects, some of the most common culprits, as well as other causative drugs such as antihistamines, antiparkinsonism drugs, benzodiazepines, and H_2-blockers.

Further evaluation, similar to the medical workup for reversible or contributing causes to dementia, should include complete blood count (CBC), electrolytes (including calcium, phosphate and magnesium), blood urea nitrogen (BUN) and liver enzymes, and thyroid function. If infection is suspected, a urinalysis and chest x-ray should be administered, as well as an electrocardiogram and troponin test to assess for underlying ischemia, myocardial infarction (MI), or arrhythmia. It is important to keep in mind that older adult patients can fail to manifest typical signs of infection (elevated white blood cell count, fever, or focal symptoms). In patients with new focal neurologic signs, unexplained confusion, or suspected head trauma, such as from a recent fall, neuroimaging (CT or MRI) is indicated. If there is worsening severity or a prolonged course with no identifiable cause or causes, a repeat workup is required to look for new precipitants or less common causes of delirium such as encephalitis, rapidly progressive dementia, or seizure disorder. Neuroimaging should be repeated; if necessary, lumbar puncture and an electroencephalogram should also be considered in these situations.

Prevention of delirium should be a priority whenever possible and part of the routine care for every hospitalized older adult or those residing in a skilled nursing facility. This should include identification and interventions to address the six risk factors that commonly contribute to delirium in older adults: cognitive impairment, sleep deprivation, immobility, visual impairment, hearing impairment, and dehydration. Other important strategies include managing pain, maintaining nutrition, and performing regular thorough medication reviews (O'Mahony et al., 2011). Discontinuation of urinary catheters, whenever possible, is important given the association of catheters with urinary tract infections. Other important aspects of the care plan include assisted feeding and positioning in bed to prevent aspiration, frequent turning to prevent skin breakdown, and avoiding the use of restraints given the association of restraints with injury and worsened delirium. Involvement of family at the bedside or hiring of a patient sitter should always be considered as preferable to the use of restraints whenever possible.

The basic tenets of the management of delirium include the following:

- High index of suspicion and early identification
- Withdrawal of suspected offending drug(s), especially anticholinergics
- Treatment of the underlying cause
- Supportive care, including a well-lit, safe, and familiar environment
- Reassurance for both the patient and the family

Even with accurate identification of the suspected cause or causes of delirium and treatment, sometimes a patient's behaviors continue to be disruptive and nonpharmacologic treatments ineffective. If there is sleep-wake disturbance or psychosis, use of medication may need to be considered. Antipsychotics can be used in limited circumstances with the understanding that the potential for side effects and the lack of robust evidence means that use of antipsychotics for symptoms of delirium is considered off-label. Typical and atypical antipsychotics are commonly employed for acute management of delirium, even though there is inconclusive evidence that these agents reduce severity or duration (Table 11.3). Potential side effects include extrapyramidal symptoms (EPSs), including parkinsonism, akathisia, dystonia, and prolongation of the QTc interval, particularly with the use of haloperidol and quetiapine. Thus there must be close monitoring of patients when placed on these medications and treatment should be for a short time, with reassessment for ongoing need and down-titration or discontinuation considered on a daily basis. The risks and benefits of treatment should be discussed before initiating antipsychotic therapy, and families should be informed about the initiation of these medications and expected duration of use.

Antipsychotics have been suggested as potentially useful in delirium prophylaxis, particularly in the postsurgical period. A meta-analysis showed that perioperative olanzapine and

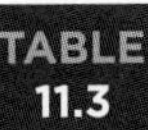

TABLE 11.3 Antipsychotics Commonly Used in Delirium Management

Medication	Dose	Common Side Effects
First generation/typical Haloperidol	0.25–0.50 Q 4 hrs IM	Extrapyramidal signs
Second generation/atypical	12.5–25 mg twice daily	Sedation, confusion, dizziness
Quetiapine	0.5 mg twice daily	Sedation, dizziness, extrapyramidal signs
Risperidol	2.5–5 mg/day	
Olanzapine	15–30 mg/day	Sedation, dizziness, restlessness
Aripiprazole	20–100 mg/day	
Ziprasidone		

None approved for use.
IM, Intramural.

TABLE 11.4 Medications That Cause or Exacerbate Urinary Incontinence

Medication Class	Mechanism of Action
ACE inhibitors	Produce cough, exacerbate stress incontinence
Alpha adrenergic agonists and antagonists	Decrease urethral tone
Anticholinergics and antihistamines	Cause incomplete bladder emptying and constipation
Calcium channel blockers	Cause constipation, which exacerbates incontinence
Diuretics	Increase frequency, exacerbate incontinence
Psychotropic agents	Cause urinary retention or constipation leading to overflow Lead to detrusor overactivity
Sedative hypnotics	Decrease movement and alertness at night, contribute to nocturia and nocturnal incontinence
Tricyclic antidepressants	Cause urinary retention or constipation leading to overflow Lead to detrusor overactivity

ACE, Angiotensin-converting enzyme.

risperidone were useful in delirium prevention, whereas no difference was found when haloperidol was compared with a placebo (Hirota & Kishi, 2013). Currently the off-label use of prophylactic antipsychotics perioperatively is not standard of care. Melatonin has also been investigated for the prevention of delirium with little support. However, its good safety profile makes melatonin a reasonable choice for use with hospitalized patients at high risk for delirium, or in established delirium as a sleep aid. Doses between 0.5 and 9 mg have been studied in delirium and in dementia patients, with 3 to 6 mg being used commonly in clinical practice (de Jonghe et al., 2010).

Urinary Incontinence

Urinary incontinence (UI), the involuntary loss of urine, is common problem in the older population due to a combination of normal changes with age, acute and chronic medical problems, medications, and functional impairment. It is more common in women, and prevalence increases in both men and women with advanced age. In the population of 60- to 79-year-olds, prevalence is 23%, or about one in four, and rises to greater than 32%, or one in three, in persons over age 80 (Nygaard et al., 2008). Nursing home residents have especially high rates of UI, ranging from 60% to 78% in women and 45% to 72% in men.

Identified risk factors that should raise the suspicion of urinary incontinence in an older adult are impaired mobility, falls, certain medications (Table 11.4), depression, stroke and transient ischemic attacks, dementia, congestive heart failure, constipation, fecal incontinence, and obesity. Arthritis and Parkinson disease are two common conditions in older adults that can exacerbate urinary incontinence. Urinary incontinence can cause significant morbidity, such as falls, fracture, and functional impairment, and among frail older adults with caregivers, it can lead to caregiver stress and institutionalization.

Classification

Accurate identification of the type of urinary incontinence is done based on history and examination findings and is

TABLE 11.5 Common Types of Chronic Urinary Incontinence (UI)

Classification	Description
Urge UI	Involuntary leakage associated with a strong need (urge) to void; often associated with overactive bladder
Stress UI	Involuntary leakage associated with pressure on the bladder, usually occurs with coughing, sneezing, lifting, or exercise
Overflow UI	Involuntary leakage associated with loss of bladder muscle contractile strength or bladder outlet obstruction, result is incomplete emptying of bladder and retention of urine
Mixed UI	Involuntary leakage associated with a combination of urge and stress UI
Functional UI	Involuntary leakage associated with cognitive, psychiatric, or mobility difficulties that impair ability to use the toilet, without impairment of the bladder's capacity for storage or elimination

Adapted from Abrams, P., Andersson, K.E., Birder, L., Brubaker, L, Cardozo. L, Chapple, C., Cottenden, A., Davila, W., de Ridder, D., Dmochowski, R., Drake, M., Dubeau, C., Fry, C., Hanno, P., Smith, J.H., Herschorn, S., Hosker, G., Kelleher, C., Koelbl, H., Khoury, S., Madoff, R., Milsom, I., Moore, K., Newman, D., Nitti, V., Norton, C., Nygaard, I., Payne, C., Smith, A., Staskin, D., Tekgul, S., Thuroff, J., Tubaro, A., Vodusek, D., Wein, A., & Wyndaele, J.J.; Members of Committees; Fourth International Consultation on Incontinence. (2010). Fourth international consultation on incontinence recommendations of the international scientific committee: Evaluation and treatment of urinary incontinence, pelvic organ prolapse, and fecal incontinence. *Neurology and Urodynamics*, *29*(1), 213–240. https://doi.org/10.1002/nau.20870; Khandelwal, C., & Kistler, C. (2013). Diagnosis of urinary incontinence. *American Family Physician*, *87*(8), 543–550.

essential to assuring the treatment and management is appropriate.

There are four classifications of urinary incontinence: urge incontinence, stress incontinence, overflow, and functional incontinence. With increasing age there can also be mixed incontinence, where urine leakage is due to the combination of two (or more) types of bladder dysfunction. Table 11.5 summarizes the different types of chronic urinary incontinence.

Stress urinary incontinence is the most common form, particularly among women as they age. It is defined as the involuntary loss of urine, usually small amounts, with increasing abdominal pressure that occurs when one coughs, laughs, or exercises. It is associated with weak pelvic floor muscles that can be the result of multiple childbirths and menopause. It can also be due to bladder outlet or urethral sphincter weakness or can be due to changes from urologic surgery.

Urge urinary incontinence is leakage of urine, often large amounts, associated with a compelling, sudden urgency to void and an inability to delay voiding after the sensation of a full bladder is perceived. It is usually associated with uninhibited bladder contractions, called detrusor overactivity (DO), and is commonly referred to as overactive bladder. Up to 40% of continent healthy older adults have DO upon urodynamic testing, thus suggesting that there are other factors involved that produce incontinence. It is often due to underlying neurologic condition such as stroke, dementia or Alzheimer disease, multiple sclerosis, Parkinson disease, or injuries. Pelvic floor atrophy in women, prostate enlargement in men, or constipation in either sex can also lead to urge incontinence.

Overflow urinary incontinence generally involves small amounts of urine leakage caused by mechanical forces on an overextended bladder, sometimes due to urinary retention. This can be due to anatomic obstruction by the prostate or a stricture of cystocele. Neurologic damage from diabetes or a spinal cord injury leading to an acontractile bladder can also produce overflow incontinence.

Functional urinary incontinence is associated with the inability to toilet due to either physical or cognitive deficits, psychological unwillingness, or environmental barriers. Severe dementia or depression in an older adult is the most common underlying reason for this form of urinary incontinence.

Evaluation

In the older population, lower urinary tract symptoms such as increased urgency, frequency, and nocturia are common (Pfisterer et al., 2006). Clinicians should routinely ask all older adults about urinary incontinence because only about half of the population affected by this condition will voluntarily report it to a medical provider (Mardon et al., 2004). History should include questions about onset, frequency, volume, timing, and associated factors or events. Patients or caregivers should be asked about the impact of urinary incontinence on daily function and associated quality of life. Simple questions can help to determine the type of UI through the symptoms; for example, the health care provider might ask, "Do you lose urine during coughing, sneezing, or lifting?" for stress urinary incontinence and "Do you experience such a strong and sudden urge to urinate that you leak before reaching the toilet?" for urge urinary incontinence.

A bladder diary can be helpful to get a better understanding of the timing and volume of urine loss. The patient, or caregiver, is advised to record the timing and circumstances of urinary incontinence, typically over 3 days.

The physical examination for an older adult with incontinence should include cognitive and functional assessments and focus on potential comorbid conditions associated with urinary incontinence. An abdominal exam should be performed with particular attention paid to the presence of palpable masses in the lower abdomen and suprapubic areas. A neurologic evaluation should include an assessment of sacral cord integrity with perineal sensation, anal "wink" (anal sphincter contraction when the perirectal skin is lightly scratched), and bulbocavernosus reflex (anal sphincter contraction when either the clitoris or glans is lightly touched). A rectal exam is essential to assess for masses, tone, and prostate nodules or firmness in men. A pelvic examination of women includes attention to vaginal mucosa for severe atrophy and an evaluation for pelvic organ prolapse (cystocele, rectocele, uterine prolapse) with straining.

Urinalysis, dipstick and microscopic, should be performed as part of the basic evaluation of urinary incontinence. Pyuria aor bacteriuria in an older woman may represent asymptomatic bacteriuria, without dysuria, fever, or other signs of urinary tract infection. Glycosuria would suggest poorly controlled diabetes, diagnosed or undiagnosed, that warrants further evaluation. Hematuria, without evidence on examination of a source, should be validated with a repeat specimen and if persistent warrants referral to a urologist for further evaluation.

For women with suspected stress urinary incontinence, a clinical stress test can help with diagnostic etiology. The patient should have a full bladder and a relaxed perineum and buttocks, and the examiner should be positioned to observe or catch any leakage when the patient gives a single vigorous cough. The test is most sensitive when the patient is upright and insensitive if the patient cannot cooperate, is inhibited, or the bladder volume is low.

Post-void residual testing (PVR) testing is not part of the routine evaluation. It is used in select patients, commonly those with diabetes, previous urinary retention or elevated PVR, recurrent urinary tract infections (UTIs), Parkinson disease, marked pelvic organ prolapse or medications known to decrease detrusor contractility (e.g., anticholinergics), persistent or worsening urge despite antimuscarinic treatment, or a prior urodynamic evaluation showing poor contractility or outlet obstruction. Routine urodynamic testing is not part of the evaluation of urinary incontinence in older adults and should be reserved for individuals who do not respond to first-line therapy.

Treatment and Management

A combination of nonpharmacologic and pharmacologic approaches is recommended for addressing urinary incontinence in older men and women. Nonpharmacologic and behavioral strategies such as noninvasive lifestyle and behavioral interventions are the first-line treatment of choice in the older adult population. Advantages of these approaches are low cost, absence of adverse effects, and ease of implementation. However, their effectiveness largely depends on patient motivation, functional capacity, and cognitive function.

Lifestyle modifications for urinary incontinence include smoking cessation, caffeine and alcohol reduction, weight loss, and modified fluid intake. Caffeine intake and overactive bladder is dose dependent, and those who consume greater than 400 mg/day of caffeine are 2.4 times more likely to experience detrusor instability. Reductions in caffeine intake should be undertaken gradually to avoid withdrawal symptoms such as headache and irritability. Weight loss in women with obesity is associated with decreased frequency of incontinence (Subak et al., 2012). Many older adult patients will restrict fluid on their own in an attempt to manage incontinence. Patient education regarding the timing of fluid intake is critical, but fluid restriction is not recommended because it may lead to dehydration and increased risk of infection.

Behavioral therapy can be effective for overactive bladder in older adults who have the cognitive ability to learn and the motivation to manage their incontinence. Bladder training is an urge suppression technique in which patients learn to resist or inhibit the sensation of urgency by gradually increasing toileting intervals. Another approach is to use a timed voiding schedule where the older adult learns to urinate according to a scheduled timetable, rather than with the symptoms of urge. Intervals are increased by 15- to 30-minute increments per week until a voiding interval of 3 to 4 hours is achieved. Bladder diaries can be a useful adjunct to bladder training.

Pelvic muscle rehabilitation (PMR), known commonly as Kegel exercises, is a treatment strategy for stress urinary incontinence. Repetitive contraction and relaxation of the pelvic floor muscles is used to improve the reflex inhibition of involuntary detrusor contractions and enhance the ability to voluntarily contract the external sphincter. Pelvic muscle rehabilitation has been shown to reduce episodes of urinary incontinence by 54% to 75% compared with reductions of 6% to 16% without treatment (Goode et al., 2010). PMR has also been shown to be an effective treatment for urinary incontinence in men after prostatectomy (MacDonald et al., 2007).

Pharmacologic treatment of urinary incontinence is symptomatic, not curative, and comes with increased risk in the older adult population. It should be employed in conjunction with lifestyle and behavioral treatment as part of a multimodality treatment plan. The most commonly prescribed drug class used for urinary incontinence is muscarinic receptor blockers.

Oxybutynin was the first approved antimuscarinic agent for urinary incontinence. The immediate-release formulation has significant anticholinergic effects (dry mouth, constipation, confusion) that should be closely monitored. Oxybutynin also comes in a longer-acting formulation and topical and transdermal formulations, which have fewer adverse effects. The transdermal patch must be applied every 3 or 4 days, whereas the gel must be applied daily. Although initially marketed as more uroselective, evidence is insufficient to support other agents (e.g., tolterodine, fesoterodine, trospium) over oxybutynin with respect to better efficacy or tolerability. All the oral antimuscarinic agents are considered by the Beers criteria as a class that exacerbates constipation and should be avoided unless no alternative is available (American Geriatrics Society, 2019).

Mirabegron is a newer medication that decreases the activity of the bladder muscle and has different side effects than antimuscarinic medications. Mirabegron can cause an increase in blood pressure and can interact with commonly used medications like metoprolol, which are commonly used medications in older adults, so a careful medication review is required before prescribing. Alpha-blockers and 5-alpha reductase inhibitors are classes of medication often used to treat men with urinary symptoms due to an enlarged prostate. Alpha-blockers can cause a drop in blood pressure in some men.

Oral and topical estrogen therapy was thought to improve the symptoms of stress urinary incontinence but has fallen out of favor. Oral estrogen has been found to increase the risk of cardiovascular adverse events, possibly worsening cognition, and increased breast cancer risk. Topical estrogens can be used for stress incontinence with less risk at recommended doses for vaginal atrophy. Duloxetine is approved in Europe for use in stress urinary incontinence, but this remains an off-label use in the United States.

Another agent being used for detrusor overactivity is Onabotulinum toxin A ("Botox"). It has FDA approval for use in patients with a neurologic condition (e.g., multiple sclerosis) and inadequate response to anticholinergic therapy but is increasingly being used off-label for urinary incontinence with detrusor overactivity even in the absence of an underlying neurologic condition. Administration is done as an office procedure with an injection of the botulinum toxin into the bladder muscle. There are few side effects, and when effective it can decrease frequency and urgency for several months.

There are several devices that can be used to decrease symptoms of urinary incontinence. Pessaries are small devices inserted into the vagina for women who have a "dropped" bladder or uterus. They work by supporting the bladder muscle and preventing urine leakage. A clinician must fit the patient with the correct size and then teach the woman patient how to remove, clean, and reinsert the device on a regular basis. Nerve stimulators are devices implanted under the skin in a manner similar to that used for a cardiac pacemaker; they send painless electrical pulses to nerves that control the bladder muscle to treat urge incontinence.

Surgical treatment of urinary incontinence is considered as a last option after trials of medications along with lifestyle and behavior management have failed. This is most commonly used for women who have stress urinary incontinence with bladder or uterine prolapse. Referral to a urologist or gynecologic surgeon would be required to assess whether a surgical procedure would provide a viable solution along with risks and benefits given other comorbidities of the older adult.

Sleep Disturbance and Insomnia

Sleep problems are not an inherent part of aging but do become more common with increasing age. More than half of older adults report sleep problems that include difficulty initiating sleep, maintaining sleep, or early morning awakening, and these complaints often go unreported (Kamel & Gammack, 2006). Older adults are less likely to complain of sleep problems than younger people, possibly because of age-related adjustments of sleep status or because they tend to be more tolerant of sleep deprivation The recognition of insomnia is especially important in the older population due to age-related increases in comorbid medical conditions and medication use, along with age-related changes in sleep structure, which shorten sleep time and impair sleep quality.

Sleep patterns change with aging. Total sleep time decreases slightly from the usual 8 to 9 hours in adulthood to 6.5 to 7 hours. Older adults often report awakening more during the night and earlier in the morning but not more difficulty falling asleep. With age there is an advanced circadian tendency, having an earlier bedtime and an earlier wake-up time. Older adults report more total time in bed but a harder time falling asleep. The transition between sleep and awakening is often abrupt, which can lead older people to believe they are lighter sleepers than when they were younger.

Sleep architecture changes with age. Older age has been shown to be associated with shorter sleep duration, reduced sleep efficiency, and increased arousal. Older adults spend less time in deep, dreamless sleep, which can lead to more frequent awakening. An increased proportion of time is spent in stages N1 and N2 sleep (i.e., the lighter stages of sleep), whereas a decreased proportion of time is spent in stage N3 sleep (i.e., a deeper stage of sleep) and in rapid eye movement (REM) sleep (Floyd et al., 2000). These changes reflect a decrease in deep, restorative sleep and an increase in light, transitory sleep.

Insomnia is defined by difficulty with sleep initiation, duration, consolidation, or quality that occurs despite adequate opportunities and situations for sleep (Vaughn & D'Cruz, 2011). Insomnia disorders that occur at least 3 nights per week for at least 3 months are classified as chronic insomnia disorder (American Academy of Sleep Medicine, 2014).

Assessment

Sleep disturbances in older adults are most often related to a number of interacting factors and are rarely due to one underlying condition. Evaluation of sleep complaints in an older adult should begin with a thorough history that calls attention to the onset of the problem, whether new or longstanding, and focuses on coexisting medical problems, current treatment, and any prior evaluations or treatments. A sleep diary is a useful tool to assess sleep patterns and usual sleep times.

Changes in medications, chronic and acute illnesses, environmental conditions, and physical/psychosocial stressors should be actively screened for. Recent changes in medications, paying particular attention to not only prescribed medications but the use of over-the-counter products, including herbal supplements, is essential. The use of caffeine, tobacco, and alcohol is often overlooked as a contributing factor. Lifelong sleep habits, working late, and using the computer and Internet and watching TV late at night can contribute to poor sleep hygiene and quality of sleep. The health care provider should also pay attention to pain and nocturia, common reasons for awakening during sleep among older adults. Screening for psychiatric diseases such as depression and anxiety should be part of the evaluation of any older adult with sleep disturbances.

The physical examination is focused on identifying conditions that could be contributing to changes in sleep or poor-quality sleep. This includes conducting a respiratory exam and cardiovascular examination for evidence of chronic obstructive pulmonary disease (COPD) and heart failure, a neurologic examination to check for parkinsonism, and a musculoskeletal examination to assess for arthritis and pain. Referral to a sleep laboratory is not generally required except when obstructive sleep apnea or REM sleep disorder (discussed later) is being considered as an underlying cause.

Differential Diagnosis

There are several primary sleep disorders that occur with increased frequency in the older adult population. Clinicians caring for older adults must be aware of these disorders, as they can often present with complaints of sleep disturbance or daytime sleepiness and fatigue due to poor quality nighttime sleep. Questions that address abnormal nocturnal behavior symptoms of possible sleep apnea syndrome (SAS), restless legs syndrome (RLS), and REM sleep behavior disorder are important to include when screening for sleep problems.

Sleep apnea is a breathing disorder caused by repetitive upper airway obstruction during sleep, whether at night or during daytime naps. Adults over age 60 have a higher risk for developing sleep apnea, and the risk of death is more than two times higher in older adults who have sleep apnea (Gooneratne & Vitiello, 2014). Primary symptoms of sleep apnea include snoring, daytime sleepiness, and decreased cognitive functioning. Risk factors for sleep apnea are listed in Box 11.5.

• BOX 11.5 Risk Factors for Sleep Apnea in Older Adults

Male gender
Obesity
Thick neck circumference
Smoking
Alcohol, sedative, or tranquilizer use
Nasal congestion

HEALTHY PEOPLE 2030 BOX 11.8

Increase the proportion of adults with sleep apnea symptoms who get evaluated by a health care provider—SH-02

According to the American Academy of Sleep Medicine, the most common form of sleep apnea is obstructive sleep apnea, which occurs when soft tissue in the back of the throat collapses and blocks the upper airway during sleep. Older adults also are at risk for central sleep apnea, a much less common form, which involves a repetitive absence of the breathing effort during sleep caused by dysfunction in the central nervous system or the heart. Sleep apnea syndrome (SAS) or obstructive sleep apnea (OSA) are best diagnosed by nocturnal polysomnography, which is performed in a sleep laboratory. During this test the patient is connected to equipment that monitors heart, lung, and brain activity; breathing patterns; arm and leg movements; and blood oxygen levels during sleep. Central positive airway pressure (CPAP) therapy is the treatment of choice for OSA. CPAP provides a steady stream of air through a mask that is worn during sleep. This airflow keeps the airway open to prevent pauses in breathing and restore normal oxygen levels.

Restless legs syndrome (RLS) is classified as a sleep-related movement disorder typified by an urge to move the legs and abnormal leg sensation, resulting in sleep-initiation or sleep-maintenance problems (American Academy of Sleep Medicine 2014). Diagnostic criteria proposed by the International Restless Legs Syndrome Study Group (IRLSSG) include four essential features: (1) there is an urge to move the legs, (2) the symptoms begin or worsen during periods of inactivity, (3) the symptoms are partially or totally relieved by movement, and (4) the symptoms occur only in the evening or at night or are worse during these times (Allen et al., 2003). Patients with RLS rarely report daytime sleepiness but may complain of an inability to "get comfortable" or strange feelings in their legs that awaken them. A family history of RLS is present in up to 50% of patients with the condition. Low-dose dopamine agonists, such as pramipexole and the rotigotine patch, and alpha-2 delta ligands, such as gabapentin, pregabalin, and gabapentin enacarbil, are effective.

REM sleep behavior disorder is characterized the acting out of dream content, including talking, shouting, punching, and kicking. These abnormal nocturnal behaviors can be associated with injury of the patients and their bed partners during sleep. Questioning a spouse or bed partner can help to identify these behaviors. Older patients with REM sleep behavior disorder should be regularly evaluated for the presence of subtle parkinsonism (tremor, rigidity, gait change) and cognitive and olfactory impairment, as this is frequently an overlooked presenting sign of underlying neurodegenerative disease (Howell & Schenck, 2015).

Management

Sleep hygiene education should be the first approach for managing sleep disturbances because the development of good sleep habits benefits all insomnia sufferers. This includes regular exercise and meals, limiting fluid intake before bedtime, avoiding stimulants such as caffeine and tobacco, and creating a comfortable sleep environment. Nonpharmacologic treatment strategies are always preferable and should be employed as a first-line approach. A warm bath, a glass of warm milk, or cup of herbal tea such as chamomile or valerian root are safe and effective approaches for most older adults.

Stimulus control involves having the patient go to bed only when sleepy and using the bed for sleep only, not reading, watching television, or eating. If unable to fall asleep within 20 minutes, the patient should get up and go to another room to do something, then return to the bedroom when sleepy. The health care provider should advise patients to get up at the same time every morning, irrespective of how much sleep they had during the night, and to avoid daytime naps. Cognitive behavioral treatment has also been found to be beneficial with older adults who have insomnia. This therapeutic approach has patients identify incorrect thoughts, beliefs, or knowledge about sleep and works with them to correct knowledge, emotions, and behaviors related to sleep.

When nonpharmacologic strategies do not work, pharmacologic treatments should be considered. Hypnotic drugs should be used at the lowest effective dose, and short-term use is recommended. These are effective for the short-term treatment of insomnia complaints but there is no evidence of their effectiveness in the long term. Because there are risks associated with the long-term use of these medications by older adults, use beyond 35 days is not recommended (National Institutes for Health, 2005). If left untreated, insomnia is known to have a negative impact on the quality of life and should therefore not be ignored.

Dizziness

Dizziness is a common complaint among older adults. It is of concern because it puts older adults at a greater risk of falling (discussed earlier). Prevalence ranges from approximately 20% to 30%, depending on the definition of dizziness and the population studied. In a population-based study, just under a quarter (22%) of people over age 72 reported experiencing dizziness (Tinetti et al., 2000). The prevalence tends to increase with age with dizziness affecting up to approximately 50% in people older than 85 (Jonsson et al., 2004).

Dizziness includes a range of sensations such as a sensation of lightheadedness, weakness, or a sense of imbalance. *Vertigo* is the term used when there is a sense that the surroundings are spinning or moving. The underlying causes in older adults vary widely and are often multifactorial. Physiologic deterioration in function of the components of the balance system occur with age, contributing to the increased prevalence of dizziness. As a geriatric syndrome, dizziness should be thought of as potentially involving multiple organ systems: neurologic, cardiovascular, visual, vestibular, and psychological. Changes in any of the factors associated with the balance system, which includes sensory, visual, vestibular, neurologic, and muscular changes, may be causing or contributing to dizziness (Fig. 11.1).

Evaluation

The key to the evaluation of a person with dizziness is to elicit a clear understanding of what the person is experiencing, how often it occurs, and in what circumstances. Is the sensation present all the time, does it come and go, and are how does it impact function? Does it occur primarily when the person is arising from bed or a chair, when getting up from the table after a meal, or during ambulation? A complete review of medications that focuses on recent additions or dose changes to existing medications, particularly antihypertensive and diabetes medications, along with over-the-counter medication use, should be conducted.

A physical examination for dizziness must include an observation of the patient's ability to arise from a chair, walk, and balance, with eyes both open and closed. A complete cardiovascular examination with positional blood pressure measurement is essential. The neurologic examination should include an observation of extraocular movements to look for nystagmus, peripheral sensory, and proprioceptive examination.

Common Causes

Underlying causes of dizziness include inner ear disturbance, motion sickness, and medication effects. Sometimes there is an underlying health condition, such as poor circulation, infection, or injury. Often it is a combination of factors rather than one single cause.

Cardiovascular disease is the most common major contributory cause of dizziness in an older person. A dramatic drop in systolic blood with change of position, orthostatic hypotension, can result in brief lightheadedness or a feeling of faintness. Dizziness can occur after sitting up or standing too quickly. Poor blood circulation in conditions such as cardiomyopathy, heart attack, heart arrhythmia, and transient ischemic attack can also cause dizziness. And a decrease in blood volume due to anemia or bleeding may cause inadequate blood flow to the brain or inner ear, causing dizziness or a sense of imbalance.

Peripheral vestibular dysfunction is one of the most frequent causes of dizziness in an older adult. Benign paroxysmal positional vertigo (BPPV) is the most frequent form of vestibular dysfunction in patients over age 65. It is thought to be due to small particles trapped in the semicircular canals. BPPV is usually diagnosed by the presence of episodic vertigo provoked by changes in head position and nystagmus observed during the positioning maneuver. Physical therapy is the most effective treatment. The use of vestibular

• BOX 11.6 Vestibular Suppressants

Anticholinergics

Transdermal scopolamine
Promethazine
Amitriptyline
Meclizine

Mycin Antibiotics

Gentamicin

suppressants, such as meclizine, or antiemetics (Box 11.6) is helpful in the week after onset, prior to physical therapy referral. For older patients who are too physically limited to perform the exercises or who do not respond to them, medications can be used, but for only a limited period of time while being closely monitored for both efficacy and side effects.

Meniere syndrome has its highest incidence among adults above 50 years of age. Meniere syndrome usually presents as spells of rapid decline in hearing, a roaring tinnitus, vertigo, and monaural fullness. For acute conditions, vestibular suppressants and antiemetics are used. Long-term treatment with a 2-gram salt diet combined with a mild diuretic may reduce the frequency of attacks. An outpatient treatment for Meniere involving injections of gentamicin through the eardrum is about 90% effective for unilateral disease.

Vestibular neuritis is a self-limited condition that usually lasts 2 to 3 days. It is characterized by vertigo, both at rest and positional, accompanied by nausea, ataxia, and nystagmus. Spontaneous nystagmus differentiates this disorder from BPPV. An antiemetic, such as Phenergan, may be used. Vestibular suppressants should be used sparingly, as they can delay central compensation to the lesion. Older patients may not recover as quickly as younger patients and may benefit from vestibular physical therapy.

Medications can be a direct cause as well as a contributory factor in dizziness. Antihypertensive medications are designed to lower blood pressure and may cause light-headedness or faintness if they lower blood pressure too much or too quickly. A common side effect of certain medications, such as antiseizure drugs, antidepressants, sedatives, and tranquilizers, is dizziness, so whenever these are prescribed one should caution patients about possible dizziness.

Dizziness can occur as a symptom in certain medical conditions. Patients with Parkinson disease may experience a progressive loss of balance and experience this as dizziness. Anxiety disorders and panic attacks can have light-headedness associated with them. Diabetic patients with hypoglycemia can experience light-headedness, faintness, or weakness.

Dehydration is a common cause of dizziness in older adults. This is a concern during the summer months but can occur throughout the year due to decreased thirst and limitation of liquid intake. Patients on certain medications, such as diuretics, and those with diabetes are at increased risk for dehydration as a contributing or causative factor.

Weight Loss/Malnutrition

Unintentional weight loss in older adults is associated with increased morbidity and mortality. It is defined as more than a 5% reduction in body weight within 6 to 12 months and occurs in 15% to 20% of older adults (McMinn et al., 2011).

The underlying pathophysiology of unintentional weight loss with advanced age is not well understood. Malignancy (19% to 36%) is the most common cause, then nonmalignant gastrointestinal disease (9% to 19%), and psychiatric conditions such as depression and dementia (9% to 24%). Overall, nonmalignant diseases are more common than malignancy (Gaddey & Holder, 2014). A variety of social factors associated with unintentional weight loss include poverty, alcoholism, isolation, financial constraints, and barriers to obtaining food such as lack of assistance in grocery shopping or meal preparation.

The role of medications as a cause or contributing factor to weight loss and malnutrition in older adults is often overlooked. Medications can affect appetite and taste, either as a direct side effect or in combination. Medications prescribed for many of the common chronic diseases that accompany aging, such as hypertension, diabetes, depression, arthritis, and osteoporosis, can alter taste and smell or cause anorexia. The effect of anticholinergic medications on taste and reduction of appetite due to dry mouth is often unrecognized.

Evaluation

It is rare that an older adult patient will complain of weight loss or decreased appetite. A more common complaint would be that food does not taste good or taste right. All patients should be asked about changes in appetite. If a patient has depression or cognitive impairment, information about food intake may need to be sought from a family member or caregiver. A change in clothing size or the added need for a belt can provide another clue. There are a number of validated nutrition screening tools that can be used with older adults. The Nutritional Health Checklist is an easy-to-use a tool for assessing nutritional status. The Nutritional Health checklist identifies noninstitutionalized older persons at risk for low nutrient intake and subsequent health problems (National Resources Center on Nutrition and Aging, 2022). The history should include a review of known chronic problems, past medical history with attention to abdominal surgical procedures, or cancer. A complete medication review with attention to those that can impact taste and appetite is essential.

Weight loss and malnutrition more often come to light in the course of the patient evaluation. Getting and recording a weight on every patient at every visit can help to establish a baseline and reference. The physical examination should start with an evaluation of the oral cavity and dentition to identify problems with chewing or swallowing. Heart, lung, gastrointestinal (including rectal), and neurologic examinations are useful to identify illnesses that may contribute to or cause weight loss. Laboratory testing should include a measure of the patient's complete blood count (CBC), serum chemistries, thyroid function tests, a C-reactive protein test, a measure of the erythrocyte sedimentation rate, and a urinalysis. Chest x-ray and a fecal occult blood test should be routinely done as part of the evaluation for weight loss. An abdominal x-ray or ultrasound may be warranted based on physical examination findings.

Underlying Causes

Many commonly occurring medical conditions in older adults can impact appetite, make eating difficult, change metabolism, and require dietary restrictions. Cancer, diabetes, and Alzheimer disease are three common conditions in older adults that frequently have associated unintentional weight loss.

Treatment

Optimal treatment depends on identification of the underlying cause or causes. A multidisciplinary team, including dentists; dietitians or nutritionists; speech, occupational, or physical therapists; and social service workers are often required over an extended period of time to stabilize and then reverse unintentional weight loss. Strategies used include dietary changes, environmental modifications, nutritional supplements, and appetite stimulants.

Dietary changes may require an adjustment of food consistency to accommodate for chewing or swallowing disabilities. Supervised or assisted feeding may be necessary for patients who cannot sustain attention to complete a full meal or who have physical disabilities that limit their ability to self-feed. Nutritional supplements can be provided to increased caloric intake. These should be used in addition to regular meals and not as substitutes. There is little evidence to support the use of appetite stimulants in older adults. Megestrol (Megace), the most commonly used medication to improve appetite, when used in older adults has shown minimal improvement in appetite and weight gain and an increased risk of thrombotic events, fluid retention, and death. The American Geriatrics Society Choosing Wisely campaign recommends that older adults avoid using prescription appetite stimulants or high-calorie supplements for treatment of anorexia or cachexia; instead, such patients should optimize social supports, discontinue medications that may interfere with eating, and seek appealing food and feeding assistance, and health care providers should clarify patient goals and expectations.

Frailty

Frailty is a syndrome of physiologic decline that is characterized by decreased physiologic reserve with increased vulnerability to stress (Fig. 11.2). It is characterized by diminished endurance, strength, and reduced physiologic function, and it is predictive of disability, institutionalization, and death. Frailty is thought of by some as accelerated aging, whereas others consider it a syndrome with a distinct underlying pathophysiology. Rockwood (2007) has proposed that frailty is based on an accumulation of deficits where "the more things that are wrong, the more likely the person is frail" (p. 758). In contrast, others view frailty as a biologic syndrome of decreased reserve due to the accumulation of deficits in multiple physiologic systems (Fried et al., 2001).

Identifying frail older adults can help target specific health interventions and services needed to improve outcomes for this vulnerable cohort. Frailty develops as a consequence of age-related decline in multiple physiologic systems, which collectively results in vulnerability to sudden health status changes triggered by relatively minor stressor events. Frailty is not an inevitable part of ageing and it should not be a barrier to interventions. If identified early enough and if appropriate interventions and services are initiate, there is the potential for improved outcome.

There is a strong relationship between frailty and chronologic age. It is most common in the oldest old and those with multiple underlying comorbidities. Ten percent of the older adult population has been found to meet the criteria for frailty based on either the Cardiovascular Health Study (CHS) or the FRAIL scale (which stands for Fatigue, Resistance, Ambulation, Illnesses, and Loss of weight) (Table 11.6). It is estimated that a quarter to a half of people over 85 years of age meet the definition of frailty, and these people have a significantly increased risk of falls, disability, long-term care, and death (Fried et al., 2001; Song et al., 2010).

Several different frailty subtypes have been identified. Physical frailty is the most frequently assessed and identified among older adults. Cognitive frailty, psychological frailty, and nutritional frailty have also been identified, which can overlap or coexist with the frailty syndrome.

Identification of frailty should heighten concerns about prognosis and indicates an increased potential for sudden changes in health status as a result of relatively minor illnesses, such as a urinary tract infection, new medication, or dehydration (see Fig. 11.1). Fit older adults will typically experience a small deterioration in function after an acute illness, recover within a brief period of time, and return to their baseline function. Frail older adults who experience a similar minor illness will take a longer time to recover and will not return to their baseline function but instead will experience a decline in function and an increased level of dependency.

Frailty occurs as the result of underlying changes in multiple interrelated physiologic systems. Fig. 11.3 presents a diagrammatic representation of this current understanding. With aging there is a gradual decline in physiologic reserve, but in frailty, this decline is accelerated and a failure of homeostatic mechanisms occurs (Ferucci et al., 2002). The central nervous system, endocrine system, immune system, and skeletal muscle are closely interrelated and are the organ systems most often found in studies to contribute to the development of frailty. Loss of physiologic reserve in other

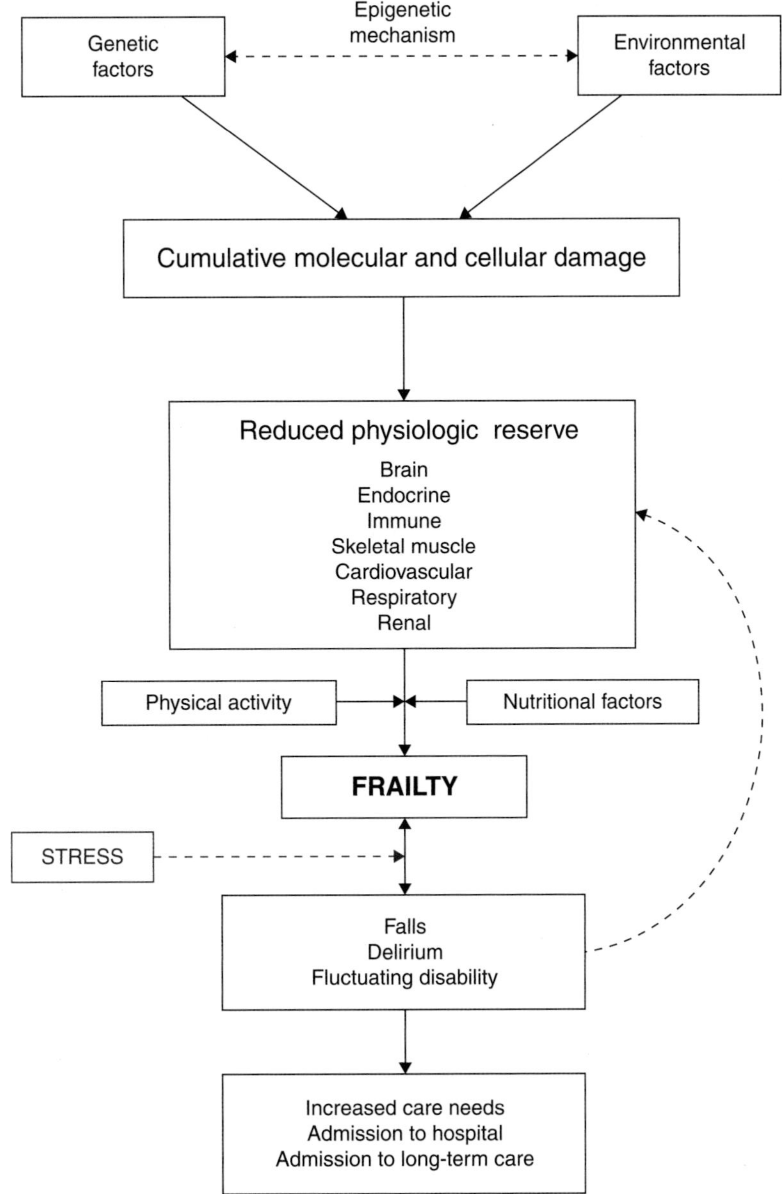

• **Fig. 11.2** Frailty Conceptualization (From Frailty in older people. [2013]. *Lancet, 381*[9868]: 752–762.)

TABLE 11.6 The FRAIL Instrument

Sign/Symptom	Assessment
Fatigue	Are you fatigued?
Resistance	Cannot walk up a flight of stairs?
Ambulation	Cannot walk one block?
Illnesses	Do you have more than five illnesses
Loss of weight	Have you lost more than 5% of your weight in the last 6 months?

1 point for yes; 1 or 2 = prefrail, >3 = frail.

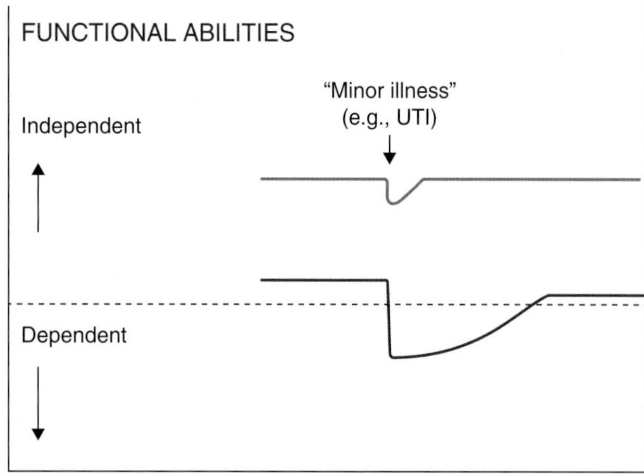

• **Fig. 11.3** Frailty (From Clegg A, Young J, Iliffe S, Rikkert MO, Rockwood K. Frailty in elderly people. [2013]. *Lancet, 381*[9868]: 752–762.)

systems, including the cardiovascular, respiratory, and renal systems, also contributes. A cumulative loss in physiologic reserve in these organ systems (along with a reduced level of physical activity) and nutritional factors combine to produce the frailty syndrome.

Assessment and Risk Factors

Identification of patients who are frail or at risk of frailty allows for interventions to reverse the syndrome, prevent further decline, and address patient preferences in light of the association of mortality with frailty. Indicators of frailty are identified and measured clinically as part of the history by self-report, which can be elicited as part of the history or by completion of questionnaires and through direct observation during the physical examination. Cardiovascular risk factors, including congestive heart failure, coronary artery heart disease, peripheral arterial disease, diabetes, and hypertension, increase the risk for frailty (Afilalo et al., 2009). Cognitive impairment has also been found, in association with vascular risk factors, to be an additional frailty indicator (Panza et al., 2006).

Signs and symptoms of frailty that have consistently been identified are unintentional weight loss, self-reported exhaustion or fatigue, low activity, slow gait speed, and weak grip strength. Unintentional weight loss is defined as more than 4 to 5 kg or more than 5% over a year. Exhaustion or fatigue is the inability to walk several hundred yards or feeling extremely tired or exhausted more than 3 to 4 days per week. Low activity is a caloric expenditure of less than 383 kcal per week for a male or less than 270 kcal per week for a female. A walking speed <0.8 m/s has been found to be a simple indicator to the diagnosis of frailty in the primary care setting (Castell et al., 2013). Grip strength is a simple objective measure that reflects decreased muscle strength. It is a quick and inexpensive measure that clinicians can employ in all settings, and it can be especially useful in patients who have limited ambulatory ability and for whom a walking test is not appropriate. A hand dynamometer is used to formally assess grip strength with differences expected in men when compared with women and a slight overall decline likely with increasing age (Bohannon et al., 2007) (Table 11.7). Using a simple handshake of the dominant hand or asking the patient to squeeze the examiner's hand can provide a clinician with a general, though less objective, sense of grip strength.

A number of tools have been developed to help clinicians identify older adults who meet the criteria for frailty and to differentiate among frail, vulnerable, and robust older adults. The Frailty Index for Elders (FIFE) uses a 10-item instrument with score of 0 to 10. A score of 0 indicates no frailty, a score 1 to 3 indicates risk for frailty, and score 4 or greater indicates frailty (Tocchi et al., 2014). The FRAIL instrument is easily used in a busy outpatient setting to identify older adults at risk for negative outcomes (see Table 11.6). As noted earlier, this instrument uses the FRAIL acronym to address five areas: Fatigue, Resistance, Ambulation, Illnesses, and Loss of weight. A positive response to three or more of the five questions identifies someone at risk for frailty and the lack of any positive response indicates robustness. The Deficit Accumulation Index (DAI) is a listing of 70 items drawn from the Canadian Study of Health and Aging (CSHA). The more items that are endorsed by an individual, the greater the likelihood of frailty. The Vulnerable Elders Survey (VES-13) is a simple function-based tool for screening community-dwelling populations to identify older persons at risk for health deterioration. The VES considers age, self-rated health, limitations in physical function, and functional disabilities (Saliba et al., 2001).

Tools for identifying frail older adults are increasingly being used across specialties and settings to guide treatment decisions and aid in the identification of patients at high risk of adverse outcomes. As the age of patients in specialty practices increases, particularly in cardiology, oncology, and surgery, there is increasing attention to the identification of frail older adults as a factor to be considered in medical decision making. There is high prevalence of frailty among older adults with cardiovascular disease, affecting between 10% and 60% depending on the frailty assessment tool (Afilalo et al., 2009). Among older adults undergoing cardiovascular surgery, there is a twofold increase in mortality among those who are identified as frail (Afilalo et al., 2014). Frailty has been identified as one of three criteria used to determine whether an older adult with symptomatic severe aortic stenosis should undergo a transcatheter aortic valve implantation (TAVI) rather than a surgical aortic valve replacement (SAVR) (Godino et al., 2010).

As the age of patients with cancer and certain specific malignancies increases, so does the importance of identifying frailty among these patients. Furthermore, frailty and cancer share many of the same presenting signs, such as weight loss and wasting, which can delay and confound early recognition and accurate diagnosis. Among oncologists the term *frailty* is often used broadly to define any high-risk older adult, whether marked by disability, functional deficits,

TABLE 11.7 Grip Strength Norms for Older Adults[a]

Women Age	Right Hand (kg)	Left Hand (kg)
60–69 years	25.3	23.6
70–79 years	23.7	22.0
80+ years	20.0	18.5
Men Age		
60–69 years	45.6	43.6
70–79 years	42.4	40.5
80 + years	34.5	32.1

[a]Jamar Dynometer.
From Desrosiers, J., Bravo, G., Hébert, R., & Dutil, E. (1995). Normative data for grip strength of elderly men and women. *American Journal of Occupational Therapy, 49*(7), 637–644.

multimorbidity, advanced age, poor nutritional status, polypharmacy, cognitive impairment, or mood disorders. An assessment of fitness and frailty can be useful to help to guide cancer treatment for older adults. Frail and prefrail cancer patients have been found to be at greater risk for all-cause mortality, postoperative mortality, chemotherapy intolerance, and postoperative complications (Handforth et al., 2015). Frailty identified through a variety of tools and measures has been found to predict poor outcomes from both surgical and chemotherapy treatment among older adults with colorectal cancer, gynecologic oncology, and glioblastoma (Huisingh-Scheetz & Walston, 2017). Nutritional intervention is the most successful when paired with exercise in the management of frailty and improvement of outcomes among cancer patients.

The American College of Surgeons (ACS) has recognized the critical importance of addressing frailty and optimizing the care of the older adult patient. Among older surgical patients, frailty has been identified as an independent risk factor for morbidity, mortality, length of stay and institutional discharge (Partridge et al., 2012). Preoperative frailty in an older adult is significantly associated with adverse clinical outcomes after emergent or nonemergent general surgery (Makary et al., 2010). Additionally, frail adults are more likely than non-frail adults to have surgical complications following elective surgery.

Emergency departments and trauma centers are other settings where tools to identify frail older adults are increasingly being employed. A 15-item Trauma Specific Frailty Index that can be completed by a patient or family member was found to be an independent predictor of poor outcomes after trauma (Joseph et al., 2014).

Treatment

The management of a frail older patient is challenging on many levels. Whether frailty can be arrested or reversed is currently debatable. Care of frail older individuals is difficult due to complex comorbidities, vulnerability to deterioration, and increased social needs. Consistent ongoing management is needed but difficult within the fragmented medical delivery system. There is a strong relationship between frailty and chronologic age, but frailty status is only one of several factors that determine outcome; others include personal resources, social support, environmental factors, and illness acuity and severity (Khatry et al., 2018). No clinical trials have been conducted to investigate specific interventions to alter or reverse frailty. The British Geriatrics Society Fit for Frailty guideline is the only current consensus best practice guidance for the management of frailty in community and outpatient settings (Turner & Clegg, 2014).

Geriatric assessment teams have repeatedly been shown to be well suited to identify frail older adults, and interprofessional geriatric team care is considered the preferred approach for managing the frail older adult in all settings. The gold standard for the care of an older adult with frailty is the Comprehensive Geriatric Assessment (CGA). The principles of CGA are used to guide the development of a comprehensive treatment plan for the older adult identified with frailty. Older frail individuals require a plan of integrated services, medical and psychosocial, that is person centered and coordinated. An individualized care plan that optimizes the treatment of medical conditions based on evidence-based practice and includes discussions with the older adult as well as the person's family and caregivers is essential.

The development of a treatment plan for an older adult who has been identified as frail, or prefrail/vulnerable, needs to be individually tailored to address that person's underlying problems and the contextual factors that influence the individual's condition, such as family, social support, and living situation. The goal of the treatment plan is to provide interventions aimed at improving physical, cognitive, and social functioning with a goal of maintaining the frail older adult's independence and self-management, while decreasing vulnerability to adverse outcomes such as falls, injury, hospitalization, and institutionalization. To be successful, the treatment plan should provide interventions over an extended period, usually months, with periodic reevaluations. Systems also need to be in place that facilitate consistent management in the presence of acute events that are likely to occur. It is often necessary to include and engage family and caregivers in the treatment plan to assure implementation and continuance over time.

Specific components of the management of frailty often focus on functional and nutritional outcomes. Physical therapy, either through home health in a person's home or as part of rehabilitation in a nursing home, is often prescribed to address the lack of endurance, strength, and mobility, which are key components of frailty. Addressing weakness through exercise programs improves frailty measures in as little as 6 weeks, and sustained improvements are evident with continued regular exercise. Nutritional support and supplementation are frequently part of the treatment plan to address weight loss.

Key Points

- Geriatric syndromes are common clinical conditions that are multifactorial, have shared risk factors, and do not fit into discrete disease categories.
- Multidisciplinary teams are usually required to optimally manage outcomes for geriatric syndromes.
- Medication interactions and side effects are commonly involved as contributing factors in geriatric syndromes.
- Dementia has an insidious onset and is slowly progressive; in comparison, delirium has a rapid onset and high risk for mortality if undetected.
- Urinary incontinence is a treatable condition with treatment dependent on the correct identification of the underlying type of incontinence.
- Sleep problems are common and need evaluation to determine if they are symptoms of an underlying disease or represent a primary sleep disorder.
- Dizziness is a common complaint that warrants a complete evaluation, including otolaryngologic, cardiovascular, and neurologic examinations.
- Unintentional weight loss should not be overlooked, as it is associated with increased morbidity and mortality.
- Frailty is characterized by physiologic decline and decreased physiologic reserve with increased vulnerability to stress.

More information about tools and the Interprofessional Education Collaborative (IPEC) competencies mentioned in this chapter can be found in Appendix 1: Tools and Appendix 2: IPEC Competencies

References

Abrams, P., Andersson, K. E., Birder, L., Brubaker, L., Cardozo, L., Chapple, C., Cottenden, A., Davila, W., de Ridder, D., Dmochowski, R., Drake, M., Dubeau, C., Fry, C., Hanno, P., Smith, J. H., Herschorn, S., Hosker, G., Kelleher, C., Koelbl, H., Khoury, S., Madoff, R., Milsom, I., Moore, K., Newman, D., Nitti, V., Norton, C., Nygaard, I., Payne, C., Smith, A., Staskin, D., Tekgul, S., Thuroff, J., Tubaro, A., Vodusek, D., Wein, A., Wyndaele, J. J., & Members of Committees; Fourth International Consultation on Incontinence. (2010). Fourth international consultation on incontinence recommendations of the international scientific committee: Evaluation and treatment of urinary incontinence, pelvic organ prolapse, and fecal incontinence. *Neurology and Urodynamics*, *29*(1), 213–240. https://doi.org/10.1002/nau.20870.

Afilalo, J., Alexander, K. P., Mack, M. J., Maurer, M. S., Green, P., Allen, L. A., Popma, J. J., Ferrucci, L., & Forman, D. E. (2014). Frailty assessment in the cardiovascular care of older adults. *Journal of the American College of Cardiology*, *63*(8), 747–762.

Afilalo, J., Kanunananthan, S., Eisenberg, M. J., Alexander, K. P., & Bergman, H. (2009). Role of frailty in patients with cardiovascular disease. *American Journal Cardiology*, *103*(110), 1616–1621.

Allen, R. P., Picchietti, D., Hening, W. A., Trenkwalder, C., Walters, A. S., & Montplaisir, J. (2003). Restless legs syndrome: Diagnostic criteria, special considerations, and epidemiology. A report from the restless legs syndrome diagnosis and epidemiology workshop at the National Institutes of Health. *Sleep Medicine*, *4*, 101–119.

Alzheimer's Association. *2019 Alzheimer's Disease Facts and Figures.* Alzheimer's Association https://www.alz.org/media/Documents/alzheimers-facts-and-figures-2019-r.pdf

American Academy of Sleep Medicine. (2014). *International classification of sleep disorders* (3rd ed.). American Academy of Sleep Medicine.

American Geriatrics Society. (2019). 2019 American Geriatrics Society Beers Criteria® Update Expert Panel (2019). American Geriatrics Society 2019 Updated AGS Beers Criteria® for Potentially Inappropriate Medication Use in Older Adults. *Journal of the American Geriatrics Society*, *67*(4), 674–694. https://doi.org/10.1111/jgs.15767.

American Geriatrics Society, British Geriatrics Society. (2010). *Clinical practice guidelines: Prevention of falls in older persons.* American Geriatrics Society. http://www.americangeriatrics.org/health_care_professionals/clinical_practice/clinical_guidelines_recommendations

American Psychiatric Association. (2013). *Diagnostic and statistical manual of mental disorders* (5th ed.). American Psychiatric Publishing.

Aranda-Gallardo, M., Enriquez de Luna-Rodriguez, M., Canca-Sanchez, J. C., Moya-Suarez, A. B., & Morales-Asencio, J. M.

(2015). Validation of the STRATIFY falls risk-assessment tool for acute-care hospital patients and nursing home residents: Study protocol. *Journal of Advanced Nursing, 71*(8), 1948–1957.

Baek, S., Piao, J., Jin, Y., & Lee, S. M. (2014). Validity of the Morse Fall Scale implemented in an electronic medical record system. *Journal of Clinical Nursing* (17–18), 2434–2340.

Berg, K., Wood-Dauphine, S. L., Williams, J. L., & Gayton, D. (1992). Measuring balance in the elderly: Validation of an instrument. *Canadian Journal of Public Health, S2*, s7–s11.

Bloch, F., Thibaud, M., Dugué, B., Breque, C., Rigaud, A. -S., & Kemoun, G. (2010). Episodes of falling among elderly people: A systematic review and meta-analysis of social and demographic pre-disposing characteristics. *Clinics (Sao Paulo), 65*, 895–903.

Bohannon, R. W., Bear-Lehman, J., Desrosiers, J., Massy-Westropp, N., & Mathiowetz, V. (2007). Average grip strength: A meta-analysis of data obtained with a Jamar dynometer from individuals 75 years of age or more. *Journal of Geriatric Physical Therapy, 30*(1), 28–30.

Bradley, S. M. (2011). Falls in older adults. *Mount Sinai Journal of Medicine, 78*(4), 590–595.

Castell, M. V., Sánchez, M., Julián, R., Queipo, R., Martín, S., & Otero, Á. (2013). Frailty prevalence and slow walking speed in persons age 65 and older: Implications for primary care. *BMC Family Practice, 14*, 86. https://doi.org/10.1186/1471-2296-14-86.

de Jonghe, A., Korevaar, J. C., van Munster, B. C., & de Rooij, S. E. (2010). Effectiveness of mela-tonin treatment on circadian rhythm disturbances in dementia. Are there implications for delirium? A systematic review. *International Journal of Geriatric Psychiatry, 25*, 1201–1208.

Ferrucci, L., Cavazzini, C., Corsi, A., Bartali, B., Russo, C. R., Lauretani, F., Corsi, A. M., Bandinelli, S., & Guralnik, J. M. (2002). Biomarkers of frailty in older persons. *Journal of Endocrinological Investigation, 25*(10 Suppl.), 10–15.

Floyd, J. A., Medler, S. M., Ager, J. W., & Janisse, J. J. (2000). Age-related changes in initiation and maintenance of sleep: A meta-analysis. *Research in Nursing & Health, 23*, 106–117.

Fried, L. P., Tangen, C. M., Walston, J., Newman, A. B., Hirsch, C., Gottdiener, J., Seeman, T., Tracy, R., Kop, W. J., Burke, G., & McBurnie, M. A. (2001). Cardiovascular Health Study Collaborative Research Group. Frailty in older adults: Evidence for a phenotype. *Journals of Gerontology: Series A Biological Sciences and Medical Sciences, 56*(3), M146–M156.

Gaddey, H. L., & Holder, K. (2014). Unintentional weight loss in older adults. *American Family Physician, 89*(9), 718–722.

Ganz, D. A., Bao, Y., Shekelle, P. G., & Rubenstein, L. Z. (2007). Will my patient fall? *Journal of the American Medical Association, 297*, 77–86.

Gates, S., Smith, L. A., Fisher, J. D., & Lamb, S. E. (2008). Systematic review of accuracy of screening instruments for predicting fall risk among independently living older adults. *Journal of Rehabilitation Research and Development, 45*, 1105–1116.

Gillespie, L. D., Robertson, M. C., Gillespie, W. J., Sherrington, C., Gates, S., Clemson, L. M., & Lamb, S. E. (2012). Interventions for preventing falls in older people living in the community. *Cochrane Database of Systematic Reviews, Issue 9*. Art. No.: CD007146. https://doi.org/10.1002/14651858.CD007146.pub3.

Godino, C., Maisano, F., Montorfano, M., Latib, A., Chieffo, A., Michev, I., Al-Lamee, R., Bande, M., Mussardo, M., Arioli, F., Ielasi, A., Cioni, M., Taramasso, M., Arendar, I., Grimaldi, A., Spagnolo, P., Zangrillo, A., La Canna, G., Alfieri, O., & Colombo, A. (2010). Outcomes after transcatheter aortic valve implantation with both Edwards-SAPIEN and Core Valve devices in a single center. *JACC: Cardiovascular Interventions, 3*(11). 1110–1021.

Goode, P. S., Burgio, K. L., Richter, H. E., & Markland, A. D. (2010). Incontinence in older women. *Journal of the American Medical Association, 303*, 2172–2181.

Gooneratne, N. S., & Vitiello, M. V. (2014). Sleep in older adults: Normative changes, sleep disorders, and treatment options. *Clinics in Geriatric Medicine, 30*(3), 591–627.

Handforth, C., Clegg, A., Young, C., Simpkins, S., Seymour, M. T., Selby, P. J., & Young, J. (2015). The prevalence and outcomes of frailty in older cancer patients: A systematic review. *Annals of Oncology, 26*(6), 1091–1101.

Hirota, T., & Kishi, T. (2013). Prophylactic antipsychotic use for postoperative delirium: A systematic review and meta-analysis. *Journal of Clinical Psychiatry, 74*, e1136–e1144.

Howell, M. J., & Schenck, C. H. (2015). Rapid eye movement sleep behavior disorder and neurodegenerative disease. *Journal of the American Medical Association, Neurology, 72*, 707–712.

Hshieh, T. T., Fong, T. G., Marcantonio, E. R., & Inouye, S. K. (2008). Cholinergic deficiency hypothesis in delirium: A synthesis of current evidence. *Journals of Gerontology: Series A Biological Sciences and Medical Sciences, 63*, 764–772.

Huisingh-Scheetz, M., & Walston, J. (2017). How should older adults with cancer be evaluated for frailty? *Journal of Geriatric Oncology, 8*(1), 8–15.

Inouye, S. K., & Charpentier, P. A. (1996). Precipitating factors for delirium in hospitalized elderly persons: Predictive model and interrelationship with baseline vulnerability. *Journal of the American Medical Association, 275*, 852–857.

Inouye, S. K., Studenski, S., Tinetti, M. E., & Kuchel, G. A. (2007). Geriatric syndromes: Clinical, research and policy implications of a core geriatric concept. *Journal of the American Geriatric Society, 55*(5), 780–791.

Inouye, S. K., van Dyck, C. H., Alessi, C. A., Balkin, S., Siegal, A. P., & Horwitz, R. I. (1990). Clarifying confusion: The confusion assessment method. A new method for detection of delirium. *Annals of Internal Medicine, 113*, 941–948.

Inouye, S. K., Westendorp, R. G., & Saczynski, J. S. (2014). Delirium in elderly people. *Lancet, 383*(9920), 911–922.

Jönsson, R., Sixt, E., Landahl, S., & Rosenhall, U. (2004). Prevalence of dizziness and vertigo in an urban elderly population. *Journal of Vestibular Research, 14*(1), 47–52.

Joseph, B., Pandit, V., Zangbar, B., Kulvatunyou, N., Hashmi, A., Green, D. J., Keeffe, T. O., Tang, A., Vercruysse, G., Fain, M. J., Randall, S., Friese, R. S., & Rhee, P. (2014). Superiority of frailty over age in predicting outcomes among geriatric trauma patients: A prospective analysis. *Journal of the American Medical Association, Surgery, 149*(8), 766–772.

Kamel, N. S., & Gammack, J. K. (2006). Insomnia in the elderly: Cause, approach, and treatment. *American Journal of Medicine, 119*, 463–469.

Kean, J., & Ryan, K. (2008). Delirium detection in clinical practice and research: Critique of current tools and suggestions for future development. *Journal of Psychosomatic Research, 65*, 255–259.

Khandelwal, C., & Kistler, C. (2013). Diagnosis of urinary incontinence. *American Family Physician, 87*(8), 543–550.

Khatry, K., Peel, N. M., Gray, L. C., & Hubbard, R. E. (2018). The utility of the frailty index in clinical decision making. *Journal of Frailty and Aging, 7*, 138–141.

MacDonald, R., Fink, H. A., Huckabay, C., Monga, M., & Wilt, T. J. (2007). Pelvic floor muscle training to improve urinary incontinence after radical prostatectomy: A systematic review of effectiveness. *British Journal of Urology, 100*, 76–81.

Makary, M. A., Segey, D. L., Pronovost, P. J., Syin, D., Bandeen-Roche, K., Patel, P., Takenaga, R., Deygan, L., Holzmueller, C. G., Tian, J., & Fried, L. P. (2010). Frailty as a predictor of surgical outcomes in older adults. *Journal of the American Geriatric Society, 210*, 901–908.

Mardon, R. E., Halim, S., Pawlson, L. G., & Haffer, S. C. (2004). Management of urinary incontinence in Medicare-managed beneficiaries: Results from the 2004 Medicare Health Outcomes Survey. *Archives of Internal Medicine, 166*, 1128–1133.

McGilton, K. S., Mahomed, N., Davis, A. M., Flannery, J., & Calabrese, S. (2009). Outcomes for older adults in an inpatient rehabilitation facility following hip fracture (HF) surgery. *Archives of Gerontology and Geriatrics, 49*, e23–e31.

McMinn, J., Steel, C., & Bowman, A. (2011). Investigation and management of unintentional weight loss in older adults. *BMJ, 342*, d1732.

National Institute for Health and Care Excellence. (2013). *Falls in older people: Assessing risk and prevention. Clinical guideline.* https://www.nice.org.uk/guidance/cg161.

National Institutes of Health, (2005). National Institutes of Health State-of-the-Science Conference Statement on manifestations and management of chronic insomnia in adults. *NIH Consensus and State-of-the-Science Statements, 22*(2), 1–3.

National Resources Center on Nutrition and Aging. (2022) *Building the capacity of senior nutrition programs.* https:/nutritionandaging.org/toolkit-the-nutrition-screening-initiatives

Nygaard, I., Barber, M. D., Burgio, K. L., Kenton, K., Meikle, S., Schaffer, J., Spino, C., Whitehead, W. E., Wu, J., & Brody, D. J. (2008). Prevalence of symptomatic pelvic floor disorders in US women. *Journal of the American Medical Association, 300*, 1311–1316.

Oliver, D., Britton, M., Seed, P., Martin, F. C., & Hopper, A. H. (1997). Development and evaluation of evidence-based risk assessment tool (STRATIFY) to predict which elderly inpatients will fall: Case-control and cohort studies. *BMJ, 315*, 1049–1053.

O'Mahony, R., Murthy, L., Akunne, A., & Young, J. (2011). Guideline Development Group. Synopsis of the National Institute for Health and Clinical Excellence guideline for prevention of delirium. *Annals of\ Medicine, 154*, 746–751.

Panel on Prevention of Falls in Older Persons. American Geriatrics Society and British Geriatrics Society, (2011). Summary of the Updated American Geriatrics Society/British Geriatrics Society clinical practice guideline for prevention of falls in older persons. *Journal of the American Geriatrics Society, 599*(10), 148–157.

Panza, F., D'Introno, A., Colacicco, A. M., Capurso, C., Del Parigi, A., Capurso, S. A., Caselli, R. J., Pilotto, A., Scafato, E., Capurso, A., & Solfrizz, V. (2006). Cognitive frailty: Predementia syndrome and vascular risk factors. *Neurobiology of Aging, 49*(7), 941–947.

Partridge, J. S. L., Harari, D., & Dhesi, J. K. (2012). Frailty in the older surgical patient: A review. *Age and Ageing, 41*(2), 142–147.

Pfisterer, M. H., Griffiths, D. J., Schaefer, W., & Resnik, N. M. (2006). The effect of age on lower urinary tract function: a study in women. *Journal of the American Geriatric Society, 54*(3), 405–409.

Piccoliori, G., Gerolimon, E., & Abholz, H. H. (2008). Geriatric assessment in general practice using a screening instrument: is it worth the effort? Results of a South Tyrol Study. *Age and Ageing, 37*(6), 647–652.

Powell, L. E., & Myers, A. M. (1995). The activities-specific balance confidence (ABD) scale. *Journals of Gerontology: Series A Biological Sciences and Medical Sciences, 50A*(10), M28–M34.

Rau, C. S., Lin, T. S., Wu, S. C., Yang, J. C., Hsu, S. Y., Cho, T. Y., & Hsieh, C. H. (2014). Geriatric hospitalizations in fall-related injuries. *Scandinavian Journal of Trauma, Resuscitation and Emergency Medicine, 22*(1), 63. https://doi.org/10.1186/s13049-014-0063-1.

Rockwood, K., & Mitnitski, A. (2007). Frailty in relation to the accumulation of deficits. *Journals of Gerontology: Series A, 62*(7), 722–727.

Rosen, T., Mack, K. A., & Noonan, R. K. (2013). Slipping and tripping: Fall injuries in adults associated with rugs and carpets. *Journal of Injury and Violence Research, 5*(1), 61–69.

Saliba, S., Elliott, M., Rubenstein, L. A., Solomon, D. H., Young, R. T., Kamberg, C. J., Roth, C., MacLean, C. H., Shekelle, P. G., Sloss, E. M., & Wenger, N. S. (2001). The Vulnerable Elders Survey (VES-13): A tool for identifying vulnerable elders in the community. *Journal of the American Geriatric Society, 49*, 1691–1699.

Segal-Gidan, F., Cherry, D., Jones, R., et al. (2011). Alzheimer's disease management guideline: Update 2008. (2008). *Alzheimers Dement, 7*, e51.

Song, X., Mitnitski, A., & Rockwood, K. (2010). Prevalence and 10-year outcomes of frailty in older adults in relation to deficit accumulation. *Journal of the American Geriatrics Society, 58*(4), 681–687.

Stenhagen, M., Ekström, H., Nordell, E., & Elmstahl, S. (2013). Falls in the general elderly population: A 3- and 6- year prospective study of risk factors using data from the longitudinal population study 'Good ageing in Skane. *BMC Geriatrics, 13*, 81. https://doi.org/10.1186/1471-2318-13-81.

Subak, L. L., Marinilli Pinto, A., Wing, R., Nakagaw, S., Kusek, J. W., Herman, W. H., Kupperman, M., & Program to Reduce Incontinence by Diet and Exercise. (2012). Decrease in urinary incontinence management costs in women enrolled in a clinical trial of weight loss to treat urinary incontinence. *Obstetrics and Gynecology, 120*, 227–283.

Tabue-Tego, M., Grasset, L., Avila-Funes, J. A., Gemuer, R., Proust-Lima, C., Peres, K., Feart, C., Amieva, H., Harmand, M. G. -C., Helmer, C., Salles, N., Rainfray, M., & Dartigues, J. F. (2017). Prevalence and co-occurrence of geriatric syndromes in people aged 75 and older in France: Results from the Bordeaux three-city study. *Journals of Gerontology: Series A Biological Sciences and Medical Sciences, 73*(1), 109–116.

Tinetti, M. E., Richman, D., & Powell, L. (1990). Falls efficacy as a measure of fear of falling. *Journal of Gerontology, 45*(6), P239–P243.

Tinetti, M. E., Williams, C. S., & Gill, T. M. (2000). Dizziness among older adults: A possible geriatric syndrome. *Annals of Internal Medicine, 132*(5), 337–344.

Tinetti, M. E., Williams, T. F., & Mayewski, R. (1986). Fall risk index for elderly patients based on number of chronic disabilities. *American Journal of Medicine, 80*, 429–434.

Tocchi, C., Dixon, J., Naylor, M., Jeon, S., & McCorkle, R. (2014). Development of a frailty measure for older adults: The frailty index for elders. *Journal of Nursing Measurement, 22*(2), 223–240.

Turner, G., & Clegg, A. (2014). Best practice guidelines for the management of frailty: A British Geriatrics Society, Age UK and Royal College of General Practitioners report. *Age and Ageing, 43*(6), 744–747.

US Preventive Services Task Force. (2011). *Prevention of falls in older adults: Draft recommendation statement.* http://www.uspreventiveservicestaskforce.org/uspstf/uspsfalls.htm

van Gool, W. A., van de Beek, D., & Eikelenboom, P. (2010). Systemic infection and delirium: When cytokines and acetylcholine collide. *Lancet, 375*(9716), 773–775.

Vaughn, B. V., & D'Cruz, O. (2011). Cardinal manifestations of sleep disorders. In M. H. Kryger, T. Roth, & W. C. Dement (Eds.),

Principles and practice of sleep medicine (5th ed., pp. 647–658). Saunders.

Vlaeyen, E., Coussement, J., Leysens, G., Van der Elst, E., Delbaere, K., Cambier, D., Denhaerynck, K., Goemaere, S., Wertelaers, A., Dobbels, F., Dejaeger, E., Milisen, K., & Center of Expertise for Fall and Fracture Prevention Flanders, (2015). Characteristics and effectiveness of fall prevention programs in nursing homes: A systematic review and meta-analysis of randomized controlled trials. *Journal of the American Geriatrics Society, 63*(2), 211–221.

Verma, S. K., Willetts, J. L., Corns, H. L., Marucci-Wellman, H. R., Lombardi, D. A., & Courtney, T. K. (2016). Falls and fall-related injuries among community-dwelling adults in the United States. *PloS One, 11*(5), e0155073.

Woolcott, J. C., Richardson, K. J., Wiens, M. O., Patel, B., Marin, J., Khan, K. M., & Marra, C. A. (2009). Meta-analysis of the impact of 9 medication classes on falls in elderly persons. *Archives of Internal Medicine, 169*, 1952–1960.

World Health Organization. (2012). *Falls*. www.who.int/mediacentre/factsheets/fs344/en/index.html

12
Sensory Changes

SOO JUNG KIM, MSN, ANP, AGPCNP-BC

OBJECTIVES

Student Learning Objectives

After completing this chapter, the student should be able to do the following:

1. Discuss the prevalence of sensory deficits in older adults, state normal age-related changes, and discuss current screening recommendations for the senses of vision, hearing, olfaction, and taste.
2. Discuss the differential diagnosis and potential risks associated with a change or loss of vision, hearing, smell, or taste.
3. Discuss treatment options for vision and hearing loss, and describe the role of nurse practitioners, physician assistants, and other health professionals in identifying and managing these symptoms.
4. Discuss the importance of effective communication and coordination of care among care providers throughout a patient's care journey.

Practitioner Objectives

After completing this chapter, the practitioner should be able to do the following:

1. Appropriately recognize signs of and screen for sensory impairment in older adults.
2. Perform assessments for patients with sensory impairments, provide treatment, and generate referrals based on assessment findings.
3. Partner with health care providers to improve patient outcomes and patient safety.
4. Provide support for the patient and caregiver to assist them in managing sensory impairments.
5. Coordinate care and facilitate effective communication with the interdisciplinary team.

Overview

Prevalence

A large number of older adult patients experience sensory impairments but do not report these conditions unless directly and specifically questioned about them. This underreporting is partly due to the insidious onset and progressive nature of these changes as individuals age. Resultantly, sensory impairments too often go unrecognized by patients, families, and providers.

Sensory impairments are common in aging individuals, and the prevalence increases with age. Among older adults ≥70 years of age in the United States, 15.4% have vision impairment and 26.3% have hearing impairment (Dillon et al., 2010). In adults 65 to 80 years of age, greater than 50% have declines in olfactory function, and this increases to 75% in those age 80 and older (Doty & Kamath, 2014; Kaufman, 2007). Gustatory disorders are also more common in aging individuals, prevalent in 5.1% of older adults ages 60 to 69 and in 14% to 22% of nursing home residents (Imoscopi et al., 2012). In the United States, men have greater prevalence of hearing impairment compared to women. Adults ≥80 years of age are more than twice as likely to have vision and hearing impairments compared to those who are younger (ages 70 to 79), and those who are living below the poverty threshold are more likely to have vision impairment. Despite the availability of sensory aids for vision and hearing impairment that may be beneficial, 60% do not use glasses (or have glasses that suboptimally correct their vision), and 70% do not use hearing aids (Dillon et al., 2010). Vision and hearing impairment, referred to as dual sensory impairment (DSI), increases risk for cognitive impairment, communication difficulties, functional dependence (in activities of daily living [ADLs] and instrumental activities of daily living [IADLs]), social isolation, depression, and mortality. Optimizing hearing and vision is essential for communication, quality of life, and independence in daily activities (Davidson & Guthrie, 2019; Gopinath et al., 2013).

Interprofessional Collaboration

The care of an older adult with sensory impairment necessitates a team-based approach to care. The interprofessional team may be composed of physicians, nurse practitioners (NPs), physician assistants (PAs), nurses, case managers, social workers, specialists for the evaluation of specific sensory impairments, occupational therapists, and speech and language pathologists. Each member of the team shares her or his expertise to develop a comprehensive, personalized care plan for the patient. Clear communication among providers, patients, and caregivers is essential to prevent fragmented care and to maintain the focus on the patient's wishes and values in order to provide optimal care.

CASE STUDY

A 78-year-old male with history of head and neck cancer (squamous cell carcinoma) who underwent prior radiation therapy, surgery, and chemotherapy presents for an initial visit to establish care. He has age-related cataracts and resultant poor vision. He also has a chronic fistula in the oropharynx due to prior treatment, permanent hearing loss on the right ear, and moderate hearing loss on the left ear as well. His medical records indicate Mandarin is his preferred language. Due to prior treatment, he has dysphagia (requiring percutaneous endoscopic gastrostomy placement) and a speech impairment. He attempts to speak but is unable to produce audible sound. He presents to visit with a Mandarin-speaking interpreter. Notably he is distressed and anxious. The interpreter attempts to communicate with the patient, but this proves to be challenging due to marked dual sensory impairment. As the provider, what would you do?

A thorough evaluation of the patient's history and exam reveals that the stronger of his senses is vision. He has lived in the United States for 30+ years and has good understanding of the English language. You bring in a white paper on a clipboard and, using a black pen and writing in large font, attempt to communicate with the patient. The patient enthusiastically responds, finally being able to express his concerns. He is referred to an ophthalmologist and undergoes cataract surgery. The following visit, he presents with new glasses and with marked improvement in vision and mood. At each subsequent encounter the clipboard and black pen are used to communicate with the patient, which proves to be the most effective method of communication. You document and share this information with the care team to enhance communication and improve the coordination of care.

The takeaway message from this case is that health care providers should evaluate for sensory impairments in older adults and once identified utilize the most effective method of communication for the individual. Always ask patients how to best communicate with them. This way, we can plan care to maximize quality of life, address potentially treatable conditions, and appropriately connect patients to needed supportive services.

Brief Description of the Roles of Several Members of the Interdisciplinary Team

Two complementary health professionals who specialize in the assessment and treatment of vision loss are optometrists and ophthalmologists:

- *Optometrists* are health care professionals who provide eye exams, perform vision tests, and prescribe corrective lens and medications to treat certain eye conditions. They can also dispense corrective lenses. They provide primary vision care by treating and managing changes in vision.
- *Ophthalmologists* are physicians who specialize in diseases of the eye. They can evaluate for and diagnose eye conditions and provide treatments such as surgery or laser treatments depending on their area of specialty (i.e., glaucoma specialists).

Other health care professionals who can assist patients facing sensory changes include the following:

- *Opticians* are technicians who are trained to fit corrective lenses using prescriptions from ophthalmologists or optometrists.
- *Otolaryngologists* are physicians who specialize in diseases of the ear, nose, and throat (ENT). Working often in collaboration with ENT specialists are audiologists.
- *Audiologists* are trained professionals who assess and diagnose hearing loss. Many times, they work with hearing aid dispensers.
- *Speech and language pathologists* are health care professionals who evaluate, diagnose, and treat disorders of language, speech, swallowing, and communication.
- *Dentists (DMD or DDS)* specialize in the prevention, treatment, and diagnosis of conditions affecting teeth, gums, and the mouth. Individuals experiencing problems with taste and smell often will need to be evaluated by a dentist.
- *Occupational therapists (OTs)* can play a role in working with older adults who have sensory loss to find adaptive equipment, alternative approaches, and environmental redesign strategies to accommodate the sensory loss and maintain function. These experts can also help by identifying activities that the patients can do within their sensory limitations that can contribute to their quality of life.

Implications for the Older Adult

Sensory loss for an older adult can have serious implications for health and well-being. An older adult patient with vision loss may be unable to appreciate obstacles such as cracks on pavement and potentially fall. With hearing loss, the older adult may be unable to hear conversations, respond inappropriately, or be considered cognitively impaired. With impaired taste or loss of taste (gustatory loss), the individual may be unable to taste spoiled food, and loss of smell (olfactory) may make the person unable to smell warnings such as smoke. Therefore, early recognition, evaluation, and effective communication among providers are all essential for optimal care management that will maximize the patient's quality of life and minimize the effects sensory impairments have on aging individuals.

HEALTHY PEOPLE 2030 BOX 12.1

Healthy People 2030 lists the following objectives relating to sensory impairment in aging individuals over the coming decade with the goal of improving quality of life and overall health:

- Reduce the number of patients who are edentulous (complete loss of teeth).
- Reduce loss of vision from age-related macular degeneration (ARMD), glaucoma, cataracts, diabetic retinopathy, and refractive errors.
- Increase utilization of vision rehabilitation services, assistive devices, and adaptive devices in those with vision loss.
- Increase the number of adults who have hearing exams in recent 5 years.
- Increase hearing aid use in adults with hearing loss.

Olfaction

In the aging population, declines in olfactory function commonly occur, and with this decline the pleasures of eating, nutrition, safety, and quality of life are affected (Kaufman, 2007). Our senses help us to engage with the world around us. In the case of the sense of smell, it allows us to detect odors that may protect us from harm (Box 12.1)—for example, the ability to smell gas, fire, or spoiled food. It also allows individuals to enjoy smells such as the fragrance from flowers or the aroma of a good meal. Hyposomnia is the reduced sense of smell, and anosmia is the loss of one's sense of smell (Lafreniere, 2020b). Evaluation of the patient with smell impairment necessitates an interdisciplinary team approach to care. This can include the primary care provider, allergist, ENT specialist, and neurologist. However, loss of the sense of smell is often underreported; patients themselves may not be aware of smell impairment, thus it is left unaddressed (Lafreniere, 2020a).

The first cranial nerve is the olfactory nerve, and its function is to transmit information connected to smell. Among the cranial nerves it is the shortest, and it passes through receptors located in the nasal mucosa to forebrain (Rea, 2014). Odorant molecules enter the nasal mucosa and interact with the olfactory receptor neurons (ORN) located in the olfactory epithelium lining the inside of the nose. Axons of the ORN extend to olfactory bulb neurons, which then extend to the pyriform cortex (located in the temporal lobe) and several other areas of the forebrain (including the amygdala and hypothalamus). From the forebrain and pyriform cortex, through the thalamus, olfactory information is sent to other areas of the cerebral cortex where smell information is further processed to identify the odorant and generate appropriate responses (emotional, motor, or visceral) to the odorant stimuli (Purves et al., 2001). Fig. 12.1 demonstrates the olfactory process. Many conditions cause anosmia, but the most common causes are obstructive and inflammatory disorders accounting for 50% to 70% of cases. These include nasal polyps, allergic rhinitis, and rhinosinusitis, all of which block odorant molecules from reaching olfactory nerves by causing inflammation of the nasal mucosa (Li, 2019). Other causes of anosmia include head trauma, damage to the olfactory nerve, smoking, and viral infections such as COVID-19. Additionally, aging-related changes including loss of numbers of cells in the olfactory bulb and loss of olfactory sensory neurons that are essential for perceiving smell may also contribute to a reduction or loss of the sense of smell. Fig. 12. 1 shows the anatomy of the olfactory system.

Box 12.2 summarizes the most common causes and consequences of anosmia. The olfactory neurons have ability to regenerate compared to other CNS nerves. However, anosmia (lack of smell) can be temporary or permanent (Kaufman, 2017; Li, 2019; Rawson et al., 2012; Rea, 2014).

• BOX 12.1 Risks Associated With Chemosensory Dysfunction (Disorders of Taste and Smell)

- Cooking-related incidents
- Unable to detect leaking gas or smell fire
- Eating spoiled food

Data from Kaufman, D. M. (2007). *Kaufman's clinical neurology for psychiatrists*. Elsevier; Lafreniere, D. (2020). Evaluation and treatment of taste and smell disorders.

Assessment

For patients complaining of anosmia, obtaining a thorough history (including the patent's social history: smoking history, illicit drug use, and medical conditions) and review of systems is essential to identify potential causes. Also ask the patient about the onset of symptoms and preceding events (i.e., head trauma or nasal complaints).

Review vital signs and medications, and a perform a thorough physical exam focusing on the nose and paranasal sinuses. Consider performing a neurologic exam that may help to identify the neurologic causes of anosmia.

Examination of the Nose

Inspect

Examine the skin; erythema may be indicative of an infectious etiology or inflammation. Ecchymosis may indicate prior injury. Using an otoscope, inspect inside the nose, examining the nasal turbinate and the nasal septum for asymmetry. Structural problems such as a deviated septum may cause difficulties with breathing and smelling. Examine the nostrils to assess for patency. Occlude one nostril at a time, and ask the patient to breathe through the open nostril with his or her mouth closed. Check both sides.

Palpate

Palpate the nose, feeling for bumps or depressions. Palpate the paranasal sinus to evaluate for swelling. Tenderness to palpation may indicate sinusitis.

Olfactory Nerve Testing

Option 1

- Patients are asked to identify selected substances by smelling from one nostril while the clinician presses the other nostril.
- Examples of substances: coffee, vanilla essence.
- Avoid volatile substances or those that can be irritating such as alcohol, as these can lead to inaccurate results.

Option 2

- University of Pennsylvania Small Identification Test (UPSIT).
- This is a scratch-and-sniff test that comes prepackaged.

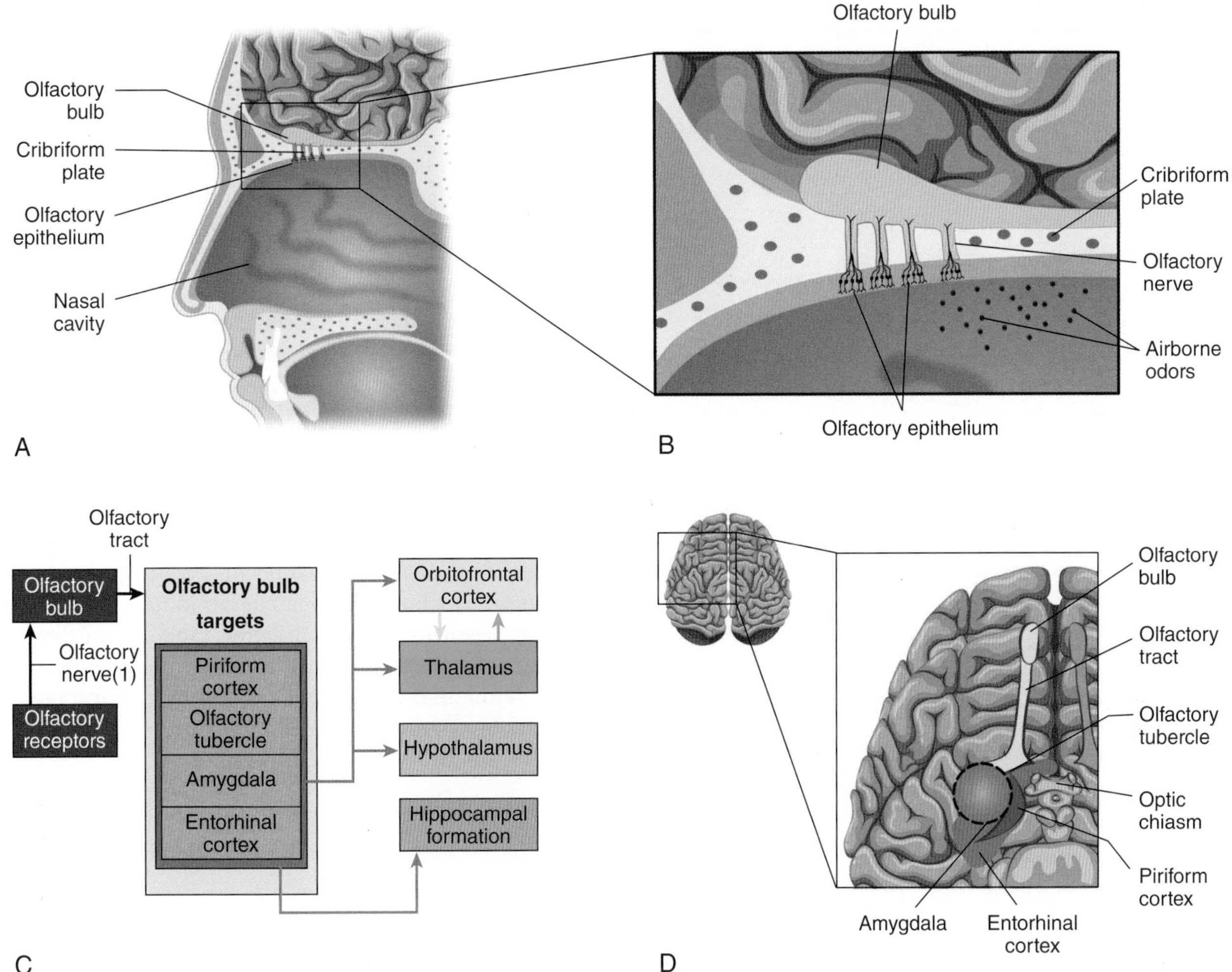

• **Fig. 12.1** Olfactory system. Diagram of the olfactory system. (A) Central and peripheral areas of olfactory pathway. (B) Closer view of boxed area in (A) shows relationship between olfactory receptor neurons (ORN) present in olfactory epithelium with the olfactory bulb. The main target for ORN is the olfactory bulb. (C) Simplified diagram of demonstrating the pathway for the processing of olfactory information. (D) Key components in the olfactory system. (From Purves, D., Augustine, G., Fitzpatrick, D., Katz, L. C., LaMantia, A.-S., McNamara, J. O., & Williams, S. M. [2001]. *Neuroscience* [2nd ed.]. Sinauer Associates.)

Treatment and Management

Anosmia is a symptom and requires further evaluation to determine its underlying etiology. Further testing will depend on the patient's symptoms but can include laboratory tests such as a complete blood count, respiratory nasopharyngeal panel (to rule out viral infection), and neuroimaging (i.e., magnetic resonance imaging [MRI] of the brain, computerized tomography [CT] scan of the brain or sinus) (Li, 2019; Rea, 2014).

Taste

Gustatory (taste) cells are found in the palate, epiglottis, tongue, pharynx, and upper third region of the esophagus. Gustatory receptor cells (Fig. 12.2) are found in taste buds that are contained in papillae on the tongue, which when stimulated transmit signals to the brain via cranial nerves VII (facial), IX (glossopharyngeal), and X (vagal nerve) to carry information that allows us to identify specific tastes (Fig. 12.3). The five basic taste qualities that can be discerned are bitter, salty, sour, sweet, and umami (savory). Additionally, the trigeminal nerve innervates the tongue to allow the sense of taste through our perception of temperature, pain (i.e., spicy, hot foods), touch, and pressure.

Contrary to common beliefs, gustatory cells (of the tongue) are not located in particular regions of the tongue but rather are distributed throughout the tongue. The experience of the sense of taste is more complex than taste quality. Sensations of taste are experienced through a chemosensory mechanism named chemesthesis, the common chemical sense involving thousands of nerve endings, particularly in the moist areas of the eyes, nose, throat, and mouth, which give rise to sensations such as cold, texture, or the burn of spicy peppers. The sensations arising from

• BOX 12.2 Causes of Anosmia

Most Common

- Inflammatory conditions and obstructive disorders including upper respiratory infection (URI), nasal polyp, allergic rhinitis, rhinosinusitis.
- Infections such as COVID-19
- Smoking (chronically)
- Head trauma
- Age-related changes

Other Causes

- Neurodegenerative conditions such as Alzheimer disease, Parkinson disease
- Exposure to toxins (i.e., paint solvent, formaldehyde, benzene, sulfuric acid, chlorine)
- Exposure to industrial agents (i.e., nickel, lead, chromium, chalk, ashes, cadmium)
- Nutritional (i.e., malnutrition, liver disease, acquired immunodeficiency syndrome, vitamin (A, B_6, B_{12}) and trace mineral deficiency (i.e., zinc, copper), renal failure (chronic)
- Cancer in the brain or nasal cavity, tumors
- Radiation therapy to head and neck
- Subarachnoid hemorrhage
- Congenital conditions (i.e., Kallmann syndrome)
- Psychiatric conditions (i.e., depression, schizophrenia)
- Endocrine disorders (i.e., diabetes mellitus, hypothyroidism)
- Cerebrovascular accident (CVA)
- Systemic lupus erythematosus
- Autoimmune disease (i.e., Sjogren syndrome)
- Medications (note that medications may cause changes in both taste and smell): Thyroid medications (i.e., methimazole), antihypertensives (i.e., enalapril, hydrochlorothiazide), cardiac medications (i.e., nitroglycerine) antibiotics (i.e., ciprofloxacin, tetracycline, azithromycin, metronidazole), anticonvulsants (i.e., phenytoin), antidepressants (i.e., Elavil, nortriptyline), antihistamines (i.e., loratadine), decongestants (i.e., pseudoephedrine), antiinflammatory medications (i.e., hydrocortisone, colchicine, dexamethasone), muscle relaxants (i.e., baclofen), chemotherapy (i.e., doxorubicin, vincristine, cisplatin), antimanic medications (lithium), antipsychotic medications (i.e., clozapine), Parkinson medications (i.e., levodopa), statins (i.e., pravastatin, lovastatin)

Consequence of Anosmia

- Risk of being unable to smell gas leaking, which can be life threatening
- Inability to smell (body) odors such as urine, which may have social consequences
- Bland-tasting food
- Reduced appetite

Data from Bromley, S. M. (2000). Smell and taste disorders: a primary care approach. *American Family Physician, 61*(2), 427–436, 438; Kaufman, D. M. (2007). *Kaufman's clinical neurology for psychiatrists*. Elsevier; Li, X. L., Forshing. (2019). *Anosomnia*. StatPearls; Rea, P. (2014). *Clinical anatomy of the cranial nerves*: Academic Press; Silvestre, F. J., Perez-Herbera, A., Puente-Sandoval, A., & Bagán, J. V. (2010). Hard palate perforation in cocaine abusers: A systematic review. *Clinical Oral Investigations, 14*(6), 621–628. https://doi.org/10.1007/s00784-009-0371-4

the five taste qualities combined with the common chemical sense, along with temperature sensations (heat/cold), texture, and aroma, give rise to the perception of flavor that lets individuals identify what they are eating—for example, whether they are eating an orange or a lemon (Gravina et al., 2013).

Gustatory Loss

Gustatory loss occurs with aging but is not as prevalent as olfactory changes. Loss of taste buds may occur after 50 years of age. Changes in gustatory function are caused by multiple etiologies. Our sense of smell affects our ability to taste. Thus they are closely connected, and many times gustatory loss is chiefly from anosmia, or the loss of smell. More commonly, there is localized gustatory dysfunction more so than generalized dysfunction, meaning the whole mouth is not affected. Poor dentition, dentures, and problems chewing can affect taste. Additionally, with increasing age, dry mouth (xerostomia) commonly occurs, which is a risk factor for dental carries and can affect taste and the pleasure of eating, which then can impact nutrition. Gustatory loss can lead to increased utilization of seasonings such as salt and sugar, which may worsen comorbidities such as hypertension, heart disease, and diabetes. Obtaining a thorough history is important because it allows the practitioner to examine the underlying etiology that may contribute to a patient's loss of taste and smell.

Gustatory Disorders

- Hypogeusia (reduced ability to respond to the five taste qualities)
- Ageusia (complete loss of taste)
- Dysgeusia (a persistent rancid, foul, salty, metallic sensation)

Common Etiology of Gustatory Disorders

Some patients have gustatory disorders from birth; however, the majority occur as a result of illness or injury. Examples include those that arise following surgery to the nose or throat, radiation therapy for head and neck cancer, upper respiratory infection, allergic rhinitis, viral infections, xerostomia (dry mouth), head trauma, cigarette smoking (chronic), dental issues, poor oral hygiene, drug use (i.e., perforated nasal septum and hard palate caused by intranasal use of cocaine), and nutritional deficiency (vitamin A, B_6, B_{12}, or trace metal deficiency [i.e., copper or zinc]). Many chronic diseases, such as diabetes, stroke, hepatic or renal dysfunction, neurodegenerative diseases (i.e., Alzheimer disease), and medications (i.e., antibiotics like metronidazole or clindamycin causing metallic taste) can also cause associated changes in taste. Sometimes no identifiable cause can be found, and these are termed *idiopathic causes* (Bromley, 2000).

Assessment

For patients complaining of gustatory loss, obtaining a good history and through review of systems is essential in order to identify potential causes. The patient's vital signs, weight,

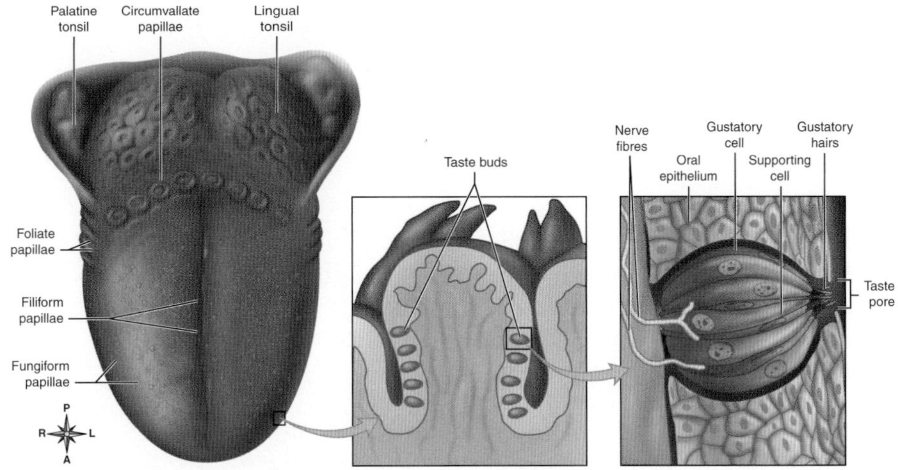

• **Fig 12.2** Anatomy of human tongue (papillae and taste buds). (From Tomkins, Z. [2021]. *Integrating systems: Clinical cases in anatomy and physiology*. Elsevier.)

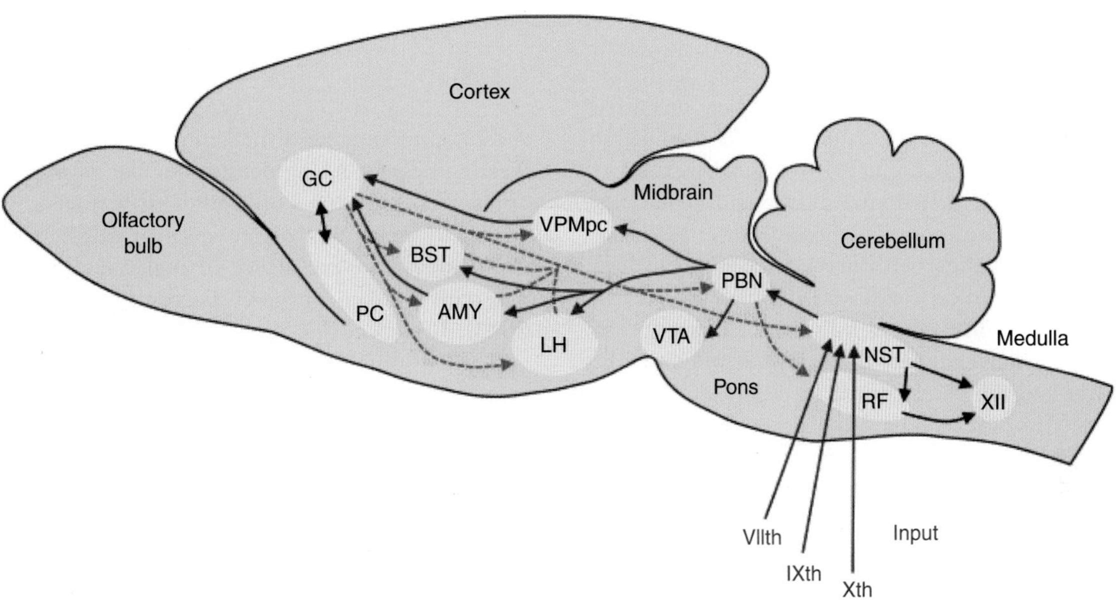

• **Fig. 12.3** Peripheral taste pathway anatomy. (From Fritzsch B: *The Senses: A Comprehensive Reference*, ed2, Elsevier, 2020, Pages 280–297.)

and medications should be reviewed. Also, a thorough physical exam should be performed, including an examination of the head and neck, mucous membranes, teeth, gums, tongue, and neurologic conditions.

The clinician should ask patients about the onset of symptoms; changes in symptoms (i.e., worsening or improving); if they have difficulty tasting salty, sweet, sour, or bitter foods; and if they have dry mouth, trouble chewing or swallowing, mouth pain, a smoking history, or a recent infection (i.e., upper respiratory infection [URI]). The clinician should also ask about their oral hygiene, any weight loss, and new medications or treatments (i.e., for cancer).

Commonly performed taste tests include the "three-drop test," which uses three drops of liquid (taste stimulus versus water with a volume of less than 0.1 mL). The threshold is defined as the concentration with which the taste is identified correctly and consecutively three times. Additional tests utilizing impregnated strips of filter paper are in development. The benefit of this test is that it has been found to help in the identification of taste deficits for patients who have burning mouth syndrome.

The diagnostic workup for gustatory loss will depend on the patient's symptoms and the examination findings. Laboratory tests can help to rule out medical conditions potentially uncovered through the history and physical exam. These may include malnutrition, upper respiratory infection, or inflammation symptoms such as nasal congestion and cough, seasonal allergies, and thyroid disease. The laboratory workup may include a comprehensive blood count, vitamin studies (i.e., B_{12}, B_6), a comprehensive metabolic panel, and thyroid function tests. Imaging tests should be considered for further evaluation as deemed appropriate, such as a CT scan to evaluate the sinus and an MRI to evaluate soft tissues or brain function.

Treatment

There are no specific therapies for aging-related declines in taste and smell. Treatment will depend on identifying and addressing the underlying etiology, such as the treatment of URI or the use of artificial saliva for xerostomia. Referrals to dental, ENT, psychiatry, or neurology specialists should be considered for further evaluation and treatment of the underlying diseases. In the case of underlying neurodegenerative processes (such as Alzheimer disease and Parkinson disease), no specific treatment is available that has been shown to improve or alter the loss of smell or taste (Bromley, 2000; Wick, 2015).

Oral Health

Studies have shown that 17% to 43% of older adults are edentulous (meaning there has been a complete or partial loss of natural teeth) (Bromley, 2000; Centers for Disease Control and Prevention [CDC], 2019c). Primary causes of this condition include periodontal disease and dental caries. It occurs more commonly in those of lower socioeconomic status and in those with limited access to medical care. Additionally, medical conditions and medications can cause a decreased production of saliva, which can lead to tooth decay. Dental changes commonly accompany the aging process and are characterized by yellowing of teeth brought about from daily use. Maxillary and mandibular bones undergo the process of resorption and bone formation. When there is loss of teeth, alveolar and jaw bone atrophy can occur. As a result, denture fitting may be more challenging. In settings of local disease, such as periodontal disease versus systemic diseases such as osteoporosis, there can be greater alveolar bone resorption (Boyce & Shone, 2006; Heckmann et al., 2003; National Institutes of Health [NIH], 2013; Razak et al., 2014; Silvestre et al., 2010; Welge-Lüssen, 2009).

About 20% older adults 65 years old and older have cavities that are untreated (CDC, 2019a, 2019b; NIH, 2018c; Razak et al., 2014). Many times, tooth decay occurs at the root as a result of receding gums and at the margins and area of prior restorations. Additionally, 41% of those 65 years old and older have periodontal disease, which is infection of the gums that are caused by plaque due to bacteria buildup (Ritchie, 2002). Plaque and calcified plaque (calculus) cause inflammation in the gums or gingiva. If this progresses to the jaw (alveolar) bone and the connective tissue, it ultimately causes loosening of teeth and eventual tooth loss due to the loss of support from these structures (Razak et al., 2014; Ritchie, 2002).

Oral candidiasis (Fig. 12.4) is more common in aging individuals due to poor dentition and denture wear. The most common cause of oral candidiasis is the continuous wearing of poor-fitting dentures or poorly cleaning dental appliances. Symptoms of candidiasis include a heightened sensitivity to foods that are spicy or acidic, mouth pain, or soreness. The prevalence of oral cancer increases with age, with the median age of diagnosis at 62 years (Ritchie, 2002). Recurrent oral cancer also increases with advanced age. Many times oral cancer causes swallowing problems, so providers should pay particular attention when an older adult presents with swallowing difficulty. Treatment-related complications from radiation therapy, such as dental caries, osteonecrosis, or xerostomia, can occur. Chemotherapy can also lead to odynophagia (tooth pain), dry mouth, and changes in taste. Additionally, oral cancer treatment–related problems may require supplemental nutrient intake such as enteral nutrition (Razak et al., 2014; Ritchie, 2002).

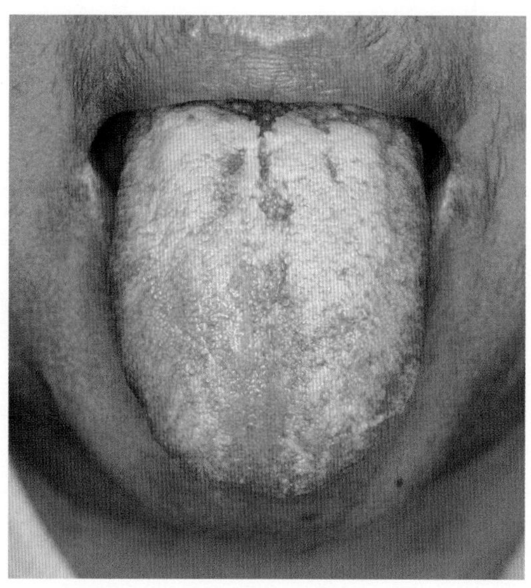

• **Fig. 12.4** Oral candidiasis. (From Millsop, J. W., & Fazel, N. [2016]. Oral candidiasis. *Clinics in Dermatology, 34*[4], 487–494. https://doi.org/10.1016/j.clindermatol.2016.02.022.)

Xerostomia (dry mouth) is a common complaint and finding among older adults. A variety of medications and medical conditions that commonly occur with older adults can cause xerostomia (Box 12.3). Xerostomia can cause a change in taste perception and experience, which in turn can cause patients to choose certain foods and avoid others such as dry foods, breads, and firmer vegetables such as carrots. This may lead to reduced caloric intake, which can have consequences on medical conditions, medication dosing, and nutritional well-being. (Richie, 2002). A diagnosis will be made after a review of the patient's history, medications, and physical exam.

Treatment for xerostomia may include the use of a saliva substitute, sips of water, chewing (sugarless) gum, and eating sour candy (lemon drops). Patients may also be instructed to avoid smoking and alcohol, obtain a dental evaluation, and maintain good oral hygiene (Bartok, 2011; Millsop & Fazel, 2016; NIH, 2018a).

• BOX 12.3 Causes of Xerostomia

Medications (hundreds)

- Diuretics (i.e., hydrochlorothiazide)
- Antidepressants (i.e., tricyclic antidepressants)
- Analgesics (i.e., opioids)
- Medications with anticholinergic properties like antihistamines (i.e., diphenhydramine) and antispasmodics (i.e., oxybutynin)

Medical Conditions

- Damage to nerves involving the mouth and salivary gland (from trauma [accident or surgical])
- Status post bone marrow transplant
- Uncontrolled diabetes
- Psychiatric disorder (i.e., anxiety or depression)
- Stress (emotional)
- Radiation therapy in head and neck area
- Autoimmune disease (i.e., Sjogren syndrome, systemic lupus, sarcoidosis)
- HIV/AIDS
- Chemotherapy

Data from Bartok, V. (2011). Drug-induced dry mouth; National Institutes of Health. (2013). *NIDCD NIDCD [National Institute on Deafness and Other Communication Disorders] fact sheet: Taste and smell taste disorders*. US Department of Health and Human Services: National Institutes of Health; Oral Cancer Foundation (OCF). (2020a). *Complications of treatment*. The Oral Cancer Foundation; Oral Cancer Foundation (OCF). (2020b). *Understanding oral cancer*. The Oral Cancer Foundation; Ritchie, C. S. (2002). Oral health, taste, and olfaction. *Clinics in Geriatric Medicine, 18*(4), 709–717. https://doi.org/10.1016/s0749-0690(02)00041-1

Vision Impairment

A number of age-related changes occur in the structures of the eye (Fig. 12.5) that contribute to changes in vision that accompany aging.

Cornea

The curvature of the cornea changes in the aging eye, and this causes changes in refraction, how light passes through from outside to the retina at the back of the eye. With increasing age the lens becomes less flexible, which leads to changes in near vision (presbyopia). The cornea is more fragile, and there is a decrease in luster and corneal sensitivity. Due to these changes, presbyopia and astigmatism become more common.

Uveal Changes

Increased resistance to aqueous humor outflow, beyond that caused by normal aging, increases the risk of glaucoma. The pupil becomes smaller, the iris becomes less reactive, and dilating the eyes grows more difficult, resulting in a longer period of time to adjust to changes in light intensity. The ciliary body shape and tone changes, the lens becomes less elastic, and accommodation decreases, causing presbyopia.

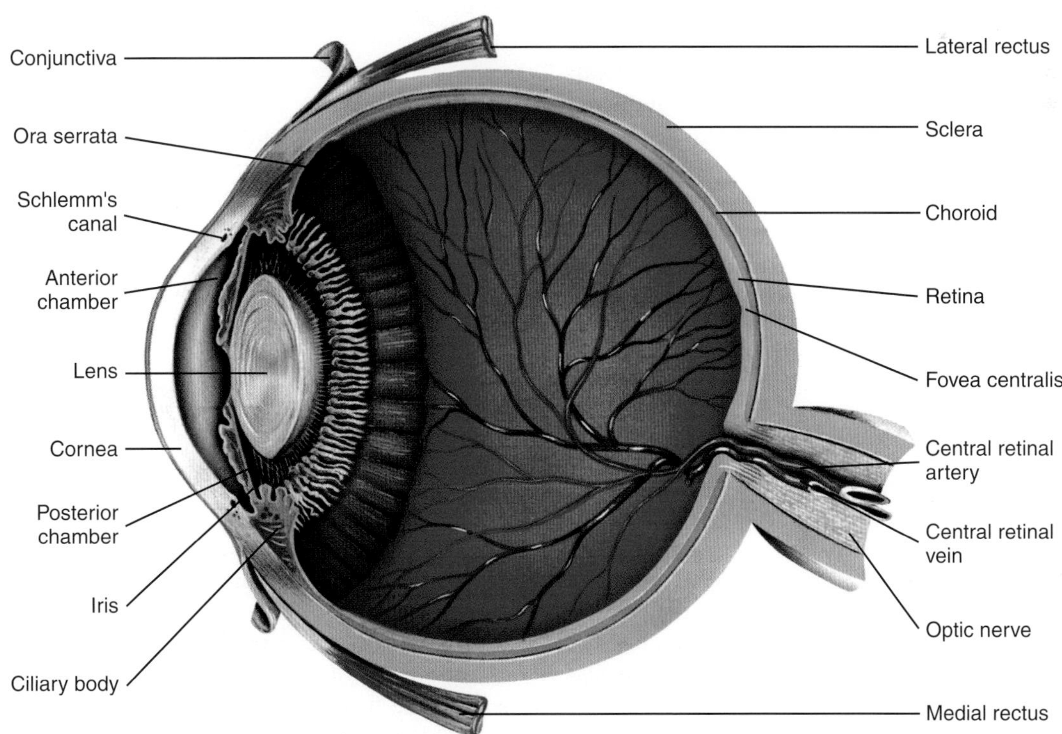

• Fig. 12.5 Anatomy of the eye. (From Lutz, R. M., Zambroski, C., & Visovsky, C. G. [2023]. *Edmund's pharmacology for the primary care provider* [5th ed.]. Elsevier.)

Lens Changes

Nuclear sclerosis (hardening) of the lens occurs due to a number of bio/photochemical changes causing cataract formation. Changes in hyaluronic acid components and collagen fibers of the vitreous humor cause floaters (which are harmless). Condensation of the vitreous gel, increased mobility and enhancement of fibrillary structures, and the formation of lacunae (which are optically empty spaces) accompany the aging eye. The vitreous body shrinks with increased vitreous liquefaction and larger cavities formed by coalescence of the lacunae. This causes posterior vitreous detachment (PVD), which manifests as a spider-like floater located in the front of the eye that moves toward the direction of the gaze. Retinal tears can occur during an acute event of PVD, which results from vitreoretinal adhesions at the peripheral retina. This condition requires laser treatment to prevent detachment of the retina. If the patient experiences floaters (caused by the dispersion of pigment from a torn retina) and new onset flashes (caused by retinal traction in the event of an acute PVD), then he or she will need prompt evaluation by an ophthalmologist to assess for a possible retinal tear associated with PVD. A new onset curtain-like shadow in a patient's visual field may be suggestive of a retinal detachment, which requires an ophthalmologic referral for surgical treatment.

Retina

Decreases in visual acuity, contrast sensitivity (with resultant reduced depth perception), visual field sensitivity decline, and an increased threshold for adaptation to darkness occur with aging. Decline in vision functions occur as a result of changes in neuronal functions of the visual system, including neuronal cell loss and degeneration. There are decreases in numbers of ganglion cells, optic nerve axons, and photo receptors. The retinal pigment epithelium (RPE) is essential for maintaining the integrity of rods and cone. With the aging process, changes occur that include decreased melanin, increased lipofuscin, decreased cytoplasm volume, increased pleomorphism, and thickening of the basement membrane. These are aging signs of the retina.

Macula

Macular changes include reduced retinal macular microcirculation. Significant changes occur in Bruch's membrane with debris accumulating from the retina. When the production of this debris surpasses the removal, as occurs with aging, deposits accumulate in macular areas manifesting eventually as drusen. Drusen appear as yellowish white specks below the retina. Although they usually do little to cause disturbances in vision, they cannot be treated. Over time, the condition can get progressively worse and is connected to age-related macular degeneration (AMD) in some older adults. Hard drusen (with small round solid deposits with distinctive borders) may progress to dry atrophic AMD, which causes progressive visual distortion and central deterioration of vision. It is not treatable and accounts for the majority of the 90% of cases of AMD. Soft drusen (with larger, pale, indistinct borders) are more likely to progress to wet AMD, which may lead to the formation of a subretinal neovascular membrane, which can cause bleeding, central visual distortion, a sudden decline in central visual acuity, and exudative maculopathy (NIH, 2018a) (Chou et al., 2016).

Considerations for Clinicians

The most common eye conditions in older adults are listed in Box 12.4, common symptoms of vision loss are listed in Box 12.5, and interventions for safety are listed in Box 12.6. It is crucial to ask patients about symptoms of vision changes and vision loss to diagnose and intervene appropriately. Additionally, safety measures can help prevent falls and potential injury.

Presbyopia, the decline in near vision, is by far the most common eye condition that affects vision in older adults. The lens becomes less elastic and accommodation decreases.

• BOX 12.4 Common Eye Conditions in Older Adults

- Presbyopia
- Astigmatism
- Cataracts
- Macular degeneration/age-related macular degeneration
- Dry eye/keratoconjunctivitis
- Glaucoma—acute angle closure and open angle
- Diabetic retinopathy

• BOX 12.5 Common Symptoms of Vision Loss

Reports of the following:

- Ocular pain
- Diplopia
- Visual distortion (straight lines appearing wavy)
- Seeing flashing lights
- Seeing halos around lights
- Trouble with night driving
- Falling
- Injuries (burns, cuts, bumping into, holding onto items) due to poor vision
- Poor balance
- Getting lost

• BOX 12.6 Interventions for Safety

- Use color contrast such as bright colors against a white/beige wall
- Vision-enhancing devices (i.e., magnifier or glasses)
- Large print
- Good lighting
- Rubber mats to prevent falling

It commonly begins in midlife, around age 45, and continues through aging into later life. The diagnosis is made by checking refraction, usually performed during an optometrist or ophthalmologist examination. Correction often necessitates the use of reading/distance glasses or contacts and may also include elective laser corrective surgery (e.g., Lasik eye surgery) for most individuals (Purves et al., 2001).

Cataracts occur with increasing frequency with advanced age. Over half of Caucasian Americans were found to have cataracts by age 75. At 80 years of age, 61% of Hispanic Americans, 53% of Blacks, and 70% Whites had cataracts (NIH, 2019). Cataracts cause progressive vision loss due to the clouding of the lens and may be unilateral or bilateral. Cataracts are caused by oxidative damage to the lens protein and lipofuscin in the lens (deposit of fat). Visual acuity gradually declines to 20/30 or below (normal vision is 20/20). Symptoms related to cataract development include blurry vision, reduced light and color perception, objects appearing with yellowish tint, reduced glare sensitivity, and the appearance of halos around objects. The treatment is surgical removal performed by an ophthalmologist. Cataract extraction is done under local anesthesia, usually as a same-day surgery, and is considered low risk for most older adults. Most patients have reports of excellent vision following surgery which entails lens removal and placement of a plastic intraocular lens. Corrective visual aids (contacts or glasses) may be needed if no plastic lens is placed, but this occurs rarely, often due to surgical complications such as infection.

Age-related macular degeneration (AMD) is a leading cause of blindness in older adults (CDC, 2020). Risk factors include normal age-related changes, genetics, lifestyle (i.e., smoking), and family history. The primary symptom is central vision loss with intact peripheral vision. The Amsler grid can be used to evaluate for AMD, monitor vision changes, and identify central vision deficits in patients. To administer this exam, the clinician will ask patients to fix their gaze on the center black dot and state whether any of the grid lines look distorted or are missing. If the patient identifies changes in the configuration of the lines, this indicates an abnormal test and warrants further evaluation with an ophthalmologist. Treatment of AMD may involve laser therapy to reduce drusen in dry AMD, which carries a potential risk of increased rates for choroidal revascularization. The benefits of this approach are not yet proven. Vascular endothelial growth factor (VEGF) inhibitors like ranibizumab and bevacizumab are used to limit progression, reverse vision loss, or stabilize vision. This involves an intravitreal injection for wet AMD and carries with it an increased risk for vascular events. Photodynamic therapy using laser plus injection to the eye for wet AMD and retreatment is generally considered a safe procedure. Laser photocoagulation used for wet AMD can lead to the formation of a permanent blind spot. Macular surgery for wet AMD has a limited role with risks including potential diplopia, retinal detachment, and proliferative vitreoretinopathy. Radiation therapy for wet AMD has unknown long-term safety. Smoking cessation, eye vitamin supplementation with products such as AREDS, Ocuvite, and PreserVision; and ongoing regular follow-up with ophthalmologists are recommended for the ongoing care of AMD in older adults (Arroyo, 2020; NIH, 2019).

Dry eye, also known as keratoconjunctivitis sicca, becomes more common in adults with increasing age. Common symptoms are increased tearing, discomfort, decreased mucus production, and a dry, irritated feeling to eyes. Common causes include medications (e.g., antihistamines, diuretics, sedative hypnotics, beta-blockers, diuretics), vitamin A deficiency, Sjogren syndrome, and sequelae of eye surgeries such as LASIK procedures. The diagnosis can be made symptomatically or by measuring the patient's tear production rate by placing a paper strip underneath the lower lid, called the Schirmer tear test. Treatment should focus on removing the causative agent, as would occur if a medication was known or suspected to cause dry eye. Artificial tears are often prescribed, which can be purchased over the counter. Patients should be cautioned that products in a dispensing bottle may contain preservatives that can irritate the eye and pose a slight increased risk for infection. Using a single-dose product, usually sold in boxes with individual plastic doses, is preferable but can be more costly.

Glaucoma involves damage to the optic nerve caused by increased intraocular pressure (IOP). It should be considered a chronic and usually progressive condition. There are two types of glaucoma: open angle glaucoma and acute angle-closure glaucoma. Acute angle-closure glaucoma symptoms are due to a quick rise in IOP that produces pain, redness around eye, headache, blurry vision, nausea, and vomiting. The underlying cause is IOP >50 mm Hg due to blockage of the pathway of aqueous humor. The normal IOP range is 11 to 20 mm Hg. It is important for the practitioner to recognize this condition promptly and refer the patient to an ophthalmologist for surgical treatment with an iridectomy. Failure to recognize and treat symptoms of acute angle-closure glaucoma can result in blindness.

The majority of glaucoma cases among older adults are open angle glaucoma. Individuals are usually asymptomatic until late in the course of the disease. The most common symptom, when it does occur, is tunnel vision due to a loss of peripheral vision. The cause is considered idiopathic with the underlying mechanism thought to be due to a blockage of natural fluids in the eye that gradually cause pressure buildup and nerve damage. Risk factors for open angle glaucoma include family history, diabetes, and prior eye injury. Medications that cause papillary dilation, vasodilators, and those with anticholinergic properties (like antihistamines) also heighten the risk for the development of glaucoma. Ophthalmologic evaluation and early diagnosis and treatment can prevent serous vision loss. A diagnosis of glaucoma requires a thorough eye examination with dilation and tonometry testing for intraocular pressure. This is usually done by an eye specialist, ophthalmologist, or optometrist. For those diagnosed with glaucoma, a routine exam (at least every 6 months) by an ophthalmologist is recommended.

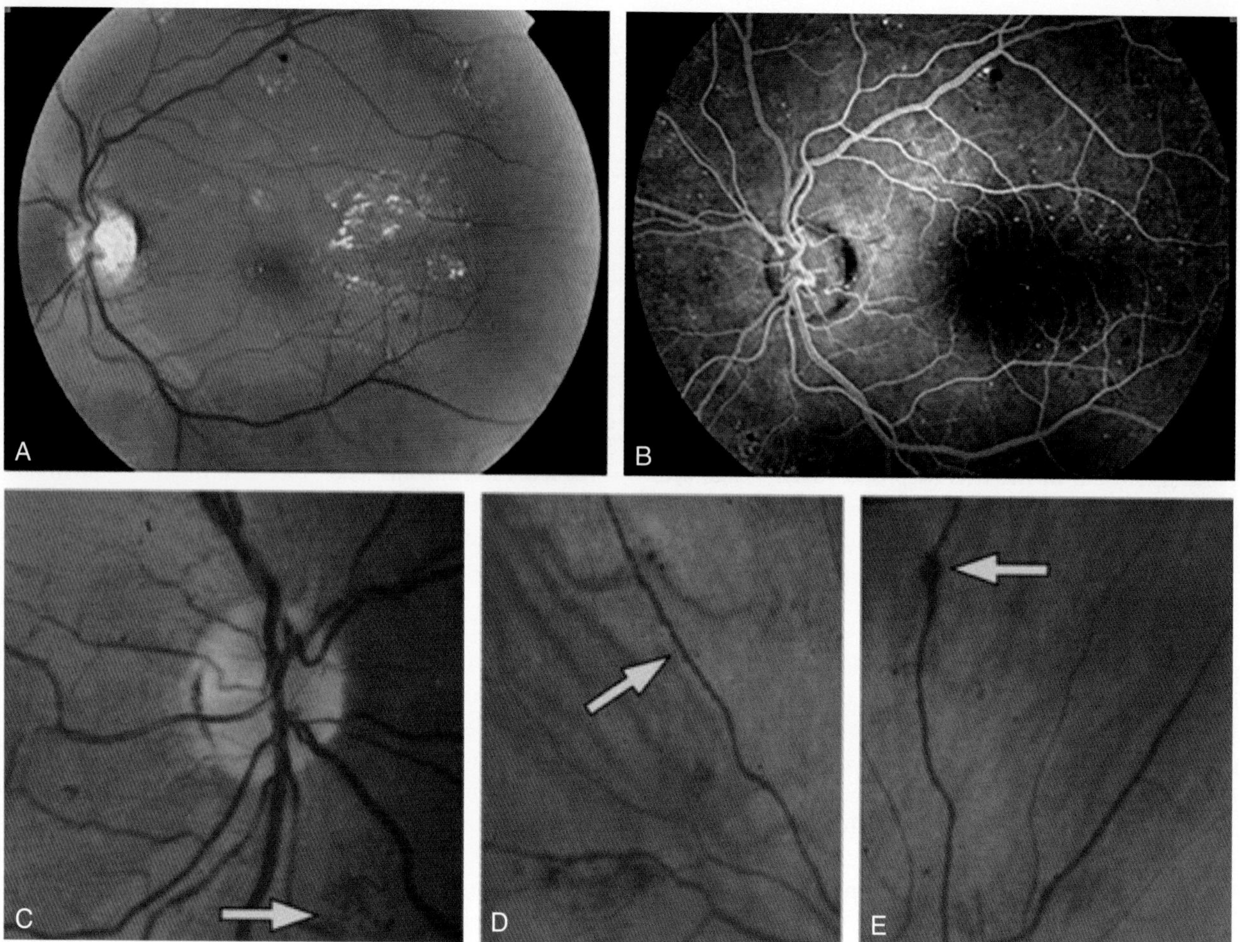

• **Fig 12.6** Nonproliferative DR Cardinal signs. (A and B) Hard exudates, retinal microaneurysms, and hemorrhages. (C) Intraretinal microvascular abnormalities *(see arrow)*. (D) Venous beading *(see arrow)*. (E) Venous loop formation *(see arrow)*. (From Cheung, N., Mitchell, P., & Wong, T. Y. [2010]. Diabetic retinopathy. *Lancet, 376*[9735], 124–136. https://doi.org/10.1016/S0140-6736(09)62124-3.)

Diabetic retinopathy (DR) is a leading cause of blindness globally, and with the increasing rates of diabetes and survival into older ages, DR can be expected to increase (Boyd, 2020; Lee, Wong, & Sabanayagam, 2015). The primary risk factor is poorly controlled diabetes. Elevated blood glucose causes microaneurysms in retinal capillaries, leading to impaired oxygenation and nutrient to the eye. Diagnosis is made by fundoscopic examination. Flame-shaped hemorrhages, dilated capillaries, hard exudate, cotton wool spots, and microaneurysms are characteristic findings (see Figs. 12.6 and 12.7). These are often difficult for providers to see on routine examination in the early stages. It is recommended that all diabetic patients have annual eye exams as part of routine care to promote early identification of retinal changes and intervention to prevent or delay vision loss. Screening for diabetic retinopathy involves a dilated eye examination performed by an eye specialist, and this should occur annually. Treatment focuses on the management of diabetes and other comorbid conditions such as hypertension. Laser photocoagulation treatment to slow the progression of disease performed by an ophthalmologist is available (Cheung et al., 2010; Fraser et al., 2019).

Ear

Age-related hearing impairment (ARHI) is common in older adults. Risk factors for hearing loss in aging individuals include genetics, male sex, environmental exposure (e.g., chemicals), lifestyle (e.g., alcohol, smoking, illicit drug use), ototoxic medications (Box 12.7), and medical conditions (e.g., hypertension, diabetes, infections). Additionally, chronic exposure to loud sounds or noise can cause damage to sensory hair cells (in the ear), which is another both causative and contributing factor. When hair cells are damaged, they are nonrepairable and hearing diminishes. ARHI begins with high frequencies and gradually increases to include the lower speech range. The major cause is the loss of cochlear neurons and hair cells.

Aging-Related Changes

Presbycusis is hearing loss that progressively occurs with aging and occurs most commonly in both ears. Changes in the inner ear as well as changes in the middle ear or the nervous system can cause changes in hearing. Fig. 12.8 shows

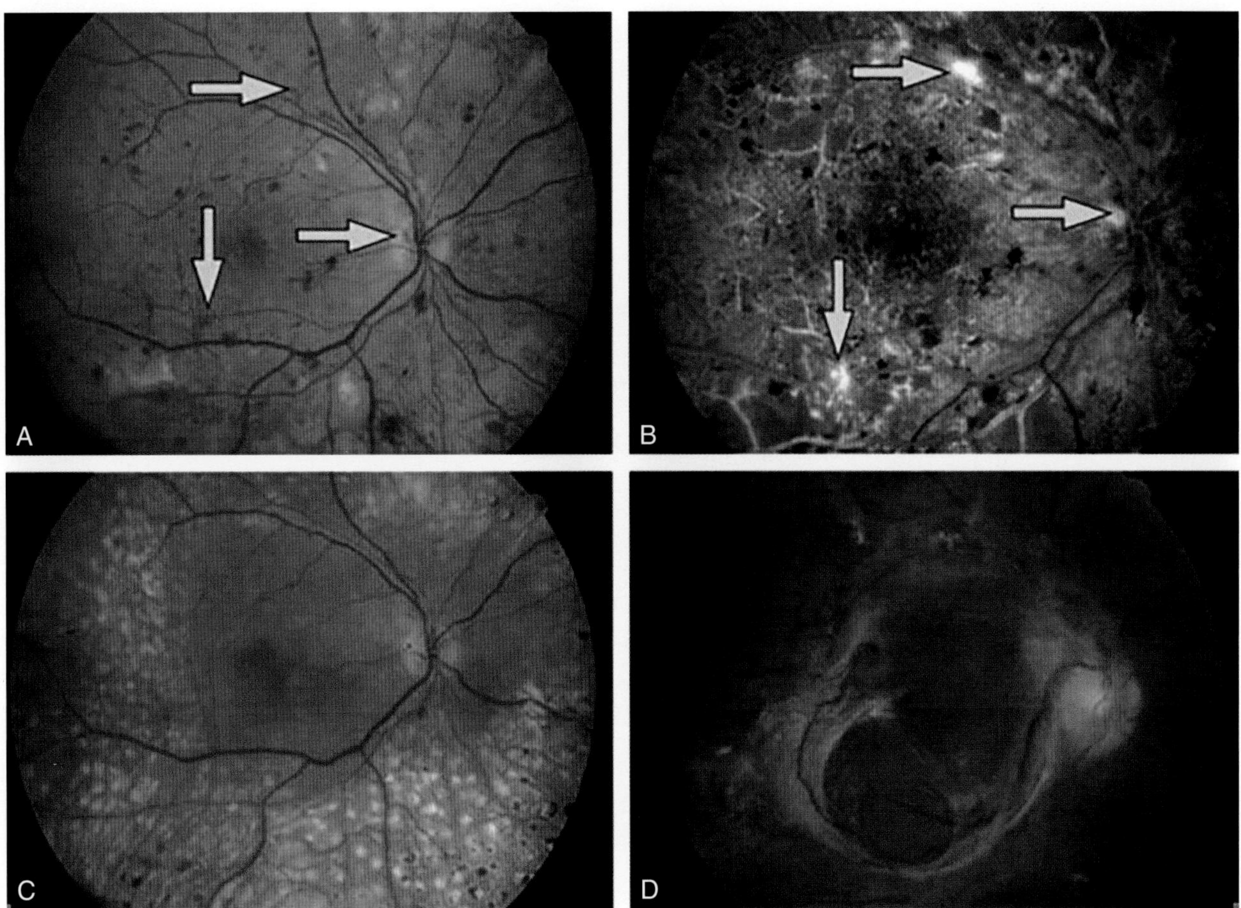

• **Fg 12.7** Proliferative diabetic retinopathy. Note the fibrosis, new vessel formation and hemorrhage. (From Cheung, N., Mitchell, P., & Wong, T. Y. [2010]. Diabetic retinopathy. *Lancet, 376*[9735], 124–136. https://doi.org/10.1016/S0140-6736(09)62124-3; Fraser, C. E., D'Amico, D. J., & Shah, M. R. [2019]. Diabetic retinopathy: Prevention and treatment. *UpToDate*.)

• BOX 12.7 Common Ototoxic Medications

- Certain antibiotics (such as gentamycin, erythromycin, tetracycline, vancomycin, metronidazole, neomycin)
- Chemotherapeutic agents (such as cisplatin, carboplatin) see Geriatric Plan for more information: http://libguides.mskcc.org/GeriatricPlan/intro
- NSAIDS
- Aspirin
- Quinine
- Loop diuretics

the anatomy of the auditory system. With aging, there are often changes such as excessive cerumen production, hair growth, collapse of the ear canal, and enlargement of the pinna. The tympanic membrane stiffens, thickens, and loses vascularity. The ossicles ossify. The Eustachian tube cartilage thickens, and muscle function declines. The cochlea loses elasticity. Vascular changes include reduced blood flow due to normal age-related degeneration. This may lead to a lack of proper functioning of the stria vascularis and an impaired ability to maintain cochlear homeostasis needed for the transduction of current and the maintenance of tissue integrity. Neurodegenerative changes occur in the brain by a similar mechanism and affect central nervous system medical conditions such as Alzheimer disease. Many times, older patients experience challenges with recognizing speech compared to an impaired ability to hear sounds. The audiograms may be within normal range, but patients still report having difficulty in noisy environments. This may be due to impairments in the processing of sound in higher auditory centers.

Evaluation

There are a number of simple tests to evaluate hearing capabilities, which can easily be performed in the clinical setting:

- *Whispered voice test:* Performed standing arm's length behind the patient (to keep the patient from lip reading). Occlude the ear canal and rub the tragus with a circular motion on one ear to mask hearing. Then whisper a short list of numbers and letters, and ask patient to repeat them.

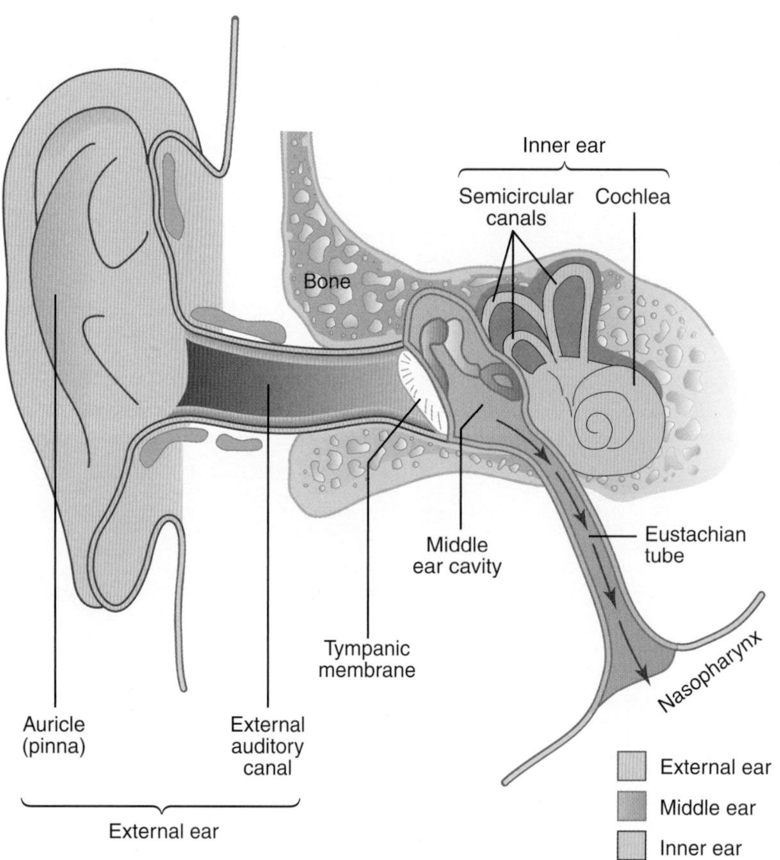

• **Fig. 12.8** Anatomy of the auditory system. (From Rosenthal, L. D., & Rosenjack, J. [2022]. *Lehne's pharmacology for nursing care* [11th ed.]. Elsevier.)

- *Weber tuning fork test:* Performed by gently pressing the handle part of the tuning fork in between the patient's eyebrows, over the nose or teeth. Then ask the patient if the sound produced is over one ear versus the other. If the sound is audible on both sides, there is either bilateral hearing loss or normal hearing.
- *Rinne test:* Performed by comparing sound when a tuning fork is placed over the mastoid bone in the rear of the ear (this would be evaluating for bone conduction) compared to holding the tuning fork close to the ear (this would be evaluating for air conduction). A normal test is when air conduction is greater than bone conduction, meaning the vibrating tuning fork sounds louder placed near the ear versus on the mastoid bone (Weber, 2019).

At present, presbycusis is not preventable or curable. More research is being conducted in this area. Hearing loss has been found to be associated with cognitive impairment and impacts mobility and the way patients engage with the environment around them (Gopinath et al., 2013).

To better understanding the etiology of hearing loss in an older adult, the clinician should be able to do the following:

- Assess for hearing loss.
- Refer the patient to an audiologist to evaluate the degree of hearing impairment or the need for a hearing aid.
- Refer the patient to an ENT specialist to address ear conditions (including chronic ear infections).
- Hearing aids are recommended rehabilitation in ARHI, but these are costly and are not covered by Medicare at present. Discuss alternatives, such as pocket amplifiers.
- Additional options such as digital hearing aids, cochlear implants, and assistive listening devices may offer a wider range of choices for patients utilizing advanced technology. These should also be considered and appropriate referrals generated if indicated (NIH, 2016).

Tests for Hearing Impairment

Formal audiology testing is the diagnostic standard for detection of hearing loss. This involves the use of audiometric equipment in a quiet environment for pure tone audiometry testing across the speech spectrum, which ranges from 500 to 4000 Hz in the upper limit for normal hearing (i.e., 25 to 30 decibels in adults). The purpose of the test is to assess whether or not hearing levels for the patient are within normal limits. Results of the test are pass (normal) or refer (denoting hearing loss). Testing is done on each ear separately.

In the primary care setting, asking patients and caregivers if the patient has difficulty hearing is the first step. Screening questionnaires may also provide more insight. The Hearing Handicap Inventory for the Elderly Screening Version (HHIE-S) is a 10-item questionnaire that was developed to assess how the person perceives the emotional and social effects of hearing loss. This is an assessment administered by staff. The questions are answered yes, sometimes, or no. Patients who score 10 or more are recommended to be evaluated by an audiologist (NIH, 2016, 2018b; Walling & Dickson, 2012; Weber, 2020).

When screening for hearing loss, the NP or PA provider must remember the following points:

- A physical exam including otoscopic exam of the ear should be performed on every patient. The Weber and Rinne are simple tests that can also be used to evaluate hearing capabilities prior to referral for audiometric testing.
- When a patient complains of hearing loss or answers a screening questionnaire positively, she or he should be assessed for treatable conditions associated with hearing loss. The patient should be questioned about a history of recent excessive noise exposure, like an explosion, something pertaining to the patient's work history (e.g., working in the military), or recent trauma. Additionally, it is important to ask about the presence of tinnitus, a ringing or buzzing in the ear, which can affect hearing. Tinnitus is relatively common among older adults, often goes nreported, and affects 10% to 30% of older adults in one or both ears (Negrila-Mezei et al., 2011).
- The clinician should also review medications that are known to have ototoxicity (see Box 12.7)

Interventions for Hearing Loss

When hearing loss is identified and an examination demonstrates occlusion of the auditory canal by cerumen, removal of cerumen to clear the auditory canal is one of the first steps that should be taken. Over-the-counter ear drops like carbamide peroxide can be prescribed for daily use over approximately 4 days, and then a return appointment for reassessment scheduled. Mechanical debridement by the clinician under visualization is often needed. This can often be performed by the NP or PA clinician but in some cases may require referral for cerumen removal by an ENT doctor.

The clinician should avoid prescribing medications that are ototoxic. If use of an ototoxic medication is identified, this should be discontinued whenever possible and hearing reevaluated once the patient is off the offending medication. If the medication has been prescribed by another clinician, it is essential for the clinician to contact that medical provider and discuss discontinuation and use of an alternate medication.

Many older adult patients with hearing loss will require augmentation with the use of a hearing aid (Fig. 12.9) or other assistive listening device. However, most (80%) do not wear them although they may be of potential benefit. Hearing aids can be challenging for older adults to use, as they require considerable fine motor dexterity to operate and adjust and for battery changes (McCormack & Fortnum, 2013). Technology has greatly improved the ability of hearing aids to be more user-friendly through connection to a cell phone that allows for varied settings. Hearing aids can be fitted and dispensed by a physician, audiologist, or licensed hearing aid dispenser. They can also be quite costly, up to several thousand dollars for each aid, which is not covered by Medicare or other medical insurance options. Other assistive listening devices include the use of ear phones on a cellular telephone connected to an amplification application or a portable amplification system called a Pocketalker. These are not as cosmetically appealing, but they are much more affordable and extremely effective. Cochlear implants should be considered in patients with moderate to severe

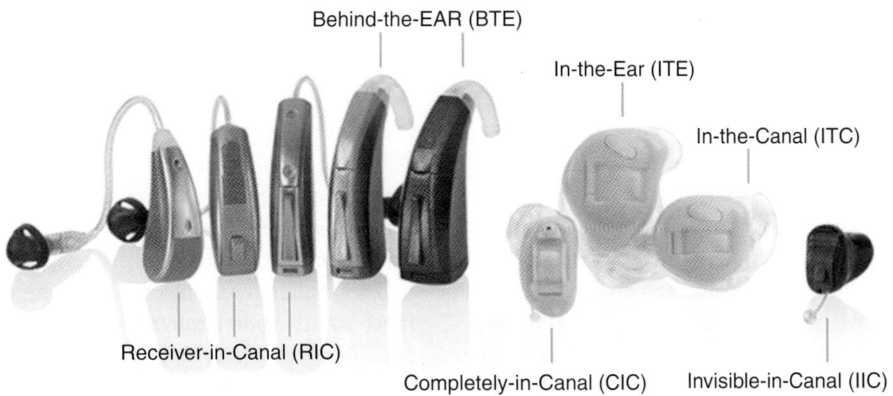

• **Fig. 12.9** Hearing aid styles. (From Scholes, M. A., & Ramakrishnan, V. R. [2016]. *Ent secrets* [4th ed.]. Elsevier.)

sensorineural hearing loss, in whom appropriately fitting hearing aids provide little benefit (Mamo et al., 2016; Weber, 2020). Referral for communication therapy by a speech therapist after evaluation with a specialist may also be considered if appropriate. This will depend on the etiology of hearing loss.

Risks Associated With Vision and Hearing Impairment

Dual sensory impairment (DSI), also known as dual sensory loss (DSL), with loss in both vision and hearing, is common in older adults. It is associated with decreased quality of life, and has negative impacts on mental health as well as physical, social, and cognitive functioning. Older adults with DSI have greater disparities in their health and social roles, greater communication difficulties, and a greater risk for cognitive decline and depression. Additionally, there is an increased need for supportive services, assistance with ADLs and IADLs, and an increased risk for medication errors, falls, and fractures. Vision loss and hearing loss have been independently found to increase the risk for mortality in older adults. However, self-reported dual sensory impairment has been found to heighten the risk of morbidity, and all cause morality compared to single sensory impairment in hearing or vision. DSI is also thought to be a marker of frailty, which is also correlated with an increased risk of morbidity and mortality. Given the known frequency of sensory impairments in older adults, DSI is often overlooked and poorly documented in the medical records. For the NP or PA assessing for DSI and sensory impairments, detecting impairments early allows for earlier intervention, such as initiating the use of sensory aids and rehabilitation to decrease the negative health impacts of DSI and potentially improve survival. There is a need for tailored support for each older adult's unique needs with DSI (Gopinath et al., 2013).

Screening Recommendations

In the primary care setting, providers are in a critical position to identify those at risk for sensory changes and loss, including vision, hearing, smell, and taste. Providers can then counsel patients and refer them for specific treatments as described in this chapter.

According to the US Preventive Services Task Force (USPSTF), there is insufficient evidence to screen for vision or hearing impairment in older adults (USPSTF, 2012, 2016). The American Academy of Ophthalmology recommends a comprehensive examination of the eye annually or every 2 years for adults age 65 and older (USPSTF, 2016). There are no routine screening tests for gustatory and olfactory dysfunction, as these are symptoms that commonly occur from other underlying pathologies.

• BOX 12.8 Communication With the Older Person With Hearing Loss

1. Address the person by their name.
2. Face the person when you speak.
3. Do not communicate from another room.
4. Try to have good lighting.
5. Avoid talking too fast or too slow.
6. Don't yell. Keep you voice at a normal pitch.
7. Avoid talking with food or gum in your mouth.
8. Do not interrupt the person when they're talking.
9. Write down important information.
10. Have the person repeat important information back to you.

Communicating With Older Adults With Sensory Deficits

To most effectively communicate with the older adult, clinicians can utilize several strategies as outlined in Box 12.8.

Promoting Safety and Improving Quality of Life

There are many ways to maximize quality of life and function in older adults with sensory impairments. For example, an occupational therapist and interior designer who specializes in living spaces for older adults (aging-in-place specialists) can be called on to modify the home environment and increase safety for patients with sensory deficits (vision, hearing, mobility) who have a greater fall risk. Additionally, coordination of care among health care providers is essential to ensure the older adult patient has the needed follow-up for sensory deficits. It is important to address potential safety concerns, and a referral for visiting nurse services to evaluate home safety and the need for caregiver assistance (such as the addition of a home health aide [HHA]) ought to be considered. The clinician has an opportunity educate patients and caregivers on home safety by suggesting these changes: good lighting, rubber-gripped mats, and night lights to prevent falls. When patients come to visit alone, the clinician can assess for home supports and identify caregivers if available. It is important to remember that each visit is an opportunity to educate/coach patients and caregivers for positive behavior changes including avoiding risk-taking behaviors (such as using improper footwear and not using sensory aids like glasses) for enhanced safety in setting of sensory impairments.

Key Points

- There are normal age-related changes in vision, hearing, olfaction, and gustatory function in older adults.
- Sensory impairment in older adults is common.
- Sensory deficits can lead to different levels of disability and are associated with depression, decreased quality of life, and impaired physical, social, and cognitive functioning.
- Older adults with dual sensory impairment (DSI) have greater disparities in their health and social roles, greater communication difficulties, a greater risk for cognitive decline and confusion, and an increased risk of mortality.
- Involving patients and families in care planning is essential to optimize care.
- Evaluating for sensory (vision, hearing, taste, smell) impairment allows the clinician to identify deficits that may otherwise go unnoticed.
- The primary care clinician's continued involvement in patients' care is of utmost importance.

More information about tools and the Interprofessional Education Collaborative (IPEC) competencies mentioned in this chapter can be found in Appendix 1: Tools and Appendix 2: IPEC Competencies.

References

Arroyo, J. (2020). Age-related macular degeneration: Treatment and prevention. *UpToDate.*

Bartok, V. (2011). Drug-induced dry mouth. Cough and cold. *Pharmacy Times, 77*(11).

Boyce, J. M., & Shone, G. R. (2006). Effects of ageing on smell and taste. *Postgraduate Medical Journal, 82*(966), 239–241. https://doi.org/10.1136/pgmj.2005.039453.

Boyd, K. (2020). Have AMD? Save your sight with an Amsler grid.

Bromley, S. M. (2000). Smell and taste disorders: A primary care approach. *American Family Physician, 61*(2), 427–436. 438.

Centers for Disease Control and Prevention (CDC). (2019a). *Edentulism and tooth retention.* Division of Oral Health, National Center for Chronic Disease Prevention and Health Promotion. https://www.cdc.gov/oralhealth/publications/OHSR-2019-edentulism-tooth-retention.html.

Centers for Disease Control and Prevention (CDC). (2019b). *Oral health for older Americans: Facts about older adult oral health.* Centers for Disease Control and Prevention. https://www.cdc.gov/oralhealth/basics/adult-oral-health/adult_older.htm.

Centers for Disease Control and Prevention (CDC). (2019c). *Oral Health Surveillance Report, 2019: Edentulism and tooth retention.* https://www.cdc.gov/oralhealth/publications/OHSR-2019-edentulism-tooth-retention.html.

Centers for Disease Control and Prevention (CDC). (2020). *Common eye disorders and diseases.* https://www.cdc.gov/visionhealth/basics/ced/index.html.

Cheung, N., Mitchell, P., & Wong, T. Y. (2010). Diabetic retinopathy. *Lancet, 376*(9735), 124–136. https://doi.org/10.1016/S0140-6736(09)62124-3.

Chou, R., Dana, T., Bougatsos, C., Grusing, S., & Blazina, I. (2016). *Screening for impaired visual acuity in older adults: A systematic review to update the 2009 U.S.* Preventive Services Task Force Recommendation.

Davidson, J. G. S., & Guthrie, D. M. (2019). Older adults with a combination of vision and hearing impairment experience higher rates of cognitive impairment, functional dependence, and worse outcomes across a set of quality indicators. *J Aging Health, 31*(1), 85–108. https://doi.org/10.1177/0898264317723407.

Dillon, C. F., Gu, Q., Hoffman, H. J., & Ko, C. W. (2010). Vision, hearing, balance, and sensory impairment in Americans aged 70 years and over: United States, 1999–2006. *NCHS Data Brief, 31*, 1–8.

Doty, R. L., & Kamath, V. (2014). The influences of age on olfaction: A review. *Front Psychology, 5*, 20. https://doi.org/10.3389/fpsyg.2014.00020.

Fraser, C. E., D'Amico, D. J., & Shah, M. R. (2019). Diabetic retinopathy: Prevention and treatment. *UpToDate.*

Gopinath, B., Schneider, J., McMahon, C. M., Burlutsky, G., Leeder, S. R., & Mitchell, P. (2013). Dual sensory impairment in older adults increases the risk of mortality: A population-based study. *PLoS One, 8*(3), e55054. https://doi.org/10.1371/journal.pone.0055054.

Gravina, S. A., Yep, G. L., & Khan, M. (2013). Human biology of taste. *Annals of Saudi Medicine, 33*(3), 217–222. https://doi.org/10.5144/0256-4947.2013.217.

Heckmann, J. G., Heckmann, S. M., Lang, C. J., & Hummel, T. (2003). Neurological aspects of taste disorders. *Archives of Neurology, 60*(5), 667–671. https://doi.org/10.1001/archneur.60.5.667.

Imoscopi, A., Inelmen, E. M., Sergi, G., Miotto, F., & Manzato, E. (2012). Taste loss in the elderly: Epidemiology, causes and consequences. *Aging Clinical and Experimental Research, 24*(6), 570–579. https://doi.org/10.3275/8520.

Kaufman, D. M. (2007). *Kaufman's clinical neurology for psychiatrists.* Elsevier.

Lafreniere, D. (2020a). Evaluation and treatment of taste and smell disorders. https://www.uptodate.com/contents/taste-and-olfactory-disorders-in-adults-evaluation-and-management

Lafreniere, D. (2020b). Overview of taste and olfactory disorders in adults. https://www.uptodate.com/contents/taste-and-olfactory-disorders-in-adults-anatomy-and-etiology

Lee, R., Wong, T. Y., & Sabanayagam, C. (2015). Epidemiology of diabetic retinopathy, diabetic macular edema and related vision loss. *Eye Vis (Lond), 2*, 17. https://doi.org/10.1186/s40662-015-0026-2.

Li, X., Lui, F., & Forshing. (2019). *Anosomnia.* StatPearls.

Mamo, S. K., Reed, N. S., Nieman, C. L., Oh, E. S., & Lin, F. R. (2016). Personal sound amplifiers for adults with hearing loss. *American Journal of Medicine, 129*(3), 245–250. https://doi.org/10.1016/j.amjmed.2015.09.014.

McCormack, A., & Fortnum, H. (2013). Why do people fitted with hearing aids not wear them. *International Journal of Audiology, 52*(5), 360–368. https://doi.org/10.3109/14992027.2013.769066.

Millsop, J. W., & Fazel, N. (2016). Oral candidiasis. *Clinical Dermatology, 34*(4), 487–494. https://doi.org/10.1016/j.clindermatol.2016.02.022.

National Comprehensive Cancer Network (NCCN). (2020). *NCCN Guidelines version 1.2020: Older adult oncology*. https://www.nccn.org/professionals/physician_gls/pdf/senior.pdf

National Institutes of Health (NIH). (2013). *NIDCD [National Institute on Deafness and Other Communication Disorders] fact sheet: Taste and smell. taste disorders*. US Department of Health and Human Services: National Institutes of Health. https://www.nih.gov/about-nih/what-we-do/nih-almanac/national-institute-deafness-other-communication-disorders-nidcd.

National Institutes of Health (NIH). (2016). *Hearing loss and older adults*. https://www.nidcd.nih.gov/health/hearing-loss-older-adults.

National Institutes of Health (NIH). (2018a). *Dry mouth*. National Institutes of Health.

National Institutes of Health (NIH). (2018b). *Hearing loss and older adults*. National Institutes of Health. https://www.nidcd.nih.gov/health/hearing-loss-older-adults.

National Institutes of Health (NIH). (2018c). *Tooth loss in seniors*. National Institutes of Health. https://www.nidcr.nih.gov/research/data-statistics/tooth-loss/seniors.

National Institutes of Health (NIH). (2019). *Cataract data and statistics*. National Institutes of Health. https://www.nei.nih.gov/learn-about-eye-health/eye-health-data-and-statistics/cataract-data-and-statistics/cataract-tables.

Negrila-Mezei, A., Enache, R., & Sarafoleanu, C. (2011). Tinnitus in elderly population: Clinic correlations and impact upon QoL. *Journal of Medicine and Life*, *4*(4), 412–416.

Oral Cancer Foundation (OCF). (2020a). *Complications of treatment*. The Oral Cancer Foundation. https://oralcancerfoundation.org/complications/.

Oral Cancer Foundation (OCF). (2020b). *Understanding oral cancer*. The Oral Cancer Foundation.

Purves, D., Augustine, G., Fitzpatrick, D., Katz, L. C., LaMantia, A. -S., McNamara, J. O., & Williams, S. M. (2001). *Neuroscience* (2nd ed.). Sinauer Associates.

Rawson, N. E., Gomez, G., Cowart, B. J., Kriete, A., Pribitkin, E., & Restrepo, D. (2012). Age-associated loss of selectivity in human olfactory sensory neurons. *Neurobiology of Aging*, *33*(9), 1913–1919. https://doi.org/10.1016/j.neurobiolaging.2011.09.036.

Razak, P. A., Richard, K. M., Thankachan, R. P., Hafiz, K. A., Kumar, K. N., & Sameer, K. M. (2014). Geriatric oral health: a review article. *Journal of International Oral Health*, *6*(6), 110–116.

Rea, P. (2014). *Clinical anatomy of the cranial nerves*. Academic Press.

Ritchie, C. S. (2002). Oral health, taste, and olfaction. *Clinics in Geriatric Medicine*, *18*(4), 709–717. https://doi.org/10.1016/s0749-0690(02)00041-1.

Silvestre, F. J., Perez-Herbera, A., Puente-Sandoval, A., & Bagán, J. V. (2010). Hard palate perforation in cocaine abusers: A systematic review. *Clinical Oral Investigations*, *14*(6), 621–628. https://doi.org/10.1007/s00784-009-0371-4.

US Department of Health and Human Services (USPSTF) Office of Disease Prevention and Health Promotion. (2020). *Healthy people 2030*. https://health.gov/healthypeople.

US Preventative Services Task Force (USPSTF). (2016). *Final recommendation statement: Impaired visual acuity in older adults: Screening*. https://www.uspreventiveservicestaskforce.org/uspstf/recommendation/impaired-visual-acuity-screening-older-adults.

Walling, A. D., & Dickson, G. M. (2012). Hearing loss in older adults. *American Family Physician*, *85*(12), 1150–1156.

Weber, P. (2020). Evaluation of hearing loss in adults. *UpToDate*.

Welge-Lüssen, A. (2009). Ageing, neurodegeneration, and olfactory and gustatory loss. *B-ENT*, *5*(Suppl. 13), 129–132.

Wick, J. Y. (2015). Drug-induced metallic taste: No irony. July 2015 Digestive Health. *Pharmacy Times*, *81*(7).

13

Chronic Conditions

JILL BEAVERS-KIRBY, DNP, MS, ACNP-BC AND THERESA KIRESUK, MSN, NP

OBJECTIVES

Student Learning Objectives

After completing this chapter, the student should be able to do the following:

1. List common chronic conditions in the older adult.
2. Describe the approach to diagnosis of common chronic conditions in the older adult.
3. Identify the unique aspects of the presentation and management of common chronic conditions in the older adult.

Practitioner Objectives

After completing this chapter, the practitioner should be able to do the following:

1. Describe the assessment and manifestations of chronic conditions in older adults.
2. Discuss the management of co-occurring chronic diseases for older adults with chronic conditions.
3. Examine the goals and management for older adults with chronic conditions.

Overview

The geriatric population can suffer from many common conditions. Many of these chronic conditions are considered "just a part of growing old." However, these chronic conditions can be avoided by making healthy lifestyle changes and sticking to those healthy habits.

This chapter reviews the pathophysiology, assessment, treatment, and lifestyle changes of diabetes, cerebral vascular accident, chronic kidney disease, peripheral artery disease, atrial fibrillation, chronic constipation, hypertension, and dyslipidemia in the older patient.

Diabetes

Diabetes mellitus (DM) is an endocrine disorder that involves inadequate insulin secretion or development of resistance to insulin. Diabetes mellitus can be type 1, where there is a lack of insulin production, or type 2, which is a result of increasing insulin resistance. Type 1 diabetes is a result of genetic predisposition and autoimmune dysfunction, whereas type 2 diabetes is thought to be acquired. Risk factors for the development of type 2 diabetes include advancing age; obesity; sedentary lifestyle; family history; ethnicity such as individuals of color, Hispanics, Asians, Native Americans, and Pacific Islanders; and the presence of certain diseases such as cardiovascular disease, polycystic ovarian syndrome (PCOS), and gestational diabetes. In addition, several medications have been found to contribute to elevated blood sugar levels and subsequent diabetes, including thiazide diuretics, antipsychotic medications, and corticosteroids. Ninety percent of adults with diabetes have type 2 diabetes.

CASE STUDY 13.1

Phil is a 72-year-old male who is a retired school bus driver. He lives with his wife in a small house on the outskirts of town. He visits his primary care provider (PCP) every 6 months for a checkup and medication refills. He has hypertension, high cholesterol, and diabetes, for which he takes 500 mg of Metformin daily. At his latest PCP appointment, his hemoglobin A1c (HgbA1c) was 8.2%; previously this was 6%. His PCP wants to change his medication for his diabetes based on his most recent HgbA1c.

Pathophysiology

Insulin is responsible for moving glucose from the bloodstream into the liver and cells where it is stored or used as energy. The inability to move the glucose into the liver or into cells results in elevated levels of blood glucose. Elevated blood sugars, or hyperglycemia, causes glucose to be carried into the urine. This causes increased amounts of water to be eliminated by the kidneys. The symptoms associated with this include polyuria and nocturia. As more water is eliminated by the kidneys, the amount of water in the vascular system is decreased, leading to polydipsia. Weight loss occurs as a result of muscle and tissue breakdown in an attempt to pull fuel from muscle and tissues. Fatigue develops due to the inadequate nutrition and energy available for the muscles and tissues to use for movement. Increased frequency of infections occurs due to the increased nutrients in the blood and body fluids where there are elevated blood sugars. Infections tend to occur in the skin and bladder, and women also get vaginal infections.

Type 2 diabetes frequently occurs with other comorbid conditions such as hypertension, lipid abnormalities particularly high-density lipoproteins (HDL), and elevations of low-density lipoproteins (LDL), total cholesterol, and triglycerides. Individuals with type 2 diabetes are also at an increased risk for metabolic syndrome, which is the presence of diabetes, hypertension, and hyperlipidemia.

Complications of diabetes mellitus are vast and can include cardiovascular disease, cerebrovascular disease, neuropathy, retinopathy, hearing problems, nephropathy, and lower extremity neuropathy. Older adults will have a reduced life expectancy, and higher rates of geriatric syndromes and vascular complications when compared to older adults without diabetes (Harper et al., 2019).

Assessment

Screening for diabetes is recommended every 1 to 3 years for adults who have risk factors, including family history, obesity, cardiovascular disease, or diabetes symptoms. Screening can be completed with a blood sugar measurement or by obtaining a hemoglobin A1C. Diabetes can be diagnosed in several ways. To receive a diagnosis of diabetes, the patient will need to have one of the following criteria that has been repeated on a separate day:

1. Hemoglobin A1C ≥ 6.5%
2. Random blood sugar ≥ 200 mg/dl with symptoms of polyuria, polydipsia, and unexplained weight loss.
3. Fasting plasma glucose (FPS) ≥ 126 mg/dl.
4. Oral glucose tolerance test (OGTT) with a blood glucose level of ≥ 200 mg/dl after ingestion of 75 mg of glucose in 300 ml of water (American Diabetes Association, n.d.)

The goals for treatment of diabetes are to control blood sugar and prevent secondary health issues associated with diabetes. Older adults are more sensitive to extreme fluctuations in blood sugar levels. Avoidance of hypoglycemia in older adults is an important component in the management of type 2 diabetes mellitus. Risks associated with hypoglycemia are especially concerning for older adults and include confusion and falls. Drug-disease and drug-drug interactions are more common in older adults as well. The goal for blood sugar management needs to be individualized based on the patient's overall health status. Younger or healthier older adults would have goals of more tight control of diabetes than older or more frail older adults with comorbid conditions (Kirkman et al., 2012).

Treatment Options for the Older Adult With Diabetes

Lifestyle modification is imperative for all patients with diabetes mellitus. Lifestyle modification should include weight management and increased exercise. See Table 13.1 for pharmacologic options for the management of type 2 DM.

Microvascular Risk Reduction

Diabetes that is not well controlled can lead to the development of one or more microvascular complications, including, nephropathy, retinopathy, and neuropathy.

Retinopathy is common and progressive. The patient with diabetes should have an evaluation by an ophthalmologist to monitor for the development of retinopathy at the time of diagnosis and annually. Persistent hyperglycemia increases the risk for the development and progression of diabetic retinopathy.

Nephropathy contributes to q progressive loss of renal function in the patient with diabetes. Older adults should undergo annual evaluation for the presence of microalbumin in the urine. Patients with microalbumin in the urine should be managed with an angiotensin-converting enzyme inhibitor (ACEI).

Neuropathy may develop due to microvascular changes that cause decreased circulation. Although neuropathy can impact multiple systems, the most common is peripheral neuropathy in the lower extremities. The declining sensation to the feet and lower extremities places the older adult with diabetes at risk for delayed recognition of wounds and injuries to the lower extremities. The older adult is also at risk for falls due to mobility impairment from decreased sensation. Decreased circulation and hyperglycemia contribute to delayed healing. Older adults may also have functional mobility or cognitive limitations that impede their ability to evaluate their feet or manage minor injuries.

Evaluation of the feet should be performed at every visit for the older adult with diabetes. This evaluation should include an assessment of the patient's ability to perform self-care of his or her feet, inspection for wounds and signs of declining circulation, assessment of sensation using microfilament testing in multiple locations, palpation for pulses, and provision of nail care or referral to a podiatrist for appropriate nail and wound management.

Concomitant Disease Risk Reduction

Older adults with diabetes often have one or more concomitant cardiovascular disorders, including hyperlipidemia, hypertension, and heart failure. The older adult also has higher risk than younger adults for the development and complications of vascular disease, including cardiovascular disease and cerebrovascular disease (Francisco et al., 2018). Risk reduction measures include lifestyle management discussed previously, including weight reduction and increased exercise. Additional measures include smoking cessation, management of hypertension, management of dyslipidemia, and the consideration of aspirin therapy. Older adults typically tolerate statins. The use of a moderate-intensity statin may increase tolerance of the therapy. (See Table 13.2.) Older adults with type 2 diabetes are highly sensitive to the complications from the various management options. Physiologic changes that happen due to aging, concomitant disease, and frailty require adjustment of diabetes management from the younger population. The goals for treatment include risk management, glycemic control, prevention of complications, and optimized management of concomitant diseases.

Cerebral Vascular Accident

Definition

A cerebral vascular accident (CVA) or stroke happens when the blood flow to the brain is reduced or interrupted. This

TABLE 13.1 Pharmacologic Options for Management of Type 2 Diabetes Mellitus

Drug	Benefits	Adverse Effects
Metformin	A1c decreased by 1.0 to 2.0%	Gastrointestinal (GI) intolerance: symptoms of nausea and diarrhea Contraindication for renal impairment
Sulfonylureas	A1c decreased by 1.0 to 2.0% Quick onset of action	Hypoglycemia
Glucagon-like peptide-a (GLP-1)	A1c decreased by 0.5 to 1.5% Weight loss Decreased cardiovascular risk	Hypoglycemia Injection only Cost GI intolerance
Thiazolidinedione	A1c decreased by 0.5 to 1.4% Decreased cardiovascular events	Cardiovascular: heart failure due to fluid retention Increased myocardial infarction potential Bladder cancer
Glinide	A1c decreased by 0.5 to 1.5% Quick onset of action	Hypoglycemia Weight gain Multiple doses/day
Sodium-glucose co-transporter 2 (SGLT2 Inhibitors)	A1c decreased by 0.5 to 0.7% Weight loss Decreased cardiovascular risk Improvement in renal function	Candidiasis Urinary tract infection (UTI) Bone cancer Increased risk for diabetic ketoacidosis (DKA) Increased incidence of lower limb amputation Short-term use; long-term risks unknown
Dipeptidyl peptidase 4 (DPP-4 Inhibitor)	A1c decreased by 0.5 to 0.8%	Cost Cardiovascular: Increased risk of heart failure
Alpha-glucosidase inhibitor	A1c decreased by 0.5 to 0.8%	GI intolerance Multiple doses/day
Pramlintide	A1c decreased by 0.5 to 1.0% Weight loss	Requires injection GI intolerance Short-term use; long-term risks unknown
Insulin	A1c decreased by 1.5 to 3.5% Multiple formulations for short acting to long acting	Cost Requires injection Hypoglycemia

TABLE 13.2 Goal Blood Pressure and Lipid Levels for Older Adults With Type 2 Diabetes Mellitus

Blood Pressure	Lipids
< 150/90 (Healthier and younger gerontology patients may have a goal of <140/90)	Total cholesterol < 200 LDL-C < 70 (Frail elderly may have a goal LDL-C of <100) HDL > 40 Triglycerides < 150

HDL, High-density lipoprotein; *LDL-C*, low-density lipoprotein cholesterol.

Data from National Cholesterol Education Program (NCEP) Expert Panel on Detection, Evaluation, and Treatment of High Blood Cholesterol in Adults (Adult Treatment Panel III) (2002). Third Report of the National Cholesterol Education Program (NCEP) Expert Panel on Detection, Evaluation, and Treatment of High Blood Cholesterol in Adults (Adult Treatment Panel III) final report. *Circulation*, *106*(25), 3143–3421.

prevents the brain from receiving the oxygen and nutrients it needs to survive, and brain cells will start to die. A stroke is considered a medical emergency (Stroke, www.mayoclinic.org).

Stroke is defined by the World Health Organization (WHO) as "rapidly developing clinical signs of focal (sometimes global) disturbance of brain function lasting more than 24 hours or leading to death, with no apparent cause that is not vascular in origin." This definition conventionally includes ischemic stroke, intracerebral hemorrhage, and subarachnoid hemorrhage. Because of advances in our knowledge of the nature, timing, and clinical presentation of stroke and its mimics,

CASE STUDY 13.2

Vickie is a 70-year-old female who was out to dinner with friends at a local restaurant. Vickie has a past medical history of hypertension that is poorly controlled. She is 5′7″ and weighs 160 pounds. She has smoked 1 pack of cigarettes a day for the past 50 years. She enjoys an occasional glass of wine. While at dinner, Vickie suddenly stated, "The right side of my face feels numb." One of her dinner companions is a registered nurse (RN). He asked Vickie if she could smile. At first, Vickie looked at him like he was confused, but he asked her again to smile. When Vickie smiled, he noticed that the right side of her smile was drooping. Vickie started to ask a question, but her words were jumbled and slurred. Scott, the RN, was concerned that Vickie may be having a stroke and he immediately called 9-1-1 on his cell phone.

as well as significant advances in neuroimaging (particularly magnetic resonance imaging [MRI]), an updated definition of central nervous system (CNS) infarction has been proposed by the American Heart Association (AHA)/American Stroke Association (ASA) (McGrath et al., 2018).

There are essentially three different types of stroke. The most common (87%) are ischemic strokes. An ischemic stroke occurs when blood flow is blocked through the artery that supplies oxygenated blood to the brain. Blockages are usually caused by blood clots.

A hemorrhagic stroke occurs when blood leaks or ruptures from an artery in the brain. The leaking blood puts too much pressure on the brain cells, damaging them. Elevations in blood pressure or an aneurysm in the brain can cause a hemorrhagic stroke (Stroke; www.cdc.gov).

A hemorrhagic stroke can be intracerebral or subarachnoid. An intracerebral hemorrhagic (ICH) stroke is caused by bleeding within the brain. In Europe and North America, a subarachnoid hemorrhage (SAH) is when the bleeding occurs when blood enters the space surrounding the brain.

A transient ischemic attack (TIA) or "ministroke" is a warning sign that a stroke may occur. A TIA differs from a stroke in that the blood flow to the brain is only blocked for a short time frame, usually less than 5 minutes. A TIA is considered a medical emergency, and 9-1-1 should be called immediately.

Pathophysiology

The WHO estimates that 15 million people have a stroke each year, of whom 5 million are left with a disability. Without further effective population-based interventions, 7.8 million people are estimated to die in 2030. A methodical review of population-based research reported that there was a 42% decline in the incidence of stroke from 1970 to 2008 in high-income countries, compared to a greater than 100% increase in the occurrence of stroke in low- and middle-income nations (McGrath et al., 2018).

McGrath et al. (2018) have noted that a large-artery ischemic stroke is typically an effect of hardening in the extracranial (vertebral or carotid) or intracranial arteries (e.g., basilar or cerebral artery), with plaque rupture and also thrombus development. An ischemic stroke might arise from a thromboembolism in an artery that leads to occlusion or, much less frequently, by a blockage that leads to hypoperfusion (e.g., watershed infarction).

Cardioembolic stroke is the existence of a possible intracardiac source of a blood clot in the lack of cerebrovascular illness in an individual with nonlacunar stroke. Cardioembolic strokes are responsible for around 20% of all ischemic strokes. A gold standard diagnostic test is not available for this diagnosis. Scientific attributes suggestive of cardioembolic etiology are atrial dysrhythmia as well as abrupt neurologic deficits. Embolic strokes might be more prone bleeding in the brain based on computerized tomography (CT). This may be because of spontaneous thrombolysis and reperfusion. Other symptoms of a cardioembolic stroke may include Wernicke aphasia, ideomotor apraxia, and hemianopia without hemiparesis (Marcoff & Homma, 2018).

Paradoxical emboli happen when emboli form in the vascular network, such as from a deep vein thrombosis, enter the arterial circulation through an arteriovenous malformation (AVM), atrial septal defect (ASD), or from a patent foramen ovale (PFO), which are present in approximately 20% of the population. A variety of empirical studies have reported a connection between the first ischemic stroke and also PFO, especially in younger people, yet PFO has actually not been revealed to be a risk variable for another ischemic stroke (McGrath et al., 2018).

Left-sided cardiac causes of emboli consist of left atrial thrombus due to atrial arrhythmias such as fibrillation or flutter (which lead to a fivefold increase in the possibility of a stroke), left ventricle clots following transmural myocardial infarction, cardiac myxomas, and anomalies of the mitral valve, including artificial valves. Heart failure can also increase the risk of having a stroke by two- to threefold. Valvular heart problems are also a risk factor for stroke. Emboli can develop from vegetation on the valve even in cases of thrombotic or infective endocarditis. Mechanical valves significantly increase the risk of having a stroke, so it is strongly recommended that the patient is on lifelong anticoagulation (McGrath et al., 2018).

Plaques in the aortic arch can be another source of emboli, which can then penetrate the cerebral circulation, which can lead to a stroke. Atheromas in the aortic arch that are > 4 mm in diameter have been found to cause a fourfold increase in stroke risk (McGrath et al., 2018).

Small-vessel infarcts or lacunar strokes account for roughly 20% of all ischemic strokes. Small-vessel infarcts happen when the smaller branches of the anterior or middle cerebral arteries become occluded. Smoking, hyperglycemia, and hypertension are known factors that can damage the vascular endothelium. McGrath et al. (2018) noted that additional "causes of small-artery occlusion include microemboli from atherosclerotic plaques, polycythemia vera, antiphospholipid antibodies, amyloid angiopathy, cerebral autosomal dominant arteriopathy with subcortical infarcts and leukoencephalopathy (CADASIL), cerebral autosomal recessive arteriopathy with subcortical infarcts and leukoencephalopathy (CARASIL), Sneddon syndrome, and various types of small-vessel arteritis."

Intracerebral hemorrhages (ICHs) represent approximately 10% to 15% of all strokes. Spontaneous ICH represents 80% to 90% of incidents and is seen in patients with hypertension or patients who on antithrombotic therapy.

A subarachnoid hemorrhage (SAH) happens when there is bleeding in the subarachnoid space, which is located between the pia mater and arachnoid spaces. Approximately 3% to 5% of all strokes are in the subarachnoid space. Most SAHs happen when there is a tear in an intracranial aneurysm (McGrath et al., 2018).

Cerebral Autoregulation

Cerebral autoregulation is the ability of the blood vessels in the brain to maintain a constant amount of pressure regardless of the changes in perfusion pressure. This autoregulation usually occurs when there is a mean arterial pressure of 60 to 150 mm Hg. The cerebral blood flow is related to the diameter of the vessel. If the vessel dilates, there will be an increase in the amount of blood flow. When blood vessels constrict, this decreases the amount of blood that is able to flow in the brain.

If the perfusion pressure decreases, the blood vessels will dilate. However, if the perfusion pressure drops to a level that inhibits adequate compensation, cerebral blood flow will be diminished. Flow rates of protein synthesis will start to decrease. If the flow rate drops below 35 mL/100 g per minute, protein synthesis stops completely. At this point, glucose consumption will momentarily be increased, but this is not sustainable. When the flow rate drops to 25 mL/100 g per minute, anaerobic glycolysis happens, which leads to acidosis and a buildup of lactic acid within the tissues. The electrical activity will fail when flow rates drop to 17 mL/100 g per minute, which then leads to homeostasis of the ions in cell membranes. This is when the infarct occurs (Majid & Kassab, 2020).

Cerebral edema can occur because of a stroke. This edema can then lead to increased intracranial pressure and mass effect, which can cause brain tissue to herniate. Approximately 10% of strokes cause cerebral edema significant enough to lead to herniation (Majid & Kassab, 2020).

Assessment

The initial assessment of the patient presenting with symptoms of stroke should be a brief, targeted assessment of airway, breathing, and circulation. Once the patient is medically stable, consideration is given to any reversible cause of the patient's symptoms.

Diagnoses other than stroke should be ruled out. These include seizure, cerebral tumor, head trauma, hypertensive encephalopathy, hypoglycemia, spinal cord disorder, and subdural hematoma, among others. It is important to ascertain if the patient has a past history of taking hypoglycemic agents or insulin or if the patient has a history of drug overdose or abuse.

For patients experiencing an acute ischemic stroke, consideration for thrombolytic therapy or endovascular thrombectomy needs to be evaluated. As with the patient who is experiencing an acute myocardial infarction, time is of the essence.

A history, physical exam, vital signs, including oxygenation, saturation, and a noncontrast computed tomography (CT) scan are adequate in most cases to start treatment. Additional testing can be ordered but is not a reason to delay treatment (Filho & Mullen, 2021). A noncontrast CT scan is highly sensitive and can determine if the patient has an intracerebral bleed.

If the patient has a decline in level of consciousness or brain hemorrhage resulting in elevated intracranial pressure, ensuring the patient's airway is protected and providing adequate ventilation is a priority. The patient may need supplemental oxygen, or even mechanical ventilation may be required with the goal of keeping the oxygen saturation at >94% (Filho & Mullen, 2021).

Evaluation of the patient includes listening for vascular bruits, heart murmurs, aberrant lung sounds, and fluid overload.

If the nurse practitioner (NP) or physician assistant (PA) suspects a neck injury, the neck should be immobilized until this possibility is thoroughly evaluated and ruled out. The NP/PA should inspect the skin for cholesterol emboli, endocarditis, or ecchymoses.

There are numerous rating scales available to evaluate the patient with a suspected stroke. This includes the National Institutes of Health Stroke Scale (NIHSS), which contains 11 items that add up to a potential score of 42. The scale, which is one of the most validated, assess the patient's level of consciousness (LOC), ability to follow commands, eye gaze, visual acuity, facial palsy, arm and leg drift, limb ataxia, sensory perception, speech, dysarthria, and attention to stimuli (Filho & Mullen, 2021).

There are several laboratory studies that should also be obtained. Initial lab studies include a noncontrast head CT or brain MRI, blood glucose, and oxygen saturation. Other labs that ought to be evaluated are a complete blood count (CBC), prothrombin time and international normalized ratio (INR), activated partial thromboplastin time (aPTT), electrocardiogram (ECG), and troponin. Treatment of the acute stroke patient should not be delayed while awaiting these results. If the patient is a candidate for thrombolytics, the only test required is the serum glucose. Additional tests that may be needed depend on the working diagnosis, and planned treatments include lumbar puncture, serum electrolytes, electrocardiography pregnancy test, blood alcohol level, chest radiograph, and electroencephalogram (Filho & Mullen, 2021).

Treatment

Ischemic Stroke

Treatment will vary depending on the type of stroke. If the patient has an ischemic stroke, thrombolytic therapy with recombinant tissue plasminogen activator (tPA) should be considered. Alteplase is the only medication that has been approved by the Federal Drug Administration (FDA) for the pharmacologic treatment of acute ischemic stroke (Goldstein, 2019). To be eligible for tPA, the patient must have a clinical diagnosis of ischemic stroke with neurologic deficit, the symptom onset must be < 4.5 hours, and the patient must be at least 18 years of age (Filho & Mullen, 2021). If the symptom onset is > 4.5 hours, then the patient would receive standard evaluation and care, which may include mechanical thrombectomy. Additional measures to decrease potential disability in the stroke patient include the administration of aspirin, prophylaxis for deep vein thrombosis, statin therapy, management of hypertension, smoking cessation, and decreasing obesity.

Hemorrhagic Stroke

Treatment of hemorrhagic stroke centers on decreasing neurologic decline and preventing the hemorrhage from increasing. Because determining the prognosis for individuals with acute intracerebral hemorrhage (ICH) is an indeterminate science, comprehensive medical care should be given for at least the first day after ICH onset. "Do Not Resuscitate" (DNR), orders should not be considered until after the first 24 hours to allow for a more complete assessment of prognosis can be performed.

Treatment may include minimally invasive procedures such as stereotactic image-guided catheter placement to aspirate the clot, especially if there is brainstem compression or neurologic decline. According to Jadhav et al. (2016), in a "phase II trial using this technique, a 46% reduction in clot volume was observed compared with a 4% reduction over the same time frame using traditional medical management." In addition, the minimally invasive approach showed a faster decrease in clot volume, and more patients have better outcomes, as well as a decrease in the length of hospital stay, which leads to a decrease in hospital costs when compared to the surgical group (Jadhav et al., 2016).

Systolic blood pressure should be reduced to 140 to160 mm Hg. Studies show that decreasing the systolic pressure can improve patient outcomes. The treatment plan should also include the reversal of any anticoagulation agents if present. In patients with intraventricular blood, a ventricular drain may be placed to avoid hydrocephalus. If the patient is on any anticoagulant medication, bleeding times should be evaluated and corrected if necessary (Goldstein, 2021). Hypoglycemia should be avoided, as this can cause vasospasm and has been shown to increase disability in patients who have had a subarachnoid hemorrhage (Naidech et al., 2010). It is also paramount to maintain euthermia, as hyperthermia has been shown to increase morbidity and mortality. According to Samudra and Figueroa (2016), hypothermia has not shown any benefit to the patient.

The patient may develop an increase in intracranial pressure (ICP) due to clot formation, edema, or hydrocephalus. There are several ways to prevent and manage ICP, such as keeping the head of the bed elevated at 30 degrees, light sedation for patient comfort, and normal saline for fluid replacement as hypotonic solutions are contraindicated. If the patient has a Glasgow Coma Scale (GCS) score of < 8, invasive monitoring of ICP may be required. Placement of a ventricular drain might be indicated if the patient has a decreased level of consciousness or hydrocephalus. Osmotic intravenous fluids such as mannitol or hypertonic saline can be given to lower ICP. If these treatments are ineffective for lowering ICP, a pharmacologic coma, hyperventilation, or neuromuscular blockade have been shown to lower ICP. Surgical evacuation of the hematoma depends on the location of the bleed (Rordorf & McDonald, 2021).

Surgical Options

Surgery is another option for treating strokes, but this will depend on the location of the stroke. If the stroke is in the cerebella area and the size of the bleeding is greater than 3 cm in diameter or if the patient's neurologic status is deteriorating or if there is brainstem compression, then surgical removal of the clot is indicated.

If the stroke is in the supratentorial region, surgical management is debatable. However, if the hemorrhage is causing a life-threatening issue, then surgery is warranted.

Strokes that extend into the intraventricular can lead to complications such as hydrocephalus. If signs of neurologic deterioration develop, an emergent CT scan should be done, and if indicated, a ventriculostomy and external ventricular drainage performed (Rordorf & McDonald, 2021).

Lifestyle Changes

Risk factors for stroke include hypertension, smoking, and diabetes among other conditions (Table 13.3). Nonmodifiable risk factors include age, having a history of TIA, male gender, ethnicity, and family history of having a stroke. The chance of having a stroke increases with age. The possibility of having a stroke doubles for each decade over the age of 55. Roughly 65% of all strokes happen in people who are older than 65 (Pathophysiology and Etiology of Stroke, n.d.).

Chronic Kidney Disease

Epidemiology

Chronic kidney disease (CKD) is a global public health issue. The number of people registered in the end-stage renal illness (ESRD) Medicare-funded program has risen from roughly 10,000 beneficiaries in 1973 to 703,243 as of 2015.

Although the exact factors for the increased enrollment in the ESRD program are unidentified, changes in the demographics of the populace, distinctions in disease burden among racial clients, and underrecognition of earlier phases of CKD along with variables for CKD may partly explain this growth.

CASE STUDY 13.3

Randy H. is a 67-year-old Caucasian male who presents to his primary care provider (PCP), Wendy, who is a physician's assistant, with complaints of polydipsia and polyuria. Randy has not been seen by his PCP for longer than 3 years. He is a former smoker. He has been drinking a glass of whiskey every day for the past 30 years, and he takes 1 mg of lorazepam twice a day for anxiety. He does not exercise routinely or follow a healthy diet. He is 6′1″, weighs 255 pounds, and his body mass index (BMI) is 33.6, which is considered obese. Labs are noted as follows:

Lab	Result	Normal Range
Hemoglobin	8.9 g/dL	13.5 to 17.5 g/dL
Creatinine	2.3 mg/dL	0.74 to 1.35 mg/dL
Serum albumin	3.2 g/dL	3.4 to 5.4 g/dL
Hemoglobin A1c	8.5%	4% and 5.6%

The PA tells Randy that he has diabetes and kidney disease. She advises Randy to stop drinking, eat a healthy diet, and to start exercising to help slow the damage that is occurring to his kidneys.

TABLE 13.3 Risk Factors for Stroke

Risk Factor	Population Attributable Risk (PAR) (99% CI)
Hypertension (self-reported history or blood pressure ≥140/90 mm Hg)	47.9% (45.1–50.6)
Current smoking	12.4% (10.2–14.9)
Diabetes mellitus	3.9% (1.9–7.6)
Ratio of apoB to apoA1	26.8% (22.2–31.9)
Obesity (waist to hip ratio)	18.6% (13.3–25.3)
Physical inactivity	35.8% (27.7–44.7)
Diet risk score	23.2% (18.2–28.9)
Alcohol consumption (current)	5.8% (3.4–9.7)
Psychosocial factors	17.4% (13.1–22.6)
Cardiac etiologies	9.1% (8.0–10.2)

From O'Donnell M. J., Chin S. L., Rangarajan S., et al. (2016). Global and regional effects of potentially modifiable risk factors associated with acute stroke in 32 countries (INTERSTROKE): A case-control study. *Lancet 388*, 761.

Patients with ESRD use a disproportionate share of health care resources. However, regardless of the magnitude of the resources dedicated to the treatment of ESRD and the significant improvements in the high quality of dialysis, these individuals remain to experience significant death and morbidity as well as a decreased lifestyle.

The overall prevalence of people with chronic kidney disease in the United States, according to the National Health and Nutrition Examination Survey (NHANES), was 14.8%. If the estimated glomerular filtration rage (eGFR) is <60 mL/min/1.73m^2, then the prevalence was 7.2%. The number of people with end-stage renal disease continues to grow. In 2015, the number of new patients receiving renal replacement therapy (RRT) was 124,114. The total number of patients receiving RRT in 2015 was 703,234, and 63% of these patients were receiving hemodialysis.

How does this compare to other countries? Worldwide, 2.618 million people were receiving RRT in 2010. The approximate number of patients who needed renal replacement therapy was between 4.902 million a 5.431 million using a conservative model (Obrador, 2020).

Pathophysiology

Chronic kidney disease (CKD) "is a heterogeneous group of disorders characterized by alterations in kidney structure and function, which manifest in various ways depending upon the underlying cause or causes and the severity of disease" (Levey & Inker, 2020).

Formal guidelines for defining and staging CKD were presented by the National Kidney Foundation (NKF) Kidney Disease Outcomes Quality Initiative (KDOQI) in 2002 and later endorsed by the Kidney Disease Improving Global Outcomes (KDIGO) organization in 2004. When a patient's kidneys are so far damaged that they require dialysis, this is referred to as kidney failure and is the end-stage of chronic kidney disease (Levey & Inker, 2020).

The official definition of chronic kidney disease was formulated by KDIGO and is defined as "a decline in glomerular filtration rate (GFR) below 60 mL/min/1.73 m^2 and/or the presence of persistent albuminuria, proteinuria, hematuria, and/or electrolyte imbalances" (Litbarg, 2018).

There are many health disorders that can cause a decrease in kidney function; nevertheless, there are commonalities that lead to CKD. These include chronic inflammation, oxidative stress, and endothelial dysfunction; these factors are also common in the development of cardiovascular disease.

Regardless of the reason for the initial insult, the development of kidney disease occurs in a consistent, uniform pattern. There is a loss of nephrons, which leads to hyperfiltration and hypertrophy of the functioning nephrons. The loss of functioning nephrons will eventually cause maladaptive changes that trigger an increase in oxidative stress, overproduction of proinflammatory cytokines and the stimulation of the renin-angiotensin-aldosterone system, premature apoptosis, deterioration of renal tubules, fibrosis, and ongoing damage to the nephrons (Litbarg, 2018).

There are four stages that lead up to chronic kidney disease. First, there is malfunction of the excretory function resulting from a buildup of endogenous and also nonessential substances. This results in modifications in pharmacokinetics and also a buildup of various medications. Breakdown happens when the glomeruli are faced with an excess of waste items, resulting in osmotic diuresis. There is also a decrease in the concentrating capability of the kidneys. The nephrons will produce three to four times the amount of urine when the kidneys are failing due to the inability to filter the additional dissolved substances.

During the second stage, the kidney's ability to regulate hormones is impaired. This can cause persistent renal failure, which impacts the endocrine system. Due to a lack of erythropoietin, there is a decrease in erythrocyte synthesis, which leads to renal anemia, then uremia results in a reduction of normal erythrocytes due to hemorrhage or hemolysis. Vitamin D production is also damaged, and phosphate excretion is decreased. Secondary hyperparathyroidism can occur and result in hyperphosphatemia. Alongside this, other pathomechanisms bring about a disturbance in bone metabolic rate and osteomalacia, especially in dialysis individuals.

During the third phase of kidney disease, there is electrolyte imbalance as well as overhydration. As kidney function declines, the ability of the glomeruli to filter decreases, and the capability of the kidneys to overcome this lessens. This will cause an increased retention of electrolytes and water.

It is during this phase of renal decline that incidental health complications appear. Complications due to water retention include pulmonary edema, hypertension, and peripheral edema. Diuretics can be prescribed in this phase, but it is important to monitor the patient's sodium level, as this can be adversely affected by the use of diuretics. Calcium-sparing diuretics (i.e., thiazides) are recommended to prevent hyperkalemia due to increased potassium secretion.

Because the kidneys cannot adequately eliminate waste due to decreased glomerular filtration, there is a risk of metabolic acidosis. When a patient has ongoing metabolic acidosis, there is an increase in bone calcium, decreased protein metabolism, and an increase in gastrointestinal problems.

During the fourth phase of kidney disease, uremia occurs. There is an increase in excreted urinary metabolites such as urea, beta-2 microglobulin, creatinine, and parathyroid hormone into the blood, which leads to azotemia. These metabolites impair normal organ function, particularly the central nervous system, circulatory system, and blood flow. This conglomeration is termed *uremic syndrome*.

The patient with uremic syndrome may demonstrate café au lait spots on the skin and can also present with peritonitis, pleurisy, and pericarditis. In addition, the uremia can cause hemolysis and dysfunction with the thrombocytes and leukocytes (Centers for Medicare & Medicaid Services, 2021).

Assessment

The symptoms of chronic kidney disease (CKD) are not apparent in the early stages of the disease and are usually evident in conjunction with medical complications such as hyperparathyroidism, hypertension, and anemia. Symptoms appear in later phases of the disease. Along with generally identified hormone and metabolic difficulties, CKD can also include enhanced risks for cardiovascular disease, toxicity from medications, infection, and cognitive disability. Issues that generally occur later on in the disease process can bring about death prior to kidney disease advancing to kidney failure. Difficulties might also arise from the unfavorable impacts of interventions used to treat the disease.

When kidney disease is identified, the practitioner must assess the degree of kidney failure and how quickly the kidney disease has progressed. The physical exam and history from the patient are important in determining the degree of kidney disease; however, the approximation of the glomerular filtration and the presence of any urinary sediment will provide key diagnostic information.

"The glomerular filtration rate (GFR) is equal to the sum of the filtration rates in all of the functioning nephrons; thus, the GFR gives a rough measure of the number of functioning nephrons." The kidney filters about 180 liters per day at a rate of 125 mL/min. A normal GFR is contingent upon body size, sex, and age and is about "130 and 120 mL/min/1.73 m^2 for men and women, respectively" (Inker & Perrone, 2020).

It is difficult and time consuming to measure the actual glomerular filtration rate, so most practitioners use an equation to provide an estimation of the GFR. In the United States, the most common equations used for GFR estimation are the Cockcroft-Gault equation and the Modification of Diet in Renal Disease (MDRD) study equation.

The Cockcroft-Gault formula is more commonly used in the general population under the age of 65. This formula is founded on the values of creatinine production from age, weight, and gender of the patient. However, it stems from results obtained in "normal, hospitalized" patients, so one could argue that it is not the best tool for determining creatinine clearance in a patient who already has CKD.

The MDRD equation was developed from a multicenter, randomized, controlled clinical study that assessed the value of dietary protein restriction and diligent blood pressure control and the progression of renal insufficiency (Table 13.4). The MDRD formula has evolved to include the patient demographics and serum values, thus omitting the serum urea nitrogen and the urine urea nitrogen. In the geriatric population, the estimated GFR should be calculated using the MDRD because the age of the patient is included as a variable. This will permit the proper doses of medications and avoid nephrotoxins in patients who have more advanced kidney disease (Arora, 2021).

The MDRD equation is endorsed by the National Kidney Disease Education Program (NKDEP) of the National Institutes of Health (NIH), the National Kidney Foundation (NKF), and the American Society of Nephrology (ASN). If, according to the MDRD equation (see Table 13.4), the patient has an estimated GRF below 60 below 60 ml/min/1.73 m^2, the patient is at an increased risk of worsening CKD and end-stage renal disease (Workeneh & Mitch, 2013).

TABLE 13.4 Creatinine Clearance Calculation Formulas

Name of Equation	Formula
Cockcroft-Gault CCr[25]	Men: CCr = [(14-age) × Weight (kg)]/SCr × 72 Women: CCr = ([(14-age) × Weight (kg)]/SCr × 72) × 0.85
MDRD Study Equation[26]	GFR (mL/min/1.73 m^2) =186× $(S_{cr})^{-1.154}$ × $(Age)^{-0.203}$ × (0.742 if female) × (1.212 if African American)

CCr, Creatinine clearance; *GFR*, glomerular filtration rate (GFR); *MDRD*, modification of Diet in Renal Disease.
From Workeneh, B. T., & Mitch, W. E. (2013). In R. J. Alpern, O. W. Moe, & M. Caplan (Eds.), *Seldin and Giebisch's the kidney* (5th ed.) Elsevier.

TABLE 13.5 Staging in Chronic Kidney Disease

GFR Category	GFR ml/min/1.73 m^2	Terms
G1	≥ 90	Normal or high
G2	60–89	Mildly decreased
G3a	45–59	Mild to moderately decreased
G3b	30–44	Moderate to severely decreased
G4	15–29	Severely decreased
G5	< 15	Kidney failure

GFR, Glomerular filtration rate.
From Kidney International Supplement (2013). *3*(1), p.27. Available at https://kdigo.org/guidelines/ckd-evaluation-and-management/

Other than the estimated creatinine clearance, other testing should be performed when the practitioner suspects chronic kidney disease, including a basic metabolic panel, complete blood count, and urinalysis. It is common to discover normocytic normochromic anemia in patients with kidney disease. An elevated serum creatinine and blood urea nitrogen (BUN) will also be elevated in patients who have chronic kidney disease.

Electrolyte levels may also be abnormal. Hyperkalemia is a common finding in someone who has CKD. The elevated potassium level is due to the reduced ability of the kidney to excrete potassium ions and also the medications the patient is taking to slow the progression of the disease. The potassium level needs to be closely monitored because hyperkalemia can lead to cardiac arrhythmias and sudden death. A low potassium diet should be initiated, and potassium-binding medications should be considered (Watanabe, 2020). Because of the risk for cardiovascular disease, all patients with CKD should have lipid panel evaluated.

Patients with CKD are also at risk of developing bone disease, so serum phosphate, 25-hydroxyvitamin D, alkaline phosphatase, and intact parathyroid hormone (PTH) levels should be checked to evaluate for renal bone disease. A renal ultrasound may be helpful in determining if hydronephrosis is present, if there is any fibrotic tissue in or around the kidney, or if there is any adenopathy. If the NP or PA suspects obstruction of the ureters, then a retrograde pyelogram without contrast would be ordered. A plain abdominal x-ray may show kidney stones in the patient (Arora, 2021).

The workup for someone with kidney disease may also include computed tomography (CT), magnetic resonance imaging (MRI), magnetic resonance angiography (MRA), or a renal radionuclide scan. A CT scan can better identify renal masses or cysts that may have been found on ultrasound. Intravenous contrast should not be used in patients with renal impairment, as this can worsen the patient's kidney function.

If the patient cannot have a CT, magnetic resonance imaging can be used to detect structural abnormalities with the kidneys. MRIs are also very good at discovering if there is a renal vein thrombosis that may be the cause of kidney disease.

An MRA can be used to detect renal artery stenosis; however, a renal arteriography is considered the standard for diagnosing stenosis. Renal radionuclide scans can also detect stenosis, but they are not reliable in patients who have a GFR of less than 30 mL/min/1.73 m^2 (Arora, 2021).

If a patient has kidney damage or severe proteinuria and the diagnosis is unclear, a percutaneous renal biopsy may be needed. This is usually done with guidance from ultrasound. The practitioner needs to be aware of the potential complications of doing a percutaneous biopsy, such as bleeding, which can be fatal. An open surgical biopsy is safer and should be considered if there is a risk of bleeding (Arora, 2021).

Differential diagnoses for patients with abnormal glomerular filtration rates include renal artery stenosis, Wegener granulomatosis, renal artery stenosis, and systemic lupus erythematosus (Arora, 2021).

Staging in chronic kidney disease is based on the estimated GFR. Table 13.5 defines the stages.

Treatment

The treatment of CKD will depend on the underlying cause, and there are several ways to delay the progression of the disease. Keeping the patient's blood pressure as close to recommended guidelines is one way to slow progression. Elevated cholesterol should also be addressed and treated per recommended guidelines. The American Diabetes Association recommends a hemoglobin A1c goal of < 7%, as elevated blood sugar can impact the glomerular filtration rate. The use of sodium-glucose cotransporter 2 (SGLT2) inhibitors has been shown to slow the progression of CKD. In addition, the patient with diabetes with proteinuria should be receiving renin-angiotensin system (RAS) blockers (ex. candesartan) (Arora, 2021).

In addition to treating the underlying cause of renal failure, there are additional health conditions that may arise due to CKD such as anemia, hyperphosphatemia, hyperparathyroidism, hypocalcemia, fluid overload, and metabolic acidosis. If the patient's hemoglobin is less than 10 g/dL, the patient should be given an erythropoiesis-stimulating agent. If the patient has a higher than normal level of phosphorus, then a phosphorus binding agent should be given. For hypocalcemia, a calcium supplement can be added to the patient's medication regimen. If the patient experiences fluid overload, diuretics or ultrafiltration can aid in the removal of excess fluid. If metabolic acidosis is present, then an oral alkali supplement would be called for (Arora, 2021).

The Eighth Joint National Committee (JNC 8) and KDIGO recommends that patients with CKD be given angiotensin-converting enzyme (ACE) inhibitors and angiotensin receptor blockers (ARBs) because these medications have been proven to decrease the rate of injury to the kidneys in the patient with CKD (recommendation grade B). Most patients with CKD will also develop generalized edema that can be treated with diuretics. The use of thiazide diuretics in patients with an estimated GFR of < 45 mL/min/1.73 m^2 is not very efficacious; however, loop diuretics such as bumetanide or furosemide are recommended for patients with stage 3, 4, and 5 kidney disease (Schoolwerth et al., 2001). A study by Lewis et al. (1993) discovered that diabetic patients who took captopril long term were able to decrease the rate of progression to end-stage renal failure. Additionally, angiotensin-converting enzyme inhibitors also slowed the rate of progression in nondiabetic patients who had CKD.

Patients who have elevated uric acid levels are at risk of rapidly progressive impairment in kidney function. Also, elevated uric acid levels have also been shown to increase the patient's risk of developing contrast-induced nephropathy. Multiple studies have shown that febuxostat had a safer toxicity profile compared to allopurinol. Guidelines also recommend that serum bicarbonate should be kept > 22 mmol/L; however, the optimal level of serum bicarbonate has not been established. This is to slow the development of renal bone disease and advancement of kidney impairment (Litbarg, 2018).

There are several medications that need to have their recommended dose adjusted based on the patient's kidney function. The most common medications that require dose adjustments are antibiotics, nonsteroidal antiinflammatory drugs (NSAIDs), and chemotherapy medications. Bowel preparations, proton pump inhibitors (PPIs), and anabolic steroids can also cause damage to the kidneys such as acute interstitial nephritis, acute phosphate nephropathy, and focal segmental glomerulosclerosis.

The NP/PA should also monitor the patient's magnesium level, as low levels of magnesium have been found to increase all-cause mortality in patients with chronic kidney disease and have been shown to add to the progression of CKD (Litbarg, 2018). An oral magnesium supplement should be given to patients who are deficient and have CKD, diabetes, and who also take diuretics, calcineurin inhibitors, and proton pump inhibitors.

Dietary Changes

A decrease in appetite is a common phenomenon in patients with end-stage kidney disease. Approximately half of the patients with CKD suffer a decline in appetite as their kidney disease progresses. A decrease in appetite can lead to poor nutritional intake, which presents a challenge for the patient with CKD.

The patient with chronic kidney disease needs to eat a healthy diet with fresh fruits and vegetables, whole grains, and a minimal intake of processed foods in order to slow the progression to end-stage disease. Poor nutrition can lead to volume overload, hypernatremia, hyperphosphatemia, hyperkalemia, and a buildup of toxic metabolites (Cho & Beddhu, 2020).

Adults with CKD stages 3 through 5 should have a consult with a registered dietician to perform a comprehensive nutrition assessment. The assessment should include evaluation of the patient's appetite, food intake log, anthropomorphic measurements, and biochemical data.

Protein restriction in the patient with kidney impairment remains controversial. The KDIGO guidelines recommend varying amounts of protein intake based on the stage of kidney disease. For the patient who is not receiving dialysis, KDIGO recommends 0.6 to 1 g/kg of protein per ideal body weight. If the patient is receiving hemodialysis, the recommended daily protein intake is ≥ 1.1 g/kg of ideal body weight. And for the patient who is receiving peritoneal dialysis, the recommended daily protein intake is 1.0 to 1.2 g/kg of ideal body weight. The need for additional protein intake must be considered if the patient is acutely ill (Naylor et al., 2013). Previously many guidelines recommended a diet low in protein, but more recent, rigorous studies have not found a benefit in a low-protein diet (Cho & Beddhu, 2020). Decreased protein intake has been shown to diminish the levels of blood urea nitrogen, serum phosphorus, and toxins. Patients need to be monitored closely for acceptable caloric intake and to determine if there is any indication of protein malnutrition. To avoid malnutrition, three criteria must be met. The patient must sustain an acceptable caloric intake that avoids processed carbohydrates, the protein source must have a high amount of essential amino acids, and at least 60% of the protein must have a high biologic value. For example, an egg has a biologic value of 100. The "biological value (BV) is a measure of the proportion of absorbed protein that is incorporated into the proteins of the body." And the breakdown of skeletal muscle should be avoided to decrease the net loss of nitrogen (Cho & Beddhu, 2020).

Sodium intake also needs to be monitored in the patient with chronic kidney disease. One gram salt of contains 0.4 g (17 mEq) of Na^+ ion. Patients with chronic kidney disease who have an estimated glomerular filtration rate of < 60 mL/min/1.73 m^2 and who have coexisting conditions such as excess protein excretion, hypertension, or volume overload will need to restrict their sodium intake to < 2 g/day or 5 g/day of salt. If the patient does not have any of these coexisting conditions, then the recommended daily sodium intake is < 2.3 g/day or 5.75 g/day of salt. A study by Suckling et al. (2010) determined that decreasing salt intake significantly decreased blood pressure in those with type 1 and type 2 diabetes (Arora, 2021).

Potassium restriction is generally not required in patients with chronic kidney disease until the eGFR < 30 mL/min/1.73 m^2 unless the patient is taking an angiotensin receptor blocker (ARB) or angiotensin-converting enzyme (ACE) inhibitor. In this case the patient may need to decrease his or her potassium intake. KDOQI advise potassium restriction of 2 to 4 g/day for patients who are in the later stages of kidney disease (Arora, 2021).

The KDOQI guidelines (2000) recommend that calcium intake not exceed 1500 mg/day. To date, there are no randomized, controlled trials that establish a safe level of calcium ingestion for patients who are not on dialysis.

Phosphorus consumption should be no more than 1 g/day. High levels of serum phosphate have shown an increase in cardiovascular disease. The risk of cardiovascular disease and elevated phosphorus does not depend on the patient's eGFR. Inorganic phosphorus that is found in processed foods should be avoided because it has a higher bioavailability than organic phosphate. Organic phosphate can be found in unprocessed food and must be hydrolyzed in the gut so it can be absorbed (Arora, 2021).

Carbohydrate and fat intake must also be considered in the patient with CKD. It is recommended that carbohydrate intake be limited to 30 to 35 kcal/kg/day for patients with an eGFR of < 60 mL/min/1.73 m^2. Fat intake should be < 30% of daily caloric intake. Patients who are obese and specifically those with central adiposity are at a greater risk of increased progression of their CKD and end-stage kidney disease. Losing weight has been shown to slow the progression of kidney disease (Arora, 2021).

Recommendations for dietary fiber intake for patients with CKD who have an eGFR ≤ 60 mL/min/1.73 m^2 is 5 to 38 g/day, which is the same as for patients who do not have CKD. Dietary fiber, or "roughage," is the part of the plant that your body cannot digest or absorb. Sources of dietary fiber include peas, beans, nuts, whole grains, and fruits (Arora, 2021).

Lifestyle Changes

There are lifestyle changes that patients with CKD can make to slow the progression of the disease. Restricting the daily intake of dietary protein and sodium is one way to slow the progression. For the patient who has diabetes in addition to CKD, it is important to decrease microvascular and cardiovascular complications. According to Whittier and Lewis (2018), "empagliflozin has been shown to lower blood pressure and weight and delay progression of CKD compared to placebo."

One of the risk factors for developing CKD is obesity. Patients who are obese (body mass index [BMI] > 30.0) and have CKD are at risk for disease progression. Chronic kidney disease leads to albuminuria, which is worsened by obesity but can be improved by weight loss. Elevated lipids can also increase disease progression because of the proinflammatory and profibrotic markers that are found in low-density lipoproteins (LDL). Both of these factors are modifiable lifestyle changes that the NP and PA should educate and encourage their patients to do. Finally, smoking is a risk factor for CKD and can also speed progression, so the patient with CKD should be urged to quit (Whittier & Lewis, 2018).

Meditation, yoga, and tai chi can lower blood pressure, promote calm, decrease sympathetic activity, lessen oxidative stress, and reduce psychological stress. These therapies have been shown to improve the quality of life and decrease stress in patients with CKD, which can slow the progression of worsening kidney function (Whittier & Lewis, 2018).

Peripheral Artery Disease

CASE STUDY 13.4

A 66-year-old female was sent from the clinic for worsening of severe right calf pain and a decrease in exercise tolerance due to the pain. She had a 3-month history of intermittent right calf pain and denied trauma, back pain, fever, and leg weakness. Otherwise, the medical history was significant for hyperlipidemia. She was a former smoker and stopped smoking 6 months ago; however, she smoked one pack of cigarettes per day for the past 40 years before quitting. The patient does not drink or use any recreational drugs. Her medications include low-dose aspirin and atorvastatin. On physical examination, her vital signs were normal. Body mass index was 29 kg/m^2. Femoral pulses were diminished bilaterally. Popliteal, right dorsalis pedis, and left posterior tibialis pulses were faint. The right dorsalis pedis and posterior tibialis pulses were not palpable. Cardiac examination was normal. Otherwise, the physical examination was unremarkable. The ankle-brachial index was 0.68 on the left and 0.92 on the right. She was enrolled in a supervised exercise program 3 months ago, but she reported no improvement despite adherence to the exercise program, and her symptoms progressed.

Epidemiology

Peripheral artery disease (PAD) refers to atherosclerotic, inflammatory, occlusive, and aneurysmal diseases involving the abdominal aorta and its branch arteries (Nguyen & Patel, 2021). Peripheral artery disease is measured by determining the ankle-brachial index (ABI). This is a noninvasive test that measures the ratio of ankle to brachial systolic blood pressure. In patients who are 65 years old and over, the ABI should be 1.0 to 1.4. There are 8 to 10 million people in the United States who have PAD, and there are more than 200 million individuals worldwide who have PAD. There are more men than women who have PAD, and Blacks are more likely to have PAD than non-Hispanic Whites (Bonaca & Creager, 2019).

Patients with PAD often have claudication. Claudication is a pain caused decreased blood flow most often in the lower extremities that usually occurs when walking because there is less oxygen available when walking or exercising. This is a common symptom of PAD. Early in PAD, the pain from claudication will go away when the person quits walking because blood flow and oxygen consumption are normal at rest. However, with time, the pain can become so severe that it does not go away at rest (Hopkins Medicine, n.d.). Studies suggest that 10% to 30% of patients with PAD have claudication (Bonaca & Creager, 2019). PAD also decreases the perfusion to calf muscles and weakens mitochondrial action (Berger & Davies, 2021).

Pathophysiology

When there is an oxygen supply-demand mismatch, which occurs in the setting of dysfunctional oxygen extraction and utilization in the muscles, ischemic pain occurs within the sensory receptors and lactate builds up, causing intermittent claudication. (See Fig. 13.1.)

When a patient has PAD, the skeletal muscles in the legs will have partial axonal denervation. The oxidative slow-twitch fibers or type 1 fibers are not damaged; however, the glycolytic fast-twitch fibers (type 2 fibers) are not preserved within the skeletal muscles due to PAD. When type 2 fibers are damaged, there is reduced exercise ability and a reduction in muscle strength. The muscles will enter anaerobic metabolism during and after exercise. This causes a buildup of lactate, which leads to an increase in acylcarnitines while exercising, which then leads to inefficient oxidative metabolism (Bonaca & Creager, 2019).

There are four different classifications of PAD: asymptomatic, intermittent claudication, critical limb ischemia, and acute limb ischemia. Asymptomatic represents 20% to 50% of patients with PAD and includes patients with uncharacteristic symptoms. The intermittent claudication classification defines 10% to 35% of patients with PAD and is given when the pain occurs during exercise or exertion but will go away within 10 minutes of rest. Critical limb ischemia occurs in 1% to 2% of PAD patients and is categorized as an ongoing period (> 2 weeks) of pain at rest with unhealing wounds, skin ulcers, or gangrene. Acute limb ischemia (ALI) will happen in 14 per 100,000 patients and is defined as significant hypoperfusion with "pain, pallor, nonpalpable peripheral pulses, paresthesias, and paralysis of the limb, which is cold to touch; duration is less than 2 weeks" (Clinical Overview, 2021; Nguyen & Patel, 2021). Acute limb ischemia is further divided into three categories: viable, threatened, and irreversible. Viable ischemia will have audible pulses and there will be no sensory or muscle loss. Threatened ischemia has mild to moderate motor or sensory damage and pulses will not be perceptible with a Doppler. Finally, irreversible ischemia will have severe motor or sensory damage and the pulses will not be heard with a Doppler (Nguyen & Patel, 2021).

Assessment

Intermittent claudication is the cardinal symptom of PAD. This pain usually occurs at the site of the nearest stenosis. If the patient has thigh, hip, or buttock claudication pain, then the area of stenosis is most likely in the aorta or iliac arteries. Pain in the calf is due to stenosis in the femoral or popliteal arteries. The calf muscle or gastrocnemius utilizes more oxygen while walking than other muscles of the legs. Because of this increased oxygen consumption, patients frequently complain of pain in the calf. If claudication occurs in the ankle or foot, then the blockage is most likely in the tibial or peroneal artery.

When getting the history, it is important for the NP/PA to ask patients how far they can walk without pain, how fast they are walking, and if the pain is worse when walking up a hill. This information will help determine any existing or potential disability and the patient's stability. Peripheral artery disease can cause mobility limitations in addition to

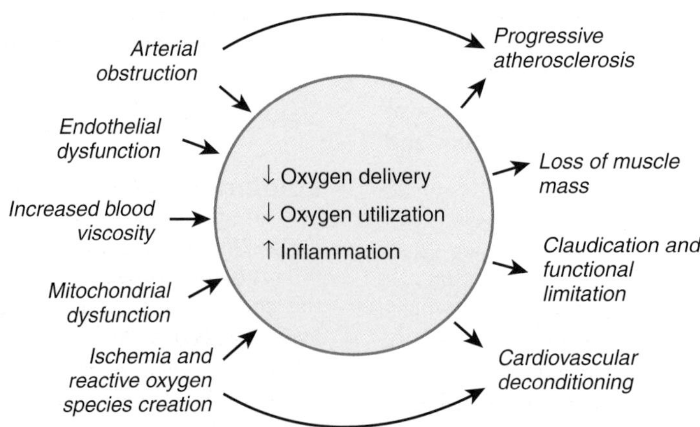

• **Fig. 13.1** Mechanisms for functional limitations in peripheral artery disease (PAD). (Modified from Bonaca, M. P., & Creager, M. A. [2015]. Pharmacological treatment and current management of peripheral artery disease. *Circulation Research, 116*, 1579–1598.)

pain. Several questionnaires have been developed to determine the severity of claudication. These questionnaires are the Edinburgh Claudication Questionnaire, the San Diego Claudication Questionnaire, and the Walking Impairment Questionnaire (Bonaca & Creager, 2019).

The NP/PA should also measure the patient's blood pressure in both arms to determine if there is an indication of subclavian stenosis. If there is a systolic blood pressure difference of more than 15 to 20 mm Hg, then subclavian stenosis should be considered. The brachial, ulnar, radial, popliteal, femoral, posterior tibialis, and dorsalis pedis pulses should be felt to ascertain the symmetry and strength. The strength of the pulse is graded on a scale of 0 to 3 with 0 being absent pulse and 3 being a bounding pulse.

Auscultation for any bruits over the pulse points should be noted. The limbs should also be palpated and inspected to assess temperature, skin integrity, hair distribution, quality of the nails if they are brittle or split, and muscle tone of the limbs should be analyzed. If the extremity is cool, pulseless, immobile, pale, or cyanotic, the practitioner should suspect acute limb ischemia. A Doppler ultrasound should be ordered to evaluate this possibility. If both the arterial and venous pulses are absent via Doppler, the affected limb may require amputation (Clinical Overview, 2021).

The Fontaine Classification of Peripheral Artery Disease is widely used to delineate the extent of disease. (See Table 13.6.)

Ankle-Brachial Index

The patient's ABI should also be calculated as part of the physical assessment. To calculate the ABI, divide the highest systolic blood pressure of the posterior tibial or dorsalis pedis by the highest systolic blood pressure taken in the right or left arm. A normal ABI is 1.0 to 1.4, abnormal is ≤ 0.9, borderline is 0.91 to 0.99, and noncompressible is > 1.4. The ABI should be determined at a resting state in both legs to obtain a baseline measurement. However, if the ABI is borderline or abnormal, then an exercise ABI should be documented. Also, patients who have PAD are at a higher risk of having an abdominal aortic aneurysm; however, routine screening for PAD is not recommended (Nguyen & Patel, 2021).

Treadmill Testing

A patient's PAD can also be evaluated by using a treadmill. Treadmill testing can assess the severity of PAD. The practitioner will record the time of onset of the claudication, which is called the "claudication onset time." When the patient cannot walk any further on the treadmill because of pain, this is noted as the "peak walking time." The treadmill walking test is a standardized test that provides a quantitative assessment of the patient's PAD. It is also a way to monitor the impact of the interventions. To perform the treadmill test, the practitioner will need a motorized treadmill that can maintain a 12% grade and various levels of incline. The speed during the test is maintained at 2 miles per hour (mph), and the grade will be increased 2% every 2 to 3 minutes (Bonaca & Creager, 2019).

Imaging

Duplex ultrasound is one of many imaging modalities that can be used to assess PAD. An advantage of duplex ultrasound imaging is that it can evaluate the anatomy and the consequence of arterial stenoses.

If the aorta or peripheral arteries need to be visualized, then a magnetic resonance angiography (MRA) would be ordered. Using a gadolinium-enhanced MRA is ideal to envision systemic vasculature before deciding on the best treatment plan for the patient.

If the patient has metal clips, stents, or a pacemaker, then a computed tomography (CT) scanner can be used to examine the vasculature. CT scanners can obtain cross-sectional imaging, which allows visualization of the peripheral arteries. The sensitivity and specificity of CT scans when compared to conventional angiography is 95% and 96%, respectively (Bonaca & Creager, 2019).

Risk Factors

Nonmodifiable risk factors for PAD include being 65 years old and older, male gender, and genetics. Some risk factors are inherited, such as diabetes or dyslipidemia. PAD is less common in Caucasian people than in people of color; PAD is two to three times higher in Black people than White people. Chronic kidney disease and chronic inflammation as documented by an elevated C-reactive protein are also risk factors for PAD.

Other risk factors for PAD include poorly controlled diabetes, smoking, high blood pressure, and uncontrolled dyslipidemia. There is a 30% risk increase for PAD for every 1% elevation of hemoglobin A1c. Hypertension can increase a person's risk for PAD by three times compared to someone who does not have PAD. Observational studies also indicate that there is a two-to-fourfold increase occurrence of PAD in people who smoke when compared to people who have never smoked (Alvarez et al., 2013). (See Table 13.7.)

TABLE 13.6 Fontaine Classification of Peripheral Artery Disease

Stage	Symptoms
I	Asymptomatic
II	Intermittent claudication
IIa	Pain free, claudication walking >200 m
IIb	Pain free, claudication walking <200 m
III	Rest and nocturnal pain
IV	Necrosis, gangrene

From Nguyen, P., & Patel, P. M. (2021). Peripheral artery disease. In F. F. Ferri (Ed.), *Ferri's clinical advisor*. Elsevier.

TABLE 13.7 Odds Ratio of Peripheral Artery Disease in Persons With Risk Factors

Risk Factor	Odds Ratio (95% CI)
Cigarette smoking	4.46 (2.25–8.84)
Diabetes mellitus	2.71 (1.03–7.12)
Hypertension	1.75 (0.97–3.13)
Hypercholesterolemia	1.68 (1.09–2.57)
Hyperhomocysteinemia	1.92 (0.95–3.88)
Chronic kidney disease	2.00 (1.08–3.70)
Insulin resistance	2.06 (1.10–4.00)
C-reactive protein	2.20 (1.30–3.60)

From Bonaca, M.P., & Creager, M.A. (2019). In D. P. Zipes, P. Libby, R. O. Bonow, D. L. Mann, G. F. Tomaselli, & E. Braunwald (Eds.), *Braunwald's heart disease: A textbook of cardiovascular medicine* (11th ed.). Elsevier.

Tobacco Cessation

One option for patients who smoke and wish to stop is by using pharmacotherapy such as varenicline. The patient may experience nausea while taking varenicline, but this will resolve with continued use. However, a study in 2018 found that varenicline may be associated with a 34% higher risk of cardiovascular events when compared to patients who were not taking varenicline (Collins, 2021).

Blood Sugar Management

Keeping a tighter control of blood sugar can also slow the progression of PAD. The NP/PA should encourage the patient to start an exercise program as a way to help control blood sugar. A retrospective study among 790 military veterans with PAD showed that managing blood glucose in African Americans reduced the risk for lower extremity bypass surgery or amputation by 67% (Collins, 2021).

Platelet Therapy

Antiplatelet treatment will decrease platelet aggregation, which can improve outcomes for patients with PAD. Numerous studies have shown that antiplatelet therapy is beneficial in the patient with a history of coronary artery disease (CAD) or cerebrovascular disease, and there is a strong association between having CAD, cerebrovascular disease, and PAD. Also, antiplatelet medications such as aspirin or clopidogrel can decrease the risk for arterial surgery and improve vascular grafts. Aspirin is preferred in the geriatric patient with stable CAD and asymptomatic PAD (Collins, 2021).

Dyslipidemia

If the patient has dyslipidemia and PAD, starting the patient on a statin medication can reduce cardiovascular events, mortality, and stroke. The American Heart Association recommends high-intensity statin therapy, such as simvastatin. Once statin therapy is maximized, evolocumab every 2 weeks or monthly depending on dose has been shown to decrease cardiovascular events in patients with peripheral artery disease (Collins, 2021).

Treatment

Hypertension Management

An additional way to decrease the risk for morbidity and mortality in patients with PAD is to maintain a blood pressure < 130/80 mm/Hg. This can be accomplished with pharmacotherapy and lifestyle modifications. Thiazide diuretics should be used first. For patients with kidney disease or with chronic heart failure, angiotensin receptor blockers (ARB) or angiotensin-converting enzyme (ACE) inhibitors should be prescribed. If the patient has resistant hypertension, the NP/PA should consider adding a calcium channel blocker. Previously, it was thought that beta-blockers worsened the symptoms of people with PAD, but this has never been proven (Collins, 2021).

Cilostazol

Cilostazol is a used to treat PAD with intermittent claudication. This drug is a phosphodiesterase type-3 antiplatelet medication that also has vasodilator properties. Cilostazol works by causing vasodilation and inhibiting platelet aggregation. A main benefit of cilostazol is that it decreases restenosis in patients who have had self-expandable nitinol stents (Collins, 2021).

Surgical Interventions

If the PAD is unresponsive to lifestyle changes and pharmacologic management, then surgical interventions may be necessary. Deciding which surgical options is suitable for the patient depends on several issues such as the "wound ischemia, foot infection" (WIfI) stage, anatomic location and amount of disease, any comorbidities the patient may have, risk of the intervention, and which procedure the patient prefers. Surgical options revolve around whether or not the affected limb is salvageable (Berger & Davies, 2021). Surgical repair can be done by endovascular therapy (EVT) or open surgery. EVT is usually the first choice for revascularization. The only study to evaluate the benefits of EVT versus open surgery is the study by Bradbury et al. (2010), which did not prove an immediate benefit of open bypass over balloon angioplasty; however, at the 2-year mark after repair, the group who had open surgical bypass had improved amputation-free survival. A visual representation of medical therapy for patients with PAD is shown in Fig. 13.2.

The Society for Vascular Surgery (SVS) has implemented objective performance goals that are patient centered. Surveillance after surgical repair focuses on major adverse cardiovascular events (MACEs), 30-day major adverse limb events (MALEs), the 30-day amputation rate, amputation-free survival, and freedom from major adverse limb events.

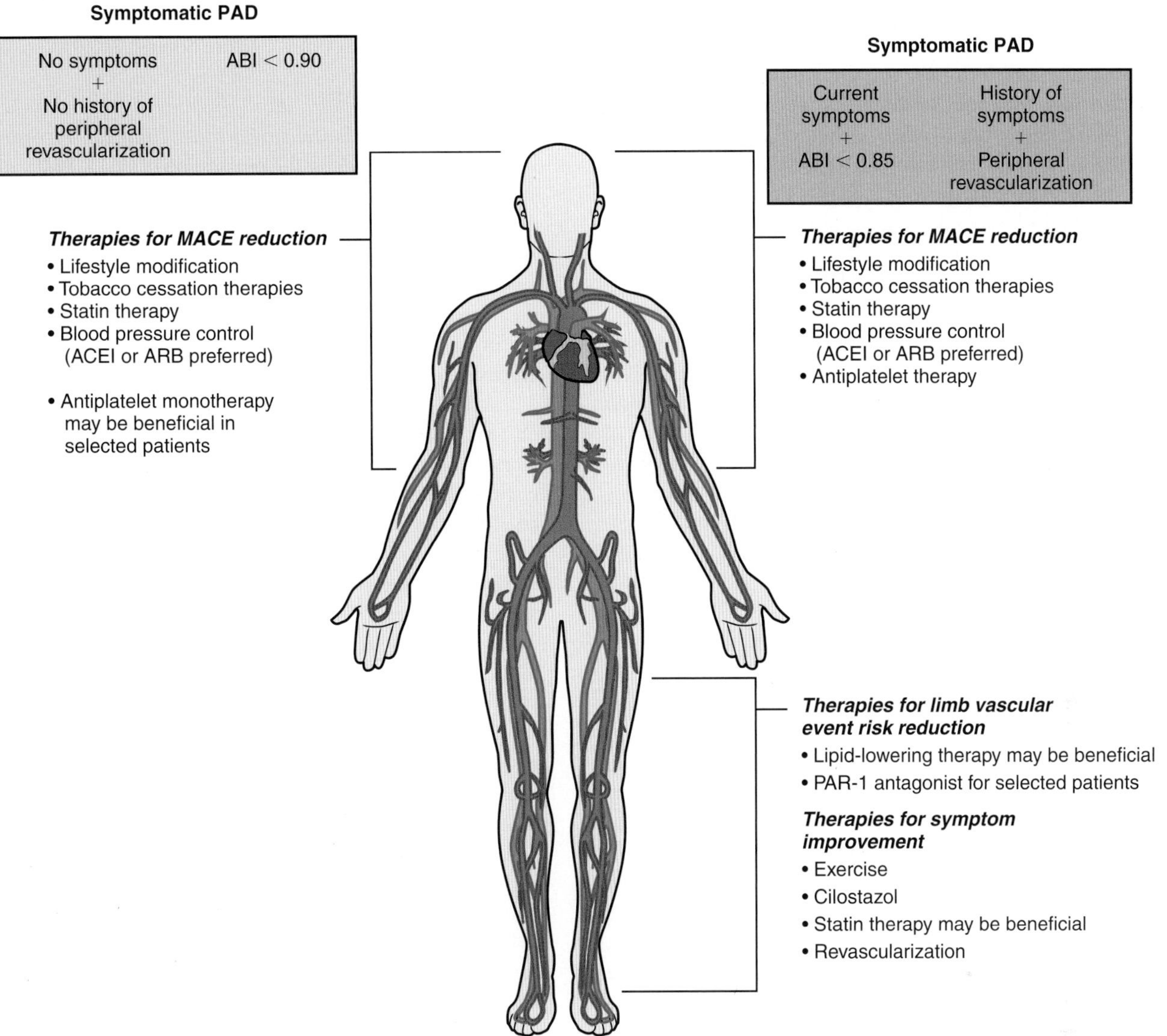
Symptomatic PAD
No symptoms + No history of peripheral revascularization
ABI < 0.90
Therapies for MACE reduction
• Lifestyle modification
• Tobacco cessation therapies
• Statin therapy
• Blood pressure control (ACEI or ARB preferred)
• Antiplatelet monotherapy may be beneficial in selected patients
Symptomatic PAD
Current symptoms + ABI < 0.85
History of symptoms + Peripheral revascularization
Therapies for MACE reduction
• Lifestyle modification
• Tobacco cessation therapies
• Statin therapy
• Blood pressure control (ACEI or ARB preferred)
• Antiplatelet therapy
Therapies for limb vascular event risk reduction
• Lipid-lowering therapy may be beneficial
• PAR-1 antagonist for selected patients
Therapies for symptom improvement
• Exercise
• Cilostazol
• Statin therapy may be beneficial
• Revascularization

• **Fig. 13.2** MACE, Major adverse cardiovascular events. (Modified from Bonaca, M. P., & Creager, M. A. [2015]. Pharmacological treatment and current management of peripheral artery disease. *Circulation Research, 116*, 1579–1598.)

Functionally, the patency of the surgical repair focuses on assessing the time to principal failure, such as occlusion or need for intervention, and the time to absolute failure after many revisions and interventions. Primary patency refers to patency that is obtained without the need for an additional or secondary surgical or endovascular procedure. Assisted primary patency refers to patency achieved with the use of an additional or secondary endovascular procedure as long as occlusion of the primary treated site has not occurred. Secondary patency refers to patency obtained with the use of an additional or secondary surgical procedure once occlusion occurs. Another outcome measure after revascularization procedures is the measurement of the ABI. An expected positive outcome would be an increase in the ABI of at least 0.15. The NP/PA needs to be aware of the main potential complications of surgical repair. Complications include thrombosis in the graft or stent, stenosis in the vein graft, and new thromboses or stenoses (Berger & Davies, 2021).

There is not a recognized interval follow-up after repair of PAD by an endovascular technique. Nevertheless, it is appropriate to follow up with patients after they have had endovascular repair. Follow-up should include a complete history and physical, evaluations of comorbid illnesses, any wounds that are due to a decrease in circulation, and ongoing measurement of the ankle-brachial indices. Also, a duplex ultrasound should be repeated within the first 30 days after EVT has been advised (Mills et al., 2022).

If the patient has had a surgical repair of PAD, the surveillance guidelines are clearly established. Four weeks after surgery, a duplex ultrasound, clinical evaluation, and ABI measurements should be done. Then follow-up will occur at the 3-, 6-, and 12-month time frame for the first 2 years.

If the patient has undergone an autologous vein graft, then duplex ultrasound, clinical evaluation, and ABI measurements should be done at 1-month, 3-month, 6-month, and 12-month follow-ups for 2 years.

The duplex ultrasound is better at detecting patency than an ABI measurement. A thorough evaluation of the distal and proximal anastomoses, the graft patency, native outflow, and inflow should be done. Grafts are considered at high risk of thromboses when either of these criteria are noted: peak systolic velocity (PSV) is > 300 cm/s and/or the velocity ratio (Vr) is > 3.5 at the site of the stenosis, or the globally low peak systolic graft flow velocity is < 45 cm/s or a drop in ABI is > 0.15 low flow velocity. If either of these conditions is noted, a diagnostic angiography should be performed.

Intrinsic vein graft stenosis is to blame for approximately 75% to 80% in the first 3 to 8 postoperative months. The rate of graft stenosis falls significantly after the first 2 years; then only annual surveillance is needed. Overall prognosis depends on the patient's specific risk factors for PAD, the vessels that were affected, and if heart disease or other comorbidities are affected (Berger & Davies, 2021). Complications of PAD include osteomyelitis, infection, wounds, and amputation.

Lifestyle Changes

Lifestyle changes for patients with peripheral artery disease are aimed at prevention and slowing the progression of the disease. Elevated cholesterol is a known factor leading to coronary artery disease and thereby peripheral artery disease. Studies show that adding statin therapy or a proprotein convertase subtilisin/kexin type 9 (PCSK9) inhibitor to a patient's medication regimen is associated with improved cardiovascular outcomes. The American College of Cardiology (ACC) and the American Heart Association (AHA) endorses that all patients with symptomatic PAD be prescribed a high-intensity statin such as atorvastatin 40 to 80 mg or rosuvastatin 20 to 40 mg. If the patient has an additional cardiovascular disease issue or two minor risk factors, the goal low-density lipoprotein should be < 70 (Bevan & White Solaru, 2020).

Antiplatelet therapy should also be initiated in patients with symptomatic PAD. In a small study conducted in 2007, low-dose aspirin (81 mg) was shown to produce a 64% relative risk in major cardiovascular events. The ACC and AHA classify antiplatelet therapy as a class I recommendation for PAD. Clopidogrel and ticagrelor can also be used instead of aspirin (Bevan & White Solaru, 2020).

Blood Pressure

Another lifestyle modification is to maintain blood pressure at < 130/80 mm Hg. This is considered a class IA recommendation from the ACC/AHA. However, the International Verapamil-SR/Trandolapril Study (INVEST) revealed a j-shaped curve of mortality and blood pressure. In patients who were diagnosed with PAD, the best mortality benefits were seen when the systolic blood pressure was 135 to 145 mm Hg and the diastolic pressure was 60 to 90 mm Hg. Because of the INVEST study, the European Society of Cardiology has endorsed the proposal that the patient's blood pressure should be < 140/90 mm Hg as a class IA recommendation (Bevan & White Solaru, 2020).

Smoking Cessation

Smoking cessation is the single most common recommendation to prevent or delay the progression of PAD. Willigendeal et al. (2004) found an increase of endothelial cell permeability, which leads to atherosclerosis, of 2.3-fold in current smokers. In addition, patients who smoke and have PAD have an increased mortality rate and smoking-related complications. Multidisciplinary endeavors encouraging and educating patients to quit smoking have been shown to be effective.

Exercise Therapy

Lack of exercise has been shown to cause plaque buildup and dysfunction of the endothelial cells, which causes the arteries to become stiff. This leads to claudication. Exercise can decrease plaque buildup and arterial stiffening. Numerous studies have shown that there is an increase in functional capacity after exercise. Therefore the ACC and AHA have categorized this as a class IA recommendation (Bevan & White Solaru, 2020).

Health Inequity

It is of utmost importance that the NP/PA emphasize health care equality for all patients, especially Black patients. Black patients have a high morbidity and mortality, and their incidence of PAD in this population is approximately two to three times that of non-Hispanic White patients. Being Black is one of the greatest risk factors for the development of PAD. Black patients are more two to four times more likely to suffer amputation when compared to non-Hispanic White patients. Additionally, graft failure is more likely to occur in Black patients (Bevan & White Solaru, 2020).

Peripheral arterial disease can be an overwhelming condition that can lead to significant morbidity and mortality. It is vital that the NP/PA be on the lookout for signs and symptoms of PAD in the geriatric patient.

Atrial Fibrillation

CASE STUDY 13.5

Sophia is a 69-year-old female who is brought to the emergency department by her daughter for complaints of dizziness, shortness of breath, and the feeling that her "heart is racing." Her heart rate is 154 beats per minute, blood pressure is 102/52 mm Hg, respiratory rate is 24 breaths per minute, and her oxygenation saturation is 87% on room air. Sophia states that she started feeling bad about 4 hours ago, and the pains are getting worse. Her past medical history is significant for coronary artery disease with stent placement and hypertension. An electrocardiogram (ECG) showed an irregularly irregular rhythm with a narrow QRS complex tachycardia. The patient is diagnosed with atrial fibrillation with a rapid ventricular response.

Pathophysiology

Atrial fibrillation (Afib) is the most prevalent arrhythmia and is a leading contributor to patient morbidity and mortality. The Centers for Disease Control and Prevention (CDC) estimates that by 2030, 12.1 million people will have atrial fibrillation (Centers for Disease Control and Prevention, 2020). The risk of atrial fibrillation increases with age and is the most prominent risk factor for Afib. Afib is designated as *recurrent* when the patient has two or more episodes. If this arrythmia ends spontaneously, then it is termed *paroxysmal atrial fibrillation* and if Afib requires electrical or pharmacologic intervention for termination then it is *persistent atrial fibrillation*. If atrial fibrillation lasts for over a year and it is not effectively terminated by any method, it is considered *permanent* (Dewar & Lip, 2007).

Afib can happen due to various pathophysiologic processes that occur in the atria. During Afib, the refractoriness of the atria leads to a loss of atrial contractility. Chronic heart disease stimulates signaling pathways that initiate cellular changes such as hypertrophy of the myocytes, proliferation of fibroblasts, and modifications to the extracellular matrix, which cause a chronic stretch of the atrial muscle, one of the risk factors for Afib. Neurohumoral activation and aging are additional causes of Afib. These alterations are referred to as *electrical remodeling*. The remodeling produces a shortened atrial effective refractory period (ERP), a shortened action potential duration (APD), and a reentry pathway (Schotten et al., 2011).

Changes to the cardiomyocytes and extracellular matrix of the atria have also been identified as an instigator of atrial fibrillation. Interstitial fibrosis can cause a delay in conduction. which produces an electrical impulse to generate a substitute pathway that will eventually encroach on tissue that has already recovered from its impulse, leading to reactivation and additional reentry circuits. If the atrial chamber is dilated, then the patient is at an increased risk of Afib.

Physical alterations other than changes to the myocytes and other molecular modifications have been identified as potential initiators of Afib. Structural remodeling has been proven to contribute to the sustainability of Afib. For example, patients with cardiomyopathy or end-stage heart failure have increased collagen in the extracellular matrix, which can cause and sustain Afib (Kourliouros et al., 2009).

Inflammation is another factor that can cause this arrythmia. Studies have shown that the cellular changes that occur in the setting of myocarditis can produce Afib. In addition, patients who have undergone cardiac surgery experience cellular inflammation, which, in turn, can trigger Afib in the postoperative period. Administration of antiinflammatory medications prior to surgery has been shown to prevent Afib in the postoperative cardiac patient (Jahangiri & Cramm, 2007).

C-reactive protein (CRP) is an acute phase reactant that is produced in the liver. High serum levels of CRP have been linked to an increased risk of cardiovascular events. CRP can cause an abnormal cell membrane that depletes energy and apoptosis, which is seen in oxidative stress and ischemia (Kourliouros et al., 2009). For a pictorial representation of the pathophysiology of atrial fibrillation, see Fig. 13.3.

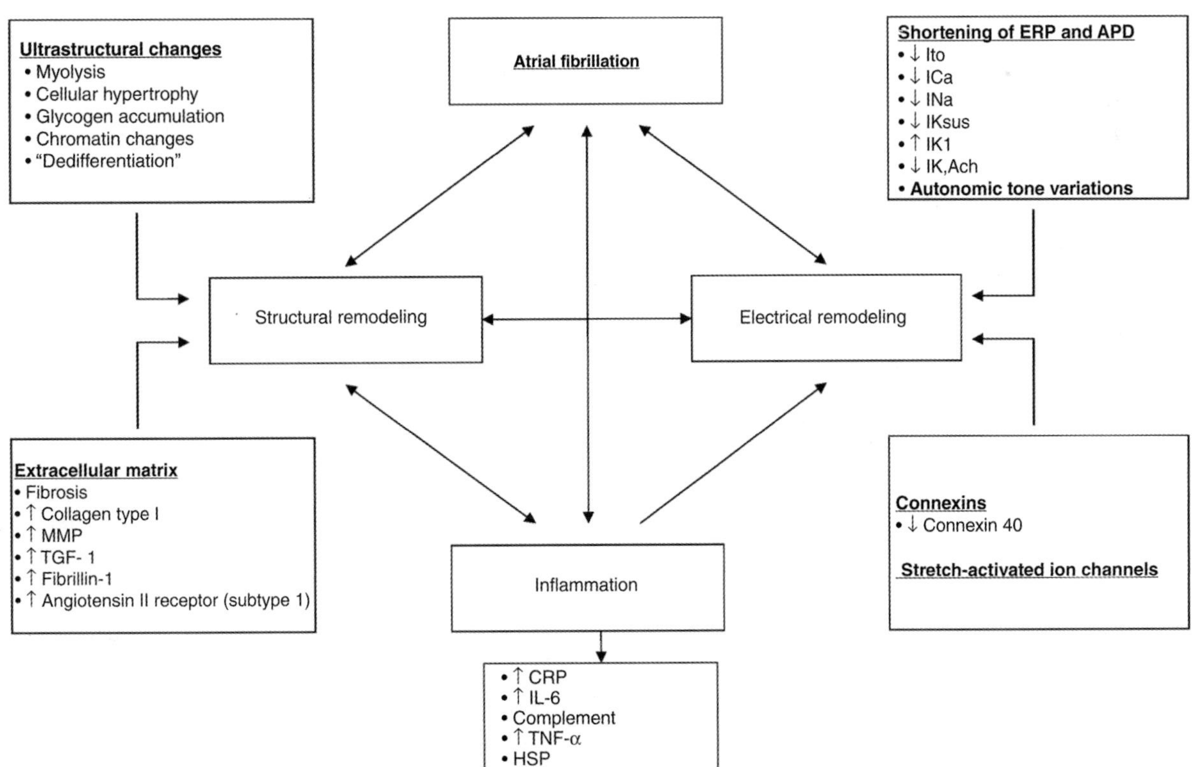

• **Fig. 13.3** Representation of pathophysiology of atrial fibrillation. (From Kourliouros, A., Savelieva, I, Kiotsekoglou, A., Jahangiri, M., & Camm, J. [2009]. Current concepts in the pathogenesis of atrial fibrillation. *American Heart Journal, 157*[2], 243–252.)

Assessment

The symptoms of atrial fibrillation can be very mild or life threatening and disabling. The most common symptoms are dizziness, dyspnea, fatigue, lightheadedness, decreased exercise capacity, and palpitations. Symptoms can come and go even if the patient is in Afib. Approximately a quarter of patients do not have any symptoms, and this is common in the older adult patient. Many of these symptoms are nonspecific; a diagnostic cardioversion may be utilized to ascertain if the patient feels better when she or he is in a normal rhythm. A diagnostic cardioversion can also be used to guide the practitioner's goal of treatment: rhythm control or rate control (Morady & Zipes, 2019).

Because symptoms of Afib are so subjective and can range from minor to severe, the European Heart Rhythm Association (EHRA) created a guide to use as an aid in classifying symptoms.

The older adult patient should be queried about the onset of symptoms, frequency and duration, and severity, and a determination should be made regarding the type of atrial fibrillation, whether it is paroxysmal or persistent. In addition, the timing of Afib episodes should also be gleaned from the patient. If this is unable to be determined, then it may be necessary to order 2 to 4 weeks of ambulatory monitoring.

The NP/PA should ask about any precipitating factors, such as alcohol consumption or exercise, and if the patient has any associated diseases, such as preexisting cerebrovascular or cardiovascular disease, hypertension, diabetes, obstructive sleep apnea, chronic obstructive pulmonary disease, or excessive alcohol intake.

Blood testing should include electrolytes, complete blood count, thyroid, liver, and kidney function. Coagulation studies such as the prothrombin time/international normalized ratio (INR) and activated partial thromboplastin time need to be ordered.

If there is a suspicion of Afib, then the patient should have an electrocardiography (ECG). Correct interpretation of the ECG is essential to confirm a diagnosis of Afib. An echocardiogram should also be performed to calculate the size of the atria and left ventricular function. Any evidence of congenital heart disease or left ventricular hypertrophy should also be assessed. If the NP/PA suspects a pulmonary component, then a chest radiography should be done. If the patient is at risk for ischemic heart disease, then it is appropriate to order a stress test (Morady & Zipes, 2019).

Atrial Fibrillation and Stroke

Atrial fibrillation is a known risk factor for a cerebrovascular accident (CVA) or stroke. Approximately 20% of all strokes are due to atrial fibrillation. In patients who are 80 years and older, this increases to 25%. Atrial fibrillation is associated with a fivefold increased risk of ischemic stroke. When a stroke is due to atrial fibrillation, patients suffer greater neurologic disability, decreased functional outcomes, and an increased rate of mortality (Kotecha et al., 2018).

When a patient has Afib, the thrombi tend to congregate in the left atrial appendage because of the decreased emptying and stagnant flow in this area. Most, but not all, thrombi are formed in this area.

The CHADS$_2$ score, which stands for congestive heart failure, age, diabetes, and previous stroke or transient ischemic attack, was created in 2001 and is used to determine stroke risk among patients over 65 years old. Each of these items are given a point score of 1 or 2. The risk for stroke is rated low if the total is 0 to 1, intermediate if the score is 1 to 2, and high if the score is ≥3.

The CHADS$_2$ score was revised in 2010 to include additional known risk factors such as age, vascular disease, any interventions (percutaneous coronary intervention, myocardial infarction, coronary artery bypass graft, pulmonary vein disease), and female gender. This revised score, CHA$_2$ DS$_2$ -VASc, is now the preferred risk stratification tool and has been validated in numerous studies (Rossi & Mounsey, 2019).

Patients with Afib have a higher risk of hypertensive stroke and atherosclerosis; these two issues are the leading risk factors for cerebrovascular events worldwide. The CHA$_2$ DS$_2$ -VASc score has been used to foresee other acute cardiovascular issues in patients.

These patients also have a higher risk of bleeding complications, and bleeding risk increases with age. If the risk of bleeding outweighs the benefits of oral anticoagulation, many patients choose to go without anticoagulation. There is a guide that has been authenticated to estimate bleeding risk. The HAS-BLED (Hypertension, Abnormal renal/liver function, Stroke, Bleeding, Labile international normalized ratio, Elderly, Drugs or alcohol use) calculation is recommended by the American College of Cardiology/American Heart Association/Heart Rhythm Society and European and Canadian Atrial Fibrillation guidelines to assess bleeding risk in older adult patients (Rossi & Mounsey, 2019).

Besides than stroke, patients with atrial fibrillation are prone to other cardiovascular and noncardiovascular outcomes. Heart failure is often a coexisting condition found in patients with Afib. When Afib causes acute heart failure, it is called tachycardiomyopathy and is caused by the fast heart rate. However, when Afib occurs after a patient has been diagnosed with heart failure, there is an increase in mortality regardless of the type of heart failure, systolic or diastolic dysfunction. In addition, females have a higher mortality rate if they have heart failure and then develop atrial fibrillation (Kotecha et al., 2018).

Treatment

The goal of treating atrial fibrillation is to avoid thromboembolic events, such as strokes, which can lead to poorer quality of life and worse patient outcomes. Treatment of acute atrial fibrillation will be determined by the patient's hemodynamic status. If the patient is hypotensive, has congestive heart failure, or angina, then the patient should receive conscious sedation and have synchronized cardioversion.

Thromboembolic episodes can be prevented with anticoagulant therapy. Also, catheter ablation is another technique that can be used to abort atrial fibrillation. Catheter ablation is highly contraindicated in patients who have a thrombus in the left atrium or in patients who are unable to receive anticoagulation for at least 6 to 8 weeks after the ablation (Karamichalakis et al., 2015).

Anticoagulation in the older adult patient requires special attention. The revised CHA_2DS_2-VASc highlights the importance of considerations of advanced age in anticoagulation therapy. According to the CHA_2DS_2-VASc, all patients over 75 years old should receive anticoagulation, except if there is a strong contraindication. The target international normalized ratio (INR) is 2.0 to 3.0. Keeping an INR > 3.0 has been shown to increase the patient's risk of bleeding. The INR needs to be checked routinely even if the patient has been stable. Vitamin K antagonists, such as warfarin, are routinely used in patients with a history of atrial fibrillation. Newer anticoagulant medications, such as dabigatran, edoxaban, apixaban, and rivaroxaban, are becoming more popular in the aging population. Dabigatran, a direct thrombin inhibitor, has been shown to reduce cerebral hemorrhage risk in patients who are 75 years and older when dosed at 110 mg twice daily. If the patient has a creatinine clearance that is less than 30 mL/min, the dabigatran should be cautiously used because it is renally eliminated. Rivaroxaban, which is a direct factor Xa inhibitor, has been shown to cause less intracranial bleeding and fatal hemorrhages but should also be used cautiously if the patient's creatinine clearance is less than 30 mL/min (Karamichalakis et al., 2015).

In the older adult patient, oral anticoagulant therapy can be difficult. Patients who are 75 years and older who present with atrial fibrillation after acute coronary syndrome with revascularization require three antithrombotic medications. Aspirin, an oral anticoagulant, and clopidogrel are required for at least 4 weeks and potentially 6 months. After the acute phase of treatment, an antiplatelet medication plus an oral anticoagulant are required for 1 year.

If the patient has atrial fibrillation and stable coronary artery disease with revascularization, then the three-medication regimen is only required for 2 to 4 weeks with dual therapy for the next 1 to 12 months. For patients who have not received revascularization, monotherapy with a vitamin K antagonist or a newer oral anticoagulant medication is sufficient (Karamichalakis et al., 2015).

Due to the potential for fatal hemorrhages in the geriatric patient, many patients are choosing to undergo a relatively new procedure called a percutaneous left atrial appendage (LAA) closure. This is an invasive procedure that is usually done under general anesthesia. The cardiologist inserts the catheter into the venous system and deploys the device into the left atrial appendage (Karamichalakis et al., 2015). In approximately 45 days, thin layers of tissue will grow over the device, which prevents thrombi from entering the bloodstream.

Contraindications to using anticoagulants include esophageal varices, active bleeding, peptic ulcer within the past 3 months, neoplasms, clotting issues, anemia, myelodysplastic syndrome, liver disease, and thrombocytopenia. It is important for the NP/PA to remember that frailty, comorbidities, and increased risk of falling does not outweigh the benefits of oral anticoagulation.

Recommended guidelines for cardioversion of atrial fibrillation can be found in Table 13.8. The risk of incurring a thromboembolism in atrial fibrillation is considered low if the Afib lasts less than 48 hours. The risk increases the longer the patient remains in Afib. If the practitioner elects to perform cardioversion and a transesophageal echocardiogram does not show an atrial thrombus, then cardioversion can be safely executed if the patient is appropriately anticoagulated. It is also acceptable to perform cardioversion up to 1 month after therapeutic anticoagulation has been achieved without conducting a transesophageal echocardiogram. The patient should remain on anticoagulation for at least 30 days after cardioversion to decrease the possibility of having a thromboembolic event. If the patient remains in sinus rhythm after the 30 days, then the anticoagulation can be discontinued as long as the patient's CHA_2DS_2-VASc is low.

Table 13.9 shows the ACC/AHA recommendations for the rate control of Afib. These recommendations are for the hemodynamically stable. Table 13.10 provides the recommendation from the ACC/AHA for maintaining sinus rhythm after atrial fibrillation.

Lifestyle Changes

There are several lifestyle changes that can be made to reduce one's risk of developing atrial fibrillation. Quitting smoking, managing high blood pressure, and reducing alcohol consumption are just a few modifications.

Smoking has been associated with causing atrial fibrillation in several studies. A study by Heeringa et al. (2008) showed that everyday smokers had a 2.1 times increased risk for Afib and former smokers had a 1.3 times increased risk of Afib. Quitting smoking can reduce the patient's risk of having Afib by 36%.

High blood pressure is another cause that is known to contribute to atrial fibrillation. James et al. (2014) discovered that poorly managed hypertension increased the patient's risk of developing Afib by 56%. Staerk et al. (2018) found that hypertension increased the incidence of Afib in patients who were 65 years old by 57% and increased the incidence of Afib in patients who were 75 years old by 70%.

Drinking alcohol has been proven to increase the prevalence of Afib. The lifetime risk of experiencing Afib if the patient consumes alcohol on a routine basis was found to be 40.9% compared to 35.1% for people who did not consume

TABLE 13.8 American College of Cardiology (ACC)/American Heart Association (AHA) Recommendations for Cardioversion of Atrial Fibrillation

Class	Indication	Level of Evidence
	Pharmacologic Cardioversion	
Class I (indicated)	Administration of flecainide, dofetilide, propafenone, or ibutilide is recommended for pharmacologic cardioversion of AF.	A
Class IIa (reasonable)	Administration of amiodarone is a reasonable option for pharmacologic cardioversion of AF.	A
	A single oral bolus dose of propafenone or flecainide ("pill-in-the-pocket") can be administered to terminate persistent AF outside the hospital once treatment has proved safe in the hospital for selected patients without sinus or AV node dysfunction, bundle branch block, QT interval prolongation, the Brugada syndrome, or structural heart disease. Before antiarrhythmic medication is initiated, a beta-blocker or nondihydropyridine calcium channel antagonist should be given to prevent rapid AV conduction in the event atrial flutter occurs.	C
	Administration of amiodarone can be beneficial on an outpatient basis in patients with paroxysmal or persistent AF when rapid restoration of sinus rhythm is not deemed necessary.	C
Class IIb (may be considered)	Administration of quinidine or procainamide might be considered for pharmacologic cardioversion of AF, but the usefulness of these agents is not well established.	C
Class III (not indicated)	Digoxin and sotalol may be harmful when used for pharmacologic cardioversion of AF and are not recommended.	A
	Quinidine, procainamide, disopyramide, and dofetilide should not be started out of the hospital for conversion of AF to sinus rhythm.	B
Direct-Current Cardioversion		
Class I (indicated)	When a rapid ventricular response does not respond promptly to pharmacologic measures for patients with AF with ongoing myocardial ischemia, symptomatic hypotension, angina, or heart failure, immediate R wave–synchronized direct-current cardioversion is recommended.	C
	Immediate direct-current cardioversion is recommended for patients with AF involving preexcitation when very rapid tachycardia or hemodynamic instability occurs.	B
	Cardioversion is recommended in patients without hemodynamic instability when symptoms of AF are unacceptable to the patient. In case of early relapse of AF after cardioversion, repeated direct-current cardioversion attempts may be made after administration of antiarrhythmic medication.	C
Class IIa (reasonable)	Direct-current cardioversion can be useful to restore sinus rhythm as part of a long-term management strategy for patients with AF.	B
	The patient's preference is a reasonable consideration in the selection of infrequently repeated cardioversions for the management of symptomatic or recurrent AF.	C
Class III (not indicated)	Frequent repetition of direct-current cardioversion is not recommended for patients who have relatively short periods of sinus rhythm between relapses of AF after multiple cardioversion procedures despite prophylactic antiarrhythmic drug therapy.	C
	Electrical cardioversion is contraindicated in patients with digitalis toxicity or hypokalemia.	C
Pharmacologic Enhancement of Direct-Current Cardioversion		
Class IIa (reasonable)	Pretreatment with amiodarone, flecainide, ibutilide, propafenone, or sotalol can be useful to enhance the success of direct-current cardioversion and to prevent recurrent AF.	B
	In patients who relapse to AF after successful cardioversion, it can be useful to repeat the procedure after prophylactic administration of antiarrhythmic medication.	C

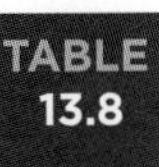

TABLE 13.8 **American College of Cardiology (ACC)/American Heart Association (AHA) Recommendations for Cardioversion of Atrial Fibrillation—cont'd**

Class	Indication	Level of Evidence
Class IIb (may be considered)	For patients with persistent AF, administration of beta-blockers, disopyramide, diltiazem, dofetilide, procainamide, or verapamil may be considered, although the efficacy of these agents to enhance the success of direct-current cardioversion or to prevent early recurrence of AF is uncertain.	C
	Out-of-hospital initiation of antiarrhythmic medications may be considered in patients without heart disease to enhance the success of cardioversion of AF.	C
	Out-of-hospital administration of antiarrhythmic medications may be considered to enhance the success of cardioversion of AF in patients with certain forms of heart disease once the safety of the drug has been verified for the patient.	C
Prevention of Thromboembolism in Patients With Atrial Fibrillation Undergoing Cardioversion		
Class I (indicated)	For patients with AF of 48-hr duration or longer, or when the duration of AF is unknown, anticoagulation (INR 2.0–3.0) is recommended for at least 3 wk before and 4 wk after cardioversion, regardless of the method (electrical or pharmacologic) used to restore sinus rhythm.	B
	For patients with AF of more than 48-hr duration requiring immediate cardioversion because of hemodynamic instability, heparin should be administered concurrently (unless contraindicated) by an initial intravenous bolus injection, followed by a continuous infusion in a dose adjusted to prolong the activated partial thromboplastin time to 1.5 to 2× the reference control value. Thereafter, oral anticoagulation (INR, 2.0–3.0) should be provided for at least 4 wk, as for patients undergoing elective cardioversion. Limited data support subcutaneous administration of low-molecular-weight heparin in this indication.	C
	For patients with AF of less than 48-hr duration associated with hemodynamic instability (angina pectoris, myocardial infarction, shock, or pulmonary edema), cardioversion should be performed immediately, without delay, for prior initiation of anticoagulation.	C
Class IIa (reasonable)	During the 48 hr after onset of AF, the need for anticoagulation before and after cardioversion may be based on the patient's risk of thromboembolism.	C
	As an alternative to anticoagulation before cardioversion of AF, it is reasonable to perform transesophageal echocardiography in search of thrombus in the left atrium or left atrial appendage.	B
	a. For patients with no identifiable thrombus, cardioversion is reasonable immediately after anticoagulation with unfractionated heparin (e.g., initiated by intravenous bolus injection and an infusion continued at a dose adjusted to prolong the activated partial thromboplastin time to 1.5–2× the control value until oral anticoagulation has been established with an oral vitamin K antagonist [e.g., warfarin] as evidenced by an INR ≥2.0).	B
	Thereafter, continuation of oral anticoagulation (INR, 2.0–3.0) is reasonable for a total anticoagulation period of at least 4 wk, as for patients undergoing elective cardioversion.	B
	Limited data are available to support the subcutaneous administration of a low-molecular-weight heparin in this indication.	C
	b. For patients in whom thrombus is identified by transesophageal echocardiography, oral anticoagulation (INR, 2.0–3.0) is reasonable for at least 3 wk before and 4 wk after restoration of sinus rhythm, and a longer period of anticoagulation may be appropriate even after apparently successful cardioversion because the risk of thromboembolism often remains elevated in such cases.	C
	For patients with atrial flutter undergoing cardioversion, anticoagulation can be beneficial according to the recommendations as for patients with AF.	C

From Zipes, D. P. (2019). *Braunwald's heart disease: A textbook of cardiovascular medicine* (11th ed.). Elsevier.

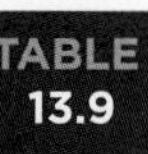

TABLE 13.9 American College of Cardiology (ACC)/American Heart Association (AHA) Recommendations for Rate Control of Afib

Class	Indication	Level of Evidence
Class I (indicated)	Measurement of the heart rate at rest and control of the rate with pharmacologic agents (either a beta-blocker or nondihydropyridine calcium channel antagonist, in most cases) are recommended for patients with persistent or permanent AF.	B
	In the absence of preexcitation, intravenous administration of beta-blockers (esmolol, metoprolol, or propranolol) or nondihydropyridine calcium channel antagonists (verapamil, diltiazem) is recommended to slow the ventricular response to AF in the acute setting, exercising caution in patients with hypotension or heart failure.	B
	Intravenous administration of digoxin or amiodarone is recommended to control heart rate in patients with AF and heart failure who do not have an accessory pathway.	B
	In patients who experience symptoms related to AF during activity, the adequacy of heart rate control should be assessed during exercise, adjusting pharmacologic treatment as necessary to keep the rate in the physiologic range.	C
	Digoxin is effective after oral administration to control the heart rate at rest in patients with AF and is indicated for patients with heart failure or left ventricular dysfunction and for sedentary individuals.	C
Class IIa (reasonable)	A combination of digoxin and either a beta-blocker or nondihydropyridine calcium channel antagonist is reasonable to control the heart rate both at rest and during exercise in patients with AF. The choice of medication should be individualized and the dose modulated to avoid bradycardia.	B
	It is reasonable to use ablation of the AV node or accessory pathway to control heart rate when pharmacologic therapy is insufficient or associated with side effects.	B
	Intravenous amiodarone can be useful to control heart rate in patients with AF when other measures are unsuccessful or contraindicated.	C
	When electrical cardioversion is not necessary in patients with AF and an accessory pathway, intravenous procainamide or ibutilide is a reasonable alternative.	C
Class IIb (may be considered)	When the ventricular rate cannot be adequately controlled both at rest and during exercise in patients with AF by a beta-blocker, nondihydropyridine calcium channel antagonist, or digoxin, alone or in combination, oral amiodarone may be administered to control the heart rate.	C
	Intravenous procainamide, disopyramide, ibutilide, or amiodarone may be considered for hemodynamically stable patients with AF involving conduction over an accessory pathway	B
	When the rate cannot be controlled with pharmacologic agents or tachycardia-mediated cardiomyopathy is suspected, catheter-directed ablation of the AV node may be considered in patients with AF to control the heart rate.	C
Class III (not indicated)	Strict rate control (<80 beats/min at rest or <110 beats/min during 6-minute walk) is not beneficial compared to a resting rate <110 beats/min in asymptomatic patients with persistent AF and an ejection fraction >40%, although uncontrolled tachycardia can lead to reversible left ventricular dysfunction over time.	B
	Digitalis should not be used as the sole agent to control the rate of ventricular response in patients with paroxysmal AF.	B
	Catheter ablation of the AV node should not be attempted without a prior trial of medication to control the ventricular rate in patients with AF.	C
	In patients with decompensated heart failure and AF, intravenous administration of a nondihydropyridine calcium channel antagonist may exacerbate hemodynamic compromise and is not recommended.	C
	Intravenous administration of digitalis glycosides or nondihydropyridine calcium channel antagonists to patients with AF and a preexcitation syndrome may paradoxically accelerate the ventricular response and is not recommended.	C

From Zipes, D. P. (2019). *Braunwald's heart disease: A textbook of cardiovascular medicine* (11th ed.). Elsevier.

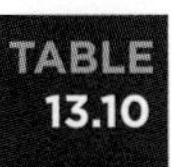

TABLE 13.10 American College of Cardiology (ACC)/American Heart Association (AHA) Recommendations for Maintaining Sinus Rhythm After Atrial Fibrillation

Class	Indication	Level of Evidence
Class I (indicated)	Before initiation of antiarrhythmic drug therapy, treatment of precipitating or reversible causes of AF is recommended.	C
	Catheter ablation by an experienced operator is useful in selected patients with symptomatic paroxysmal AF who have failed treatment with an antiarrhythmic drug and have a normal or mildly dilated left atrium and normal or mildly reduced left ventricular function.	A
Class IIa (reasonable)	Pharmacologic therapy can be useful in patients with AF to maintain sinus rhythm and to prevent tachycardia-induced cardiomyopathy.	C
	Infrequent, well-tolerated recurrence of AF is reasonable as a successful outcome of antiarrhythmic drug therapy.	C
	Outpatient initiation of antiarrhythmic drug therapy is reasonable in patients with AF who have no associated heart disease when the agent is well tolerated.	C
	In patients with lone AF without structural heart disease, initiation of propafenone or flecainide can be beneficial on an outpatient basis in patients with paroxysmal AF who are in sinus rhythm at the time of drug initiation.	B
	Sotalol can be beneficial in outpatients in sinus rhythm with little or no heart disease, prone to paroxysmal AF, if the baseline uncorrected QT interval is shorter than 460 milliseconds, serum electrolyte values are normal, and risk factors associated with class III drug–related proarrhythmia are not present.	C
	Catheter ablation is a reasonable for treatment of symptomatic persistent AF.	A
Class IIb (may be considered)	Catheter ablation may be reasonable for patients with symptomatic paroxysmal AF and significant left atrial dilation or significant left ventricular dysfunction.	A
Class III (not indicated)	Antiarrhythmic therapy with a particular drug is not recommended for maintenance of sinus rhythm in patients with AF who have well-defined risk factors for proarrhythmia with that agent.	A
	Pharmacologic therapy is not recommended for maintenance of sinus rhythm in patients with advanced sinus node disease or AV node dysfunction unless they have a functioning electronic cardiac pacemaker.	C

From Zipes, D. P. (2019). *Braunwald's heart disease: A textbook of cardiovascular medicine* (11th ed.). Elsevier.

alcohol. Only one drink a day can statistically increase the patient's risk of incurring Afib by 10% (Staerk et al., 2018).

Lack of sleep has been shown in several studies to be a modifiable risk factor for Afib. Patients with obstructive sleep apnea (OSA) have a four times higher risk of developing atrial fibrillation regardless of age, obesity, heart failure, or hypertension. Also, 49% of people with Afib also have OSA. Neilan et al. (2013) found that patients with OSA are at a higher risk of recurrent Afib after cardioversion or catheter ablation. They also found that OSA should be adequately treated to reduce the risk of atrial fibrillation in these patients.

Patients who suffer from insomnia for reasons other than OSA are also at an increased risk for experiencing Afib. A study by Kayrak et al. (2013) discovered that even acute loss of sleep can increase a patient's risk of developing Afib by 3.6 times.

Diabetes mellitus can also be a factor in developing atrial fibrillation because of the many systemic effects of high blood sugar. Dublin et al. (2010) discovered that the higher the patient's hemoglobin A1c and the longer the patient has had diabetes, the higher the risk of Afib.

Other modifiable risk factors are an unhealthy diet and obesity. The Women's Health Study Study (Tedrow et al., 2010) and the Atherosclerosis Risk in Communities (ARIC) study (Huxley et al., 2014) discovered that weight gain is linked to an increased risk of Afib. Patients who have chronic atrial fibrillation can decrease the burden of Afib and symptom severity by losing weight and eating a healthier diet. Pathak et al. (2014) found that losing weight improves the long-term success of Afib ablation, better control of symptoms, and recurrence-free survival.

A positive mental outlook is another modifiable risk factor that has been studied extensively. Lampert et al. (2014) found that atrial fibrillation occurred 85% less on days that patients recorded as "happy days." Emotions such as sadness, stress, anger, anxiety, and impatience have been shown to trigger symptomatic atrial fibrillation. Also, practicing yoga has been proven to decrease the incidence of Afib by almost 24%.

Atrial fibrillation is the most common dysrhythmia in developed countries. The NP/PA needs to be well-informed of the signs and symptoms, assessment, treatment, and lifestyle modifications as they pertain to the geriatric patient to decrease the patient's morbidity and mortality.

• BOX 13.1 Rome IV Criteria for Functional Constipation

Must include two or more of the following: (Criteria fulfilled for the past 3 months with symptom onset at least 6 months prior to diagnosis.)

- Loose stools are rarely present without the use of laxatives
- Insufficient criteria for irritable bowel syndrome
  a. Straining during more than 25% of defecations
  b. Lumpy or hard stools
  c. Sensation of incomplete evacuation during more than 25% of defecations
  d. Sensation of anorectal obstruction/blockage during more than 25% of defecations
  e. Manual maneuvers (e.g., digital evacuation, support of the pelvic floor) to facilitate more than 25% of defecations
  f. Fewer than three spontaneous bowel movements per week

From Lacy, B. E., Mearin, F., Chang, L. (2016). Bowel disorders. *Gastroenterology*. 150:1393–1407.e5.

Chronic Constipation

CASE STUDY 13.6

A 67-year-old male presents to the emergency department with complaints of generalized abdominal pain and distention. He reports that his last bowel movement was 7 days ago. He states that he usually has a bowel movement every day. He denies fever, vomiting, or diarrhea. He has a history of high cholesterol and hypertension. Otherwise he is in good physical condition. His heart rate is 100 beats per minute, blood pressure is 146/90, his respiratory rate is 16 breaths per minute, and his temperature is 98.4 °F. His abdomen is distended and large, with tympanic bowel sounds in all four quadrants. There is diffuse tenderness to palpation throughout.

Pathophysiology

Constipation is a common complaint for patients that can occur at any age. However, the complaint is more prevalent due to diminished rectal sensation, decreased resting anal pressures, and decreased rectal compliance (Gaines, 2021).

Constipation is a term used to describe a patient's opinion of his or her bowel movements. It is important to ask patients what they mean when they say that they are constipated. Patients may describe their bowel habit as having hard stools, pain with defecation, and a feeling that they still have stool in the rectal vault. In the medical community, constipation is defined as three or fewer bowel movements per week. However, among patients the definition can vary. Because of this, the Rome Criteria was developed in 1992 but has been revised to its current version, the Rome IV Criteria for Functional Constipation (see Box 13.1) (Lacy et al., 2016).

Constipation is considered chronic when these symptoms persist for at least 3 consecutive months. Chronic constipation can have many causes such as neurologic issues or metabolic conditions, and it can even be due to certain medications. Chronic constipation can be divided into three categories. These categories involve the rate of transition through the colon are are referred to as slow-transit, normal-transit, and rectal evacuation disorder (Iturrino & Lembo, 2021).

Approximately 30% of people will experience constipation at some point in their life. Older adult men, as well as women of all ages, are more commonly affected. However, most people rely on the advice of television commercials, pharmacists, and friends (De Giorgio et al., 2015). The overall prevalence is projected to be 14%. Interestingly, when the Rome Criteria are utilized to define constipation, it is estimated to be lower than 14%; when constipation is self-reported, it is estimated to be higher than 14%. "According to data from the National Emergency Department Sample, the frequency of emergency department visits for constipation in the United States increased by 41.5% between 2006 and 2011, and the associated costs increased by 121.4%" (Iturrino & Lembo, 2021).

Slow Transit Constipation

Slow transit constipation is when the time for the stool to pass through the colon is slower than normal. This is often accompanied by reduced sensation in the rectum. The motor activity is irregular. The colonic waves should allow the lumina in the colon to absorb water and electrolytes by propulsive waves, but in slow transit constipation this does not happen. In addition, the gastro-colic reflex is defective in these patients. This modified motility is the major reason for the slowdown of gastrointestinal contents in people who have slow transit constipation.

There are endocrine, metabolic, and structural disorders that can lead to slow transit constipation. Hypercalcemia, hypothyroidism, and diabetes mellitus can delay transit time. Structural abnormalities can include myopathies and neuropathies. In older adults there are two applicable characteristics that contribute to slow transit constipation. There is an abundance of collagen in the ascending colon and there are more binding sites for plasma endorphins. These two mechanisms can impact fecal transit time (De Giorgio et al., 2015).

Outlet Obstruction

Outlet obstruction can happen due to miscoordination between the pelvic floor muscles relaxing and the contraction of the abdominal muscles. Outlet obstruction can also happen due to an obstruction in the perineal area, urogynecologic conditions, or anorectal abnormalities.

Loss of muscle mass and contractility and injury to the pudendal nerve can cause a decrease in the pressure of the anal sphincter at rest and while trying to have a bowel movement. In the older adult patient, there is a decrease in elasticity of the rectal wall and added thickness of the internal anal sphincter. Anal fissures, rectocele, hemorrhoids, pelvic floor dysfunction, anal stenosis, and urogynecologic ailments can not only cause constipation but also incontinence in the older adult patient (De Giorgio et al., 2015).

Secondary Causes of Constipation

Other causes of constipation can include medications, especially narcotics, which slow transit time in the colon. Neuropathic conditions such as amyloidosis, central nervous system lesions, and multiple sclerosis can also be factors. Idiopathic diseases can also cause constipation; some of these conditions include Parkinson disease, dementia, spinal tumors, ischemia, and paraneoplastic syndromes.

Assessment

The patient with constipation will usually complain of gas, abdominal distention, bloating, hard stools, difficulty having a bowel movement, and abdominal pain. The NP/PA should perform a physical exam, including a check of vital signs and weight. All quadrants of the abdominal area should be auscultated, percussed, and palpated. A digital rectal exam should also be conducted to assess for rectal tone, anorectal disorders, impaction, or rectal mass.

In addition, the clinician should test serum electrolytes, hemoglobin, and thyroid stimulating hormone. Any red flag symptoms such as sudden, unplanned weight loss, abdominal cramping, acute onset, rectal bleeding, nausea or vomiting, and fever will require a computed tomography, barium enema, or endoscopy of the abdomen and pelvis. If there is suspicion of pelvic floor dysfunction or defecatory issues, then an anorectal examination with manometry and a rectal balloon expulsion test should take place. If slow transit constipation problems are suspected, then transit rates with radiopaque markers should be evaluated using serial abdominal x-rays over 4 to 7 days (Gaines, 2021).

Treatment

The goals of treatment should be discussed with the patient at the beginning of treatment. The first goal should be to decrease the patient's symptoms, and the second goal should be to resolve the patient's constipation so the patient is having a bowel movement at least three times a week.

Unless the patient is dehydrated, giving the patient fluids is not indicated. Probiotics have not shown any benefit either. Patients can be advised to place their feet on a small stool while sitting on the toilet to help straighten out the anorectal junction (Mounsey et al., 2015).

Advising patients to start an exercise regimen or to increase the amount of exercise that they are already doing has not been shown to provide benefits in relieving constipation either. However, increasing fiber intake to 30 g/day has been found to provide some benefit. Patients can increase their fiber by increasing their intake of fruit, vegetables, and nuts. In addition, taking a fiber supplement in the form of gummies, crackers, or tablets can aid in relieving constipation.

There are pharmacologic agents that can relieve symptoms of constipation. See Table 13.11 for a list of medicinal treatments.

Suppositories or enemas are good options for patients who cannot take an oral medication. Mineral oil enemas are much safer than phosphate enemas, as they do not cause significant electrolyte problems. Warm water enemas are also acceptable, as are glycerin suppositories (Mounsey et al., 2015).

Psyllium, bran, methylcellulose, and polycarbophil are bulking agents that are safe to use in the older patient. These treatments work by absorbing water into the digestive system and softening the stool. Psyllium and bran have been shown to increase stool frequency in patients. Psyllium has side effects such as gas, distention, and bloating, which may prove bothersome for the geriatric patient. Do not use bulk-forming laxatives if there is a fecal impaction (Mounsey et al., 2015).

Osmotic laxatives are another choice of treatment when the goal is to draw water into the intestine. Sorbitol and lactulose will increase the frequency of bowel movements and are absorbed by the mucosa of the colon. Polyethylene glycol (PEG) is another laxative that has been used for many years and has fewer side effects than sorbitol or lactulose.

Magnesium preparations such as magnesium salts have not been thoroughly studied for use in the older patient population. Side effects of magnesium-based laxatives include ileus formation and can even make constipation worse. Due to the lack of clinical data, it is best to not use magnesium salts, such as magnesium hydroxide and magnesium citrate, in this population (Mounsey et al., 2015).

Stimulant laxatives are another option for older adult patients. These work by promoting intestinal motility and increasing the fluid in the bowel. Long-term use of stimulant

TABLE 13.11 **Medicinal Management of Constipation**

Class	Drug Name (Brand)	Adult Dosing	Mechanism of Action	Time to Onset (H)	Adverse Effects
Fiber	Bran Psyllium (Metamucil) Methylcellulose (Citrucel) Calcium polycarbophil (FiberCon)	1 cup/day 1 tsp 1 tbsp or 1 tab twice daily 2–4 tabs/day	Increase water content and bulk of stool decreasing transit time	Unknown	Bloating excessive gas
Hyperosmolar agent	Sorbitol 70% Lactulose (Chronulac)	15–30 mL twice daily	Disaccharide metabolized by colonic bacteria into acetic acid and short-chain fatty acids	24–48	Sweet tasting, transient abdominal cramps, flatulence
Hyperosmolar agent	PEG-ES (GoLytely,[1] CoLyte[1]) PEG (MiraLAX)	8–32 oz daily 17 g (1 tbsp) qd	Osmotic effect increasing intraluminal fluids	0.5–1	Incontinence
Guanylate cyclase-C agonist	Plecanatide (Trulance) Linaclotide (Linzess)	CIC and IBS-C: 3 mg once daily CIC: 72–145 mcg once daily IBS-C: 290 mcg once daily	Osmotic effect increasing intraluminal fluids, increase transit time	Cannot be calculated	Diarrhea Abdominal pain, diarrhea
Chloride channel activator	Lubiprostone (Amitiza)	CIC and OIC: 24 mcg twice daily IBS-C in women ≥18 y: 8 mcg twice daily	Increase intestinal fluid secretion and improve fecal transit	Unknown	Headache, nausea, diarrhea
Stimulant	Glycerin suppository Bisacodyl (Dulcolax) Senna (Senokot, Perdiem) Senna/docusate (Peri-Colace)	1 daily 10 mg suppository or 5–10 mg PO three times a week 2–4 tabs twice daily	Local rectal stimulation, secretory and prokinetic effect	8–12	Degeneration of Meissner and Auerbach plexus
Enemas	Mineral oil retention enema Tap water enema Sodium phosphate enema (Fleet)	199–250 mL daily PR 500–1000 mL PR 1 unit PR	Evacuation induced by distended colon and mechanical lavage	6–8 for a mineral oil enema 5–15 min for all other enemas	Mechanical trauma, incontinence, rectal damage
Opioid antagonist	Methylnaltrexone (Relistor)	8–12 mg 1 dose SC every other day as needed for OIC with advanced illness. 450 mg PO once daily or 12 mg SC once daily for OIC with chronic noncancer pain.	Opioid mu receptor antagonist in gut decreasing transit time	4	Diarrhea, intestinal perforation
Opioid antagonist	Naloxegol (Movantik)	12.5–25 mg PO daily	Same as Relistor	6–36	Abdominal pain, opioid withdrawal reported

CIC, Chronic idiopathic constipation; *IBS-C*, irritable bowel syndrome with constipation; *OIC*, opioid-induced constipation; *PEG-ES*, polyethylene glycol and electrolyte solution; *PR*, per rectum; *SC*, subcutaneously.

From Gaines, M. (2021). In R. D. Kellerman & D. P. Rakel (Eds.), *Conn's current therapy*. Elsevier.

laxatives can lead to dehydration, electrolyte imbalances, and potential harm to the gastrointestinal track. Because of these possible adverse reactions, stimulant laxatives should only be used after osmotic laxatives and fiber have been tried (Mounsey et al., 2015).

Lifestyle Changes/Risk Factors

Changes in lifestyle and dietary habits should be recommended to the patient as first-line therapy for constipation. Patients should set a regular time for bowel movements and set aside enough time so they do not feel rushed to defecate. Physical activity should be encouraged, and use of medications such as anticholinergics, iron supplements, and opioid agonists should be avoided if possible because they can lead to constipation (Iturrino & Lembo, 2021).

Constipation is a frequently encountered complaint in the older adult population. It has a significant impact on a patient's quality of life and health care. Many factors are to blame for constipation, including medications, limited mobility, other coexisting conditions, and motor or sensory dysfunction.

A digital rectal exam and clinical history may help to identify causes of constipation, but more than one mechanism might be involved. Diet and lifestyle modifications are often ineffective to manage constipation in older adults and a multifactorial approach is suggested. Laxatives remain a mainstay to solve the problem, but safety concerns in the frail older adult should be addressed. For cases of laxative-resistant constipation, several new agents that target different underlying pathophysiologic mechanisms have proved to be safe and effective in adults but only partially validated in older adults.

Hypertension

CASE STUDY 13.7

A 66-year-old female with type 2 diabetes presents with concerns about high blood pressure. She recently had a dental exam, and the dentist told her that her blood pressure was "a little elevated." She does not remember what her blood pressure was at the time. She tells the physician assistant that she does not "have any symptoms of high blood pressure" but she wanted to mention the comment from the dentist. She has never taken medications for high blood pressure, but she does take 500 mg of metformin daily for type 2 diabetes. Her current blood pressure is 148/96 in the right arm while sitting. Her physical exam is unremarkable except for obesity. Her electrocardiogram (ECG) is unremarkable.

Epidemiology

The risk for the development of high blood pressure increases with advancing age. Hypertension (HTN) is a significant risk factor for the development of end organ diseases. These diseases include cardiovascular disorders such as myocardial infarction, coronary artery disease, heart failure, renal failure, cerebrovascular disorders such as stroke and transient ischemic attack, and multi-infarct dementia. Hypertension is typically asymptomatic or has symptoms that can be attributed to many other conditions, which can contribute to delays in the establishment of a diagnosis. This delay in diagnosis of HTN increases the risk for the development of secondary conditions as well as conditions that are more severe at the time of diagnosis. Hypertension is classified as primary, which includes isolated systolic HTN and diastolic HTN or secondary HTN.

The prevalence of arterial hypertension for men and women ages 64 to 77 is 77% and 75%, respectively when using the 2017 diagnosis threshold criteria established by the American College of Cardiology (ACC) and the American Heart Association (AHA) (Ripley & Barbato, 2019).

In 2016, the European Union had 27.3 million people who were aged 80 years and older, compared to only 20 million in 2006. By the year 2050, there is expected to be 7.4% of the entire population of the United States will be 80 years and older; this is double the percentage of those 80 years old and older in 2006 (Benetos et al., 2019).

Even though the chance of becoming hypertensive increases with age, clinical studies specifically geared toward this population remain sparce. These studies include the Systolic Hypertension in the Elderly Program (SHEP) trial, the Hypertension in the Very Elderly Trial (HYVET), the Syst-Eur trial, the SPRINT trial, and the Medical Research Council (MRCO) trial. The Framingham Heart Study and the National Health and Nutrition Examination Survey (NHANES) are landmark trials where much of the data regarding hypertension diagnosing and managing come from.

Assessment

Hypertension is diagnosed when there are three elevated readings on three separate occasions that are at least 1 week apart. Staging of hypertension severity varies among the committees and study authors. The VIII Joint National Committee (JNC8) does not identify hypertension staging by blood pressure (BP), instead focusing on the management of target thresholds. The American College of Cardiology (ACC) and the American Heart Association (AHA) have identified four levels of hypertension severity staging as normal, elevated, stage 1, and stage 2. Normal blood pressure is considered to be < 120/80 mm Hg. Elevated blood pressure is a systolic reading of 120 to 129 mm Hg and a diastolic < 80 mm Hg. Stage 1 hypertension is a systolic reading of 130 to 139 mm Hg and a diastolic reading of 80 to 89 mm Hg. Stage 2 hypertension is a systolic reading of > 140 mm Hg and a diastolic reading of > 90 mm Hg. The blood pressure target threshold is < 130/80 mm Hg. If the systolic measurement and diastolic measurement fall in different categories, the highest classification for diagnosis is used.

Hypertension can be primary or secondary. Primary, or essential hypertension, is caused by an alteration in the sympathetic nervous system response for blood pressure regulation. Secondary hypertension occurs with an elevation in blood pressure is due to another diagnosis, illicit drug use, excessive alcohol intake, or medications. Isolated systolic hypertension (ISH), when the systolic blood pressure is >160 while the diastolic blood pressure is <90, is more common in older adults (Ripley & Barbato, 2019). Hypertension can also occur as a "white coat effect," where the blood pressure is elevated for a short term due to the patient's anxiety or reaction in the clinical setting, or it can be pseudohypertension due to stenosis, calcification, or stiffening of the arterial vasculature making the vessels uncompressible to the extent that the sphygmomanometer cannot provide an accurate measurement of the blood pressure.

The clinician should verify that HTN is present through accurate BP measurement. The correct method of measuring blood pressure includes using the correct size blood pressure cuff, ensuring the sphygmomanometer is calibrated and functioning, and verifying that the patient is sitting or lying with the feet and legs uncrossed. When the BP readings are elevated, it is reasonable to recheck the blood pressure later in the visit to verify the elevated reading.

Once HTN is established, it is important to rule out secondary causes of HTN. Most older adults will have primary HTN, though HTN caused by renovascular disease is the most common secondary cause of HTN in older adults. The patient should be assessed for the presence of target organ damage. This may include obtaining labs such as a basic metabolic panel to evaluate renal function or diagnostics such as an ECG, baseline neurologic exam, or funduscopic eye exam. The patient should be assessed for any comorbid conditions. Lastly, the patient should have a risk assessment completed using a risk stratification tool such as a cardiovascular risk calculator.

Treatment

Effective treatment for the older adult with HTN has been demonstrated in multiple research trials. It is important to identify the target blood pressure. Adults have a general target blood pressure goal of <130/80 as recommended by JNC8. Aggressive blood pressure goals have been associated with higher mortality when applied to older adults. The recommended target blood pressure goal for older adults is a systolic blood pressure of <140 mm Hg with the systolic blood pressure being identified as the priority (James et al., 2014). Treatments to target blood pressure thresholds were associated with a reduction in the occurrence of morbidity and mortality from cardiovascular events by 26%, cerebrovascular events by 30%, and overall morbidity and mortality from all causes at 13% (Wright et al., 2014). The HYVET, which focused on adults over the age of 80, showed similar or better outcomes on morbidity and mortality in cardiovascular, cerebrovascular, and overall morbidity and mortality in the treatment group as compared to the placebo group. The benefits were to the extent that the trial was stopped early. The SPRINT trial also showed a decrease in cardiovascular events by 33%. There is evidence that pursuing a diastolic blood pressure level below threshold levels may contribute to increased mortality, therefore recommendations focus on targeting the systolic blood pressure in the older adult, whereas a focus on lowering the systolic blood pressure is associated with improved outcomes (Park, 2019). These studies support the belief that management of high blood pressure that targets blood pressure levels should be pursued for older adults as it is in younger patient populations. The second goal for treatment of hypertension is to reduce risk or prevent target organ damage. Target organ damage can develop with longstanding uncontrolled HTN and with prolonged hypertensive crises, emergency, or urgency. Target organ damage may include acute myocardial infarction, pulmonary edema, cerebrovascular event, aortic dissection, papilledema, and encephalopathy.

Patient characteristics when determining a treatment plan should also be considered. These characteristics include a focus on frailty. The hypertension studies reviewed in this chapter do not support the theory that lowering the blood pressure to target goals increases the incidence of falls.

Pharmacologic Therapy

Patients who are in stage 1 or higher with a risk stratification score of >10% should be treated with both lifestyle management and pharmacologic therapy. The selection of pharmacologic agents is based on the patient's profile along with other medications and concomitant diseases such as diabetes, coronary artery disease and heart failure, chronic kidney disease, and cerebrovascular disorders such as stroke. Other factors to consider is include efficacy of the pharmacologic agent on cardiovascular morbidity and mortality as well as all cause morbidity and mortality (James et al., 2014).

Thiazide Diuretics

The drop in blood pressure immediately following the initiation of thiazide diuretics is due to the decrease in plasma volume. The initial drop in plasma volume is often self-compensated by the activation of the renin-angiotensin system when plasma volume decreases. This compensatory action may be blocked through concurrent prescribing of an angiotensin-converting enzyme inhibitor (ACEI) or angiotensin receptor blocker (ARB). Weeks after initiation of diuretic therapy, the lowering of blood pressure is thought to be due to decreased vascular resistance.

Angiotensin-Converting Enzyme Inhibitors (ACEIs)

Angiotensin II causes vasoconstriction and elevations in blood pressure. The ACEIs block conversion of angiotensin I to angiotensin II, thus facilitating vasodilation and decreased blood pressure.

Angiotensin Receptor Blockers (ARBs)

The ARB medications lower blood pressure by blocking the action of angiotensin II at the receptor.

Calcium Channel Blockers (CCBs)

CCBs decrease or slow the rate of calcium movement through the slow channels, resulting in relaxation of the smooth muscle and lowering of the blood pressure.

Beta-Blockers or Beta Receptor Antagonists

These medications block beta 1 receptors, causing slowing of the heart rate and thus decreasing the blood pressure. Beta-blockers are no longer used as first-line agents for hypertensive management. They have decreased cerebrovascular protection in older adults and can be associated with impaired glucose tolerance. Beta-blockers continue to have benefit in patients with recent myocardial infarction, heart failure, rate control needs, and migraine prophylaxis.

Pharmacologic selection is best when tailored to the patient profile. Consideration of concomitant disease, cost, frailty, and compliance ability should be incorporated into the individualized management plan. For example, a patient with diabetes should receive an ACEI or an ARB, and a patient with chronic obstructive pulmonary disease should avoid beta-blockers. Patients who also have heart failure do better with ACEIs, ARBs, beta-blockers, or thiazide or spironolactone diuretics. Patients who also have coexisting coronary artery disease would benefit from an ACEIs, ARBs, beta-blockers, thiazide diuretics, or a calcium channel blocker.

Guidelines from JNC8 for individuals over the age of 60 with hypertension and a blood pressure of >150/90 recommend following these steps. Advance a step if the blood pressure has not reached the goal blood pressure (James et al., 2014).

1. Implement lifestyle changes.
2. Start the first-line single medication (based on concomitant disease).
3. Titrate single medication up, or add low doses of a second medication.
4. Titrate current medication(s) up, or start low doses of an additional medication.
5. Refer to a specialist.

Acute issues of hypertension include hypertensive crisis, hypertensive emergency, and hypertensive urgency. A hypertensive crisis can occur with significant elevations in blood pressure. Hypertensive emergency occurs when the blood pressure is >180/120 with symptoms of end organ damage. The target organ damage can be new or worsening. Hypertensive urgency should be managed with frequent monitoring and adjustment of current antihypertensive pharmacotherapy. A sudden lowering of the BP is contraindicated due to the potential for complications from hypoperfusion effects of a rapidly lowering blood pressure. Hypertensive emergencies require inpatient management where the blood pressure can be lowered safely with the patient on continuous monitoring. The practice of lowering the blood pressure rapidly through the use of nifedipine or clonidine is not supported due to the potential complications that may occur from inadequate perfusion as the blood pressure drops rapidly.

It is reasonable to follow up in 4 to 6 weeks when treatment is first initiated or if an adjustment has been made to an existing treatment plan. Progressing to 12-week intervals once the blood pressure is optimally managed is acceptable. The clinician should monitor for and identify adverse effects from the pharmacotherapy and should check the status of the patient's concomitant conditions to ensure proper condition management. A decrease in dosing should be attempted at yearly intervals once the patient has been stable for 12 months.

Lifestyle Changes

Treatment should always start and continue to include lifestyle modifications followed by pharmacologic therapies. Lifestyle modifications should focus on weight loss for patients who are overweight or obese, limited alcohol consumption, regular exercise, and a decrease in sodium intake such as the Dietary Approaches to Stop Hypertension (DASH) diet. It is important to note that in patients with stage 1 hypertension and have a risk stratification score that is < 10%, lifestyle modifications alone have been found to be sufficient for blood pressure management. Moderate weight loss of 8 to 10 pounds can decrease the need for initiation of pharmacologic therapy. Sodium restriction is even more beneficial with a reduction of systolic blood pressure by 3.7 mm Hg for a 2.4-g reduction in sodium. Females over the age of 50 have an average daily sodium intake of 2.7 g and males over the age of 50 average 3.7 g of sodium daily (What We Eat in America, 2013–2014). Diets with reduced or limited sodium are an important component of lifestyle modification for managing hypertension.

Although hypertension is a common disease of older adults, lifestyle modifications and pharmacologic measures can bring hypertension under control and prevent end organ damage.

Dyslipidemia

CASE STUDY 13.8

Francis is a 68-year-old African American female with a family history of atherosclerotic cardiovascular disease. She is taking 50 mg of metoprolol for hypertension. She also takes a calcium supplement because she heard it was "good" for her. She tries to eat a healthy diet by eating low carbohydrate foods, and she walks around her block for 30 minutes most days of the week. Her BMI is 30 kg/m^2, she does not drink alcohol, and she has never smoked. Most of her labs are normal except for total cholesterol is 245 mg/dL; high-density lipoprotein cholesterol (HDL-C) is 45 mg/dL, triglycerides are 120 mg/dL, low-density lipoprotein cholesterol (LDL-C) is 135 mg/dL, and non-HDL-C is 60 mg/dL.

Pathophysiology

Lipids and lipoproteins are important components of cell composition in the body. They are expressed as cholesterol, triglycerides, low-density lipoproteins (LDL), high-density lipoproteins (HDL), and very low density lipoproteins (VLDL). Dyslipidemia is the alteration in lipid regulation seen as an overproduction of lipoprotein. Abnormalities in lipid regulation may include elevations in total cholesterol, triglycerides, cholesterol, low-density lipoprotein, and decreased high-density lipoproteins. Dyslipidemia is known to be a significant risk factor for the development of cardiovascular disease and cerebrovascular disease. Cardiovascular diseases are the leading cause of morbidity and mortality in the United States (US Preventive Services Task Force [USPSTF], 2016). Management of lipid disorders is an effective method for reducing cardiovascular and cerebrovascular morbidity and mortality risk.

Assessment

Cholesterol levels rise with aging, then trend down again starting around age 60. Elevated lipid levels are just one of the risk factors for coronary artery disease (CAD). Other risk factors for CAD include male gender, tobacco use, obesity, sedentary lifestyle, family history, diabetes, and hypertension. The US Preventive Services Task Force (USPSTF) recommends use of a statin for treating adults up to age 75 with elevated lipids and at least one additional risk factor or a calculated 10-year cardiovascular disease risk of >10%. The benefit for initiation of statin therapy for adults over the age of 75 has not been supported by evidence (US Preventive Services Task Force, 2016). Continuing the use of statins for older adults to age 85 with CAD and already on lipid lowering therapy is beneficial (Harper et al., 2019).

Screening for dyslipidemia is aimed at identifying those at risk for cardiovascular disease and cardiac events with the goal of reducing the risk through appropriate treatment. Annual screening for dyslipidemia up to age 74 is an important component for diagnosing dyslipidemia. Starting statin therapy for individuals age 75 years and older who have not previously been on a statin has not been shown to be beneficial (Chou et al., 2016). Thus it follows that annual screening for dyslipidemia would end at the age of 74. Continuation of statin therapy for adults over the age of 74 has been found to be beneficial. Dyslipidemia can be broken down to the type of lipid or lipoprotein that is out of the normal range. These subtypes include hypercholesterolemia, which involves an elevation in total cholesterol, hypertriglyceridemia, which involves an elevation in triglycerides, hyperlipoproteinemia, which involves an elevation in the low-density lipoprotein (LDL), and combined dyslipidemia where there is an elevation of both LDL and triglycerides. Lowering of LDL has been shown to be the most beneficial for reducing the risk of cardiovascular events (Pignone, 2021). (See Table 13.12.)

Treatment

Following lifestyle modification, statins are the mainstay of treatment for dyslipidemia. The decision to start statin therapy is based on individual patient characteristics as well as 10-year cardiovascular risk. For younger patients, a 30-year cardiovascular risk can also be calculated. Cardiovascular risk can be estimated using a risk calculator of which several are available. Cardiovascular risk calculators factor some or all of the following data: total cholesterol, LDL cholesterol, age, gender, ethnicity, presence of hypertension, and diabetes. One of the first cardiac risk calculators is the Framingham calculator, which was developed from the Framingham Heart Study. The Framingham calculator has largely been replaced by other calculators that factor in ethnicity, as well as variations of calculators tailored to geographic regional practices. The American College of Cardiology (ACC) and the American Heart Association (AHA) together developed the Cardiovascular Risk Assessment in Adults (to assess an individual's risk for the upcoming 10 years), which incorporates ethnicity and regional location. In addition, the ACC/AHA calculator focuses on disorders that can benefit from statin therapy.

Pharmacologic therapy is typically considered for patients with low-density lipoprotein-cholesterol (LDL-C) levels up to 190 mg/dl based on the level of elevation and cardiovascular risk. The first-line pharmacologic agents are the statins. Statins are hydroxymethylglutaryl (HMG) CoA reductase inhibitors. They will block binding of HMG CoA reductase to the receptor site on enzymes, which limits cholesterol biosynthesis. Statins also lower low-density lipoprotein receptor turnover, increase high-density lipoprotein (HDL), and decrease triglyceride concentration through decreased

TABLE 13.12 Normal Levels of Lipids and Lipoproteins

	Normal	Borderline High	High
Total Cholesterol	<200	201–239	240 and above
LDL	<130	131–159	160 and above
Triglycerides	<150	151–200	201–499: high 500 and above—very high
	Major risk	Acceptable	Less risk
HDL	<40	40–60	>60

TABLE 13.13 Low-Density Lipoprotein Cholesterol Treatment Recommendations

LDL-C up to 190 mg/dl			
Estimated Cardiovascular Risk	**Initiate Statin Therapy**	**Follow-up (F/U)**	
>10%	Yes Start moderate dose statin	F/U labs in 6 weeks	
5%–10%	Possibly Discuss statin therapy with patient	Statin therapy started F/U in 6–8 weeks to assess therapy	Statin therapy not started F/U in 6–12 months based on preventive screening protocols
<5%	No	F/U with annual screening	
LDL-C ≥ 190 mg/dl			
Cardiovascular risk not assessed	High-dose statin	F/U 6–8 weeks	

very low density lipoprotein (VLDL) synthesis. Statins are the most effective pharmacologic agent for the reduction of LDL cholesterol. Statins have some effect for increasing HDL cholesterol, though this effect is not correlated with effects of LDL cholesterol. For patients with a cardiovascular risk factor of >10% and the threshold LDL-C of 190 mg/dl, a moderate-dose statin is recommended. For patients with a cardiovascular risk factor of 5% to 10%, the decision is made based on individual patient characteristics. Patients with a cardiovascular risk factor of <5% should be monitored periodically for ongoing elevated lipids. Patients with LDL-C ≥ 190 mg/dl should be started on a high-dose statin regardless of the 10-year cardiovascular risk. (See Table 13.13.)

For patients with LDL-C > 190 mg/dl statin therapy is initiated without calculating a 10-year cardiovascular risk. These patients should be evaluated for familial hypercholesteremia. If present, follow treatment guidelines for familial hypercholesteremia. If not present, start high intensity statin therapy.

Adverse effects of statins include myalgia and hepatic dysfunction. Patients who develop myalgias can be taken off the statin; then it can be determined if the myalgia was true rhabdomyolysis with myoglobinuria or acute renal failure. If not true rhabdomyolysis, it is reasonable to retry statin therapy with an alternate agent or lower dose. In the case of hepatic dysfunction, aspartate aminotransferase (AST) and alanine aminotransferase (ALT) levels up to three times the limit of normal are acceptable. If hepatic function continues to rise, a trial of dose reduction or an alternate agent should be considered. (See Table 13.14.)

Nonstatin Treatment Options

Bile acid sequestrants work to reduce LDL-C by binding to bile acids in the intestine. This leads to decreased reabsorption of bile acids. Bile acid sequestrants can also promote a slight elevation in HDL-C. Bile acid sequestrants are rarely used alone; they are usually used in combination with other agents, most often a statin. The main side effects of the bile acid sequestrants include nausea, bloating, and constipation. The bile acid sequestrants interact with other medication through a process of binding to the agents. Concomitant use with digoxin, blood thinners, and fat-soluble vitamins can lead to unpredictable blood levels of these agents.

TABLE 13.14 Statin Drug Options and Dose

	Low to Moderate Dosing	High Dosing
Atorvastatin	10–20 mg	40–80 mg
Lovastatin	40 mg	n/a
Pravastatin	40 mg	n/a
Rosuvastatin	5–10 mg	20–40 mg
Simvastatin	40 mg	n/a

Fibric acid derivatives, such as gemfibrozil, work in multiple ways. Fibric acid derivatives are nuclear transcription factor agonists for peroxisome proliferator-activated receptor-alpha. They decrease the inhibition lipoprotein lipase through downregulation of apoprotein C-III and stimulate synthesis of apolipoprotein, fatty acid transport protein, and lipoprotein A-I. This causes an increase in VLDL catabolism and fatty acid oxidation, and it results in the elimination of triglyceride-rich particles. These actions result in decreased triglycerides, increased HDL, and decreased VLDL (Brothers & Daniels, 2015).

Niacin (Nicotinic acid)

Nicotinic acid gets broken down in the body to the enzymes responsible for lipid metabolism and glycogenolysis. This ultimately allows for a decrease in total cholesterol, apolipoprotein, triglycerides, VLDL, LDL-C, and lipoprotein, as well as an increase in HDL-C.

Omega 3 Fatty Acids

The omega-3 polyunsaturated fatty acids (*n*-3 PUFAs) reduce the production and synthesis of triglycerides and very low density lipoproteins in the liver. Omega-3 polyunsaturated fatty acids should be recommended to patients who are at high risk of cardiovascular disease (Pizzini et al., 2017).

PCSK9 Inhibitors

High levels of proprotein convertase subtilisin/kexin type 9 (PCSK9) have been found to be linked to an increase in LDL-C and worse cardiovascular outcomes (Stroes et al., 2021). When used in combination with statins, administration of monoclonal antibodies PCSK9 inhibitors can lower LDL-C by up to 60%. PCSK9 administration causes suppression of unbound PCSK9 proteins. This suppression results in an increased clearance of LDL-C from the blood by increasing the expression of LDL surface receptors. PCSK9 inhibitors are used in resistant hypercholesterolemia.

Lifestyle Changes

The Adult Treatment Panel II (ATP II) guidelines recommend lifestyle changes for patients with elevated cholesterol. Patients should be encouraged to eat a low saturated fat diet, increase physical activity, limit alcohol intake, and maintain a healthy weight. Nurse practitioners and physician assistants should recommend these lifestyle changes on an ongoing basis (National Center for Chronic Disease, 2020).

High cholesterol is a common chronic condition, especially in the older adult patient. Guidelines recommend evaluating a patient's cholesterol levels up to the age of 75. The NP/PA is in a prime position to educate patients about the impact of untreated high cholesterol and should counsel patients on lifestyle changes, pharmacologic treatments, and nonpharmacologic options.

Key Points

- The assessment and manifestations of chronic conditions differ in the older adult, and specialized assessment techniques may be required.
- The aspects of the presentation and management of common chronic conditions in the older adult are different than that of the general population.
- The management of coexisting chronic conditions in the older adult requires the provider to consider all aspects of disease management.
- The health care practitioner must carefully consider the older adult's goals and objectives for disease management as part of the patient's treatment and care plan.

More information about tools and the Interprofessional Education Collaborative (IPEC) competencies mentioned in this chapter can be found in Appendix 1: Tools and Appendix 2: IPEC Competencies.

References

Alvarez, L. R., Balibrea, J. M., Surinach, J. M., et al. (2013). FRENA Investigators. Smoking cessation and outcome in stable outpatients with coronary, cerebrovascular, or peripheral artery disease. *European Journal of Preventive Cardiology, 20*, 486–495.

American Diabetes Association (n.d.). *Understanding A1C: Diabetes.* https://www.diabetes.org/a1c/diagnosis.

Arora, P. (2021). Chronic kidney disease. *Medscape.* https://emedicine.medscape.com/article/238798-overview.

Benetos, A., Petrovic, M., & Strandberg, T. (2019). Hypertension management in older and frail older patients. *Circulation Research, 124*, 1045–1060. https://www.ahajournals.org/doi/full/10.1161/CIRCRESAHA.118.313236.

Berger, J. S., & Davies, M. G. (2021). *Overview of lower extremity peripheral artery disease.* https://www.uptodate.com/contents/overview-of-lower-extremity-peripheral-artery-disease?search=pathophysiology%20peripheral%20artery%20disease&source=search_result&selectedTitle=1~150&usage_type=default&display_rank=1.

Bevan, G. H., & White Solaru, K. T. (2020). Evidence-based medical management of peripheral artery disease. *Arteriosclerosis, Thrombosis, and Vascular Biology, 40*(3), 541–553.

Bonaca, M. P., & Creager, M. A. (2019). Diabetes and the cardiovascular system. In D. P. Zipes, P. Libby, R. O. Bonow, D. L. Mann, G. F. Tomaselli, & E. Braunwald (Eds.), *Braunwald's heart disease: A textbook of cardiovascular medicine* (11th ed.). Elsevier.

Brothers, J. A., & Daniels, S. R. (2015). In C. M. Ballantyne (Ed.), *Clinical lipidology: A companion to Braunwald's heart disease.* Elsevier.

Centers for Disease Control and Prevention. (2020). *Atrial fibrillation.* https://www.cdc.gov/heartdisease/atrial_fibrillation.htm.

Centers for Medicare & Medicaid Services (CMS.gov.). (2021). *Chronic conditions.* https://www.cms.gov/Research-Statistics-Data-and-Systems/Statistics-Trends-and-Reports/Chronic-Conditions/CC_Main.

Cho, M. E., & Beddhu, S. (2020). *Dietary recommendations for patients with nondialysis chronic kidney disease.* https://www.uptodate.com/contents/dietary-recommendations-for-patients-with-nondialysis-chronic-kidney-disease?search=pathophysiology%20chronic%20kidney%20disease&source=search_result&selectedTitle=7~150&usage_type=default&display_rank=7.

Chou, R., Dana, T., Blazina, I., Daeges, M., Bougatsos, C., Grusing, S., & Jeanne, T. L. (2016). Statin use for the prevention of cardiovascular disease in adults: A systematic review for the U.S. Preventive Services Task Force. *Agency for Healthcare Research and Quality (US)*; Report No. 14-05206-EF-2.

Clinical Overview. (2021). *Atherosclerotic peripheral artery disease*. Elsevier.

Collins, T. C. (2021). Peripheral artery disease. In R. D. Kellerman & D. P. Rakel (Eds.). *Conn's current therapy*. Elsevier.

De Giorgio, R., Ruggeri, E., Stanghellini, V., Eusebi, L. H., Bazzoli, F., & Chiarioni, G. (2015). Chronic constipation in the elderly: A primer for the gastroenterologist. *BMC Gastroenterology, 15*(130).

Dewar, R. I., & Lip, G. Y. H. (2007). Identification, diagnosis and assessment of atrial fibrillation. *Heart, 93*(1), P25–P28.

Dublin, S., Glazer, N. L., Smith, N. L., Psaty, B. M., Lumley, T., Wiggins, K. L., & Heckbert, S. R. (2010). Diabetes mellitus, glycemic control, and risk of atrial fibrillation. *Journal of General Internal Medicine, 25*(8), 853–858.

Filho, J. O., & Mullen, M. T. (2021). Initial assessment and management of acute stroke. *UpToDate*. https://www.uptodate.com/contents/initial-assessment-and-management-of-acute-stroke?search=assessment%20of%20stroke&source=search_result&selectedTitle=1~150&usage_type=default&display_rank=1.

Francisco, P., Segri, N., Borim, F., & Malta, D. (2018). Prevalence of concomitant hypertension and diabetes in Brazilian older adults: Individual and contextual inequalities. *Ciência & Saúde Coletiva, 23*(11), 3829–3840. https://doi.org/10.1590/1413-812320182311.29662016.

Gaines, M. (2021). In R. D. Kellerman & D. P. Rakel (Eds.), *Conn's current therapy*. Elsevier.

Goldstein, J. (2021). In R. D. Kellerman & D. P. Rakel (Eds.), *Conn's current therapy*. Elsevier.

Goldstein, L. (2019). Prevention and management of stroke. In D. P. Zipes, P. Libby, R. O. Bonow, D. L. Mann, G. F. Tomaselli, & E. Braunwald (Eds.), *Braunwald's heart disease: A textbook of cardiovascular medicine* (11th ed.). Elsevier.

Harper, G. M., Lyons, W. L., & Potter, J. F. (2019). Geriatric review syllabus: *American Geriatrics Society*. American Geriatrics Society.

Heeringa, J., Kors, J. A., Hofman, A., van Rooji, F. J., & Witteman, J. C. (2008). Cigarette smoking and risk of atrial fibrillation: The Rotterdam study. *American Heart Journal, 156*(6), 1163–1169.

Hopkins Medicine (n.d.). *Claudication*. https://www.hopkinsmedicine.org/health/conditions-and-diseases/claudication.

Huxley, R. R., Misialek, J. R., Agarwal, S. K., et al. (2014). Physical activity, obesity, weight change, and risk of atrial fibrillation: The Atherosclerosis Risk in Communities study. *Circulation: Arrhythmia and Electrophysiology, 7*, 620–625.

Inker, L. A., & Perrone, R. D. (2020). Assessment of kidney function. *UpToDate*. https://www.uptodate.com/contents/assessment-of-kidney-function?search=chronic%20kidney%20disease%20definition&topicRef=16406&source=see_link.

Iturrino, J. C., & Lembo, A. J. (2021). Constipation. In M. Feldman, L. S. Friedman, & L. J. Brandt (Eds.), *Sleisenger and Fordtran's gastrointestinal and liver disease* (11th ed.). Elsevier.

Jadhav, A. P., Ares, W. J., Jovin, T. G., Jankowitz, B. T., & Ducruet, A. F. (2016). Acute surgical and endovascular management of ischemic and hemorrhagic stroke. In H. R. Winn (Ed.), *Youmans & Winn Neurological Surgery* (7th ed.). Elsevier.

Jahangiri, M., & Cramm, J. (2007). Do corticosteroids prevent atrial fibrillation after cardiac surgery? *Nature Clinical Practice, 4*, 592–593.

James, P. A., Oparil, S., Carter, B. L., Cushman, W. C., Dennison-Himmelfarb, C., Handler, J., & Ortiz, E. (2014). 2014 evidence-based guideline for the management of high blood pressure in adults: Report from the panel members appointed to the Eighth Joint National Committee (JNC8). *Journal of the American Medical Association, 311*(5), 507–520.

Karamichalakis, N., Letsas, K. P., Vlachos, K., Georgopoulos, S., Bakalakos, A., Efremidis, M., & Sideris, A. (2015). Managing atrial fibrillation in the very elderly patient: Challenges and solutions. *Vascular Health Risk Management, 11*, 555–562.

Kayrak, M., Gul, E. E., Aribas, A., Akilli, H., Alibasic, H., Abdulhalikov, T., & Ozdemir, K. (2013). Self-reported sleep quality of patients with atrial fibrillation and the effects of cardioversion on sleep quality. *Pacing and Clinical Electrophysiology, 36*(7), 823–829.

KDOQI Nutrition in Chronic Renal Failure Guidelines. (2000). *Dietary energy intake (DEI) for nondialyzed patients*. https://www.kidney.org/sites/default/files/docs/kdoqi2000nutritiongl.pdf

Kidney International Supplement. (2013). CKD evaluation and management. *The Lancet, 3*(1), 27. https://www.kdigo.org/guidelines/ckd-evaluation-and-management/.

Kirkman, M. S., Briscoe, V. J., Clark, N., Florez, H., Haas, L. B., Halter, J. B., Huang, E. S., & Swift, C. S. (2012). Diabetes in older adults. *Diabetes Care, 35*, 2650. https://doi.org/10.2337/dc12-1801.

Kotecha, D., Senoo, K., & Lip, G. Y. H. (2018). Atrial fibrillation. In R. Hoffman, E. J. Benz, L. E. Silberstein, H. E. Heslop, J. I. Weitz, & J. Anastasi (Eds.), *Hematology: Basic principles and practice* (7th ed.). Elsevier.

Kourliouros, A., Savelieva, I., Kiotsekoglou, A., Jahangiri, M., & Camm, J. (2009). Current concepts in the pathogenesis of atrial fibrillation. *American Heart Journal, 157*(2), 243–252.

Lacy, B. E., Mearin, F., Chang, L., Chey, W. D., Lembo, A. J., Simren, M., & Spiller, R. (2016). Bowel disorders. *Gastroenterology, 150*(6), 1393–1407, e5.

Lampert, R., Jamner, L., Burg, M., Dziura, J., Brandt, C., Liu, H., & Soufer, R. (2014). Triggering of symptomatic atrial fibrillation by negative emotion. *Journal of the American College of Cardiology, 64*(14), 1533–1534.

Lecturio Medical Concept Library. (2020, October 2). *Chronic kidney disease—Pathophysiology and diagnosis*. https://www.lecturio.com/magazine/chronic-renal-failure/#pathophysiology.

Levey, A. S., & Inker, L. A. (2020). Definition and staging of chronic kidney disease in adults. *UpToDate*. https://www.uptodate.com/contents/definition-and-staging-of-chronic-kidney-disease-in-adults?search=chronic%20kidney%20disease%20definition&source=search_result&selectedTitle=1~150&usage_type=default&display_rank=1#H27258404.

Lewis, E. J., Hunsicker, L. G., Bain, R. P., et al. (1993). The effect of angiotensin-converting- enzyme inhibition on diabetic nephropathy: The Collaborative Study Group. *New England Journal of Medicine, 329*, 1456–1462.

Litbarg, N. O. (2018). Chronic kidney disease. In D. Rakel (Ed.), *Integrative medicine* (4th ed.). Elsevier.

Majid, A. M., & Kassab, M. (2020). Pathophysiology of ischemic stroke. *UpToDate*. https://www.uptodate.com/contents/pathophysiology-of-ischemic-stroke?search=pathophysiology%20of%20stroke&source=search_result&selectedTitle=1~150&usage_type=default&display_rank=1#H1222833.

Marcoff, L., & Homma, S. (2018). Embolism, cardiac and aortic. In R. Daroff & M. Aminoff (Eds.), *Encyclopedia of neurological sciences* (2nd ed.). Elsevier.

McGrath, E., Canavan, M., & O'Donnell, M. (2018). Stroke. In R. Hoffman (Ed.), *Hematology: Basic principles and practice* (7th ed.). Elsevier.

Mills, J. L., Zachary, S., & Pallister, S. (2022). Peripheral arterial disease. In C. M. TownsendJr., R. D. Beauchamp, B. M. Evers, & K. L. Mattox (Eds.), *Sabiston textbook of surgery*. Elsevier.

Morady, F., & Zipes, D. P. (2019). In D. P. Zipes, P. Libby, R. O. Bonow, D. L. Mann, G. F. Tomaselli, & E. Braunwald (Eds.), *Braunwald's heart disease: A textbook of cardiovascular medicine* (11th ed.). Elsevier.

Mounsey, A., Raleigh, M., & Wilson, A. (2015). Management of constipation in older adults. *American Family Physician, 92*(6), 500–504.

Naidech, A. M., Levasseur, K., Liebling, S., Garg, R. K., Shapiro, M., Ault, M. L., et al. (2010). Moderate hypoglycemia is associated with vasospasm, cerebral infarction, and 3-month disability after subarachnoid hemorrhage. *Neurocritical Care, 12*(2), 181–187. https://doi.org/10.1007/s12028-009-9311-z.

National Center for Chronic Disease Prevention and Health Promotion, Division for Heart and Stroke Prevention. (2020). *Preventing high cholesterol.* https://www.cdc.gov/cholesterol/prevention.htm.

National Cholesterol Education Program (NCEP) Expert Panel on Detection, Evaluation, and Treatment of High Blood Cholesterol in Adults (Adult Treatment Panel III). (2002). Third Report of the National Cholesterol Education Program (NCEP) Expert Panel on Detection, Evaluation, and Treatment of High Blood Cholesterol in Adults (Adult Treatment Panel III) final report. *Circulation, 106*(25), 3143–3421.

Naylor, H. L., Jackson, H., Walker, G. H., Macafee, S., Magee, K., Hooper, L., Stewart, L., MacLaughlin, H. L., & on behalf of the Renal Nutrition Group of the British Dietetic Association. (2013). British Dietetic Association evidence-based guidelines for the protein requirements of adults undergoing maintenance haemodialysis or peritoneal dialysis. *Journal of Human Nutrition and Dietetics, 26*, 315–328. https://doi.org/10.1111/jhn.12052.

Neilan, T. G., Farhad, H., Dodson, J. A., Shah, R. V., Abbasi, S. A., Bakker, J. P., & Kwong, R. Y. (2013). Effect of sleep apnea and continuous positive airway pressure on cardiac structure and recurrence of atrial fibrillation. *Journal of the American Heart Association, 25*(6), e000421.

Nguyen, P., & Patel, P. M. (2021). Peripheral artery disease. In F. F. Ferri (Ed.), *Ferri's clinical advisor*. Elsevier.

Obrador, G.T. (2020). *Epidemiology of chronic kidney disease.* https://www.uptodate.com/contents/epidemiology-of-chronic-kidney-disease?search=chronic%20kidney%20disease%20definition&topicRef=16406&source=see_link.

O'Donnell, M. J., Chin, S. L., Rangarajan, S., et al. (2016). Global and regional effects of potentially modifiable risk factors associated with acute stroke in 32 countries (INTERSTROKE): A case-control study. *Lancet, 388*, 761.

Park, S. (2019). Ideal target blood pressure in hypertension. *Korean Circulation Journal, 49*(11), 1002–1009. https://doi.org/10.4070/kcj.2019.0261.

Pathak, R. K., Middeldorp, M. E., & Lau, D. H. (2014). Aggressive risk factor reduction study for atrial fibrillation and implications for the outcome of ablation: The ARREST-AF cohort study. *Journal of the American College of Cardiology, 64*, 2222–2231.

Pathophysiology and Etiology of Stroke (n.d.). http://www.strokecenter.org/professionals/stroke-management/for-pharmacists-counseling/pathophysiology-and-etiology/.

Pignone, M. (2021). Management of elevated low density lipoprotein-cholesterol (LDL-C) in primary prevention of cardiovascular disease. *UpToDate.* https://www.uptodate.com/contents/management-of-elevated-low-density-lipoprotein-cholesterol-ldl-c-in-primary-prevention-of-cardiovascular-disease.

Pizzini, A., Lunger, L., Demetz, E., Hilbe, R., Weiss, G., Ebenbichler, C., & Tancevski, I. (2017). The role of omega-3 fatty acids in reverse cholesterol transport: A review. *Nutrients, 9*(10), 1099. https://doi.org/10.3390/nu9101099.

Ripley, T., & Barbato, A. (2019). Hypertension: *PSAP 2019 Book 1: Cardiology. (2019).* United States: *American College of Clinical Pharmacy*. https://www.accp.com/docs/bookstore/psap/p2019b1_sample.pdf.

Rordorf, G., & McDonald, C. (2021). Spontaneous intracerebral hemorrhage: Treatment and prognosis. *UpToDate.* https://www.uptodate.com/contents/spontaneous-intracerebral-hemorrhage-treatment-and-prognosis?search=treatment%20of%20hemorrhagic%20stroke&source=search_result&selectedTitle=1~150&usage_type=default&display_rank=1#H1282843263.

Rossi, J. S., & Mounsey, J. P. (2019). Atrial fibrillation: Stroke prevention. In G. A. Stouffer, M. S. Runge, C. Patterson, & J. S. Rossi (Eds.), *Netter's cardiology* (3rd ed.). Elsevier.

Samudra, N., & Figueroa, S. (2016). Intractable central hyperthermia in the setting of brainstem hemorrhage. *Therapeutic Hypothermia and Temperature Management, 6*(2), 98–101. https://doi.org/10.1089/ther.2016.0004.

Schoolwerth, A. C., Sica, D. A., Ballermann, B. J., & Wilcox, C. S. (2001). Renal considerations in angiotensin converting enzyme inhibitor therapy. *Circulation, 104*(16), 1985–1991.

Schotten, U., Verheule, S., Kirchof, P., & Goette, A. (2011). Pathophysiological mechanisms of atrial fibrillation: A translational appraisal. *Physiological Reviews, 91*(1), 265–325.

Staerk, L., Wang, B., Preis, S. R., Larson, M. G., Lubitz, S. A., Ellinor, P. T., McManus, D. D., Ko, D., Weng, L. C., Lunetta, K. L., Frost, L., Benjamin, E. J., & Trinquart, L. (2018). Lifetime risk of atrial fibrillation according to optimal, borderline, or elevated levels of risk factors: cohort study based on longitudinal data from the Framingham Heart Study. *BMJ (Clinical research ed.), 361*, k1453. https://doi.org/10.1136/bmj.k1453.Stroes.

Stroes, E. S. G., Stiekema, L. C. A., & Rosenson, R. S. (2021). PCSK9 inhibitors: Pharmacology, adverse effects, and use. *UpToDate.* https://www.uptodate.com/contents/pcsk9-inhibitors-pharmacology-adverse-effects-and-use.

Stroke. *What is a stroke? A Mayo Clinic expert explains.* https://www.mayoclinic.org/diseases-conditions/stroke/symptoms-causes/syc-20350113.

Suckling, R. J., He, F. J., & Macgregor, G. A. (2010). Altered dietary salt intake for preventing and treating diabetic kidney disease. *Cochrane Database of Systematic Reviews*, CD006763.

Tedrow, U. B., Conen, D., Ridker, P. M., et al. (2010). The long- and short-term impact of elevated body mass index on the risk of new atrial fibrillation the WHS (Women's Health Study). *Journal of the American College of Cardiology, 55*, 2319–2327.

US Preventive Services Task Force. (2016). Final recommendation statement: Statin use for the primary prevention of cardiovascular disease in adults: Preventive medication. https://www.uspreventiveservicestaskforce.org/Page/Document/RecommendationStatementFinal/statin-use-in-adults-preventive-medication.

Watanabe, R. (2020, January 13). Hyperkalemia in chronic kidney disease. Revista da Associacao Medica Brasileira, *66*, 1. https://doi.org/10.1590/1806-9282.66.s1.31.

What we eat in America. (2013–2014). *NHANES data tables 2013–2014.* https://www.ars.usda.gov/ARSUserFiles/80400530/pdf/1314/Table_1_NIN_GEN_13.pdf.

Whittier, W. L., & Lewis, E. (2018). Kidney disease in the elderly. In S. Gilbert (Ed.), *National Kidney Foundation primer on kidney diseases* (7th ed.). Elsevier.

Willigendeal, E. M., Teijink, J. A., Bartelink, M. L., Kuiken, B. W., Boiten, J., Moll, F. L., et al. (2004). Influence of smoking on incidence and prevalence of peripheral arterial disease. *Journal of Vascular Surgery, 40,* 1158–1165. https://doi.org/10.1016/j.jvs.2004.08.049.

Wright, J. T., Fine, L. J., Lacklund, D. T., Ogedegbe, G., & Dennison Himmelfarb, C. R. (2014). Evidence supporting a systolic blood pressure goal of less than 150 mm Hg in patients aged 60 years or older: The minority view. *Annals of Internal Medicine, 160*(7), 499–503. https://doi.org/10.7326/M13-2981.

Workeneh, B. T., & Mitch, W. E. (2013). Chronic kidney disease: Pathophysiology and the influence of dietary protein. In R. J. Alpern, O. W. Moe, & M. Caplan (Eds.), *Seldin and Giebisch's the kidney* (5th ed.). Elsevier.

14

Infectious Diseases

DANIEL PODD, BS, MPAS

OBJECTIVES

Student Learning Objectives

After completing this chapter, the student should be able to do the following:

1. Describe the infectious diseases that are prevalent among the geriatric population.
2. Assess the unique aspects of the presentation of an infectious disease in a geriatric patient.
3. Summarize the approach to diagnosing the geriatric patient who has an infectious disease.

Practitioner Objectives

After completing this chapter, the practitioner should be able to do the following:

1. Use evidence-based practice to improve the quality of care given to the older adult patient with an infectious disease.
2. Comprehend and appraise the risk factors, pathologic process, and epidemiology for management of an infectious disease.
3. Develop clinical approaches based on patient information, scientific evidence, and informed clinical judgment, and integrate research, theory, and knowledge for the older adult client with an infectious disease.

Introduction

Infectious diseases occur in the geriatric population with greater frequency and duration when compared with other patient age groups. Also, patient outcomes and prognoses are less favorable in geriatric patients (Gavazzi & Krause, 2002); infections are a major cause of morbidity and mortality in older adults. The most common causes of death due to infection include influenza, pneumonia, and bacteremia. The most encountered infections are those of the urinary, upper and lower respiratory tracts, gastroenteritis, skin, and soft tissue (Mody et al., 2014). HIV and AIDS are also of increased importance in the geriatric population and will be further explored in this chapter.

Considering that the management of infections may require inpatient care, patients are at a heightened risk of exposure to infectious agents. Increased hospitalization rates occurring in the geriatric population contribute to the elevated risk of acquired nosocomial infections. Additionally, older adult patients have an increased number of infections per day of stays in an institution, including nursing home, day care, senior center, and rehabilitation settings. Infection by antibiotic-resistant bacteria becomes increasingly commonplace in institutional settings versus community dwellings (Bradley, 1999; Kupronis et al., 2003; O'Fallon et al., 2009).

Malnutrition is an important risk factor linked to the development of infection (Gavazzi & Krause, 2002). Strong epidemiologic evidence exists that links protein-energy malnutrition to the development of infection. Individuals with even mild reductions in albumin levels have an impaired response to immunizations. Specifically, deficiencies in vitamins B_{12}, D, and E can induce immune diminution (High, 2017).

Anatomic and physiologic changes also contribute to infections in older adults. Mechanisms include maladaptive changes to the protective barrier provided by the various mucosal linings in the body, skin, lungs, and gastrointestinal tract (Gomez et al., 2005). These alterations permit the penetration of invasive organisms. Changes in the geriatric population that require the presence of foreign bodies and prostheses significantly increase the risk for acquired infection. Such entities include urinary catheters, joint prostheses, pacemakers, and synthetic heart valves (Juthani-Mehta & Quagliarello, 2010; Wang et al., 2012).

Interprofessional Collaboration

The successful management of infectious diseases in the geriatric population centers on timely recognition of disease syndromes, employing an appropriate diagnostic workup, and an efficient, synergistic relationship among all involved health care providers. Physicians, physician assistants (PAs), and nurse practitioners (NPs) function as integral components in the comprehensive care of patients with infectious disorders.

Interprofessional Approach and Management of Infectious Diseases

Vital aspects of the medical history to ascertain include two main areas: an exposure history that may identify microorganisms with which the patient may have come into contact and host-specific factors that may predispose to the development of an infection. An exposure history comprises consideration of previous infections or exposure to drug-resistant agents, a social history (inclusive of high-risk behaviors), dietary habits, animal exposures, and a travel history. Host-specific factors pertain to the overall host immunocompetence. Elements detrimental to the normal functioning of the immune system due to underlying immunosuppressive states should be elucidated: these include concurrent or underlying disease conditions (such as malignancy, HIV infection, malnutrition, or primary immunodeficiency), medications (e.g., chemotherapy, glucocorticoids, monoclonal antibodies treatments), other treatments (e.g., total body irradiation or splenectomy), and current immunization status (Surana & Kasper, 2018).

Although infectious disease can affect any bodily system, particular attention should be paid to the physical exam systems that infectious diseases most often manifest or influence; these include the general survey, vital signs, dermatologic, otolaryngic, cardiovascular, pulmonary, lymphatic, gastrointestinal, and genitourinary systems. The conscientious provider should be mindful of the presence of foreign bodies as a source of infection; these account for apertures in the normal epithelial barrier present. The presence of intravenous lines, surgical drains, or tubes (such as endotracheal tubes and Foley catheters) all potentially permit microbiota to colonize sites where they would otherwise not be found.

Findings should be accurately and precisely documented in the medical record. NPs and PAs will then order and perform all laboratory and imaging relevant to the assessment of an underlying infectious process. Diagnostic testing should serve as a supplement to, not a replacement for, a complete history and physical examination; the selection of initial tests should be based on the antecedent clinical encounter. Generally, the medical provider may consider certain diagnostic tests valuable in the assessment of infectious diseases. A leukocyte count with a differential is helpful to delineate bacterial versus viral diseases. Bacteria are associated with a greater proportion of polymorphonuclear neutrophils, often with increased earlier formative forms (bands); viruses are associated with a lymphocytosis. Parasites are often associated with an eosinophilia. Other laboratory tests of consideration include those that assess the erythrocyte sedimentation rate (ESR) and the C-reactive protein (CRP). Although both acute phase reactants are a sensitive measure of inflammation (with a possible underlying cause being infection), neither is specific. An extremely elevated ESR (i.e., > 100 mm/hr) has a 90% predictive value for a serious underlying disease (e.g., a significant infection). Additionally, the serial monitoring of ESR and CRP following diagnosis may be useful in establishing the evolution or resolution of disease.

Analysis of the cerebrospinal fluid (CSF) is essential in all cases of suspected meningitis or encephalitis. Parameters measured include the color, opening pressure, glucose, pH, protein levels, abnormal cell presence, antibodies, viral DNA, bacteria, Gram stain, and culture.

The principal mode of infection diagnosis is culture of infected tissue or fluid. Preferably, cultures should be obtained prior to the initiation of antimicrobial therapy. Cultures permit the identification of the etiologic agent(s), allow the practitioner to determine the antimicrobial susceptibility profile, and isolate typing. If culturing is not possible, microscopic analysis utilizing alternative means (such as Gram-staining or potassium hydroxide preparation) is especially critical.

Beyond cultures, additional pathogenic-specific tests are available. These include serology, antigen testing, and PCR testing. Benefits of employing these tests include the obtaining the ability to identify pathogens not amendable to culture or further microscopic assessment and to accurately and more precisely diagnosticate infectious etiologies overall. Whenever possible, cultures should be procured prior to the implementation of any antimicrobial therapy; antibiotic therapy usually complicates diagnosing an infectious disease.

Ancillary diagnostic testing may encompass the use of diagnostic imaging. Various modalities are available to the provider in this setting. These include x-rays, CT scans, MRI, ultrasound, nuclear medicine, and the use of contrast. The assessment of associated lymphadenopathy, visualization of infected internal organs, and assistance in the image-guided sampling of bodily areas are all invaluable functions of imaging exams in this setting. In practicing within the team management paradigm, the physician assistant or nurse practitioner should consult with the diagnostic radiologist regarding the appropriateness, indications, and interpretations of such imaging exams.

Often, the clinician must weigh the necessity of empiric treatment with the patient's current clinical status. Although most empiric treatments generally provide a broad spectrum of microbial coverage, it is recommended that regimens be narrowed following conclusive diagnosis. Appropriate management also includes the implementation of infectious control measures. Such actions are imperative to prevent the transmission of infectious agents to other patients and providers alike. Postexposure prophylaxis is available and should be offered to those exposed to specific entities (e.g., *N. meningitidis*, HIV, *Bacillus anthracis*).

Collaboration with an infectious disease specialist should be considered under certain circumstances. These include challenging cases with difficult-to-diagnose or rare etiologies, patients who do not respond to treatment as expected, and patients with complex underlying conditions such as organ transplant recipients or the immunosuppressed. Consultation with an infectious disease specialist results in improved patient outcomes, shorter hospital stays, and reduced health care costs. Beneficial services provided by these specialists include the implementation of infectious control strategies, application antimicrobial stewardship, appropriate management of outpatient antibiotic therapy, and coordination and practice of occupational exposure programs (Interprofessional Education Collaborative, 2016; Surana & Kasper, 2018).

INFECTIOUS DISEASE CASE REPORT

The Case of Mrs. Jones

Mrs. Jones, a 76-year-old female with a past medical history of Alzheimer dementia, hypertension, hyperlipidemia, urinary incontinence, chronic pain secondary to generalized arthritis, and chronic pulmonary disease, is evaluated at her bedside during morning rounds. She is a long-term resident at the local nursing home. According to the overnight nurse, the patient had exhibited acutely progressive unawareness, inattention, decreased alertness, and lethargy. She demonstrated impairment of short-term memory, slower and increasingly sparse speech, and motor activity more sluggish than normal. Mrs. Jones' vital signs were assessed and included a temperature, blood pressure of 106/68, heart rate of 96 beats per minute, and a respiratory rate of 16 per minute; her blood glucose was measured as 140 mg/dL. No other remarkable findings were reported, and her physical exam was otherwise normal.

The clinical presentation provided suggests a state of acute delirium. More specifically, Mrs. Jones exhibited hypoactive delirium. Other forms of delirium include hyperactive and mixed delirium. Hypoactive delirium occurs most commonly in the older adult and is the most commonly missed subtype of delirium. Many comorbid factors exist; these include an age greater than 65, underlying dementia, major depression, chronic pain, polypharmacy, visual and hearing impairments, poor nutrition, and hepatic or renal failure. Infection is the most common precipitating factor of delirium; infectious etiologies contribute to 50% of all cases of delirium in the older adult. Notable infections implicated include pneumonia, urinary tract infections, intraabdominal infections, soft-tissue infections (including infected pressure sores), and central nervous system infections (meningitis and encephalitis).

The recognition and diagnosis of an infection in the older adult patient is challenging. Atypical presentations of infectious disease such as in the case of Mrs. Jones are more common in the older adult population. Additionally, the presence of cognitive impairment also frequently coexists and is exacerbated in geriatric patients during infection. These aspects have the significant potential to confound the differential diagnostic picture. Pathophysiologic changes responsible for this presentation emanate from dehydration that occurs because of infection; reduced perfusion to the brain as well as the compounding of central nervous system-related medication side effects ensue. Causation of an altered sensorium may also be explained by inflammation, hyper or hypothermia, or subsequent infection-related metabolic derangements.

All patients should have a comprehensive metabolic panel, complete blood count, urinalysis, and urine culture. At the discretion of the provider, additional laboratory tests to consider include those that evaluate blood cultures, thyroid function, vitamin B_{12} levels, arterial blood gas, serum ammonia, toxicology screening, serum medication levels, C-reactive protein, the erythrocyte sedimentation rate, and a lumbar puncture. A chest x-ray should be performed to assess for occult pneumonia, whereas a CT scan for evaluation of the head is indicated for the following: states of altered mental status, focal neurologic deficits, head trauma, or fever associated with encephalopathy findings. An electrocardiogram will be beneficial in the assessment of dysrhythmias present (Moses, 2018).

Pulmonary Infections

Infectious respiratory diseases including pneumonia, influenza, and other infections are common in the older adult. Various risk factors are responsible for the development of respiratory tract infections; these will be discussed next.

Pneumonia

Pneumonia, defined as an infection of the pulmonary parenchyma, is a cause of significant morbidity and mortality in the older adult. Adults ages 65 years and older account for greater than 50% of all pneumonia cases. Pneumonia may be classified as community acquired (CAP), hospital acquired (HAP), or ventilator associated (VAP). More recently, a fourth category has been coined, health care–associated pneumonia (HCAP).

Several protective mechanisms are present in the prevention of pneumonia. These include the arrest of inhaled particles in the more proximal respiratory tree by hairs and turbinates of the nares, preventing further dissemination to the lower airways. Furthermore, the branching nature of the tracheobronchial tree aids in sequestering microbes in the airway lining, allowing mucociliary clearance and local anti-antigenic activity to neutralize potentially harmful antigens. Alveolar macrophages are especially adept in the neutralization of foreign agents; in conjunction with surfactant proteins A and D, they phagocytose and eliminate bacteria and viruses via the mucociliary elevator or local lymphatics. Finally, within the respiratory tree, local resident bacterial flora maintains a steady residence, further impeding the attachment of pathogenic agents. Pneumonia becomes clinically apparent only when the ability of alveolar macrophages to ingest or kill the microorganisms is exceeded by the pathogenicity of the offending agent.

The pathophysiology of pneumonia involves the growth of microbes at alveoli as well as exceeding the host immune response. The most common route of infection is aspiration of microorganisms from the oropharynx. Low levels of aspiration occur frequently during sleep and especially in the older adult and in patients with decreased levels of consciousness; patients with an impaired gag or cough reflex are more susceptible to aspiration. Pneumonia may also occur due to deleterious changes in host defense that permit the proliferation of one or more components of the normal bacterial flora (Mandell & Wunderink, 2019). With age, the lung parenchyma loses its elastic recoil resulting in reduced chest wall compliance, along with a loss of alveoli and alveolar ducts, all of which can increase the risk of pneumonia in the setting of functional disability and acute illness.

Established risk factors cited in the development of pneumonia include older age, male gender, history of aspiration, functional disability, history of smoking, chronic bronchitis or emphysema, heart disease, malignancy, neurologic conditions such as cerebrovascular diseases, recent surgery or intensive care unit stay, and the presence of a feeding tube (Mody et al., 2014).

Community-Acquired Pneumonia (CAP)

Community-acquired pneumonia is defined as a pneumonia that presents outside the hospital setting. It may be further differentiated into health care–associated pneumonia (HCAP) provided any of the following criteria are met: (1) hospitalization for 2 days or more in the preceding 90 days, (2) residence in a nursing home or extended care facility, (3) home infusion therapy (including antibiotics), (4) chronic dialysis within 30 days, (5) home wound care, or (6) family member with a multidrug-resistant pathogen (del Castillo & Sánchez, 2019).

The rate of CAP rises with increased age; the incidence nearly triples from those ages 65 to 69 to those older than 85 years of age. Annually, approximately 1 in 20 people older than 85 will develop CAP, with more than 900,000 cases occurring overall in the older adult population (https://emedicine.medscape.com/article/234240-overview#a4 CAP). Increased age is associated not only with a higher incidence of CAP but also with more severe disease, greater need for hospitalization, and higher mortality (Mandell et al., 2007; Teramoto et al., 2008).

The typical etiologic agents include *Streptococcus pneumoniae, Haemophilus influenza*, and *Moraxella catarrhalis*, with *S. pneumoniae* being the most common cause overall. The atypical bacterial causes of CAP generally decrease with advancing age; these include *Chlamydia psittaci* (psittacosis), *Francisella tularensis* (tularemia), *Coxiella burnetii* (Q fever), *Legionella pneumophila* (Legionnaires disease), *Mycoplasma pneumoniae*, and *Chlamydia pneumoniae*. Although the atypical bacteria demonstrate a decrease in incidence with age, a relative increase in the incidence of pneumonia due to *Haemophilus influenzae* and gram-negative bacilli (GNB) has been observed in this cohort. Finally, respiratory viruses also contribute to atypical causes in 12% to 18% of all cases. Of these, influenza virus, respiratory syncytial virus (RSV), and human metapneumovirus (HPV) are the most clinically significant, factoring between 8% and 14% of all pneumonia cases in older adults (especially during seasonal outbreaks) (del Castillo & Sánchez, 2019).

Older patients with a history of dementia, cerebrovascular accident, or a diminished level of consciousness have a higher risk of aspiration; there is also an increased incidence of oral aerobic, anaerobic, and gram-negative enteric bacterial pulmonary infections (https://emedicine.medscape.com/article/234240-overview#a4 CAP; Mandell & Wunderink, 2019).

Patients who meet the requirements for HCAP have a higher rate of methicillin-resistant *Staphylococcus aureus* (MRSA) or resistant gram-negative bacilli infections, such as from *Pseudomonas aeruginosa*. For risk factors that favor the development of lesser common bacterial etiologies, refer to Table 14.1.

In the older adult, pneumonia often manifests with asymptomatic or atypical symptoms and signs. These include the exacerbation of any chronic medical condition, generalized weakness or fatigue, dizziness, dehydration, incontinence, loss of appetite, falls, acute functional decline, or acute confusion. Importantly, up to quarter of this population may not mount a fever and they are less likely to present with chills or pleuritic chest pain when compared with other population demographics. Furthermore, older adult patients are less likely to have tachycardia; an elevated respiratory rate and altered level of consciousness may be the only initial signs of pneumonia in older patients. The absence of fever, hypoxemia, or respiratory symptoms does not rule out a pneumonia diagnosis. Despite these limitations and when present, an increased respiratory rate of greater than 25 breaths/min and hypoxia do portend a poorer prognosis and are useful tools for risk assessments (del Castillo & Sánchez, 2019; Mody et al., 2014).

Approach to Pneumonia

The evaluation of the geriatric patient with suspected pneumonia should begin with a computation of the patient's severity status. Two tools are available and recommended by the 2007 Infectious Diseases Society of America/American Thoracic Society Consensus Guidelines (Mandell et al., 2007) to facilitate the clinical decision making, namely to determine to need for hospital admission or admission to the intensive care unit (ICU). The Pneumonia Severity Index (PSI) and CURB-65 (confusion, uremia, respiratory rate, blood pressure age >65 years) are used to calculate the need for admission and the probability of death due to pneumonia based on specific patient characteristics, physical exam findings, and laboratory findings at presentation.

Patients with a > CURB-65 score or PSI classes IV to V may necessitate hospitalization or more aggressive in-home services. ICU is recommended for any patient who requires mechanical ventilation or vasopressors. ICU consideration should be made for patients with three or more minor risk factors, including a respiratory rate of 30 or more, $PaO_2/FiO_2 < 250$, multilobar infiltrates, confusion, uremia, leukopenia, thrombocytopenia, hypothermia, and hypotension requiring aggressive fluid replenishment (https://emedicine.medscape.com/article/234240-overview#a4 CAP). More severe cases of pneumonia should also raise the suspicion of infection by resistant or especially organisms such as *Pseudomonas aeruginosa*, methicillin-resistant *S. aureus*, or extended-spectrum β-lactamase-producing *Enterobacteriaceae*. In these scenarios, more expanded-spectrum antibiotic coverage should be initiated (del Castillo & Sánchez, 2019).

The diagnosis of pneumonia in the older adult patient cannot be reliably made on the history and physical exam alone; the clinical presentation should be confirmed rapidly with diagnostic testing, including chest imaging and laboratory analysis (del Castillo & Sánchez, 2019; Mody et al., 2014). Chest x-rays should be ordered for all patients with suspected CAP to evaluate possible differential diagnoses and to corroborate the presence of an infiltrate consistent with CAP (https://emedicine.medscape.com/article/234240-overview#a4 CAP). It is noteworthy that initial chest x-rays may not be revealing in up to a third of all

TABLE 14.1 Risk Factors for the Development of Uncommon Pneumonia Etiologies

Bacteria	Risk Factors
Pseudomonas aeruginosa	Severe COPD with FEV_1 < 35% COPD > 4 cycles of antibiotic treatment in the last year Bronchiectasis with previous colonization Nasogastric enteral feeding Intensive care unit admission
Enterobacteriaceae and/or anaerobic organisms	Functional impairment Risk factors for aspiration Dysphagia Gastroesophageal reflux History of vomiting Cerebrovascular diseases Dementia Periodontal disease Poor oral hygiene
Extended spectrum β-lactamase producing *Enterobacteriaceae*	Previous antibiotic Hemodialysis Long-term indwelling urinary catheter Residence in long stay center Recent hospitalization Diabetes mellitus Recurrent urinary tract infections
MRSA	Undergoing care for bedsores or wounds Clinically serious illness + recent hospitalization + prior intravenous antibiotics + institutionalization Previous colonization Superinfection of pneumonia virus influenza during influenza epidemic

From del Castillo, J., & Martín Sánchez, F. (2019). Pneumonia. In J. B. Halter, J. G. Ouslander, S. Studenski, K. P. High, S. Asthana, M. A. Supiano, & C. Ritchie (Eds.), *Hazzard's geriatric medicine and gerontology* (7th ed.). McGraw-Hill. http://accessmedicine.mhmedical.com/content.aspx?bookid=1923§ionid=144563755

cases; this is more likely to occur in the case of underlying dehydration or neutropenia.

Viral pneumonias may display few or no infiltrates, but when present, infiltrates are generally bilateral, perihilar, symmetric, and interstitial. Meanwhile, bacterial pneumonias have a chiefly focal segmental or lobar distribution, with or without associated pleural effusions (refer to Fig. 14.1 for a radiograph of CAP). Atypical bacterial agents cause varying patterns; focal segmental to bilateral interstitial findings are possible. *P. jiroveci* (PJP) pneumonia typically presents as bilateral patchy interstitial infiltrates. Of importance, radiographic findings alone are not dependable in the differentiation of specific etiologies of CAP (https://emedicine.medscape.com/article/234240-overview#a4 CAP). If the clinical suspicion remains high and initial imaging is unremarkable, a repeat radiograph in 24 to 48 hours is warranted. CT scanning has a greater accuracy in the diagnosis of pneumonia; it may be considered if there are uncharacteristic chest x-ray findings or if there is a failure to respond to conventional therapy.

The acquisition of blood cultures has generally been recommended, as it facilitates confirmation of the underlying agent. This is especially valuable in atypical presentations, which are common in the older adult. Unfortunately, the

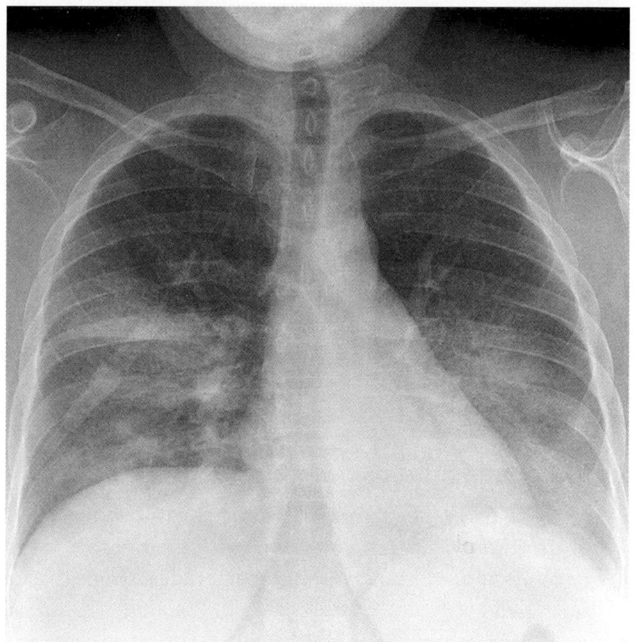

• **Fig. 14.1** Community-acquired pneumonia PA chest radiograph. (From Santiago, M. J., Rosado-de-Christenson, M. L. [2002]. *Diagnostic imaging: Chest* [3rd ed]. Elsevier.)

diagnostic yield from blood cultures is low, with only up to 15% of all hospitalized patients with CAP testing positive. Moreover, most of these are found to be *S. pneumoniae*; most empiric antibiotics provide *S. pneumoniae* coverage regardless. In consideration of these findings, the merit of blood cultures is unclear. Nonetheless, blood cultures should be obtained in cases of neutropenia/leukopenia, asplenia, complement deficiencies, chronic and severe liver disease, alcoholism, severe presentations of CAP, those with cavitary infiltrates, pleural effusion, or a positive urine antigen for *S. pneumoniae* (del Castillo & Sánchez, 2019; Mandell & Wunderink, 2019).

Additional testing includes the collection of sputum Gram stain and culture and the detection of bacteria in urine (pneumococcal and *Legionella* immunochromatographic test). Sputum collection may be difficult due to functional impairment or dehydration; a sufficient sample is obtained in approximately one-third of all patients (del Castillo & Sánchez, 2019). A satisfactory specimen contains >25 neutrophils and <10 squamous epithelial cells per low-power field. A greater percentage may be achieved with more invasive collection techniques such as employing hypertonic saline induction or bronchoscopy. Microbial yield is increased in ICU patients when collecting a deep-suction aspirate or bronchoalveolar lavage sample via a bronchoscope (Mandell & Wunderink, 2019). Fluid replenishment in the dehydrated patient is anticipated to increase sputum production and infiltrate appearance on the chest x-ray (del Castillo & Sánchez, 2019; Mandell & Wunderink, 2019). The provider should be cognizant that the Gram stain will reveal few or no predominant organisms in patients with atypical CAP (https://emedicine.medscape.com/article/234240-overview#a4 CAP) and that there is a greater presence of gram-negative bacilli, *S. aureus*, and multidrug resistant organisms as part of the normal flora of the oropharynx in the functionally impaired. Obtaining sputum is significant in that antimicrobial treatment may be adjusted based on bacterial identification and susceptibility results; it is important to identify *S. aureus*, *Pseudomonas*, and *Klebsiella pneumoniae* when selecting the proper antibiotics, as these agents typically necessitate broad-spectrum coverage. When these bacteria have been excluded, the antibiotic spectrum may be appropriately narrowed.

Urinary antigen testing is applicable to the identification of pneumococcus and *L. pneumophila*. The specificity of this test exceeds 90% for either organism, whereas sensitivity rates for pneumococcal detection range from 50% to 80% and over 90% for *L. pneumophila* (https://emedicine.medscape.com/article/234240-overview#a4 CAP; del Castillo & Sánchez, 2019). Benefits of this exam include application to pleural fluid samples and that results are not altered by prior antibiotic treatment or pneumococcal vaccination. However, a positive result may remain for up to 3 months following the resolution of pneumonia; there is therefore limited utility in patients with recurrences or in the assessment of treatment response. Also, the urinary antigen test for legionellosis only detects *L. pneumophila* serogroup I, which accounts for 80% of all cases of legionellosis (del Castillo & Sánchez, 2019). Finally, urine testing may be negative within the first 48 hours of a case of legionellosis (https://emedicine.medscape.com/article/234240-overview#a4 CAP).

Other laboratory tests are of limited utility owing to senile immunosenescence. The curtailed immune response may result in a diminution of the leukocyte count and inflammatory markers such as C-reactive protein (CRP), erythrocyte sedimentation rate, and procalcitonin (PCT). CRP values may be of greater help in the assessment of worsening disease or treatment failure (Mandell & Wunderink, 2019). PCT readings have not demonstrated acceptable sensitivity in older populations for the diagnosis of acute bacterial infection; rather, they may be of greater use for severity assessment. Other potential uses identified include the ability to distinguish between bacterial and viral etiologies, determine the necessity of antibacterial therapy, or help determine when to discontinue treatment. PCT testing can result in reduced antibiotic use in CAP with no concomitant increase in treatment failure or mortality risk (Mandell & Wunderink, 2019). A serum lactate level >2 mmol/L is considered a reliable predictor of 30-day mortality in older adults. MR-proADM has been shown to be a useful prognostic indicator in respiratory infection; it is a peptide produced by the endothelium released in a state of bodily stress (del Castillo & Sánchez, 2019).

Nasopharyngeal swab collection for polymerase chain reaction (PCR) testing has emerged as the diagnostic test of choice for respiratory viral infections. PCR can also detect the presence of *S. pneumoniae*, *Legionella* species, *M. pneumoniae*, *C. pneumoniae*, and mycobacteria. In patients with pneumococcal pneumonia, a higher PCR burden is associated with septic shock, the need for mechanical ventilation, and death. However, its definitive use in the assessment of pneumonia is not validated owing to a lack of cost effectiveness (Mandell & Wunderink, 2019). Because of limited specificity in the workup of pneumonia, a positive test for a respiratory virus cannot supplant an underlying bacterial diagnosis and its treatment (del Castillo & Sánchez, 2019).

Treatment of CAP begins with the consideration of hospitalization. A computation a PSI score greater than or equal to III or a CURB-65 greater than or equal to 2 meets the criteria for hospital admission. CAP infections due to *S. aureus*, Enterobacteriaceae, and *Pseudomonas aeruginosa* are typically more significant and require admission to the hospital. Once the diagnosis of pneumonia is confirmed, the provision of empiric antibiotic treatment should be expedited. In the outpatient setting, the older adult without frailty, comorbidities, or suspected resistance may be empirically treated with macrolide (azithromycin, clarithromycin, or erythromycin) or doxycycline. Although doxycycline remains an alternative to a macrolide, stronger data support the use of a macrolide provided resistance is not a concern. For older adults with comorbidities such as chronic lung, renal or liver disease, diabetes, asplenia, alcoholism, malignancy, or immunosuppression, a beta-lactam agent (high-dose amoxicillin or amoxicillin-clavulanate) or second- or third-generation cephalosporin (e.g., ceftriaxone, cefpodoxime, or cefuroxime) plus a macrolide or a respiratory fluoroquinolone (such as moxifloxacin or levofloxacin 750 mg) will be suitable. In this cohort, those who received an antibiotic from a particular drug class within the previous 3 months should receive an alternative antimicrobial from a different drug class (del Castillo & Sánchez, 2019; Mandell et al., 2007; Mody et al., 2014).

Inpatients without frailty or ICU disposition should receive either amoxicillin/clavulanate, ceftriaxone, cefotaxime, or ceftaroline, plus azithromycin or a fluoroquinolone. In cases of severe pneumonia, these patients should receive ceftriaxone, cefotaxime, ceftaroline, or ertapenem, plus azithromycin or fluoroquinolone. Should ICU admission be required, combination therapy is indicated as follows: an antipneumococcal beta-lactam (cefotaxime, ceftriaxone, or ampicillin-sulbactam) and azithromycin, or an antipneumococcal beta-lactam (cefotaxime, ceftriaxone, or ampicillin-sulbactam) and a respiratory fluoroquinolone. Penicillin-allergic patients may be treated with a respiratory fluoroquinolone (moxifloxacin, levofloxacin) plus aztreonam (Mandell et al., 2007).

If risk factors for *S. aureus* are present, adding linezolid or vancomycin to the regimen is warranted. An antipseudomonal β-lactam should be used if risk factors for *Pseudomonas aeruginosa* are applicable. Consideration of influenza may be of pertinence during seasonal outbreaks; the addition of oseltamivir may be justified, especially in cases of severe pneumonia. It is well established that colonization by *S. aureus* is more frequent when there has been a prior episode of influenza (del Castillo & Sánchez, 2019).

Inpatients designated as prefrailty should be considered for treatment with amoxicillin/clavulanate, ceftriaxone, cefotaxime, or ceftaroline, plus azithromycin or a fluoroquinolone. Those with multiple comorbidities or frailty should be treated with ertapenem, amoxicillin/clavulanate, or ceftriaxone plus clindamycin. The clinician should scrutinize local resistance rates of *Enterobacteriaceae* to amoxicillin-clavulanic and ceftriaxone as well as anaerobes to clindamycin when selecting treatment regimens. The treatment of specific organisms is identified in Table 14.2 (del Castillo & Sánchez, 2019).

Consideration of antibiotic resistance is crucial in the medical management of pneumonia. Resistance to *S. pneumoniae* and *S. aureus* is the central resistance concerns. The most important risk factor in penicillin-resistant pneumococcal infection is antimicrobial therapy within the previous 3 months. Additional factors include an age of >65 years, attendance at day care centers, recent hospitalization, and HIV infection. Resistance to macrolides and fluoroquinolones has been reported; these rates are increasing. MRSA resistance may occur in the community-acquired (CA-MRSA) or hospital-acquired (HA-MRSA) forms, with CA-MRSA generally being more susceptible to the classical antibiotic coverage provided by trimethoprim-sulfamethoxazole, clindamycin, tetracycline, vancomycin, and linezolid (Mandell & Wunderink, 2019).

TABLE 14.2 Organism-Specific Antimicrobial Treatment

Bacteria	Recommended Antibiotic Regimen
Enterobacteriaceae/ anaerobes	Ertapenem or amoxicillin/ clavulanate or ceftriaxone; plus clindamycin
Extended-spectrum β-lactamase producing *Enterobacteriaceae*	Ertapenem
Methicillin resistant *Staphylococcus aureus*	Add linezolid or vancomycin to selected treatment
Pseudomonas aeruginosa	Piperacillin/tazobactam, or imipenem or meropenem, or cefepime; plus, levofloxacin or ciprofloxacin or amikacin or tobramycin

From del Castillo, J., & Martín Sánchez, F. (2019). Pneumonia (Chapter 126). In J. B. Halter, J. G. Ouslander, S. Studenski, K. P. High, S. Asthana, M. A. Supiano, & C. Ritchie (Eds.), *Hazzard's geriatric medicine and gerontology* (7th ed.). McGraw-Hill. http://accessmedicine.mhmedical.com/content.aspx?bookid=1923§ionid=144563755.

Prevention

Pneumococcal vaccines have been shown to be effective in preventing pneumococcal pneumonia, bacteremia, and invasive disease. The vaccination is, however, not effective against all etiologies of community-acquired pneumonia (Bonten et al., 2015; Kim et al., 2016).

Two pneumococcal vaccines have been approved in the United States; 13-valent polysaccharide conjugate vaccine (PCV13; Prevnar 13) has been approved for children ages 6 weeks to 17 years and adults age 50 years or older. The 23-valent pneumococcal polysaccharide vaccine (PPSV23; Pneumovax 23) has been approved for adults age 65 years or older and persons ages 2 years or older who are at increased risk for pneumococcal disease. The Advisory Committee on Immunization Practices (ACIP) recommends routine use of PCV13 in addition to PPSV23 for adults older than 65 years. It is recommended that an initial dose of PCV13 be given, followed by PPSV23 at least 1 year later. If PPSV23 has already been given, it should be followed by PCV13 a year later. A second dose of PPSV23 is not needed in immunocompetent hosts. If PPSV23 is inadvertently given prior to 1 year after PCV13, it does not need to be repeated (Baer, 2018).

Influenza

Viral influenza is of paramount concern in the geriatric population. Yearly, the syndrome contributes to approximately

36,000 deaths in older adults. Outbreaks are common in long-term care venues, including nursing homes. Despite aggressive immunization efforts, influenza substantially impacts geriatric morbidity and mortality.

Pathophysiology

The primary site of infection acquisition is respiratory with large amounts of viral burden existing in the respiratory sections of infected hosts. Infection can be transmitted via sneezing and coughing, both of large respiratory droplets and smaller particle aerosols.

Three influenza virus subtypes exist: influenza A, B, and C. Clinically, only variants A and B are significant. The influenza virus maintains a viral envelope with a nucleic acid core consisting of a single-stranded RNA. The RNA directs the production of the major structural proteins of the virus including hemagglutinin and neuraminidase. Hemagglutinin is the surface protein that facilitates binding to respiratory epithelial cells, thereby permitting its entrance to cells via endosome production. Yearly mutations to hemagglutinin occur; this antigenic shifting is central to the promulgation of new influenza vaccines annually. Influenza neuraminidase is responsible for stimulating the release of virions from infected cells (High, 2017). The typical incubation period for influenza is 1 to 4 days, with an average of 2 days (Centers for Disease Control and Prevention, 2010; Cox & Subbarao, 1999).

Epidemiology

Influenza outbreaks occur annually, most often between November and April in the Northern Hemisphere. During outbreaks, several strains of influenza may be concurrently present and contribute to infection. Although those in the geriatric population, especially residents of long-term care facilities, are equally likely to contract influenza as younger, healthy adults, older patients are at a higher risk for complications of influenza. Rates of hospitalization due to influenza range from 136 to 508 per 100,000 persons in older adults. This contrasts with significantly lower levels observed in patients 5 to 49 years old. In the latter, 10 to 25 per 100,000 persons are hospitalized. Several studies have also concluded that an age older than 65 years alone is independently associated with an increased risk for influenza complications. Beyond the age-related risk factor, the presence of several chronic conditions increases the risk for complications following infection with influenza. These include chronic lung disease, congestive heart failure, metabolic disorders, and illnesses that predispose to aspiration, such as cerebrovascular accident (High, 2017).

Clinical Manifestations

The clinical presentation of influenza in older adults differs from that in younger adults. Although younger adults classically present with an abrupt onset of fever, cough, myalgia, sore throat, and headache, those in the older adult population manifest a relative paucity of respiratory symptoms. Cough, fever, and altered mental status predominate as presenting findings in older adults hospitalized with documented influenza. Other general symptoms such as anorexia, malaise, weakness, and dizziness are common. Moreover, the presentation may be more subtle, with solely the presence of cough and a change in baseline temperature being apparent. Older adults with influenza may have more gastrointestinal symptoms when compared with those who have other respiratory viruses.

Archetypally, decompensation of other bodily systems commonly occurs during the evolution of influenza; manifestations of worsening of comorbid conditions are then experienced. Examples include exacerbations of chronic obstructive pulmonary disease and congestive heart failure (High, 2017; Mody et al., 2014).

Physical findings are generally lacking in cases of uncomplicated influenza. The patient may appear hot and flushed; oropharyngeal abnormalities may reveal hyperemia. Mild cervical lymphadenopathy may be present but is more frequent in younger patients. Physical examination of the chest is generally unremarkable in uncomplicated cases, although mild ventilatory defects and increased alveolar-capillary diffusion gradients have been documented (Hall et al., 1976).

In assessing the possibility of influenza in the clinical setting of cough and fever, it is important to consider the clinical presentation in the context of local influenza activity. Cough and fever in conjunction with high influenza activity in a community more likely suggests an underlying diagnosis of influenza. In settings where the presentation is nonspecific (commonly observed in nursing homes), diagnostic testing is of paramount concern. Many other viruses, such as respiratory syncytial virus, may be concurrent. Following a definitive diagnosis, medical treatment and prophylactic measures can be appropriately implemented (High, 2017).

Diagnosis

Classically, the diagnosis of influenza has been made on clinical grounds. The presentation is further assessed with diagnostic tests such as rapid antigen testing, viral cultures and serology, reverse-transcriptase polymerase chain reaction (PCR) testing, and immunologic assays. Rapid tests that can detect influenza A, B, or both are available and can detect influenza viruses within 30 minutes. The sensitivity and specificity of these tests increase when they are performed close to the illness onset (Mody et al., 2014). Conventionally, viral cultures of nasopharyngeal or pharyngeal secretions had been the mainstay of diagnosing influenza. Practically, limitations exist utilizing this modality; these include reduced diagnostic accuracy as well as delays receiving the results.

Rapid tests include direct fluorescent antigen (DFA) or direct immunofluorescence. These tests contain monoclonal antibodies labeled with fluorescent material that are specified to influenza cell coat antigens. Typically, results are available within hours.

Rapid enzyme-linked immunoassay (ELISA) tests are commercially available. Sensitivity, however, can approach only 20% in geriatric patients. Beyond viral culture, another criterion standard in the diagnosis of influenza is nucleic acid amplification testing (e.g., reverse transcription polymerase chain reaction [RT-PCR]). This exam yields over 95% specificity and sensitivity; it additionally offers the advantage of a rapid turnaround time. One shortcoming is that not all laboratories can perform PCR daily at this time (High, 2017).

Other laboratory findings are generally not helpful to establish the diagnosis of influenza. Leukopenia or normal leukocyte counts are common early in the course of the illness but may become elevated later in the illness. A leukocytosis of >15,000 cells/mcl should suggest bacterial superinfection (Cohen & Dolin, 2015).

Treatment

Presently, six antivirals have been approved for treating influenza. These agents include oral adamantanes (amantadine and rimantadine), the neuraminidase inhibitors (oseltamivir, peramivir, and zanamivir), and a cap-dependent endonuclease inhibitor, baloxavir marboxil. Zanamivir is an inhaled medication. Peramivir, a neuraminidase inhibitor approved by the Food and Drug Administration (FDA) in 2015, is delivered intravenously. Amantadine and rimantadine are only active against influenza A. Unfortunately, currently circulating influenza A strains are largely resistant to both amantadine and rimantadine. The neuraminidase inhibitors zanamivir and oseltamivir are active against influenza A and B. These are 70% to 90% effective for prophylaxis in preventing influenza and when used as treatments to reduce the clinical severity and duration of illness when given within 48 hours of symptom onset. These agents are most effective if started within the first 24 hours of symptoms and less effective if begun 24 to 48 hours after symptoms appear. However, the feasibility of using these agents for treatment is reduced because the majority of patients in the community present over 48 hours following symptom onset. It is noteworthy that doses of treatment and prophylaxis are different; the provider must use therapeutic strength for patients with an active illness. Zanamivir and oseltamivir are generally well tolerated without significant adverse reactions. Zanamivir may, however, worsen or provoke respiratory distress in those with underlying obstructive disease. Oseltamivir should be dosed based on renal function (High, 2017).

Baloxavir marboxil was approved by the FDA in October 2018 for use in adults and adolescents age 12 years or older as a single weight-based oral dose for use within 48 hours of symptom onset. It is a prodrug that inhibits cap-dependent endonuclease, an enzyme specific to influenza, resulting in inhibition of viral replication. Single-dose baloxavir has been found to be safe and effective in treating patients with uncomplicated influenza with demonstrated influenza A and B, including strains resistant to neuraminidase inhibitors (Nguyen, 2019).

Prevention

Prevention of influenza centers on immunization. Older adults and individuals with underlying health problems are at increased risk for complications of influenza, including death. Influenza vaccination not only reduces the risk of influenza infection but also reduces the severity of illness in those who are infected (Castilla et al., 2013; Ehrlich et al., 2012). Annual influenza vaccination has also been shown to decrease pneumonia diagnoses, hospitalizations, and cardiac events in certain populations (Phrommintikul et al., 2011; Powner et al., 2014; Talbot et al., 2013; Udell et al., 2013).

Presently, three inactivated vaccines are licensed for adults age 65 years or older. At this time, use of any of these three vaccines is recommended by the US ACIP. Vaccines available include a trivalent inactivated vaccine, a quadrivalent vaccine, and a newer higher-dosage variant of the trivalent vaccine. Compared to the regular strength vaccines, the higher-dose vaccine has been shown to generate higher antibody levels in older adults than the traditional trivalent vaccine and is 24% more effective for the prevention of illness due to influenza (High, 2017). A multicenter trial that included 31,989 adults ≥65 years of age also demonstrated that the Fluzone High-Dose was modestly more effective than standard-dose Fluzone (DiazGranados et al., 2014). Statistically significant rates of seroconversion improvement and an increase in mean influenza hemagglutination-inhibition antibody titers occurred 1 month following vaccination in individuals who received the high-dose vaccine as opposed to the standard-strength dose (Falsey et al., 2009). Superior immunogenic responses were also realized in frail, older adult residents of long-term care facilities using the enhanced formulation (Nace et al., 2015).

Another larger study compared the mortality rates of >6 million US Medicare beneficiaries ≥65 years with high-dose versus the standard-dose influenza vaccine during the 2012 to 2013 and 2013 to 2014 influenza seasons. It concluded that the high-dose vaccine was more effective than the standard-dose vaccine for preventing postinfluenza death during the 2012 to 2013 influenza season. During that year, the more severe H3N2 influenza A strain was predominant. Interestingly, the high-dose form was not more effective for preventing postinfluenza death during the following season: during the subsequent year, the milder H1N1 influenza A strain was more common. It was concluded that mortality reductions are not as apparent during a mild influenza season, when death is altogether a rarer outcome. Nonetheless, use of the high-dose vaccine was associated with a reduced risk of hospitalization during both seasons (Shay et al., 2017). Reductions in hospital admissions from nursing home residents were also observed in those given the high-dose vaccine versus those who received the standard-dose vaccine (Gravenstein et al., 2017). Significant reductions in influenza-related hospital admissions were also demonstrated in in another large study of Medicare patients receiving high-dose inactivated influenza when compared with those who received the standard-dose vaccine. The high-dose inactivated influenza vaccine was significantly more effective than the standard-dose vaccine in preventing influenza-related medical encounters (Izurieta et al., 2015).

An additional adjuvanted vaccine has been approved by the FDA for use in individuals ≥65 years of age. Its use is not recommended, however, due to no reported clinical efficacy trials of this vaccine in older adults.

Compared to other patient populations, older adults respond less well to influenza immunizations. Data from systematic review studies across multiple countries have demonstrated that influenza immunization plays an important but modest role in prevention; during years of strain matching, influenza prevention rates ranged from 38% to 70%, whereas during years of mismatching, rates were reduced to 15% to 59%.

During nursing home and long-term care facility influenza outbreaks, several strategies can be applied to help mitigate and manage the spread of influenza. These include isolating infected residents, strict adherence to hand hygiene, chemoprophylaxis with antiviral agents, and immunization of all unvaccinated residents and staff alike. Several studies have demonstrated the benefit of these interventions. Evidence has supported the use of oseltamivir versus placebo and zanamivir versus rimantadine in the chemoprophylaxis of influenza. Significantly lower rates of influenza were observed in the neuraminidase inhibitor groups (Hayden et al., 1999; High, 2017). Immunizing health care workers against influenza reduces mortality in residents of long-term care facilities; it also prevents deaths, reduces the need for health services, and reduces influenza-like illnesses in nursing home residents (Hayward et al., 2006).

Complications

The causes of death in geriatric patients with influenza include viral pneumonia, myocardial infarction, cerebrovascular accident, and exacerbation of underlying comorbid conditions. Additionally, bacterial infections commonly complicate influenza infection. Patients with influenza are predisposed to *Streptococcus pneumoniae* or *S. aureus* infections, most commonly manifesting as bacterial pneumonia. A causal factor is the deficit of innate immune cell function within phagocytes and natural killer cells and deficiencies of acquired immunity of T cells, cytokine activity, and antibody responses.

Coronavirus-19

The severe acute respiratory syndrome coronavirus 2 (SARS-CoV-2), the causative agent of the coronavirus infectious disease-19 (COVID-19), is responsible for the worldwide pandemic of coronavirus disease (COVID-19) that originated in Wuhan, China, in late 2019. Eighty percent of all hospitalizations and approximately three-quarters of total deaths attributed to the infection occur in persons 65 years or older; increased age is the single most important risk factor for death related to COVID-19. More specifically, poorer outcomes correlated to advancing age include the following: physiologic changes of aging; multiple age-related comorbid conditions such as heart and lung disease, diabetes, and dementia; and associated polypharmacy. Geriatric residents of senior living institutions are at greatest risk because of the combination of chronic medical disorders in conjunction with a convoking living environment.

Pathophysiology

Coronaviruses (CoV) are a family of large positive-strand RNA viruses. Coronaviruses have caused diseases ranging from common-cold-like processes to severe respiratory diseases caused by β-coronaviruses like the severe acute respiratory syndrome (SARS)-CoV-1 (SARS-1) and Middle East respiratory syndrome (MERS)-CoV. The behavior of SARS-CoV-2 is more consistent with SARS-1 and MERS as opposed to coronaviruses causing common-cold processes.

SARS-CoV-2 is spread through respiratory droplets or by direct contact. Upon entry via the nose, mouth, or eyes, the virus then migrates to the posterior nasal channels. There, it adheres to and enters the host cell through dimerization of the host cell angiotensin-converting enzyme 2 (ACE2) receptor. It continues to migrate along the mucosal layers of the pharynx, larynx, and bronchial tubes, ultimately infiltrating the lungs where it invades pneumocytes (type 2 alveolar epithelial cells). This can then propagate a deficiency of lung surfactant and an increase in oxidative stress culminating in acute respiratory distress syndrome (ARDS). The ACE2 receptor is present extensively on the surface of both epithelial and microvascular pericytes, cell types that are found within a multitude of organs. Thus, systemic infection by the virus of both cell types is easily facilitated, enabling a widespread distribution of clinical manifestations.

Concurrently, inflammation and endothelial dysfunction of the lung, heart, kidney, liver, and brain occur as a consequence of the recruitment of immune cells to sites of infection. A cytokine release syndrome can quickly evolve, leading to disseminated intravascular coagulation (DIC) with ensuing liver damage, renal dysfunction, cardiovascular inflammation, coagulopathy, and death (Neumann-Podczaska et al., 2020; Nikolich-Zugich et al., 2020).

Clinical Manifestations

COVID-19 manifests similarly to both SARS and influenza and unlike coronavirus infections causing the common cold. The most common symptom experienced is fever. Although common, it is noteworthy that a febrile response is frequently attenuated in geriatric patients, especially those with multiple infirmities. As such, it is recommended that health care providers employ a lower calibration of fever definition in the geriatric patient (e.g., a single oral temperature of 100 °F or two repeated oral temperatures of >99 °F). Following fever, the second most common symptom is a nonproductive cough. The neurologic manifestations anosmia and dysgeusia may precede respiratory disease in up to two-thirds of patients; additional neurologic findings are headache or dizziness. Other prevalent symptoms include shortness of breath and dyspnea, fatigue, chest tightness, and myalgias. Gastrointestinal symptoms such as diarrhea may herald fever and pulmonary symptoms; other possible gastrointestinal symptoms include anorexia, nausea, or vomiting. Possible dermatologic manifestations include a maculopapular or wheal-like rash, pernio-like findings with associated erythema, and swelling of the toes, acrocyanosis, and livedo reticularis.

As compared to classic COVID-19 complaints, atypical presentations common to the older adult may occur. Cough and shortness of breath causing hypoxemia may manifest as a decline in function, an acute impairment of mobility or a new fall, confusion or altered mental status, or an exacerbation of heart failure or chronic obstructive pulmonary disease (COPD). Sequestration interventions and the clinical assessment of COVID-19 in the geriatric patient with dementia are especially onerous.

Geriatric males with comorbidities are at highest risk for severe disease. Overall, multiple studies have identified the principal comorbidities observed in COVID-19 patients. Listed in descending order of frequency these are hypertension, cardiovascular disease, diabetes, hypercholesterolemia, chronic lung disease, and malignancy. Other risk factors for severe disease include obesity, chronic kidney disease, concurrent immunosuppression, or dependence on a medical device (such as a gastrostomy tube, tracheostomy, or non-COVID-related noninvasive positive pressure ventilation) (Moses, 2022; Neumann-Podczaska et al., 2020; Nikolich-Zugich et al., 2020; Severe Acute Respiratory Syndrome—Coronavirus 2019 SARS-CoV-2, 2021).

Milder presentations may spontaneously remit without interventions. Alternatively, progression to pneumonia and respiratory failure may ensue, necessitating inpatient care. Especially in geriatric populations, deterioration observed in severe cases of the disease are characterized by acute lung injury compatible with ARDS; this is demonstrated by diffuse alveolar damage with hyaline membrane formation. In addition to ARDS, multiorgan dysfunction and ultimately death may occur (Neumann-Podczaska et al., 2020; Nikolich-Zugich et al., 2020).

Diagnosis

Overall, there should be a low threshold for suspicion and testing for SARS-2 in older adults. Efforts should be made to avoid the emergency department and to conduct testing and management in rapidly accessible areas with a low risk of exposure to mitigate spread and avoid overwhelming the health care system (Nikolich-Zugich et al., 2020 Apr).

Many studies have reported neutropenia, an absolute leukopenia, lymphopenia, and an increased neutrophil to lymphocyte ratio as common laboratory findings. Additional laboratory findings, especially evident in severe disease, include elevations of inflammatory markers. C-reactive protein levels are commonly above 10 mg/L, whereas erythrocyte sedimentation rates often exceed 35 mm/hr. Inflammatory laboratory findings are further supported by increases in ferritin, lactate dehydrogenase, procalcitonin, and interleukin (IL) 6. Although studies have generally identified hepatic measurements within the normal ranges, more advanced disease will result in increased liver function tests including total bilirubin. Cardiac indicators are usually within the normal ranges, whereas elevations were noted in the creatinine and BUN renal indices.

Coagulation findings include an elevated von Willebrand factor (VWF) antigen, elevated D-dimer, and fibrin/fibrinogen degradation products. Prothrombin time, partial thromboplastin time, and platelet counts are usually unaffected initially; however, coagulation times may increase with advancement. On occasion, thrombocytopenia was evident (Neumann-Podczaska et al., 2020; Severe Acute Respiratory Syndrome—Coronavirus 2019 SARS-CoV-2, 2021). Plain chest radiographs as well as chest CT scans may be normal or may demonstrate findings similar to those noted with other viral pulmonary infections. With disease progression, the most common radiographic abnormalities on CT scan are bilateral ground glass opacities and multilobular infiltrates with consolidations in a peripheral, posterior, and lower lobe distribution (refer to Fig. 14.2 for CT scan images demonstrating diffuse ground glass findings in an older adult patient with COVID-19 pneumonia).

Chest ultrasonography, MRI, and positron emission tomography (PET)/CT findings often corroborate the afore-

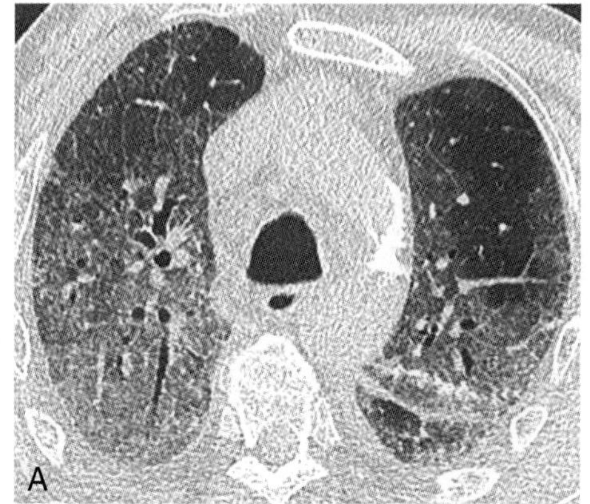

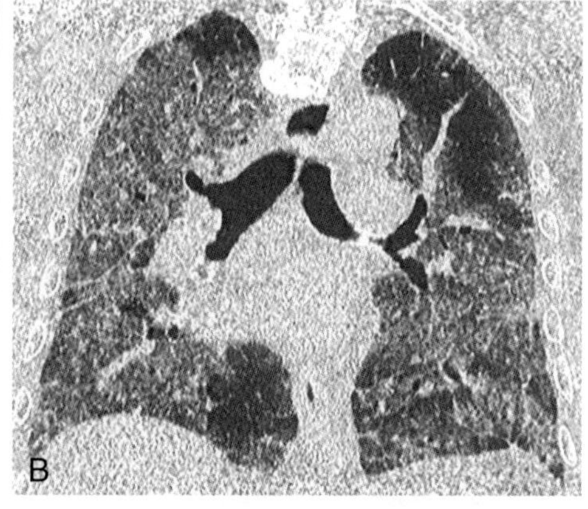

• Fig. 14.2 Axial (A) and coronal (B) CT images demonstrating extensive ground-glass opacities in an older adult male with COVID-19 pneumonia. (From Hani, C., Trieu, N. H., Saab, I., Dangeard, S., Bennani, S., Chassagnon, G., & Revel, M. P. [2020, May]. COVID-19 pneumonia: A review of typical CT findings and differential diagnosis. *Diagnostic Interventional Imaging, 101*[5], 263–268. *COVID-19 pneumonia: A review of typical CT findings and differential diagnosis*, ClinicalKey.)

mentioned radiologic patterns consistent with an organizing pneumonia process (Neumann-Podczaska et al., 2020; Severe Acute Respiratory Syndrome—Coronavirus 2019 SARS-CoV-2, 2021).

COVID-19 testing should be performed for all symptomatic patients (regardless of vaccination history or prior COVID-19 infection), asymptomatic patients admitted to hospitals, patients having procedures performed, and asymptomatic patients with a known positive exposure (Moses, 2022). Fully vaccinated older adult patients without COVID-19 symptoms do not need testing following exposure to a person with COVID-19. Geriatric patients not fully vaccinated and without symptoms should undergo testing if they are in close contact with someone with confirmed COVID-19 or reside in congregate venues such as nursing homes or acute care facilities. Finally, geriatric patients who have tested positive for COVID-19 within the previous 3 months and have recovered do not need testing following an exposure as long as they remain asymptomatic (Centers for Disease Control and Prevention, 2021a).

The preferred, initial diagnostic test of COVID-19 consists of nucleic acid amplification testing (NAAT). Most commonly, the detection of SARS-CoV-2 RNA by NAAT is accomplished by reverse transcription polymerase chain reaction (RT-PCR). As compared to throat samples, nasopharynx (via deep nasal swab) samples are preferred. Lower respiratory specimens may offer better positive yields than upper respiratory samples and have higher viral loads. SARS-CoV-2 RNA has also been isolated from stool and blood. Although the presence of SARS-CoV-2 RNA in blood may be indicative of severe disease, the assessment of SARS-CoV-2 RNA in nonrespiratory samples has a limited function in diagnosing disease. Older patients and those with serious manifestations necessitating inpatient care may shed viral RNA on a protracted interval; the median span has been reported as 12 to 20 days.

Antigen testing is accomplished via a nasopharyngeal or oropharyngeal swab. The benefits of antigen testing include a rapid turnaround time and cost effectiveness. Limitations of antigen testing include a lower overall sensitivity as compared to RT-PCR and an increased risk of false negatives, especially between day 5 and 12 following symptom onset. Negative testing may require additional testing in certain situations.

Antibody testing should not replace virologic testing nor should it be used to establish the presence or absence of acute SARS-CoV-2 infection. Persons suspected of having COVID-19 and who test positive by NAAT or antigen detection tests typically begin to produce antibodies 7 to 14 days after the illness onset; by 3 weeks the majority of patients will have positive antibody measurements. Both IgM and IgG may be detected around the same time after infection. Although IgM is most useful for determining recent infection as it usually becomes undetectable weeks to months following infection, IgG may remain detectable for longer periods. Assays that measure total antibody or IgG may have higher sensitivity as the time between infection and antibody testing increases. Serologic tests with very high sensitivity and specificity and that have been granted emergency use authorization by the Food and Drug Administration are preferred because they are more likely to exhibit high expected predictive values when administered at least 3 weeks following the onset of illness (Centers for Disease Control and Prevention, 2021a).

Management

Although management of COVID-19 is primarily supportive, a number of proposed specific therapies are being investigated. Older adults and their caretakers should be cognizant of the updated recommendations regarding changes to their usual medications. In admitted patients, the monitoring for signs of disease progression, decompensation, and exacerbation of a chronic illness is essential. Owing to the need to minimize the risk of aerosolization of the virus and airborne spread, standard respiratory therapies are being used cautiously in COVID-19 patients. These include the use of high-flow nasal oxygen, noninvasive positive-pressure ventilation, nebulized medications, and airway clearance therapies. Treatment guidelines of a recovering and a recovered patient are not well established and need to be explored early, as hospitals and acute care settings are expected to be overwhelmed, especially with susceptible older adult patients (Nikolich-Zugich et al., 2020).

Older adult patients with mild to moderate disease (those without viral pneumonia or hypoxia) may not initially require hospitalization, and most patients will be able to manage their illness at home. The decision to monitor a patient in the inpatient or outpatient setting should be made on a case-by-case basis. This decision will depend on the clinical presentation, requirement for supportive care, potential risk factors for severe disease, and the ability of the patient to self-isolate at home.

Patients 65 years of age and older are at risk for severe disease requiring hospitalization for management. Inpatient medical care includes supportive management of the most common complications of severe COVID-19: pneumonia, hypoxemic respiratory failure/ARDS, sepsis and septic shock, cardiomyopathy and arrhythmia, acute kidney injury, and complications from prolonged hospitalization, including secondary bacterial and fungal infections, thromboembolism, gastrointestinal bleeding, critical illness polyneuropathy/myopathy, and pressure wounds.

In hospitalized geriatric patients without contraindications, anticoagulation should be initiated. Laboratory anomalies frequently associated with COVID-19-associated coagulopathy include mild thrombocytopenia, increased D-dimer levels, increased fibrin degradation products, and a prolonged prothrombin time. In particular, elevated D-dimer levels have been strongly associated with a greater risk of death (Centers for Disease Control and Prevention, 2021b). Hypercoagulability increases the risk for venous and arterial thrombosis of large and small vessels.

The use of specific medications in the management of COVID-19 has been studied. To date, the Infectious Diseases

Society of America (IDSA) guidelines recommend against the use of either hydroxychloroquine or chloroquine alone or in combination with azithromycin in the hospital setting for COVID-19 due to potential harms of this regimen. In particular, the risk of the QTc prolongation is increased. The IDSA guideline panel also recommends against the use of the combination lopinavir/ritonavir for hospitalized patients. Gastrointestinal side effects, skin eruptions, and QTc prolongation have all been reported. Among hospitalized critically ill patients or those with severe but noncritical COVID-19, the IDSA guideline panel recommends dexamethasone. Glucocorticoids are not recommended for patients with COVID-19 without hypoxemia requiring supplemental oxygen.

Several investigational treatments have been studied in the management of COVID-19. These include monoclonal antibodies, convalescent plasma, and remdesivir. The use of the anti-IL 6 monoclonal antibody tocilizumab is suggested as adjunctive treatment in addition to the standard of care (i.e., steroids) rather than the standard of care alone. Tocilizumab demonstrated a trend toward reduced mortality at 28 days compared to no tocilizumab treatment; tocilizumab showed a lower relative risk of clinical deterioration, defined as death, need for mechanical ventilation, extracorporeal membrane oxygenation (ECMO), or ICU admission compared to placebo/usual care. Among ambulatory patients with mild to moderate COVID-19 at high risk for progression to severe disease, the guideline panel suggests use of the additional monoclonal antibodies bamlanivimab/etesevimab, casirivimab/imdevimab, or sotrovimab. Among hospitalized patients with severe COVID-19, the IDSA guideline panel recommends against bamlanivimab monotherapy. Regarding passive immunotherapy, the use of convalescent plasma is currently not supported by the IDSA as a conditional recommendation with a low certainty of evidence. Convalescent plasma may be considered among ambulatory patients with mild to moderate COVID-19 only in the context of a clinical trial. Remdesivir, an RNA polymerase inhibitor, should not be used in the routine treatment of patients with oxygen saturation levels >94% and not using supplemental oxygen. The guideline panel suggests remdesivir for the treatment of severe COVID-19 in hospitalized patients with an oxygen saturation <94% on room air. However, the guideline panel suggests against the routine initiation of remdesivir among patients on invasive ventilation or ECMO. The panel strongly urges continued study of remdesivir through recruitment into randomized controlled trials.

Baricitinib, a selective Janus kinase 1 and 2 inhibitor currently FDA approved for the treatment of rheumatoid arthritis (RA), is being investigated in multiple studies for treatment of COVID-19. The proposed benefits of baricitinib in the management of COVID-19 may relate to both its antiinflammatory and potential antiviral activity. For patients hospitalized with severe COVID-19 with increased inflammatory markers but not receiving invasive mechanical ventilation, the panel suggests baricitinib. Furthermore, in those who are hospitalized with severe infection who cannot receive the standard of care with a corticosteroid due to a contraindication, the IDSA guideline panel suggests use of baricitinib with remdesivir rather than remdesivir alone. Side effects of baricitinib include an increased risk of infections (especially upper respiratory tract infections), thrombosis, lymphopenia, anemia, increases in lipids, elevations in liver enzymes, and elevations in creatinine phosphokinase.

The panel recommends against the use of both famotidine and ivermectin for the sole purpose of treating COVID-19 outside of the context of a clinical trial (Bhimraj et al., 2021). Empiric antibiotic treatment should be implemented for cases complicated by bacterial pneumonia.

Complications

A multitude of ensuing complications may arise as a result of COVID-19 infection. Studies have identified renal impairment and injury as the most remarkable complication with an occurrence of approximately 25%. The second and third most commonly reported complications were co-infection and hepatic impairment and injury, respectively. Additional complications such as ARDS and cardiovascular-related complications such as acute heart injury, cardiac insufficiency, and arrhythmia were also reported (Neumann-Podczaska et al., 2020).

The most common thrombotic complications include deep venous thrombosis and pulmonary embolism. Others include microvascular thrombosis causing a swollen, erythematous to violaceous pernio-like eruption of the fingers or more commonly toes ("COVID toes"; Fig. 14.3), the clotting of intravascular catheters, myocardial injury with ST-segment elevation, and large vessel cerebrovascular accidents (Centers for Disease Control and Prevention, 2021b). Some patients who recover from pneumonia have pulmonary limitations of yet-to-be-determined etiology. It is unclear whether older adults are disproportionately affected long term (Nikolich-Zugich et al., 2020).

Prevention

In the effort to mitigate the introduction and spread of COVID-19, certain general preventive measures should be undertaken. To reduce transmission, diligent hand washing (especially following the touching of surfaces in public) or the use of hand sanitizer containing at least 60% alcohol if the hands are not visibly dirty is recommended. Other measures include practicing respiratory hygiene (which should be regularly practiced by covering a cough or sneeze), avoiding touching the face (especially the eyes, nose, and mouth), cleaning and disinfecting objects and surfaces that are frequently touched, providing sufficient ventilation of indoor spaces, wearing masks in the community, practicing social/physical distancing at a minimum of 6 feet, avoiding public gatherings and travel, identifying aggressive cases, isolating cases, contact tracing, and quarantine (McIntosh, 2021).

In nursing homes, these include vaccination of residents and staff, the employment of certain visitor restrictions, the application of source control (e.g., the use of masks),

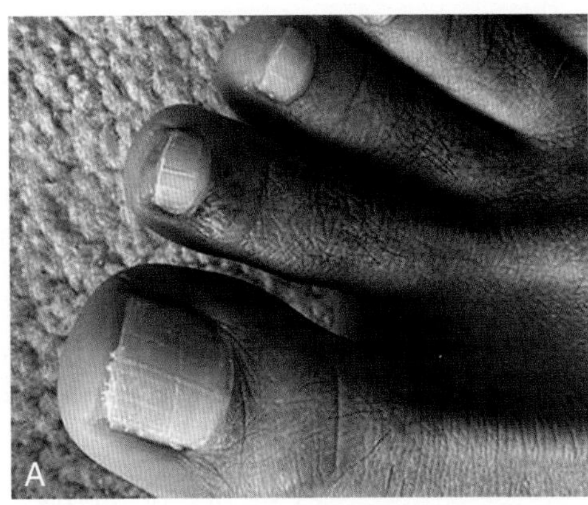

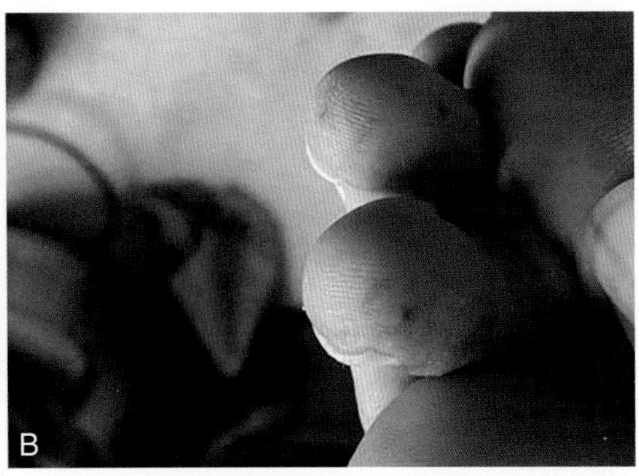

• Fig. 14.3 The pernio-like eruption, "COVID toes," is most often associated with asymptomatic or mildly symptomatic presentations. The digits may initially appear as swollen and erythematous, progressing to violaceous and purpuric lesions. Papules, plaques, or vesicles may all occur. (From Daneshjou, R., Rana, J., Dickman, M., Yost, J. M., Chiou, A., & Justin, K. [2020]. *JAAD Case Reports, 6*[9], 892–897. Copyright © 2020 American Academy of Dermatology, Inc. https://www.clinicalkey.com/#!/content/journal/1-s2.0-S2352512620304987?scrollTo=%231-s2.0-S2352512620304987-f14-07-9780323608459.)

symptom screening, and testing of both residents and health care persons. It is essential that these procedures be generally implemented because asymptomatic and presymptomatic spread can occur and symptom screening alone may not identify all cases of COVID-19 (Yurkofsky & Ouslander, 2021).

Adults 65 years old and older who were fully vaccinated with an mRNA COVID-19 vaccine (Pfizer-BioNTech or Moderna) had a 94% reduction in risk of COVID-19 hospitalizations, and vaccination was 64% effective among those who were partially vaccinated (Pfizer-BioNTech or Moderna) (Yurkofsky & Ouslander, 2021). The single-dose Johnson & Johnson Janssen vaccine was found to prevent severe COVID-19 requiring ICU admission or infection resulting in death in 85% of patients (Moses, 2022).

The COVID-19 global pandemic is ongoing and uncertainties regarding the various aspects of the disease exist, especially related to the long-term consequences, emergence of variants, and efficacy of the various treatment options.

GASTROINTESTINAL INFECTIONS

Clostridium difficile Colitis

Clostridium difficile is an anaerobic gram-positive, spore-forming toxigenic bacillus that is responsible for pseudomembranous colitis. The organism is regarded as the single most important cause of nosocomial infectious diarrhea in the United States (Greenwald, 2017) as it occurs primarily in hospitalized patients. In the United States, infection causes approximately 3 million cases of diarrhea annually and causes 14,000 deaths per year. While the rate of other nosocomial infections declines, new cases of *C. difficile* colitis continue to rise. Additionally, more cases are being reported in community populations affecting nontraditional demographics, such as pregnant patients, those with inflammatory bowel disease, and those without antecedent antibiotic exposure (Aberra, 2018).

Pathophysiology

Pathogenic strains of *C. difficile* produce two protein-toxins. Toxin A is an enterotoxin, and toxin B is a cytotoxin; both are capable of binding to specific receptors on the intestinal mucosal cells. A hypervirulent strain of *C. difficile*, NAP1/BI/027, is associated with the most serious sequelae of infection, causing severe and fulminant colitis marked by leukocytosis, renal failure, and toxic megacolon (Pant et al., 2011). Its development has been linked to the overuse and resistance of fluoroquinolones; it has additionally been isolated from several recent infectious outbreaks in Canada and the United States (Loo et al., 2005; McDonald et al., 2005; Pant et al., 2011; Pépin et al., 2005a, 2005b).

The preeminent event in the development of *C. difficile* colitis is exposure to antibiotics. Antimicrobial use is the most modifiable risk factor for infection (Guh et al., 2017; Kelly et al., 1994; Loo et al., 2011). Although any antibiotic may lead to infection, the most notorious agents include fluoroquinolones, clindamycin, cephalosporins, and penicillins. Less common agents include the macrolides, sulfonamides, tetracyclines, trimethoprim, and chloramphenicol (Greenwald, 2017). It is noteworthy that some of the medications used to treat *C. difficile* colitis may also initiate infection, including metronidazole and vancomycin (Kelly et al., 1994).

Colonization by the bacteria occurs because of exposure of the gut microflora to antibiotics. Antibiotics alter the normal resident bacterial barrier, facilitating the growth of *C. difficile*.

Other risk factors promoting the development of infection include older age, nasogastric tube use or enteral feeding, a recent gastrointestinal procedure, use of digestive acid suppression agents, stay in an intensive care unit, obesity, severe comorbidities, especially a history of chronic kidney disease, necrotizing enterocolitis, intestinal ischemia, cancer, Hirschsprung disease, hemolytic-uremic syndrome, and increased hospitalization length. Other risks include hematopoietic stem cell transplantation, chemotherapeutic use, inflammatory bowel disease, and cirrhosis (Aberra, 2018; Bishara et al., 2013; Kamthan et al., 1992; Loo et al., 2011; Reigadas et al., 2018; Rodemann et al., 2007; Yan et al., 2017).

C. difficile infection may result in an asymptomatic carrier state; this is most likely to occur in immunocompetent individuals with an inability to mount an immune response to the *C. difficile* toxin. *C. difficile* is highly transmissible via the fecal-oral route by ingestion of spores. The organism can be cultured readily from the hospital environment, including items in patient rooms as well as the hands, clothing, and stethoscopes of health care workers (Gerding et al., 1995; Kim et al., 1981).

C. difficile colitis should be suspected in any patient with diarrhea who has received antibiotics within the previous 3 months, has been recently hospitalized, or has an occurrence of diarrhea 48 hours or more after hospitalization (McDonald et al., 2007). However, it has been observed that *C. difficile* can cause diarrhea in adults in the community without a recent hospitalization or antibiotic use (Khanna et al., 2012).

Clinical Manifestations

The clinical manifestations of *C. difficile* colitis can range from asymptomatic to mild to moderate self-limiting diarrhea to life-threatening pseudomembranous colitis and fulminant colitis. Symptoms typically begin soon after colonization. Manifestations of watery, nonbloody diarrhea most often begin during or after just beginning an antibiotic regimen. Watery diarrhea (at least three loose stools in 24 hours) is the cardinal symptom of infection (Bagdasarian et al., 2015). In up to 40% of patients, however, symptoms may not commence for up to 10 weeks following completion of an antibiotic course. More severe illness is characterized by fever and cramping abdominal pain. Mucus or occult blood may also be present, but the presence of hematochezia should suggest an alternative diagnosis. Patients with a more severe presentation may develop colonic ileus or toxic dilation without diarrhea.

In patients with mild *C. difficile* infection, the physical examination is generally unremarkable. When findings are apparent, they consist of fever, signs of dehydration, and lower abdominal tenderness. Findings suggestive of complications such and colonic perforation and peritonitis will increase the likelihood of rebound tenderness. More significant complications such as toxic megacolon and bowel perforation are heralded by marked dehydration, marked abdominal tenderness, abdominal distention, decreased bowel sounds, and marked rigidity (Aberra, 2018; Greenwald, 2017).

Diagnosis

The diagnosis of *C. difficile* infection should be suspected in patients with acute diarrhea (≥3 loose stools in 24 hours) with no obvious alternative explanation (such as laxative use), particularly in the setting of known risk factors.

A complete blood count will commonly identify a leukocytosis; white blood cell elevations signify more significant disease. Serum chemistries should also be assessed, as patients with *C. difficile* infection are subject to acute kidney injury; increased creatinine findings also indicate a more serious presentation (Aberra, 2018; Greenwald, 2017). Specific laboratory criteria proposed by the Infectious Diseases Society of America (IDSA) and Society for Healthcare Epidemiology of America (SHEA) for nonsevere infection include a white blood cell count ≤15,000 cells/mL and serum creatinine <1.5 mg/dL (McDonald et al., 2018).

The diagnosis is confirmed when the cytotoxin is present in the patient's stool sample. The SHEA and IDSA recommend stool toxin testing for *C. difficile* in symptomatic patients only on diarrheal stool unless there is suspicion of ileus due to *C. difficile*. Furthermore, stool toxin testing is not recommended for asymptomatic patients (unless for study purposes) nor is repeat testing recommended following successful treatment in a patient recently treated for *C. difficile*.

Cytotoxin testing's sensitivity range is between 70% and 100%, with a specificity of 90% to 100%. Several limitations exist; the test results are reported only as positive or negative, it is expensive, and it requires overnight incubation and a tissue culture facility.

Stool cultures are the most appropriate studies in asymptomatic patients (Cohen et al., 2010; Martinez-Melendez et al., 2017); stool cultures are the most sensitive tests for detecting *C. difficile* and its toxins (Cohen et al., 2010). Although it is the criterion standard, drawbacks to culture include a long turnaround time and increased resource allocation. Instead, the most widely used is an enzyme linked immunoassay (ELISA). This assay detects *C. difficile* toxin A or B. Although the main advantages are speed, cost, ease of testing, and high specificity, this immunoassay has relatively low sensitivity (Greenwald, 2017), with a reported range between 79% and 80%, but excellent specificity (98%). Repeat testing is needed if the initial test is negative. The reduced sensitivity of the ELISA may be offset by obtaining repeat stool specimens or by combining ELISA with a polymerase chain reaction (PCR) assay or *C. difficile* antigen (glutamate dehydrogenase [GDH]) ELISA. *C. difficile* antigen GDH ELISA is sensitive (sensitivity approaches 100% and specificity up to 98%). This test detects the presence of GDH produced by *C. difficile;* however, positive test results need to be confirmed by another assay modality.

Another diagnostic test includes the PCR for the detection of toxin genes. It is regarded as an alternative gold standard test to the stool culture, with some studies demonstrating excellent sensitivity and specificity, as well as test-retest reliability; it possesses high positive and negative predictive values. Additional benefits offered include a rapid turnaround time and cost effectiveness (Aberra, 2018; Greenwald, 2017).

Colonoscopy, or more often flexible sigmoidoscopy, may be helpful in making the diagnosis of *C. difficile* colitis but is usually not necessary in the diagnosis or management of disease. Compared to stool testing, endoscopy has reduced sensitivity; findings may be normal in patients with mild disease or may demonstrate nonspecific colitis in moderate cases. Furthermore, sigmoidoscopy will likely be unremarkable if disease is localized to the right colon. Endoscopy is most useful when the diagnosis is in doubt or when disease severity demands rapid diagnosis. The finding of colonic pseudomembranes in a patient with antibiotic-associated diarrhea is almost pathognomonic for *C. difficile* colitis (Greenwald, 2017). Findings common to infection are elevated, yellowish white, 2- to 10-mm plaques overlying an erythematous, edematous mucosa. These are referred to as pseudomembranes, which are demonstrable in 14% to 25% of patients with mild disease and 87% of patients with fulminant disease (Fig. 14.4).

Biopsy of the characteristics plaques reveals an inflammatory exudate composed of mucinous debris, fibrin, necrotic epithelial cells, and polymorphonuclear cells. The underlying crypts show disruption by mucous and inflammatory debris. The interposing mucosa shows edema but is otherwise unremarkable (Fig. 14.5) (Aberra, 2018).

An abdominal computed tomography (CT) scan is the imaging modality of choice for *C. difficile* colitis when pseudomembranous colitis, other complications of *C. difficile* infection, or other intraabdominal pathology is suspected (Grant et al., 2008). The most common radiographic finding is marked colonic wall thickening. Additional features include ascites, irregularity of the bowel wall, and pericolonic stranding. An abdominal plain film may be ordered instead of CT scan in patients with sepsis to identify megacolon more rapidly (Aberra, 2018).

Treatment

Factors guiding treatment decisions include the assessment of severity of infection, local epidemiology, and the type of *C. difficile* strains present. The first step in the management of *C. difficile* colitis is to remove any unnecessary contributory antibiotics. Additionally, antidiarrheal agents (e.g., diphenoxylate with atropine) should be avoided, as they have been reported to increase the duration and severity of symptoms. Asymptomatic carriers should not be treated (Greenwald, 2017).

For patients with severe or complicated infection suggested by leukocytosis or renal impairment, oral vancomycin 125 mg four times per day for 10 to 14 days is recommended as first-line therapy; treatment should be

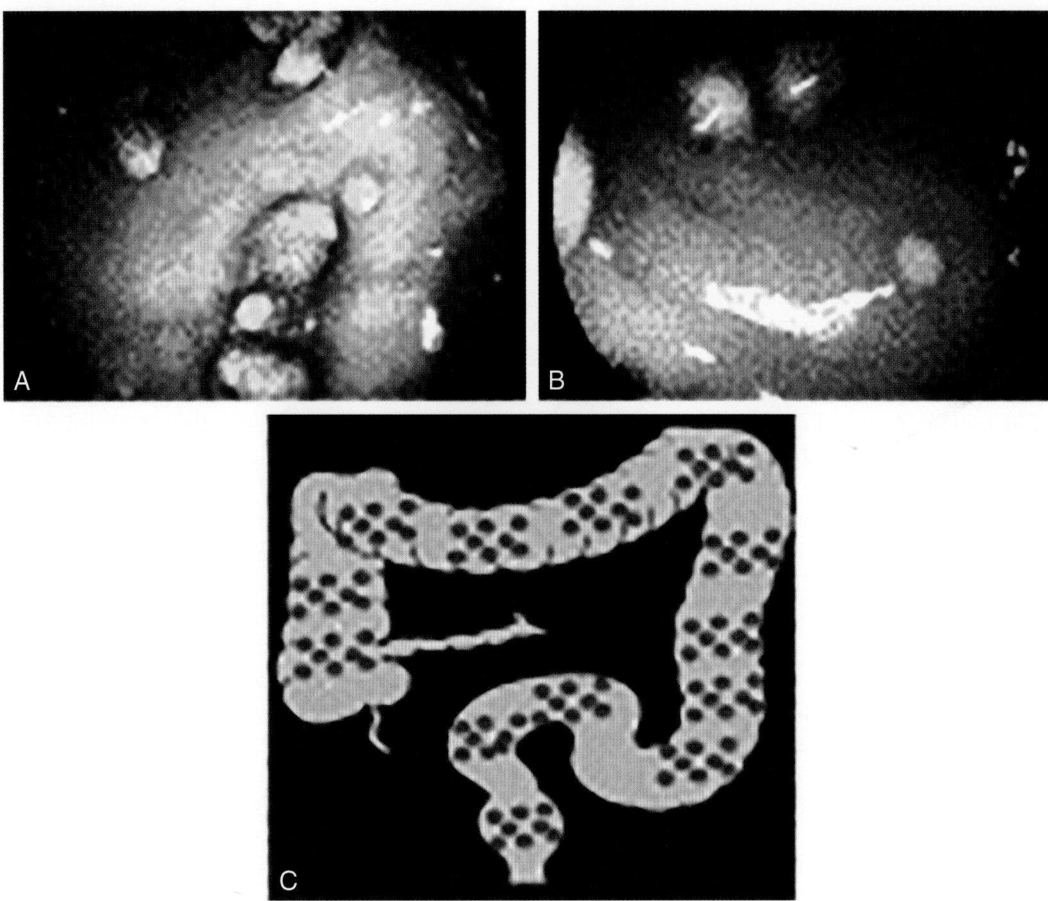

• Fig. 14.4 Colonoscopic view of pseudomembranous colitis. (A and B) Discrete lesions surrounded by normal-appearing mucosa are seen early in disease. Hemorrhage is seen at the edges of some pseudomembranes in A in this patient with underlying leukemia. (C) Anatomic location of the lesions. (From Bennett, J. E., et al. [2015]. *Mandell, Douglas, and Bennett's principles and practice of infectious diseases* [8th ed.]. Elsevier. https://doi.org/10.1016/B978-1-4557-4801-3.00245-9.)

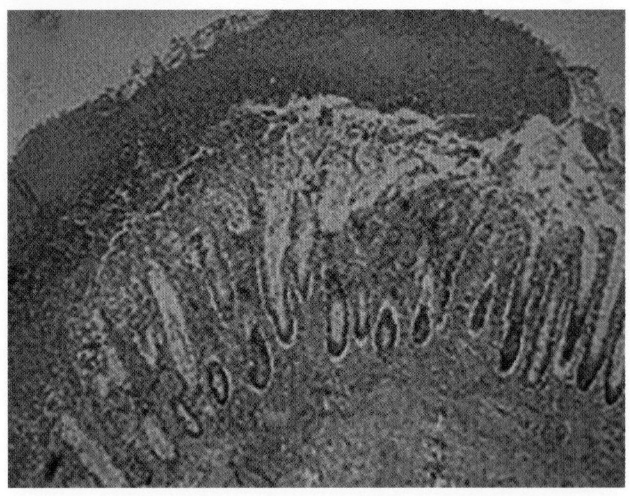

• **Fig. 14.5** Histopathology of pseudomembranous colitis. There is significant polymorphonuclear infiltrate, a fibrinous exudate, and epithelial damage. (From Bennett, J. E., et at. *Mandell, Douglas, and Bennett's principles and practice of infectious diseases* [8th ed.]. Elsevier. https://doi.org/10.1016/B978-1-4557-4801-3.00245-9.)

begun empirically. Implementation with vancomycin results in more rapid symptom resolution and fewer treatment failures as compared to metronidazole. In fulminant cases, combined therapy with intravenous metronidazole and vancomycin (PO or PR) is the treatment of choice (Cohen et al., 2010). Intravenous vancomycin is ineffective, as it does not penetrate the colonic lumen and should not be used for *C. difficile* (Greenwald, 2017). Therefore, the recommended regimen is intravenous metronidazole 500 mg every 8 hours with oral vancomycin 500 mg four times per day (and/or 500 mg every 6 hours in 100 mL as a retention enema) (Cohen et al., 2010).

Fidaxomicin 200 mg orally every 12 hours is approved in the treatment of primary *C. difficile* colitis and is equally efficacious with a lower relapse rate versus vancomycin. Further study also demonstrated a lower relapse rate in older adults, but providers generally do not prescribe it as first-line therapy because it is much more expensive than metronidazole or vancomycin. The treatment duration is 10 days (Cornely et al., 2012; Feher et al., 2017).

According to the SHEA and IDSA, for patients with mild to moderate disease (i.e., white blood cell counts <15,000 μL, creatinine < 1.5 × baseline) or for patients without fever, sepsis, or megacolon, the primary treatment is metronidazole 500 mg orally three times daily for 10 to 14 days (Cohen et al., 2010; Little, 2018). The use of vancomycin for mild to moderate disease may induce vancomycin-resistant enterococci (Greenwald, 2017). It should be noted, however, that due to increased resistance to metronidazole approaching 30% in some regions, vancomycin has been increasingly recommended by the IDSA as first-line therapy for mild to moderate disease (Moses, 2019a).

A strong recommendation from the IDSA citing high-quality evidence now favors a 10-day course of vancomycin or fidaxomicin rather than metronidazole for first-line therapy of mild/moderate *C. difficile* in adults. This new recommendation was based on several clinical trials demonstrating greater cure rates and less frequent recurrence following vancomycin compared with metronidazole (Kociolek, 2018).

C. difficile recurs in approximately a quarter of patients and manifests 3 days to 3 weeks after the treatment is discontinued. Antibiotic exposure, failure to eradicate the organism from the colon, and reinfection from the environment are cited as reasons for reinfection; however, any established risk factor for the disease may be implicated in its recurrence (Aberra, 2018). Because resistance to metronidazole or vancomycin is rarely a causative factor in recurrence, patients with recurrent disease generally are given a repeat trial with the antibiotic used to treat the initial infection. Subsequent infection is typically treated with a tapered vancomycin course (Box 14.1).

Metronidazole can be used for recurrent mild to moderate infection; however, it should not be used for more than once recurrence or over a chronic period owing to an accumulated risk of neurotoxicity.

Probiotics such as *Lactobacillus* GG and *Saccharomyces boulardii* are not recommended for the treatment of active infection owing to limited data supporting their benefits and a potential risk for septicemia. However, a meta-analysis upheld previous study findings that found probiotics prevented diarrhea associated with antibiotic use (Videlock & Cremonini, 2012).

Fecal microbiota transplantation (FMT) has been shown to be highly effective in the treatment of recurrent *C. difficile* infection and is also a very effective therapy for selected patients with severe or fulminant disease (Greenwald, 2017). This treatment transfers stool from a healthy donor to a patient with *C. difficile* infection for the purposes of reestablishing the normal colonic microbial flora. Multiple studies across varied age demographics have demonstrated successful treatment and culmination of infection utilizing this approach. Resolution was achieved for recurrent, refractory, or severe disease. A risk of infection transmission (HIV, hepatitis, and retrovirus) does exist (Laidman, 2013; van Nood et al., 2013; Kling, 2013).

An overview of improper procedures (i.e., do nots) in the prevention and management of *C. difficile* colitis is identified in Box 14.2 (Little, 2018).

Surgical consultation is recommended in patients with suspected fulminant colitis, toxic megacolon, or peritonitis. Surgery may include colectomy with preservation of the rectum under such conditions. Determining the need for surgery referral may be guided by any of the criteria identified in Box 14.3 (Bhangu et al., 2012; Ferrada et al., 2014; Hall & Berger, 2008; Sailhamer et al., 2009; van der Wilden et al., 2017).

Gastroenteritis

Gastroenteritis is common in the older adult. Consistent with other infectious syndromes, morbidity and mortality affect older adults disproportionately; older adult patients more commonly experience severe presentations and

• BOX 14.1 Oral Vancomycin Tapered/Pulse Regimen

Oral Vancomycin Tapered/Pulse Regimen for *C. difficile* Recurrence

- 125 mg 4 times daily for 10–14 days, then
- 125 mg 3 times daily for 7 days, then
- 125 mg twice daily for 7 days, then
- 125 mg daily for 7 days, then
- 125 mg every 48 hours for 7 days, then
- 125 mg every 72 hours for 7 days

Data from Little, M. (2018). Treating and preventing clostridium difficile infection in long-term care facilities. *Annals of Long-Term Care, 26*(7), P25–P27.

• BOX 14.2 Items to Avoid in Patients With *C. difficile* Colitis

In the management of *C. difficile* colitis, do not do the following:

- Test stool in asymptomatic residents to look for carriers
- Test stool after treatment to assess for cure
- Prescribe antiperistaltic agents to treat *C. difficile* colitis diarrhea
- Forget to wash hands with soap and water
- Use alcohol-based cleaners
- Share multiuse equipment prior to vigorous cleaning with 10% bleach or 1:10 hypochlorite solution
- Use antibiotics for asymptomatic bacteriuria or acute viral illnesses
- Allow asymptomatic patients to use public or shared toilets
- Use a prolonged metronidazole course, combination oral treatment, high-dose vancomycin or toxin-binders

Data from Little, M. (2018). Treating and preventing clostridium difficile infection in long-term care facilities. *Annals of Long-Term Care, 26*(7), P25–P27.

• BOX 14.3 Criteria for Surgical Consultation in *C. difficile* Colitis

Indications for surgical consultation in the management of *C. difficile* infection (CDI) can be any one of the following:

- Hypotension with or without required use of vasopressors
- Fever ≥ 38.5°C
- Ileus or significant abdominal distention
- Peritonitis or significant abdominal tenderness
- Mental status changes
- WBC ≥ 20,000 cells/mL
- Serum lactate levels > 2.2 mmol/L
- Admission to intensive care unit for CDI
- End organ failure (mechanical ventilation, renal failure, etc.)
- Failure to improve after three to five days of maximal medical therapy

From Bhangu et al., 2012; Ferrada et al., 2014; Hall & Berger, 2008; Sailhamer et al., 2009; van der Wilden et al., 2017.

complications of infection. Various factors increase the risk of gastroenteritis in this population. Factors that enhance the predisposition to diarrheal illnesses in older adults include hypochlorhydria and achlorhydria, impaired gastric motility, inappropriate use of antibiotics, and waning immunity.

Etiology

Viral gastroenteritis may be caused by rotavirus and enteroviruses, including norovirus (previously called Norwalk-like viruses) (Mody et al., 2014); viruses are responsible for a significant percentage of cases affecting patients of all ages. In the United States, viruses are the leading cause of acute gastroenteritis (Chiejina and Samant, 2018, January). Most cases of epidemic viral gastroenteritis in adults are caused by the caliciviruses. Examples include Norovirus (previously called Norwalk-like viruses). The most common causes of sporadic viral gastroenteritis are caliciviruses, non–group A rotavirus, astrovirus, and adenovirus. Bacterial gastroenteritis may be induced by *C. difficile, Bacillus cereus, Escherichia coli, Campylobacter, Clostridium perfringens,* or *Salmonella.* Additionally, parasites are well-known causes of diarrhea in skilled nursing facilities (Mody et al., 2014). Among bacterial causes of acute diarrhea, nontyphoidal Salmonella and Campylobacter species are the most common causes in the United States. Other causes include exposure to parasitic agents, toxins, and drugs.

Pathophysiology

Infection is generally by fecal-oral transmission of contaminated food and water. Some viruses like noroviruses may be transmitted by an airborne route. The pathophysiology of infectious agents is highly varied. There are a multitude of causes of watery (non-inflammatory) diarrhea. Common viral etiologies include norovirus, and other enteric viruses. The norovirus incubation is approximately one to two days with common sources of infection being shellfish, contaminated prepared foods, fruits and vegetables. Disease often occurs in those frequenting restaurants, medical settings, schools, cruise ships and within military installations. The enteric viruses, such rotavirus, enteric adenovirus, astrovirus and sapovirus, have an average incubation period of two days whose etiology is fecally-contaminated food or water causing acute gastroenteritis in children attending daycare or in immunocompromised adults. The *Clostridioides* bacteria may also cause diarrhea, with *Clostridium difficile* able to cause both inflammatory or non-inflammatory diarrhea. Risk factors for *Clostridium difficile* include antibiotic use, recent hospitalization, receiving cancer chemotherapy, gastric acid inhibition and a history of inflammatory bowel disease. *Clostridium perfringens* diarrhea is generally watery, accompanied by abdominal cramping and occurs within 6 – 24 hours following the consumption of contaminated meat, poultry, gravy, or home-canned items. Enterotoxigenic *Escherichia coli* is the most common cause of tourist's diarrhea. The typical incubation period is 10 – 72 hours whose symptoms include a rapid onset of voluminous watery, nonbloody diarrhea accompanied by little or no fever. It is contracted by the consumption of fecally-contaminated foods or drinks. *Giardia lamblia*, a pear-shaped flagellated protozoan, also causes watery diarrhea via fecal contamination. It is the most common parasitic infection in the world and the leading waterborne illness in the United States. Its onset is a week to up to one month following exposure. Risk factors include poor sanitation, close contact with an infected individual, oral-anal intercourse and wilderness travel that is associated with intake of contaminated water. Manifestations include a non-inflammatory diarrhea, steatorrhea, flatulence, abdominal pain, eructation, malabsorption and weight loss. Nausea, vomiting and dehydration are uncommon; fever suggests an alternative diagnosis. *Cryptosporidium parvum*, a coccidian protozoan, is a common cause of traveler's diarrhea and waterborne illness outbreaks. Fecal-oral contamination occurs through contaminated drinking water or uncooked foods; infection is common in day care settings as well as afflicting those with human immunodeficiency virus. Manifestations occur from 2 – 10 days after infection and consists of abdominal pain, diarrhea, nausea, vomiting and fever. Immunocompromised patients may experience chronic watery secretory diarrhea and cough. Another coccidian parasite, *Cyclospora cayetanensis*, is transmitted as a waterborne or foodborne (e.g., from fresh produce) illness and infects the small intestine in humans. Following an incubation period of 2 – 14 days, the following symptoms may occur: anorexia, weight loss, fatigue, low-grade fever, nausea, vomiting, explosive, non-bloody diarrhea, abdominal cramping and bloating, and excessive flatus. A final major cause of non-inflammatory diarrhea is *Listeria monocytogenes*, a gram positive bacillus. Risk factors include those that are immunocompromised, pregnant, newborns and the elderly. Clinical listeriosis occurs between 9 to 48 hours following incubation and manifests as a gastroenteritis following intake of contaminated deli meats, frozen vegetables, unpasteurized milk and soft cheese. Self-limited diarrhea, fever, nausea and myalgias are typical manifestations in the immunocompetent; invasive bacteremia, meningitis or endocarditis may complicate cases in the immunocompromised.

Inflammatory diarrhea, characterized by fever, mucoid or bloody stools, is chiefly caused by bacterial agents. Nontyphoidal *Salmonella* (*Salmonella typhimurium* and *Salmonella enteritidis*) are gram-negative rods that cause abdominal cramping, fever, vomiting, bloody stools and diarrhea. Symptoms manifest approximately up to three days following exposure to eggs, cheese, dry cereal, unpasteurized milk or juice, ice cream, poultry, unpeeled fruits, vegetables or pets (especially birds or reptiles). *Campylobacter* species, also gram-negative rods, cause bloody diarrhea, nausea, abdominal cramping and pain, and fever within two to five days after exposure to the bacteria. Infection occurs upon consuming raw or undercooked poultry, seafood, meat, produce, by contact with animals, and by drinking untreated water. *Shigella* species, causing the clinical syndrome of shigellosis, is the most common cause of bloody diarrhea in the United States. Once consumed through contaminated water or raw produce, the bacteria invades the bowel mucosa and produces an enterotoxin in the colon. Following an incubation period of 1 to 7 days, a multitude of significant manifestation ensue. These include: severe bloody diarrhea often with accompanying mucus, tenesmus, abdominal pain and cramping, nausea, vomiting, lassitude, fever and dehydration. Enterohemorrhagic *E. coli* is another cause of inflammatory bloody diarrhea as a result of acute hemorrhagic colitis. Most strains are capable of producing Shiga-like toxins. The foodborne illness usually commences rapidly (within 12 – 72 hours) following the consumption of undercooked meat products (especially hamburgers, pork, poultry and lamb), mayonnaise, sausage, salami, raw milk, alfalfa sprouts and unpasteurized apple cider and apple juice. *Yersinia enterocolitica* causes enterocolitis, acute bloody diarrhea, terminal ileitis, mesenteric lymphadenitis, and pseudoappendicitis. In addition to bloody diarrhea, other manifestations include a low-grade fever, abdominal pain (often localizing to the right lower quadrant), erythema nodosum and vomiting. The incubation period is typically 4 – 7 days and is transmitted by contaminated unpasteurized milk and milk products, raw pork, tofu, meats, raw vegetables, oysters, and fish. Since *Yersinia* can proliferate at refrigerated temperatures, outbreaks can occur as a result of consumption of pasteurized milk and dairy products as well. *Vibrio parahemolyticus* diarrhea may be watery or bloody and accompanied by abdominal cramping, nausea, vomiting, fever and a headache. Infection usually occurs within 24 hours after ingesting the bacteria from shellfish or raw seafood consumption. Risk factors for *Entamoeba histolytica* infection include mental health institution or crowded living settings, poor sanitation, travel to endemic areas (e.g., Asia, Africa or Latin America), oral-anal intercourse food preparation contaminated by poor hygiene and the use of human waste as crop fertilizer. *Entamoeba histolytica* causes enterocolitis following an incubation period of 1 – 3 weeks. Enterocolitis results from intraluminal intestinal disease and is characterized by diarrhea, distal intestinal ulceration and intestinal bleeding. Systemic dissemination in the form of liver, lung or brain abscess formation is possible. The acute, fulminant phase of the illness caused by the *Entamoeba* trophozoite is characterized by profuse bloody and mucoid diarrhea, moderate to severe abdominal pain and cramping, tenesmus, malaise, fever, dehydration, and malabsorption; the chronic cyst phase typically results in normal stool formation and is generally asymptomatic (fever and tenderness and cramping of the cecum and ascending colon may occur in a minority of patients during the chronic illness period). Table 14.3 lists types of food frequently associated with bacterial causes of gastroenteritis.

Noroviruses

Noroviruses are transmitted person to person via direct contact, exposure to aerosols, or fecal–oral routes. Noroviruses are highly contagious with an incubation period of approximately 1 to 2 days, and symptoms typically last 1 to 3 days with expanded time frames in immunocompromised individuals. Viral shedding occurs for up to 3 weeks following infection. Infection is characterized by blunting damage to the microvilli in the small intestine. Pathogenically, there is

TABLE 14.3 Common Foodborne Pathogens and Their Food Source

Pathogens	Food Source
Salmonella	Raw eggs, undercooked meat or poultry, unpasteurized milk or juice, unpasteurized soft cheese
Campylobacter spp	Undercooked meat or poultry, unpasteurized milk or juice, unpasteurized soft cheese
Clostridium botulinum	Homemade canned goods
Clostridium perifringens	Undercooked meat or poultry
Shiga toxin producing *Escherichia coli* (STEC)	Undercooked meat or poultry, unpasteurized milk or juice, unpasteurized soft cheese
Listeria monocytogenes	Unpasturized soft cheese, raw hot dogs, deli meat
Norwalk-like virus	Raw seafood
Vibrio spp	Raw seafood
hepatitis A	Raw seafood

increased epithelial cell apoptosis and damage to tight junction proteins, with diarrhea occurring as a complication of D-xylose and fat malabsorption, with enzymatic dysfunction observed at the brush border, along with leak flux and anion secretion. Vomiting is related to virus-mediated changes in gastric motility and delayed gastric emptying (Khan, 2018).

Rotaviruses

Rotaviruses attach and enter mature enterocytes at the tips of small intestinal villi. They cause structural changes to the small bowel mucosa, including villus shortening and mononuclear inflammatory infiltrate in the lamina propria. Malabsorption of carbohydrates and other nutrients occurs within the intestinal lumen. The increased accrual of these components in conjunction with the inhibition of water reabsorption leads to a malabsorption component of diarrhea. Furthermore, rotavirus secretes an enterotoxin promoting the secretion of chloride causing diarrhea (Lin, 2018).

Escherichia coli O157:H7 and Other Enterohemorrhagic *E. Coli*

The enterohemorrhagic *E. coli* (EHEC) strain includes more than 100 serotypes that produce Shiga and Shiga-like toxins. The Shiga toxin–producing *E. coli* (STEC) is also known as verotoxin-producing *E. coli* (VTEC). *E. coli* O157:H7 is the most common STEC in North America. However, non-O157 STEC serotypes (particularly O26, O45, O91, O103, O111, O113, O121, O128, and O145) may also cause enterohemorrhagic illness, particularly outside the United States. *E. coli* O 157:H7 and other forms of STEC have a bovine reservoir. Transmission is via the fecal-oral route and results from food or water contaminated with cow manure, as in the outbreaks and sporadic cases that typically occur after the ingestion of undercooked beef (especially ground beef) or unpasteurized milk. Other sources are additionally possible; the 2011 European O104:H4 outbreak was transmitted by contaminated raw bean sprouts.

Following ingestion, *E. coli* O157:H7 and similar STEC serotypes produce high levels of toxins in the large intestine; these toxins are closely related to the potent cytotoxins produced by *Shigella dysenteriae* type 1. These toxins appear to directly damage mucosal cells and vascular endothelial cells in the gut wall. If absorbed, they exert toxic effects on other vascular endothelia (e.g., renal). About 5% to 10% of cases (especially of the age extremes) are complicated by hemolytic-uremic syndrome, which typically develops in the second week of illness. Death may occur, especially in the older adult, with or without this complication (Bush et al., 2018).

Clinical Manifestations of Viral Gastroenteritis

In the adult, acute gastroenteritis is defined as diarrheal disease (three or more times per day or at least 200 g of stool per day) of rapid onset that lasts less than 2 weeks and may be accompanied by nausea, vomiting, fever, or abdominal pain. Although both vomiting and diarrhea are typically apparent, either can occur alone. Associated respiratory symptoms such as sore throat, cough, and rhinorrhea can occur in approximately 10% of patients. Other constitutional symptoms such as weight loss and fatigue are possible.

Common findings suggesting a viral etiology of acute gastroenteritis include an intermediate incubation period (24 to 60 hours), a short infection duration (12 to 60 hours), and a high frequency of vomiting. Norovirus infection usually lasts a median of 2 days; rotavirus infection follows a minimally more protracted course at 3 to 8 days. Bloody diarrhea is overall an atypical finding in viral gastroenteritis.

A common abdominal physical exam finding in acute viral gastroenteritis includes mild but diffuse abdominal tenderness on palpation. Generally, the abdomen is soft, but there may be voluntary guarding. Fever (38.3 to 38.9°C [101 to 102 °F]) occurs in approximately 50% of patients.

The provider should be cognizant of clinical manifestations that suggest moderate to severe dehydration; these are not common (less than 10% of patients). These objective findings consist of dry mucous membranes, decreased skin turgor, tachycardia, hypotension, or altered mental status (Alexandraki & Smetana, 2019).

Clinical Manifestations of Bacterial Gastroenteritis

Symptoms of nontyphoidal salmonellosis generally occur within a period of 8 to 72 hours following exposure. Diarrhea, nausea, vomiting, and fever are typical in symptomatic infection, but diarrhea is not usually grossly bloody (LaRocque & Harris, 2019a; LaRocque & Harris, 2019b). Abdominal cramping, headache, and myalgias also occur, and fever usually resolves within 48 hours. Rarely, *Salmonella* infections cause large-volume cholera-like diarrhea or may be associated with tenesmus. The diarrhea is typically self-limiting and resolves within 3 to 7 days. It is noteworthy that focal disease may also manifest in any organ due to transient or continual bacteremia (Klochko, 2018).

Symptom onset consistent with enterohemorrhagic *E. coli* (EHEC) infection usually occurs 3 to 4 days (ranging from 1 to 9 days) following exposure, with bloody diarrhea and abdominal pain. At times, the diarrhea may initially be watery but often progresses to become bloody. Fever is often absent or low grade (LaRocque & Harris, 2019a; LaRocque & Harris, 2019b).

Clinical manifestations of bacterial gastroenteritis can be suggested by the timeline of symptom development. The ingestion of preformed toxins, as in the case of infection from *S. aureus* and *Bacillus cereus*, commonly causes symptomatology within hours of exposure. Conversely, bacteria that produce toxin following an extended period, such as enterotoxigenic *E. coli*, or that directly damage or invade across the intestinal epithelial cell membranes (e.g., *Salmonella, Campylobacter, Shigella*) usually result in symptoms after approximately 24 hours or longer. Protozoal pathogens such as *Cryptosporidium parvum* generally produce manifestations following an incubation period of about 7 days.

Identification of the dietary history can be an asset in the implication of a possible bacterial cause. A list of associated etiologies and associated food sources has been presented in Table 14.3. Various postinfectious syndromes associated with enteric infections are found in Fig. 14.6.

Diagnosis

The diagnosis of acute viral gastroenteritis is made by a characteristic history of diarrheal disease, defined as three or more times per day or at least 200 g of stool per day of rapid onset that lasts less than 1 week and may be accompanied by nausea, vomiting, fever, or abdominal pain and a characteristic physical examination of mild, diffuse, abdominal tenderness (Alexandraki & Smetana, 2019).

Routine laboratory and stool studies for the presence of fecal leukocytes, occult blood, or lactoferrin are generally not required for the diagnosis of acute viral gastroenteritis, as it is not necessary to determine a specific viral diagnosis.

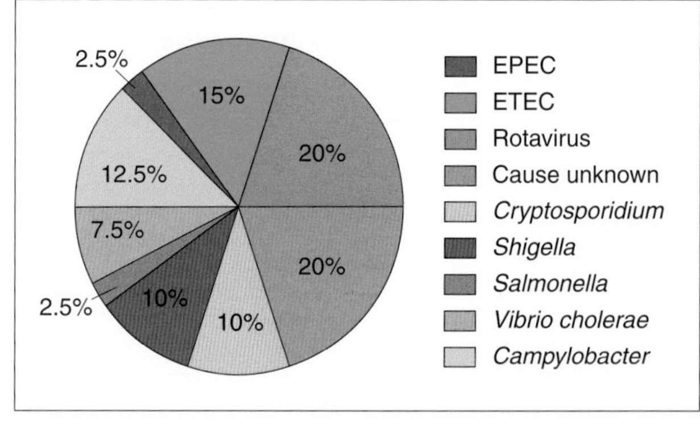

• **Fig. 14.6** Postinfectious Manifestations Associated with Enteric Pathogen. In Roitt et al: *Mims' Medical Microbiology*, ed4, 2008, Elsevier. (Data from the WHO.)

Additionally, these parameters will be negative for fecal leukocytes and occult blood, and a stool culture will not yield any bacterial pathogens. An inflammatory, nonviral gastroenteritis is suggested by the presence of fecal leukocytes, occult blood, lactoferrin, or positive stool cultures. However, stool studies should be obtained in these conditions: adults presenting with persistent fever, dehydration, blood or pus in the stool, or other alarm symptoms and signs listed in Box 14.4 and based on the algorithm found in Fig. 14.7. Stool studies are also indicated if the provider suspects a nonviral, inflammatory etiology of acute gastroenteritis (Alexandraki & Smetana, 2019). The workup for parasitic etiologies should be contemplated in cases of persistent diarrhea of at least 10 days duration or for whom diarrhea does not improve with standard antibiotic therapy (LaRocque & Harris, 2019a; LaRocque & Harris, 2019b).

• BOX 14.4 Alarm Symptoms and Signs in Gastroenteritis

- Dry mucous membranes (dry mouth)
- Decreased skin turgor
- Increased thirst
- Altered mental status (confusion, lethargy)
- Dizziness, lightheadedness
- Headache
- Tachycardia, palpitations
- Hypotension, orthostasis
- Presyncope or syncope
- Weakness, fatigue
- Decreased urine output, concentrated urine (deep yellow or amber color)
- Bloody stool/rectal bleeding
- Weight loss
- Severe abdominal pain
- Prolonged symptoms (more than a week)
- Recent hospitalization or antibiotics
- Age ≥65 years
- Comorbidities such as HIV and diabetes (immunocompromised status)
- Pregnancy

From Jones, R., & Rubin, G. (2009). Acute diarrhoea in adults. *BMJ. 338*, b1877; Thielman, N. M., & Guerrant, R. L. (2004). Clinical practice: Acute infectious diarrhea. *New England Journal of Medicine, 350*(1), 38.

The complete blood count is not useful in distinguishing between viral and bacterial etiologies of gastroenteritis. Leukocytosis may or may not be observed; however, a leukocytosis is common the diagnosis of *C. difficile* infection (Alexandraki & Smetana, 2019; LaRocque & Harris, 2019a; LaRocque & Harris, 2019b). In patients with acute viral gastroenteritis with volume depletion, the red cell counts may indicate hemoconcentration findings. Thrombocytopenia may herald the development of the hemolytic-uremic syndrome. Blood cultures should be obtained in patients with high fevers or who appear systemically ill (LaRocque & Harris, 2019a; LaRocque & Harris, 2019b).

Treatment

Acute viral gastroenteritis is usually a self-limited process and is treated supportively with fluid repletion and unrestricted nutrition. Fluid replenishment is the mainstay of therapy. Empiric antibiotic treatment is not warranted in cases clearly suggestive of viral gastroenteritis (Alexandraki & Smetana, 2019).

For geriatric patients with acute viral gastroenteritis without signs of volume depletion, adequate volume can be maintained with sport drinks and broths. Soft drinks and fruit juices that are high in sugar content should be avoided owing to increased dehydration these agents induce. In cases characterized by mild to moderate hypovolemia, over-the-counter replacement oral solutions may be more beneficial than sport drinks and broth in replenishing electrolytes and fluid rehydration (e.g., ceralyte, oralyte, and Pedialyte). Although most patients can be treated in an outpatient setting, those with alarm manifestations should be considered for the possibility of admission to a hospital. Patients with severe hypovolemia, or an inability to tolerate oral rehydration, resuscitation with intravenous normal saline or Ringer's lactate is necessary (Alexandraki & Smetana, 2019).

Patients should be encouraged to eat as tolerated, with smaller volume meals being less likely to induce vomiting than larger ones. For healthy adults with acute viral gastroenteritis without signs of dehydration, sport drinks, diluted fruit juices, and other flavored soft drinks enhanced with broths or soups can meet the fluid and salt needs in almost all cases. Other appropriate foods include broiled starches/cereals (potatoes, noodles, rice, wheat, and oat), saltine crackers, bananas, yogurt, soups, and boiled vegetables.

Although the BRAT diet (consisting of bananas, rice, applesauce, and toast) is often recommended, evidence to support it is weak. Evidence is also lacking regarding the advice to patients to exclude milk and dairy products from their diet during and immediately following an illness. Concerning probiotics, several studies have demonstrated a modest reduction in the duration of infectious diarrhea with use.

Although antimotility agents may be implemented to assuage fluid losses, providers should exercise with caution when prescribing these. Antimotility medications may conceal the amount of fluid lost, as fluid may collect in the intestine. The antimotility agent loperamide (Imodium) is available and should be used cautiously in patients in whom the dysenteric findings such as fever or bloody or mucoid stools are absent. An alternative agent, bismuth salicylate (as Pepto-Bismol) can be administered when the use of loperamide is deemed potentially harmful. Bismuth salicylate is somewhat less effective than loperamide, and there is a risk of salicylate toxicity (especially in patients already taking aspirin). Diphenoxylate (Lomotil) is another antimotility agent, but evidence supporting its use is lacking and it may also cause opiate or cholinergic side effects (LaRocque & Harris, 2019a; LaRocque & Harris, 2019b).

Antiemetic medications such as prochlorperazine or ondansetron can be used to treat patients who cannot tolerate oral rehydration secondary to excessive vomiting. Generally, treatment lasts 1 to 2 days as needed to facilitate oral fluid replenishment (Alexandraki & Smetana, 2019).

Antibiotics should be reserved for select patients with more symptomatic disease or with risk for more severe disease. In these circumstances, empiric antibiotic treatment is appropriate for the purpose of symptom reduction. Empiric antibiotics are suitable for patients with severe disease with manifestations such as fever, greater than six stools per day, or volume depletion severe enough to warrant hospital admission. Another indication is a presentation that suggests invasive bacterial infection with bloody or mucoid stools (except in nonsevere disease or with low to absent fever). A third consideration is the presence of complicating host conditions that could potentially enhance the risk of complications such as an age of 70 years old and older and the presence of cardiovascular disorders and immunocompromised states. Not all cases of bacterial gastroenteritis should be treated with antimicrobial therapy; one example is infection caused by enterohemorrhagic (Shiga toxin producing) *E. coli* (LaRocque & Harris, 2019a; LaRocque & Harris, 2019b). Although *E. coli* is sensitive to most commonly used antibiotics, antibiotics have not been shown to alleviate symptoms, reduce carriage of the organism, or prevent hemolytic-uremic syndrome. Furthermore, the use of fluoroquinolones is suspected of increasing the release of enterotoxins and the risk of hemolytic-uremic syndrome (Bush et al., 2018). For patients whose diarrhea persists for greater than 10 to 14 days, or for diarrhea that does not improve with antibiotic therapy, less common or drug-resistant etiologies should be suspected. Parasitic causes should be especially considered (LaRocque & Harris, 2019a; LaRocque & Harris, 2019b).

Infective Endocarditis

Infective endocarditis (IE) can occur within the community or in a health care setting. The rates of illness have increased to approximately 15 per 100,000 population (Sexton & Chu, 2018a). The illness increasingly involves older patients: more than one-third of these patients are over 70 years old in Western countries; mortality also tends to be higher than in the general population (Forestier et al., 2016).

In the United States and most developed countries, *S. aureus* is the most common cause of infection and is a common cause of health care–associated endocarditis. Streptococcal endocarditis is a common cause of community-acquired endocarditis in geriatric patients (Sexton & Chu, 2018a); however, *S. aureus* has now emerged as the predominant cause (Forestier et al., 2016). Related to the increased incidence of hospital-acquired IE, MRSA is often found in older patients (Forestier et al., 2016). To a lesser extent, the HACEK organisms (comprising *Haemophilus, Actinobacillus, Cardiobacterium, Eikenella*, and *Kingella*) may cause endocarditis. Owing to geriatric comorbidities, an etiologic shift is observed in the older population. Due to the increased prevalence of prosthetic devices in the older adult, a greater proportion of genitourinary and gastrointestinal enterococci and gram-negative rods has become evident in native valve endocarditis (High, 2017). Because of the higher incidence of colonic lesions in older adult patients, streptococci colonizing the digestive tract like *Streptococcus gallolyticus* and enterococci have also increased (Forestier et al., 2016). Coagulase-negative staphylococci are a frequent cause of prosthetic valve endocarditis; this occurs due to intraoperative infection of from bacteremia during hospitalization. Other nosocomial bacteremias, often with more resistant organisms (e.g., *Enterobacter* spp.), can also result in prosthetic valve endocarditis.

The risk factors for developing endocarditis are multifactorial. More than half of all cases are diagnosed in patients greater than 60 years of age. Older adults are more likely to develop degenerative valve disease and to require valve replacement, both of which are associated with an increased risk of endocarditis (Sexton & Chu, 2018a). Mitral regurgitation, nonrheumatic aortic stenosis, prosthetic valve, and intracardiac devices are the most frequent conditions

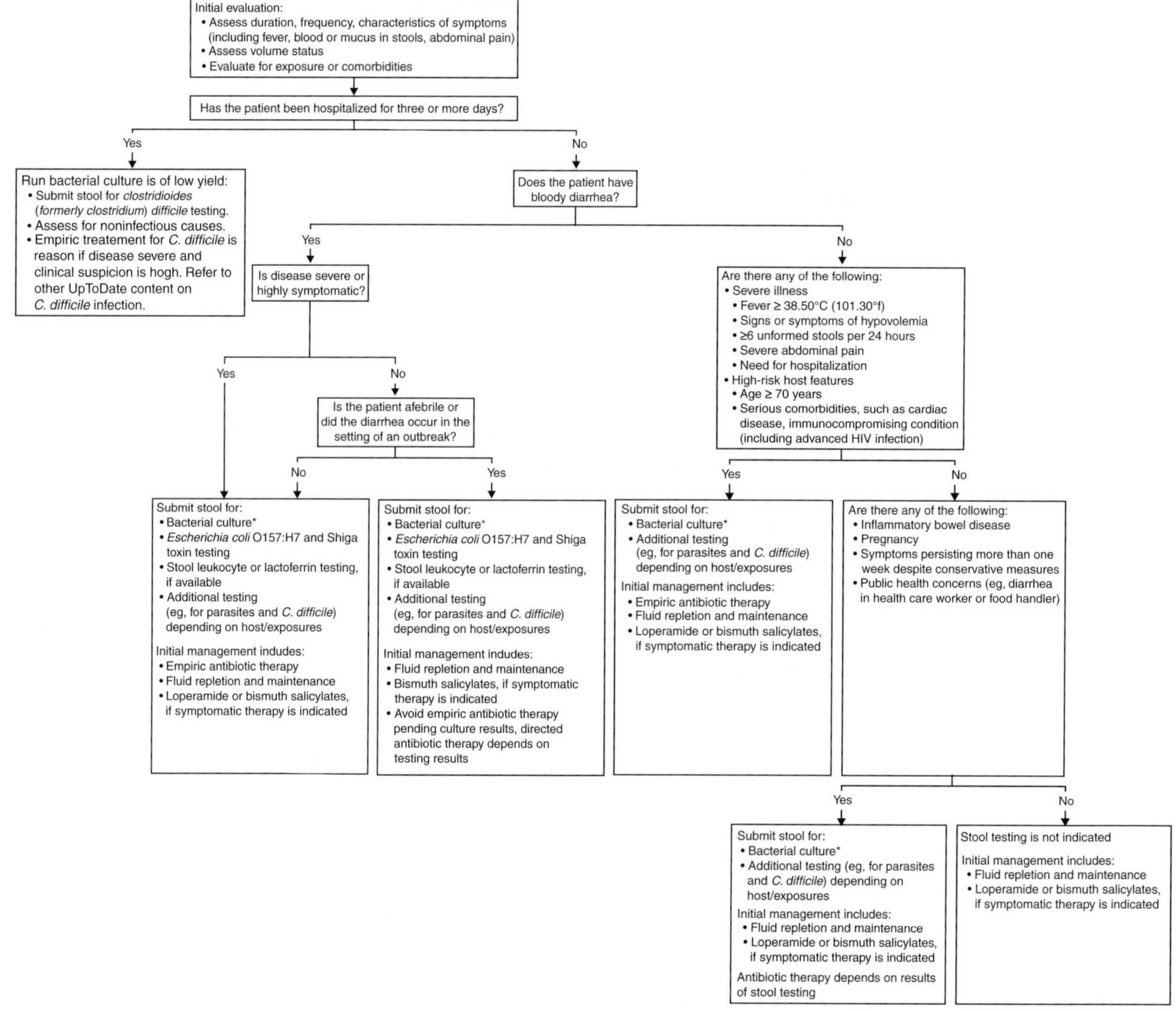

• **Fig. 14.7** Approach to the workup and initial management of acute diarrhea. (Data from Riddle, M. S., DuPont, H. L., & Connor, B. A. [2016]. ACG clinical guideline: Diagnosis, treatment, and prevention of acute diarrheal infections in adults. *American Journal of Gastroenterology, 111*[5], 602. Shane, A. L., Mody, R. K., Crump, J. A., et al. [2017]. 2017 Infectious Diseases Society of America clinical practice guidelines for the diagnosis and management of infectious diarrhea. *Clinical Infectious Diseases*, *65*[12], e45–e80; Thielman, N. M., & Guerrant, R. L. [2004]. Clinical practice: Acute infectious diarrhea. *New England Journal of Medicine, 350*[1], 38.)

predisposing to IE in this population. In the older adult, the increasing number of cardiovascular electronic devices, prosthetic valve implants, and transcatheter aortic valve implantation (TAVI), along with frequent invasive diagnostic or therapeutic procedures performed, may also contribute to the rise of IE in this population (especially of the health care–associated type) (Forestier et al., 2016).

Additional risk factors include male gender, injection drug use, poor dentition or dental disease, underlying structural heart disease (including valvular disorders and congenital heart defects), prosthetic heart valves, transcatheter aortic valve replacement, a previous history of infective carditis, implanted cardiac defibrillators, chronic hemodialysis, and HIV infection (Sexton & Chu, 2018a). Age-related degenerative valvular damages are now the most frequently involved underlying heart lesions. Diabetes, gastrointestinal or genitourinary cancer, or multiple chronic illnesses are found in more than half of older adult patients with IE (Forestier et al., 2016).

Clinical Manifestations

The diagnosis of endocarditis is challenging given the nonspecific and highly variable manifestations of the infection. It may present as an acute, rapidly progressive fulminant infection, a subacute syndrome, or a chronic disease with unremarkable symptoms. The most common symptom is fever, which is often associated with chills, anorexia, and weight loss. Other symptoms include malaise, headache, myalgias, arthralgias, nocturnal diaphoresis, abdominal pain, dyspnea, cough, and pleurisy. Patients may also note tooth pain significant of an underlying dental infection. Cardiac murmurs are present of most patients. Supportive signs include splenomegaly and petechial findings in the skin or on mucosal membranes. Within the skin, petechiae most commonly form on the extremities, whereas mucous membrane locations are usually found on the palate or conjunctivae. Splinter hemorrhages (Fig. 14.8), which consist of nonblanching linear reddish brown lesions under the nail bed, may also occur.

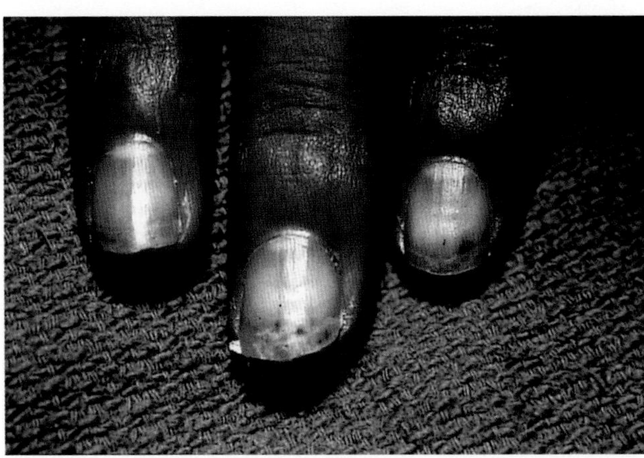

• **Fig 14.8** Splinter hemorrhages. Subungual or splinter hemorrhages in a patient with endocarditis. (From Crawford, M. H., et al. [2003]. Clinical presentation of infective endocarditis. *Cardiology Clinic*, *21*[2], 159–166, 2003, Fig. 14.1.)

More suggestive but less common findings of endocarditis are Janeway lesions (Fig. 14.9), Osler nodes (Figs. 14.10 and 14.11), and Roth spots. Janeway lesions are nontender erythematous macules on the palms and soles. Osler nodes are tender subcutaneous, violet nodules usually found on the pads of the fingers and toes as well as the thenar and hypothenar eminences. Exudative, edematous hemorrhagic lesions of the retina with pale centers describe Roth spots (Fig. 14.12).

Although some findings may be subtle, broad, systemic presentations causing a multitude of manifestations may occur. These complications are often due to septic embolization, which may be associated with localized thrombosis, bleeding, infection, or the development of immune reactions. These may be present at the time of initial presentation or may develop subsequently. The most common

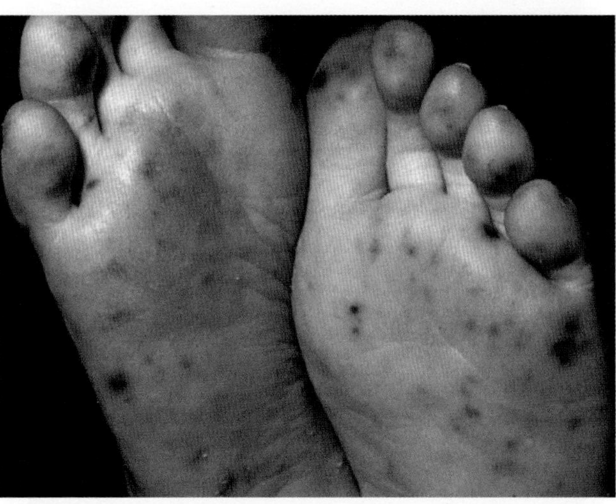

• **Fig. 14.9** Bacterial endocarditis. Acute bacterial endocarditis with necrotic and purpuric area of sepsis due to *Staphylococcus aureus* (Janeway lesions) (John Aeling Collection). (From Ferri, F. F. [2019]. *Ferri's fast facts in dermatology: A practical guide to skin diseases and disorders.* [2nd ed.]. Elsevier.)

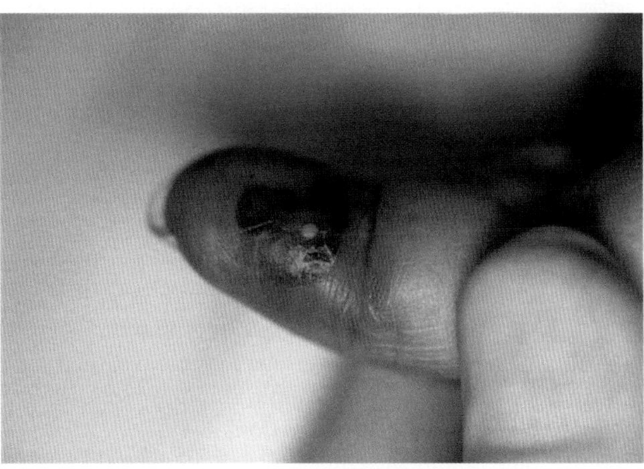

• **Fig. 14.10** Osler node or septic embolus. (From Nguyen, T. T., et al. [2004]. Complication of subacute bacterial endocarditis. *Journal of Clinical Neuroscience, 11*[8], 872–873.)

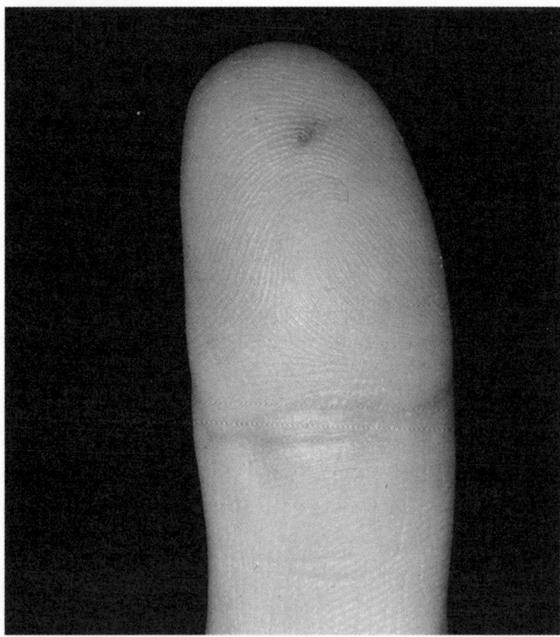

• **Fig. 14.11** Osler node. (From Adams, J. G., et al. [2013]. *Emergency medicine, clinical essentials* [2nd ed.]. Elsevier.)

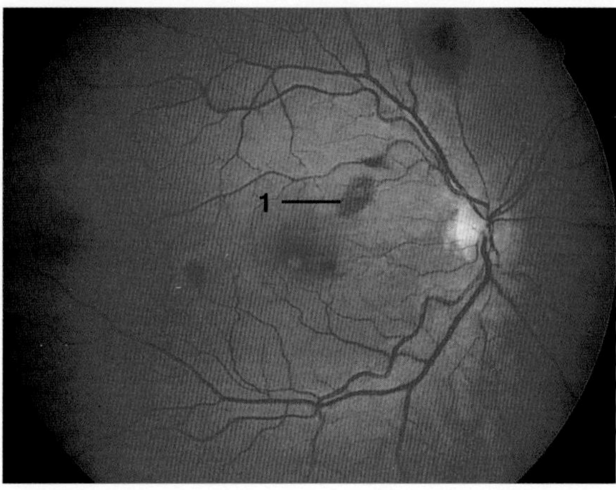

• **Fig. 14.12** Roth spots. Eye of a patient with subacute bacterial endocarditis. A classic Roth spot, or white-centered hemorrhage, is present within the superotemporal arcade. (From Olsen, T. W. (2005). Retina. In D. A. Palay, et al. [Eds.]. *Primary care ophthalmology* [2nd ed.]. Mosby.)

complications are cardiogenic in nature and may include valvular incompetence and congestive heart failure. Other systems may also be affected. These include the neurologic (causing embolic stroke, central nervous system abscesses, and parenchymal hemorrhage), septic emboli (resulting in embolism of many organs including the kidneys, spleen, and lungs), infections (e.g., vertebral osteomyelitis, septic arthritis, psoas abscess), and systemic immunoreactions such as glomerulonephritis (Chu & Sexton, 2018).

In the older adult, the clinical presentation of IE is often nonspecific, consisting of general symptoms such as fatigue, weight loss, or confusion. Fever seems to be as common as in younger patients, and time between onset of symptoms and diagnosis was rather shorter in patients older than 75 years. The immunologic events (Osler nodules, Roth spots, and Janeway lesions) and embolic complications such as strokes, intracranial hemorrhages, or mycotic aneurysms are likely less frequent in the older adult population (Forestier et al., 2016).

Finally, a dental examination should be performed. Findings may reveal signs of periodontal inflammation, pocketing around teeth, and caries that may result in pulpal infection and subsequent abscess (Chu and Sexton, 2018).

Diagnosis

The diagnosis of infective endocarditis should be suspected in patients with fever (with or without bacteremia) or associated cardiac risks (e.g., prior episodes of endocarditis, presence of a prosthetic valve or cardiac device, history of valvular or congenital heart defect) or noncardiac risk factors (intravenous drug use, indwelling intravenous lines, immunosuppression, or a recent dental or surgical procedure). Delay in diagnosis and treatment may be associated with complications, including valvular regurgitation, heart failure, embolic events, and sepsis.

The diagnosis is made based on clinical manifestations, blood cultures (or other microbiologic data), and echocardiography. The modified Duke criteria are the criteria standard for the diagnosis of IE (Boxes 14.5 and 14.6) (Chu & Sexton, 2018). In Box 14.5, the category of "possible IE" represents a modification from the previously published Duke criteria. Box 14.6, which denotes the major and minor criteria, also contains modifications.

Laboratory parameters in IE are relatively nonspecific; they may include elevated inflammatory markers such as erythrocyte sedimentation rate or elevated C-reactive protein, a normochromic-normocytic anemia, and positive rheumatoid factor (Chu & Sexton, 2018). A leukocytosis is often evident in acute IE, and rheumatoid factor becomes negative following successful treatment (Brusch, 2019). Hyperglobulinemia, cryoglobulinemia, circulating immune complexes, hypocomplementemia, and false-positive serologic tests for syphilis occur in some patients. The urinalysis may demonstrate microscopic hematuria, proteinuria, or pyuria. The presence of red blood cell casts on urinalysis is generally indicative of glomerulonephritis (Chu & Sexton, 2018).

The gold standard for the diagnosis of IE is documentation of a continuous bacteremia (>30 minutes in duration) based on blood culture results; in acute IE, three sets should be drawn over 30 minutes to help document a continuous bacteremia (Brusch, 2019). Each set of blood cultures should be obtained from separate venipuncture sites; this will facilitate the detection of over 95% of all bacteremia (Chu & Sexton, 2018). Two sets of blood cultures are expected to demonstrate greater than 90% sensitivity when bacteremia is present (Brusch, 2019). To diagnose subacute endocarditis, three to five sets of blood culture samples should be drawn over 24 hours.

A minority of cases (5%) will be characterized as culture negative. Utilizing the standard collection procedures,

• BOX 14.5 **Modified Duke Criteria for Diagnosis of Infective Endocarditis**

Definite IE Established

Pathologic Criteria

- Pathologic lesions identified: vegetation or intracardiac abscess demonstrating active endocarditis on histology, Or,
- Microorganism demonstrated by culture or histology of a vegetation or intracardiac abscess

Clinical Criteria (refer to table 14.6 for a list of clinical criteria)

- 2 major clinical criteria, Or,
- 1 major and 3 minor clinical criteria, Or,
- 5 minor clinical criteria

Possible IE

- Presence of 1 major and 1 minor clinical criteria, Or presence of 3 minor clinical criteria

Rejected IE

- A firm alternate diagnosis is made, Or,
- Resolution of clinical manifestations occurs after ≤4 days of antibiotic therapy, Or,
- No pathologic evidence of infective endocarditis is found at surgery or autopsy after antibiotic therapy for four days or less, Or,
- Clinical criteria for possible or definite IE not met

IE, Infective endocarditis.

From Li, J. S., Sexton, D. J., Mick, N., et al. (2000). Proposed modifications to the Duke criteria for the diagnosis of infective endocarditis. *Clinical Infectious Diseases*, *30*(4), 633–638.

culture-negative IE is characterized by negative cultures after 5 days of incubation and subculturing. The most common cause is prior antimicrobial therapy that can inhibit bacterial growth within the vegetation but is incapable of eliminating the valvular infection. It should be considered when blood cultures are negative despite persistent fever with one or more clinical findings consistent with IE, or in patients with vegetations identified on echocardiogram. Fungal endocarditis must also be considered in the clinical setting of culture-negative IE that fails to respond to appropriate antibiotic therapy. Candida species are detectable only approximately in 50% of blood cultures, whereas Histoplasma and Aspergillus are almost never isolated from the blood (Brusch, 2019; Chu & Sexton, 2018).

Echocardiography should be performed in all patients with suspected IE. Positive findings indicative of IE include the presence of vegetation, abscess, or new dehiscence of a prosthetic valve. Echocardiogram can assess the extent of valvular dysfunction, underlying ventricular function, and the identification of associated abnormalities such as shunts. In addition, echocardiography is an important tool for follow-up evaluation of patients with persistent or recurrent bacteremia or other clinical deterioration (Chu & Sexton, 2018). It is specific as it identifies the mitral valve being more frequently affected, with vegetations and valve defects

• BOX 14.6 **Clinical Criteria: Modified Duke Criteria for Diagnosis of Infective Endocarditis**

Major Criteria

Positive Blood Cultures for IE (one of the following)

Typical Microorganisms Consistent With IE From Two Separate Blood Cultures

Staphylococcus aureus
Viridans streptococci
Streptococcus gallolyticus (formerly *S. bovis*), *including nutritional variant strains (Granulicatella* spp and *Abiotrophia defectiva)*
HACEK group: *Haemophilus spp, Aggregatibacter* (formerly *Actinobacillus actinomycete comitants), Cardiobacterium hominis, Eikenella* spp, and *Kingella kingae*
Community-acquired enterococci, in the absence of a primary focus; **OR**

Persistently Positive Blood Culture

For organisms that are typical causes of IE: At least two positive blood cultures from blood samples drawn >12 hours apart
For organisms that are more commonly skin contaminants: Three or a majority of ≥4 separate blood cultures (with first and last drawn at least one hour apart)
Single Positive Blood Culture for *Coxiella burnetii* or Phase I IgG Antibody Titer >1:800*

Evidence of Endocardial Involvement (one of the following)

Echocardiogram Positive for IE

Vegetation (oscillating intracardiac mass on a valve or on supporting structures, in the path of regurgitant jets, or on implanted material, in the absence of an alternative anatomic explanation) **OR**
Abscess **OR**
New partial dehiscence of prosthetic valve

New Valvular Regurgitation

Increase in or change in preexisting murmur not sufficient

Minor Criteria

Predisposition: Intravenous drug use or presence of a predisposing heart condition (prosthetic heart valve or a valve lesion associated with significant regurgitation or turbulence of blood flow)
Fever: Temperature ≥ 38.0°C (100.4 °F)
Vascular phenomena: Major arterial emboli, septic pulmonary infarcts, mycotic aneurysm, intracranial hemorrhage, conjunctival hemorrhages, or Janeway lesions
Immunologic phenomena: Glomerulonephritis, Osler nodes, Roth spots, or rheumatoid factor
Microbiologic evidence: Positive blood cultures that do not meet major criteria **OR** serologic evidence of active infection with organism consistent with IE
(Echocardiographic minor criteria eliminated)*

IE, Infective endocarditis; *TEE*, transesophageal echocardiography; *TTE*, transthoracic echocardiography.
*Modifications from the previous published Duke criteria are noted by the asterisk.

From Li, J. S., Sexton, D. J., Mick, N., et al. (2000). Proposed modifications to the Duke criteria for the diagnosis of infective endocarditis. *Clinical Infectious Diseases*, *30*(4), 633–638.

being less frequently present and perivalvular abscesses more often found. The first diagnostic test for patients with suspected cases is a transthoracic echocardiography (TTE); sensitivity rates are approximately 75%, whereas specificity approaches 100% (refer to Figs. 14.13 and 14.14).

Although sensitive and specific, the absence of vegetation on TTE does not fully exclude the diagnosis of IE. Transesophageal echocardiography (TEE) has an increased sensitivity of greater than 90% in detection of valve vegetations and is superior to TTE for the detection of cardiac complications such as abscess, leaflet perforation, and pseudoaneurysm.

False-positive readings are possible with cardiac tumors, mural thrombi, or fibrous strands on the aortic valve. Patients with a negative TEE but a high clinical suspicion for IE should undergo repeat TEE approximately 1 week subsequent to the first test. Repeat TEE is also warranted after an initial positive TEE if new developments of an intracardiac complications manifest (Chu & Sexton, 2018).

Transesophageal echocardiography is considered to have greater diagnostic utility in older patients. Drawbacks include the possibility of limited cooperation among older adult patients undergoing TEE due to cognitive disorders or agitation. Employing sedation or general anesthesia presents risks to patients already exhibiting polypharmacy or who possess multiple illnesses (Forestier et al., 2016).

Chest radiographs may demonstrate solid, cavitary, or pyogenic abscess lesions due to pulmonary emboli; these findings strongly suggest tricuspid disease (Brusch, 2019). Radiographs are also useful in the evaluation of infiltrates (with or without cavitation), congestive heart failure, and possible alternative causes of fever and systemic symptoms (Chu & Sexton, 2018).

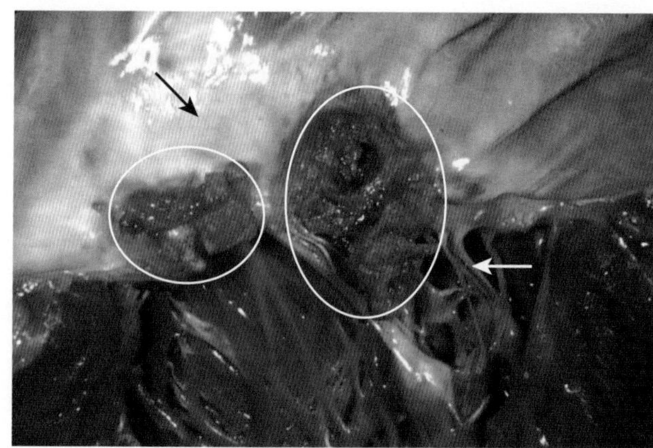

• **Fig. 14.14** Large vegetations *(circles)* at the edge of this mitral valve *(black arrow)*. Chordae tendineae *(white arrow)* connect the mitral valve to papillary muscles in the left ventricle. (From Adams, J. G. [2014]. *Emergency medicine: Clinical essentials* [2nd ed.]. Elsevier.)

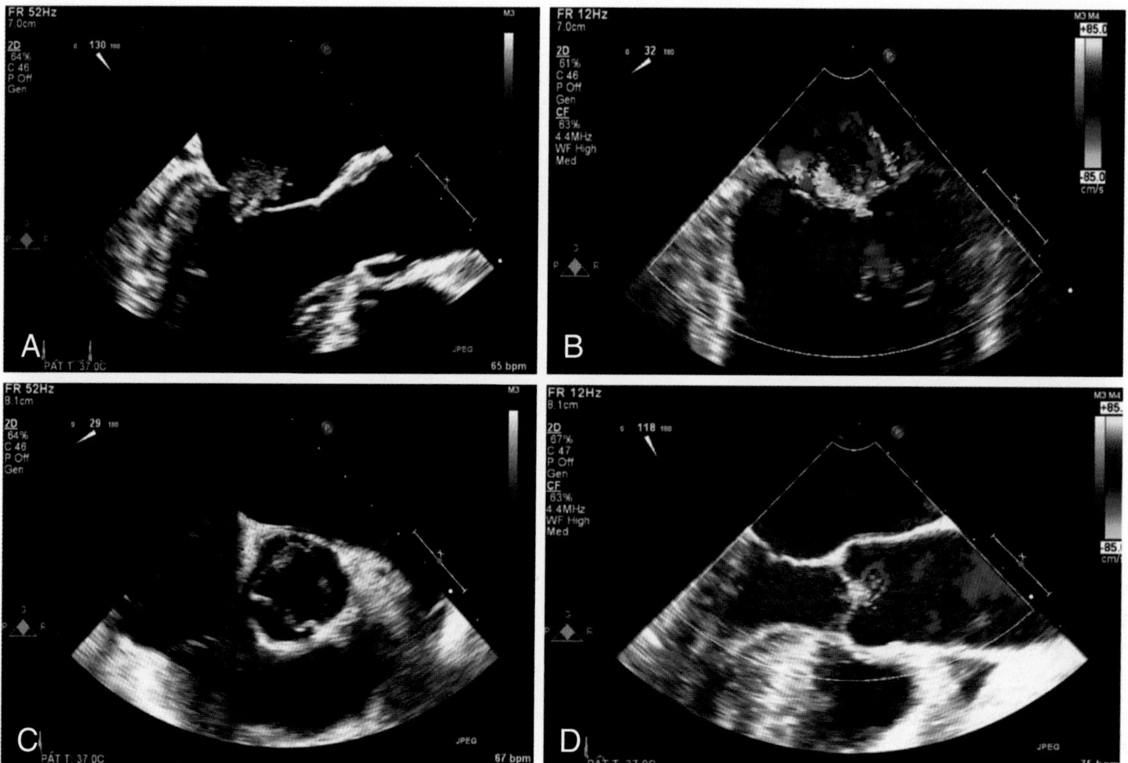

• **Fig. 14.13** Transesophageal echocardiography in a patient with antiphospholipid antibody syndrome with both mitral and aortic vegetations. A, Midesophageal long-axis view demonstrates a large 1.5-cm × 1.4-cm heterogeneous echogenic mass attached to the posterior mitral valve leaflet. B, Color Doppler midesophageal bicommissural view of the mitral valve demonstrates mild mitral regurgitation associated with the valvular mass. C, Midesophageal short-axis view of the aortic valve demonstrates masses on the noncoronary (0.9 × 0.5 cm) and right coronary (0.4 × 0.3 cm) cusps. D, Color Doppler. (From Goldstein et al, *ASE's Comprehensive Echocardiography*, ed3, 2022, Elsevier.)

Treatment

In the setting of acute, symptomatic IE, antibiotic therapy should be initiated as soon as possible to minimize valvular damage. For patients with suspected IE who present without acute symptoms, empiric therapy may not always be necessary; treatment can be deferred until blood culture results are available because an accurate microbiologic assessment is integral to successful treatment. Otherwise, the initial antibiotic choice is empiric in nature, determined by clinical history and physical examination findings and based on the most likely infecting organisms (refer to Box 14.7 for a comprehensive list of appropriate therapies). In general, empiric therapy consists of agents covering methicillin-susceptible and methicillin-resistant staphylococci, streptococci, and enterococci.

Patients with a history of intravenous (IV) drug use have been treated with nafcillin and gentamicin to cover for methicillin-sensitive staphylococci. The evolution of MRSA and penicillin-resistant streptococci has, however, resulted in a substitution with vancomycin instead of penicillin-based antibiotics for empiric treatment. A significant concern is that MRSA may become resistant to vancomycin (Brusch, 2019; Chu & Sexton, 2018). Linezolid and daptomycin are options for patients with an intolerance to vancomycin or resistant organisms. Treatment with linezolid has proven to be superior to treatment with vancomycin in methicillin-sensitive *S. aureus* (MSSA) and MRSA infections; its use should be strongly considered in patients who are seriously ill (Brusch, 2019).

According to the European Society of Cardiology (ESC) and the American Heart Association (AHA), antibiotic therapy of IE relies on monotherapy or a combination (as appropriate) of intravenously administered antibiotics at high doses, up to 6 weeks in duration. The objective is to eradicate the slow-growing bacteria present in vegetations and biofilm. Conversely, aging is associated with various physiologic changes corresponding to aging of each organ and induces pharmacokinetic modifications. Important pharmacokinetic implications that can impact antibiotic selection in the older adult include an increase in fat mass, nephron loss with decreased renal clearance, and decreased albumin level. Renally excreted and nephrotoxic antibiotics, such as aminoglycosides or vancomycin, may induce acute injury in older adult patients if dosing is not appropriately adjusted. Geriatric patients suffering from diabetes or using diuretics or ACE inhibitors are more susceptible to developing acute kidney injury under these conditions. Overdose, resulting in a neurotoxic effect in patients with cognitive disorders, can also occur because of altered pharmacokinetics.

In the older adult, penicillins are the antibiotics of choice against susceptible strains of staphylococci and streptococci. Higher dosages may be required, and the dosing interval should be reduced to 4 hours to target stable serum concentration above a minimal inhibitory concentration (MIC) over 24 hours (Forestier et al., 2016).

In cases of staphylococcal prosthetic valve endocarditis, vancomycin and gentamicin may be used for treatment, regardless of renal dysfunction concern. In conjunction with vancomycin and gentamicin, synergistic rifampin is required in the treatment in these cases as well as other cardiac devices. The addition of rifampin is critical as it penetrates infectious biofilm associated with most of the causative bacteria (especially *S. aureus* and coagulase-negative staphylococcus) (Brusch, 2019).

Meta-analysis has demonstrated no benefit from combination therapy with aminoglycosides compared to β-lactam monotherapy for treating IE, whereas renal function decline was more likely with combination therapy. In patients older than 75 years, aminoglycoside treatment longer than 3 days is associated with increased nephrotoxicity; the synergistic benefit of aminoglycosides with β-lactams therefore may only be appropriate in the older adult only in cases of staphylococcal prosthetic valve endocarditis (Chu & Sexton, 2018). In the older adult or those with renal impairment, should the use of an aminoglycoside be required, a single daily injection is now preferred according to the most recent European guidelines because it is associated with lower nephrotoxicity versus multiple administrations. Notwithstanding, the efficacy and toxicity of aminoglycosides are assessed by monitoring peak and trough concentrations. Furthermore, according to the 2015 guidelines for IE due to enterococcus, the combination of amoxicillin and ceftriaxone could be considered a viable alternative, especially in older adult patients at risk of or with renal impairment. This regimen was deemed to be effective and safe, and much less toxic than aminoglycoside-containing regimens (i.e., gentamycin-containing therapies) (Baddour et al., 2015; Habib et al., 2015).

Options for outpatient therapy for IE include once or twice daily ceftriaxone or daptomycin (preferred), but continuous cloxacillin or vancomycin could also be used alternatively. Venous access is accomplished by a peripherally inserted central catheter (PICC) or direct intravenous injection. Maintaining venous access for weeks could be a concern in older adults. Challenges to this approach include cognitive disorders or confusion, which may compromise the sustainability of the catheter. Chronic indwelling intravascular devices can be complicated with thrombosis or superinfection. A few observational studies have suggested that an oral antibiotic regimen might also be considered after initial intravenous therapy. A fluoroquinolone plus rifampin or linezolid will retain good bioavailability and diffusion properties, making this combination a consideration for outpatient sequent therapy (Chu & Sexton, 2018). Orally administered antibiotics have otherwise been used as suppressive therapy for incurable valvular infections (Brusch, 2019).

Although thrombosis is a component of IE, anticoagulation is controversial. According to available limited data, neither anticoagulant therapy nor antiplatelet therapy reduces the risk of embolism in patients with IE (Ortel and Gaasch, 2019, March). In patients with IE and a separate indication for antithrombotic therapy (such as the presence of a prosthetic valve, coronary artery disease, deep venous

• BOX 14.7 Treatment Options for Infective Endocarditis

Methicillin-Sensitive *S aureus* (MSSA)

- Nafcillin or oxacillin at 2 g IV every 4 hours for 4–6 weeks, Or,
- Cefazolin at 2 g IV every 8 hours for 4–6 weeks
- Either of above with rifampin at 300 mg orally every 8 hours for 6 weeks or longer and with gentamicin at 1 mg/kg (based on ideal body weight) IM or IV every 8 hours for the first 2 weeks*
- Penicillin-allergic: vancomycin at 30 mg/kg (usually, do not to exceed 2 g/24 h unless serum levels are monitored) for 4–6 weeks; (peak level of 30–45 mcg/mL 1 hour after completion IV infusion

MRSA

- Vancomycin at 30 mg/kg (not to exceed 2 g/d unless serum levels are monitored) for 6 weeks or longer combined with rifampin and gentamicin as outlined above; target peak vancomycin range of 30–45 mcg/mL, 1 hour after completion of the IV infusion
- Linezolid or daptomycin may be substituted for vancomycin in patients with compromised renal function or in cases of staphylococci infection with an MIC of greater than 1.5–2 mcg/mL

Culture-Negative NVE

- Vancomycin and gentamicin
- In patients who have previously received antibiotics
  - Ampicillin-sulbactam plus gentamicin (3 mg/kg/d), Or,
  - Vancomycin plus gentamicin and ciprofloxacin

Culture-Negative NVE

- In patients with suspected PVE who have previously received antibiotics
  - Vancomycin, gentamicin, cefepime, and rifampin

Options for Resistant Streptococci

- Penicillin G at 18 million U/d IV, via continuous pump or in six equally divided doses, for 4 weeks, and,
- Cefazolin at 6 g/d IV in three equally divided doses for 4 weeks, Plus,
- Gentamicin at 1 mg/kg (based on ideal body weight) IM or IV every 8 hours for the first 2 weeks of therapy
- Allergic to penicillin: vancomycin 30 mg/kg/d IV in two equally divided doses (not to exceed 2 g/d unless serum levels are monitored) for 4 weeks; target peak vancomycin levels of 30–45 mcg/mL 1 hour after completion of the intravenous infusion)

Penicillin-Sensitive *S viridans* PVE should be treated with the following:

- Penicillin G for 2 weeks, Or,
- Ceftriaxone combined with gentamicin, followed by 4 weeks of penicillin G or ceftriaxone

S viridans PVE with a penicillin MIC of 0.2 mcg/mL or more:

- Penicillin G or ceftriaxone combined with gentamicin combination for 4–6 weeks.
- If the combination therapy is administered for only 4 weeks, penicillin G or ceftriaxone should be continued for an additional 2 weeks.
- Vancomycin is substituted for penicillin or ceftriaxone if the there is a risk of severe, immediate penicillin hypersensitivity

Nonresistant enterococci, *resistant S viridans*, or nutritionally *variant S viridans* and PVE caused by penicillin-G–susceptible *S viridans* or *S bovis:*

- Penicillin G at 18–30 million U/d IV, by continuous pump or in six equally divided doses daily, plus gentamicin at 1 mg/kg IM or IV every 8 hours for 4–6 weeks, Or,
- Ampicillin at 12 g/d by continuous infusion or in six equally divided doses daily, plus gentamicin at 1 mg/kg IM or IV every 8 hours for 4–6 weeks
- Allergic to penicillin: vancomycin at 30 mg/kg/d in two equally divided doses (not to exceed 2 g/24 h unless serum levels are monitored); may add gentamicin for 4–6 weeks of treatment (target peak vancomycin level of 30–45 mcg/mL 1 hour after completion of the intravenous infusion)

Enterococci susceptible to penicillin and gentamicin (if creatinine clearance <50 mL/min):

- Double beta-lactam therapy (ampicillin 2 g IV every 4 hours and ceftriaxone 2 g IV every 12 hours)

Enterococci PVE resistant to both gentamicin and streptomycin:

- Preferred agent is ampicillin (to achieve serum level of 16 mcg/mL administered for 8–12 weeks by continuous infusion
- Alternatives: Imipenem, ciprofloxacin, or ampicillin with sulbactam

No effective therapy is known for vancomycin-resistant enterococcus PVE

• BOX 14.7 Treatment Options for Infective Endocarditis—cont'd

Treatment of HACEK Microorganisms

- Ceftriaxone at 2 g/d IV for 4 weeks, Or
- Ampicillin at 12 g/d by continuous pump or in six equally divided doses daily; this may be combined with gentamicin at 1 mg/kg (based on ideal body weight) IM or IV every 8 hours for 4 weeks
- P aeruginosa: ceftazidime, cefepime, or imipenem, combined with high-dose tobramycin at 8 mg/kg/d in three divided doses, to attain peak blood levels of 15–20 mcg/mL, for 6 weeks
- Enteric gram-negative rods (e.g., *E. coli, Proteus mirabilis*): Ampicillin, ticarcillin-clavulanic acid, piperacillin, piperacillin-tazobactam, ceftriaxone, or cefepime combined with gentamicin or amikacin for 4–6 weeks
- Streptococcus pneumoniae: ceftriaxone at 2 g/d IV or vancomycin (if penicillin allergy or high-level penicillin G resistance [MIC of 2 mcg/mL or more]) for 4 weeks
- Diphtheria: administer penicillin G at 18–24 million U/d in six divided doses or vancomycin combined with gentamicin for 4 weeks
- Q fever (*C burnetii* infection), administer doxycycline combined with rifampin, trimethoprim-sulfamethoxazole, or a fluoroquinolone for 3–4 years
- Candida and Aspergillus fungal endocarditis requires surgical excision of infected valves in conjunction with amphotericin B therapy

MRSA, Methicillin-resistant *Staphylococcus aureus*.

thrombosis, or atrial fibrillation), a standard regimen of anticoagulation should be followed (Brusch, 2019).

Surgical interventions become required in addition to antibiotic therapy to treat IE under conditions of severe valvular damage that causes heart failure, extended vegetation at risk of systemic embolism, or with uncontrolled infection. It is also mandated in prosthetic valve endocarditis, especially caused by *S. aureus*; removal of an infected intravascular device is strongly recommended. Surgery is rarely employed in cases of IE complicating TAVI, which is used as a substitute to open heart surgery in the disabled older adult. For life-threatening complications, immediate valvular surgery is necessary (Chu & Sexton, 2018). The indications for surgery in patients with native valve endocarditis (NVE) are identified in Box 14.8. Congestive heart failure is the chief requirement for surgical intervention.

Other conditions that may necessitate surgery include the presence of a paravalvular abscess and an intracardiac fistula, the presence of a culture-negative NVE with a persistent fever of more than 10 days, persistent hypermobile vegetations, especially in those with a history of embolization beyond 7 days of antibiotic therapy, and the presence of multiresistant organisms (e.g., enterococci). The indications for surgery in patients with prosthetic valve endocarditis (PVE) are the same as those for patients with NVE, with the addition of the conditions of valvular dehiscence and early PVE. Orally administered antibiotics have been used as suppressive therapy for incurable valvular infections (i.e., inoperable PVE).

Age is not a contraindication to surgery; the older adult could benefit from surgery with mortality, with one study concluding reduced mortality in patients undergoing surgery as opposed to being managed medically (Durante-Mangoni et al., 2008). One must be cognizant of the fact that patients undergoing surgery are more likely in optimal health as compared to those managed medically.

• BOX 14.8 Indications for Surgery in Native Valve Endocarditis (NVE)

- Congestive heart failure recalcitrant to standard medical therapy
- Fungal infective endocarditis (except due to *Histoplasma capsulatum*)
- Persistent sepsis after 72 hours despite appropriate antibiotic treatment
- Recurrent septic emboli, especially after 2 weeks of antibiotic treatment
- Rupture of an aneurysm of the sinus of Valsalva
- Conduction disturbances caused by a septal abscess
- Kissing infection of the anterior mitral leaflet in patients with infective endocarditis of the aortic valve

From Brusch, J. L. (2019). *Infective endocarditis*. https://emedicine.medscape.com/article/216650

Endocarditis Prophylaxis

Prophylaxis against endocarditis is recommended for patients with the highest risk of adverse effects from endocarditis. These patients are identified in Box 14.9 (Nishimura et al., 2017; Wilson et al., 2007), whereas high-risk procedures are noted in Box 14.10 (Sexton & Chu, 2018b). Adaptation and Alternatives to 2015 Guidelines on IE Suggested According to Elder's Comorbidities and Functional Status are shown in Table 14.4.

In general, the risk of IE is considered to be most significant for dental procedures that involve manipulation of gingival tissue or the periapical region of the teeth or perforation of the oral mucosa, such as tooth extractions or drainage of a dental abscess; this includes routine dental cleaning. By contrast, vaginal or cesarean delivery is not an indication for routine antibiotic prophylaxis as the rate of bacteremia associated with these procedures is low. For a list of acceptable antibiotic regimens in the prophylaxis of IE, refer to Table 14.5. In general, most antibiotics should be administered 30 to 60 minutes prior to the procedure. However, vancomycin should be administered 120 minutes prior to the procedure. Where applicable, cefazolin or ceftriaxone are alternative agents for patients with a nonsevere,

• BOX 14.9 High-Risk Conditions Requiring Prophylactic Antibiotics in Infective Endocarditis

- Prosthetic heart valves, including mechanical, bioprosthetic, and homograft valves (transcatheter-implanted as well as surgically implanted valves are included)
- Prosthetic material used for cardiac valve repair, such as annuloplasty rings and chords
- A prior history of infective endocarditis
- Unrepaired cyanotic congenital heart disease
- Repaired congenital heart disease with residual shunts or valvular regurgitation at the site or adjacent to the site of the prosthetic patch or prosthetic device
- Repaired congenital heart defects with catheter-based intervention involving an occlusion device or stent during the first 6 months after the procedure
- Valve regurgitation due to a structurally abnormal valve in a transplanted heart

Data from Nishimura, R. A., Otto, C. M., Bonow, R. O., et al. (2017). AHA/ACC focused update of the 2014 AHA/ACC guideline for the management of patients with valvular heart disease: A report of the American College of Cardiology/American Heart Association task force on clinical practice guidelines. *Journal of the American College of Cardiology*; Wilson, W., Taubert, K. A., Gewitz, M., et al. (2007). Prevention of infective endocarditis: Guidelines from the American Heart Association: A guideline from the American Heart Association Rheumatic Fever, Endocarditis, and Kawasaki Disease Committee, Council on Cardiovascular Disease in the Young, and the Council on Clinical Cardiology, Council on Cardiovascular Surgery and Anesthesia, and the Quality of Care and Outcomes Research Interdisciplinary Working Group. *Circulation*, *116*(15), 1736.

• BOX 14.10 High Risk Procedures That Put Patients at Risk for Infective Endocarditis

- Intravenous drug use
- Having an artificial heart valve
- Presence of pacemaker leads
- Mitral valve prolapse
- History of having infective endocarditis
- Bicuspid aortic valve
- Age-related aortic stenosis
- Valve issues due to rheumatic fever
- Valve issues due to degenerative conditions
- Congenital heart disease

non-IgE-mediated penicillin allergy who cannot take oral therapy (Wilson et al., 2007).

Skin and Soft-Tissue Infections

Cellulitis

Cellulitis can occur in adults and the older adult. Risk factors include defective cutaneous immunity associated with aging (from immunosenescence or immunosuppression), diabetes, peripheral vascular disease, obesity, underlying skin conditions (such as eczema, varicella, tinea pedis, impetigo, venous stasis, and edema), or frequent trauma. Additionally, older adults have a greater likelihood of being bed bound and hence at an increased risk for pressure ulcers. The incidence of cellulitis ranges from 1% to 9%, with the most common cause of cellulitis being beta-hemolytic streptococci (groups A, B, C, G, and F). Most commonly, group A *Streptococcus* or *Streptococcus pyogenes* is the offending organism. *S. aureus* (including methicillin-resistant strains) is a less common cause, whereas gram-negative aerobic bacilli cause a minority of cases.

Clinical Manifestations

Cellulitis manifests as areas of skin erythema, edema, and warmth; they develop because of bacterial entry via breaches in the skin barrier. Petechiae or hemorrhage can be seen in erythematous skin, and superficial bullae can occur. Fever and other systemic manifestations of infection may also be present. Cellulitis is nearly always unilateral, with the lower extremities being the most common site of involvement. A bilateral distribution is atypical; the provider should consider other diagnoses under such circumstances. Cellulitis involves the deeper dermis and subcutaneous fat. Cellulitis may present with or without purulence (Figs. 14.15 and 14.16) (Mody et al., 2014; Spelman & Baddour, 2019).

The presence of abscesses or purulent drainage is a hallmark of *S. aureus* (Moses, 2019b). Cellulitis cases usually have a more slowly progressive course with development of localized symptoms over a few days.

Additional manifestations of cellulitis include lymphangitis and enlargement of regional lymph nodes. Edema surrounding the hair follicles may lead to dimpling in the skin, creating an appearance reminiscent of an orange peel texture ("peau d'orange"; Fig. 14.17).

Vesicles, bullae, and ecchymoses or petechiae may also occur. Cutaneous hemorrhage is possible with major skin inflammation (Mody et al., 2014; Spelman & Baddour, 2019) the presence of bullae and hemorrhage suggest infection by group A Streptococcus, Pseudomonas, *Vibrio vulnificus*, *Clostridium perfringens*, or *Aeromonas hydrophila* (Moses, 2019b).

Clostridia and other anaerobic species may also induce the formation of crepitus and gangrene cellulitis. Severe manifestations with systemic toxicity should prompt an investigation for additional underlying sources of infection.

The interdigital toe spaces should be examined for fissuring or maceration. Minimizing these conditions may reduce the likelihood of recurrent lower-extremity cellulitis.

Other forms of cellulitis include orbital cellulitis, abdominal wall cellulitis (in morbidly obese individuals), buccal cellulitis, and perianal cellulitis (Mody et al., 2014; Spelman & Baddour, 2019).

Diagnosis

The diagnosis of cellulitis is primarily clinical. Uncomplicated infections generally do not require laboratory testing. If completed, the laboratory finding of cellulitis is nonspecific and may include a leukocytosis and the elevation of ESR and CRP inflammatory markers. Blood cultures or cultures of debrided elements should be considered in the following situations: severe local infection, systemic signs of infection,

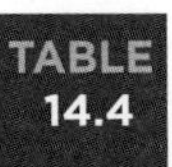

TABLE 14.4 Adaptation and Alternatives to 2015 Guidelines on Infective Endocarditis (IE) Suggested According to Elder's Comorbidities and Functional Status

	Guidelines	Suggested in Elderly
Transesophageal echography	In all cases except negative **TTE** and low clinical	In case of major confusion and agitation exposing to excess
	suspicion	risk of the procedure, consider only repeated **TTE** in patients contraindicated to surgery
Aminoglycosides	Combined to penicillin A or **G** or vancomycin	Consider aminoglycoside free regimens to avoid renal
	in case of streptococcal or enterococcal or	toxicity
	staphylococcal endocarditis as stated	
Vancomycin	First-line therapy in i-lactam allergic patients or in case of MRSA	Consider daptomycin to avoid renal toxicity
Therapeutic drug monitoring	Only for vancomycin and aminoglycosides	Consider also for all β-lactams to avoid overdose and underdose adverse effects (neurological toxicity) and inefficacy, respectively
Intravenous therapy	Throughout the antibiotic therapy in all cases	Consider oral or subcutaneous route for antibiotic therapy if infection is under control and in case of poor venous access and/or agitation
Outpatient parenteral therapy	Only in reliable and compliant patients living	Consider in patients for whom the hospital stay is the most
	close to the hospital	deleterious regarding their functional and cognitive decline, especially for elderly living in long-term care facilities

From Forestier, E., Fraisse, T., Claire Roubaud-Baudron, C., Selton-Suty, C., & Pagani, L. (2016). Managing infective endocarditis in the elderly: New issues for an old disease. *Clinical Interventions in Aging, 11*, 1199–1206.

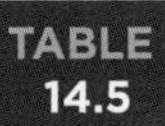

TABLE 14.5 Infective Endocarditis (IE) Prophylactic Regimens

Route	Agent	Adult Single Dose
Oral	Amoxicillin	2 gm
Unable to take oral medication	Ampicillin or	2 gm IM or IV
	Cefazolin or ceftriaxone	1 gm IM or IV
Allergic to penicillins - oral	Cephalexin	2 gm
	Clindamycin	600 mg
	Azithromycin or clarithromycin	500 mg
Allergic to penicillins and unable to take oral medication	Cefazolin or ceftriaxone	1 g IM or IV
	Clindamycin	600 mg IM or IV
	Vancomycin	15–20 mg/kg, to a maximum of 2 gm per dose

Data from Wilson, W., Taubert, K. A., Gewitz, M., et al. (2007). Prevention of infective endocarditis: Guidelines from the American Heart Association: A guideline from the American Heart Association Rheumatic Fever, Endocarditis, and Kawasaki Disease Committee, Council on Cardiovascular Disease in the Young, and the Council on Clinical Cardiology, Council on Cardiovascular Surgery and Anesthesia, and the Quality of Care and Outcomes Research Interdisciplinary Working Group. *Circulation, 116*(15), 1736. Epub 2007 Apr 19.

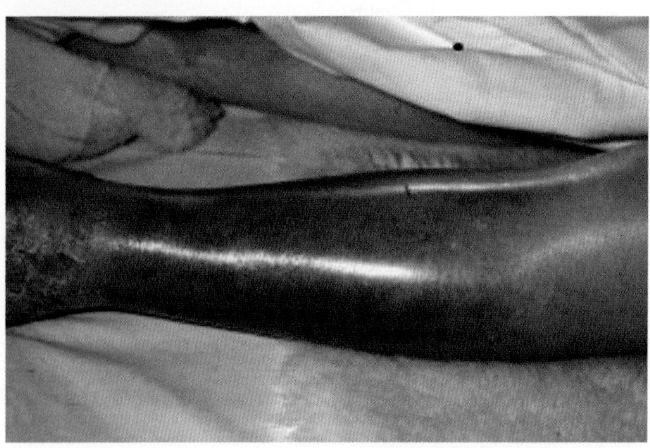

• **Fig. 14.15** Cellulitis, a common cause of painful swollen leg. (From Lowe, G., et al. [2008]. Limb pain and swelling. *Medicine, 37*[2], 96–99, Fig. 14.1B.)

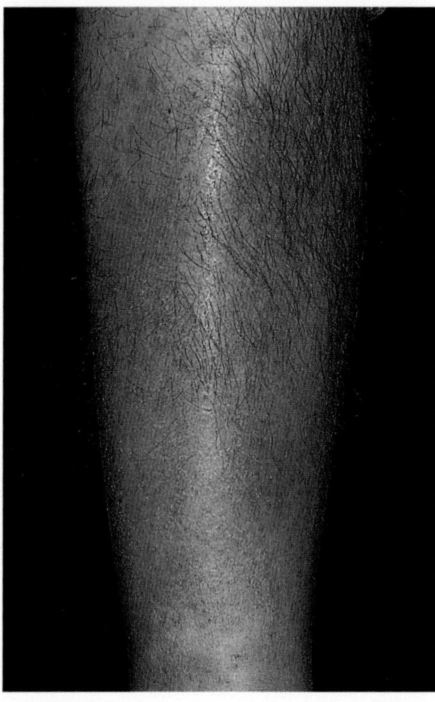

• **Fig. 14.16** Cellulitis, an early case with diffuse erythema and minimal swelling. Pain was elicited with palpation. (From Habif, T. P., et al. [2011]. Bacterial infections. In T. P. Habif, et al. [Eds.], *Skin disease* [3rd ed.]. Elsevier.)

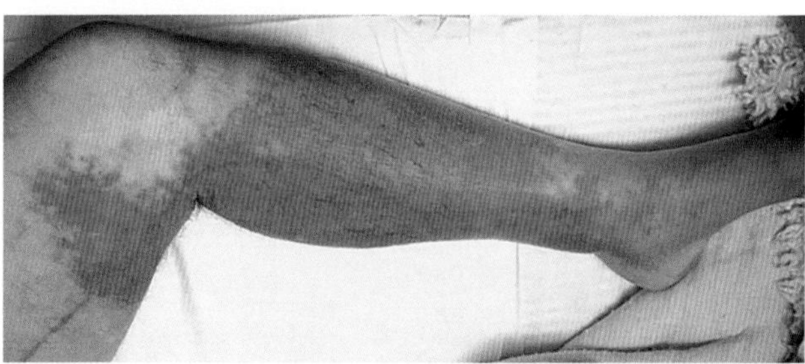

• **Fig. 14.17** Cellulitis. Note the erythema and edema with dimpling (peau d'orange). (From Hirschmann, J. V., et al. [2012]. Lower limb cellulitis and its mimics. *Journal of the American Academy of Dermatology* 67[2], 163.e1–163.e12. © 2019.)

a history of recurrent or multiple abscesses, the failure of initial antibiotic therapy, the presence of underlying comorbidities (lymphedema, malignancy, neutropenia, immunodeficiency, splenectomy, diabetes), the presence of special exposures (e.g., animal bite, water-associated injury), and the presence of an indication for prophylaxis against infective endocarditis or community patterns of *S. aureus* susceptibility. Blood cultures, however, have a low yield, with less than 10% cases reporting positive results. A skin biopsy may be required should the diagnosis not be definite.

Ultrasound can aid in the determination of skin abscess presence via ultrasonography. Alternatively, magnetic resonance imaging can distinguish cellulitis from osteomyelitis. Radiographic evaluation may be indicated in patients meeting the criteria for culture (refer to preceding paragraph). It is noteworthy that radiographic imaging cannot reliably discern cellulitis from necrotizing fasciitis or gas gangrene; should these alterative diagnoses be considered, radiographic imaging should not supersede surgical treatment.

In patients with recurrent cellulitis, serologic assay testing for beta-hemolytic streptococci may prove beneficial. Tests include the antistreptolysin-O (ASO) reaction, the antideoxyribonuclease B test (anti-DNAse B), the antihyaluronidase test (AHT), and the Streptozyme antibody assay. Anti-DNase B and AHT responses are more reliable than the ASO response following group A streptococcal skin infections (Spelman & Baddour, 2019).

Treatment

Because most cases of cellulitis are usually caused by *Streptococci* species or *S. aureus*, antibiotic regimens directed against these agents are indicated. Viable antimicrobials include first-generation cephalosporins, vancomycin, and clindamycin. In cases where community acquired-MRSA is suspected, therapy with vancomycin, daptomycin, clindamycin, or linezolid should be employed. Furthermore, the severity at presentation and the presence of comorbidities should govern whether oral or intravenous therapy will be utilized (Mody et al., 2014). Specific regimens and durations are found in Table 14.6 (Moses, 2019b).

Necrotizing Fasciitis

Necrotizing soft tissue infections (NSTIs) include necrotizing forms of fasciitis, myositis, and cellulitis. These infections result in fulminant tissue destruction, systemic signs of toxicity, and high mortality. Although portions of the epidermis, dermis, subcutaneous tissue, fascia, and muscle may all be affected, necrotizing fasciitis primarily involves fascia. Infections are stratified by both microbiology and the presence or absence of gas in the tissues.

Polymicrobial (type I) necrotizing infection usually occurs in older adults or in individuals with underlying comorbidities; the most important predisposing factor is diabetes, especially in association with peripheral vascular disease. It is caused by aerobic and anaerobic bacteria. Usually, at least one anaerobic species is present, with *Bacteroides*, *Clostridium*, or *Peptostreptococcus* most likely. These are

TABLE 14.6 Antibiotic Regimens for Cellulitis

First-Line Therapies	Mild to moderate (uncomplicated cellulitis coverage) for Streptococcus and MSSA coverage	• Cephalexin 500 mg orally four times per day • for 7–10 days or • Dicloxacillin 500 mg orally four times per day • for 7–10 days or • Amoxicillin-Clavulanate (Augmentin) 875 mg orally twice per day for 7–10 days
	Severe infections	• Cefazolin 1 gram IV every 8 hours or • Nafcillin 2 grams IV q4 hours or • Oxacillin 2 grams IV q4 hours
	Cellulitis with abscess	• Incision and drainage is primary therapy • Antibiotics as above
	MRSA coverage for mild to moderate infections	• Septra DS 1–2 tabs twice daily for 7–10 days or • Use 2 tabs if normal renal function, serious infections or weight >100 kg • Minocycline of doxycycline 100 mg twice daily for 7–10 days or • Linezolid 600 mg PO bid (very expensive) • Clindamycin is no longer recommended for MRSA coverage due to growing resistance
	MRSA Coverage for severe infections	• Vancomycin 15 mg/kg IV every 12 hours (adjusted for Renal Function) • Linezolid 600 mg IV q12 hours (very expensive) • Daptomycin • Telavancin • Ceftaroline fosamil
	Outpatient parenteral (adults, narrower spectrum parenteral protocol)	• Cefazolin 2 gram IV q24 hours Plus Probenacid 1 gram PO q24 hours (decreases cefazolin excretion) for 7–10 days
Second-Line Therapies for Complicated, Refractory or Pustular Cellulitis Coverage for Streptococcus and MRSA Coverage	Mild to moderate	• Septra DS 1 tab orally twice daily • Use with Penicillin, Amoxicillin, or Cephalexin • Clindamycin 300 mg orally four times per day for 7–10 days (increasing MRSA resistance) or • Linezolid 600 mg orally twice daily
	Severe	• Vancomycin 15 mg/kg IV every 12 hours (adjusted for Renal Function) or • Linezolid 600 mg IV q12 hours or • Clindamycin 600–900 mg IV q8 hours

IV, Intravenous; *MRSA*, methicillin-resistant *Staphylococcus aureus; MSSA*; methicillin-sensitive S aureus.

From Moses, S. (2019, April 6). *Cellulitis*. https://fpnotebook.com/Derm/Bacteria/Cllts.htm; Moses, S. (2019c, April 6). *Group A streptococcal cellulitis*. https://fpnotebook.com/Derm/Bacteria/GrpAStrptcclCllts.htm

present in combination with Enterobacteriaceae (such as *Escherichia coli*, *Enterobacter*, *Klebsiella*, or *Proteus*) and one or more facultative anaerobic streptococci (other than group A *Streptococcus*). Rarely, obligate aerobes (such as *Pseudomonas aeruginosa*) and fungi (e.g., *Candida* species) are found in type I infections.

Monomicrobial (type II) necrotizing infection may occur in any age group and in individuals without any underlying contributory illnesses. It is usually caused by group A *Streptococci* (GAS), other beta-hemolytic streptococci, or *Staphylococcus aureus*. About half of these infections are without a distinct genesis. The presumed route of infection in these cases is likely the bloodborne spread of GAS originating from asymptomatic or symptomatic pharyngitis and deposited to an area of blunt trauma or muscle strain. Infrequently, *Vibrio vulnificus* is associated with seawater exposure, whereas *Aeromonas hydrophila* is associated with fresh water; these are possible in the setting of traumatic injury. *V. vulnificus* may also occur as a consequence of underlying cirrhosis and ingestion of contaminated oysters.

Type III gas gangrene refers to clostridial myonecrosis. Most commonly, *Clostridium perfringens* is the causative agent when necrotizing fasciitis occurs spontaneously. When underlying colon cancer or leukemia is present, *C. septicum* is the most likely bacterial cause (Schulz, 2018).

General risk factors for the development of NSTIs include factors that induce a disruption of the normal protective dermal layers; examples are major penetrating trauma; minor laceration or blunt trauma from muscle strains, sprains, or contusions; skin breaching from varicella lesion; insect bites; injection drug use; recent surgery (colonic, urologic, and gynecologic procedures as well as neonatal circumcision); and mucosal disruptions from hemorrhoids, rectal fissures, or episiotomy. Additional risk factors are underlying immunodeficiency from diabetes, cirrhosis, neutropenia, or HIV infection and the presence of major comorbidities such as malignancy, obesity, or alcoholism. Diabetes is an especially important risk factor for the development of necrotizing fasciitis throughout the body; beyond this, the use of sodium-glucose cotransporter 2 inhibitors in the treatment of adults with type 2 diabetes has been associated with infections of the perineum (Fournier gangrene). Finally, females who are pregnant, have given birth or experienced pregnancy loss, or have had a gynecologic procedure are at an increased risk.

Although data are somewhat inconsistent, the use of nonsteroidal antiinflammatory drugs (NSAIDs) may be associated with the development or progression of streptococcal infections. The theorized mechanism involves the concealment of NSAID-mediated signs and symptoms of inflammation in patients, thereby contributing to a delayed diagnosis.

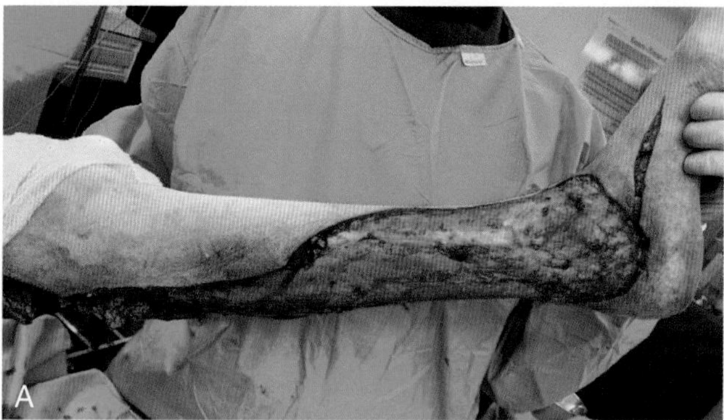

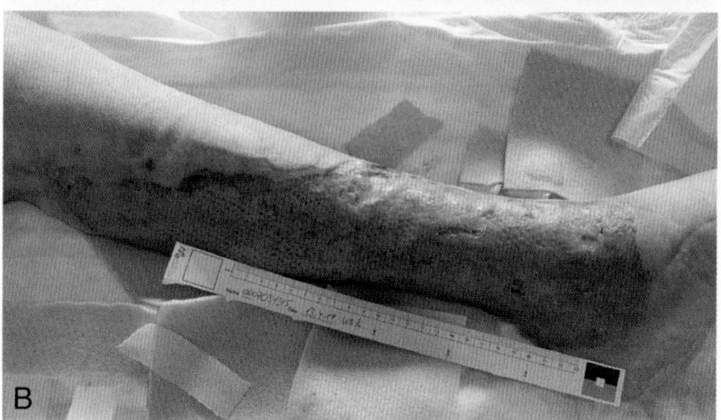

• **Fig. 14.18** Necrotizing Fasciitis. Post-radical debridement (A) and post skin grafting (B). The so-called flesh-eating bacteria, group A β-hemolytic Streptococcus, can cause significant tissue destruction rapidly. This patient had pain, erythema, and swelling of the foot followed by necrotic ulceration over a week without any history of trauma. (From I.P.E. Bayard, A.O. Grobbelaar, M.A. Constantinescu,Necrotizing fasciitis caused by mono-bacterial gram-negative infection with E. coli – the deadliest of them all: A case series and review of the literature, *JPRAS Open*, Volume 29, 2021,Pages 99-105.)

Clinical Manifestations

Findings most commonly involve the extremities (lower extremities more so than upper extremities). Commonly, the presentation is acute, spanning hours, whereas a subacute presentation over days is atypical. Rapid progression to extensive destruction can occur, leading to systemic toxicity, limb loss, or death.

Clinical findings significant of systemic toxicity may be present. These include fever of up to 105°F, tachycardia, and hypotension. The physical exam may also reveal erythema without distinct margins, edema extending beyond the visible erythema, severe pain that is out of proportion to exam findings, and palpable crepitus. Subcutaneous gas causing crepitus is often present in the polymicrobial (type I) subtype, especially in diabetic patients. Skin pigmentary changes rapidly progress from red-purple ecchymotic lesions to patches of blue-gray. Three to five days following the onset, skin breakdown ensues with bullae formations containing thick pink or purple fluid (Fig. 14.18). Overt cutaneous gangrene then becomes evident. Prior to skin necrosis, a diminished sensation to pain may develop in the involved area due to vascular thrombosis and the destruction of superficial nerves in the subcutaneous layer (Stevens & Baddour, 2018). A foul smell in the lesion strongly suggests the presence of anaerobic organisms (Schulz, 2018).

Other symptoms include malaise, myalgias, diarrhea, and anorexia. The subcutaneous tissue may be firm and indurated, not permitting the underlying muscle groups to be discernable. Compartment syndrome may be a consequence of the pronounced edema. Lymphangitis and lymphadenitis are infrequently found. Concomitant diabetic or peripheral vascular disease findings may also be apparent.

Necrotizing fasciitis of the perineum, known as Fournier gangrene, can occur due to a discontinuity of the gastrointestinal or urethral mucosal surfaces. It is more common in men. Fournier gangrene is a form of polymicrobial (type I) infection. It is characterized by an abrupt, severe pain with rapid dissemination to the anterior abdominal wall and the gluteal muscles. In males, infection may extend to involve the scrotum and penis, whereas in females, affliction of the labia can occur (Figs. 14.19 and 14.20).

Diagnosis

The diagnosis may be suspected in patients with soft tissue infection (with erythema, edema, warmth) and signs of systemic illness (fever, hemodynamic instability) in association with crepitus, rapid progression of clinical manifestations, or severe pain that is out of proportion to skin findings. Early recognition of necrotizing infection is critical; rapid progression to extensive destruction can occur, leading to systemic toxicity, limb loss, or death. As such, laboratory tests and imaging studies should not delay surgical intervention (Schulz, 2018).

Surgical exploration is the only way to establish the diagnosis of necrotizing infection. Positive findings upon visualization are a swollen and dull gray appearance of the fascia, thin exudate without clear purulence, and uncomplicated disjunction of the tissue planes upon dissection.

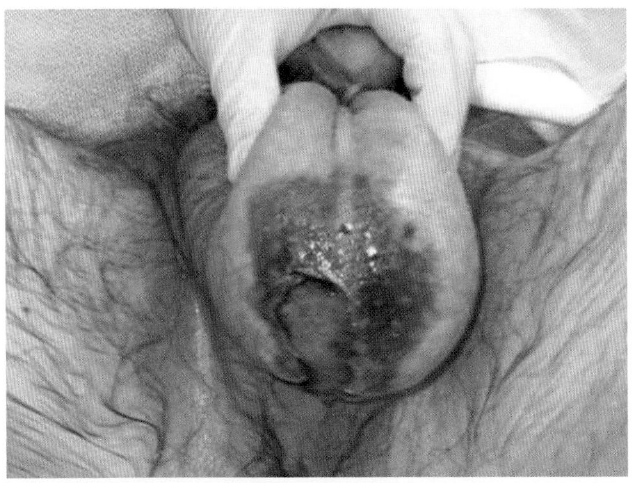

• **Fig. 14.19** Fournier's gangrene and its emergency management. Example of extent of debridement sometimes needed in Fournier's gangrene. (From Aho T, Canal A, Neal DE. Fournier's gangrene. *Nat Rev Urol*. 2006;3(1):54-57.)

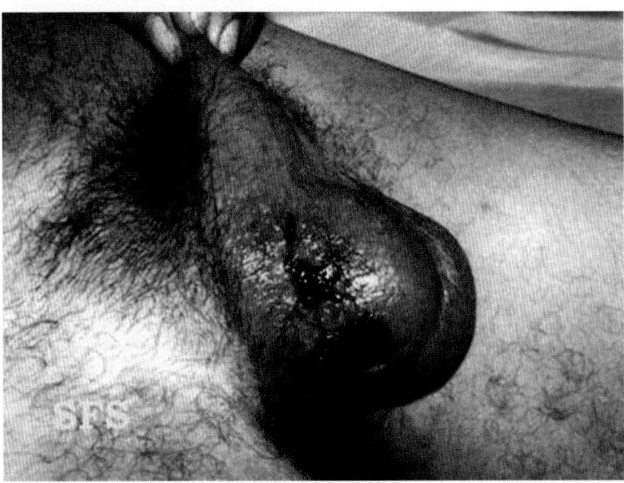

• **Fig. 14.20** Necrosis on scrotum in early Fournier's gangrene. (From http://www.health-pictures.com/conditions3/fourniers-gangrene-picture.htm. Found in Summers, Anthony, MSc... Published September 1, 2014, *10*[8], 582–587, Fig. 14.2. © 2014.)

Limited diagnostic accuracy is afforded by skin and superficial tissue biopsy because these samples may not be infected. Furthermore, obtaining specimens for biopsy is not essential for the diagnosis. Deeper tissue histologic findings suggestive of infection include extensive tissue destruction, thrombosis of blood vessels, profuse bacteria spread along fascial planes, and intrusion of acute inflammatory cells. Characteristic pathologic features of necrotizing myositis include degeneration and necrosis of skeletal muscle fibers, granulocyte permeation, and abundant bacterial populations within necrotic areas of muscle (Stevens & Baddour, 2018).

New techniques include the use of rapid streptococcal diagnostic kits and a polymerase chain reaction (PCR) assay for tissue specimens that test for the genes for streptococcal pyrogenic exotoxin (SPE; e.g., SPE-B) produced by group A *Streptococci* (Schulz, 2018).

Laboratory testing includes a complete blood count with differential, chemistries, as well as tests to evaluate liver function, creatinine levels, coagulation studies, creatine kinase (CK), serum lactate, and inflammatory markers such as C-reactive protein and erythrocyte sedimentation rate.

Laboratory tests should not be used to establish the diagnosis of NSTIs, as findings are generally nonspecific. Observed aberrations may include leukocytosis with left shift (with counts exceeding 14,000/μL), acidosis, coagulopathy, hyponatremia, an elevated blood urea nitrogen (BUN) level (possibly to greater than 15 mg/mL), elevated inflammatory markers, and elevations in serum creatinine, lactate, CK, and aspartate aminotransferase (AST) concentrations. Elevations in serum CK or AST concentrations suggest deep infection of the muscle or fascia as opposed to more superficial infections.

An assessment instrument known as the Laboratory Risk Indicator for Necrotizing Fasciitis (LRINEC) score is available; it is based on laboratory parameters such as the white cell count, hemoglobin, sodium, glucose, creatinine, and C-reactive protein (Stevens & Baddour, 2018). One study identified it as a useful diagnostic and prognostic tool; patients with an LRINEC score of 6 or above had a greater tendency toward diabetes mellitus, *Pseudomonas aeruginosa* infection, and a higher Sequential Organ Failure Assessment (SOFA) score. They also tended to have a longer period of intensive care, a longer hospital stay, and higher septic shock and mortality rates (Schulz, 2018). However, evidence is conflicting regarding its use in the diagnosis and prognosis in patients with NSTIs; the scores have a limited sensitivity and should not be used to rule out NSTI (Stevens & Baddour, 2018). Further limitations include that it is inaccurate when used in the emergency department assessment of necrotizing fasciitis risk stratification and in the differentiation of cellulitis from necrotizing fasciitis. Furthermore, in emergency department patients with confirmed cellulitis, the LRINEC score had a high false-positive rate. Additionally, emergency department patients with confirmed necrotizing fasciitis also had LRINEC scores with a high false-negative rate. In cases of both cellulitis and necrotizing fasciitis, the misclassification rate was higher for nondiabetic patients than for patients with diabetes (Schulz, 2018).

B-mode and possibly color Doppler ultrasonography, contrast-enhanced computed tomography (CT) scanning, or magnetic resonance imaging (MRI) are beneficial in the early diagnosis of necrotizing infections. These facilitate the visualization of the location of the rapidly spreading infection. Of vital utility is the ability for MRI or CT scans to define the extent of necrotizing infection as to guide rapid surgical debridement.

The best initial radiographic imaging exam is a computed tomography (CT) scan; the most important and specific revelation is the occurrence of gas in soft tissues, signifying clostridial infection or polymicrobial (type I) necrotizing fasciitis. Surgical treatment should then follow the identification of this finding. Other radiographic findings may include fluid collections, absence or heterogeneity of tissue enhancement with intravenous contrast, and inflammatory changes beneath the fascia. MRI is not as valuable as compared to CT in the detection of gas in soft tissues. In addition, MRI can be overly sensitive; it tends to overestimate deep tissue involvement and therefore cannot accurately be used to discern between necrotizing cellulitis and deeper infection. Although ultrasound may be used to detect localized abscesses and gas in tissues, this modality is not well studied in necrotizing fasciitis (Schulz, 2018).

Treatment

The course of necrotizing fasciitis can be especially severe in the older adult population. In addition to being the diagnostic gold standard, surgical intervention is the gold standard treatment modality in cases of necrotizing fasciitis (Mody et al., 2014c). Early and aggressive surgical exploration and debridement of necrotic tissue together with broad-spectrum empiric antibiotic therapy and hemodynamic support are the mainstays of therapy (See Fig. 14.20).

Interventions that do not include surgical debridement are universally fatal. Debridement involves the serial removal of all nonviable tissue, revealing healthy and intact tissue. Within the extremities, treatment may necessitate amputation to achieve definitive infection control. Empirical antibiotics should be initiated after procuring blood cultures. Suggested regimens include the combination therapeutics listed in Box 14.11.

Clindamycin is included to cover streptococci, staphylococci, gram-negative bacilli, and anaerobes. Additionally, it possesses antitoxin and other effects against toxin-elaborating strains of streptococci and staphylococci. Alternatives to ampicillin-sulbactam belonging to the beta-lactam–beta-lactamase inhibitors include piperacillin-tazobactam, ampicillin-sulbactam, and ticarcillin-clavulanate; patients with an intolerance to these agents may be treated with either an aminoglycoside or a fluoroquinolone, plus metronidazole. Patients with Fournier gangrene should receive intensive intravenous fluid replenishment and parenteral broad-spectrum triple antimicrobial therapy using a third-generation cephalosporin combined with metronidazole or an aminoglycoside prior to the surgical resection of necrotic tissues. Finally, penicillin-allergic patients can be treated with clindamycin 600 mg IV every 8 hours plus vancomycin 15 mg/kg IV every 12 hours or linezolid 600 mg PO or IV every 12 hours plus aztreonam 1 to 2 g IV every 6 to 8 hours or gentamicin 3 to 5 mg/kg/day IV in three divided doses or ciprofloxacin 400 mg IV every 12 hours.

Aggressive fluid resuscitation and vasopressors may be required owing to significant capillary leaking, which can occur during NSTIs. With cases of streptococcal toxin-mediated NSTIs, nutritional support with albumin may be needed due to excessive catabolism that occurs due to the presence of large open wounds. Implementation should follow correction of hemodynamic instability and, if necessary, may be achieved utilizing enteral feeding. The addition of intravenous immune globulin (IVIG) following treatment with clindamycin has been shown to reduce mortality due to streptococcal toxin NSTI (Schulz, 2018; Stevens & Baddour, 2018). Hyperbaric oxygen therapy as an adjunctive treatment remains controversial, although some studies have suggested a benefit when combined with the standard treatments (Schulz, 2018).

• BOX 14.11 Empiric Antibiotic Regimens for the Treatment of Necrotizing Fasciitis

- Penicillin G 1–4 million U IV every 4 hours + an aminoglycoside (if renal function permits) + clindamycin 600–900 mg intravenously every eight hours in adults; 40 mg/kg per day divided every eight hours in children and neonates
- Carbapenem (e.g., imipenem-cilastatin 1 g IV every 6–8 hrs, or meropenem 1 g IV every 8 hrs, or ertapenem 1 g IV every 24 hrs), or a beta-lactam-beta-lactamase inhibitor (ampicillin-sulbactam 1.5–3 g IV every 6–8 hrs) + an antibiotic with activity against MRSA (e.g., vancomycin 15–20 mg/kg/dose every 8 to 12 hours, not to exceed 2 g per dose, daptomycin 4 mg/kg IV once daily or linezolid 600 mg IV every 12 hrs), + clindamycin

From Stevens & Baddour, 2018; Schulz, 2018; Schwartz, 2019.

Scabies

Scabies is a common illness characterized by an infestation of the skin by the mite *Sarcoptes scabiei* (Fig. 14.21). The global prevalence is approximately 100 million people, and it affects persons across wide age and socioeconomic strata.

Direct and extended skin-to-skin bodily contact is the most common mode of transmission. Thus, outbreaks among family members or sexual partners are common.

Fomite transmission (e.g., via clothing, bedclothes, or other objects) is an uncommon route for the classic form of scabies because the female mite cannot survive away from the host for >24 to 36 hours. Risk factors include nursing home residence, HIV and AIDS, and crowded living conditions such as occurs in long-term care facilities and prisons.

A less common form of scabies is referred to as crusted scabies. It occurs with reduced cellular immunity such as occurs in those with AIDS, human T cell lymphotropic virus type 1 (HTLV-1) infection, leprosy, and lymphoma; it is more likely to be transmitted through fomites. It is typically caused by a heavy mite burden.

Clinical Manifestations

The most common and classic form of scabies may be distributed to the sides and webs of the fingers, flexor wrists, extensor elbows, anterior and posterior axillary folds, areolae, periumbilical skin, waist, extensor knees, lower buttocks and adjacent thighs, genitalia, and lateral and posterior aspects of the feet. Except for when this occurs in young

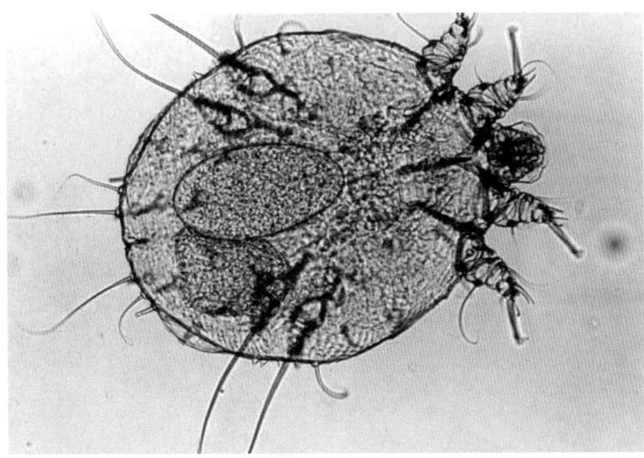

• **Fig. 14.21** Scabies mite. Note the eggs within the body of the mite. (Live scabies mite, ×40 magnification.) (From Paller AS, Mancini AJ: *Hurwitz clinical pediatric dermatology: a textbook of skin disorders of childhood and adolescence*, ed 5, Philadelphia, 2016, Elsevier.)

children, the patient's head and back are relatively spared from involvement.

Symptoms typically begin 3 to 6 weeks after the primary infestation. In patients with previous episodes, however, symptoms may commence within 1 to 3 days after infestation owing to prior sensitization.

The hallmark clinical characteristic of classic scabies is pruritus. It is often intractable, debilitating, and severe; it is usually exacerbated at night. Pruritus is secondary to a delayed-type hypersensitivity reaction to the mite, its excreta (scybala), and eggs. The characteristic dermatologic findings include multiple small, erythematous papules with excoriations. Mite burrows may be visible as 2 to 15 mm, thin, gray, red, or brown serpiginous lines. Burrows are a distinctive feature but are not often visible due to the presence of excoriations or secondary infection. Diminutive wheals, vesicles, pustules, and, rarely, bullae also may be present. There is a greater degree of inflammation to the lesions in children when compared with adults, and a greater preponderance vesicular or bullous findings exist when compared with older patients. Generalized urticarial findings are rare in scabies.

Crusted scabies will manifest chiefly as thickened scales, crusts, and fissures. Scales may progress to wartlike lesions, especially overlying bony prominences. Additionally, skin lesions are malodorous, and nails are often thickened, discolored, and dystrophic. Compared to classic scabies, pruritus may be marginal or absent. The most common locations of affliction are the scalp, hands, and feet. Refer to Figs. 14.22 to 14.25.

Nodular scabies is an uncommon presentation. Findings include enduring firm, erythematous, intensely pruritic, dome-shaped papules 5 or 6 mm in diameter. These are commonly found in the groin, genitalia, buttocks, and axillary folds. It is theorized that this form represents a hypersensitivity reaction to a prior or currently active scabies condition (Fig. 14.26).

Diagnosis

Although the diagnosis is confirmed by the observation of mites, eggs, or fecal scybala using direct microscopy of skin

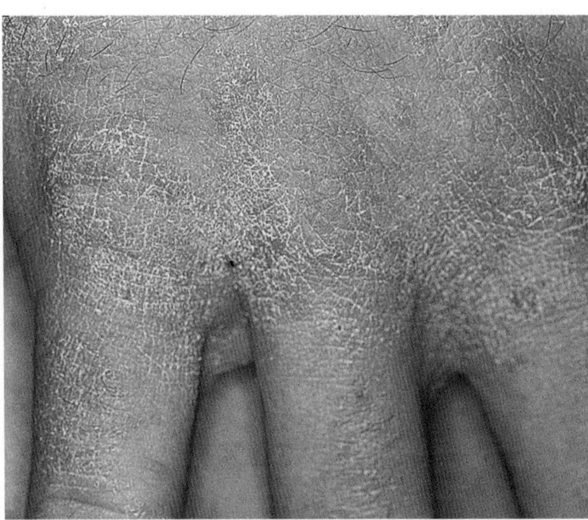

• **Fig. 14.22** Scabies: secondary lesions result from infection or are caused by scratching. Scaling, erythema, and all stages of eczematous inflammation occur as a response to excoriation or to irritation caused by overzealous attempts at self-medication. (From Zug KA, Dinulos JGH: *Skin Disease: Diagnosis and Treatment,* ed4, 2018, Elsevier.)

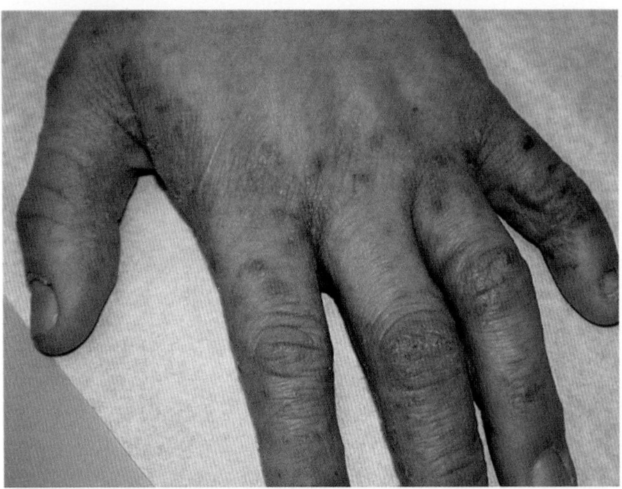

• **Fig. 14.23** Scabietic vesicle involving the web space between the thumb and forefinger. (From Hills, J. L., et al. [2007]. Head lice and scabies. In L. B. Zaoutis, et al. [Eds.], *Comprehensive pediatric hospital medicine* [pp. 976–980]. Mosby.)

scrapings in a simple bedside test, the clinical presentation is often sufficient for diagnosis. Central findings that suggest the diagnosis include the presence of widespread itching that is worse at night, sparing the head (except in infants and young children) and seemingly out of proportion to visible changes in the skin, a pruritic eruption with characteristic lesions and distribution, and other household members exhibiting the characteristic findings.

Dermoscopy (examination of the skin surface with a handheld dermatoscope) allows for the observation of mites and burrows and guides the placement of the confirmatory skin scrapings. A drawback of this tool is reduced specificity compared with scabies preparation if it is the sole diagnostic test utilized. Mites are also frequently difficult or impossible to detect via dermoscopy in patients with highly pigmented skin.

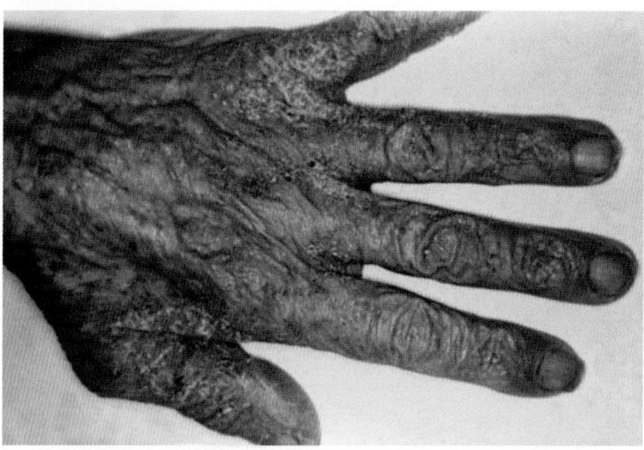

• **Fig. 14.24** Dorsal view of an older patient's hand demonstrating a crusted scabies infestation by the scabies mite, *Sarcoptes scabiei*. Note the localized crusting in the interdigital web spaces. (From Centers for Disease Control and Prevention [CDC], Atlanta, GA. CDC Public Health Image Library, image 4800.)

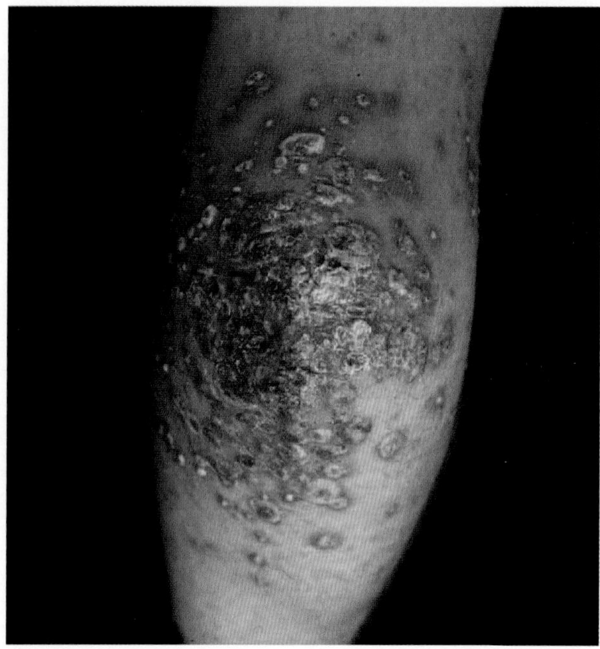

• **Fig. 14.25** Crusted (Norwegian) scabies on the extensor surface of the elbow secondarily infected with *Staphylococcus aureus*. Note the confluence of the crusts and pustules and the similarity of the lesion to psoriasis, both in its hyperkeratotic appearance and in its location on an extensor surface. Risk factors for crusted scabies include immunocompromise by advanced age, prolonged glucocorticoid therapy, cancer chemotherapy, and human immunodeficiency virus or human T-cell lymphotropic virus type 1 infection. (From Fitzpatrick TB, Johnson RA, Wolff K, Suurmond D. Color Atlas and Synopsis of Clinical Dermatology. 4th ed. New York: McGraw-Hill; 2001:841.)

The principal finding on dermoscopic examination is a dark, triangular shape that represents the head of the mite within a burrow ("delta wing" sign); the burrows themselves are also easily visualized. A noodle-like pattern representing aggregates of burrows has been described in the crusted form of scabies.

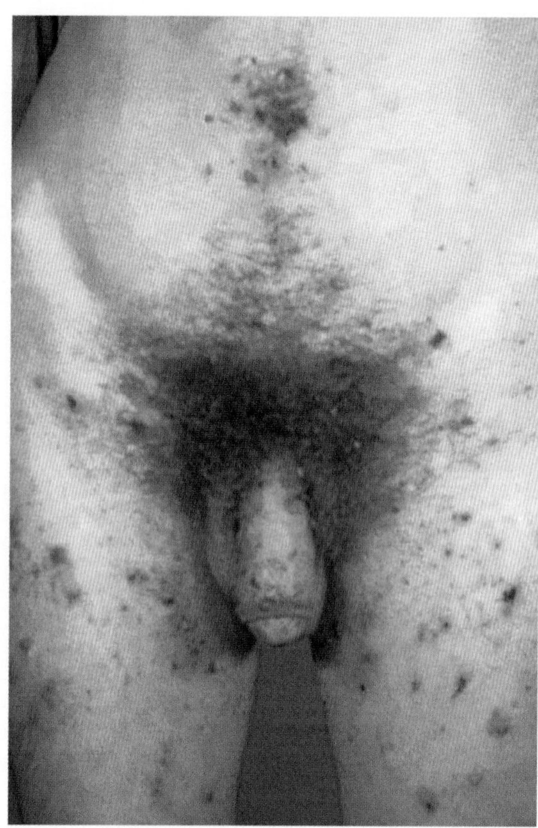

• **Fig. 14.26** Sexually transmitted nodular scabies infestation in a male caused by the scabies mite, *Sarcoptes scabiei*. Note the nodular pustular lesions clustered around the umbilicus and inner thighs. (From Centers for Disease Control and Prevention [CDC], Atlanta, GA. CDC Public Health Image Library, image 6538.)

Skin scraping collection involves the sampling and microscopic examination of the epidermis from those sites that may harbor scabies mites. The sensitivity of scabies preparation ranges from 46% to 90%; the specificity is 100%.

Scrapings should be performed with a blade on skin lesions in multiple sites; burrows or erythematous papules are ideal. Anesthesia is not necessary; scraping should not result in significant bleeding. In children, a disposable curette is an alternative tool that may be helpful instead of a blade. The removal of mites, scale, and debris is facilitated by the addition of a small amount of mineral oil to the sites. Following preparation, the clinician then examines the specimen for scabies mites, eggs, or feces.

Alternatively, a scabies preparation can be performed using a piece of transparent tape with a strong adhesive such as clear packing tape (i.e., "the adhesive tape test"). The tape is firmly applied to a skin lesion and then is rapidly pulled off. After applying the tape to a glass slide, a microscope is used to examine the tape for mites and eggs. An advantage of the adhesive tape test is the lack of a need for equipment beyond a microscope. The procedure may also be useful in children who demonstrate an aversion to skin scrapings (Urman & Loo, 2014).

Treatment

The objectives of therapy include mite eradication, symptomatic treatment of pruritus, and prevention of transmission. The patient and all close contacts should be treated simultaneously, including those who are asymptomatic. The scabicidal agent permethrin 5% cream is the most effective topical treatment. A 60-g tube is prescribed for whole-body application. Patients can be instructed to take a bath or shower and completely dry before application. It should be applied to the entire skin surface (from the neck down), with particular attention to finger web spaces, feet, genitals, and intertriginous sites. The cream should be washed off in 8 hours. This regimen is repeated in 1 week. Compliance typically results in over a 90% cure rate. Another option is ivermectin. Ivermectin, 0.2 mg/kg, is administered as an oral dose and repeated at 10 to 14 days. It is a safe and efficacious alternative to topical treatment. However, two doses 2 weeks apart must be used, as the drug only kills the mite and not the eggs (Schwartz, 2019).

Additional topical treatment options for scabies include benzyl benzoate (10% or 25%), topical sulfur (6% to 33%), lindane (1%), crotamiton, and malathion (0.05%); these medications, however, have not been shown to be more effective than topical permethrin. Lindane is not a preferred agent due to the risk of systemic toxicity resulting in seizures or death); it should be used only as an alternative therapy in patients who cannot tolerate other therapies or when other therapies have failed.

Because pruritus can persist for up to 1 month following successful mite elimination, patients may receive repeated treatment for scabies in the mistaken belief that infestation persists. For this symptom, a class 1 steroid ointment can be applied two to three times daily for 2 to 4 weeks or until the complete resolution of pruritus. An oral prednisone taper may be required to manage patients with debilitating pruritus.

All clothes worn within 2 days of treatment, towels, and bedsheets should be machine washed in hot water or dry cleaned. Management of nursing home outbreaks requires clinical and epidemiologic expertise and possibly the involvement of public health experts (Schwartz, 2019).

Complications

Complications of scabies infestations include secondary staphylococcal or streptococcal infections (such as impetigo, ecthyma, paronychia, and furunculosis). Additionally, fissures associated with crusted scabies provide for a route of ingress for bacteria. Sepsis may ensue in older adults and the immunocompromised. Streptococcal infections may lead to poststreptococcal glomerulonephritis; it has been suggested that the scabies mite possesses the complement inhibitor (SMSB4), increasing the likelihood of secondary streptococcal infections. Rarely, scabies may cause secondary generalized urticaria as a consequence (Urman & Loo, 2014).

Herpes Zoster

Varicella-zoster virus (VZV) infection exists as two discrete entities. Initial infection by VZV causes varicella (chickenpox), whereas herpes zoster (shingles) manifests as a reactivation of latent VZV from the sensory ganglia during the varicella stage.

In the United States, VZV causes infection in greater than 1.2 million patients yearly, resulting in significant morbidity; according to the Centers for Disease Control and Prevention (CDC), about 30% of all persons in the United States will experience an episode. Worldwide, the incidence of herpes zoster has been increasing (Albrecht & Levin, 2019a), and nearly all older adults are seropositive and latently infected with VZV (Schmader, 2017).

Pathophysiology

VZV virus is transmitted from person to person via direct contact or airborne or droplet nuclei when a virus-naive individual is exposed to the vesicular rash of varicella or herpes zoster (Schmader, 2017). In general, however, VZV is much less transmissible from a person with herpes zoster than from a person with varicella. Patients with herpes zoster can transmit VZV to individuals who have not had varicella and have not received the varicella vaccine (Albrecht, 2018). All cases of herpes zoster are caused by the reactivation of endogenous VZV (Schmader, 2017).

During the initial phase of varicella, airborne droplets of VZV infiltrate lymph tissue of the nasopharynx in a suitable host. As a result, T cells become infected with VZV and are subsequently disseminated throughout the body.

Varicella-zoster virus is a double-stranded DNA herpesvirus that exhibits substantial pathogenicity through various mechanisms. It can inhibit several host defenses, such as downregulating major histocompatibility complex (MHC) class I expression as well as inhibiting interferon response genes, thereby augmenting the host immune response. The protracted incubation period in advance of the eruption of skin lesions in varicella indicates the time requirement of VZV to overcome local immune-mediated defenses, such as alpha interferon (IFN-a) produced by epidermal cells. VZV DNA, mainly found in T lymphocytes, is present 11 to 14 days before rash onset; VZV viremia is detected 6 to 8 days before rash appears and ceases 1 to 2 days later.

Once the rash develops, liberated virus particles are present only in skin vesicles. At this juncture it is theorized that the virus then infects nerve endings in skin and migrates retrograde along sensory axons. Once there, the virus becomes dormant within the regional ganglia. VZV may also infect neurons because of viremia. VZV-specific cell-mediated immune responses that develop during varicella are required to end the infection, and they play a critical role in controlling VZV latency and limiting the potential for reactivation to cause herpes zoster.

During the quiescent stage, transcription of one or a small number of VZV genes occurs; however, the virus is not found within the ganglia. Upon reactivation, VZV disseminates within the ganglion to involve multiple sensory neurons and subsequently spreads in an antegrade manner down the sensory nerve to cause infection in the skin, resulting in the classic rash (Albrecht & Levin, 2019a). The exposure of a latently infected individual to herpes zoster does not cause herpes zoster or varicella (Schmader, 2017).

Following VZV reactivation and continuing VZV replication, the involved sensory ganglion typically exhibits intense inflammation associated with the hemorrhagic necrosis of neurons. These changes to neurons are the origin of the usually neurologic symptoms experienced during zoster. An ensuing loss of neurons occurs at the ganglion with consequent fibrosis of afferent nerve fibers, especially type C nociceptors.

Risk Factors

The occurrence of herpes zoster is strongly related the immune status of the host. Reactivation is influenced by age-related immunosenescence, disease-related immunodeficiency secondary to underlying disease, or other modes immunosuppression.

Age is the most important risk factor for the development of herpes zoster; this risk factor is identified as the principal risk factor in up to 90% of all cases of herpes zoster. A significant increase in the incidence of herpes zoster begins at approximately 50 years of age, with 20% of cases occurring between the ages of 50 and 59 years and 40% in patients at least 60 years of age. Approximately 50% of patients 85 years of age and older will have had at least one episode of herpes zoster.

Globally, older adults constitute the majority of medical consultations and hospitalizations for herpes zoster. Furthermore, the severity of disease and the likelihood of complications, such as postherpetic neuralgia (PHN), increases with advancing age (Albrecht & Levin, 2019a).

Immunocompromised patients are at risk for herpes zoster and its complications. Notable conditions include a human immunodeficiency virus (HIV) infection, Hodgkin disease, non-Hodgkin lymphomas, leukemia, hematopoietic stem cell or solid organ transplant, systemic lupus erythematosus, and the use of immunosuppressive medications such as glucocorticoids, nonbiologic disease-modifying antirheumatic drugs (DMARDs), tumor necrosis factor (TNF)-alpha inhibitors, and Janus kinase (JAK) inhibitors. Other risk factors include White race, female sex, psychological stress, and physical trauma. Health care workers and staff in nursing homes and hospitals and children who have not received the varicella vaccine may not have had VZV primary infection and are also potentially at risk for varicella (Schmader, 2017).

Clinical Manifestations

The main presenting features of herpes zoster is a rash and symptoms of acute neuritis. Initially the rash commences most typically as erythematous papules, usually in a single, unilateral dermatome or several contiguous dermatomes. This dispersion of the vesicular rash corresponds to the sensory area of the affected ganglion (or adjacent ganglia). Although any dermatome may manifest lesions, the thoracic and lumbar dermatomes are the most commonly involved (Figs. 14.27 and 14.28). In some patients, a few scattered vesicles may be found remote from the primary dermatome(s); this likely reflects VZV viremia occurring initially in herpes zoster.

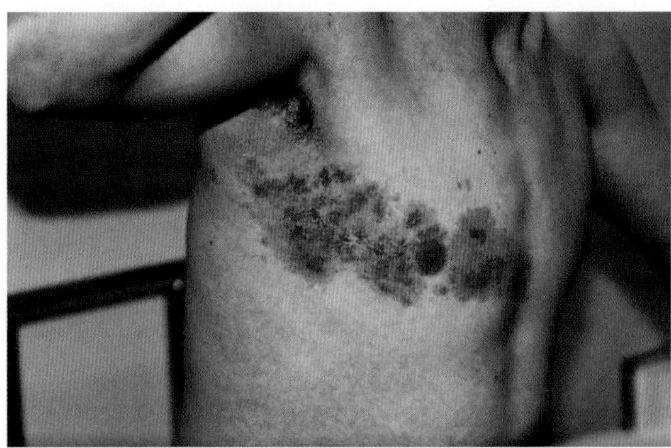

• **Fig. 14.27** Herpes zoster infection, typically involving a single unilateral dermatome. (From White, G., & Cox, N. [2006]. *Diseases of the skin* [2nd ed.]. Mosby.)

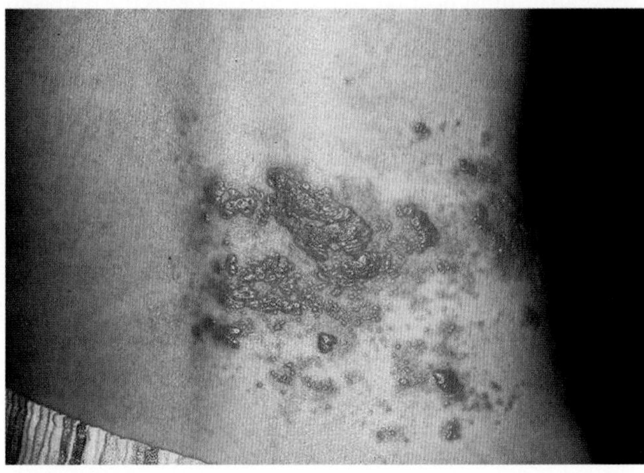

• **Fig. 14.28** Herpes zoster involving the lumbar dermatome. (From Bennett, J. E., Dolin, R., & Blaser, M. J. [2020]. *Mandell, Douglas, & Bennett's principles and practices of infectious diseases* [vol. 2, 2nd ed.]. Elsevier.)

Herpes zoster ophthalmicus occurs because of VZV reactivation of the ophthalmic division of the fifth cranial nerve. It is a serious vision-threatening condition. The presentation starts as a prodrome of headache, malaise, and fever. Following this, unilateral pain or hypesthesia in the affected eye, forehead, and top of the head occurs. Vesicular lesions on the lateral aspects or tip of the nose (i.e., Hutchinson sign) are highly associated with eye involvement; findings in this area of the face imply affliction of the nasociliary branch of the trigeminal nerve, which also supplies the globe (Fig. 14.29).

Within several days, grouped vesicles or bullae are the most prevalent feature. Following 3 to 4 days, the rash evolves to become pustular. In the older adult or immunocompromised individual, the rash can also be hemorrhagic in nature. In patients with intact immune systems,

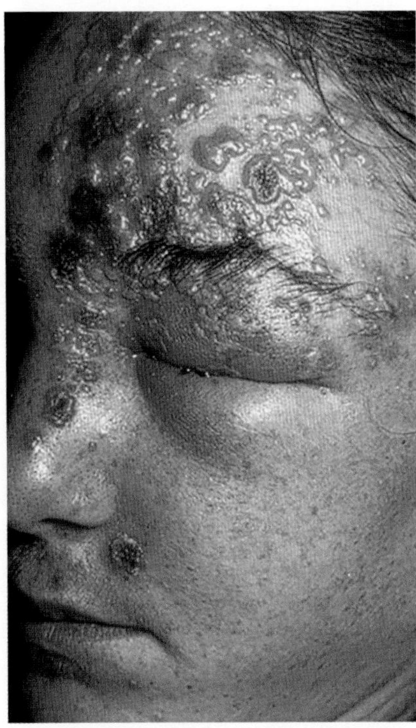

• **Fig. 14.29** Herpes zoster ophthalmicus. Ophthalmologic zoster vesicles and crusting of the top and side of the nose in herpes zoster implies involvement of the nasociliary branch of the trigeminal nerve and eye involvement. (From White, G., & Cox, N. [2006]. *Diseases of the skin* [2nd ed.]. St. Louis, MO: Mosby.)

the lesions crust by a week to 10 days and patients are no longer considered infectious. Long-term sequelae such as scarring and hypo/hyperpigmentation may persist months to years after resolution of the illness. Should new lesions develop more than a week after the initial presentation, providers should consider an underlying immunodeficient state.

Pain as acute neuritis is the most common symptom of herpes zoster; it is most often characterized as a range from a superficial itching, tingling, paresthesia, hyperesthesia, or burning to severe, deep, boring throbbing or a lancinating/stabbing sensation. Pain also tends to be more severe in older patients. Acute neuritis is a distinct process from postherpetic neuralgia (PHN). In most patients, pain exists as a prodrome, preceding the rash in the dermatome where the rash appears. Pain may be constant or intermittent and usually heralds the rash by 2 to 3 days, although longer periods are possible; periods of up to a month can occur in approximately 20% of patients. Commonly, the prodromal dermatomal pain is often misinterpreted as another disease, such as angina, pleurisy, cholecystitis, glaucoma, trigeminal neuralgia, appendicitis, spinal disc or vertebral diseases, renal colic or unappreciated trauma. Consideration of alternative diagnoses depends on the location of neuritis and is more likely prior to rash eruption (Albrecht & Levin, 2019a; Schmader, 2017). Zoster sine herpete occurs when patients experience acute dermatomal neuralgia without ever developing a skin eruption (Schmader, 2017).

Diagnosis

In most immunocompetent patients, the diagnosis of herpes zoster is primarily clinical. In older patients or in the immunocompromised, the presence of atypical VZV skin lesions or herpes simplex virus lesions can be misperceived as herpes zoster (zosteriform herpes simplex), and laboratory analysis is warranted. Diagnostic tests include polymerase chain reaction (PCR) testing, direct fluorescent antibody (DFA) testing, and viral culture. PCR is the optimal diagnostic test because it has the highest sensitivity (more than 95%) in diagnosing herpes zoster; additionally, testing is highly specific, and results are realized rapidly (up to 1 day) compared with traditional culture procurement. Additional benefits include the ability to test lesions during all stages, including the late stage during which ulcers and crusts might predominate. PCR use may be expanded to encompass areas beyond the dermal layers, such as the CSF, blood, vitreous humor, and bronchoalveolar lavage.

DFA and is an alternative to PCR; scrapings may be harvested from vesicular skin lesions that have yet to crust. Compared to PCR, DFA sensitivity is approximately 55%; accurate results require both a sufficient quantity and a sufficient quality of infected cells collected.

Viral cultures and DFA may both be accomplished from unroofed vesicles or recently ruptured vesicles. Viral cultures can also be performed on sterile body fluid samples (e.g., CSF). Although DFA testing can achieve results in roughly 2 hours, VZV culture usually necessitates about 1 week of cultivation. Culture sensitivity depends on the lesion's stage (range of 50%–75%); virus levels precipitously decline as the VZV lesion advances to healing. A false-negative culture results can occur if antiviral therapy has begun prior to testing.

Treatment

The management of herpes zoster focuses on antiviral and analgesic therapy. Antivirals are employed to augment the healing of cutaneous lesions, prevent the occurrence of new lesions, prevent postherpetic neuralgia (PHN), reduce viral shedding to limit disease transmission, and decrease the duration and severity of symptoms (especially pain). Analgesia is utilized for patients with moderate to severe acute neuritis.

Antiviral agents are recommended for patients with uncomplicated herpes zoster who present within 72 hours of clinical symptoms. Initiating antiviral treatment during this window serves to maximize the potential benefits of treatment. The maximum benefit is achieved in patients older than 50 years of age in whom the pain of zoster generally persists longer. Although the efficacy of antiviral therapy in patients younger than 50 years of age has not been as well studied, the risk of adverse events secondary to antiviral therapy is extremely low. Time frames beyond 72 hours may be considered for antiviral therapy if new lesions are appearing at the time of presentation; this marks ongoing viral replication. However, the clinical utility of initiating antiviral therapy more than 72 hours after the onset of lesions

• BOX 14.12 Oral Treatment of Uncomplicated Herpes Zoster

- Valacyclovir: 1000 mg three times daily for 7 days
- Famciclovir: 500 mg three times daily for 7 days
- Acyclovir: 800 mg five times daily for 7 days

in immunocompetent persons is not known. For patients in whom encrusted lesions are present, a marginal benefit from antiviral therapy use is expected.

The nucleoside analogues acyclovir, valacyclovir, and famci-clovir are the preferred antivirals for treatment of acute herpes zoster infection (Box 14.12). These agents are used to treat herpes simplex infections as well; however, higher dosages are required to treat herpes zoster.

Oral antiviral therapy is general adequate for the primary therapy of uncomplicated herpes zoster. Should evidence of complicated disease exist (in the form of acute retinal necrosis, encephalitis, zoster ophthalmicus, Ramsay Hunt syndrome, or other central nervous system complications), oral antiviral therapy is not a sufficient treatment.

Drawbacks of acyclovir include frequent daily dosing and poor bioavailability. Rather, valacyclovir and famciclovir have improved bioavailability and a lower dosing frequency requirement. Overall, the antiviral class has an excellent safety record at the currently recommended doses with adverse reactions uncommon. When present, they can include nausea, vomiting, diarrhea, or headache.

For immunocompromised patients with herpes zoster, antiviral therapy should be instituted, even if the presentation is beyond 72 hours. Therapy should be hastened, especially in the severely immunocompromised patient; those with disseminated zoster should be hospitalized for intravenous acyclovir treatment.

The use of adjuvant agents such as gabapentin, tricyclic antidepressants, and corticosteroids in the treatment of acute uncomplicated herpes zoster is controversial insomuch as they do not prevent PHN when compared to placebo or acyclovir (Schmader, 2017). Furthermore, the use of tricyclic antidepressants in the older adult is associated with a concerning adverse effect profile, which includes anticholinergic properties, orthostasis, and dysrhythmias. Glucocorticoids can also potentially increase the risk of secondary bacterial skin infection in patients with zoster (Albrecht, 2018). However, some clinical trials have demonstrated diminutions in acute pain and benefits with sleep, return to routine activities, and the elimination of analgesic medications among patients with no relative contraindications to corticosteroids. Therefore, corticosteroids may have utility in the reduction of moderate to severe acute pain not relieved by antivirals and analgesics. Corticosteroids are used to treat VZV-induced facial paralysis, cranial polyneuritis to improve motor outcomes and provide pain relief, zoster ophthalmicus, and retinal necrosis. If prescribed, corticosteroids should always be used in conjunction with antiviral agents (Schmader, 2017).

Complications

Secondary bacterial infections of the zoster rash can occur. Patients should receive staphylococcal and streptococcal antibiotic coverage in addition to antiviral therapy should a bacterial infection be suspected. Patients should contact their provider if there are findings significant of bacterial superinfection such erythema, warmth, or purulence that surround any zoster lesions.

Although antiviral therapy reduces pain associated with acute neuritis, pain syndromes associated with herpes zoster can still be debilitating. Approximately 10% to 15% of patients may develop PHN (Albrecht, 2018). Tricyclic antidepressants (TCAs), gabapentin, pregabalin, lidocaine patch, and opioids are considered first-line therapies because one or more high-quality randomized controlled trials demonstrated efficacy with these agents. Gabapentin, pregabalin, the topical lidocaine patch 5%, and the topical capsaicin patch 8% have been approved by the FDA for the treatment of PHN. Often, a combination of analgesic therapies may prove to be beneficial when single agents fail to achieve satisfactory analgesia.

Topical lidocaine therapy has not been shown to result in systemic toxicity in patients. Concerning the topical capsaicin patch, many patients may not be able to tolerate the burning sensation it causes; it should be considered as a second-line treatment of PHN because it may be effective in certain patients. Capsaicin requires application by clinicians who are trained in its correct administration. The anticonvulsant gabapentin is indicated in the treatment of PHN; patients without at least partial relief at 1800 mg of daily gabapentin are unlikely to derive meaningful benefit. Frail geriatric persons usually require reduced doses due to worsening adverse medication effects, which include somnolence, dizziness, ataxia, peripheral edema, and cognitive impairment. Additionally, the regimen should be adjusted for creatinine clearance. Pregabalin works similarly to gabapentin and is associated with a similar side effects profile; these include dizziness, somnolence, peripheral edema, dry mouth, and gait disturbances. The medication has limited drug-drug interactions, can be given less frequently than gabapentin, and has a relatively rapid onset of action. Other anticonvulsants (such as phenytoin, levetiracetam, oxcarbazepine, tiagabine, topiramate, zonisamide, and valproate) are possibly useful but cannot be considered first-line agents because of limited data for efficacy or significant adverse effects. The tricyclic antidepressants (TCAs) modulate nerve transmission. TCAs have demonstrated significant pain relief in patients with PHN, with nortriptyline providing an equivalent efficacy yet better tolerated when compared to amitriptyline in a PHN. Nortriptyline and desipramine are preferred over amitriptyline because they have fewer anticholinergic effects, resulting in less dry mouth, sedation, constipation, cognitive impairment, and orthostatic hypotension. However, tricyclic antidepressants are contraindicated in patients with QT prolongation, familial histories of long-QT syndromes, atrioventricular block, bundle-branch block, or a recent acute myocardial infarction. A screening ECG should be performed to evaluated for QT prolongation or heart block prior to instituting therapy and with each change in dose. Caution should be exercised in the coadministration of TCAs and selective serotonin reuptake inhibitors (SSRIs); toxic TCA plasma concentration could result in this situation (Schmader, 2017).

Nonsteroidal antiinflammatory drugs and acetaminophen are also indicated for mild pain, either alone or in combination with a weak opioid analgesic such as codeine or tramadol. For patients suffering with moderate to severe pain that disturbs sleep or causes significant impairment of quality of life, stronger opioid analgesics such as oxycodone or morphine may be required (Albrecht, 2018). Although studies have demonstrated a patient preference for opioids compared to TCAs and placebo in the management of PHN, concerning adverse effects of opioids must be recognized. These are constipation, nausea, sedation, impaired cognitive function, falls, and fractures; these are more likely to occur in older patients when prescribed opioids. Patients should have adequate bowel preparation when taking opioids, and prescribers should begin regimens at a low dose and slowly titrate the dose to mitigate any undesired adverse effects. Tramadol, a mu-opioid agonist and a norepinephrine and serotonin reuptake inhibitor, has demonstrated pain reductions in patients with PHN; however, prescribers should be cautious of the standard opioid side effects and the possibility of additional effects; these are orthostatic hypotension, an increased risk of epilepsy in patients with a history of seizures, and a risk for serotonin syndrome in patients who use serotonergic medications (especially SSRIs and monoamine oxidase inhibitors) (Schmader, 2017).

With the evolution of the rash of herpes zoster ophthalmicus, hyperemic conjunctivitis, uveitis, episcleritis, and keratitis may all be possible. VZV keratitis affects the epithelial, stromal, or endothelial layers of the cornea; those with epithelial or stromal involvement are most at risk for vision loss (Albrecht & Levin, 2019a). Treatment is with the standard oral antiviral therapy to curtail VZV reproduction and the use adjunctive topical steroid drops to inhibit inflammation and to contain immune-mediated keratitis and iritis. If, however, the patient is immunocompromised or requires hospitalization for sight-threatening disease, then intravenous acyclovir 10 mg/kg three times daily for 7 days is proper (Albrecht, 2018). Ocular involvement mandates ophthalmologic consultation. Additional treatments may include antibiotic ophthalmic ointment to prevent bacterial infection of the ocular surface, mydriatics as needed for iritis, and ocular pressure-lowering drugs as needed for glaucoma (Schmader, 2017).

VZV is the most common cause of acute retinal necrosis (ARN). ARN occurs in both immunocompetent and immunocompromised hosts. Clinically, patients initially present with unilateral acute iridocyclitis, vitritis, necrotizing retinitis, occlusive retinal vasculitis with rapid loss of vision, and ultimately retinal detachment. Blurry vision is a hallmark symptom, and pain is present in the involved eye due to progressive necrotizing retinitis. Bilateral disease can occur in up to half of all patientsof patients; those with advanced AIDS are subject to rapid progression and severe disease (Albrecht & Levin, 2019a).

For immunocompetent patients with acute retinal necrosis (ARN), intravenous acyclovir 10 mg/kg every 8 hours for 10 to 14 days is given followed by oral valacyclovir 1 g three times daily (or equivalent) for approximately 6 weeks. Adjunctive treatment with empiric systemic glucocorticoids is a consideration, especially if there is decreased visual acuity secondary to inflammation or optic nerve involvement. Again, patients should be evaluated by an ophthalmologist to determine the need for intraocular therapy /or vitrectomy.

The chief otologic complication of VZV reactivation is the Ramsay Hunt syndrome, which manifests as the triad of ipsilateral facial paralysis, ear pain, and vesicles in the auditory canal and auricle. Valacyclovir 1 g three times per day for 7 to 10 days in conjunction with prednisone 1 mg/kg for 5 days, without a taper, is an acceptable regimen for most patients. In severe cases characterized by vertigo, tinnitus, or hearing loss, IV therapy can be initiated. The patient can then be converted to an oral antiviral agent upon lesion encrustation.

Patients with VZV may also be subjected to central and peripheral nervous system dissemination causing the following: aseptic meningitis, encephalitis, peripheral motor neuropathy, cerebrovascular accidents, Guillain-Barré Syndrome, and myelitis. For these patients, intravenous acyclovir should be administered. The course of treatment is typically 10 to 14 days. Severe complications include cutaneous dissemination and visceral involvement, which can occur in the immunocompromised. Fulminant and rapidly progressive pneumonitis or hepatitis can occur in this patient subset.

Prevention

Geriatric patients with localized zoster are not infectious before vesicles appear and are no longer infectious once the lesions have re-epithelized. For patients with active lesions, no specific precautions within the community setting are recommended. However, patients should be instructed about the risk of viral transmission to others. In addition, until the lesion has crusted, patients should keep the rash covered if possible and should wash their hands often to prevent the spread of virus to others. Older adult patients should also avoid contact with pregnant women who have never had chickenpox or the varicella vaccine, premature or low-birth-weight infants, and immunocompromised individuals (Albrecht, 2018). The herpes zoster vaccination is indicated for individuals ≥50 years of age to reduce the risk of developing herpes zoster and postherpetic neuralgia. Vaccination is not indicated for the treatment of herpes zoster or postherpetic neuralgia. Presently, two forms of the vaccine are available, a nonlive recombinant glycoprotein E vaccine and the second, a live attenuated vaccine. The recombinant zoster vaccine is preferred in older adult

TABLE 14.7 Key Urinary Definitions

Bacteriuria	The presence of bacteria in the urine	
Pyuria	>10 WBCs (WBC/mm^3) per high-power field (hpf) in a urine sample, suggesting inflammation of the genitourinary tract	
ASB	General	the presence of bacteria in the urine, with or without pyuria, in the absence of genitourinary signs or symptoms
	Females	two consecutive voided urine specimens with isolation of the same uropathogen of counts >10^5 colony forming units/milliliter (cfu/mL)
	Males	a single clean-catch voided urine specimen with 1 uropathogen isolated in quantitative counts greater than or equal to 10^5 cfu/mL
	Catheterized	a single catheterized urine specimen with one uropathogen isolated in a quantitative count greater than or equal to 10^2 cfu/mL
Symptomatic UTI	Both pyuria and bacteriuria are present in a patient with at least two signs and symptoms of a genitourinary tract infection (e.g., dysuria, frequency, urgency, suprapubic pain/tenderness, costovertebral angle pain/tenderness or hematuria)	
Acute uncomplicated cystitis	A symptomatic UTI that is limited to the lower urinary tract (i.e., bladder, urethra) in otherwise healthy adults without structural or functional abnormalities of the urinary tract	
Complicated UTI	infection of the upper tract (e.g., pyelonephritis), or symptomatic UTI in patients with either functional or structural genitourinary abnormalities, urinary catheters, or in patients with systemic illness (e.g., chronic kidney disease, diabetes, or other immunodeficiency)	
Recurrent UTI	three or more symptomatic UTIs within a 12-month period or two or more symptomatic UTIs in a 6-month period following clinical resolution of each UTI with antimicrobial treatment	
Catheter-associated UTI (CAUTI)	patients with an indwelling urethral, suprapubic, or intermittent catheterization with signs or symptoms compatible with UTI (i.e., new onset or worsening of fever, rigors, altered metal status, malaise, or lethargy with no other identified cause; flank pain; costovertebral angle tenderness; hematuria; pelvic discomfort;OR dysuria, urgency or frequency in patients whose catheters have been removed within the previous 48 hours with no other identified source of infection), along with greater than or equal to 10^3 cfu/mL of one or more bacterial species in a single catheter urine specimen	

From Rowe, T., & Juthani-Mehta, M. (2019). Urinary tract infections. In J. B. Halter, J. G. Ouslander, S. Studenski, K. P. High, S. Asthana, M. A. Supiano, & C. Ritchie (Eds.). *Hazzard's geriatric medicine and gerontology* (7th ed.). McGraw-Hill. http://accessmedicine.mhmedical.com/content.aspx?bookid=1923§ionid=144563864.

patients, as it has demonstrated greater efficacy in patients 70 years of age and older, whereas the efficacy of the live zoster vaccine was superior in the cohort of patients ages 60 to 69 (Albrecht & Levin, 2019b).

Urinary Tract Infections

Urinary tract infection (UTI) is the most frequent bacterial infection in the older adult. Although asymptomatic bacteriuria (ASB) in older adults is usually regarded as a colonization state, symptomatic infection to the contrary is associated with morbidity and, uncommonly, mortality. The ideal treatment of UTI in geriatric patients is difficult owing to diagnostic ambiguity, concerns of antibiotic stewardship, and increasing bacterial resistance in the community and long-term care setting. Within these two arenas, the influence and treatment of UTIs diverges; compounding the spectrum are multiple patient variables that dictate an unstandardized approach in the management of UTIs; additionally, the presence of indwelling catheters in some geriatric patients further complicates the approach. Several key definitions are explained in Table 14.7 (Rowe & Juthani-Mehta, 2019).

Epidemiology: UTIs

UTI is responsible for more than 8 million outpatient and emergency department visits in the United States yearly. It is one of the most frequently listed diagnoses among hospitalized patients at least 50 years old in the United States, accounting for almost 25% of infectious disease hospitalizations in this cohort.

Epidemiology: Asymptomatic Bacteriuria

The prevalence of asymptomatic bacteriuria (ASB) increases with age and is more prevalent in long-term care (LTC) residents. Rates of ASB among healthy, older adult women ranges from 5% to 20% in women ages 65 to 90 years; however, in females over 90 years of age, this increases to nearly 45%. ASB is relatively uncommon in younger men, but as with women, it increases significantly with age. This is especially true in men with prostatic hypertrophy. The rate of ASB is approximately 5% in men living in the community, but the rate rises to 20% in men greater than 80 years of age. ASB is highly prevalent in long-term care residences, with several studies authenticating rates for men and women to be approximately 15% to 50%. Importantly, ASB in this population is probably higher than the documented rates; adults with urinary incontinence and dementia are more likely to have ASB, but they are also more likely not to be included in studies owing to a greater complexity in securing a urine sample in these conditions. Almost exclusively, chronically catheterized older adults develop bacteriuria within 1 month of catheterization. However, ASB often resolves spontaneously, without antimicrobial intervention (Rowe & Juthani-Mehta, 2019).

The incidence of UTI in postmenopausal women is 0.07 per person-year according to a large population-based study. Because there is a large disparity on the definition of UTI, criteria used to define a UTI may not accurately reflect the correct incidence of disease across the population. In long-term care residents, the rate of UTI appears to remain high with an estimated rate of 0.15 per patient-year for older women and 0.11 per patient-year for older men. One study of nursing home residents with advanced dementia reported that 27% of older adults were diagnosed with UTI over a 2-year period (Rowe & Juthani-Mehta, 2019).

Pathophysiology

The urinary tract, composed of the urethra, bladder, ureters, and kidneys, is sterile under normal circumstance. With advancing age, however, this veracity becomes altered owing to increased colonization, inducing the high rates of ASB. Normally, physiologic factors prevent contamination and infection of the urinary tract from bacteria. Most importantly, urination is the primary defense mechanism for preventing bacterial invasion of the urinary tract from gastrointestinal flora. Other properties include low urinary acidity, ureter peristalsis, a functional vesicoureteral valve, and a host of additional mucosal and immunologic impediments. UTIs most commonly occur via an ascending pathway. Organisms populate the periurethral region and ascend proximally into the bladder and, at times, the kidneys. Determinants of renal infection include virulence characteristics of the offending agent or the presence of genitourinary anomalies such as obstruction or urinary reflux. Seldomly, infection may occur because of hematogenous dissemination rather than the ascending route; this presents as a UTI due to bacteremia from an extraurinary source (such as the isolation of *S. aureus* in patients without an indwelling catheter).

Etiology

The most common form of bacteria isolated in both asymptomatic and symptomatic ambulatory older women is *Escherichia coli*, making up from 75% to 95% of all infections. In uncomplicated UTI, over 95% of cases are due to a single pathogen. In geriatric females with uncomplicated infection, the range of virulence factors of *E. coli* isolates is comparable to that shown in younger females. Agents causing complicated infections (i.e., pyelonephritis) contain more complex virulence factors such as possessing fimbriae, a capsule, adhesins, and various disease-enhancing proteins (e.g., iron-binding proteins and hemolysins). Other bacteria causing disease in this demographic include other Enterobacteriaceae (*Klebsiella pneumoniae, Proteus mirabilis*) and *Enterococcus* species. *Pseudomonas aeruginosa* or group B and D streptococci are rarely causative. The presence of common skin flora in isolates suggests contamination, particularly if multiple organisms are noted.

Risk factors for non-*E. coli* UTIs in the community setting in older adults include male gender, a severe clinical presentation (such as a protracted course of greater than 7 days, documented or reported fever, nausea or vomiting, flank pain), a previous diagnosis of a UTI in the past year, diabetes mellitus, previous treatment failure using TMP/SMX, or functional or anatomic abnormalities.

E. coli is also the most common bacterial cause of UTI in long-term care facility (LTCF) patients. Other common agents (identified in order of reducing occurrence) include *Proteus* spp., *Klebsiella* spp., *Enterococcus* spp., *Staphylococcus* spp., and *Pseudomonas* spp. Uncommon causes of UTI in LTCF patients are *Acinetobacter*, *Candida* spp., and methicillin-resistant *S. aureus* (MRSA). Older adults with MRSA urinary infections should also be evaluated for underlying staphylococcal bacteremia. Polymicrobial bacteriuria occurs in up to a quarter of long-term care facility patients; this is especially apparent in those with chronic urinary catheter placement.

Risk Factors

Multiple risk factors contribute to the development of a UTI. Reduced B- and T-cell function due to advancing age (i.e., immunosenescence) continues to be a recurring theme in the older adult population infectious disposition. Environmental factors via hospitalization or residence in a long-term care facility) increases patient contact to potentially virulent nosocomial pathogens. Hospitalization often is characterized by genitourinary instrumentation; introduction of an indwelling catheter has regularly been shown to be a strong risk factor for development of symptomatic UTI in both genders. Older adults are also at an increased risk of having anatomic or functional abnormalities, which predisposes these patients to urinary stasis, leading to an impairment of the normal expulsion of urine and pathogens from the body. In males, benign prostatic hypertrophy is implicated, whereas in females, the presence of cystoceles should be considered. Paradoxically, however, a high postvoid residual (PVR) volume has not reliably been shown to increase the risk of developing a symptomatic UTI in either ambulatory women or long-term residents.

In older adults, the most common risk factor associated with developing a UTI is having history of UTIs. In postmenopausal women, sexual activity, urinary incontinence, and estrogen deficiency have all been associated with developing UTIs and are additional risk factors. Pathogenically, reductions of estrogen levels facilitate increased colonization of the vagina with potential urobacteria; with fewer commensal lactobacilli colonizing the vagina, a greater number of *E. coli* and *Enterococci* spp. become apparent. These changes in vaginal flora, coupled with a higher pH and an environment devoid of lactobacilli, dramatically increase the risk of UTIs in older women. A review of randomized controlled trials, however, found that evidence was lacking in the use of oral estrogens to reduce the recurrence of UTIs in this population.

Multiple comorbid illnesses have been associated with the development of UTIs in older adults. The greatest risk is diabetes mellitus; in postmenopausal women, those with diabetes mellitus were almost three times as likely to develop a UTI compared to women without diabetes. Furthermore, geriatric patients with diabetes are also at an increased risk for developing a UTI from a more atypical bacteria such as *Pseudomonas* spp. and *Proteus* spp., and they are more likely to experience upper tract disease (e.g., pyelonephritis). Other common comorbidities include benign prostate hypertrophy, prior UTIs, cerebrovascular disease, Alzheimer disease, and Parkinson disease.

Clinical Manifestations in Community Patients

Older adults present in a highly variable manner; the clinical manifestations are reliant on the patient's age, presence of underlying illnesses (such as diabetes, cerebrovascular disease, Parkinson disease), anatomic or functional urinary system aberrations, living situation (long-term care facility versus community), and presence of a urethral or suprapubic urinary catheter. The wide array of presentations and varying definitions of a symptomatic UTI contributes to difficulty in arriving at a definitive diagnosis and effective treatment of the disorder.

In geriatric patients with an intact cognitive state, symptomatic UTI clinical findings are reminiscent to those of young adults. In these cases, infection is initiated with the presence of new or deteriorating genitourinary symptoms. Acute uncomplicated UTI, referred to as cystitis, is the leading presentation of symptomatic UTI in older women; characteristics include dysuria (with or without frequency), urgency, suprapubic pain, or hematuria. In postmenopausal women, urgency, nocturia, incontinence, and generalized nonspecific symptoms (low-back pain, low abdominal pain, constipation, cold, and chills) are also common. It is also important to note that in older women without a urinary infection, symptoms of urinary urgency and incontinence can often occur, as does bacteriuria. It is therefore a diagnostic dilemma in determining if a true symptomatic UTI exists in this group and as a corollary would benefit from antibiotic therapy. Patients with upper tract disease (such as pyelonephritis) typically have additional symptoms such as fever, chills, fatigue and malaise beyond an established baseline, nausea or vomiting, flank pain, and costovertebral angle tenderness (Hooton & Gupta, 2019; Rowe & Juthani-Mehta, 2019).

Clinical Manifestations in Long-Term Care Facility Patients

The demonstration of symptomatic urinary infections in long-term care populations is vastly more obscure as compared to community patients. Residents in long-term care settings do not commonly present with the classical characteristics of a genitourinary tract infection (such as dysuria, frequency, or flank pain). Much like outpatients, these patients have chronic noninfectious urinary symptoms such as urinary incontinence, frequency, nocturia, and urgency, making it more difficult to identify a symptomatic UTI that would benefit from treatment. Long-term care patients additionally have varying degrees of cognitive compromise limiting their ability to effectively convey genitourinary manifestations of a potential symptomatic UTI. In a study of suspected UTI in residents of long-term facilities with advanced dementia, the most common symptom for suspected UTI was change in mental status (44.3%). Other symptoms of a suspected UTI in this demographic include a change in the character of the urine, fever, declining functional status, and hematuria.

Currently, it is not well established as to the utility of nonspecific symptoms (mental status change or changes in functional state) in identifying symptomatic UTIs in geriatric patients, especially those residing in long-term care or patients with cognitive impairment. At this time, there is also no definitive association with delirium or change in functional status alone to symptomatic UTI in adults without an indwelling catheter. Geriatric falls have also not been conclusively linked to bacteriuria, pyuria, or a diagnosis of symptomatic UTI; health care providers should pursue an alternative underlying diagnosis in an older adult patient whose only manifestation of a possible UTI is a fall event.

Clinical Manifestations in Geriatric Patients with Indwelling Catheters

Catheter-associated urinary tract infection (CAUTI) is the most common health care–associated infection and the most common indication for antibiotic prescriptions in sthe geriatric demographic. In LTCFs, the prevalence of indwelling urethral catheters ranges from 7% to 10%; in the acute care setting, the overall CAUTI incidence rate is 14.7/1000 device days. CAUTI is challenging to correctly diagnose, as geriatric patients' catheters often present with nongenitourinary such as fever and mental status changes. Additionally, almost all patients with a chronic catheter will have some degree of bacteriuria and pyuria, resulting in a complicated differentiation between catheter-associated asymptomatic bacteriuria (CA-ASB) and CAUTI in patients with nonspecific symptoms.

Diagnostic Approach in Community Patients

Although the use of a urinary dipstick (in assessing leukocyte esterase and nitrites), urinalysis, and urine culture are not routinely recommended in younger patients with reliable histories, in older adults, this approach presents significant challenges. The high prevalence of chronic urinary symptoms, such as incontinence, urgency, and nocturia may all confound the diagnosis of symptomatic UTI in the older adult. Diagnosing and treating UTI with antibiotics in geriatric patients without an additional assessment of bacteriuria and pyuria can result in unnecessary and harmful antibiotic treatment. Several studies in older women have recommended employing a delayed empiric prescription approach and use of urinary diagnostic testing (such as a urine dipstick and urine culture) to reduce overall unnecessary antibiotic use without causing worse outcomes or significant morbidity. Beyond this, most patients reported clinical improvement or cure without any antibiotic therapy whatsoever. Worsening or progression of urinary disease to pyelonephritis or bacteremia was not observed as a repercussion of delaying antibiotic treatment. It is therefore practical to delay empiric antibiotics in women whose diagnosis of UTI is unclear, especially in women with chronic urinary symptoms, while awaiting further diagnostic testing. Usually, the evaluation for symptomatic UTI in patients with new localized genitourinary symptoms should be initiated with a urinary dipstick to evaluate for the presence of nitrite or leukocyte esterase. If either nitrite or leukocyte esterase is positive, a urine culture and consideration of empiric oral antibiotics should follow (Fig. 14.30).

The urine culture is the diagnostic test of choice to delineate and quantify bacteriuria in sufficient quantities as well as to govern antibiotic selection. In geriatric patients with chronic incontinence, frequency, or urgency without localized genitourinary signs or symptoms, urinary testing with dipstick, urinalysis, or urine culture should not routinely be performed. Health care clinicians instead should recommend hydration, scrutinize medications for potential side effects (e.g., diuretics, antipsychotics), and contemplate the possibility of other illnesses.

If a UTI is suspected in a frail older adult patient with cognitive impairment, based on alterations in mental status (manifestations of delirium, disorganized speech, lethargy) or a change in the character of the patient's urine (hematuria, change in odor or color), the clinician should encourage hydration, perform a medication reconciliation, and observe the patient closely for 24 to 48 hours in order to evaluate for other causes of symptoms. Should symptoms persist or new localized genitourinary symptoms develop, a urinary dipstick can then be performed. If remarkable findings are evident on the urinary dipstick and further testing with a urinalysis and urine culture reveals bacteriuria plus pyuria, then treatment with antimicrobials for symptomatic UTI should be strongly considered. For patients who experience falls, the clinician should only send urine studies after considering alternative diagnoses and wait to initiate empiric antibiotics following the results.

When obtaining a urine sample, a clean catch voided collection is ideal to curtail contagion; if possible, a midstream specimen is preferred. Women should use an antiseptic cloth to first clean the inner folds of the labia, wiping from front to back. A second wipe should then be used to clean the opening of the urethra. Although uncommon, symptomatic sexually active women who present with dysuria without pyuria or bacteriuria should be evaluated for a sexually transmitted infection (STI). Should concerning subjective findings suggest a possible STI, a diagnostic evaluation for chlamydia, gonorrhea, trichomoniasis, HSV, and HIV is indicated.

Diagnostic Approach in Long-Term Facility Care Patients

The diagnosis of UTI in LTC patients is especially problematic due to the lack of a standard definition of symptomatic UTI. Guidelines have attempted to demystify the need to prescribe antimicrobials for UTIs in this population. The McGeer criteria of 1996 and the Loeb criteria published in 2001 sought to account for the variations present in the community and LTC population in forming a clinical diagnosis of UTI.

The McGeer criteria identified conditions for infection surveillance purposes, and the Loeb criteria were developed to help clinicians identify patients who would benefit from empiric antimicrobial therapy. Both guidelines, however, still require the presence of localized genitourinary symptoms in adults without an indwelling catheter (Box 14.13).

Although many professional societies and health care agencies have recognized these criteria, clinicians have generally not applied these into clinical practice. A significant weakness of both guidelines is that they are largely based on expert opinion, and many of the recommendations from these guidelines are formulated based on the conclusions from studies in younger adults. In one prospective study of nursing home residents in Connecticut, the sensitivity of both the McGeer criteria and Loeb criteria

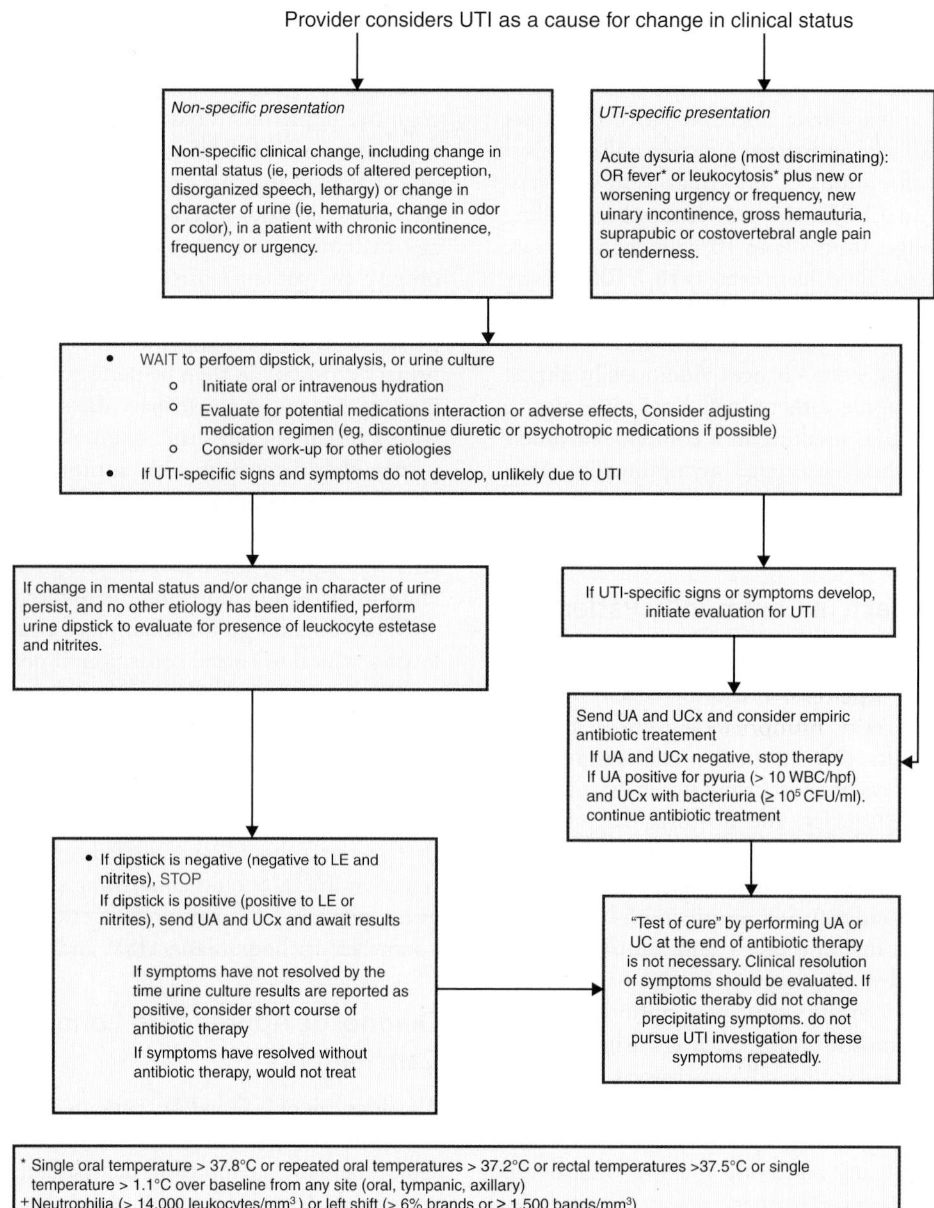

• **Fig. 14.30** Urinary tract infection evaluation and treatment protocol. (From Rowe, T., & Juthani-Mehta, M. [2019]. Urinary tract infections. In J. B. Halter, J. G. Ouslander, S. Studenski, K. P. High, S. Asthana, M. A. Supiano, & C. Ritchie [Eds.]. *Hazzard's geriatric medicine and gerontology* [7th ed.]. McGraw-Hill. http://accessmedicine.mhmedical.com/content.aspx?bookid=1923§ionid=144563864.)

were low at 30% and 19%, respectively. To help improve diagnostic accuracy, the same investigators attempted to identify clinical features that were predictive of bacteriuria plus pyuria (which indicates urinary tract inflammation and is necessary for diagnosis of a clinical infection) in nursing home residents. It was found that dysuria alone predicted 39% of cases of confirmed bacteriuria plus pyuria; however, when used in combination with other symptoms such as change in mental status or change in the constitution of the urine, the predicted probability increased to 63%. This predicted probability is higher than both the McGeer and Loeb criteria, which both had positive predictive values of 57%.

In 2012, an expert consensus panel for the Society for Healthcare Epidemiology (SHEA) proposed revised guidelines designed specifically for LTCFs (Table 14.8). The new guidelines broadened the diagnostic requirements of UTI and included a new prerequisite for etiologic confirmation with urine culture.

Although these guidelines were designed for all patients in the long-term setting (inclusive of those with cognitive impairment), localizing genitourinary signs and symptoms is still nonetheless necessary to satisfy criteria standards. Following this, the application of these criteria to patients with advanced dementia remains exigent. As in observed in the community, older adults residing in LTC environments

• BOX 14.13 McGeer and Loeb Consensus Criteria for Diagnosis of Urinary Tract Infection in Long-Term Care Residents Without an Indwelling Catheter

McGeer Criteria	Loeb Criteria
1. Fever ≥ 38°C or chills 2. New or increased burning pain on urination, frequency, or urgency 3. New flank or suprapubic pain or tenderness 4. Change in character of the urine (e.g., new bloody urine, foul smell, or amount of sediment) 5. Worsening of mental or functional status (may be new or increased)Three of the above must be present	1. Acute dysuria aloneor 2. Fever ≥ 37.9°C or 1.5° increase above baseline temperature *plus* ≥ 1 of the following new or worsening symptoms: a. Urgency b. Frequency c. Suprapubic pain d. Gross hematuria e. Costovertebral angle tenderness f. Urinary incontinence

From Rowe, T., & Juthani-Mehta, M. (2019). Urinary tract infections. In J. B. Halter, J. G. Ouslander, S. Studenski, K. P. High, S. Asthana, M. A. Supiano, & C. Ritchie (Eds.). *Hazzard's geriatric medicine and gerontology* (7th ed.). McGraw-Hill. http://accessmedicine.mhmedical.com/content.aspx?bookid=1923§ionid=144563864

with vague, nonspecific symptoms (such as disorientation, delirium, disorganized speech, lethargy, or change urine characteristics) should first be observed for 24 to 48 hours for the advancement of symptoms. Further steps include the optimization of hydration, consideration of different diagnoses, and withholding of medications (such as antipsychotics or diuretics) to see if symptoms convalesce.

Should symptoms continue and an alternative cause is not explanatory, urinary dipstick testing for the presence of leukocyte esterase and nitrite should be performed. Dipstick testing is readily accessible in LCTFs and is easily performed with findings rapidly available. The sensitivity and specificity for a positive urine dipstick in the older adult are 82% and 71%, respectively, for diagnosis of bacteriuria with pyuria. Negative leukocyte esterase and nitrate testing has demonstrated a negative predictive value of 88% to 100% in long-term care settings.

Patients with nonspecific symptoms in conjunction with a negative leukocyte esterase and nitrites on dipstick testing should no longer have UTI considered as a diagnosis (i.e., empiric antibiotics directed at UTI are unlikely to be beneficial in these cases). If leukocyte esterase or nitrites are positive, additional testing with urinalysis and urine culture may then be indicated.

Obtaining a clean catch urine is preferred when analyzing urine specimens. Those with severe dementia or urinary incontinence and a high likelihood of a UTI should have an in-and-out catheterization performed if a specimen is otherwise unable to be collected via standard voiding. For residents without an indwelling catheter and who can provide a voided urine specimen, at least 10^5 cfu/mL of no more than two species of

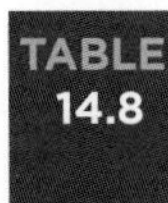

TABLE 14.8 2012 Society for Healthcare Epidemiology of America/Centers for Disease Control and Prevention Surveillance Definitions for Urinary Tract Infection in Long-Term are Residents Without an Indwelling Catheter

≥ One of the following signs or symptoms: Acute dysuria or acute pain, swelling, or tenderness of the testes, epididymis, or prostate,Or, Fever[a] or leukocytosis[b] and ≥ 1 of the following: a. Acute costovertebral angle pain or tenderness b. Suprapubic pain c. Gross hematuria d. New or marked increase in incontinence e. New or marked increase in urgency f. New or marked increase in frequency *Or,* ≥ Two of the following: a. Suprapubic pain b. Gross hematuria c. New or marked increase in incontinence d. New or marked increase in urgency e. New or marked increase in frequency	Plus	At least 105 cfu/mL of ≤ 2 species of microorganisms in a voided urine sample or at least 10^2 cfu/mL of any number of organisms in a specimen collected by an in-and-out catheter.

[a]Single oral temperature > 37.8°C *or* repeated oral temperatures > 37.2°C or rectal temperatures > 37.5°C or single temperature > 1.1°C over baseline from any site (oral, tympanic, axillary).
[b]Neutrophilia > 14,000 le3ukocytes/mm^3 or left shift (> 6% bands or ≥ 1,500 bands/mm^3).

microorganisms will be required for the diagnosis of symptomatic UTI. For specimens collected by in-and-out catheterization, fewer microorganisms are required, of at least 10^2 cfu/mL. Lower numerical counts should be presumed as being contaminated with colonizing periurethral agents.

Diagnostic Approach in Geriatric Patients With Indwelling Catheters

The Infectious Disease Society of America (IDSA) revised its guidelines in 2009 about the diagnosis, treatment, and prevention of CAUTI in adults for the purposes of limiting unwarranted antibiotics in this cohort. Inclusive patients are those with indwelling urethral catheters, those with indwelling suprapubic catheters, or those needing intermittent catheterization. The IDSA identifies CAUTI as patients with a catheter who develop manifestations consistent with UTI as defined in Box 14.14.

The 2012 SHEA guidelines for diagnosis of CAUTI are similar, although they require the presence of a urinary catheter culture with at least 10^5 cfu/mL of any organism(s). As for residents without a catheter, routing screening for CA-ASB should not be undertaken, with the exception of those patients being evaluated for invasive urologic instrumentation or procedures. The presence or absence of urine odor or cloudiness should not be used as a sole determinant in differentiating CA-ASB from CAUTI.

Diagnostic Approach for Asymptomatic Bacteriuria (ASB)

Providers should not screen older adults for ASB, and those with ASB should not be treated with antibiotics. Several prospective randomized studies found no differences in morbidity or mortality in geriatric patients treated with antibiotics compared to those who did not receive treatment in ASB. Beyond this, persistent asymptomatic colonization of the urinary tract has not been linked to an increased risk of the development of renal failure or hypertension. As a result, the US Preventive Services Task Force (USPSTF), Society for Healthcare Epidemiology of America (SHEA), Infectious Diseases Society of America (IDSA), and American Geriatrics Society's Choosing Wisely initiative all recommend against screening and treating for ASB in geriatric patients (Table 14.9). ASB testing is, however, a viable consideration in patients scheduled for invasive urologic procedures.

Treatment of UTI in older adults within the community setting follows the young adult protocols. Because geriatric patients are at an increased risk of multidrug-resistant organisms (MDROs), a urine culture should be performed in order to refine antibiotic treatment. Fluoroquinolones (FQs) are the most prescribed antibiotic class for the treatment of UTI in the community. They are favored by clinicians owing to a comparably lower adverse reaction profile, increased oral bioavailability, and uncomplicated dosing schedule.

A randomized control trial of ciprofloxacin or trimethoprim/sulfamethoxazole (TMP/SMX) in ambulatory and nursing home patients demonstrated that a 10-day course of ciprofloxacin was superior a 10-day regimen of TMP/SMX. The ciprofloxacin group also reported fewer side effects.

However, pervasive use of FQs, particularly in the treatment of UTI, has resulted in higher frequencies of FQ resistance in the older adult. This is especially observed LTCFs. In most clinical settings, resistance is often in excess of 30%; FQs are therefore not endorsed as the initial empiric antibiotic choice for UTI. For older women with acute uncomplicated cystitis, the International Clinical Practice Guidelines issued by the European Society for Microbiology and Infectious Diseases and the IDSA recommend as first-line treatment either nitrofurantoin monohydrate/macrocrystals, 100 mg twice daily for 5 days, or TMP/SMX 160/800 mg for 3 days. Oral fosfomycin (3 g as a single dose) is an acceptable alternative; however, several studies have established inferiority in efficacy versus nitrofurantoin or TMP/SMX for the treatment of uncomplicated UTI. In geriatric patients, TMP/SMX or fosfomycin may be favored

• BOX 14.14 Infectious Diseases Society of America IDSAFindings Suggestive of Catheter-Associated Urinary Tract Infection (CAUTI)

- New onset or worsening of fever, rigors, altered mental status, malaise, or lethargy with *no* other known cause; flank pain; costovertebral angle tenderness; acute hematuria; pelvic discomfort, Or
- Dysuria, urgency, or frequency in patient whose catheters have been removed in the previous 48 hours with no other identified source of infection, along with greater than or equal to 10^3 cfu/mL of one or more bacterial species in a single catheter urine specimen or in a midstream voided urine specimen from a patient whose catheter has been removed in the previous 48 hours.

TABLE 14.9 Management: Community-Dwelling Geriatric Patients

Organization	Recommendation
IDSA	Screening for and treatment of ASB is not recommended for the following persons: (1) diabetic women; (2) older women living in the community; (3) older, institutionalized subjects; (4) persons with spinal cord injury; and (5) catheterized patients while catheter remains in situ.
USPSTF	Against screening for ASB in men and nonpregnant women
American Geriatrics Society Choosing Wisely	Against using antimicrobials to treat bacteriuria in older adults unless specific urinary tract symptoms are present

because of a reduced treatment course (1- or 3-day therapy) when matched against nitrofurantoin (5 days).

Because UTI is generally considered complicated when occurring in men, most experts endorse a 7- to 14-day course. However, a study of male veterans concluded that a shorter-course treatments for UTI (< 7 days) is as effective compared to an extended treatment period (>7 days). When UTI is linked with acute bacterial prostatitis, a minimum 14-day course of antibiotics is generally warranted in patients with mild symptoms who respond expeditiously to therapy. In severe cases, treatment recommendations of least 28 to 42 days are appropriate. Second-line antibiotics for empiric antibiotic treatment include amoxicillin/clavulanate 500/125 mg orally twice daily for 3 to 7 days, or cefpodoxime 200 mg orally twice daily for 3 to 7 days, or cefixime 400 mg orally for 3 to 7 days.

In all cases of pyelonephritis/complicated UTI, urine culture and sensitivity testing should be obtained to guide antibiotic selection. Although age older than 60 years has been recognized as a relative indication for admission to a hospital, geriatric patients with acute pyelonephritis may be considered for outpatient treatment if the following conditions are present: mild to moderate disease, sufficient social support, and clinical stability. In this cohort, management is likely to be as safe and effective as hospitalization. Admission with hospitalization should be implemented in patients with severe pyelonephritis characterized by persistent vomiting, progression of uncomplicated UTI, suspected sepsis or critical illness, an unclear diagnosis or evidence of urinary tract obstruction. Other indications for inpatient management include persistently high fever (e.g., >101 °F/>38.4°C) or pain, marked debility, inability to maintain oral hydration or take oral medications, or concerns regarding adherence to therapy.

The FQ class is the sole oral antibiotic treatment recommended as empiric treatment of acute uncomplicated pyelonephritis (Rowe & Juthani-Mehta, 2019). Empiric therapies with acceptable FQs are ciprofloxacin 500 mg twice daily, ciprofloxacin 1000 mg extended release once daily, or levofloxacin 750 mg once daily, with either agents given for 5 to 7 days (Hooton & Gupta, 2019).

Due to a rise in resistance observed in many clinical locations, authorities do not recommend the use of FQs as first-line empiric treatment in areas with resistance rates noted to be higher than 10%. Additionally, nitrofurantoin and fosfomycin are not appropriate choices owing to inadequate renal penetration (Rowe & Juthani-Mehta, 2019). For patients who have contraindications to fluoroquinolones, where resistance rates exceed 10%, or in situations where there are other preclusions regarding fluoroquinolone use and there is mild infection, treatment should begin with a single dose of a long-acting parenteral agent followed by a nonfluoroquinolone oral agent. Examples of a single-dose agent include ceftriaxone (1 gram IV or IM once), ertapenem (1 gram IV or IM once) as an alternative for patients with an allergy, or aminoglycosides (gentamicin or tobramycin 5 mg per kg IV or IM once); aminoglycosides should be reserved for patients who cannot use the other two agents. Following the dose of the parenteral agent, options include any antimicrobial identified in Box 14.15 (Hooton & Gupta, 2019).

• BOX 14.15 Treatment of Uncomplicated UTIs

- Levofloxacin: 250mg orally once daily for 3 days
- Cephalexin: 500mg orally twice to four times daily for 3-7 days
- Amoxicillin/Clavulanate: 500mg orally twice daily for 3-7 days
- Ciprofloxacin: 250mg orally (immediate-release) twice daily for 3 days; 500mg orally (extended-release) once daily for 3 days

Patients with severe presentations or clinically deteriorating conditions following a course of oral antibiotics should also receive parenteral therapy. Acceptable agents achieving broad empiric coverage include piperacillin/tazobactam, a fourth-generation cephalosporin (cefepime or ceftazidime), or a carbapenem (meropenem, ertapenem, or doripenem). The aminoglycosides (gentamicin or tobramycin) are sometimes used synergistically with β-lactams and to expand coverage; however, they are more toxic when compared to other antimicrobials in the geriatric populations. This is especially of concern in patients with renal insufficiency. However, evidence has supported the unlikely probability of ototoxicity and nephrotoxicity if duration of treatment does not exceed 48 to 72 hours. If identified, urinary obstructive causes should be managed. Those with an anatomic or functional urinary tract abnormality (such as a neurogenic bladder, an indwelling bladder catheter, nephrostomy tubes, or ureteral stents) may require more frequent catheterization to improve urinary flow, exchange of a catheter, or urologic or gynecologic consultation; these interventions are in addition to antimicrobial administration.

Management: Long-Term Facility Care Patients

Currently, no specific guidelines exist for treatment of UTI of geriatric adults in LTCFs. As a result, most providers employ the guidelines applied in younger outpatient adults. Although this approach is generally acceptable, there are several situations in which medical professionals should digress from these protocols. Because the rates of antibiotic resistance are generally greater in LTCFs, clinicians should prescribe empiric antibiotic regimens based on these resistance trends. Urine culture and sensitivity reports should be utilized to guide appropriate management. Additionally, changes in antibiotic pharmacokinetics in the older adult LTC population occur; these include an increased volume of distribution and decreased renal clearance. Therefore, providers should assess the glomerular filtration rate (GFR) when dosing antibiotics. Third, polypharmacy and drug-drug interactions should always be examined. Relative to UTIs, there are several significant interactions with anticoagulants; international normalized ratio (INR) monitoring is recommended in patients who are already taking warfarin. In most cases, warfarin strengths will need to be diminished by at least 50% through the entire duration of infective treatment. Nitrofurantoin is listed on the American Geriatric Society's Beers criteria for potentially inappropriate medication use in older adults. Pulmonary toxicity and a lack of effectiveness in patients with CrCl less than 60 mL/min are possible concerns when applied in older adult LTC patients. Nonetheless, nitrofurantoin remains a suitable empiric antibiotic choice for UTI caused by *E. coli*, as it has regularly demonstrated lower rates of resistance. Beyond this, studies have indicated that nitrofurantoin may be carefully prescribed when creatinine clearance is at least 40 mL/min and is as effective as other agents in treating uncomplicated UTI.

Infections caused by highly resistant organisms (such as vancomycin-resistant *enterococci* [VRE] and extended-spectrum β-lactamase [ESBL] producing organisms) are most effectively treated with fosfomycin; there is no reported resistance at this time. Following fosfomycin, nitrofurantoin can be considered as well, owing to a relatively low resistance rate of 15%. ESBL-producing organisms are generally resistant to TMP/SMX, FQs, and amoxicillin/clavulanic acid.

Although the recommended duration of antibiotic treatment in this age group is not definitely established, some experts advise lengthier intervals while classifying these patients as having complicated UTI. Based on expert judgment, SHEA recommended a 7-day course of antibiotics for women with cystitis. However, a systematic review found no differences in short-term outcomes in treatments of brief durations (3 to 6 days) and expanded durations (7 to 14 days). As a result, shorter courses of antibiotics for UTI are likely to be sufficient in a majority of clinical scenarios. Should a favorable reaction to antiinfective agents not be observed in a timely manner, protracted treatments are warranted.

Prevention

The objectives of nonpharmacologic UTI preventive therapies are to minimize excessive antibiotic prescriptions and associated morbidity and mortality of the infection. Cranberry juice has been widely touted as a preventive and treatment agent. Higher strengths of the active component in cranberry, noted as cranberry proanthocyanidin (PAC), may be beneficial, although further studies are needed. A study examining 36 to 108 mg of PAC found a tendency of reduced bacteriuria and pyuria in LTC residents. Furthermore, a systematic review and meta-analysis of only randomized controlled trials (RCTs) found that cranberry products reduced UTI recurrence in women with at least three UTIs in a 1-year period. In conclusion, additional investigation of cranberry supplementation in geriatric patients is needed to fully endorse it as a prevention strategy.

In older females, the reduction of estrogen is hypothesized to cause fewer lactobacilli in the vaginal tract and therefore an increase in colonization of the perineal area with pathologic bacteria such as *E. coli*. A randomized controlled trial (RCT) was undertaken to compare the effectiveness of supplemented lactobacilli (*Lactobacillus rhamnosus GR-1* and *Lactobacillus reuteri RC-14*) to daily antibiotic prophylaxis with TMP/SMX in preventing recurrent UTI. Although lactobacilli was not found to be noninferior to antibiotics, lower rates of antibiotic resistance in the group assigned to lactobacilli were observed. Additionally, topical estrogen appears to be a safe and potentially effective method for preventing UTI in postmenopausal women. RCTs identified that vaginal estrogen cream containing 0.5 mg of estriol or vaginal rings with 2 mg estradiol significantly reduced the risk of UTI in postmenopausal women; however, their pooled effect was not significant.

The current rate of inappropriate catheter use is between 20% and 50%. The most effectual strategy for the prevention of CAUTI includes the avoidance of catheterization. If a catheter is necessary, it should be removed as soon as possible. The Healthcare Infection Control Practices Advisory Committee as part of the Centers for Disease Control (CDC) issued guidelines in 2009 to prevent CAUTI and to diagnose and manage persons with CAUTI. For geriatric patients who require catheters, recommendations include inserting catheters aseptically by trained personnel, using the smallest diameter catheter feasible, hand washing prior to and after handling the catheter, maintaining a closed catheter system, avoiding irrigation unless obstruction of the catheter exists, keeping the collecting bag below the level of the bladder, and encouraging sufficient hydration of patients. The use of antimicrobial-coated catheters has demonstrated a delayed bacterial colonization with a reduction of the incidence of bacteriuria. Disappointingly, an RCT assessing two antibiotic-coated catheters did not find meaningful benefit in the prevention of CAUTI. Furthermore, these catheters are more expensive and therefore unlikely to benefit most patients. A computerized clinical decision support intervention for reducing the duration of catheter use has been shown to be useful in curtailing the duration of catheter presence and associated CAUTIs in hospitalized patients, although this approach may be more difficult to execute in LTCF settings.

Key Points

- Multiple factors contribute to the development of infections in the geriatric population. These center on epidemiologic factors, immunosenescence, malnutrition, and age-related transformations in physiology and anatomy.
- In the older adult, pneumonia often manifests with asymptomatic or atypical symptoms and signs, including the exacerbation of any chronic medical condition, generalized weakness or fatigue, dizziness, dehydration,

incontinence, loss of appetite, falls, acute functional decline, and acute confusion. Patients do not have a fever and are less likely to present with chills, pleuritic chest pain, or tachycardia; an elevated respiratory rate and altered level of consciousness may be the only initial signs.

- The diagnosis of pneumonia in the older adult patient cannot be reliably made based solely on the history and physical exam; the clinical presentation should be confirmed rapidly with diagnostic testing, including chest imaging and laboratory analysis.
- The Pneumonia Severity Index (PSI) and CURB-65 are clinical assessment tools useful for calculating the need for hospital admission and the probability of death due to pneumonia based on specific patient characteristics, physical exam findings, and laboratory findings at presentation.
- *C. difficile* colitis should be suspected in any patient with diarrhea who has received antibiotics within the previous 3 months, has been recently hospitalized, or has an occurrence of diarrhea 48 hours or more after hospitalization. Antimicrobial use is the most important, renowned, and modifiable risk factor of infection; most cases involve use of fluoroquinolones, clindamycin, cephalosporins, and penicillins.
- The Severe Acute Respiratory Syndrome coronavirus 2 (SARS-CoV-2) is the causative agent of the COVID-19 pandemic. The most important risk factor contributing to death related to the virus is increased age.
- In the older adult, manifestations of COVID-19 include fever, cough, shortness of breath, anosmia, dysgeusia, headache, dizziness, dyspnea, fatigue, chest tightness, myalgias, and diarrhea. Atypical presentations such as a decline in function, an acute impairment of mobility or a new fall, confusion or altered mental status, or an exacerbation of heart failure or COPD may also occur.
- Common diagnostic test results consistent with COVID-19 are neutropenia, leukopenia, lymphopenia, elevations of inflammatory markers, ferritin, lactate dehydrogenase, procalcitonin, interleukin (IL)-6, D-dimer, and fibrin/fibrinogen degradation products. With disease progression, the most common radiographic abnormalities on CT scan are bilateral ground glass opacities and multilobular infiltrates with consolidations. The preferred, initial diagnostic test of COVID-19 consists of nucleic acid amplification testing (NAAT).
- In the United States, viruses are the leading cause of acute gastroenteritis. Most cases of epidemic viral gastroenteritis in adults are caused by the caliciviruses (norovirus). The most common causes of sporadic viral gastroenteritis are caliciviruses, non–group A rotavirus, astrovirus, and adenovirus.
- Acute viral gastroenteritis is marked by diarrhea of a rapid onset that lasts less than 1 week, accompanied by nausea, vomiting, fever, or abdominal pain and a characteristic physical examination of mild, diffuse, abdominal tenderness. Stool cultures, fecal leukocytes, occult blood, or lactoferrin results are negative.
- An inflammatory, nonviral gastroenteritis is suggested by the presence of fecal leukocytes, occult blood, lactoferrin, or positive stool cultures.
- The presentation of endocarditis is nonspecific and highly variable; the most common symptom observed is fever; associated findings include chills, anorexia and weight loss, malaise, headache, myalgias, arthralgias, nocturnal diaphoresis, abdominal pain, dyspnea, cough, pleurisy, cardiac murmurs, splenomegaly, petechiae, and splinter hemorrhages. More suggestive but less common findings of endocarditis are Janeway lesions, Osler nodes, and Roth spots.
- The diagnosis of endocarditis is made using the modified Duke criteria.
- Cellulitis can occur as a result of a multitude of immunogenic, vascular, and dermatologic risk factors. They manifest as areas of skin erythema, edema, and warmth; petechiae, hemorrhage, bullae, fever, and other systemic manifestations of infection may also be present.
- Necrotizing soft tissue infections (NSTIs) include necrotizing forms of fasciitis, myositis, and cellulitis. These infections result in fulminant tissue destruction, systemic signs of toxicity, and high mortality; the illness primarily involves fascia. Necrotizing fasciitis of the perineum is known as Fournier gangrene.
- Early and aggressive surgical exploration and debridement of necrotic tissue, together with broad-spectrum empiric antibiotic therapy and hemodynamic support, are the mainstays of the therapy for NSTIs.
- The hallmark clinical characteristic of classic scabies is pruritus. The dermatologic findings are distributed to the sides and webs of the fingers, flexor wrists, extensor elbows, anterior and posterior axillary folds, areolae, periumbilical skin, waist, extensor knees, lower buttocks and adjacent thighs, genitalia, lateral, and posterior aspects of the feet.
- All cases of herpes zoster are caused by the reactivation of endogenous VZV; advancing age is the most important risk factor in the development of the illness.
- The main presenting features of herpes zoster is a rash and symptoms of acute neuritis. Initially the rash commences most typically as erythematous papules, usually in a single, unilateral dermatome or several contiguous dermatomes. The vesicular rash corresponds to the sensory area of the affected ganglion.
- The management of herpes zoster focuses on antiviral and analgesic therapy. Antiviral agents are recommended for patients with uncomplicated herpes zoster who present within 72 hours of clinical symptoms. Analgesia is utilized for patients with moderate to severe acute neuritis.
- Urinary tract infection (UTI) is the most frequent bacterial infection in the older adult, with *E. coli* being the most common bacterial cause of UTI.
- Residents of long-term care settings do not commonly present with the classical characteristics of a genitourinary tract infection (such as dysuria, frequency, or flank pain); the most common symptom for suspected UTI in

LTCFs was a change in mental status. Other symptoms of a suspected UTI in this demographic include a change in the character of the urine, fever, declining functional status, and hematuria. Catheter-associated UTI commonly presents as fever or altered mental status.

- Providers should not screen older adults for asymptomatic bacteriuria (ASB), and those with ASB should not be treated with antibiotics. For community patients, the evaluation of symptomatic UTI in patients with new localized genitourinary symptoms should be initiated with a urinary dipstick to evaluate for the presence of nitrite or leukocyte esterase. If either nitrite or leukocyte esterase is positive, a urine culture and consideration of empiric oral antibiotics should follow.

More information about tools and Interprofessional Education Collaborative (IPEC) competencies mentioned in this chapter can be found in Appendix 1: Tools and Appendix 2: IPEC Competencies.

References

Aberra, F. N. (2018, October 10). *Clostridium difficile colitis*. https://emedicine.medscape.com/article/186458-overview.

Albrecht, M. A. (2018, December 10). *Treatment of herpes zoster in the immunocompetent host*. https://www.uptodate.com/contents/treatment-of-herpes-zoster-in-the-immunocompetent-host?search=herpes%20zoster&source=search_result&selectedTitle=1~150&usage_type=default&display_rank=1.

Albrecht, M. A., & Levin, M. J. (2019a, January 21). *Epidemiology, clinical manifestations, and diagnosis of herpes zoster*. https://www.uptodate.com/contents/epidemiology-clinical-manifestations-and-diagnosis-of-herpes-zoster?search=herpes%20zoster&source=search_result&selectedTitle=2~150&usage_type=default&display_rank=2.

Albrecht, M. A., & Levin, M. J. (2019b, February 6). *Vaccination for the prevention of shingles (herpes zoster)*. https://www.uptodate.com/contents/vaccination-for-the-prevention-of-shingles-herpes-zoster?search=zostavax%20vaccine&source=search_result&selectedTitle=1~150&usage_type=default&display_rank=1.

Alexandraki, I., & Smetana, G. W. (2019). *Acute viral gastroenteritis in adults*. https://www.uptodate.com/contents/acute-viral-gastroenteritis-in-adults?search=acute%20gastroenteritis&source=search_result&selectedTitle=1~150&usage_type=default&display_rank=1.

Baddour, L. M., Wilson, W. R., Bayer, A. S., et al. (2015). Infective endocarditis in adults: diagnosis, antimicrobial therapy, and management of complications: A scientific statement for healthcare professionals from the American Heart Association. *Circulation, 132*(15), 1435–1486.

Baer, S. L. (2018, October 5). *Community-acquired pneumonia (CAP)*. https://emedicine.medscape.com/article/234240-overview#a19

Bagdasarian, N., Rao, K., & Malani, P. N. (2015). Diagnosis and treatment of Clostridium difficile in adults: A systematic review. *Journal of the American Medical Association, 313*(4), 398.

Bhangu, A., Nepogodiev, D., Gupta, A., Torrance, A., Singh, P., & West Midlands Research Collaborative. (2012). Systematic review and meta-analysis of outcomes following emergency surgery for Clostridium difficile colitis. *British Journal of Surgery, 99*(11), 1501. Epub 2012 Sep 13.

Bhimraj, A., Morgan, R. L., Shumaker, A. H., Lavergne, V., Baden, L., Cheng, V. C., Edwards, K. M., Gandhi, R., Gallagher, J., Muller, W. J., O'Horo, J. C., Shoham, S., Murad, M. H., Mustafa, R. A., Sultan, S., & Falck-Ytter, Y. (2021). *Infectious Diseases Society of America guidelines on the treatment and management of patients with COVID-19. Infectious Diseases Society of America 2021; Version 4.4.1.* https://www.idsociety.org/practice-guideline/covid-19-guideline-treatment-and-management/

Bishara, J., Farah, R., Mograbi, J., Khalaila, W., Abu-Elheja, O., Mahamid, M., & Nseir, W. (2013). Obesity as a risk factor for Clostridium difficile infection. *Clinical Infectious Diseases, 57*(4), 489.

Bonten, M. J., Huijts, S. M., Bolkenbaas, M., Webber, C., Patterson, S., Gault, S., et al. (2015). Polysaccharide conjugate vaccine against pneumococcal pneumonia in adults. *New England Journal of Medicine, 372*(12), 1114–1125.

Bradley, S. F. (1999). Issues in the management of resistant bacteria in long-term-care facilities. *Infection Control & Hospital Epidemiology, 20*, 362.

Brusch, J. L. (2019, January 3). *Infective endocarditis*. https://emedicine.medscape.com/article/216650

Bush, L. M., Schmidt, C. E., & Perez, M. T. (2018, April). *Infection by Escherichia coli O157:H7 and other enterohemorrhagic E. coli (EHEC)*. From Merck Manual Professional Version. https://www.merckmanuals.com/professional/infectious-diseases/gram-negative-bacilli/infection-by-escherichia-coli-o157-h7-and-other-enterohemorrhagic-e-coli-ehec

Castilla, J., Godoy, P., Domínguez, A., Martínez-Baz, I., Astray, J., Martín, V., Delgado-Rodríguez, M., Baricot, M., Soldevila, N., Mayoral, J. M., Quintana, J. M., Galán, J. C., Castro, A., González-Candelas, F., Garín, O., Saez, M., Tamames, S., Pumarola, T., & CIBERESP Cases and Controls in Influenza Working Group Spain. (2013). Influenza vaccine effectiveness in preventing outpatient, inpatient, and severe cases of laboratory-confirmed influenza. *Clinical Infectious Diseases, 57*(2), 167.

Centers for Disease Control and Prevention. (2010). *Interim guidance on the use of influenza antiviral agents during the 2010–2011 influenza season*. http://www.cdc.ov/flu/professionals/antivirals/guidance/summary.htm

Centers for Disease Control and Prevention. (2021a, February 16). *Interim clinical guidance for management of patients with confirmed coronavirus disease (COVID-19)*. https://www.cdc.gov/coronavirus/2019-ncov/hcp/clinical-guidance-management-patients.html.

Centers for Disease Control and Prevention. (2021b, March 21). *Interim guidelines for Covid-19 antibody testing*. https://www.cdc.gov/coronavirus/2019-ncov/lab/resources/antibody-tests-guidelines.html.

Centers for Disease Control and Prevention. (2021c, August 2). *Covid 19 testing overview*. https://www.cdc.gov/coronavirus/2019-ncov/symptoms-testing/testing.html.

Centers for Disease Control and Prevention. (2021d, August 2). *Test for current infection*. https://www.cdc.gov/coronavirus/2019-ncov/testing/diagnostic-testing.html.

Chiejina, M., Samant, H. (2018, January). Diarrhea, viral. *NCBI StatPearls* [Internet]. https://www.ncbi.nlm.nih.gov/books/NBK470525/.

Chu, V.H., & Sexton, D.J. (2018, April 27). *Clinical manifestations and evaluation of adults with suspected native valve endocarditis.* https://www.uptodate.com/contents/clinical-manifestations-and-evaluation-of-adults-with-suspected-native-valve-endocarditis?search=endocarditis&source=search_result&selectedTitle=2~150&usage_type=default&display_rank=2.

Cohen, S. H., Gerding, D. N., Johnson, S., et al. (2010). Clinical practice guidelines for Clostridium difficile infection in adults: 2010 update by the society for healthcare epidemiology of America (SHEA) and the infectious diseases society of America (IDSA). *Infection Control & Hospital Epidemiology, 31*(5), 431–455.

Cohen, Y. Z., & Dolin, R. (2015). Influenza. In D. L. Kasper, A. S. Fauci, & S. L. Hauser (Eds.), *Harrison's principles of internal medicine* (19th ed., pp. 1209). McGraw Hill.

Cornely, O. A., Crook, D. W., Esposito, R., et al. (2012). Fidaxomicin versus vancomycin for infection with Clostridium difficile in Europe, Canada, and the USA: A double-blind, non-inferiority, randomised controlled trial. *Lancet Infectious Diseases, 12*(4), 281–289.

Cox, N. J., & Subbarao, K. (1999). Influenza. *Lancet, 354*(9186), 1277.

del Castillo, J., & Martín Sánchez, F. (2019). Pneumonia. In J. B. Halter, J. G. Ouslander, S. Studenski, K. P. High, S. Asthana, M. A. Supiano, & C. Ritchie (Eds.), *Hazzard's geriatric medicine and gerontology* (7th ed.). McGraw-Hill. http://www.accessmedicine.mhmedical.com/content.aspx?bookid=1923§ionid=144563755.

DiazGranados, C. A., Dunning, A. J., Kimmel, M., Kirby, D., Treanor, J., Collins, A., Pollak, R., Christoff, J., Earl, J., Landolfi, V., Martin, E., Gurunathan, S., Nathan, R., Greenberg, D. P., Tornieporth, N. G., Decker, M. D., & Talbot, H. K. (2014). Efficacy of high-dose versus standard-dose influenza vaccine in older adults. *New England Journal of Medicine, 371*(7), 635–645.

Durante-Mangoni, E., Bradley, S., Selton-Suty, C., et al. (2008). Current features of infective endocarditis in elderly patients: results of the International Collaboration on Endocarditis Prospective Cohort Study. *Archives of Internal Medicine, 168*(19), 2095–2103.

Ehrlich, H. J., Singer, J., Berezuk, G., Fritsch, S., Aichinger, G., Hart, M. K., El-Amin, W., Portsmouth, D., Kistner, O., & Barrett, P. N. (2012). A cell culture-derived influenza vaccine provides consistent protection against infection and reduces the duration and severity of disease in infected individuals. *Clinical Infectious Diseases, 54*(7), 946–954. Epub 2012 Jan 19.

Falsey, A. R., Treanor, J. J., Tornieporth, N., Capellan, J., & Gorse, G. J. (2009). Randomized, double-blind controlled phase 3 trial comparing the immunogenicity of high-dose and standard-dose influenza vaccine in adults 65 years of age and older. *Journal of Infectious Diseases, 200*(2), 72.

FDA approves Merck's ZINPLAVA (bezlotoxumab) to reduce recurrence of Clostridium difficile infection (CDI) in adult patients receiving antibacterial drug treatment for CDI who are at high risk of CDI recurrence [press release]. (2016, October 21). *MerckNewsroom.com.* http://www.mercknewsroom.com/news-release/corporate-news/fda-approves-mercks-zinplava-bezlotoxumab-reduce-recurrence-clostridium-

Feher, C., Munez Rubio, E., Merino Amador, P., et al. (2017). The efficacy of fidaxomicin in the treatment of Clostridium difficile infection in a real-world clinical setting: A Spanish multi-centre retrospective cohort. *European Journal of Clinical Microbiology & Infectious Diseases, 36*(2), 295–303.

Ferrada, P., Velopulos, C. G., Sultan, S., Haut, E. R., Johnson, E., Praba-Egge, A., Enniss, T., Dorion, H., Martin, N. D., Bosarge, P., Rushing, A., & Duane, T. M. (2014). Timing and type of surgical treatment of Clostridium difficile-associated disease: A practice management guideline from the Eastern Association for the Surgery of Trauma. *Journal of Trauma and Acute Care Surgery, 76*(6), 1484.

Forestier, E., Fraisse, T., Claire Roubaud-Baudron, C., Selton-Suty, C., & Pagani, L. (2016). Managing infective endocarditis in the elderly: New issues for an old disease. *Clinical Interventions in Aging, 11*, 1199–1206.

Gavazzi, G., & Krause, K. H. (2002). Ageing and infection. *Lancet Infectious Diseases, 2*(11), 659–666.

Gerding, D. N., Johnson, S., Peterson, L. R., Mulligan, M. E., & Silva, J., Jr. (1995). Clostridium difficile-associated diarrhea and colitis. *Infection Control & Hospital Epidemiology, 16*(8), 459.

Gomez, C. R., Boehmer, E. D., & Kovacs, E. J. (2005). The aging innate immune system. *Current Opinion in Immunology, 17*, 457.

Grant, T. H., Rosen, M. P., Fidler, J. L., for the Expert Panel on Gastrointestinal Imaging. (2008). *ACR appropriateness criteria: Acute abdominal pain and fever or suspected abdominal abscess.* [online publication]. American College of Radiology (ACR).

Gravenstein, S., Davidson, H. E., Taljaard, M., Ogarek, J., Gozalo, P., Han, L., & Mor, V. (2017). Comparative effectiveness of high-dose versus standard-dose influenza vaccination on numbers of US nursing home residents admitted to hospital: A cluster-randomised trial. *Lancet Respiratory Medicine, 5*(9), 738. Epub 2017 Jul 20.

Greenwald, D. A. (2017). Common large intestinal disorders. In J. B. Halter, J. G. Ouslander, S. Studenski, K. P. High, S. Asthana, M. A. Supiano, & C. Ritchie (Eds.), *Hazzard's geriatric medicine and gerontology* (7th ed.). McGraw-Hill. http://www.accessmedicine.mhmedical.com/content.aspx?bookid=1923§ionid=144526642.

Guh, A. Y., Adkins, S. H., Li, Q., Bulens, S. N., Farley, M. M., Smith, Z., Holzbauer, S. M., Whitten, T., Phipps, E. C., Hancock, E. B., Dumyati, G., Concannon, C., Kainer, M. A., Rue, B., Lyons, C., Olson, D. M., Wilson, L., Perlmutter, R., Winston, L. G., Parker, E., Bamberg, W., Beldavs, Z. G., Ocampo, V., Karlsson, M., Gerding, D. N., & McDonald, L. C. (2017). Risk factors for community-associated Clostridium difficile infection in adults: A case-control study. *Open Forum Infectious Diseases, 4*(4), ofx171.

Habib, G., Lancellotti, P., Antunes, M. J., et al. (2015). 2015 ESC guidelines for the management of infective endocarditis: The Task Force for the Management of Infective Endocarditis of the European Society of Cardiology (ESC). Endorsed by: European Association for Cardio-Thoracic Surgery (EACTS), the European Association of Nuclear Medicine (EANM). *European Heart Journal, 36*(44), 3075–3128.

Hall, J. F., & Berger, D. (2008). Outcome of colectomy for Clostridium difficile colitis: A plea for early surgical management. *American Journal Surgery, 196*(3), 384.

Hall, W. J., Douglas, R. G. Jr, Hyde, R. W., Roth, F. K., Cross, A. S., & Speers, D. M. (1976). Pulmonary mechanics after uncomplicated influenza A infection. *American Review of Respiratory Disease, 113*(2), 141.

Hayden, F. G., Treanor, J. J., Fritz, R. S., et al. (1999). Use of the oral neuraminidase inhibitor oseltamivir in experimental human influenza: randomized controlled trials for prevention and treatment. *Journal of the American Medical Association, 282*(13), 1240–1246.

Hayward, A. C., Harling, R., Wetten, S., et al. (2006). Effectiveness of an influenza vaccine programme for care home staff to prevent death, morbidity, and health service use among residents: cluster randomised controlled trial. *BMJ, 333*, 1241.

High, K. P. (2017). Infection: General principles. In J. B. Halter, J. G. Ouslander, S. Studenski, K. P. High, S. Asthana, M. A. Supiano, & C. Ritchie (Eds.), *Hazzard's geriatric medicine and gerontology* (7th ed.). McGraw-Hill. http://www.accessmedicine.mhmedical.com/content.aspx?bookid=1923§ionid=144563653.

Hooton, T.M., & Gupta, K. (2019). *Acute complicated urinary tract infection (including pyelonephritis) in adults*. https://www.uptodate.com/contents/acute-complicated-urinary-tract-infection-including-pyelonephritis-in-adults?search=urinary%20tract%20infection%20adult&source=search_result&selectedTitle=1~150&usage_type=default&display_rank=1 https://emedicine.medscape.com/article/234240-overview#a4 CAP.

Interprofessional Education Collaborative. (2016). *Core competencies for interprofessional collaborative practice: 2016 update*. Interprofessional Education Collaborative.

Izurieta, H. S., Thadani, N., Shay, D. K., Lu, Y., Maurer, A., Foppa, I. M., Franks, R., Pratt, D., Forshee, R. A., MaCurdy, T., Worrall, C., Howery, A. E., & Kelman, J. (2015). Comparative effectiveness of high-dose versus standard-dose influenza vaccines in US residents aged 65 years and older from 2012 to 2013 using Medicare data: A retrospective cohort analysis. *Lancet Infectious Diseases, 15*(3), 293.

Jones, R., & Rubin, G. (2009). Acute diarrhoea in adults. *BMJ, 338*, b1877.

Juthani-Mehta, M., & Quagliarello, V. J. (2010). Infectious diseases in the nursing home setting: Challenges and opportunities for clinical investigation. *Clinical Infectious Diseases, 51*, 931–936.

Kamthan, A. G., Bruckner, H. W., Hirschman, S. Z., & Agus, S. G. (1992). Clostridium difficile diarrhea induced by cancer chemotherapy. *Archives of Internal Medicine, 152*(8), 1715.

Kelly, C. P., Pothoulakis, C., & LaMont, J. T. (1994). Clostridium difficile colitis. *New England Journal of Medicine, 330*(4), 257.

Khan, Z. Z. (2018, September 27). *Norovirus*. https://emedicine.medscape.com/article/224225-overview.

Khanna, S., Pardi, D. S., Aronson, S. L., et al. (2012). The epidemiology of community-acquired Clostridium difficile infection: A population-based study. *American Journal of Gastroenterology, 107*(1), 89–95.

Kim, D. K., Bridges, C. B., Harriman, K. H., Advisory Committee on Immunization Practices (ACIP), & ACIP Adult Immunization Work Group. (2016). Advisory Committee on Immunization Practices Recommended Immunization Schedule for Adults Aged 19 Years or Older--United States, 2016. *MMWR Morb Mortal Wkly Rep, 65*(4), 88–90.

Kim, K. H., Fekety, R., Batts, D. H., Brown, D., Cudmore, M., Silva, J., Jr, & Waters, D. (1981). Isolation of Clostridium difficile from the environment and contacts of patients with antibiotic-associated colitis. *Journal of Infectious Diseases, 143*(1), 42.

Kling, J. (2013, October 16). Fecal transplant an option even in the immunocompromised. *Medscape Medical News*. http://www.medscape.com/viewarticle/812685.

Klochko, A. (2018, September 13). *Salmonella infection*. https://emedicine.medscape.com/article/228174-overview.

Kociolek, L. K. (2018, February 16). *Updated C difficile infection clinical guidance from IDSA/SHEA*. https://www.infectiousdiseaseadvisor.com/home/topics/gi-illness/clostridium-difficile/updated-c-difficile-infection-clinical-guidance-from-idsa-shea/.

Kupronis, B. A., Richards, C. L., Whitney, C. G., & Active Bacterial Core Surveillance Team. (2003). Invasive pneumococcal disease in older adults residing in long-term care facilities and in the community. *Journal of the American Geriatric Society, 51*, 1520.

Laidman, J. (2013, January 16). Fecal transfer proves potent clostridium difficile treatment. [serial online]. *Medscape Medical News*. http://www.medscape.com/viewarticle/777772.

LaRocque, R., & Harris, J. B. (2019a). *Causes of acute infectious diarrhea and other foodborne illnesses in resource-rich settings*. https://www.uptodate.com/contents/causes-of-acute-infectious-diarrhea-and-other-foodborne-illnesses-in-resource-rich-settings?search=bacterial%20gastroenteritis%20adult&topicRef=2717&source=see_link.

LaRocque, R., & Harris, J. B. (2019b). *Travelers' diarrhea: Clinical manifestations, diagnosis, and treatment*. https://www.uptodate.com/contents/travelers-diarrhea-clinical-manifestations-diagnosis-and-treatment?sectionName=Antibiotics&search=gastroenteritis%20adult&topicRef=2717&anchor=H1037167584&source=see_link#H1037167584.

Li, J. S., Sexton, D. J., Mick, N., et al. (2000). Proposed modifications to the Duke criteria for the diagnosis of infective endocarditis. *Clinical Infectious Diseases, 30*(4), 633–638.

Lin, B. (2018, January 8). *Viral gastroenteritis*. https://emedicine.medscape.com/article/176515-overview.

Little, M. (2018). Treating and preventing clostridium difficile infection in long-term care facilities. *Annals of Long-Term Care, 26*(7), P25–P27.

Loo, V. G., Bourgault, A. M., Poirier, L., Lamothe, F., Michaud, S., Turgeon, N., Toye, B., Beaudoin, A., Frost, E. H., Gilca, R., Brassard, P., Dendukuri, N., Béliveau, C., Oughton, M., Brukner, I., & Dascal, A. (2011). Host and pathogen factors for Clostridium difficile infection and colonization. *New England Journal of Medicine, 365*(18), 1693–1703.

Loo, V. G., Poirier, L., Miller, M. A., Oughton, M., Libman, M. D., Michaud, S., Bourgault, A. M., Nguyen, T., Frenette, C., Kelly, M., Vibien, A., Brassard, P., Fenn, S., Dewar, K., Hudson, T. J., Horn, R., René, P., Monczak, Y., & Dascal, A. (2005). A predominantly clonal multi-institutional outbreak of Clostridium difficile-associated diarrhea with high morbidity and mortality. *New England Journal of Medicine, 353*(23), 2442.

Mandell, L. A., & Wunderink, R. (2019). Pneumonia. In J. Jameson, A. S. Fauci, D. L. Kasper, S. L. Hauser, D. L. Longo, & J. Loscalzo (Eds.), *Harrison's principles of internal medicine* (20th ed). McGraw-Hill. http://accessmedicine.mhmedical.com/content.aspx?bookid=2129§ionid=184041853.

Mandell, L. A., Wunderink, R. G., Anzueto, A., Bartlett, J. G., Campbell, G. D., Dean, N. C., et al. (2007). Infectious Diseases Society of America/American Thoracic Society consensus guidelines on the management of community-acquired pneumonia in adults. *Clinical Infectious Diseases, 44*(Suppl. 2), S27–S72.

Martinez-Melendez, A., Camacho-Ortiz, A., Morfin-Otero, R., Maldonado-Garza, H. J., Villarreal-Trevino, L., & Garza-Gonzalez, E. (2017). Current knowledge on the laboratory diagnosis of Clostridium difficile infection. *World Journal of Gastroenterology, 23*(9), 1552–1567.

McDonald, L. C., Coignard, B., Dubberke, E., Song, X., Horan, T., & Kutty, P. K. (2007). Recommendations for surveillance of Clostridium difficile-associated disease. *Infection Control & Hospital Epidemiology, 28*(2), 140–145.

McDonald, L. C., Gerding, D. N., Johnson, S., Bakken, J. S., Carroll, K. C., Coffin, S. E., Dubberke, E. R., Garey, K. W., Gould, C. V., Kelly, C., Loo, V., Shaklee Sammons, J., Sandora, T. J., & Wilcox, M. H. (2018). Clinical practice guidelines for clostridium difficile infection in adults and children: 2017 update by the Infectious Diseases Society of America (IDSA) and Society for Healthcare

Epidemiology of America (SHEA). *Clinical Infectious Diseases, 66*(7), e1.

McDonald, L. C., Killgore, G. E., Thompson, A., Owens, R. C., Jr., Kazakova, S. V., Sambol, S. P., Johnson, S., & Gerding, D. N. (2005). An epidemic, toxin gene-variant strain of Clostridium difficile. *New England Journal of Medicine, 353*(23), 2433.

McIntosh, K. (2021, August 4). *COVID-19: Epidemiology, virology and prevention.* https://www.uptodate.com/contents/covid-19-epidemiology-virology-and-prevention?sectionName=Personal%20preventive%20measures&search=coronavirus&topicRef=128349&anchor=H1466934285&source=see_link#H1466934285.

Mody, L., Riddell, J., IV, Kaye, K. S., & Chopra, T. (2014). Common infections—Skin and soft tissue infections. In B. A. Williams, A. Chang, C. Ahalt, H. Chen, R. Conant, C. Landefeld, C. Ritchie, & M. Yukawa (Eds.), *Current diagnosis & treatment: Geriatrics* (2nd ed.). McGraw-Hill. http://accessmedicine.mhmedical.com/content.aspx?bookid=953§ionid=53375671.

Moses, S. (2018, December 2). *Delirium.* https://fpnotebook.com/Neuro/Cognitive/Dlrm.htm.

Moses, S. (2019a, March 3). *Clostridium difficile.* https://fpnotebook.com/GI/ID/ClstrdmDfcl.htm.

Moses, S. (2019b, April 6). *Cellulitis.* https://fpnotebook.com/Derm/Bacteria/Cllts.htm.

Moses, S. (2019c, April 6). *Group A streptococcal cellulitis.* https://fpnotebook.com/Derm/Bacteria/GrpAStrptcclCllts.htm.

Moses, S. (2022). *Corona virus 19.* https://fpnotebook.com/Lung/ID/CrnVrs9.htm.

Musher, D. M., & Musher, B. L. (2004). Contagious acute gastrointestinal infections. *New England Journal of Medicine, 351*(23), 2417.

Nace, D. A., Lin, C. J., Ross, T. M., Saracco, S., Churilla, R. M., & Zimmerman, R. K. (2015). Randomized, controlled trial of high-dose influenza vaccine among frail residents of long-term care facilities. *Journal of Infectious Diseases, 211*(12), 1915. Epub 2014 Dec 17.

Neumann-Podczaska, A., Al-Saad, S. R., Karbowski, L. M., et al. (2020). COVID 19—Clinical picture in the elderly population: A qualitative systematic review. *Aging and Disease, 11*(4), 988–1008. https://www.ncbi.nlm.nih.gov/pmc/articles/PMC7390523/.

Nguyen, H. H. (2019, February 15). *Influenza treatment and management.* https://emedicine.medscape.com/article/219557-overview

Nikolich-Zugich, J., Knox, K. S., Rios, C. T., et al. (2020 Aprr). SARS-CoV-2 and COVID-19 in older adults: what we may expect regarding pathogenesis, immune responses, and outcomes. *GeroScience, 42*(2), 505–514. https://www.ncbi.nlm.nih.gov/pmc/articles/PMC7145538/.

Nishimura, R. A., Otto, C. M., Bonow, R. O., Carabello, B. A., Erwin, J. P., 3rd, Fleisher, L. A., Jneid, H., Mack, M. J., McLeod, C. J., O'Gara, P. T., Rigolin, V. H., Sundt, T. M., 3rd, & Thompson, A. (2017). 2017 AHA/ACC Focused Update of the 2014 AHA/ACC Guideline for the Management of Patients With Valvular Heart Disease: A Report of the American College of Cardiology/American Heart Association Task Force on Clinical Practice Guidelines. *Circulation, 135*(25), e1159–e1195. https://doi.org/10.1161/CIR.0000000000000503.

O'Fallon, E., Schreiber, R., Kandel, R., & D'Agata, E. M. (2009). Multidrug-resistant gram-negative bacteria at a long-term care facility: Assessment of residents, healthcare workers, and inanimate surfaces. *Infection Control & Hospital Epidemiology, 30,* 1172.

Ortel, T.L. & Gaasch, W.H. (2019, March). *Antithrombotic therapy in patients with infective endocarditis.* https://www.uptodate.com/contents/antithrombotic-therapy-in-patients-with-infective-endocarditis?search=endocarditis&topicRef=118215&source=see_link.

Pant, C., Sferra, T. J., Deshpande, A., & Minocha, A. (2011). Clinical approach to severe Clostridium difficile infection: Update for the hospital practitioner. *European Journal of Internal Medicine, 22*(6), 561–568.

Pépin, J., Saheb, N., Coulombe, M. A., Alary, M. E., Corriveau, M. P., Authier, S., Leblanc, M., Rivard, G., Bettez, M., Primeau, V., Nguyen, M., Jacob, C. E., & Lanthier, L. (2005a). Emergence of fluoroquinolones as the predominant risk factor for Clostridium difficile-associated diarrhea: a cohort study during an epidemic in Quebec. *Clinical Infectious Diseases, 41*(9), 1254.

Pépin, J., Valiquette, L., & Cossette, B. (2005b). Mortality attributable to nosocomial Clostridium difficile-associated disease during an epidemic caused by a hypervirulent strain in Quebec. *Canadian Medical Association Journal, 173*(9), 1037.

Phrommintikul, A., Kuanprasert, S., Wongcharoen, W., Kanjanavanit, R., Chaiwarith, R., & Sukonthasarn, A. (2011). Influenza vaccination reduces cardiovascular events in patients with acute coronary syndrome. *European Heart Journal, 32*(14), 1730–1735.

Powner, J., Gallaher, T., Colombo, R., Baer, S., Huber, L., Kheda, M., et al. (2014). Influenza vaccination reduced pneumococcal disease in incident dialysis patients. *American Society of Nephrology*

Reigadas, E., Alcalá, L., Gómez, J., Marín, M., Martin, A., Onori, R., Muñoz, P., & Bouza, E. (2018). Breakthrough Clostridium difficile infection in cirrhotic patients receiving rifaximin. *Clinical Infectious Diseases, 66*(7), 1086.

Riddle, M. S., DuPont, H. L., & Connor, B. A. (2016). ACG clinical guideline: Diagnosis, treatment, and prevention of acute diarrheal infections in adults. *American Journal of Gastroenterology, 111*(5), 602.

Rodemann, J. F., Dubberke, E. R., Reske, K. A., Seo, D. H., & Stone, C. D. (2007). Incidence of Clostridium difficile infection in inflammatory bowel disease. *Clinical Gastroenterology and Hepatology, 5*(3), 339.

Rowe, T., & Juthani-Mehta, M. (2019). Urinary tract infections. In J. B. Halter, J. G. Ouslander, S. Studenski, K. P. High, S. Asthana, M. A. Supiano, & C. Ritchie (Eds.), *Hazzard's geriatric medicine and gerontology* (7th ed.). McGraw-Hill. http://www.accessmedicine.mhmedical.com/content.aspx?bookid=1923§ionid=144563864.

Sailhamer, E. A., Carson, K., Chang, Y., Zacharias, N., Spaniolas, K., Tabbara, M., Alam, H. B., DeMoya, M. A., & Velmahos, G. C. (2009). Fulminant Clostridium difficile colitis: patterns of care and predictors of mortality. *Archives of Surgery, 144*(5), 433.

Schmader, K. E. (2017). Herpes zoster. In J. B. Halter, J. G. Ouslander, S. Studenski, K. P. High, S. Asthana, M. A. Supiano, & C. Ritchie (Eds.), *Hazzard's geriatric medicine and gerontology* (7th ed.). McGraw-Hill. http://www.accessmedicine.mhmedical.com/content.aspx?bookid=1923§ionid=144564025.

Schulz, S. A. (2018, October 17). *Necrotizing fasciitis.* https://emedicine.medscape.com/article/2051157-overview.

Schwartz, R. A. (2019, April 19). *Necrotizing fasciitis empiric therapy.* https://emedicine.medscape.com/article/2012058-overview.

Severe Acute Respiratory Syndrome—Coronavirus 2019 (SARS-CoV-2). (2021). In M. A. Papadakis, S. J. McPhee, & J. Bernstein (Eds.), *Quick medical diagnosis & treatment.* McGraw-Hill. https://accessmedicine.mhmedical.com/content.aspx?bookid=2986§ionid=251104764.

Sexton, D. J., & Chu, V. H. (2018a, October 26). *Epidemiology, risk factors, and microbiology of infective endocarditis.* https://www.

uptodate.com/contents/epidemiology-risk-factors-and-microbiology-of-infective-endocarditis?search=geriatric%20endocarditis&source=search_result&selectedTitle=2~150&usage_type=default&display_rank=2.

Sexton, D. J., & Chu, V. H. (2018b, December 14). *Antimicrobial prophylaxis for the prevention of bacterial endocarditis.* https://www.uptodate.com/contents/antimicrobial-prophylaxis-for-the-prevention-of-bacterial-endocarditis?sectionName=Time-trend%20studies&search=geriatric%20endocarditis&topicRef=2151&anchor=H3266634949&source=see_link#H11.

Shane, A. L., Mody, R. K., Crump, J. A., et al. (2017). 2017 Infectious Diseases Society of America clinical practice guidelines for the diagnosis and management of infectious diarrhea. *Clinical Infectious Diseases, 65*(12), e45–e80.

Shay, D. K., Chillarige, Y., Kelman, J., Forshee, R. A., Foppa, I. M., Wernecke, M., Lu, Y., Ferdinands, J. M., Iyengar, A., Fry, A. M., Worrall, C., & Izurieta, H. S. (2017). Comparative effectiveness of high-dose versus standard-dose influenza vaccines among US Medicare beneficiaries in preventing postinfluenza deaths during 2012-2013 and 2013-2014. *The Journal of infectious diseases, 215*(4), 510–517. https://doi.org/10.1093/infdis/jiw641.

Spelman, D., & Baddour, L. M. (2019, March 28). *Cellulitis and skin abscess: Clinical manifestations and diagnosis.* https://www.uptodate.com/contents/cellulitis-and-skin-abscess-clinical-manifestations-and-diagnosis?search=cellulitis%20geriatric&source=search_result&selectedTitle=1~150&usage_type=default&display_rank=1.

Stevens, D. L., & Baddour, L. M. (2018, December 6). *Necrotizing soft tissue infections.* https://www.uptodate.com/contents/necrotizing-soft-tissue-infections?search=necrotizing%20fasciitis&source=search_result&selectedTitle=1~134&usage_type=default&display_rank=1

Surana, N. K., & Kasper, D. L. (2018). Approach to the patient with an infectious disease. In J. Jameson, A. S. Fauci, D. L. Kasper, S. L. Hauser, D. L. Longo, & J. Loscalzo (Eds.), *Harrison's principles of internal medicine* (20th ed.). McGraw-Hill. http://accessmedicine.mhmedical.com/content.aspx?bookid=2129§ionid=192019106.

Talbot, H. K., Zhu, Y., Chen, Q., Williams, J. V., Thompson, M. G., & Griffin, M. R. (2013). Effectiveness of influenza vaccine for preventing laboratory-confirmed influenza hospitalizations in adults, 2011–2012 influenza season. *Clinical Infectious Diseases, 56*(12), 1774–1777.

Teramoto, S., Yamamoto, H., Yamaguchi, Y., Hanaoka, Y., Ishii, M., Hibi, S., et al. (2008). Lower respiratory tract infection outcomes are predicted better by an age >80 years than by CURB-65. *European Respiratory Journal, 31*(2), 477–478.

Thielman, N. M., & Guerrant, R. L. (2004). Clinical practice: Acute infectious diarrhea. *New England Journal of Medicine, 350*(1), 38.

Udell, J. A., Zawi, R., Bhatt, D. L., Keshtkar-Jahromi, M., Gaughran, F., Phrommintikul, A., et al. (2013). Association between influenza vaccination.n and cardiovascular outcomes in high-risk patients: a meta-analysis. *Journal of the American Medical Association, 310*(16), 1711–1720.

Urman, C. O., & Loo, D. S. (2014). Common skin disorders. In B. A. Williams, A. Chang, C. Ahalt, H. Chen, R. Conant, C. Landefeld, C. Ritchie, & M. Yukawa (Eds.), *Current diagnosis & treatment: Geriatrics* (2nd ed.). McGraw-Hill. http://accessmedicine.mhmedical.com/content.aspx?bookid=953§ionid=53375673.

van der Wilden, G. M., Velmahos, G. C., Chang, Y., Bajwa, E., O'Donnell, W. J., Finn, K., Harris, N. S., Yeh, D. D., King, D. R., de Moya, M. A., & Fagenholz, P. J. (2017). Effects of a new hospital-wide surgical consultation protocol in patients with Clostridium difficile colitis. *Surgical Infection (Larchmt), 18*(5), 563. Epub 2017 May 30.

van Nood, E., Vrieze, A., Nieuwdorp, M., et al. (2013). Duodenal infusion of donor feces for recurrent Clostridium difficile. *New England Journal of Medicine, 368*(5), 407–415.

Videlock, E. J., & Cremonini, F. (2012). Meta-analysis: probiotics in antibiotic-associated diarrhoea. *Alimentary Pharmacology & Therapeutics, 35*(12), 1355–1369.

Wang, L., Lansing, B., Symons, K., Flannery, E. L., Fisch, J., Cherian, K., et al. (2012). Infection rate and colonization with antibiotic-resistant organisms in skilled nursing facility residents with indwelling devices. *European Journal of Clinical Microbiology & Infectious Diseases, 31*, 1797–1804.

Wilson, W., Taubert, K. A., Gewitz, M., et al. (2007). Prevention of infective endocarditis: Guidelines from the American Heart Association: A guideline from the American Heart Association Rheumatic Fever, Endocarditis, and Kawasaki Disease Committee, Council on Cardiovascular Disease in the Young, and the Council on Clinical Cardiology, Council on Cardiovascular Surgery and Anesthesia, and the Quality of Care and Outcomes Research Interdisciplinary Working Group. *Circulation, 116*(15), 1736. Epub 2007 Apr 19.

Yan, D., Chen, Y., Lv, T., Huang, Y., Yang, J., Li, Y., Huang, J., & Li, L. (2017). Clostridium difficile colonization and infection in patients with hepatic cirrhosis. *Journal of Medical Microbiology, 66*(10), 1483. Epub 2017 Sep 25.

Yurkofsky, M., & Ouslander, J.G. (2021, June 29). *COVID-19: Management in nursing homes.* https://www.uptodate.com/contents/covid-19-management-in-nursing-homes?search=coronavirus&topicRef=127759&source=see_link#H4272478442.

15

Acute, Emergent, and Urgent Conditions

JILL BEAVERS-KIRBY, DNP, MS, ACNP-BC, ANP-BC

OBJECTIVES

Student Learning Objectives

After completing this chapter, the student should be able to do the following:

1. List the common acute and chronic conditions impacting the older adult
2. Describe the approach to diagnosis of acute and urgent conditions in the older adult.
3. Identify the unique aspects of the presentation and management of acute and urgent conditions in the older adult

Practitioner Objectives

After completing this chapter, the practitioner should be able to do the following:

1. Provide an appropriate clinical evaluation for an older adult presenting with hypertension, ischemic heart disease and heart failure.
2. Develop and execute a management plan for the treatment of an older adult who presents with one of the acute or urgent conditions (Alzheimer's Disease, dementia, cardiac issues, etc.)
3. Work collaboratively with other team members to maximize outcomes for an older adult who presents with acute or urgent geriatric conditions.

Overview

This chapter details the most common chronic diseases that members of the geriatric population are diagnosed with. Each diagnosis will include its definition, the pathophysiology, how to diagnose the condition, the evidence-based treatment, and acute conditions that can arise.

Introduction

Because older people seem to suffer from a myriad of chronic diseases, it is wrongly assumed that diabetes, arthritis, and the like are only part of getting old and that nothing can be done about it. The truth is that most of these diseases and conditions are treatable and should be treated by a health care provider.

Eighty percent of seniors have at least one health issue, and 68% have two or more. According to the National Council on Aging (NCOA, 2017), the top nine conditions of adults ages 65 and older that can present as acute or urgent issues are as follows:

- Hypertension: 58%
- High cholesterol: 47%
- Arthritis: 31%
- Ischemic heart disease: 29%
- Diabetes: 27%
- Heart failure: 14%
- Depression: 14%
- Alzheimer disease and dementia: 11%
- Chronic obstructive pulmonary disease (COPD): 11%

Hypertension

CASE STUDY 15.1

C.H. is a 74-year-old African American male whose body mass index (BMI) is 28.6. He has a history of hypertension and type 2 diabetes mellitus. His blood sugars are well controlled with diet and exercise. He presents to the physician assistant (PA) for his annual physical exam. C.H. has been monitoring his blood sugar at home, but he only checks his blood pressure when he sees the machine at the drug store. He tells the PA that his average blood pressure is 158/94. What should the PA do about his blood pressure?

High blood pressure continues to be one of the most common medical diagnoses in the geriatric population as well as one of the reasons for the most prescribed class of drugs. Lifestyle changes can prevent or delay the onset of hypertension. Nevertheless, hypertension is much more widespread in both established and establishing nations, and it remains improperly recognized and poorly controlled in the United States as well as abroad (Zipes et al., 2019).

High blood pressure is the leading risk factor for cardiovascular fatalities, causing around 7.6 million sudden deaths each year worldwide. More than 1 billion people including greater than 50 million Americans have hypertension, making it the most common chronic disease. Blood pressure (BP) typically increases with age as well; in the United States, approximately 50% of individuals 60 to 69 years old as well as 75% of individuals 70 years and older have high blood pressure. In nonindustrialized areas, however, BP does not rise with aging, and only a small fraction of the people will develop high blood pressure (Alpern et al., 2013).

A direct favorable relationship between BP and cardiovascular disease (CVD) danger has actually been observed in males and females of all ages, races, ethnic teams, and countries, no matter other risk factors for CVD exist. Observational studies suggest that fatality from CVD enhances considerably as BP increases above 115 mm Hg systolic as well as 75 mm Hg diastolic stress. For each 20 mm Hg systolic or 10 mm Hg diastolic increase in BP, there is a doubling of death from heart disease and stroke in all age groups that include those from 40 to 89 years of age (Alpern et al., 2013).

Appropriate treatment of high blood pressure treatment yields large decreases in the danger for stroke, cardiac arrest, renal failure, aortic dissection, coronary events, and death. Clients with the greatest cardiovascular (CV) risk-benefit the most. With the essential exemption of some types of secondary high blood pressure, many cases of high blood pressure cannot be cured. Although interventions such as kidney denervation or baroreflex activation therapy stay in development, interventions such as lifestyle adjustments and antihypertensive medications lead to improvement of hypertension. This section discusses the use of these devices based on the readily available proof. With hypertension standards in ongoing change because of various results from major new trials, meta-analyses, observational research studies, and specialist opinions, we give a useful clinical method to the management of hypertensive clients.

Disease Process

Primary hypertension defines about 95% of all instances of high blood pressure and is typically specified as elevated BP for which an evident additional reason (e.g., renovascular condition, aldosteronism, pheochromocytoma, or genetic mutations) cannot be identified. Although primary hypertension is a heterogeneous disorder, several of the major variables are recognized. For instance, overweight and obesity may make up as much as 65% to 75% of the possibility for primary hypertension. Other elements, such as less active lifestyle, excess usage of alcohol or salt, and reduced potassium intake, are likewise believed to contribute to enhanced BP in many individuals.

Blood pressure control relies on the combined activities of several cardiovascular, renal, neural, endocrine, and regional cells' control systems. Although hypertension is normally thought of as a condition of the typical level at which BP is regulated, there is rising interest in various other measures of BP, including peak arterial pressure, BP irregularity, circadian blood pressure data, and the responses of BP to stress, which might heighten the risk of cardiovascular disease (Alpern et al., 2013).

The multifaceted regional control, neural, hormonal, and renal systems that manage BP are often reviewed in terms of exactly how they affect cardiac workload or vascular resistance due to the formula used to determine mean arterial pressure (cardiac output × peripheral resistance). This conceptual framework, with the addition of variables that affect vascular capacity and transcapillary liquid exchange, suffices to describe short-term BP regulation, but not persistent high blood pressure. Two extra ideas work when thinking about persistent BP law: (1) BP control devices are time dependent, and (2) the renal excretion of water and electrolytes play a vital function in lasting BP regulation (Alpern et al., 2013).

Blood pressure control is time dependent. This means that if something happens that causes a sudden change in blood pressure (i.e., significant blood loss), then the mechanisms that regulate blood pressure start to work. Three crucial neural control systems begin to operate within a few seconds: (1) the baroreceptors in the arteries identify changes in BP and send out autonomic response signals back to the heart and blood vessels to return the blood pressure to normal; (2) the chemoreceptors discover alterations in the oxygen or CO_2 in the blood and send feedback that affects BP; and (3) the main nerve system responds quickly to ischemic signals within the vasomotor centers in the medulla, particularly when BP falls below about 50 mm Hg. Each of these nervous control devices works rapidly and have powerful effects on BP. It is important to note that the gains in blood pressure stabilization reduce with time, as long as interruptions of blood pressure homeostasis are sustained.

Within a few minutes or hours after a BP disturbance, other control systems spur to action, including (1) there is a shift of fluid from the interstitial spaces into the blood in response to decreased BP or a shift of fluid out of the blood into the interstitial spaces due to elevated BP, (2) the renin-angiotensin-aldosterone system (RAAS) is triggered when BP falls but is inhibited when BP raises above normal, and (3) numerous vasodilator systems are suppressed when BP decreases and then are enacted when BP rises above normal.

There is also a renal–body fluid feedback mechanism that helps control blood pressure. Extracellular fluid volume is identified by the balance between consumption and excretion of salt and water by the kidneys. Even a momentary imbalance between consumption and outcome can cause a change in extracellular volume, as well as a potential change in BP.

There must be an accurate balance between consumption and the excretion of salt and water; otherwise there would be a continued buildup or loss of liquid that could lead to circulatory collapse within a couple of days. A vital component of this system for controlling salt as well as water equilibrium "is pressure natriuresis—the effects of raised BP to increase sodium excretion" (Alpern et al., 2013). This mechanism is used to maintain BP in several situations. Under several problematic conditions, this device maintains BP (such as when BP is raised above the kidney set point due to increased complete peripheral resistance or an enhanced heart).

Lifestyle Changes

Lifestyle choices as well as medical treatment can provide a foundation for the prevention and treatment of hypertension. The existing evidence pertaining to dietary patterns and certain dietary components has sufficient strength to merit suggestions on both a population and a public health level, as well as for the management of patients. Evidence regarding physical activity recommendations has straggled behind the evidence of dietary strategies to impact the treatment of hypertension. Limitations in the proof regarding lifestyle require consideration. First, few research studies have looked at the effects of standard of living interventions on cardiovascular results; most depend on the patient's blood pressure as a surrogate endpoint. Second, the result of lifestyle modification on BP as well as cardiovascular results might vary depending on sex, age, and ethnicity (Zipes et al., 2019).

Lifestyle changes that can improve hypertension include smoking cessation, control blood glucose and lipids control, and dietary changes such as the DASH diet. However, a weight reduction in patients >80 years easily induces a loss of muscle mass (sarcopenia) and can even cause cachexia unless an intensive physical training program and adequate protein supplementation are concomitantly applied (Benetos et al., 2019; thepafp.org).

Decreasing sodium intake to no more than 2400 mg/day is also recommended to aid in blood pressure reduction, but it is important for the advanced practice provider to determine if an excessive salt reduction might induce hyponatremia, malnutrition, and orthostatic hypotension along with an increased risk of falls (Benetos et al., 2019; thepafp.org).

Moderate alcohol consumption and increasing physical activity, which means moderate-to-vigorous activity 3 to 4 days a week averaging 40 minutes per session, are additional lifestyle recommendations. But the physical activity suited to the functional capabilities of older adults and to their preferences is of great significance, even if it does not correspond to the level recommended by current guidelines, which is similar for older and younger adult subjects. Lastly, excessive consumption of alcohol should be avoided, not only because of the pressure effect, but above all because of the increased risk of falling and confusion (Benetos et al., 2019; thepafp.org).

Treatment of Hypertension

In older adult populations, where polypharmacy (including antihypertensive drugs) is a common occurrence, drug-related issues are directly related to the quantity of drugs, so starting monotherapy should be the norm.

The predominance of arterial hypertension, especially systolic hypertension, is steadily increasing globally. This is primarily the clinical manifestation of arterial stiffening as a result of the aging population. Chronically elevated blood pressure is an important risk factor not only for cardiovascular morbidity and mortality but also for cognitive decline and loss of independence in later life.

Clinical evidence obtained in older adults in the population with few comorbidities and sustained independence supports the favorable consequences of blood pressure reduction in older adult hypertensive individuals, even after the age of 80. Observational research in frail older adults treated for hypertension has demonstrated greater morbidity and mortality rates compared to those with lower blood pressure. It is obvious that in very old subjects, the standard approach cannot be implemented because of the tremendous heterogenic differences in these individuals.

Geriatric medicine proposes to consider the functional ability of older people. For the obtained functional profile, the treatments proposed for younger old adults should be used. For the loss of function/sustained activities of daily living, a more comprehensive approach should be used based on the strategies proposed for younger older adults. For the loss of function/sustained activities of daily living, a more in-depth geriatric assessment is needed to define the benefit-risk ratio and the needs for adaptation of the different therapeutic strategies. Finally, therapeutic strategies for loss of function and altered activities of daily living should be thoroughly reevaluated (Benetos et al., 2019).

The European guidelines 2013, based on the Hypertension in the Very Elderly Trial (HYVET) criteria, propose the introduction of a blood pressure-lowering strategy in individuals ≥80 with a systolic blood pressure (SBP) >160 mm Hg and the alignment of the SBP to <150 mm Hg. The newer North American guidelines recommend that therapeutic goals based on age and infirmity level should not be changed. However, it is very challenging to identify compatible BP targets in the various national and international guidelines (Benetos et al., 2019).

The Canadian 2017 guidelines recommend a target SBP of <120 mm Hg for all persons over 75 years of age. The 2017 guidelines of the American College of Cardiology/American Heart Association state that a blood pressure <130/80 mm Hg should be aimed for after the age of 65. The 2018 guidelines suggest a BP target of <140/90 mm Hg for people over the age of 65. Lastly, the 2017 guidelines of the American College of Physicians/American Association of Family Physicians suggest a blood pressure target of <150/90 mm Hg (Benetos et al., 2019).

The United States guidelines for treating hypertension in patients >60 years of age list the negative effects of drug categories but do not explicitly endorse a particular drug category. The British National Institute for Health Care Excellence (NICE) guidelines do not mention BB as a frontline treatment for older adults. The European guidelines usually recommend a calcium channel blocker or a thiazide diuretic in the absence of a clear disease-specific condition and recommendations for lifestyle changes if the latter is not sufficient to reach blood pressure management. In addition, others have suggested that angiotensin-converting enzyme (ACE) inhibitors should be the first choice of medicines in patients >80 years of age, as they constitute one of the two classes of medicines used in HYVET. However, the results of some clinical trials oppose the use of ACE inhibitors as a first-line treatment in older adults and suggest replacing them with angiotensin receptor blockers (ARBs) (Benetos et al., 2019). (See Table 15.1.)

It is essential to check routinely for all possible clinical and biologic secondary effects and the impact of these treatments on the functional status and quality of life of older adult patients. Table 15.1 shows the most common adverse effects of these drugs and the safeguards to be observed in older adults. Nevertheless, the clinician should always remember that in this population, medication-induced side effects are more common, more severe, and less specific than in younger individuals. Therefore all antihypertensive medications may be responsible for some frequent clinical symptoms and conditions such as fatigue, confusion/delirium, orthostatic hypotension, and falls.

Antihypertensive combination therapy to control blood pressure should only be considered during the course of treatment if the indication appears relevant after a reasonable risk-benefit assessment. A third medication may be included after a reassessment of the medication in order to prevent drug-induced side effects. Furthermore, great caution is required when more than three antihypertensive agents are combined in persons over 80 years of age (Benetos et al., 2019).

Hypertensive Emergencies

A hypertensive urgency is a significant BP elevation without acute target organ dysfunction. A hypertensive emergency exists when extreme high blood pressure is associated with severe end-organ damage such as hypertensive encephalopathy, severe lung edema, or aortic dissection. A prompt yet cautious decrease in high blood pressure is generally suggested in these settings. Nonetheless, an excessive hypotensive situation is potentially hazardous, possibly bringing about ischemic problems such as stroke, heart attack, or blindness among other issues. Hence in people who are experiencing a hypertensive urgency, however asymptomatic, slower reductions in elevated blood pressure may be attained with oral medications (Elliot & Varon, 2019). In hypertensive emergencies, blood pressure should be decreased usually by 20 to 40 mm Hg (or no greater than 25%) over minutes to an hour, making use of parenteral drug treatment in a critical care unit (ICU) to restrict end-organ damage (Feehally et al., 2019).

Hypertensive urgencies and emergencies can develop in normotensive people or can complicate underlying benign primary or secondary hypertension. In some situations, an unknown health issue can be the cause of a hypertensive urgency or emergency. Or, in patients with glomerulonephritis or renal artery stenosis, serious elevations in blood pressure may be caused by the action of the renin-angiotensin system (RAS). For patients who have been diagnosed with pheochromocytoma, cocaine abuse, or central neurologic injury, extremely high blood pressure is the outcome of too much catecholamine release. In other people, ongoing hypertension is the inciting issue and can lead to hypertensive encephalopathy or severe high blood pressure with left ventricular failure and lung edema. In many cases, it may be challenging to differentiate whether elevated blood pressure is the reason or the outcome of a hypertensive emergency situation. For instance, in a client with intracerebral hemorrhage, an acute elevation of blood pressure may be the primary reason; conversely, a hemorrhage due to other reasons (i.e., coagulation deficiency) might have happened, followed by an episode of hypertension to protect the cerebral blood supply. Therefore a careful exam and diagnostic assessment of hypertension are important to direct correct therapy (Feehally et al., 2019).

Assessment of Hypertensive Emergencies

The main objective of the evaluation is to discern an actual hypertensive emergency from a hypertensive urgency because of the different treatment plans. The second objective is rapid evaluation of the kind as well as the seriousness of continuous target organ damages. In some hypertensive emergency situations, the history or overt symptoms and indications can steer the diagnosis, whereas in other instances the analysis needs to be more thorough.

The assessment needs to consist of a complete history, which includes an analysis of pain (quality, duration, location, etc.), a determination of whether there is any dyspnea, a psychological history to evaluate acute mental condition changes, a look at the possibility of illegal drug use, and a review of the patient's previous history of high blood pressure noting if the hypertension was controlled and if the patient was compliant with medications. The assessment should also include a precise blood pressure measurement; a funduscopic assessment for any papilledema, hemorrhages, or exudates; a neurologic evaluation to examine for any signs of a stroke; a complete cardiac and pulmonary assessment to look for findings consistent with heart failure; a dissecting aorta; and a determination of fluid overload.

If the assessment is unclear and there is a possibility of unidentified organ damage, radiologic imaging may be needed for further examination. An electrocardiogram can show if there is an indication of cardiac dysfunction.

Laboratory Evaluation

The laboratory evaluation should include kidney function tests to assess for a kidney problems, a complete blood count to appraise for platelet issues or anemia, and a peripheral smear to look for schistocytes as well as lactic dehydrogenase levels to assess for microangiopathic hemolytic anemia. The lactic acid level can indicate reduced perfusion. To evaluate for illicit drug use, a urine drug screen that looks for drugs such as PCP and cocaine should be performed. Lastly, a pregnancy test can eliminate preeclampsia as a cause of

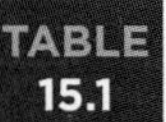

TABLE 15.1 **Antihypertensive Drugs: Adverse Effects and Precautions in Individuals Age 80+ Years**

Drug Class	Most Common Adverse Effects	Special Precautions/Considerations in Older Individuals
CCB dihydropyridine CCB Nondihydropyridine CCB	Signs related to sympathetic activation (flushing, headache, tachycardia) are less frequent than in younger subjects Lower limb edema (frequent since many other factors for LLE). Bradycardia, AV block, worsening heart failure, constipation (verapamil), fatigue, dyspnea	LLE, which is relatively frequent with these drugs, can be erroneously interpreted as a clinical sign of heart failure. In addition, LLE can contribute to the decrease in social and physical activities for practical reasons (difficulties in walking with shoes). Second-line selection; diltiazem can also cause LLE. With verapamil, LLE is unusual, but constipation may be a major problem in very old individuals, as it can lead to fecal impaction, with nausea, anorexia, delirium, and functional decline. Never combine verapamil with β-blockers.
Diuretics Thiazide Loop diuretic	Hyponatremia, hypokalemia, hyperuricemia and gout attacks, hypotension, dehydration Similar to thiazides	For both thiazide and loop diuretics: Diuretic should be titrated according to the patient's volemic status. The latter may be difficult to assess in very old and frail individuals. Creatinine and electrolyte monitoring are warranted after each dose change. Association with SSRI antidepressants increases the risk of severe hyponatremia. Risk of aggravation of urine incontinence. For this reason, diuretics may have an impact on the social life of the patient and can contribute to his/her isolation. Other patients often do not take their treatment if they want to have outdoor activities. Thiazide-like indapamide has been tested in the only RCT specific for subjects >80 y. Small doses (up to 25 mg of HCTZ or equivalent) are safe and well tolerated. Loop diuretics are not indicated for hypertension unless there is severe renal insufficiency (estimated creatinine clearance <30 mL/[min·1.73 m^2]). In the presence of both hypertension and heart failure, loop diuretics can be used for both diseases, either alone or in combination with thiazides.
ACE inhibitors	Dry cough, hyperkalemia, rash, angioedema, dizziness, fatigue, acute renal failure	ACE inhibitors have been tested in the only RCT specific for subjects >80 y. Avoid if you suspect dehydration, do not simultaneously increase diuretics to avoid a worsening in renal function. Regular control of creatinine and potassium levels.
Angiotensin II receptor antagonists	Hyperkalemia, rash, dizziness, fatigue, acute renal failure	The same as for ACE inhibitors: Do not combine ARB with ACE inhibitor or renin inhibitor. Be cautious with aldosterone antagonist because of increased risk of hyperkalemia.
β-adrenoreceptor antagonists (β-blockers)	Bradycardia, cardiac decompensation, peripheral vasoconstriction, bronchospasm, fatigue, depression, dizziness, confusion, hypoglycemia	Fatigue, which is multifactorial in older subjects, can be accentuated. Nightmares, sleep disturbances, depression, and confusion may be present especially for the β-blockers crossing the blood brain barrier. Cardiac conduction problems can also be aggravated. Caution when used in combination with acetylcholinesterase inhibitors (for Alzheimer disease): risk of major bradycardia.

Continued

TABLE 15.1 **Antihypertensive Drugs: Adverse Effects and Precautions in Individuals Age 80+ Years—cont'd**

Drug Class	Most Common Adverse Effects	Special Precautions/Considerations in Older Individuals
Aldosterone antagonists	Hyperkalemia, hyponatremia, and gastrointestinal disturbances, including cramps and diarrhea, gynecomastia	Aldosterone antagonist should not be given in instances of severe renal insufficiency, estimated creatinine clearance <30 mL/(min·1.73 m²) or hyperkalemia. Creatinine and electrolyte monitoring is warranted after each dose change.
α-adrenoreceptor antagonists (α-blockers)	Dizziness, fatigue, nausea, urinary incontinence, orthostatic hypotension, syncope	Usually not indicated. Risk of hypotension (orthostatic, postprandial) and syncope.
Central α-adrenoreceptor agonists	Drowsiness, dry mouth, dizziness, constipation, depression, anxiety, fatigue, urinary retention or incontinence, orthostatic hypotension, confusion, and delirium	High risk of delirium and confusion. Depression, which is atypical and frequent in older subjects (and tricky to diagnose vs cognitive disorders), can be aggravated.

ACE, Angiotensin-converting enzyme; ARB, angiotensin receptor blockers; AV, atrioventricular; CCB, calcium channel blockers; HCTZ, hydrochlorothiazide; LLE, lower limb edema; RCT, randomized controlled trial; and SSRI, selective serotonin reuptake inhibitors.

From Benetos, A., Petrovic, M., & Strandberg, T. (2019). Hypertension management in older and frail older patients. *Circulation Research 124*, 1045–1060. https://doi.org/10.1161/CIRCRESAHA.118.313236

hypertension for an undiscovered pregnancy (Brathwaite & Reif, 2019).

Papilledema and retinal hemorrhages can result from intracerebral hypertension. Papilledema is commonly found in hypertensive encephalopathy, yet either feature can happen apart from the other. Acute coronary disorders can trigger a hypertensive emergency but subsequently can be the outcome of drastically elevated blood pressure. Left ventricular failure from pulmonary edema can cause high blood pressure, and the increase in coronary afterload weakens the performance of the left ventricle (Brathwaite & Reif, 2019).

Treatment of Hypertensive Emergencies

It is ill advised to decrease high blood pressure too rapidly because the patient can suffer from ischemic injury in the vascular tissues that have ended up being habituated with higher blood pressure. For many hypertensive emergency situations, mean arterial pressure ought to be lowered slowly by roughly 10% to 20% in the first hour and 5% to 15% over the following 23 hours (Elliott & Varon, 2020).

However, in some circumstances lowering the blood pressure in a gradual manner is not advised. These situations include when a patient is in the acute phase of a stroke, unless the blood pressure is ≥185/110 mm Hg in patients who are candidates for reperfusion therapy or if the blood pressure is ≥220/120 mm Hg in patients who are not going to have reperfusion therapy.

If the patient is experiencing an aortic dissection, then the blood pressure should be lowered rapidly (less than 20 minutes) to a goal of a systolic pressure 100 to 120 mm Hg. This will aid in decreasing the aortic shearing forces and slow the spread of the dissection.

Patients should be started on parenteral antihypertensive medications in the emergency department and then admitted to the intensive care unit (ICU) for ongoing clinical assessment and constant measurement of the patient's blood pressure. Once the patient is stable, she or he can be transitioned to oral medications. It is important to remember that it is not the specific blood pressure reading that garners an admission to the ICU, it is the patient's clinical situation (Elliott & Varon, 2020).

There are several parenteral medications that can be used in a hypertensive emergency. The choice of drug will depend on the type of hypertensive emergency and the hospital formulary. Nitrates, calcium channel blockers, dopamine-1 agonists, adrenergic-blocking agents, enalaprilat, phentolamine, and hydralazine are the medications used most often.

Vasodilators

Vasodilators like nitroprusside and nitroglycerin supply nitric oxide that generates vasodilatation (of both arterioles as well as blood vessels) via the production of cyclic guanosine monophosphate (GMP). This then turns on the potassium channels in the cells that are calcium sensitive. Sodium nitroprusside, when given via an intravenous drip, starts to work within 60 seconds or less, and when discontinued its results go away within 10 minutes. The patient receiving sodium nitroprusside must be monitored frequently given that this medicine can create an abrupt and extreme decrease in blood pressure.

Nitroglycerin is also administered by intravenous drip and is comparable to nitroprusside except that it causes more venodilation than arteriolar dilation. Nitroglycerin also has less antihypertensive efficiency as compared to other drugs used to manage hypertensive emergencies, and its impacts on high blood pressure vary from patient to patient. Nonetheless, it may be beneficial in people who have symptomatic coronary disease and in those with high blood pressure after coronary bypass. Prolonged intravenous drips are normally avoided to prevent tachyphylaxis (Elliott & Varon, 2020).

Calcium Channel Blockers

Calcium channel blockers such as clevidipine and nicardipine have been approved by the Food and Drug Administration (FDA) for use as intravenous medications to reduce blood pressure when oral medications are not feasible. Clevidipine reduces high blood pressure without impacting the pressures needed for cardiac filling; however, it triggers response tachycardia. Clevidipine is not appropriate for use in individuals with severe aortic stenosis (due to the fact that it increases the threat of serious hypotension), impaired metabolism of lipids (because it is carried out in a lipid-laden solution), or with soy or egg allergies (due to the fact that these are utilized to make the solution). It has actually not been compared with other medications such as nitroprusside or nitroglycerin in the setting of a hypertensive emergencies, yet it was as effective as nitroglycerin, nitroprusside, and nicardipine in hypertensive clients throughout and after heart surgery.

Nicardipine is a calcium channel blocker (similar to nifedipine) that can be provided via an intravenous drip. Nicardipine has a much better safety profile as well as a comparable antihypertensive outcome when compared with nitroprusside. Drawbacks to using nicardipine is that it has a longer onset of action and the half-life is 3 to 6 hours.

Other Agents

There is one dopamine-1 receptor agonist, fenoldopam, which can maintain or improve kidney perfusion while it reduces high blood pressure. Fenoldopam may be advantageous in patients with kidney disease and, when compared to nitroprusside, can improve the patient's urine output, glomerular filtration rate, and elimination of sodium. Fenoldopam should be used with caution in patients with glaucoma. Also, because this medication is premixed in a sodium base, it should be used with caution in patients who have a sensitivity to sulfite.

Labetalol is considered a beta-adrenergic as well as an alpha-adrenergic blocker. Its quick onset of action (less than 5 minutes) makes it a valuable intravenous medicine for treating a hypertensive emergency. Nevertheless, one study discovered that labetalol has less antihypertensive effect as compared to nicardipine. Labetalol is approved to use in clients with active coronary disease given that it does not cause tachycardia. Despite that, labetalol is contraindicated in people with bronchial asthma, chronic obstructive pulmonary disease (COPD), bradycardia, heart failure, and heart block that is greater than first degree. Labetalol can be administered as a bolus or as a continuous intravenous infusion.

Though not a first-line agent, hydralazine is an arterial vasodilator that can be used in hypertensive emergency situations. Individuals with coronary disease or aortic dissection require preventive measures by the administration of a beta-blocker to be given simultaneously to reduce stimulation of the sympathetic reflex. The hypotension reaction to hydralazine is unpredictable when compared with other parenteral medications. Although intravenous hydralazine is commonly administered to patients who are in the hospital when their blood pressure is higher than acceptable limits, there is little proof that this practice enhances outcomes. Parenteral hydralazine is clinically proven to be useful in pregnant patients. Hydralazine is usually administered by means of an intravenous bolus. The decrease in blood pressure can be abrupt, starts within 10 to 30 minutes, and can last as long as 4 hours (Elliott & Varon, 2020).

High Cholesterol

CASE STUDY 15.2

B.R. is a 69-year-old female who presents to the nurse practitioner (NP) for her annual exam. She is taking 40 mg of Celexa daily and acetaminophen as needed for arthritis pain. Her body mass index (BMI) is 23.2, heart rate is 80 beats/min, and blood pressure is 132/75 mm Hg. Her basic metabolic panel and complete blood count are all within normal limits. Her cholesterol panel reveals the following: total cholesterol is 150 mg/dL, low-density lipoprotein (LDL) cholesterol is 178 mg/dL, high-density lipoprotein (HDL) cholesterol is 48 mg/dL, and triglycerides are 140 mg/dL. Are these results within normal limits? If not, what is abnormal and what, if anything, should be done about the abnormal results?

Elevated cholesterol or hypercholesterolemia occurs when blood cholesterol is ≥200 mg/dl. Ferri (2021) made the following observations:

- More than 105 million (37%) adults in the United States have total blood cholesterol levels higher than 200 mg/dl. Of this group, more than 36 million adults have extremely high-risk cholesterol levels over 240 mg/dl (13%).
- For men over the age of 20 years, approximately 48% of White men, 45% of Black men, and 50% of Hispanic men have high blood cholesterol.
- For women over the age of 20, approximately 50% of White women, 42% of Black women, and 50% of Hispanic women have hypercholesterolemia.
- The prevalence of hypercholesterolemia increases with increasing age.

According to the National Health and Nutrition Examination Survey (NHANES) data for 2009 to 2010, about 47% of adults had at least one of three risk factors for cardiovascular disease: uncontrolled high blood pressure, uncontrolled high levels of low-density lipoproteins (LDL) cholesterol, or current smoking.

The physical exam should include a thorough history, including family history that may highlight a genetic basis for hypercholesterolemia. The exam should also include measurements of blood pressure, body mass index, and auscultation of carotid arteries and peripheral pulses. A comprehensive medication overview may reveal medications such as thiazides, corticosteroids, beta-blockers, and estrogens that may impact cholesterol levels (Ferri, 2021).

Countless research studies have determined high-density lipoprotein (HDL) cholesterol to be an independent risk factor for heart disease. Among men and women ages 49 to 82 and without heart disease at the time they were enlisted into the Framingham Heart Study, HDL was a much more powerful risk factor for heart disease than was low-density lipoprotein (LDL) cholesterol, total cholesterol (TC), or plasma triglycerides (TGs).

High-Density Lipoprotein

HDL is a type of lipoprotein that contains equal quantities of healthy protein as well as a lipid component. The numerous HDL subclasses differ in their content of triglycerides, apolipoproteins apo-A1 and apo-AII, and lipid transfer enzymes as well as healthy proteins, consisting of paraoxonase-1, platelet-activating variable acetylhydrolase (PAF-AH or Lp-PLA2), lecithin cholesteryl acetyltransferase (LCAT), cholesteryl ester transfer protein (CETP), and phospholipid transfer protein (PLTP). In addition, HDL contains liposoluble vitamins and antioxidants. The safety benefits of HDL have actually mainly been credited to its inverse cholesterol transportation; however, HDL is believed to have numerous other antiatherogenic properties (Link et al., 2007). (See Table 15.2.)

The metabolic process of HDL includes five primary procedures: (1) apo A-I synthesis as well as secretion right into plasma as inceptive HDL; (2) uptake of complimentary cholesterol from the perimeter; (3) maturation right into large spherical fragments with cholesterol esterification; (4) shipment of cholesteryl ester to the liver, steroidogenic body organs, as well as apo B-containing lipoproteins; and (5) catabolism of apo A-I. See Fig. 15.1.

The protein of HDL is apo A-I, which is manufactured in the liver and is launched in plasma free from lipid as nascent HDL. Nascent HDL quickly occupies totally free cholesterol from cells. This causes the development of discoidal HDL bits. Apo A-1 functions as a signal transduction healthy protein to set in motion cholesterol ester efflux from intracellular pools. LCAT can then engage with the cholesterol substratum, creating esterification of the free-cholesterol bound to the discoidal HDL. The esterified cholesterol then moves into the hydrophobic HDL core, altering the HDL conformation from discoidal to spherical, which represents HDL in its mature stage.

TABLE 15.2 Lipoprotein Subfractions

Chylomicrons	Large particles that carry dietary lipid. Associated with apo A-I, A-II, A-IV, B-48, C-I, C-II, C-III, and E.
VLDL	Carries TG made by the liver and some LDL particles. Associated with apolipoproteins B-100, C-II, C-III, and E.
IDL	Breakdown product of VLDL-C. Carries cholesterol esters and TGs.
LDL	Core of cholesterol esters, small TGs surrounded by free cholesterol, phospholipids, and apolipoprotein B-100. Delivers cholesterol to tissues.
HDL	Carries cholesterol esters, associated with apo A-I, A-II, C-I, C-II, C-III, D, and E.

Apo, Apolipoproteins; *TG*, triglycerides.
From Link, J. J., Rohatgi, A, & de Lemos, J. A. (2007). HDL cholesterol: Physiology, pathophysiology, and management. *Current Problems in Cardiology, 32*(5), 268–314. https://www.clinicalkey.com/#!/content/journal/1-s2.0-S0146280607000059?scrollTo=%23top

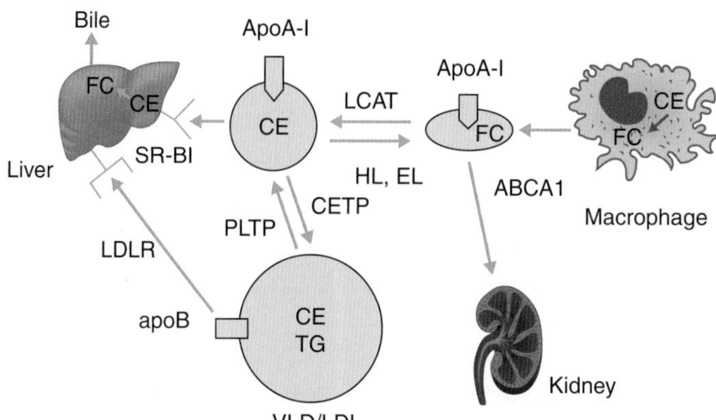

• **Fig. 15.1** Formation of spherical (mature) HDL from nascent HDL. ABCA1/G1, Adenosine triphosphate-binding cassette protein A1/G1; ApoA-I, apolipoprotein; FC, free cholesterol; LCAT, lecithin cholesteryl acetyltransferase; PL, phospholipids; SR-B1, scavenger receptor class-B1. (Adapted from Barter, P. J., et al. [2006]. Targeting cholesteryl ester transfer protein for the prevention and management of cardiovascular disease. *Journal of the American College of Cardiology, 47*[3], 492 499.)

The cholesterol is then released to the liver in an esterified form within the HDL. In the liver it can be processed and excreted as bile or converted into cholesterol-containing steroids (Link et al., 2007).

Low-Density Lipoprotein

The LDL particle consists of a monolayer of phospholipid. Unesterified cholesterol forms the surface membrane, and fatty acid esters of cholesterol form the hydrophobic core. A copy of the hydrophobic apo-B protein is embedded in the membrane and mediates the binding of the LDL particles to specific cell surface receptors (Pirahanchi & Huecker, 2019).

Problems in LDL receptor function can create hypercholesterolemia, known as familial hypercholesterolemia, an autosomal dominant condition. Due to the fact that LDL receptors, which are located externally on hepatocytes, are required for binding as well as consequent uptake of LDL particles in the blood, a hereditary reduction in the LDL receptor number would certainly create a reduced capacity of hepatocytes to soak up LDL and would raise the LDL in the blood. If this anomaly is heterozygous, some LDL receptors will exist on the hepatocytes, hence LDL is normally around 300 mg/dL. Nonetheless, a homozygous anomaly will certainly lead to the total lack of LDL receptors on hepatocytes, enhancing the LDL cholesterol degrees as much as 1000 mg/dL (Pirahanchi & Huecker, 2019).

Dyslipidemia

Dyslipidemia refers to a complex group of diseases characterized by elevated lipid levels in the blood. It is usually symptom-free until serum cholesterol or triglyceride levels are significantly elevated and well beyond the range in which cardiovascular morbidity and mortality are elevated.

Lifestyle changes (e.g., weight reduction, exercise, nutritional changes) are essential for long-term treatment; the clinician should consider medications to reduce lipid levels (e.g., statins) when lifestyle changes alone do not achieve lipid-lowering goals. Statins are the drug of first choice for high cholesterol levels. The treatment of elevated triglycerides is indicated when the triglyceride concentration exceeds 500 mg/dL (Link et al., 2007).

Treatment of High Cholesterol

Over time, high cholesterol can lead to atherosclerotic cardiovascular disease (ASCVD); therefore it is important to know who to screen and when to treat. The American Association of Clinical Endocrinologists (AACE) recommends screening of males >45 years and females >55 years of age every 1 to 2 years and those >65 years of age every year up to 75 years of age regardless of coronary artery disease (CAD) risk status. Patients older than 75 years of age with multiple CAD risk factors should continue to get screened annually. The US Preventive States Task Force (USPSTF) supports routine screening for men >35 years and women >45 years of age by measurement of a nonfasting total and HDL cholesterol alone (Ferri, 2021).

A fasting lipid panel has historically been preferred to a nonfasting lipid profile, but this recommendation has been challenged and consensus statements from experts in Europe and Canada have endorsed nonfasting lipid tests as the new standard for lipid measurement. In patients who are not fasting, triglyceride levels ≥175 mg/dl should be considered elevated compared to those <150 mg/dl for fasting panels. Fasting lipid panels are preferred for patients with triglycerides above 400 mg/dl. If clinically relevant, the clinician should perform an assessment of secondary causes (e.g., thyroid stimulating hormone, metabolic profile, liver function tests, and fasting glucose) (Ferri, 2021).

The US Adult Treatment Panel (ATP) III guidelines for the management of individuals with hyperlipidemia did not contain age restrictions but stipulated that "clinical judgment" is needed to manage patients over the age of 65.

The 2013 the American College of Cardiology (ACC)/American Heart Association (AHA) Guideline for the Treatment of Blood Cholesterol is premised on the knowledge gained over the prior decade and advocates the reduction of atherogenic particles in people ages 65 to 75 years. Nevertheless, the guideline often mentions the need to use clinical judgment when recommending a statin dose. There is a clear advantage of cholesterol reduction by statins for cardiovascular prevention in patients who are deemed at risk and are between the ages of 65 and 75. In patients who are ages 75 years or older, not only is there a gap in clinical trial data, but epidemiologic data also indicate a link between low cholesterol and all-cause mortality and no prevention of the risk of developing cardiovascular events.

In 2018, the AHA, ACC, American Association of Cardiovascular and Pulmonary Rehabilitation (AACVPR), Association of Black Cardiologists (ABC), American College of Preventive Medicine (ACPM), American Diabetes Association (ADA), American Geriatrics Society (AGS), American Pharmacists Association (aPhA), American Society for Preventive Cardiology (ASPC), National Lipid Association (NLA), and Preventive Cardiovascular Nurses Association (PCNA) created updated guidelines on the management of cholesterol.

The key recommendations of the guideline for lowering the risk of atherosclerotic cardiovascular disease through cholesterol management are discussed here.

For patients with clinical atherosclerotic cardiovascular disease (ASCVD), lower low-density lipoprotein cholesterol (LDL-C) levels with higher-dose statin therapy or the maximum tolerated statin dose should be given. In individuals with high-risk ASCVD, an LDL-C cutoff of 70 mg/dL (1.8 mmol/L) should be used to determine the benefit of adding nonstatins to statin treatment.

Clinicians should start high-intensity statin therapy in patients with severe primary hypercholesterolemia (LDL-C levels ≥190 mg/dL [≥4.9 mmol/L]). In people ages 40 to 75 years with diabetes mellitus and LDL-C levels of ≥70 mg/dL, clinicians should begin medium-intensity statin therapy without calculating the 10-year risk of ASCVD.

There are key issues to consider when deciding to prescribe a lipid-altering drug to an older adult patient. In both the older and younger age groups, the only proven effective lipid-altering drug therapy for reducing cardiovascular disease is reducing the levels of cholesterol-containing atherogenic particles through lipid-altering therapies. The definition of the term "older people" may be ambiguous, but most clinicians refer to older patients as those ages 65 years or older. From the point of view of lipid lowering, older patients can be classified into two groups:

- People ages 65 to 74 years in whom there is strong evidence of a benefit of cholesterol reduction. In such patients, the determination of medication depends only on the assessment of cardiovascular risk in patients without known cardiovascular disease and benefit versus risk in people with substantial noncardiovascular comorbidity.
- Individuals ages 75 years and older in whom there is no immediate evidence of a benefit or lack of a benefit for cholesterol lowering. In such patients, the advanced practice provider makes a recommendation to the individual based on an assessment of several factors, including risk of atherosclerotic versus nonatherosclerotic cardiovascular disease, the burden of comorbidity, socioeconomic/lifestyle status, and the presence of frailty. In this group, the final decision for lipid-altering treatment is based on individual's preference (Streja & Streja, 2017).

Ethical considerations must be considered when selecting a preventive management plan for older people. The primary problem is how to balance the value of life against the quality of life. There are few data on the desires and apprehensions of people in this age group. At what stage is the value of cardiovascular prevention lost? What is the greatest fear of the people in this group, their death or disability? If the fear of physical impairment predominates, is it the fear of physical impairment or that of cognitive impairment? At the social level, there is also the cost to the society of extending a life of dubious quality for the person who has the disability. All of these factors may influence the decision to treat patients in the older age group with lipid-lowering drugs.

A detailed examination and thorough understanding of the clinical and pathophysiologic effects of lipid-lowering therapy in the older age group, taking into account ethical and socioeconomic factors, is essential to help clinicians make informed treatment recommendations for lipid treatment in this population (Streja & Streja, 2017).

The latest average values of lipoproteins in the US population are listed in the publications of the National Health and Nutrition Examination Survey (NHANES). There are some ethnic distinctions in the allocation of lipoprotein levels in the US population: Hispanic individuals of both sexes have increased total cholesterol and triglyceride levels and decreased high-density lipoprotein cholesterol (HDLc), whereas African American women who are not Hispanic have increased HDLc and decreased triglyceride levels. Over time, there has also been a gradual decline in total cholesterol levels, and from 1960 to 2002 there was a trend toward higher triglyceride levels. These trends are especially evident in older subjects and are most likely due to the growing popularity of treatment with lipid-lowering drugs and the increased prevalence of obesity.

Socioeconomic determinants account for alterations in lipoproteins in older people. In 2003, 10.2% of individuals over 65 years of age lived below the country's threshold of poverty. Of these, 41.6% reported that they had no teeth. Measured by the Healthy Eating Index, only 9% of older adults ages 65 and over who are affected by poverty have a "good" rating for eating healthy. Socioeconomic determinants are, in most cases. also associated with the burden of comorbidity. Psychiatric or neurologic conditions can cause a deterioration in socioeconomic status and eventually lead to malnutrition. Chronic kidney disease, congestive heart failure, rheumatoid arthritis, cancer, and multiple hospitalizations also add to the deterioration in nutritional status. As a result, malnutrition leads to a significant decrease in the concentration of atherogenic substances (Streja & Streja, 2017).

Osteoarthritis

CASE STUDY 15.3

J.D. is a 70-year-old male who presents to his physician assistant (PA) for his annual physical. The patient complains of pain and stiffness in his knees, especially in the morning when rising out of bed. He reports that "it takes a while for my knees to get woke up and moving." He has been taking acetaminophen 1000 mg four times a day for the pain. He states that this does help but he "doesn't like swallowing all those pills." What drug classes treat arthritis pain? What would be the best choice of treatment for this patient?

Although getting older is the main risk factor for osteoarthritis (OA), it is not an unavoidable result of getting older. OA is the leading form of arthritis and often involves the hands, knees, feet, and hips. Pain is usually the symptom of OA, which leads people to present to their health care provider and receive a diagnosis of OA.

The Centers for Disease Control and Prevention (CDC) analyzed data from the National Health Interview Survey (NHIS) years 2013–2015 Sample Adult Core components to estimate average annual arthritis prevalence in the civilian, noninstitutionalized US adult population ages 18 years or older. The data revealed an estimated 22.7% (54.4 million) of adults had doctor-diagnosed arthritis, with a significantly higher age-adjusted prevalence in women (23.5%)

than in men (18.1%). Arthritis prevalence increased with age (CDC Arthritis, 2018).

Arthritis impairs the overall performance and flexibility of a person, which can lead to activity and other limitations. It is one of the main causes of disability among adults in the United States. The CDC's Arthritis Program analyzes data from the NHIS to evaluate the national prevalence estimates for arthritis and arthritis-attributable activity limitations.

Based on the analysis of 2013 to 2015 data from the National Health Interview Survey (NHIS), an estimated 54.4 million (22.7%) of adults aged 18 years or older have self-reported doctor-diagnosed arthritis and 23.7 million (43.5%) of adults aged 18 years or older with arthritis have arthritis-attributable activity limitation.

Based on the analysis of 2010 to 2012 data from the National Health Interview Survey (NHIS), it is projected that by 2040, 78 million (26%) adults aged 18 years or older will have doctor-diagnosed arthritis and of the adults with arthritis, an estimated 44% (35 million adults) will report arthritis-attributable activity limitations. (CDC, 2019).

There are certain activities that are more difficult for people with arthritis to do. These activities include grasping small objects, reaching above one's head, sitting for about 2 hours, climbing a flight of stairs without resting, and walking one-quarter of a mile (CDC, 2019).

OA is associated with significant morbidity, including disability and reduced quality of life. OA is the primary cause of lower limb disability in older adults, and cases of knee and hip OA account for 2.4% of all years lived with disability, a general measure of the burden of disease. Global Burden of Disease (GBD) studies consistently cite OA as one of the leading causes globally of years living with disability (YLDs) (March & Cross, 2019).

OA affects some 240 million people worldwide, including more than 30 million in the United States, whose number increased from 21 million in 1990 to 27 million in 2005. Considering the differences between rural and urban areas and between high- and low-to-middle income areas, the worldwide prevalence of OA at the hip and knee in adults over the age of 18 is approaching 5%. This rate is predicted to climb as the population ages and obesity incidence grows. The occurrence of OA rises with age, with around 10% of men and 18% of women over 60 experiencing clinical OA (March & Cross, 2019).

Risk Factors

Osteoarthritis is a complex interplay of mechanical, cellular, and biomechanical factors that lead to the pathology in the final stage. Multiple risk factors have been linked to OA. Age is one of the biggest predictors of OA, with the prevalence of hand, hip, and knee OA increasing with age, especially after the age of 50. A flattening occurs at all joint sites at around 80 years of age. About 34% of adults ages 65 years and older have OA. Global projections suggest that 10% of men and 18% of women over the age of 60 suffer from symptomatic OA.

The factors behind this increased risk with age are not well understood. Potential triggers include sarcopenia, loss of proprioception, and joint laxity, which can affect joint function and predispose the joint to injury. Alterations that affect joint tissue include loss of normal bone structure, greater stiffness of ligaments and tendons, and meniscal degeneration. Being female is associated with a higher prevalence and severity of OA. The cause for the increased risk of OA in women remains unknown but it may be related to hormones, genetics, or other undetermined variables (March & Cross, 2019).

Genetics also play a role in osteoarthritis. All forms of OA seem to be strongly genetically determined; however, the genetic involvement is complicated, as associations may vary according to factors such as the affected joint, the history of trauma, and gender. Despite the importance of genetics, not a single gene is involved in the formation of OA. Multiple genes could play a part in the manifestation of the disease, which could yield objectives for future pharmacologic treatments. Joint injuries are associated with the development of OA and are commonly referred to as posttraumatic OA. The knee is one of the most commonly affected joints, and rupture of the anterior cruciate ligament (ACL) is related to early knee OA in 13% of cases after 10 to 15 years. When such rupture is accompanied by compromised cartilage, subchondral bone, collateral ligaments, or menisci, the incidence of knee OA is higher, with estimates varying between 21% and 40% (March & Cross, 2019).

Lifestyle factors also play a role in the development of OA. Obesity is one of the major risk factors for both the incidence and progression of OA in strained joints such as the knee and hip as well as the hand. According to March and Cross (2019), "individuals with a BMI >30 kg/m^2 were 6.8 times more likely to develop knee OA than normal-weight controls."

An individual's occupation can also impact one's chance of developing OA. For example, people who repetitively bend their knees in their job are at a higher risk of developing OA in the knee. Miners have also been known to have a higher incidence of spine OA, possibly due to frequent extreme positions or a high load being placed on the spine (March & Cross, 2019).

Pathogenesis of Osteoarthritis

Osteoarthritis has always been thought of as a disease of "old age" due to wear and tear on the joints. However, we now know that OA is more than just wear and tear on the joints.

Osteoarthritis results from the age-related loss of the ability of cells and tissues in the body to maintain homeostasis, especially when they are under stress. In OA, extreme or aberrant mechanical stress clearly plays a role in the evolution of the disease. Under conditions of stress in an anatomically normal joint, the joint tissues appear to be able to adapt to the stress without causing OA. But joint stress resulting from abnormal load balance or joint anatomy adds to the development of OA.

Because OA is uncommon in young adults, and even severe joint injuries typically manifest themselves as OA years later, it appears that young joint tissues can accommodate abnormal mechanical stress. However, the ability to compensate for stress decreases with age. If the basic cellular pathways that maintain tissue homeostasis decrease with age, then the reaction to stress or joint injury is inadequate, resulting in destruction and loss of joint tissue.

There is growing evidence that the changes that occur in articular cartilage during the development of OA are the result of a loss of natural homeostasis. The chondrocyte is the only cell type present in articular cartilage and is therefore responsible for both the degradation and synthesis of the cartilaginous extracellular matrix. Impulses generated by cytokines, growth factors, and the matrix regulate the metabolic activity of the chondrocytes. In OA cartilage, the inflammatory and catabolic signals seem to exceed the antiinflammatory and anabolic signals. This signal imbalance promotes the increased production of matrix-degrading enzymes by the chondrocytes, including matrix metalloproteinases (MMP), aggrecanases, and other proteases that degrade the cartilage matrix. Aging modifications that occur in the chondrocyte seem to add to the loss of homeostasis (Anderson & Loeser, 2010).

There are probably several age-related factors that encourage the progression of age-related diseases such as OA. A key feature of OA is the disparity of catabolic and anabolic signal transmission in cartilage, which leads to progressive destruction of the matrix. Studies provide some indication that age-related oxidative stress is a key factor in this catabolic-anabolic imbalance. Studies of the molecular structure show excessive oxidation of the major antioxidant networks in chondrocytes, including glutathione and the peroxiredoxins. The oxidative deactivation of the antioxidant systems allows an increase in intracellular reactive oxygen species, which causes a disturbance in physiologic signal transmission. The inability of simple antioxidants to influence the aging process and age-related diseases may be related to their inability to specifically act on this disturbed signal transmission (Loeser, 2017).

Treatment of Osteoarthritis

Pain due to osteoarthritis stems from a diverse biopsychosocial system comprising noncartilaginous components, including subchondral bone, synovial, and periarticular components, and is impacted by both environmental and psychosocial factors. Central and peripheral sensitization of the nociceptive tracts may eventually control pain persistence and play a role in the chronic aspects of the disease. Pain associated with OA has negative effects on sleep and mood and often interferes with participation in professional and leisure activities.

There are several components to the treatment of OA. They vary from managing common OA-related conditions such as social problems, sleep disorders, and depression to joint-specific treatments, including nonpharmacologic, pharmacologic, and surgical options. Eventually, most aim to improve the pain and functional impairment that are characteristic of this widespread disease. Despite numerous efforts, treatments to modify the course of the disease have not yet reached the threshold of efficacy to be approved (Deveza, 2020).

Treatment for osteoarthritis needs to be unique to the individual based on the individual's signs, values, needs, and objectives, as well as their specific response to treatments. There is no single therapy for OA that takes care of all symptoms for all patients. For that reason, a mix of restorative methods is utilized to maximize function, lessen discomfort, and in some cases alter the pathophysiology of joint damage. It is always good practice to utilize safer treatments first before trying treatments that may have a higher risk for the patient. There are four treatment categories for OA: nonpharmacologic, pharmacologic, nonsurgical, and surgical treatments.

Patient follow-up, compliance with advice, and behavioral changes are key components of the management of osteoarthritis and can be maximized through OA education and self-management, setting treatment objectives, and periodic monitoring. Patients should be adequately educated about the cause of OA, risk factors (especially ones that can be changed), and the expected prognosis. Precise information on management options along with their benefits, harms, and costs should also be considered. The provision of this information helps to counteract frequent misunderstandings and to focus the treatment on the patient, thus encouraging an active frame of mind in dealing with one's own disease.

Patient awareness is an integral part of enhancing OA management. A significant proportion of noncompliance with treatment, especially where lifestyle adjustments are involved, may be due to the limited time clinicians have available to explain the purpose of interventions and what the patient can expect in relation to the relief of pain (Deveza, 2020).

Regular clinical appraisals should be conducted on a routine basis to measure the impact of treatment on signs, functionality, and status and to measure objective variations in metrics associated with interventions such as muscle strength. Periodic assessment of the patient allows for frequent feedback and reinforcing the treatment plan. This also allows monitoring of therapeutic effectiveness, side effects, and changes in the plan depending on the outcome (Deveza, 2020).

Holistic Assessment

A holistic assessment of the individual with osteoarthritis creates a partnership between the patient and health care professional and promotes collaborative care, where individuals and health care professionals jointly make decisions about treatment and rely on each other to improve outcomes. Osteoarthritis is a complex disease in which the structural signs of joint damage often do not correspond to the presence and severity of joint pain and disability. In addition, patients with OA are predominantly older adults who often have different types of preferences and desires, and this affects the choice of treatment.

The perceived nature and implications of the disease vary greatly from person to person and are impacted by several factors that, if undetected, make it difficult to develop an appropriate, customized plan and reduce the effectiveness of treatment. Some of the important issues that clinicians should be aware of include the patient's knowledge of OA, how pain is limiting the patient's function and quality of life, any problems with sleeping, the results of a falls risk assessment, and expectations (Deveza, 2020).

Nonpharmacologic Treatment

As with many other conditions, nonpharmacologic options are at the foundation of treatment for OA. These treatments include education, exercise, weight management, assistive gadgets, psychological treatments, and alternative therapies. Nonpharmacologic therapies represent the essentials of treatment for OA initially. These treatments include education and learning, exercise, weight management, supports, assistive gadgets, psychological treatments, hand-operated medications, and different therapies.

It is important to educate individuals concerning their diagnosis, any risk factors that can be modified for their type of OA, and their prognosis. Information needs to be provided concerning possible alternative treatments including their benefits, risks, costs, and other options. Patients' participation in setting goals as well as self-managing their condition enhances compliance and can improve their overall understanding of their condition.

Exercise is another nonpharmacologic way to treat OA. The goal of working out is to reduce pain and improve function in the joint. Numerous types of workout regimens exist, and exercise as a whole should be recommended, keeping in mind that the patient's symptoms should guide the type of exercise. The types of workouts that are most beneficial, especially in knee OA, are cardiovascular exercise and resistance training. One of the most and easily available exercises is walking. Structured walking programs have actually been proven to greatly improve the symptoms of OA and strengthen the quadriceps muscles. Water exercise has additionally been shown to be helpful and has the added advantage of reduced weight-bearing on the joints.

In obese and overweight individuals, a loss of just 10% of their body weight has demonstrated a reduction in OA-related joint discomfort. This holds true for individuals with knee and hip osteoarthritis. Using a cane, walking stick, or knee braces can help some patients who have malalignment.

Chronic pain due to OA can have considerable effects on an individual's capability to manage activities of daily living. It is common for patients to become depressed when they cannot participate in activities they enjoy due to their OA; the lack of movement then causes their OA symptoms to be exacerbated. There is some indication that cognitive therapy can be valuable in this situation (Kellerman & Rakel, 2020).

Pharmacologic Treatment

Although nonpharmacologic treatment is the initial therapy, several individuals with OA will need drug therapy as part of their treatment. It is important to keep in mind that there are no medications that can reverse or slow the development of OA; however, some medications do minimize discomfort and swelling, which can improve the patient's quality of life.

One of the most typical nonnarcotic analgesic agents currently utilized for OA is acetaminophen. Adverse side effects are uncommon, but acetaminophen should be used cautiously in individuals who have preexisting kidney or liver disease.

Selective serotonin and norepinephrine reuptake inhibitors (SNRIs) may also be beneficial. Duloxetine (Cymbalta) 60 mg once a day is authorized by the US FDA for use on mild to moderate pain due to OA.

The use of opioids to treat OA pain is not recommended. Tramadol (Ultram) is generally used specifically in patients who cannot take nonsteroidal antiinflammatory medicines (NSAIDs); however, the nurse practitioner (NP)/physician assistant (PA) should keep in mind that individuals can develop a tolerance to tramadol. Opioids were once thought to improve lifestyle and function in patients who suffered from chronic OA pain. Opioids may be required occasionally for extreme discomfort, but the dangers of tolerance, opioid abuse, addiction, overdose, and death greatly outweigh the benefits.

Analgesics usually do not adequately control the pain that people with OA experience, whereas NSAIDs can give substantial pain relief from OA. The 2013 American Academy of Orthopaedic Surgeons (AAOS) Standards on managing knee OA without surgery advise the use of NSAIDs that have clinically been shown to reduce OA pain. If simple anesthetics fail to provide appropriate relief, an NSAID medication should be prescribed. Scientific tests with naproxen, diclofenac, and sulindac revealed substantially greater pain relief when compared to high-dose acetaminophen. The primary drawback in using NSAIDs is the possibility of the patient developing gastric ulcers, facing impaired kidney function, and experiencing cardiac events. Additionally, clients with OA might be taking other platelet inhibitors, and this potential synergistic action needs to be weighed against the risks. Clients who are 75 and older should be given topical NSAIDs instead of oral medications to reduce the possibility of toxic side effects. Price and the patient's ability to comply with the dosing instructions should be considered. Most NSAIDs are now offered in dosage strengths that can be administered one or two times daily, which can improve compliance.

COX-2 inhibitors hinder prostaglandin synthesis, which can ease inflammation and pain while keeping COX-1 effects intact and protecting stomach mucosa. In the United States, the only approved NSAID COX-2-inhibitor is celecoxib (Celebrex). When comparing celecoxib to traditional nonselective NSAIDs, celecoxib is similar in regard to effectiveness; however, the potential for gastrointestinal injury as well as damage to platelet aggregation is decreased.

The potential for kidney damage is similar to traditional NSAIDs. Studies have shown that patients taking celecoxib did have a somewhat higher risk of suffering from a cardiovascular event, but this was noted at doses >400 mg/day. Celecoxib is also safe to use with other medications such as warfarin and low-dose aspirin.

Invasive procedures, such as intraarticular corticosteroid injections, should not be done until nonpharmacologic treatment options have been exhausted. Steroids are powerful medications that decrease pain and swelling but they are considered a temporary fix. Some practitioners continue to think that corticosteroid injections destroy the joint cartilage and contribute to the destruction of the joint by osteoarthritis. Corticosteroid injections should be added to the patient's treatment plan when nonpharmacologic measures are not controlling the patient's pain or when the patient is having an OA flare. According to expert opinion (not evidence-based science), corticosteroid injections are considered safe to administer up to four times a year. As with any invasive procedure, there is a slim possibility of causing an infection at the injection site; however, this risk can be minimized by using an aseptic approach. In addition, corticosteroids that are injected into a joint are less likely than systemic steroids to increase the patient's serum blood glucose levels. Nonetheless, prudence should be given to patients with preexisting diabetes (Kellerman & Rakel).

Using hyaluronic acid (HA) injections for osteoarthritis began in the 1990s. The exact mechanism of action remains unclear, but it is believed to enhance the elasticity of the cells within the synovial fluid of the joint. HA has also been shown to reduce inflammation and protect chondrocytes. Despite that benefit, HA does not cure or delay the progression of OA (Kellerman & Rakel, 2020).

At first, all hyaluronic acid products were derived from the comb of a rooster; however, this is not true anymore. In roughly 2% to 8% of people who were given an intraarticular injection of hyaluronic acid, a pseudoseptic reaction could occur, which resembled a joint infection. Products manufactured today are not animal derived. In the United States, these products are endorsed only for osteoarthritis of the knee.

Surgical Treatment

Surgical treatment of arthritis varies depending on which joint is impacted. Arthritis of the knee is the most commonly affected joint, followed by arthritis of the hip. Arthrodesis, arthroplasty, and realignment osteotomy are the most common procedures performed. Knee arthroscopy is not recommended for the treatment of osteoarthritis of the knee because there is little evidence to prove that arthroscopy works better than exercise. If the patient has unicompartmental knee arthritis, then hemiarthroplasty should be considered. Total joint arthroplasty is a costly surgical treatment, though it is typically well covered by insurance. Surgical procedures, such as cardiovascular events, infections, and deep vein thrombosis, carry significant risks. Not all people will experience pain relief or improved functional ability (Kellerman & Rakel, 2020).

Arthritis-Related Emergency: Septic Arthritis

Septic arthritis is considered an urgent medical condition. Septic arthritis (SA) is still a common enough occurrence that the NP/PA should be alert to a suspicious process when the patient presents with symptoms. The diagnosis of septic arthritis is verified by an arthrocentesis. A culture of the fluid should also be performed, but the sensitivity is not 100%. A Gram stain should also be done, but it is important to keep in mind that a negative Gram stain does not eliminate the possibility of an infection. Repeated therapeutic procedures may need to be performed when treating SA to monitor any progression of the infection (Roberts et al., 2019).

Septic arthritis is usually caused by bacteria or viruses; fungi are less commonly the cause of SA. Septic arthritis normally includes a single large joint, like a knee; however, smaller joints can also suffer from SA. The occurrence rate of SA in the general population is 0.01%, but the incidence increases to 0.07% in people who have a prosthetic joint, rheumatoid arthritis, diabetes, or who are immunosuppressed. Other risk factors include age >80, renal or liver disease, HIV, alcoholism, cancer, recent joint surgery, skin infection, or intraarticular corticosteroid injection (Wu et al., 2017).

The older population is more prone to SA due to the fact that they have more risk factors. Older patients also have a higher mortality rate because of delayed diagnosis and treatment, associated comorbid conditions, and a decline in physiologic reserve.

A research study by Wu et al. (2017) revealed that the senior population with SA had a significantly greater risk of mortality than those without septic arthritis. The underlying comorbidities in the geriatric patients with SA were osteoarthritis, diabetes mellitus, coronary artery disease, and COPD, among others. The mortality risk was higher during the initial 6 months after being diagnosed with SA, and this impact continued for the first 1 to 2 years after diagnosis. This research additionally revealed that the lower extremities were diagnosed with SA more often than the upper extremities, but a diagnosis of SA in the lower extremities carried a lower mortality rate than when SA was diagnosed in the upper extremities.

A joint can become infected by various means such as preexisting bacteremia, infective endocarditis, an infectious source near the joint, surgical contamination, urinary tract infection, or trauma. The noninfectious differential medical diagnoses include crystal-induced joint inflammation, fracture, hemarthrosis, osteoarthritis, osteomyelitis, and monoarticular rheumatoid arthritis. In many instances, a joint that is swollen due to gout cannot clinically be distinguished from an infected joint. Nevertheless, an early medical diagnosis is necessary to inhibit complications such as joint destruction, soft tissue infection, or osteomyelitis (Roberts et al., 2019).

The most common causes of infection in the older adult population are *Staphylococcus aureus* and *Streptococcus*. These account for up to 91% of all cases. Gram-negative bacillus is more commonly seen in the geriatric population. In older adults, the clinical changes due to infection are usually nonspecific and subtle. Signs that may indicate sepsis include mental status changes, cognitive decline and functional impairment, and systemic issues such as anorexia, weight loss, and falls. "Gavet, Tournadre, Soubrier, and Ristori, et al. (2005) demonstrated that in a cohort of 335 patients, 206 of whom were over 60 years old and 42 were over 80 years old, 23% were afebrile and half of the patients mounted no leukocytosis" (Matthews, 2010).

If the NP/PA suspects septic arthritis, then aspiration of the joint fluid and microscopic analysis is required prior to the initiation of antibiotics. Cultures of the joint fluid and blood cultures may increase the diagnostic probability of a septic joint, but some patients will be culture negative. Interestingly, the morbidity of patients with unidentified or culture-negative septic arthritis is the same as it is for patients with a positively identified cultured organism. Any type of fluid aspirated should additionally be reviewed under polarized light for the existence of crystals—from either urate or pyrophosphate. Crystal arthritis can also cause joint inflammation, and it is important to note that crystal arthritis can coincide with a septic joint.

The only approved contraindication to joint aspiration is if the patient has an intraarticular prosthesis. In this situation, an orthopedic surgeon should be consulted to perform the procedure. In addition to joint aspiration, the white cell count, erythrocyte sedimentation rate, or C-reactive protein should be assessed, keeping in mind that if these results are within normal limits, the diagnosis of septic arthritis cannot be ruled out. In the older population, leukocytosis is present less often as an indication of sepsis (Matthews, 2010).

Plain radiographic films should be taken to rule out osteomyelitis, fractures, chondrocalcinosis, or inflammatory arthritis. Computed tomography (CT) scans can be used to diagnose infections of the spine, hips, and sternoclavicular and sacroiliac joints. Ultrasound can help to uncover effusions in joints that are more difficult to examine, such as a hip joint (Ferri, 2021).

Treatment of Septic Arthritis

A joint that is affected by SA needs to be aspirated daily to remove the necrotic debris. Serial white blood cell counts and cultures should also be followed. The appropriate antibiotics are the mainstays of treatment for patients with presumed or proven septic arthritis.

The choice of antibiotic therapy is usually based on the results of the Gram stain of the aspirated fluid (Table 15.3). In the geriatric population, numerous additional aspects work together to make the decision of the appropriate antibiotic complicated. Choosing the best antibiotic should be made with care, thinking about possible polypharmacy with medication interactions, decreased renal function, and age-related changes in both pharmacokinetics and pharmacodynamics. Every one of these factors can add to the possibility of drug events and toxicity in the older patient. Several studies have shown that a large percentage of hospital admissions in the older population are due to medication issues. One meta-analysis revealed that the number of hospital admissions associated with medication toxicity was four times greater in older versus younger populations, and it is estimated that 88% of these admissions were avoidable.

Several comorbidities in older patients place them at a greater threat of drug interactions. Additionally, this population is at risk to the supposed "prescribing cascade," when additional medication is prescribed to neutralize the side effects of a first prescription (Matthews, 2010).

TABLE 15.3 Recommendation of Antibiotic Therapy

Gram Stain	Preferred Antibiotic	Alternative Antibiotic
Gram-positive cocci	Vancomycin, 15–20 mg/kg (ABW) daily every 8–12 hr	Daptomycin, 6–8 mg/kg daily *or* linezolid, 600 mg IV or PO every 12 hr
Gram-negative cocci	Ceftriaxone, 1 g every 24 hr	Cefotaxime, 1 g every 8 hr
Gram-negative rods	Ceftazidime, 2 g every 8 hr *or* cefepime, 2 g every 8 hr *or* piperacillin-tazobactam, 4.5 g every 6 hr	Aztreonam, 2 g every 8 hr *or* fluoroquinolone *or* carbapenem
Gram stain negative	Vancomycin plus ceftazidime *or* cefepime	Daptomycin *or* linezolid plus piperacillin-tazobactam *or* aztreonam *or* fluoroquinolone *or* carbapenem

From Ferri, F. F. (2021). *Ferri's clinical advisor*. Elsevier.

CASE STUDY 15.4

V.K. is a79-year-old female who arrives in the emergency department via ambulance with complaints of chest pain. She states she "is embarrassed" because she is "only having a bad case of indigestion." She is slightly diaphoretic and denies any shortness of breath. Her blood pressure is 180/90 mm Hg, heart rate is 104 beats/min, and respiratory rate is m16 breaths/min. She states the pain does not radiate and she keeps asking for "a Tums." An ECG is done and shows ST elevation in several leads.

As a basic guideline, given that numerous adverse medication events are dosage associated, it is practical to start medication at the minimal dosage required to achieve clinical benefit. Where feasible, existing medication treatment should be assessed, and any unneeded drugs must be stopped or replaced with safer alternatives (Matthews, 2010).

Ischemic Heart Disease

Ischemic cardiovascular disease (IHD) is a complex illness that is often caused by coronary artery disease (CAD). The frequency of ischemic heart disease and atherosclerotic vascular condition in the United States enhances dramatically with age. According to some, 30% of clients who go through a surgical procedure each year in the United States have ischemic heart disease (Hines & Marschall, 2018). Even though the death rate connected with IHD has decreased because of therapeutic healing and avoidance campaigns minimizing the incidence of fatal and nonfatal heart attack, the prevalence of IHD continues to rise. In individuals with ST-segment elevation myocardial infarction (STEMI), death remains significant, with in-hospital death as well as 1-year mortality rates as much as 10%. Survivors of a first heart attack are thought to pass away of IHD at later ages as a result of cardiac arrest and late cardiac deaths. Various other additional factors are more people being diagnosed with type 2 diabetes, physical inactivity, and obesity (Adam et al., 2021).

Pathophysiology of Ischemic Heart Disease

Ischemic heart disease is usually caused by coronary artery disease. When the coronary blood flow is dramatically damaged, signs of myocardial ischemia happen. This can occur when the coronary artery lumen is gradually impacted by developing calcification, when a coronary artery plaque ruptures, or when a clot is formed causing lumen occlusion and leading to acute coronary syndrome. Another less common cause of ischemic heart disease is spasming of a coronary artery.

There are also nonplaque or obstructed causes of ischemic heart disease. These include reduced coronary blood flow because of hypotension that can be seen in septic shock, diminished oxygen content in the blood that is often seen with anemia or chronic obstructive pulmonary disease (COPD), and tachycardias that cause an increase in myocardial oxygen demand (Yelle, n.d.).

Myocardial stunning is a sensation that is caused by a brief episode of ischemia followed by reperfusion. It is often seen when there is a spontaneous episode of ischemia, such as after having a percutaneous coronary intervention (PCI) or after a coronary artery bypass. The pathophysiology of myocardial stunning is due to the creation of oxygen-free radicals, changes in the homeostasis of calcium and the metabolized oxygen, and changes to the protein-based muscle structure.

Studies have shown more sugar uptake with decreased glycogen synthesis in the postischemic myocardial sensational designs of rats 24 hours after ischemic injury. This means that this is an essential function of improved glycolysis in the recovery from a stunned myocardium.

The ischemic cascade is the concept that progressive myocardial oxygen supply and demand trigger a constant sequence of events that begins with changes in metabolism and then problems with myocardial perfusion and anomalies in wall movement, deviations in the ECG, and, finally, angina. See Fig. 15.2.

Ischemic heart disease can lead to other serious health conditions such as acute myocardial infarction (AMI), fatal arrhythmia, and stable angina pectoris or heart failure (Moran et al., 2012). According to the American Heart Association (2016), "an estimated 85.6 million American adults (>1 in 3) have 1 or more types of coronary vascular disease. Of these, 43.7 million are estimated to be ≥60 years of age." For women ≥65 years of age, heart disease is the leading cause of death. The average age of having a first heart attack is 65.1 years for men and 72 years for women.

A study by Krumholz, Normand, and Wang (2019) reviewed 4.3 million Medicare beneficiaries ages 65 or older who were discharged after having an AMI and found that admissions for AMI have decreased 38.1%. The study showed a significant improvement in short-term mortality and readmissions.

Coronary Artery Disease: Angina

Coronary artery disease (CAD) is usually caused by ischemic heart disease. CAD can then lead to myocardial ischemia. When the coronary blood flow is dramatically decreased, signs and symptoms of myocardial ischemia occur. This may occur when the coronary artery lumen is progressively impinged by a developing atherosclerotic plaque (known as a chronic stable plaque), when a coronary artery plaque tears (or, much less frequently, during plaque disintegration), or when a thrombus develops with a sudden occlusion of the lumen, creating acute coronary syndrome. Additionally, and less usual, root causes of myocardial anemia are coronary artery spasm and microcirculatory dysfunction (Adam et al., 2021).

Two of the most common sequelae of CAD is angina and an acute myocardial infarction (AMI). The coronary artery blood flow typically provides sufficient blood circulation to satisfy the demands of the myocardium in reaction

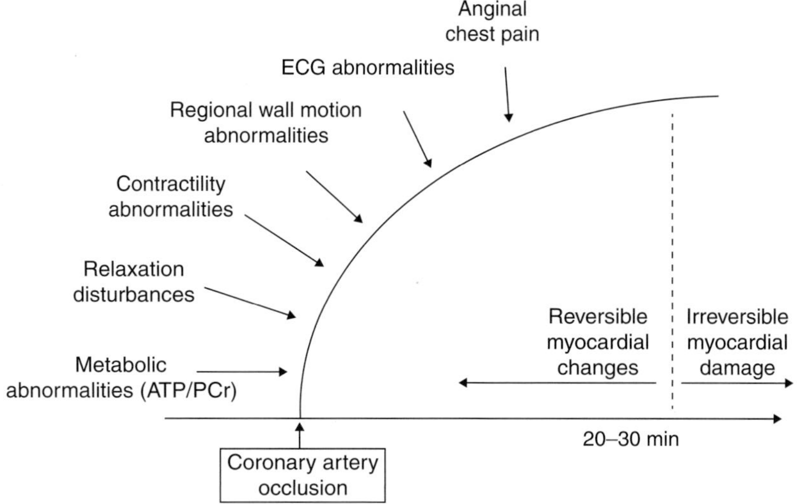

• **Fig. 15.2** The Ischemic Cascade (From Adam, A., Dixon, A. K., Gillard, J. H., & Schaefer-Prokop, C. M. [2021]. *Grainger & Allison's diagnostic radiology*. Elsevier.)

to need. An inequality between coronary blood circulation and myocardial oxygen intake can lead to the development of ischemia, which is characterized as chest discomfort and angina. When a coronary artery is >70% occluded, the patient can experience chest pain or discomfort, which would be diagnosed as angina. When the demand is more than the supply, myocardial infarction or electric instability with cardiac dysrhythmias might result.

Angina pectoris occurs due to the release of bradykinin, adenosine, and other chemicals. These chemicals promote cardiac nociceptive and mechanosensitive receptors whose afferent neurons affect the top five thoracic ganglia and somatic nerve fibers in the spine and eventually produce thalamic and cortical stimulation that causes the typical chest pain of angina pectoris. These materials are slow-moving atrioventricular transmissions, which lead to decreased cardiac contractility, and then boost the equilibrium between myocardial oxygen supply and need. Atherosclerosis is one of the most typical causes of damaged coronary blood flow leading to angina pectoris, yet it may additionally happen due to the lack of coronary obstruction because of myocardial hypertrophy, aortic constriction, or aortic regurgitation. It might additionally accompany paroxysmal tachydysrhythmias, marked anemia, or hyperthyroidism.

Diagnosis

Angina pectoris is usually called chest discomfort, pressure or as "a weight" on the chest. This pain frequently spreads to the neck, left shoulder, left arm, or jaw and sometimes to the back or down both arms. Angina might also be regarded as acid indigestion. Some clients explain angina as shortness breath, misidentifying a feeling of chest constriction as dyspnea. If the client feels that he or she needs to take a deep breath rather than take a rapid, quick breath, then the client probably has angina and not just dyspnea. Angina usually lasts several mins and usually comes in waves of severe to moderate chest pain. A pain that lasts just a couple of seconds or an ache that lasts for hours is hardly ever triggered by myocardial ischemia. Physical exertion, psychological tension, and cold weather might induce angina. Relaxation or nitroglycerin can alleviate angina (Hines & Marschall, 2018).

Treatment

The goals of treating angina pectoris are to alleviate symptoms, delay the natural course of the disease, and minimize the likelihood of having a myocardial infarction or early death. Quitting smoking can greatly reduce the side effects on the heart and can revert or at least delay atherosclerosis. Patients should be encouraged to stop smoking, and providers should take an active role in assisting them to achieve this goal. The provider should also address risk factors such as high blood pressure, diabetes mellitus, obesity, and high cholesterol (Alaeddini, 2018).

Medications used to treat angina include nitrates, beta-blockers, calcium channel blockers, and ranolazine. Nitrates work by relaxing the smooth vascular muscle tissue by stimulating intracellular intermittent GMP production. The result is a decrease in blood pressure.

Nitrates also decrease left ventricular pre- and postload by venous and arterial dilatation, which subsequently lowers myocardial oxygen intake and eliminates angina pectoris. In addition, nitrates create dilatation of the epicardial coronary arteries, which is useful in individuals with coronary spasm. Nitroglycerin has antiplatelet and antithrombotic properties in people with angina pectoris. There is no proof that nitrates enhance survival or slow the progression of CAD (Alaeddini, 2018).

Beta-blockers decrease the heart rate, blood pressure, and the force of the heart's contractions, thereby reducing the oxygen needs of the heart. In addition to nitrates, beta-blockers are generally the front runner for the therapy of secure angina and are advantageous in individuals who have angina during daily activities or exercise.

Beta-blockers have been shown to improve survival and stop another heart attack in individuals who have endured a recent cardiac arrest. Many beta-blockers are available as a long-acting preparation that are taken daily (Aroesty & Kannam, 2020).

Calcium channel blockers enlarge arteries, lower the force of the heart's contractions, and reduce blood pressure. They additionally enlarge veins, decreasing the volume of blood returning to the heart, which decreases the workload of the heart. Some calcium channel blockers slow down the heart rate, which also decreases the workload of the heart.

First-line therapy for people with stable angina includes nitrates or beta-blockers. Calcium channel blockers are another option if there are adverse effects or other conditions that limit the use of beta-blockers and nitrates. Calcium channel blockers may additionally be used if nitrates as well as beta-blockers do not control angina when used together (Aroesty & Kannam, 2020).

Ranolazine was authorized by the US FDA in 2006 for the treatment of stable angina. Originally, it was thought that ranolazine worked by partially restraining fat oxidation. However, studies have shown that it only partially restrains fat oxidation at serum levels that are unobtainable with normal dosing recommendations.

Ranolazine has been shown to stop calcium overload and the subsequent increase in diastolic tension because of inhibition of the late internal sodium network. Considering that this salt channel often falls short to inactivate in a variety of crucial myocardial illness states such as anemia and hypertrophy, additional access of sodium ions leads to activation of the sodium/calcium exchanger, consequently increasing calcium levels (Aroesty & Kannam, 2020).

Coronary Artery Disease: Acute Myocardial Infarction

Acute coronary syndrome is a term used to describe a range of disorders due to sudden, reduced blood flow to the heart. One such condition is an acute myocardial infarction (AMI):

The Joint Task Force of the European Society of Cardiology, American College of Cardiology Foundation, the American Heart Association, and the World Heart Federation (ESC/ACCF/AHA/WHF) defined acute MI (2018) as the presence of acute myocardial injury detected by abnormal cardiac biomarkers in the setting of evidence of acute myocardial ischemia. (Reeder & Kennedy, 2020)

AMI can be further classified based on the ECG changes. Patients who present with an ST elevation on their ECG are classified as having an ST elevated myocardial infarction (STEMI). Patients who present with ST-segment

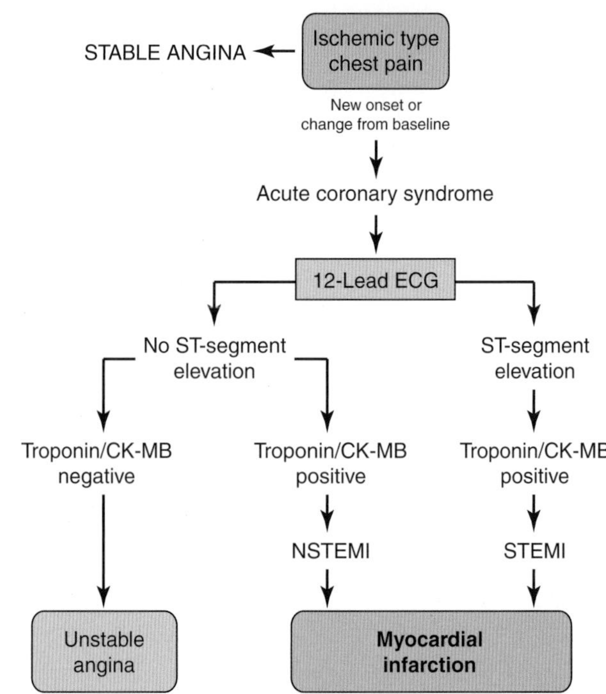

• **Fig. 15.3** Terminology of acute coronary syndrome. *CK-MB*, Creatine kinase, myocardial-bound isoenzyme; *ECG*, electrocardiogram; *NSTEMI*, non–ST-segment elevation myocardial infarction; *STEMI*, ST-segment elevation myocardial infarction. (Adapted from Alpert, J. S., Thygesen, K., Antman, E., et al. [2000]. Myocardial infarction redefined—A consensus document of the Joint European Society of Cardiology/American College of Cardiology Committee for the redefinition of myocardial infarction. *Journal of the American College of Cardiology, 36*, 959–969.)

depression or nonspecific changes on the ECG are classified based on the level of cardiac-specific troponin levels. If the troponin level is higher than normal, the patient is diagnosed as having a non-ST elevated myocardial infarction (NSTEMI). If the patient presents with complaints of chest pain and there are nonspecific changes on the ECG and his or her cardiac-specific enzymes (such as troponin) are normal, then the patient is diagnosed with unstable angina (UA). See Fig. 15.3.

Diagnosis of Acute Myocardial Infarction

The earlier the diagnosis of AMI is made, the better the chances of survival. The health care provider should maintain a high index of suspicion. Any patient presenting with complaints of chest pain, dyspnea, new-onset heart failure, sudden cardiac arrest, or new changes on an ECG should be evaluated for AMI (Reeder & Kennedy, 2020).

Although most of myocardial infarctions (MIs) in the senior population will have ECGs that are nondiagnostic or have a depressed ST-segment, STEMI is not unusual. It is approximated that 60% to 65% of STEMIs take place in clients ≥65 years of age, and 28% to 33% take place in people ≥75 years of age. Also, up to 80% of all fatalities associated with MI occur in persons ≥65 years old (Reeder & Kennedy, 2020).

When the nurse practitioner or physician's assistant suspects an AMI, a brief, focused history and physical should be obtained, followed by an ECG and a measurement of the patient's serum troponin level. These interventions should take place within 10 minutes of presentation.

Treatment for ST Elevated and Non-ST Elevated Myocardial Infarctions

Treatment for STEMI and non-STEMI consists of nonpharmacologic and pharmacologic therapies. Nonpharmacologic therapy includes restriction of the patient's activity and bed rest with a bedside commode for the first 12 to 24 hours. Activities can gradually be increased as the patient's condition improves.

The patient should not have anything to eat until stable. The health care provider should then start the patient on clear liquids and progressively advance to a diet plan customized to the patient's other medical conditions such as hypertension or diabetes. Nonpharmacologic treatment also includes patient education regarding healthy living habits such as tobacco cessation and routine exercise (Ferri, 2021).

Pharmacologic treatment for a STEMI differs slightly than that of a non-STEMI. A patient who has had a STEMI should be given supplemental oxygen if her or his oxygen saturation is <90%. Then the next step in treatment is to evaluate the patient to see if he or she is eligible for percutaneous coronary intervention (PCI).

Numerous scientific prognostic variables are accessible to the health care provider based on the preliminary history, ECG, and chest radiograph. Given the speed with which reperfusion treatment is carried out in individuals with STEMI, their professional use in clinical decision making in the emergency department is often limited.

High-risk variables consist of advanced age, hypotension, tachycardia, heart failure, and a former MI. The Thrombolysis in Myocardial Infarction (TIMI) score for ST elevation acute myocardial infarction is used to determine the chance of in-hospital mortality (Reeder & Kennedy, 2020).

Thrombolysis in Myocardial Infarction Risk Score Calculator for ST Elevated Myocardial Infarctions

Age 65 to 74 years? Yes (+2) – or – Age ≥75 years? Yes (+3)
Diabetes, hypertension, or angina? Yes (+1)
Systolic BP < 100 mm Hg? Yes (+3)
Heart rate > 100? Yes (+2)
Killip classes II through IV
Jugular venous distention (JVD) or any pulmonary exam findings of congestive heart failure? Yes (+2)
Weight < 67 kg (147.7 lbs)? Yes (+1)
Anterior ST elevation or left bundle branch block (LBBB)? Yes (+1)
Time to treatment > 4 hours? Yes (+1)

What Does This Score Mean?

0 Points	0.8% risk of all-cause mortality at 30 days.
1 Point	1.6% risk of all-cause mortality at 30 days.
2 Points	2.2% risk of all-cause mortality at 30 days.
3 Points	4.4% risk of all-cause mortality at 30 days.
4 Points	7.3% risk of all-cause mortality at 30 days.
5 Points	12.4% risk of all-cause mortality at 30 days.
6 Points	16.1% risk of all-cause mortality at 30 days.
7 Points	23.4% risk of all-cause mortality at 30 days.
8 Points	26.8% risk of all-cause mortality at 30 days.
9 Points	35.9% risk of all-cause mortality at 30 days.
10 Points	35.9% risk of all-cause mortality at 30 days.
11 Points	35.9% risk of all-cause mortality at 30 days.
12 Points	35.9% risk of all-cause mortality at 30 days.
13 Points	35.9% risk of all-cause mortality at 30 days.
14 Points	35.9% risk of all-cause mortality at 30 days.
15 Points	35.9% risk of all-cause mortality at 30 days.
16 Points	35.9% risk of all-cause mortality at 30 days.

(TIMI Study Group. https://timi.org/timi-risk-score-calculator-for-stemi/)

If the hospital does not have the capability to provide reperfusion therapy, the following is recommended:

For patients who present within two hours of the onset of symptoms, we suggest full-dose fibrinolytic therapy and transferal to a PCI center. This assumes that primary PCI cannot be performed in less than 90 minutes at a local PCI center. For patients who present with symptoms that last longer than 2 to 3 hours, we suggest transferal for primary PCI. However, there are times when the patient presents after 2 hours, and PCI cannot be accomplished in less than 120 minutes. In this setting, clinical judgement needs to be exercised; fibrinolytic therapy may be appropriate in patients with up to 12 hours of symptoms. (Reeder & Kennedy, 2020)

Primary percutaneous coronary intervention (PCI) is the preferred treatment over fibrinolysis. Multiple studies have shown that patients who underwent PCI had improved survival, a lower rate of intracranial hemorrhage, and a decreased chance of having another MI compared to patients who underwent fibrinolysis. However, if PCI is not available, fibrinolysis should be attempted.

Medications used to treat the patient with a STEMI include antiplatelet therapy with aspirin, a P2Y receptor blocker such as clopidogrel, or a GP iIb/IIIa inhibitor if the patient had PCI. An anticoagulant such as unfractionated heparin, enoxaparin, or fondaparinux should also be started. The choice of anticoagulant depends on the patient's treatment plan.

Nitroglycerin should be given to the STEMI or non-STEMI patient who has persistent chest pain, hypertension, or heart failure. Nitrates have a crucial function in the management of clients with a severe coronary syndrome, regardless of the absence of a mortality benefit. Nitrates can be of value in decreasing or potentially removing discomfort (either recurring or preliminary) because of myocardial ischemia, improving signs and symptoms of pulmonary congestion, and decreasing high blood pressure in hypertensive clients (Reeder, 2019).

For the patient who has had a STEMI or non-STEMI, the use of morphine in the setting of an acute myocardial infarction is no longer considered the standard of care. Two studies have shown that morphine may lead to decreased survival; however, the mechanism is unknown. The hypothesis is that morphine may interfere with the action of antiplatelet agents.

Beta-blockers are given to STEMI and non-STEMI patients who have had a myocardial infarction because of the numerous benefits that outweigh the risks. Beta-blockers decrease myocardial oxygen demand, decrease the risk of ventricular fibrillation, and increase the electrophysiologic threshold that slows conduction and permits bradycardia.

Finally, if the patient is not on a statin, then statin therapy should begin as soon as possible regardless of the baseline low-density lipoprotein-cholesterol level. Atorvastatin at 80 mg daily or rosuvastatin at 20 or 40 mg daily are the recommended dosages (Rosenson, 2020).

Diabetes

K.S. is a 63-year-old female who presents to her nurse practitioner (NP) for her physical exam. She tells the NP that her blood pressure has been averaging 140/89 mmHg and she measures it every day. She complains of her right hip being "stiff in the morning, but after I've been up for about 20 minutes it starts to feel better." The NP reviews the patient's lab work done 1 week earlier and notes that the HgbA1c result is 7.0. Is this result within the recommended guidelines? If not, what should the NP prescribe for this patient?

Diabetes occurs when the pancreas cannot make enough insulin or when the body cannot fully utilize the insulin that it does make. There are three main types of diabetes: type 1, type 2, and gestational diabetes. For the purposes of this text, we will only cover type 1 and type 2 diabetes.

Type 1 is the most serious form of diabetes. In type 1 diabetes, the pancreas does not make insulin. Approximately 5% of people who have diabetes have type 1, also known as insulin-dependent diabetes. Type 1 diabetes was previously synonymous with juvenile diabetes because it usually develops in children and teenagers. However, individuals of all ages can develop type 1 diabetes (International Diabetes Foundation [IDF], 2020).

Type 2 diabetes is more common in adults and accounts for around 90% of all diabetes cases. In type 2 diabetes, the body does not utilize the insulin that it produces. The foundation of type 2 diabetes treatment is healthy lifestyle, which entails increased physical activity and healthy eating habits. Unfortunately, most people with type 2 diabetes will eventually need oral medications or insulin to keep their blood glucose levels within acceptable limits.

Type 2 diabetes occurs most often in middle-aged and older adults, but it can also affect children. The likelihood of getting type 2 diabetes is higher if there is coexisting obesity, physical inactivity, or a family history of diabetes. Women with a history of gestational diabetes also have a greater chance of developing type 2 diabetes later in life ("An overview of," 2020; IDF, 2020; National Institute on Aging [NIA], 2019).

Pathophysiology of Diabetes

Type 1A diabetes is generally believed to be brought on by the immune-associated destruction of insulin-producing pancreatic beta cells. As noted earlier, type 1 diabetes was once mostly regarded as a condition affecting adolescents and youngsters, but this opinion has transformed so that age at symptom onset is no longer a limiting aspect. Polydipsia, polyphagia, and polyuria (the classic triad of symptoms) in addition to obvious hyperglycemia are still diagnostic trademarks in the younger population and to a lesser level in grownups. An urgent need for insulin is additionally a characteristic of type 1A diabetes, for which lifetime treatment is required (Atkinson et al., 2014).

Type 1B diabetes is an uncommon form of phenotypic type 1 diabetes with a virtually total insulin deficiency, a strong inherited element, and no evidence of autoimmunity. Type 1B diabetes is mostly seen in Africa and Asia. To be diagnosed with type 1B diabetes, the patient needs to meet the following criteria: there is no serum evidence of the immune system attacking beta cells and there must be times when the patient needs insulin and times when the patient does not need insulin ("What is type 1 diabetes?" n.d.).

Type 2 diabetes has several complicating factors in its pathophysiology. Environmental and genetic factors play an important role in the development of diabetes. Excess caloric intake and today's sedentary lifestyles can have an important impact on the development of type 2 diabetes.

Individuals can present with a mix of variable levels of insulin resistance, an insulin deficit, or an increased glucose production. It is possible that all three factors contribute to the development of type 2 diabetic. Additionally, all of these characteristics can occur via hereditary or environmental pathways, making it challenging to establish the specific cause. Additionally, hyperglycemia itself can hinder pancreatic beta-cell functionality as well as worsen insulin resistance, bringing about a cycle of hyperglycemia and causing a worsening of the metabolic condition.

Many times, a patient with type 2 diabetes has multiple comorbidities such as hypertension, high-serum low-density lipoprotein (LDL) cholesterol concentrations, and low-serum high-density lipoprotein (HDL) cholesterol levels, which increase cardiovascular risk. Persons with type 2 diabetes can also have metabolic syndrome (McCulloch & Robertson, 2019). Metabolic syndrome is present when at least three of the following risk factors exist: excess fat around the abdominal area, hypertension, elevated triglyceride level, a low HDL cholesterol level, and an elevated fasting blood sugar (National Heart, Lung, and Blood Institute, n.d.).

One of the earliest symptoms of type 2 diabetes is insulin resistance. Insulin resistance is a condition in which physiologic insulin concentrations elicit a decreased biologic response in target tissues (Kahn, 1978). Not only does insulin resistance lead to diabetes, but it has also been shown to increase cardiovascular disease risk.

Diagnosis of Diabetes

Diabetes can be diagnosed in several ways. One way is to check the patient's fasting plasma glucose (FPG). Fasting is defined as no caloric intake for at least 8 hours. If the FPG is greater than 126 mg/dL (7.0 mmol/L), then the patient would be given a diagnosis of diabetes.

A second way to evaluate for diabetes is to give the patient an oral glucose tolerance test (OGTT). During this test, the patient's baseline serum glucose level is checked. Then the patient drinks a liquid that contains 75 grams of glucose. Next, the patient has her or his serum glucose checked every 30 minutes. This test usually takes 3 hours. If the patient's serum glucose is ≥200 mg/dL (11.1 mmol/L) during the OGTT, the patient is diagnosed with diabetes.

The third diagnostic test for diabetes is a check of the patient's serum hemoglobin (Hgb) A1c level. The A1c test is a blood test that measures the patient's average blood sugar over the previous 3 months. A HgbA1c ≥6.5% (48 mmol/mol) indicates that the patient has diabetes (ADA, 2020). The sensitivity and specificity of the HgbA1c test is 87.2% and 98.5%, respectively (Yoon et al., 2018).

Treatment of Diabetes

Exogenous insulin is the mainstay of type 1 diabetes. It is important to remember that some patients with type 1 diabetes still produce insulin. If this is the case, it is important to try to preserve this function for the patient. Even though it is only a small amount of insulin, studies have shown it is associated with less retinopathy and less severe hypoglycemia at later stages of the disease (Steffes et al., 2003).

Continuous insulin pumps or sensor-augmented pump therapy has been shown to help the patient with type 1 diabetes reach targeted HgbA1c levels (Atkinson et al., 2014). Continuous glucose monitors (CGMs) measure blood glucose every 1 to 5 minutes. The HgbA1c goal for older adults is set higher (<7.5% or <8%) than for younger patients. The objective of insulin treatment is to provide a physiologic profile of insulin by management of a basal insulin plus mealtime boluses of a rapid-acting or short-acting insulin. The amount of the before-meal bolus is calculated by the patient's blood sugar result before the meal, the amount and make-up of the dish, physical activity after eating, and the patient's blood sugar trends that can be calculated by a CGM (Weinstock, 2019).

The treatment of type 2 diabetes is similar to the treatment of type 1 diabetes; the goal is to attain optimal glycemic control. Glucose targets are customized to each patient and must consider the following: life span, disease period, presence or lack of microvascular or macrovascular issues, presence of cardiovascular disease, any additional health issues, and if the patient is at risk for hypoglycemia (Davies et al., 2018). For older adult patients and those with comorbidities or limited life expectancy who are unlikely to benefit from intensive therapy, glycemic targets are generally set somewhat higher.

Metformin remains the preferred first-line medication for the treatment of type 2 diabetes in the adult. This is because metformin has a broad clinical profile that proves it is safe, affordable, low cost, and effective at lowering HgbA1c levels.

SGLT2 inhibitors are oral drugs that reduce plasma glucose by improving the urinary excretion of glucose. The glucose-lowering efficacy of these drugs depends on kidney function. GLP-1 receptor agonists are given subcutaneously. These drugs activate insulin release and decrease glucagon excretion in a glucose-reliant fashion, improve fullness, and enhance weight loss. DPP-4 inhibitors are oral drugs that improve insulin production and decrease glucagon release dependent on glucose. They have a modest glucose reduction effect. DPP-4 inhibitors are tolerable, have a minimal impact on weight, and have a low risk of hypoglycemia when used as a single-agent. Thiazolidinediones (TZDs) are oral drugs that enhance insulin response and have a potent glucose-lowering effect. Among glucose-lowering drugs, TZDs are associated with the best evidence of glycemic stability. These significant benefits, however, must be weighed against safety concerns about congestive heart failure, fluid retention, weight gain, bone fragility, and potential bladder cancer. Sulfonylureas are oral drugs that reduce glucose by activating insulin excretion from beta cells of the pancreas. They are affordable, commonly prescribed, and have a high glucose-lowering effect. Sulfonylureas are related to weight gain and the likelihood of low blood sugar, thus lowering the dose to reduce the risk of hypoglycemia results in higher HbA1c levels. Sulfonylureas are associated with a lack of sustained effect on glucose lowering (Davies et al., 2018).

Treatment of Diabetic Emergencies

Diabetic ketoacidosis (DKA) and hyperosmolar hyperglycemic state (HHS) are acute complications of diabetes. Diabetic ketoacidosis is a potentially lethal complication of diabetes identified by ketonuria, hyperglycemia, and ketoacidosis. It arises when insulin insufficiency prevents the capability of sugar to get in cells for application as fuel for metabolism, the outcome being that the liver creates ketones from the breakdown of fat. The ketones are then used as fuel. The surplus of ketones occurs, causing them to gather in the blood and urine, which then transforms the blood into an acidic environment. DKA happens mainly in individuals with type 1 diabetes; however, it can occur in some individuals with type 2 diabetes (Hamdy, 2019). The diagnostic criteria for DKA includes a "serum glucose >250 mg/dL, arterial pH <7.3, serum bicarbonate <18 mEq/L, and at least moderate ketonuria or ketonemia. Normal laboratory values vary; check local lab normal ranges for all electrolytes" (Hirsch & Emmet, 2020).

Hyperosmolar hyperglycemic state (HHS) occurs less often than DKA but has a much higher mortality rate and is mostly seen in patients with type 2 diabetes. HHS usually occurs when there is a preceding illness such as an infection or other medical problem such as a myocardial infarction that will ultimately lead to the patient becoming dehydrated. For this reason it is sometimes difficult to distinguish HHS from the coexisting condition. The majority of individuals with HHS do not end up with substantial ketoacidosis. Insulin stays readily available in quantities adequate to hinder lipolysis and ketogenesis but inadequate to avoid hyperglycemia. Hyperosmolarity might also reduce lipolysis, thus restricting the quantity of free fatty acids available for ketogenesis (Avichal, 2019). The diagnostic criteria required for HHS are "serum glucose >600 mg/dL, arterial pH >7.3, serum bicarbonate >15 mEq/L, and minimal ketonuria and ketonemia" (Hirsch & Emmet, 2020).

The rapid replacement of fluid with isotonic crystalloids is a mainstay of treatment. If the patient is comatose, he or she will need to be intubated for airway protection. Insulin replacement is recommended to be at 0.1 unit/kg/hr via a regular insulin IV. It is also important to replace electrolytes such as potassium, sodium, magnesium, and phosphorous. Correction of acidosis with sodium bicarbonate is only indicated in the severely academic patient and the acidosis is life threatening (Hamdy, 2019; Maloney & Glauser, 2018). If an infection is present, treatment will also include the appropriate antibiotic based on cultures and sensitivity results. Initiating empiric antibiotics is also acceptable (Hamdy, 2019).

Treatment of HHS also entails fluid replacement with isotonic crystalloids. It should be noted that it was previously thought that replacing fluid too rapidly could lead to cerebral edema. However, there have not been any studies that show a direct correlation between fluid replacement in HHS and cerebral edema. If the patient is in hypovolemic shock, then aggressive fluid resuscitation is indicated. In older adult patients, there may be coexisting conditions such as heart failure or renal failure, so the balance between fluid overload and fluid replacement must be calculated.

Electrolyte replacement is also part of the treatment algorithm in HHS. Due to dehydration, the potassium level may be falsely normal or even elevated. As the patient's hydration status is corrected, a true hypokalemic situation may appear, and potassium supplementation will be required.

For both DKA and HHS, the diabetic emergency is considered to be corrected when the following goals have been met: the ketoacidosis has been alleviated and the patient's anion gap is back to normal (less than 12 mEq/L), the patient with HHS is mentally alert and serum osmolality is less than 315 mOsmol/kg, and the patient is able to eat (Hirsch & Emmet, 2020).

Heart Failure

CASE STUDY 15.5

P.S. is a 71-year-old male who presents to the emergency department (ED) with complaints of acute shortness of breath. He states the symptoms began about 3 days ago but have been getting worse. He denies any fever, chills, cough, sputum production, wheezing, or chest pain. He says he is short of breath at rest, forgetful, fatigued, and has swelling in his bilateral lower legs. He uses a bilevel positive airway pressure machine (BiPap) at night to sleep. His weight in the ED is 15 pounds higher than what he weighs at home. What is his diagnosis, and what are the next steps in his treatment?

Heart failure is an ongoing, progressive clinical syndrome in which there is structural or functional damage causing the heart muscle to become weakened and incapable of pumping the required amount of blood to maintain adequate perfusion to fulfill metabolic requirements.

Heart failure is graded by different classifications and stages. The New York Heart Association (NYHA) sorts heart failure by class, and classes range from class I to class IV. The American College of Cardiology/American Heart Association (ACC/AHA) heart failure guidelines supplement the NYHA classification to indicate the progression of the disease; these are divided into four stages.

The NYHA classes are as follows:

- "Class I patients have no limitation of physical activity
- Class II patients have slight limitation of physical activity
- Class III patients have marked limitation of physical activity
- Class IV patients have symptoms even at rest and are unable to carry on any physical activity without discomfort" (Dumitru, 2018).

Pathophysiology of Heart Disease

Congestive heart failure or heart failure (HF) may be considered a dynamic disorder that is started after a specific event either harms the heart muscle, with a loss of working cells within the heart muscle, or, conversely, interrupts the capability of the myocardium to produce force, consequently preventing the heart from behaving normally. This inciting event may have a sudden onset, as in the case of a myocardial infarction (MI); it may have a slow or perilous onset, as when it comes to increased blood pressure or excess fluid in the circulatory system, or it could be due to genetics. No matter the nature of the event, there is one commonality: in some way, they all lead to a decrease in the pumping ability of the heart. "In the United States, heart failure is the leading cause of hospitalization in patients older than age 65 years, and once a patient is hospitalized for heart failure, the 30-day risk of rehospitalization is 25%, with a 10% risk of 30-day postdischarge mortality" (Goldman & Shafer, 2020).

In many circumstances, clients will continue to be minimally symptomatic or asymptomatic after the first decrease in the heart's pumping capacity, or symptoms may develop only after the dysfunction has existed for a period of time. Even though the exact reasons why people who have impaired left ventricular (LV) function are asymptomatic have not been discovered, one possibility is that a variety of other mechanisms become activated when there is myocardial injury or a decrease in cardiac output. With development to symptomatic HF, there is remodeling of the left ventricle (Zipes et al., 2019). Fig. 15.4 demonstrates how heart failure is a progressive disease that begins after an initial or *index event* to the myocardium.

Other than a specific inciting event such as myocardial infarction, which accounts for 70% of cases, there are many other issues that can contribute to HF. Some of these issues include coronary artery disease, hypertension, valve disease, obesity, and chemotherapy, to name a few (Goldman & Shafer, 2020).

Heart failure can impact the left ventricle, the right ventricle, or both. If heart failure is due to LV dysfunction, then it will be classified based on the ejection fraction (LVEF) of the left ventricle. If the LVEF is ≤40%, then this is known as "Heart Failure reserved Ejection Fraction" (HFrEF); this has also been called systolic heart failure. If the ejection fraction is ≥50%, then this is known as "Heart Failure preserved Ejection Fraction" (HFpEF), which was previously called "diastolic heart failure." Finally, if the patient has an LVEF of 41% to 49%, this is known as "Heart Failure with mid-range Ejection Fraction" (HFmrEF) (Colucci, 2020).

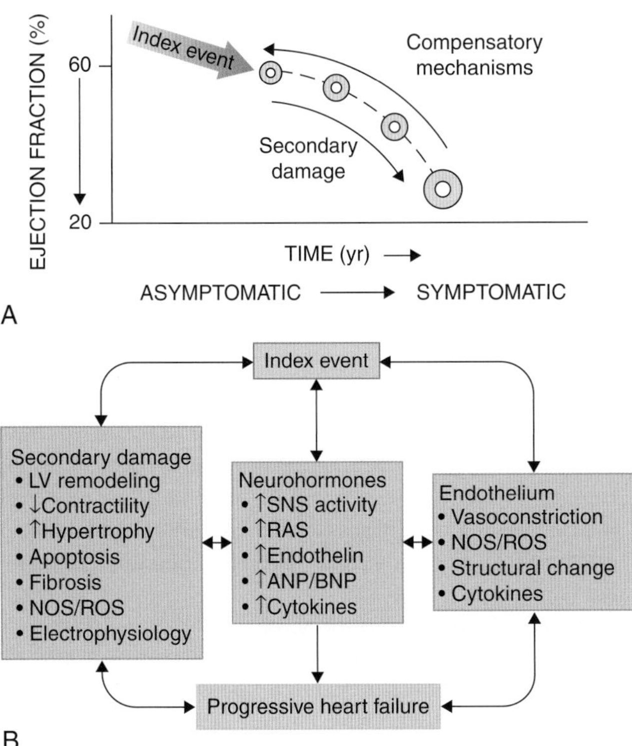

• **Fig. 15.4** Progression of heart failure. (From Zipes, D. P., Libby, P., Bonow, R. O., et al. [2019]. *Braunwald's heart disease: A textbook of cardiovascular medicine* [11th ed.]. Elsevier.)

Signs and Symptoms

As heart failure advances, the patient may experience a variety of signs and symptoms. If the patient has a history of a myocardial infarction or hypertension, the clinician's suspicions should be raised. Symptoms of advanced heart failure can include weight loss, dyspnea, fatigue, fluid overload, and hypotension. Sleep disorders such as obstructive sleep apnea, orthopnea, paroxysmal nocturnal dyspnea, and central sleep apnea can also be observed in the patient with HF (Goldman & Shafer, 2020).

Diagnosis of Heart Failure

Diagnostic results may yield hyponatremia, decreased glomerular filtration rate, hypoalbuminemia, elevated serum bilirubin, elevated B-type natriuretic peptide (BNP), or N-terminal pro-BNP. A chest x-ray will show evidence of fluid retention or congestion (Colucci, 2020). Other tests that should be considered are a cardiac catheterization, cardiac MRI, exercise capacity, hemodynamics (systemic vascular resistance, cardiac output, central venous pressure, pulmonary artery wedge pressure, and cardiac index), and pulse oximetry (Goldman & Shafer, 2020).

Three different diagnostic guidelines are used to diagnose heart failure: the Framingham, Boston, and National Health and Nutrition Examination Survey (NHANES). The Framingham criteria is used most often. There are seven major criteria and six minor criteria. The patient must have one or more of the major criteria and two or more of the minor criteria listed in Box 15.1 (Family Practice Notebook, n.d.).

Once heart failure is suspected, additional diagnostic tests may include a transthoracic echocardiogram to evaluate changes in heart valve functioning, a 6-minute walk test to evaluate exercise capacity, and a right heart catheterization to aid in confirming the diagnosis of heart failure (this test is also useful to evaluate for possible cardiac transplant) (Colucci & Dunlay, 2020).

Nonpharmacologic Treatment of Heart Failure

The treatment of heart failure involves nonpharmacologic and pharmacologic methods. Minimalizing precipitating causes (such as increased sodium intake and noncompliance with medication) and lifestyle modifications (such as

• BOX 15.1 Framingham Criteria for Diagnosis of Heart Failure

Major Criteria (one or more)	Minor Criteria (two or more)
Acute pulmonary edema	Ankle edema
Cardiomegaly	Dyspnea on exertion
Hepatojugular reflex	Hepatomegaly
Neck vein distention	Nocturnal cough
Paroxysmal nocturnal dyspnea or orthopnea	Pleural effusion
Pulmonary rales	Tachycardia (rate >120 beats/min)
Third heart sound (S3 gallop)	

tobacco and alcohol cessation, weight reduction, and avoiding nonsteroidal antiinflammatory drugs [NSAIDs] because they can cause sodium retention) are important steps.

The patient's medications should also be reviewed for any that can worsen the symptoms of heart failure such as antiarrhythmic drugs, calcium channel blockers, and thiazolidinediones. A consultation with a dietician can help the patient avoid high-sodium, overprocessed foods and provide dietary advice for the patient who may be suffering from weight loss (Ferri, 2021).

Pharmacologic treatment includes a variety of medications to treat the symptoms associated with heart failure. Diuretics are used to alleviate fluid overload and improve filling pressures. Angiotensin-converting enzyme inhibitors (ACEIs) have been shown to increase survival and reduce hospitalizations due to heart failure in patients with HFrEF (Kellerman & Rakel, 2020).

Angiotensin receptor blockers (ARBs) are indicated for those who cannot tolerate an ACEI. ARBs have also shown to decrease morbidity and mortality as a substitute to ACEIs for first-line therapy in patients who have HFrEF (Ferri's, 2021).

Angiotensin receptor neprilysin inhibitors are a newer drug in the treatment of HF. Sacubitril valsartan is a mix of two drugs that separates into the individual drugs after absorption. Adding valsartan to sacubitril causes more vasodilation and natriuresis (Waller & Sampson, 2018). The valsartan-sacubitril drug combination has been shown to decrease hospitalizations from HF and improve cardiovascular all-cause mortality (Kellerman & Rakel, 2020).

Some beta-blockers have been shown to improve survival in heart failure. These beta-blockers are carvedilol, bisoprolol, and metoprolol succinate. These drugs are usually given to patients who are euvolemic and started with renin-angiotensin agonist drugs or began using them soon after earlier treatments.

For patients with HFrEF, spironolactone and eplerenone improve survival and decrease hospitalizations. To help the patient avoid hyperkalemia, the NP/PA needs to monitor serum potassium and renal function.

Hydralazine and isosorbide dinitrate are recommended for patients who are African American and have been classified as NYHA class III or IV. This drug combination has also been shown to decrease morbidity and mortality in patients who are intolerant to ACEI and ARBs. For the patient who has heart failure with preserved ejection fraction (HFpEF), organic nitrates should be avoided (Borlaug & Calucci, 2019).

Digoxin has been shown to decrease hospitalizations in patients who have symptoms of NYHA classes II and III and can be helpful in patients with HFrEF. Digoxin levels should be monitored and kept between 0.5 to 0.9 ng/mL. A loading dose is not indicated (Ferri, 2021; Kellerman & Rakel, 2020). For patients with heart failure with preserved ejection fraction (HFpEF), digoxin should be avoided (Borlaug and Calucci, 2019).

Cardiac resynchronization therapy (CRT) is focused on individuals with heart failure who have a delay in ventricular transmission (QRS prolongation on ECG). A transmission delay will hinder ventricular function and can impair prognosis. CRT, also referred to as biventricular pacing, is the implantation of a dual-chamber pacemaker (right atrial and ideal ventricular leads), with a third lead presented by means of the coronary sinus into an epicardial coronary vein and progressed until it gets to the lateral wall surface of the left ventricle. With this lead in place as well as the timing adjusted, the heart can pump more efficiently, which leads to increased cardiac output. CRT has actually been endorsed for patients with NYHA class III or IV disease with an LVEF less than 35% as well as a QRS duration of 120 to 150 ms. Current trials have shown that CRT may even benefit individuals with an ejection fraction over 30% as well as individuals with mild signs of heart failure (Hines & Marschall, 2018).

Heart Failure Emergency: Acute Heart Failure

Acute heart failure is generally defined as a sudden onset of new or intensifying symptoms and signs of HF. It is possibly a lethal condition that requires admission to the hospital and emergent treatment to manage the patient's fluid overload and vital signs. The treatment goals of acute heart failure are straightforward: quickly obtain the diagnosis, treat life-threatening conditions, treat the symptoms, and recognize and treat the cause and triggers for the acute heart failure (Zipes et al., 2019).

There are three types of acute heart failure. These are decompensated heart failure, acute hypertensive heart failure, and cardiogenic shock. Decompensated heart failure is found in patients who have chronic heart failure and then have an acute worsening of symptoms. This is usually due to infections or medication noncompliance. The patient will present with peripheral edema, dyspnea with exertion (DOE), and orthopnea. The NP/PA will want to monitor blood pressure for hypotension and obtain a chest x-ray, which may show clear lung fields despite DOE. The patient's ejection fraction may be reduced, but his or her cardiac output will be acceptable. Patients with acute decompensated heart failure are at high risk for hospital readmission, and this group of patients represents the biggest share of patients hospitalized for acute heart failure (Zipes et al., 2019).

Hypertensive heart failure presents with a sudden onset and can be triggered by hypertension, acute coronary syndrome, or an atrial arrhythmia. The patient's physical exam may reveal dyspnea, hypoxemia, tachycardia, and rales upon auscultation of the lungs. The patient may also be hypertensive, usually >180/100 mm/Hg. A chest x-ray will most likely show pulmonary edema. Vasodilators and noninvasive ventilation are essential for the treatment (Ferri, 2021).

Some patients with advanced heart failure will eventually suffer from cardiogenic shock. Cardiogenic shock is considered the most severe form of heart failure. In this subset of patients, advanced heart failure, myocarditis, or an acute myocardial infarction can be the insult that tips the patient into cardiogenic shock. Cardiogenic shock (CS) is "defined as systemic tissue hypoperfusion secondary to inadequate cardiac output despite adequate intravascular volume and filling pressures" (Guererro-Miranda & Hall, 2020).

The clinical assessment of the patient in cardiogenic shock will show a low systolic blood pressure, normal left ventricular function, and severely depressed right ventricular function. Laboratory findings may show evidence of end-organ damage especially in the kidneys and liver. Unfortunately, patients with cardiogenic shock have a high inpatient mortality and they have a poor prognosis unless they receive a heart transplant (Ferri, 2021).

Chronic Obstructive Pulmonary Disease

CASE STUDY 15.6

B.F. is a 68-year-old female who presents to the nurse practitioner with complaints of a persistent, mild, occasionally productive cough for the past 3 to 4 months. She has been smoking one pack of cigarettes a day for the past 45 years. She denies fever or chills. She does note that she is more short of breath when climbing stairs or exercising. What are the appropriate next steps for the nurse practitioner to take to diagnose this patient?

Chronic obstructive pulmonary disease (COPD) is a chronic respiratory disease that is characterized by limited airflow exchange. COPD impacts more than 5% of the population and has a high morbidity and mortality. The Global Initiative for Chronic Obstructive Lung Disease (GOLD) defines COPD as follows:

COPD is a common, preventable, and treatable disease that is characterized by persistent respiratory symptoms and airflow limitation that is due to airway and/or alveolar abnormalities usually caused by significant exposure to noxious particles or gases. The chronic airflow limitation that characterizes COPD is caused by a mixture of small airways disease (e.g., obstructive bronchiolitis) and parenchymal destruction (emphysema), the relative contributions of which vary from person to person. Chronic inflammation causes structural changes, small airways narrowing, and destruction of lung parenchyma. A loss of small airways may contribute to airflow limitation and mucociliary dysfunction, a characteristic feature of the disease (Global Strategy, 2019).

Pathophysiology

Chronic obstructive pulmonary disease is an inflammation of the lung tissue that prohibits open gas exchange. In COPD, neutrophils, CD8+ lymphocytes, and macrophages predominate in the bronchioles thus causing a discrepancy between these cells and the defense method of the pulmonary system. Several inflammatory mediators are associated with damaging the lung parenchyma in COPD and causing mucus hypersecretion, such as tumor necrosis factor, leukotriene B4, and interleukin-8. Smoking cigarettes stimulates the release of proinflammatory mediators and then deactivates many of the antiproteases leading to an imbalance in inflammation and antiinflammation. This imbalance can be permanent. These differences in the type of the inflammatory response in COPD may explain its somewhat poor response to antiinflammatory medications.

Obstruction might occur from numerous mechanisms: airway smooth muscle mass constraint; small airway inflammation, wall surface thickening, as well as scarring; loss of little air passages owing to parenchymal devastation; and airway collapse. A concomitant alteration might due to decreased elastic recoil resulting from parenchymal tissue damage. This air obstruction causes an increased expiratory time, which can be seen as reduced flow rates over time on a spirogram. If there is a shortened expiratory time, there will be an increase in respiratory rate. This sensation, termed *dynamic hyperinflation*, causes a rise in end-expiratory lung quantity (EELV). The rise in EELV can cause a feeling of dyspnea regardless of hypoxemia (Goldman & Shafer, 2020).

Chronic Bronchitis

Chronic bronchitis and emphysema fall under the category of COPD. Chronic bronchitis can be defined as a persistent cough that is productive of sputum for 3 months in each of 2 succeeding years in an individual in whom other diagnoses of persistent coughing (e.g., bronchiectasis) have been ruled out. It might follow or precede the development of airflow restriction. This interpretation has actually been used in several types of research, regardless of the duration of symptoms. Signs and symptoms of chronic bronchitis can occur in cigarette smokers as young as 36 years old and have been related to more frequent exacerbations, even if there is minute evidence of airflow obstruction. Existing and former smokers have actually enhanced air passage mucin focus (MUC5AC as well as MUC5B), compared to those who have never smoked cigarettes (Han et al., 2020).

Emphysema

Emphysema defines several of the architectural changes that are occasionally linked with COPD. These changes consist of long-term and persistent enlargement of the bronchioles that are farthest from the bronchus. However, there will be no overt fibrosis that can be seen with the naked eye. The omission of noticeable fibrosis was meant to differentiate the alveolar devastation due to emphysema from that due to interstitial pneumonias. Nevertheless, many research studies have discovered that some patients with mild COPD can have an increased amount of collagen in the lungs, suggesting that fibrosis can exist within emphysematous changes. Although emphysema can exist in people who do not have an airflow blockage, it is much more usual among patients who have a severe or moderate airflow blockage (Han et al., 2020).

Asthma–Chronic Obstructive Pulmonary Disease Overlap

There are some instances when asthma is considered a part of COPD. Asthma is a chronic inflammatory condition that impacts the airways. However, there can be an asthma–COPD overlap (ACO). ACO is not considered a disease or a syndrome; it is a cluster of symptoms from both diseases. It is important to differentiate between the two as this impacts the treatment. There is not a standardized definition of ACO, but most of the proposed definitions include a patient older than 40 years who has persistent obstruction of airflow and a history of asthma or a bronchodilator response to albuterol (Han & Wenzel, 2020). Patients at risk for ACO are usually those with asthma who smoke and have a genetic predisposition to having an allergic inflammatory response to inhaled particles.

Symptoms of Chronic Obstructive Pulmonary Disease

The trademark signs and symptom of COPD are shortness of breath with exertion, chronic cough, and sputum production. The number one risk factor for developing COPD is cigarette smoking. Individuals can establish considerable COPD prior to becoming symptomatic due to the fact that the topmost physical effort usually is not restricted by ventilatory capability. The steady development of the disease—combined with the reality that other conditions like cardiac issues, being overweight, and deconditioning can likewise cause dyspnea on physical effort—frequently results in people having symptoms for months or even years before being diagnosed with COPD.

In many cases, individuals are diagnosed with COPD when they have worsening dyspnea, increased cough, and a change or an increase in the nature of sputum production; it might or might not be accompanied by high temperature and constitutional signs symptomatic of infection. The growth of these signs might prompt these individuals to see their primary care provider, at which time the medical history might show habits that boost the threat of COPD (commonly chronic cigarette smoking) and antecedent dyspnea on effort. In some patients, there will be a pattern of recurring exacerbations noted in the medical history.

Patients with advanced illness may have hypercarbia or hypoxemia. Hypoxemia can lead to symptomatic cyanosis, headaches, shortness of breath, and acidosis. Hypercarbia, which might be suggested by a high bicarbonate level, should be verified by an arterial blood gas. Likewise, COPD can have systemic symptoms. Individuals with emphysema often lose body mass as well as sarcopenia. Pulmonary hypertension may also be present and can cause a decrease in exercise and even a decrease in independent activities of daily living. Anxiety is a common comorbidity associated with COPD (Goldman & Shafer, 2020).

Diagnosis of Chronic Obstructive Pulmonary Disease

Components of the history appropriate to developing the medical diagnosis include a history of smoking tobacco, other inhalational or ecologic exposures, a longstanding history of frequent lung infections or preterm birth, cough (chronicity, regularity), and excess sputum creation. Particular focus should be given to which restrictions are brought on by dyspnea because clients might progressively limit activity gradually to evade the awkward feeling of being short of breath and might not report the dyspnea associated with their activities of daily living. Clients should be questioned about any family member's history of lung diseases as well as regarding the existence of comorbid conditions.

The assessment findings seen in COPD consist of whether or not the client has cyanosis, the use of pursed-lip breathing, and the use of accessory muscles to breathe or other signs of breathing distress. The persistent hyperinflation of lungs related to COPD might lead to an increased anteroposterior to thoracic measurement (barrel chest), use of the upper extremities to enable the usage of accessory muscles with respiration (tripod setting), and inward movement of the lower chest with inspiration because of the changed biomechanics of a flat but functioning diaphragm (Hoover sign). The visibility of paradoxical abdominal wall activity with respiration suggests respiratory muscular tissue exhaustion. Percussion of the upper chest might note enhanced vibration. Auscultation might show diminished breath sounds in individuals who mainly have emphysema; asymmetry increases the chance of a pneumothorax. People with airway disease might display rhonchi with inspiration and wheezing with exhalation.

COPD can also impact the heart. In this case, it usually relates to right heart failure. The heart tones may be reduced because of increased retrosternal airspace. Jugular venous pressure, a louder than normal closure of the pulmonic valve (P2), a heave of the right ventricular, hepatic congestion, and edema all increase the opportunity of pulmonary hypertension (cor pulmonale). Smoking is an additional risk for lung cancer and individuals who have COPD have a twofold greater chance of lung cancer compared with cigarette smokers who do not have COPD. If the patient has hemoptysis a physical exam should occur to establish whether the person has lung cancer (Goldman & Shafer, 2020).

The NP/PA should suspect COPD in all individuals with shortness of breath, sputum production, cough, or exposure to tobacco smoke. A careful history must include questions regarding the amount and duration of cigarette smoking and direct exposure to involuntary inhalation or other work or direct environmental exposure. The individual should be queried about his or her ability to complete daily activities; complete tasks that result in mucous, dyspnea, and cough manufacturing; and alleviate or get rid of secretions. Family members or close friends may have valuable input because the patient may have ended up being desensitized to dyspnea. On monitoring, the patient may be sitting in the "tripod" position, which puts the accessory muscles in a position to enhance breathing. Clients might also use pursed-lip breathing, or exhale via pursed lips, which increases the force in the airways, expanding them open, allowing a fuller expiration and diminishing air trapping as well as hyperinflation. Percussion may disclose evidence of hyperinflation. Auscultation might expose wheezing or protracted expiration that occurs from respiratory tract obstruction, along with rhonchi from maintained secretions in the respiratory tracts. Regular breath sounds come from terminal airways, and emphysematous damage of these respiratory tracts causes decreased breath sounds.

Spirometry is the keystone of a medical diagnosis of COPD. Respiratory tract obstruction is defined by an FEV1/FEC of <70%. Individuals with respiratory tract obstruction may have the ability to breathe out much of their essential capability (VC), yet as a result of respiratory tracts narrowing, they can refrain from doing it quickly, resulting in the reduced proportion. The severity of obstruction is determined by the FEV1 percentage of the predicted calculation (Kellerman & Rakel, 2020). (See Fig. 15.5.)

In addition to pulmonary function testing, the diagnostic workup for COPD should include a chest x-ray to evaluate the hyperinflation and to determine possible differential diagnoses, an arterial blood gas, and an alpha-1-antitrypsin (A1A), which should be done once to assess for alpha-1 antitrypsin deficiency; however it is important to remember that A1A is a genetic risk factor and an acute-phase reactant, so it should be checked when the patient is clinically stable (Ferri, 2021; Kellerman & Rakel, 2020).

A complete blood count (CBC) will not diagnose COPD but may reveal leukocytosis during an acute exacerbation. Studies have shown that eosinophilia may predict the patient's response to corticosteroids. A sputum culture may be evaluated if the patient is refractory to antibiotic treatment.

Differential Diagnoses

Chronic obstructive pulmonary disease might be diagnosed as other obstructive airway diseases, mostly bronchial asthma. Asthma will usually be present in a younger person, although it might be detected at any age. Asthmatics typically have more reversibility and less obstruction, yet overlap is observed. Asthma and COPD patients may have hyperinflation and a decrease in forced expiratory flows during spirometry, yet a decrease in diffusing capability would usually be more typical of COPD. Expired nitrous oxide (NO) will frequently be high in asthma. Eosinophils are notably elevated in the bronchoalveolar lavage (BAL) fluid in asthmatics, albeit neutrophils are generally elevated in clients with COPD. Considerable overlap takes place in every one of these areas. In a small percentage of individuals, COPD and bronchial asthma cannot be distinguished; this would be defined as *overlap syndrome*. Additional differential diagnoses can also include heart failure, tuberculosis, bronchiectasis, anemia, cystic fibrosis, obstructive sleep apnea, and neuromuscular diseases (Ferri, 2021).

SEVERITY	SPIROMETRY
Stage I: mild	FEV1/FVC <70% FEV1 ≥80%
Stage II: moderate	FEV1/FVC <70% 50% ≤FEV1 <80%
Stage III: severe	FEV1/FVC <70% 30% ≤FEV1 <50%
Stage IV: very severe	FEV1/FVC <70% FEV1 <30%

Abbreviations: FEV1 = forced expiratory volume in 1 second; FVC = forced vital capacity

• **Fig. 15.5** Severity of lung function calculation. (From Corriveau, M. L., & Fagan, J. B. [2019]. *Conn's current therapy* [pp. 837–841]. Elsevier.)

Staging

Once the diagnosis of COPD is made, the disease needs to be staged to aid in the treatment plan. Three staging systems are currently in use, however; the Global Initiative for Chronic Obstructive Lung Disease (GOLD) is probably the most widely used. The GOLD system places patients with COPD into four groups (A, B, C, D) determined by (1) the degree of airflow restriction, (2) a patient symptom score using one of two symptom questionnaires (COPD Assessment test [CAT] or modified Medical Research Council dyspnea scale [mMRC]), or (3) the number of COPD exacerbations in 1 year.

The BODE index, is another way to stage mortality after a diagnosis of COPD. The BODE system (BMI, Obstruction, Dyspnea, Exercise) is determined based on weight (body mass index [BMI]), the amount of airway obstruction (FEV_1), dyspnea (mMRC dyspnea score), and how the patient performs on the 6-minute walk test for exercise capacity. This index offers more accurate prognostic information than determining prognosis based solely on the FEV_1 and can be used to evaluate the therapeutic response to medications, pulmonary rehabilitation therapy, and other treatments.

The final staging system was created by the COPD Foundation and entails seven domains of severity. The domains are determined based on the physical exam and include spirometry results, symptoms, how many exacerbations the patient has had in the preceding 12 months, oxygen saturation, degree of emphysema present on imaging, if there is any presence of chronic bronchitis, and any comorbidities.

The benefit of the COPD Foundation system is that it makes the spirometry results easier to understand and classify, whereas with the GOLD staging, the FEV_1 is used to measure severity (Han et al., 2020).

Nonpharmacologic Treatment

Like many conditions, nonpharmacologic treatment begins with lifestyle changes. Smoking cessation is the foundation of COPD management. Patients can use a variety of methods to quit smoking such as nicotine replacement in the form of gums, patches, etc., behavior therapy, medication, or a combination of these treatments. Supplemental oxygen and smoking cessation are the only treatments that have been shown to extend life in COPD patients (Kellerman & Rakel, 2020).

In addition to smoking cessation, vaccinations for pneumonia and annual influenza are also recommended. Pulmonary rehabilitation needs to be a consideration in patients with COPD who still have breathing issues after medical treatment. Patients who are overweight should try to lose weight.

If depression is suspected, this should be identified immediately because it can lead to problems with medication compliance. Finally, use of continuous positive airway pressure (CPAP) can also improve survival in patients with COPD and reduce hospital admissions (Ferri, 2021).

Pharmacologic Treatment

Pharmacologic treatment should be given in a sequential manner according to the extent of the patient's condition as well as the patient's tolerance for particular medications. According to the GOLD criteria, a short-acting or long-acting anticholinergic or beta-2 agonist should be prescribed for occasional, mild symptoms. If the patient is in GOLD group B, long-acting anticholinergics or long-acting beta-2 agonists should be included in the treatment regimen. If the symptoms continue, then the patient should be placed on both medications. For patients who are in GOLD group C or D, a long-acting anticholinergic or a duo medication regimen consisting of either an inhaled corticosteroid and long-acting beta-2 agonist or a long-acting bronchodilator and long-acting anticholinergic should be prescribed for persistent symptoms. Patients in group C or D are also at high risk for exacerbations. Patients in group D present a challenge, as their cases are also complex and require numerous medications as well as a consideration of the administration of azithromycin and roflumilast (Ferri, 2021).

The use of bronchodilators for COPD patients allows the patient to improve her or his lifestyle, enhance exercise, and lower the incidence of exacerbations. Aerosolized bronchodilators should be prescribed for patients with stable COPD as well as FEV 1 in level 60% to 80% of predicted. For patients with an FEV 1 of <60% of predicted, long-acting bronchodilators are recommended. Current standards from ACP, ACCP, ATS, and ERS advise that medical professionals endorse monotherapy utilizing either long-acting beta agonists or inhaled anticholinergics for symptomatic individuals with COPD as well as FEV 1 <60% of predicted. NPs and PAs need to base the choice of monotherapy on individual preference, price, and any adverse outcomes that may occur. When taken as required, long-acting inhaled bronchodilators are preferred to short-acting bronchodilators.

Short-acting beta-2 agonists or short-acting anticholinergic medications are acceptable in patients with mild, variable symptoms. Anticholinergics are also used and are available in combination with albuterol. Long-acting inhaled agents (long-acting antimuscarinic agents [LAMAs]) are favored in patients with mild to moderate or ongoing symptoms. Tiotropium is a superb long-acting bronchodilator and only requires daily dosing. In clinical trials, tiotropium works better than salmeterol for patients with moderate to severe COPD. There are various other long-acting bronchodilators (LABAs) for ongoing management of bronchospasm associated with COPD. LABAs should be avoided if the patient is on other sympathomimetic drugs, medications that can prolong the QT interval, or beta-blockers.

The decision to add inhaled steroids such as budesonide, fluticasone, or triamcinolone is made to reduce flareups in individuals with moderate to severe COPD. Steroids are scheduled for clients with either ≥ two exacerbations in a year or if their FEV 1 <50% of that anticipated. The exact mechanism of action of inhaled corticosteroids (ICSs) in COPD is questionable. Although some studies have shown moderate improvement in clients' signs as well as a reduced occurrence of exacerbations, the majority of pulmonologists believe that these medicines are ineffective in many people with COPD; however, ICSs need to be prescribed for individuals with moderate to severe airflow restriction who have persistent signs regardless of ideal bronchodilator therapy.

Chronic antibiotic treatment and glucocorticoid treatment should be considered on a patient-by-patient basis. Persistent antibiotic treatment, especially a macrolide such as azithromycin, needs to be taken into consideration in people with frequent severe exacerbations of COPD regardless of optimum treatment with bronchodilators and anti-inflammatory agents. Persistent systemic glucocorticoid therapy is normally not suggested even in serious cases of COPD due to the associated rise in death and morbidity (Ferri, 2021).

Acute Exacerbations of Chronic Obstructive Pulmonary Disease

When a patient's dyspnea worsens above that patient's baseline, or there is an increase in cough or a change in the quality of the patient's mucus, the patient is having an exacerbation of the COPD. Exacerbations are considered medical emergencies; they bring about short-term mortality and can have a detrimental impact on a patient's quality of life. Exacerbations can also be costly, resulting in about 60% of the medical bills for COPD.

According to empirical studies, the risk of having an exacerbation COPD is associated with age, productive cough, how long the patient has had COPD, if there is a history of previous antibiotic treatment, a COPD-related a hospital stay within the previous year, persistent mucous production, a peripheral blood eosinophil count >0.34 × 109 cells per liter, and theophylline treatment, as well as having several comorbidities (e.g., heart disease, heart failure, or diabetes mellitus). As a whole, the deterioration of airflow (reduced forced expiratory quantity in 1 second [FEV1]) is connected with a greater chance of having an exacerbation of COPD (Stoller, 2019). The Evaluation of COPD Longitudinally to Identify Predictive Surrogate End-points (ECLIPSE) study found that "the single best predictor of exacerbations was a history of prior exacerbations, regardless of COPD severity" (Vestbo et al., 2008).

The typical path for an exacerbation, no matter the stimulus, is an inflammatory reaction identified by airway edema, mucous hypersecretion, and respiratory tract smooth muscle constriction that produces the traditional triad of cough, sputum, and dyspnea. Microbial or viral pathogens can be linked in 75% to 80% of acute exacerbations of COPD. The most common viruses to cause exacerbations are influenza, parainfluenza, rhinovirus, adenovirus, respiratory syncytial virus, and coronaviruses. Patients with persistent respiratory disease are usually colonized with microbial varieties that have been linked to these exacerbations, especially *Streptococcus pneumoniae, Hemophilus influenzae, Moraxella catarrhalis*, and, to a lesser level, *Pseudomonas aeruginosa*. In additional studies of patients with persistent colonization, procurement of a new genotype of these varieties is related to an elevated risk of exacerbation and the growth of new strain-specific antibodies that add to the inflammation (Goldman & Shafer, 2020).

The symptoms of acute exacerbations are normally similar to those of bronchitis. Severe flareups of COPD are often associated with a high temperature or happen after contact with other ill people. The individual must be queried about acute signs and symptoms, history of previous exacerbations, any comorbidities such as heart problems, any history of exposure to other infections, a decline in the patient's functional status, past reaction to treatment (if any), and if somnolence is present or if there is a change in the patient's mentation that may imply hypercarbia. Along with severe exacerbations of COPD, other issues that need to be examined include decompensated heart failure, pneumonia, pulmonary embolus, and pneumothorax. Less possible would be a tumor of the bronchus.

The physical examination ought to consist of the patient's vitals, signs of respiratory distress (i.e., use of accessory muscle mass, intercostal retractions, tachypnea, and the inability to talk in full sentences). The cardiac assessment should include the examination for tachycardia, irregular rhythm, and indicators of right or left heart failure, including bibasilar rales, a raised jugular venous stress, hepatic congestion, edema, and an S3 gallop. An irregular mental condition must elevate issues for hypercarbia.

Lab examination needs to consist of pulse oximetry as well as, in individuals with respiratory distress or other symptoms of suspected hypercarbia, an arterial blood gas. Tachycardia, increased jugular venous pressure, and peripheral edema can be seen in both right and left heart failure: an evaluation of brain natriuretic peptide (BNP) in individuals might aid in identifying patients with considerable left heart failure. Evaluation of C-reactive healthy protein to aid the prescribing of antibiotics can reduce the overuse of antibiotic prescriptions.

A chest radiograph will show abnormalities in around 15% of patients but likely change therapy in just 5% of instances. A chest radiograph should be ordered in all patients with chest discomfort, leukocytosis, a background of cardiovascular disease, or various other complicating comorbidities. A chest CT scan does not need to be ordered routinely; however, a CT scan with contrast is preferred for the assessment of patients who may have a pulmonary embolism. In the majority of cases, a sputum culture is not likely to change treatment (Goldman & Shafer, 2020).

Corticosteroids and antibiotics are helpful for people when they have exacerbations of their COPD. Indications for a hospital stay include hypercarbia, acidemia, or substantial trouble with breathing regardless of bronchodilator treatment. In other situations, the choice is subjective and the practitioner needs to consider patients' social support, their living situation, if they have reliable transportation, and their capacity to manage activities of daily living. Likewise, in people who are admitted for inpatient therapy, the timing of discharge relies on these exact same factors.

Bacterial infection is present in approximately 50% of severe exacerbations of COPD. Prescription antibiotics, which need to be broad spectrum to cover the most common viruses (i.e., *Hemophilus influenza, Streptococcus pneumoniae*, and *Moraxella catarrhalis*), decrease the length of symptoms, especially in individuals with the classic trio of symptoms: coughing, worsening dyspnea, and sputum. In individuals with significant COPD, a history of hospitalizations or a history of bacterial colonization with *Pseudomonas aeruginosa*, an antibiotic with antipseudomonal properties should be considered. When choosing an antibiotic, the NPs and PAs should consider the antibiogram appropriate for their region.

Glucocorticoids need to be prescribed to patients with signs and symptoms of severe respiratory distress or impending respiratory failure. However, it should be noted that parenteral corticosteroids are not considered to be more effective and have been found to lead to medical complications and morbidity. Patients also need a short-acting bronchodilator to alleviate dyspnea. Antimuscarinics as well as beta agonists are similarly efficacious in this situation. Methylxanthines are not advised.

Supplemental oxygen should be given to patients with hypoxemia with the goal of maintaining an SaO_2 >90%. Some patients may see a small increase in PCO_2 due to modifications in their breathing pattern and V/Q matching; however, this phenomenon ought not to be the justification for reserving supplemental oxygen. In individuals with persistent respiratory distress, severe acidemia, or hypercarbia, noninvasive positive pressure ventilation (NIPPV) can improve hypercarbia and lower the necessity for intubation, and decrease the length of time spent in the intensive care unit (ICU). For patients who have persistent hypoxemia, ongoing hypercarbia, or acidemia in spite of NIPPV, invasive mechanical ventilation is indicated if such a treatment is consistent with the patient's living will. The NP/PA should order a lower respiratory rate to avoid dynamic hyperinflation (also known as *auto-positive end expiratory pressure* [*auto-PEEP*]) in the case of airflow blockage at expiratory. Exogenous PEEP can be used to reduce the chest wall muscle work associated with initiating inspiration if the assessment shows the presence of auto-PEEP.

In people with COPD, the FEV1 is used to predict mortality and other health issues. The BODE index is more accurate at predicting mortality than the FEV1 result alone. The BODE index integrates patient-reported dyspnea, spirometry outcomes, 6-minute walk distance, and body mass index to produce a result that ranges between 0 to 10, with the higher numbers signifying a higher risk of death. Scores varying from 7 to 10 have a 48-month mortality of approximately 80%.

Exacerbations are independent factors of the patient's quality of life and are associated with a rise in short-term mortality (approximately 10% for clients who are inpatients with an exacerbation) and longer-term death (43% at 1 year, 49% at 2 years). Hypoxemia at rest, weight-loss, a low body mass index, significant dyspnea, and reduced exercise resistance are independent predictors of death in individuals with COPD. Having COPD also increases the patient's chance of being diagnosed with lung cancer. Considering that most people with COPD have a substantial cigarette smoking history, the risk of having heart disease is also increased.

For clients with resting hypoxemia, supplementary oxygen treatment minimizes mortality. For patients with predominately upper lobe COPD who have considerable exercise limitations, lung volume reduction surgery minimizes mortality. End-of-life care after a diagnosis of end-stage COPD consists of palliative treatment and the prudent use of opioids for dyspnea (Goldman & Shafer, 2020).

Key Points

- Many chronic conditions in an older adult patient can also have an acute, episodic flare that requires special attention.
- Multidisciplinary teams are needed to manage acute and chronic medical conditions that impact the geriatric patient.
- Lifestyle changes can have a positive impact on many chronic conditions.

More information about tools and the Interprofessional Education Collaborative (IPEC) competencies mentioned in this chapter can be found in Appendix 1: Tools and Appendix 2: IPEC Competencies.

References

Adam, A., Dixon, A. K., Gillard, J. H., & Schaefer-Prokop, C. M. (2021). *Grainger & Allison's diagnostic radiology*. Elsevier.

Alaeddini, J. (2018). Angina pectoris treatment & management. *Medscape*. https://emedicine.medscape.com/article/150215-treatment.

Alpern, R. J., Moe, O. W., & Caplan, M. (2013). *Seldin and Giebisch's the kidney*. Elsevier.

American Diabetes Association (ADA). (2020). Classification and diagnosis of diabetes: Standards of medical care in diabetes—2020, 43(Supplement 1): S14–S31. https://doi.org/10.2337/dc20-S002.

American Heart Association. (2016). *Older Americans and cardiovascular disease*. https://www.heart.org/idc/groups/heart-public/@wcm/@sop/@smd/documents/downloadable/ucm_483970.pdf.

An overview of diabetes types and treatments. (2020). *Medical News Today*. https://www.medicalnewstoday.com/articles/323627.

Anderson, A. S., & Loeser, R. F. (2010). Why is osteoarthritis an age-related disease? *Best Practice & Research: Clinical Rheumatology*, *24*(1), 15. https://doi.org/10.1016/j.berh.2009.08.006.

Aroesty, J. M., & Kannam, J. P. (2020). Patient education: Medications for angina (Beyond the basics). *UpToDate*. https://www.uptodate.com/contents/medications-for-angina-beyond-the-basics#H13.

Atkinson, M. A., Eisenbarth, G. S., & Michaels, A. W. (2014). Type 1 diabetes. *Lancet, 383*(9911), 69–82. https://doi.org/10.1016/S0140-6736(13)60591-7.

Avichal, D. (2019). Hyperosmolar hyperglycemic state. *eMedicine Medscape*. https://emedicine.medscape.com/article/1914705-overview#a3.

Barter, P. J., et al. (2006). Targeting cholesteryl ester transfer protein for the prevention and management of cardiovascular disease. *Journal of the American College of Cardiology, 47*, 492–499.

Benetos, A., Petrovic, M., & Strandberg, T. (2019). Hypertension management in older and frail older patients. *Circulation Research, 124*, 1045–1060. https://doi.org/10.1161/CIRCRESAHA.118.313236.

Borlaug, B.A., & Calucci, W.S. (2019). Treatment and prognosis of heart failure with preserved ejection fraction. *UpToDate.com*. https://www.uptodate.com/contents/treatment-and-prognosis-of-heart-failure-with-preserved-ejection-fraction?search=treatment%20of%20heart%20failure&source=search_result&selectedTitle=6-150&usage_type=default&display_rank=3#H885140013.

Centers for Disease Control and Prevention (CDC). (2018, February 7). *Arthritis*. https://www.cdc.gov/arthritis/data_statistics/national-statistics.html.

Centers for Disease Control and Prevention (CDC). (2019, February 27). *Arthritis data and statistics*. https://www.cdc.gov/arthritis/data_statistics/disabilities-limitations.htm.

Colucci, W. S. (2020). Overview of the management of heart failure with reduced ejection fraction in adults. *UpToDate.com*. https://www.uptodate.com/contents/overview-of-the-management-of-heart-failure-with-reduced-ejection-fraction-in-adults?search=what%20is%20heart%20failure&source=search_result&selectedTitle=2-150&usage_type=default&display_rank=2.

Colucci, W. S., & Dunlay, S. M. (2020). Clinical manifestations and diagnosis of advanced heart failure. *UpToDate*. https://www.uptodate.com/contents/clinical-manifestations-and-diagnosis-of-advanced-heart-failure?search=diagnosis%20heart%20failure&source=search_result&selectedTitle=5-150&usage_type=default&display_rank=4#H3670655013.

Davies, M. J., D'Alessio, D. A., Fradkin, J., et al. (2018). Management of hyperglycemia in type 2 diabetes, 2018: A consensus report by the American Diabetes Association (ADA) and the European Association for the Study of Diabetes (EASD). *Diabetes Care, 41*(12), 2669–2701. https://doi.org/10.2337/dci18-0033.

Deveza, L. A. (2022). Overview of the management of osteoarthritis. *UptoDate.com*. https://www.uptodate.com/contents/overview-of-the-management-of-osteoarthritis?search=treatment%20of%20osteoarthritis&source=search_result&selectedTitle=1-150&usage_type=default&display_rank=1.

Dumitru, I. (2018). Heart failure. *eMedicine Medscape*. https://emedicine.medscape.com/article/163062-overview#a2.

Elliott, W. J., & Varon, J. (2020). Evaluation and treatment of hypertensive emergencies in adults. *UpToDate*. https://www.uptodate.com/contents/evaluation-and-treatment-of-hypertensive-emergencies-in-adults?search=hypertensive%20emergency&source=search_result&selectedTitle=1-150&usage_type=default&display_rank=1#H70455682.

Family Practice Notebook. (n.d.). *Framingham heart failure diagnostic criteria*. https://fpnotebook.com/cv/exam/FrmnghmHrtFlrDgnstcCrtr.htm.

Feehally, J., Floege, J., Tonelli, M., & Johnson, R. J. (2019). *Comprehensive clinical nephrology* (6th ed.). Elsevier.

Ferri, F. F. (2021). *Ferri's Clinical Advisor 2021*. Elsevier.

Gavet, F., Tournadre, A., Soubrier, M., Ristori, J. M., & Dubost, J. J. (2005). Septic arthritis in patients aged 80 and older: A comparison with younger adults. *Journal of the American Geriatric Society, 53*(7), 1210–1213.

Global Strategy for the Diagnosis, Management and Prevention of Chronic Obstructive Pulmonary Disease: 2019 Report. (2019). *Global Initiative for Chronic Obstructive Lung Disease (GOLD)*. www.goldcopd.org.

Goldman, L., & Shafer, A. I. (2020). *Goldman-Cecil medicine* (26th ed.). Elsevier.

Guerrero-Miranda, C. Y., & Hall, S. A. (2020). Cardiogenic shock in patients with advanced chronic heart failure. *Methodist Debakey Cardiovascular Journal, 16*(1), 22–26. https://doi.org/10.14797/mdcj-16-1-22.

Hamdy, O. (2019). Diabetic ketoacidosis. *eMedicine Medscape*. https://emedicine.medscape.com/article/118361-overview.

Han, M. K., Dransfield, M. T., & Martinez, F. J. (2020). Chronic obstructive pulmonary disease: Definition, clinical manifestations, diagnosis, and staging. *UpToDate.com*. https://www.uptodate.com/contents/chronic-obstructive-pulmonary-disease-definition-clinical-manifestations-diagnosis-and-staging?search=copd%20pathophysiology&source=search_result&selectedTitle=1-150&usage_type=default&display_rank=1#H263049240.

Han, M. K., & Wenzel, S. (2020). Asthma and COPD overlap (ACO). *UpToDate.com*. https://www.uptodate.com/contents/asthma-and-copd-overlap-aco?search=asthma%20copd%20overlap&source=search_result&selectedTitle=1-19&usage_type=default&display_rank=1.

Hines, R. L., & Marschall, K. E. (2018). *Stoelting's anesthesia and co-existing disease* (7th ed.). Elsevier.

Hirsch, I. B., & Emmet, M. (2020). Diabetic ketoacidosis and hyperosmolar hyperglycemic state in adults: Treatment. *UpToDate*. https://www.uptodate.com/contents/diabetic-ketoacidosis-and-hyperosmolar-hyperglycemic-state-in-adults-treatment?search=treating%20hyperosmolar%20hyperglycemic%20state&source=search_result&selectedTitle=1-106&usage_type=default&display_rank=1#H4565770.

International Diabetes Foundation (IDF). (2020). *What is diabetes?* https://www.idf.org/aboutdiabetes/what-is-diabetes.html.

Kahn, C. R. (1978). Insulin resistance, insulin insensitivity, and insulin unresponsiveness: A necessary distinction. *Metabolism, 27*, 1893–1902.

Kellerman, R. D., & Rakel, D. P. (2020). *Conn's current therapy: 2020*. Elsevier.

Krumholz, H. M., Normand, S. T., & Wang, Y. (2019). Twenty-year trends in outcomes for older adults with acute myocardial infarction in the United States. *JAMA Network Open, 2*(3), e191938. https://doi.org/10.1001/jamanetworkopen.2019.1938.

Link, J. J., Rohatgi, A., & de Lemos, J. A. (2007). HDL cholesterol: Physiology, pathophysiology, and management. *Current Problems in Cardiology, 32*(5), 268–314. https://www.clinicalkey.com/#!/content/journal/1-s2.0-S0146280607000059?scrollTo=%23top.

Loeser, R. F. (2017). The role of aging in the development of osteoarthritis. *Transactions of the American Clinical and Climatological Association, 128*, 44–54. https://www.ncbi.nlm.nih.gov/pmc/articles/PMC5525396/.

Maloney, G. E., & Glauser, J. M. (2018). Diabetes mellitus and disorders of glucose homeostasis. In R. M. Walls, R. S. Hockberger, & M. Gausche-Hill (Eds.), *Rosen's emergency medicine: Concepts and clinical practice* (9th ed.). Elsevier.

March, L., & Cross, M. (2019). Epidemiology and risk factors for osteoarthritis. *UptoDate.com*. https://www.uptodate.com/contents/epidemiology-and-risk-factors-for-osteoarthritis?search=epidemiology%20of%20osteoarthritis&source=search_result&selectedTitle=1-150&usage_type=default&display_rank=1.

Matthews, C. J. (2010). Septic arthritis in the elderly. *Medscape Aging Health, 6*(4), 495–500.

McCulloch, D. K., & Robertson, R.P. (2019). Pathogenesis of type 2 diabetes mellitus. *UpToDate*. https://www.uptodate.com/contents/pathogenesis-of-type-2-diabetes-mellitus?search=diabetes%20pathophysiology&source=search_result&selectedTitle=1~150&usage_type=default&display_rank=1#H3.

Moran, A. E., Oliver, J. T., Mirzaie, M., Forouzanfar, M. H., et al. (2012). Assessing the global burden of ischemic heart disease. *Global Heart, 7*(4), 315–329. https://doi.org/10.1016/j.gheart.2012.10.004.

National Council on Aging (NCOA). (2017). *The top 10 chronic conditions in adults 65+ and what you can do to prevent or manage them*. https://www.ncoa.org/blog/10-common-chronic-diseases-prevention-tips/.

National Heart, Lung, and Blood Institute. (n.d.). *What is metabolic syndrome?* https://www.nhlbi.nih.gov/health-topics/metabolic-syndrome.

National Institute on Aging (NIA). (2019). *Diabetes in older people*. https://www.nia.nih.gov/health/diabetes-older-people#:~:text=In%20Type%201%20diabetes%2C%20the,then%20have%20diabetes%20for%20life.

Pirahanchi, Y., & Huecker, M. R. (2019). Biochemistry, LDL cholesterol. *StatPearls*. https://www.ncbi.nlm.nih.gov/books/NBK519561/.

Reeder, G.S. (2019). Nitrates in the management of acute coronary syndrome. *UpToDate*. https://www.uptodate.com/contents/nitrates-in-the-management-of-acute-coronary-syndrome?search=treatment%20of%20stemi&topicRef=66&source=see_link#H13.

Reeder, G. S., & Kennedy, H. L. (2020). Diagnosis of acute myocardial infarction. *UpToDate*. https://www.uptodate.com/contents/diagnosis-of-acute-myocardial-infarction?search=stemi%20diagnosis&source=search_result&selectedTitle=1~150&usage_type=default&display_rank=1.

Roberts, J. R., Custalow, C. B., & Thomsen, T. W. (2019). *Roberts and Hedges' clinical procedures in emergency medicine and acute care* (7th ed.). Elsevier.

Rosenson, R. S. (2020). Low density lipoprotein-cholesterol (LDL-C) lowering after an acute coronary syndrome. *UpToDate*. https://www.uptodate.com/contents/low-density-lipoprotein-cholesterol-ldl-c-lowering-after-an-acute-coronary-syndrome?sectionName=OUR%20APPROACH%20TO%20IN-HOSPITAL%20THERAPY&search=treatment%20of%20stemi&topicRef=66&anchor=H97544243&source=see_link#H97544243.

Steffes, M. W., Sibley, S., Jackson, M., & Thomas, W. (2003). Beta-cell function and the development of diabetes-related complications in the diabetes control and complications trial. *Diabetes Care, 26*, 832–836.

Stoller, J. K. (2019). Management of exacerbations of chronic obstructive pulmonary disease. *UpToDate*. https://www.uptodate.com/contents/management-of-exacerbations-of-chronic-obstructive-pulmonary-disease?search=acute%20exacerbation%20of%20copd&source=search_result&selectedTitle=1~150&usage_type=default&display_rank=1#H542687361.

Streja, D., & Streja, E. (2017). Management of dyslipidemia in the elderly. *Endotext [Internet]*. https://www.ncbi.nlm.nih.gov/books/NBK279133/.

Vestbo, J., Anderson, W., Coxson, H. O., Crim, C., & Tal-Singer, R. (2008). Evaluation of COPD longitudinally to identify predictive surrogate end-points (ECLIPSE. *European Respiratory Journal, 31*, 869–873. https://doi.org/10.1183/09031936.00111707.

Waller, D. G., & Sampson, A. P. (2018). *Medical pharmacology and therapeutics* (5th ed.). Elsevier.

Weinstock, R. S. (2019). Management of blood glucose in adults with type 1 diabetes mellitus. *UpToDate*. https://www.uptodate.com/contents/management-of-blood-glucose-in-adults-with-type-1-diabetes-mellitus?search=treating%20type%201%20diabetes&source=search_result&selectedTitle=1~150&usage_type=default&display_rank=1.

What is type 1 diabetes? (n.d.). *UCSF Diabetes Education Online*. https://dtc.ucsf.edu/types-of-diabetes/type1/understanding-type-1-diabetes/what-is-type-1-diabetes/.

Wu, C. J., Huang, C. C., Weng, S. F., Chen, P. J., Hsu, C. C., Wang, J. J., Guo, H. H., & Lin, H. J. (2017). Septic arthritis significantly increased the long-term mortality in geriatric patients. *BMC Geriatrics, 17*, 178. https://doi.org/10.1186/s12877-017-0561-x.

Yelle, D. (n.d.). Ischemic heart disease. *McMaster Pathophysiology Review*. http://www.pathophys.org/acs/#Mechanisms_of_ischemia.

Yoon, J. S., So, C. H., Lee, H. S., & Hwang, J. S. (2018). *Journal of Pediatric Endocrinology and Metabolism, 31*(5), 503–506. https://doi.org/10.1515/jpem-2017-0463.

Zipes, D. P., Libby, P., Bonow, R. O., et al. (2019). *Braunwald's heart disease: A textbook of cardiovascular medicine* (11th ed.). Elsevier.

16

Musculoskeletal and Rheumatologic Conditions in the Older Adult

DENISE GOBERT, PT, PHD, NCS, CEEAA AND DEBRA MCDOWELL, BS, MSHP, PHD

OBJECTIVES

Student Learning Objectives

After completing this chapter, the student should be able to do the following:

1. The student will be able to explain the attributes of the physiology of the musculoskeletal system in the older adult.
2. The student will be able to demonstrate the normal process of aging and how this impact the musculoskeletal and rheumatological systems.
3. The student will be able to identify the roles of all providers in an interprofessional approach to the older adult.

Practitioner Objectives

After completing this chapter, the practitioner should be able to do the following:

1. The practitioner will be able to describe the benefits of functional training in older adults.
2. The practitioner will be able to outline the musculoskeletal and rheumatological conditions that impact the older adult.
3. The practitioner will be able to define how interprofessional collaboration can benefit the older adult's musculoskeletal and rheumatologic systems.

Introduction

The definition and epidemiology of musculoskeletal and rheumatologic conditions in the older adult are vast. Comprehensive nursing care of the older adult includes the combination of best practice skills and the integration of the awareness of common musculoskeletal and rheumatologic conditions. For the purposes of this chapter, the term *older adult* will include adults ages 65 years and older. However, the term might also be appropriately applied to adults ages 50 to 64 with clinical conditions or impairments that limit movements (American College of Sports Medicine [ACSM], 2018).

Physiologic aging may include changes such as muscle weakness, which can present with joint instability leading to a sequela that may compromise functional movement. Common clinical presentations include three primary nursing concerns or categories, which are pain, fall risk, and functional decline and disability.

CASE STUDY

Scenario

An 83-year-old female is brought to emergency department (ED) after she fell at home. On arrival to the ED, she reports that she thinks she hit her head against the bedroom nightstand but did not lose consciousness. The patient lives alone and was found on the floor by neighbors who check her every day. She has one son who lives about 45 miles away. She had been previously active and independent with her activities of daily living (ADLs) in a two-story home and walked the neighborhood regularly. She has type 2 diabetes mellitus (DM) and takes glyburide (5 mg/day) and nonvalvular atrial fibrillation treated with apixaban (5 mg BID).

Problem

On exam, she appears thin and frail and reports severe spasms and pain in right hip. There is shortening and external rotation of the right lower extremity. Her neurologic exam and CT scan of head are unremarkable. Plain radiographs of her pelvis and right hip show a displaced fracture of the midcervical section of the right femur. Intravenous (IV) morphine (2 mg) is given with good effect, and IV morphine (2 to 4 mg every 2 hours as needed for pain) is ordered. The orthopedic service is consulted, and arrangements are made to admit her to the ortho unit of the hospital to prepare for surgical repair of the hip fracture.

Discussion

Discussion points include the following:

- Patient lives alone in two-story home, frail body type, post–head injury, diabetic, atrial fibrillation

Possible consults include the following:

- Nursing, case management, inpatient occupational therapy and physical therapy, pharmacology, neurology

Pain

Pain is the number one subjective measurement used to gauge a patient's health status or response to treatment. However, there are several aspects to pain in the older adult that need to be considered. First of all, changes in the neural system become compromised through the aging process;

therefore the patient's sensation of pain might be less than optimal.

In addition, adults with symptoms of fibromyalgia may have hypersensitivity and altered subjective pain sensations. Therefore a comprehensive medical history along with physical signs and symptoms also need to be considered when documenting pain.

Fall Risk

Older adults are at higher risk for falls due to changes that include lower vital capacity, longer reaction times, decreased flexibility, decreased muscle strength, decreased bone mass, less fat-free mass, a higher percentage body fat, and longer recovery times from bouts of activity (ACSM, Table 7.2). Changes in the sensory systems include decreased vision as well as somatosensory and vestibular feedback; all of these changes provide updates about the body in space during static and dynamic balance activities.

Functional Limitation and Disability

Participation in activities of daily living (ADLs) become increasingly more difficult for older adults due to progressive changes in physical function, which include decreases in overall strength, balance, and mobility. The decline in physical function becomes classified as a "disability" when function does not meet the basic demands of specific activity required to participate in any previous social role. The World Health Organization (WHO) defines disability as "the ecological gap between what an environment demands of a person and what that person is capable of doing."

Although there are several models of disability in the older adult, the most popular and commonly known is the World Health Organization's International Classification of Functioning (ICF), which describes three primary themes including the interaction between bodily function and activities or ability to participate as indications of impairment or disability with eventual evolution to handicap. (See Fig. 16.1.)

Prevention of Musculoskeletal and Rheumatologic Conditions in Older Adults

Evidence suggests that physiologic aging occurs at different rates depending on several factors including genetic history, environment, and personal health behaviors (ACSM, 2018, Table 7. 2; Skinner, 2005). Common musculoskeletal deficits include low aerobic capacity, muscle weakness, and general deconditioning, which all result in lower functional mobility. Older adults with a rheumatologic condition may also experience accelerated changes in musculoskeletal impairments.

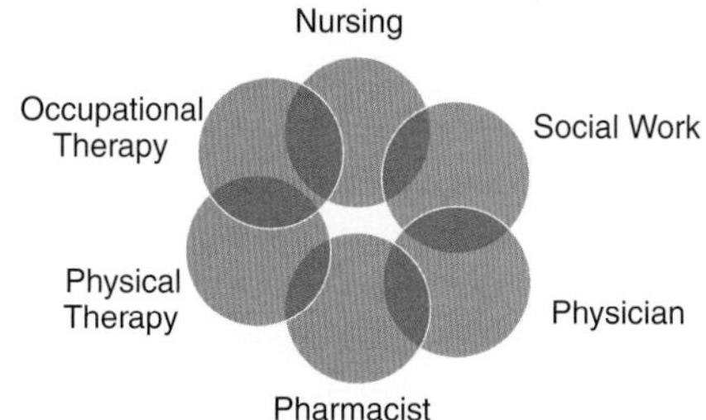

• **Fig. 16.1** Interprofessional patient-centered care.

Pharmacologic Intervention

Pharmacologic interventions become of greater consideration in older adults due to issues relating to changes in tissue integrity, pain, or longer recovery times. In addition, changes in metabolic rates may also interfere with how the body interacts with medications. This becomes more of a concern with long-term use. Evidence gathered between 2005 to 2011 indicates that 88% of older adults take at least one prescription drug and 36% take five or more prescription drugs (Qato et al., 2016).

Exercise

Although the benefits of exercise or physical activity are well known, only 11% of older adults engage in aerobic or muscle-strengthening exercise at levels recommended by US federal guidelines, and only 5% of adults 85 and older participate at recommended levels.

Recommended exercise includes the following:

1. *Stretching or flexibility exercise:* ≥ 2× per week. Stretch to the point of feeling tightness or slight discomfort, hold 30 to 60 seconds; any type of physical activity that allows slow movements to a static hold pattern.
2. *Strengthening exercise:* ≥ 2× per week. Light intensity for beginners with progression to moderate/vigorous intensities tolerated, 8 to 10 exercises involving major muscle groups, one to three sets with 8 to 12 repetitions each, any activity that includes major muscle groups.
3. *Aerobic or endurance exercise:* ≥ 5× per week for moderate intensity, 3× per week for vigorous intensity, or 3 to 5× per week for combined moderate and vigorous intensity; 30 to 60 minutes for moderate intensities and 20 to 30 minutes for vigorous intensities; type of activity includes any that do not impose undue orthopedic stress (ACSM, 2018, Table 7. 2).

Balance and Gait Training

Balance and gait training should be considered for all older adult patients. Changes in balance and gait or walking skills may occur with the aging process, therefore patient considerations should include a review of the patient's mobility skills.

There are simple physical performance screenings that can be used to see how well a patient is able to balance and walk. Evidence suggests that gait speed can be used as an indicator of general health, balance, and even mortality in older adults.

Gait speed is mostly stable between the ages of 20 and 60 years for a self-selected pace of 86 meters per minute or 1.37 to 1.43 meters per second (Bohannon, 1997). Gait speed may decrease with aging, especially in females. A slower gait speed has been associated with decreased toe clearance, decreased arm swing, and pelvic rotation.

In addition, older adults have been found to demonstrate decreased step length with increased step frequency to compensate. Changes in gait and balance have been identified to represent an important "sixth sense" because they are highly related to functional status and can predict health status, rehabilitation potential, and fall risk (Fritz, 2009). Common clinical tests are the 6-Minute Walk Test, the 10-Meter Walk Test, and the Timed Up and Go Test.

The 6-Minute Walk Test (6MWT) is a simple timed walk test in which the patient is asked to walk back and forth over 100 meters of level surface for 6 minutes. Results of the test are the total distance walked. Age-related normal values have been set and validated.

The 10-Meter Walk Test (10MWT) is another simple walk test; however, the primary outcome is gait speed. The patient is asked to walk over a set distant of 20 meters one way at a self-selected pace. The middle 10-meter portion is timed with a stopwatch and used to calculate walking speed. Age-related normal values have been set and validated.

The Timed Up and Go Test is a very good test used because it only requires a standard chair, a stopwatch, and an uncluttered, level space at least 3 to 4 meters in front of the chair. The test includes timing the patient as he or she rises from the chair, then walks 3 meters, turns, and returns to the chair and sits down. A timed walk greater than 10 seconds indicates a higher risk for falls.

Functional Training

Generalized changes in physical capacity can result in changes in an older adult's ability to perform activities of daily living, which include several levels of functional physical performance.

The World Health Organization defines functional activities as "tasks typically executed by an individual on a daily basis" or that are key to participating in work or leisure activities (WHO, 2020). Therefore the older adult may require functional training or training that mimics activities of daily living in a controlled and therapeutic environment.

Functional activities include total body movement such as changing one's body position or transferring from one surface to another. Therefore functional training might be classified into five basic categories according to body position and transitions involved, including horizontal mobility and sitting, transitional movements and transfers, ambulation and stair navigation, wheelchair mobility, and, lastly, upper extremity tasks. Examples of training might include bed mobility, transfers from sitting to standing, balancing on one leg to pull on pants, or reaching for a top-shelf item.

Interprofessional Collaboration in the Management of Musculoskeletal and Rheumatologic Conditions

It is important to develop interprofessional teams of different disciplines to provide coordinated, integrated care of older adults to promote common goals, shared resources, and responsibilities. It is especially beneficial when patients have complex medical, psychologic, and social needs, because clinical teams are better positioned to assess patient needs and create effective care plans than are practitioners who work alone.

Interdisciplinary teams can more effectively assure that the following occurs:

- Patients move safely and easily from one care setting to another and from one practitioner to another
- The most qualified practitioner provides care for each problem
- Care is not duplicated
- Care is comprehensive

A team typically includes physicians, nurses, nurse practitioners, physician assistants, pharmacists, social workers, psychologists, and sometimes a dentist, a dietitian, physical and occupational therapists, an ethicist, or a palliative care or hospice physician to name a few. Team members should have a knowledge of geriatric medicine, familiarity with the patient, dedication to the team process, and good communication skills. (See Fig. 16.2.)

Nurse Practitioner and Physician Assistant Roles

Gerontological nurse practitioners (GNPs) are advanced practice nurses with specialized education in the diagnosis,

Interprofessional Yet Mutually Exclusive Patient Care

Discipline	Diagnostics	Treatment	Social Integration	Prescriptive Care
Physician	X	X	X	Medical/Surgical
Nursing	X	X	X	Medical
Pharmacist		X		Medical
PT/OT Therapy	X	X	X	Therapeutic Exercise
Social Work			X	

• **Fig. 16.2** Interprofessional yet mutually exclusive patient care.

treatment, and management of acute and chronic conditions often found among older adults and generally associated with aging. The GNP has the clinical expertise to care for such aging persons. Practice sites of GNP include traditional ambulatory care clinics, care management companies, acute and subacute hospitals, private homes, and all levels of long-term care. Other GNPs work in specialty areas with expanded scopes of practice that require specialized education and close collaboration with other health care providers (American Association of Colleges of Nursing [AACN], 2016).

At least 160,000 physician assistants (PAs) practice in the United States (National Commission on Certification of Physician Assistants [NCCPA], 2018). These health care professionals practice medicine with physician supervision. Their use is widespread in all areas of medical care delivery, including geriatrics.

The role of PAs in American medicine has expanded and, as of 2003, PAs account for at least 10% of all outpatient contact. Most work in ambulatory care settings with significant numbers (27%) in specialty and subspecialty areas (NCCPA, 2018).

Nurse practitioners (NPs) and PAs perform *substitute* roles when they provide patients with the same range of services and perform the same functions as a physician—that is, they act as the usual providers of care. In contrast, PAs and NPs perform *supplemental* roles when they complement the services provided by physicians, such as delivering chronic disease care to patients within a practice.

NPs and PAs make up 17% of the primary care providers but act as the usual providers on only 13% of the panels. Nurse practitioners constitute the largest group (31.5%; n = 4806), followed by PAs (24.7%; n = 3767), mostly in rural areas in the south (Coombs et al., 2019).

Roles of Other Members of the Interprofessional Team

Physician

1. Primary care physician
2. Internist
3. Rheumatologist
4. Endocrinologist
5. Orthopedic surgeon
6. Radiologist

Pharmacist

Geriatric pharmacy specialists are pharmacists who have special knowledge in the care of older adults. Most curriculums offer some introductory information on geriatric pharmacy and disease states that often affect older adults; other schools may offer geriatrics-focused electives that allow students to become familiar with the approach to care for older adults.

Commonly, pharmacists who practice in long-term care are considered experts in geriatrics. These pharmacists provide a thorough review of medications for patients on a monthly basis and are trained to be aware of the needs of institutionalized older adults. Other pharmacists may choose to practice in ambulatory care settings where they work alongside prescribers to treat older adults still living in their communities. In the acute care setting, other pharmacists work in acute care for the elderly (ACE) units where geriatric patients receive care for emergent issues.

Rehabilitation Team

Physical Therapist

Geriatric physical therapy covers a wide area of issues concerning people as they go through the normal adult aging process, but it usually focuses on the older adult. Many conditions can affect people as they grow older; they include, but are not limited to, the following: arthritis, osteoporosis, cancer, Alzheimer disease, hip and joint replacement, balance disorders, and incontinence. Geriatric physical therapists specialize in providing therapy for such conditions in older adults (American Physical Therapy Association [APTA], 2019).

Occupational Therapist

Occupational therapy helps older adults develop, recover, or maintain the skills they need to do meaningful and necessary daily activities. Occupational therapists can help older adults overcome daily challenges caused by diminished ranges of motion and mobility. Occupational therapy is key during early stages of memory loss. Therapists assess a client's cognitive ability and help address any changes in the person's behavior or personality through behavioral modification.

Speech Therapist

Speech and language pathologists are important in the care of older adults because the aging process includes normal changes in speech, language, memory, and swallowing. In addition, the risk of these changes increases due to stroke, developing dementia, or Parkinson disease, as do the chances of acquiring a communication or swallowing disorder related to these diseases.

Social Worker or Case Manager

Social workers are crucial on the interdisciplinary team because they address the basics of biopsychosocial functioning and the design of interventions to treat a wide variety of challenges facing older adults. This updated edition includes content on the abuse and neglect of older adults, drug and alcohol abuse, and the social worker's role in dying, bereavement, and advance directives.

Certified case managers are specialists who assist seniors, people with special needs, and their families in planning for and implementing ways to allow for the greatest degree of health, safety, independence, and quality of life.

Musculoskeletal and Rheumatologic Disease Processes

Arthritis

Arthritis is a musculoskeletal disease that affects joints causing edema and tenderness, usually in multiple joints. A person's overall function and mobility are affected by arthritis, which most often results in decreased activity and social interaction, limitations with activities of daily living, and disability (Centers for Disease Control and Prevention, 2019).

The risk factors for arthritis increase with age, as 49.6% of provider-diagnosed cases from 2013 to 2015 were made for persons age 65 years or older (Barbour et al., 2017). As the US population ages and becomes more obese, the prevalence of provider-diagnosed arthritis is projected to increase, and two-thirds of those diagnosed with arthritis will be women. With the high prevalence of arthritis among older adults, it often occurs along with other chronic diseases and therefore complicates the management of the common chronic conditions due to the decreased activity associated with arthritis (Hootman et al., 2012, 2016). The most common forms of arthritis in older adults include osteoarthritis, crystal-associated arthritis, and rheumatoid arthritis (Centers for Disease Control and Prevention, 2019).

Approach to the Older Adult With Arthritis.

Osteoarthritis

Osteoarthritis (OA), also known as degenerative joint disease, is a chronic degenerative, late-onset disorder that appears to initially affect the articular cartilage of synovial joints then progresses to bony remodeling of the underlying bone with changes in soft tissues and synovial fluid. The loss of articular cartilage and synovial inflammation leads to signs and symptoms of joint stiffness, edema, pain, and loss of mobility (Musumeci, 2019).

Osteoarthritis is generally divided into two classifications: primary and secondary. The etiology of primary OA is unknown but is associated with risk factors that are related to the defect in the articular cartilage and it is considered to have a genetic component. Secondary OA occurs due to another disease or condition. Common conditions that can lead to secondary OA include obesity, joint trauma, surgery, congenital abnormalities, and hormonal disorders (Michael et al., 2010).

Osteoarthritis is the most common provider-diagnosed joint condition in adults 60 years of age and older, with approximately 10% of men and 18% of women in this age group affected. Globally, it is the most common joint disease and is a chief source of pain, disability, and socioeconomic cost (Barbour et al., 2017). The knee joints are most frequently affected, followed by the hand joints and the hip joints. Hip and knee versions of OA are chronic, painful, and slowly progressive degenerative joint diseases that usually lead to ambulatory dysfunction and are independent risk factors for falls. Older adults have an increased potential for falling than does the general population, with falls being one of the main causes of injuries, physical disability, and often death. The increased fall risk associated with OA can lead to irreversible social, health, and psychological consequences (Dore et al., 2014).

Etiology and Pathophysiology

Because of the etiology of OA, it is now considered to be a complex and multifactorial disease affected by systemic and local factors. Systemic factors include genetic and epigenetic predisposition, diet, estrogen deficiency, immune system response, bone metabolism, gender, age, and ethnicity.

Local risk factors are primarily biomechanical and include muscle strength, physical activity, soft tissue injury, repetitive mechanical loading, joint alignment, and bone inequality (Musumeci et al., 2015). Obesity is well established as a strong risk factor of OA with the relationship between obesity (body mass index >30) and hip OA being weaker than that between obesity and knee OA (Grotle et al., 2008; Litwic et al., 2013).

The older adult female presents an increased risk of OA due to decreased estrogen production after menopause. Numerous clinical studies have indicated that OA is directly related to lower estrogen levels. In addition, experimental and observational studies evidence the important role for estrogens in the homeostasis of joint tissues, with estrogen levels having a direct effect on joint cartilage, subchondral bone, and the synovium (Sowers et al., 2006).

Muscle weakness and ligament laxity are also directly related to OA. Estrogen has metabolic effects on skeletal muscle and is beneficial for muscle mass and strength. In postmenopausal women, higher rates of muscle protein synthesis and breakdown occur as compared to men of the same age (Chidi-Ogbolu & Baar, 2019; Smith et al., 2014). Because the primary function of ligaments is to provide stability to a joint during movement, ligamentous laxity is directly related to joint instability. Studies indicate that joint instability leads to abnormal mechanical loading that increases the risk of developing OA (Blalock et al., 2015; Farrokhi et al., 2014).

Much of the OA in older men is associated with occupational demands, especially kneeling and squatting, heavy lifting, and long-term use of heavy machinery. Jensen (2008) evaluated evidence for an association between hip osteoarthritis and physical work demands. Systemic literature reviews examined epidemiologic studies for an association between hip OA and heavy lifting, farming, construction work, and climbing stairs. The research concluded that there was a significant increase of hip OA in men whose activities involved heavy lifting, construction work, or farming. A positive association was determined between OA and stair climbing (Jensen, 2008).

Participating in sports has numerous health benefits by delaying the onset of chronic disease, modifying depression, increasing bone density, and improving metabolic health, especially as it relates to obesity. Evidence indicates an increased risk of OA in those who participate in elite sports that involve high-intensity impact, such as soccer (Arlianai et al., 2014; Tran et al., 2016).

Sports that involve direct joint impact and joint trauma, such as football and ice hockey, also have a significant correlation with a later onset of OA (Salzmann et al., 2017; Spahn et al., 2015). Research further indicates there is not a significant relationship between regular, moderate running and an increased risk of OA of the knees and hips in healthy people. In addition, existing evidence is currently insufficient to associate long-term long-distance running with OA (Cymet & Sinkov, 2006).

Pathogenesis of OA was historically understood to be a disease of mechanical cartilage degradation due to wear and tear on the cartilage. More recent research indicates that the cartilage, subchondral bone, and synovium all have key roles in the disease pathogenesis, and systemic inflammation plays an important role in the resultant symptoms and disease progression (Glyn-Jones et al., 2015).

Normal adult cartilage consists of an extracellular matrix made up of water, collagen, and proteoglycans. The main structural protein of cartilage is type II collagen that is regulated by chondrocytes in response to changes in the chemical and mechanical environment. Chondrocytes are influenced by several inflammatory response proteins, such as cytokines.

Research indicates that with the progression of OA, the production and operation of various cytokines vary depending on the stage of the disease process. The cytokine change disturbs the carbolic and anabolic process in the tissues subject to high mechanical load. Osteoarthritis then results from failure of the chondrocytes to maintain homeostasis between synthesis and degradation of the extracellular matrix components (Wojdasiewicz et al., 2014).

Articular cartilage provides a smooth, friction-free surface between the articulating bony ends while attenuating the mechanical load transmitted through the joint. Typical osteoarthritic cartilage is associated with increased anabolic and catabolic activity that leads to chondropathy with the cartilage softening and diminished cartilage thickness that becomes more pronounced with time. As the cartilage continues to break down, there is thinning and loss of the articular cartilage, resulting in exposure of the subchondral bone (Glyn-Jones et al., 2015).

With the excessive mechanical stress on the subchondral bone, sclerotic changes occur with subchondral bone plate thickness and the formation of new bone at the joint margins (osteophytes), leading to mechanical joint failure and loss of function. In addition, thickening of the synovial lining, increased vascularity, and infiltration of the synovial membranes with inflammatory cells all occur, particularly in the later stages (Neogi, 2012; Sanchez et al., 2012).

As OA progresses, cartilage loss, hypertrophic changes in the neighboring bone and joint capsule, mild synovial inflammation, and degenerative changes in the menisci, ligaments, and tendons all contribute to the patient's pain and loss of joint function with joint failure (Shakoor & Loeser, 2008).

Rheumatoid Arthritis

Rheumatoid arthritis (RA) is a systemic multifactorial autoimmune disorder, with chronic, inflammatory articular and extraarticular manifestations. Rheumatoid arthritis is a type of inflammatory polyarthritis because the disease process typically involves many joints in a symmetrical pattern, affecting the synovial lining of joints, articular cartilage, and juxtaarticular bone and can result in severe deformity and disability.

The disease can affect all joints but mainly involves the small joints of the foot and hand with erosive changes. For most persons diagnosed with RA, the disease process is aggressively progressive, commonly leading to bone erosion and joint deformity; the result is decreased function and quality of life with increased morbidity and mortality (Kobak & Bes, 2018). The disease typically progresses from the periphery to more proximal joints, resulting in significant disability within 10 to 20 years in patients who do not respond well to treatment (Venables & Chir, 2019).

The progression of RA is characterized by a fluctuating course with periods of exacerbation and remission of the symptoms. It is a complex disease that is one of the most common autoimmune disorders, even more prevalent than psoriasis, Crohn disease, and lupus. Because RA is a systemic disease, the cardiovascular, pulmonary, and gastrointestinal systems may be involved. Other possible extraarticular conditions may include eye lesions, infection, anemia, salivary gland issues, and osteoporosis.

Rheumatoid arthritis affects 1% of the US population with the average annual incidence approximately 70 per 100. Prevalence increases with age, with 5% of women over the age of 55 diagnosed with RA. The term used for RA that is diagnosed after the patient is 65 years of age is *elderly-onset RA (EORA)* (Kato et al., 2017).

The increase of RA within the geriatric population is attributed to two main factors. Patients with young-onset RA (YORA) are living longer with improved medical management, and the number of patients who are diagnosed with EORA is increasing. Although the onset of RA can occur at any age, the peak age at onset is in the fourth to fifth decades for females, and the prevalence increases in the sixth to eighth decade for males. Both the incidence and the prevalence of RA are two to three times higher in females than males (Kato et al., 2017; Kobak & Bes, 2018).

Patients with RA often have balance impairments as a result of impaired joint proprioception secondary to foot deformities, lower extremity muscle weakness, and limited joint range of motion that increases fall risk in this population. Static and dynamic balance disorders lead to inactivity and a more sedentary life, which increases the potential for an increased risk of falls, osteoporosis, fracture, and cardiovascular disease (Toprak et al., 2018).

Etiology and Pathophysiology

The cause of RA is unknown; however, gender, heredity, genetics, and environmental influences are known risk factors that increase the potential for the diagnosis of RA. An abnormal response of the immune system is the primary determinant for developing the disease process.

Characteristic of autoimmune diseases, RA develops in a genetically susceptible person. Research indicates that persons with a specific genetic marker, the HLA-DR shared epitope, have a five times increased chance of developing rheumatoid arthritis than do persons without the marker. Other genes are associated with the etiology of RA, including the STAT4 gene, which has an important role in the regulation and activation of the immune system; the TRAF1 and C5 genes, which have a role in chronic inflammation; and the PTPN22 gene, which is associated with both the development and the progression of RA. However, not all persons with these genes are diagnosed with RA, and not all persons who develop the disease have these genes (Seror et al., 2019).

Research additionally indicates that B cells produce autoantibodies: rheumatoid factor (RF) and cyclic citrullinated peptide (CCP). Both of these autoantibodies react with immunoglobulin antibodies in the blood and activate the complement system within the synovia that results in the triggering the production of proinflammatory cytokines and the inflammatory reaction is initiated. In addition, the B cells directly release cytokines with the deposit of immune complexes in the synovium. Lymphocytes, primarily T cells, are also activated in persons with RA, infiltrating the synovial tissue and contributing to inflammation and cytokine release in the joints (McInnes & Schett, 2007).

In affected joints, the synovium that is usually thin proliferates and thickens with an influx of leukocytes from the peripheral circulation and clinical synovitis results. Macrophages migrate to the diseased synovium in the early stages of the disease when there is vessel inflammation. These changes result in hyperplastic synovial tissue called pannus that no longer functions to lubricate the joint and provide nutrients to the avascular articular cartilage. This inflamed pannus intrudes upon the joint space and at the margins where the hyaline cartilage and synovial lining do not adequately cover the bone. This destructive vascular granulation tissue releases inflammatory mediators that erode cartilage, subchondral bone, articular capsule, and ligaments (McInnes & Schett, 2007).

There is controversy regarding the role of hormonal factors in the development of RA. However, overall, research indicates that the decline of estrogens is a risk factor for RA and high exposure to estrogens is a protective factor. Postmenopause has a direct association with an increased risk of developing seronegative RA. The incidence of RA in persons using antiestrogen agents was researched in a US national database for breast cancer. The use of these agents was associated with RA, with a dose- and duration-dependent effect (Alpizar-Rodriguez & Finckh, 2017; Beydoun et al., 2013; Pikwer, 2012).

Environmental factors are also associated with the etiology of RA; these include tobacco smoking, body mass index (BMI), and chronic infections. Several previous epidemiologic studies have identified smoking tobacco as an important risk factor for developing RA (Costenbader et al., 2014; Di Giuseppe et al., 2014). The risk of developing RA is approximately two times as high for smokers than nonsmokers, and there is evidence that smoking is a strong risk factor for developing seropositive RA (Chang et al., 2014; Seror et al., 2019; Zaccardelli et al., 2019). Liu et al. (2019) researched smoking cessation and reducing the risk of rheumatoid arthritis among women. The results confirmed that a behavior change of sustained smoking cessation could delay or prevent seropositive RA.

Zaccardelli et al. (2019) reviewed literature for cross-sectional studies, case-control studies, cohort studies, and clinical trials investigating modifiable lifestyle factors and RA risk. Meta-analyses of observational studies confirmed that obesity and overweight may increase overall RA risk. Patients with RA who underwent bariatric surgery showed significant improvements of symptoms of RA after substantial weight loss. However, more research is needed to provide correlations between weight loss and reduced RA risk.

Clinical studies suggest that there is an increased frequency of periodontal disease in patients with RA when compared to the general population. Findings support the hypothesis that chronic periodontal disease may be related to the initiation and maintenance of the autoimmune inflammatory responses correlated with RA (Zaccardelli et al., 2019). In addition, large retrospective cohort studies have indicated that the risk of myocardial infarction is 1.5 times higher in persons with RA when compared to controls with resulting increased cardiovascular mortality (Cheung & McInnes, 2017).

Crystal-Associated Arthritis (Gout)

Gout is a heterogeneous group of metabolic disorders; however, because the clinical presentation closely resembles arthritis, gout is also classified as a form of crystal-induced arthritis. Research evidence has determined that age is a risk factor for crystal-associated arthritis (Gamala et al., 2018).

Gouty arthritis is common in older adults, affecting 4.7 million people 60 years of age and older in the United States alone. The prevalence of gout increases with age in association with an increase in the incidence of several associated comorbidities. In addition, older adults who are diagnosed with gout are more likely to have comorbidities that often impair quality of life and reduce longevity (Abhishek, 2017).

Kuo et al. (2016) researched more than 39,000 charts from the UK Clinical Practice Research Data-link of patients diagnosed with gout to determine the burden of comorbidities in patients with gout at diagnosis and the risk of developing new comorbidities post diagnosis. The study concluded that the majority of patients with gout had worse preexisting health status at diagnosis and the risk of developing comorbidity continued to rise following diagnosis.

Women develop gout 7 to 10 years later than men, with a mean age ranging from 60 to 70 years as compared to the mean age in men, which ranges from 50 to 58 years. Menopause increases the risk of gout with the incidence of gout among postmenopausal women increasing secondary to the uricosuric effect of progesterone. However, regardless of gender, literature supports the belief that the risk for gout increases with age (Abhishek, 2017; Mirmiran et al., 2018). In Western countries, the prevalence of gout is 3% to 6% in men and 1% to 2% in women. Prevalence increases to 10% in men and 6% in women older than 80 years. The worldwide incidence of gout has increased gradually, primarily due to poor dietary habits such as the consumption of fast foods, lack of exercises, increased incidence of obesity, and metabolic syndrome (Ragab et al., 2017).

Older adults are also more likely to have tophaceous gout, with tophi typically forming at the hand interphalangeal joints, metacarpophalangeal joints, olecranon bursa, knee, and the Achilles tendon as subcutaneous white chalk deposits. In association, gout flares may manifest differently in the older population than in the young. The clinical presentation when first diagnosed in persons of all ages is characterized by symptoms in the first metatarsophalangeal (MTP1) joint. With geriatric patients, more joints than the first metatarsophalangeal joint are symptomatic at disease onset (Abhishek, 2017).

Older women often develop painful knees due to the formation of calcium pyrophosphate dihydrate (CPPD) crystals in the joint in a condition named chondrocalcinosis and often called pseudogout. With CPPD crystals in the synovial fluid, symptoms are identical to those associated with acute gout. Chondrocalcinosis may also cause polyarticular involvement and is associated with several metabolic disorders including hypothyroidism, hyperparathyroidism, hemochromatosis, and diabetes mellitus.

Etiology and Pathophysiology

Gouty arthritis is the most common crystallography in the United States. The development of gout in the majority of patients is associated with a continuous elevation of serum urate levels that results in a deposition of monosodium urate crystals in the musculoskeletal, soft tissues, and kidneys.

If inadequately treated, the deposition of these crystals produces recurrent acute flares, chronic arthritis, joint damage, and disfiguring tophi, large, visible bumps made of urate crystals. Furthermore, gout is a systemic disease that results from the deposition of the monosodium urate (MSU) crystals in tissues. Increased serum uric acid (SUA) above an identified threshold causes the formation of uric acid crystals. Hyperuricemia is most commonly defined as serum urate concentration >6.8 mg/dL. However, only approximately half of those with serum urate concentrations greater than 10 mg/dL develop clinically diagnosed gout over 15 years, implying that additional factors with prolonged hyperuricemia play roles in the pathogenesis of gout (Dalbeth et al., 2018).

There are three main classifications of gout, all of which most often begin at the first metatarsophalangeal joint causing sudden pain, swelling, and erythema. Primary hyperuricemia is an inherited condition with abnormal uric acid metabolism. Secondary hyperuricemia develops as a result of another metabolic disorder, medications that block uric acid excretion, or neoplasms. The third category, idiopathic hyperuricemia, includes conditions that are not characteristic of the other category symptoms.

Uric acid is a substance that results as the final product of purine nucleotide catabolism. At the normal physiologic pH of 7.4, uric acid circulates in the blood in the ionized form of urate. About two-thirds of uric acid is excreted through the nephrons in the kidneys, and the remaining third is excreted into the intestine. In the kidneys, approximately 90% of uric acid is reabsorbed (George & Minter, 2019). Urate production is enhanced by purine-rich diets, endogenous purine production, and high cell breakdown. Foods rich in purine include all meats but especially organ meats, game meats, and some seafood. Beer is purine rich and thus additionally increases uric acid levels by reducing kidney excretion. Endogenous production of purine may be accelerated by increased phosphoribosylpyrophosphate (PRPP) synthetase activity and by a deficiency in the regulatory enzyme hypoxanthine phosphoribosyltransferase (HPRT). Accelerated cell breakdown can occur due to rhabdomyolysis, hemolysis, and tumor lysis, which leads to increased urate production (Williams, 2019).

Steps for Diagnosing Arthritis

Osteoarthritis

Due to its high prevalence, OA is one of the leading reasons for office visits in the primary care setting. The diagnosis of osteoarthritis is primarily determined with a thorough history and physical examination findings, clinical symptoms, laboratory tests, and radiography to confirm the clinical diagnosis and rule out other conditions such as rheumatic disease. The Arthritis Foundation recommends that health care providers obtain the following information, along with the patient's health history and list of symptoms: a description of the symptoms; details about when and how the pain or other symptoms began; details about other medical problems that exist; locations of the pain, stiffness, or other symptoms; a description of how the symptoms affect daily activities; and a list of current medications.

The nurse practitioner (NP) or physician assistant (PA) relies on findings from the physical examination to determine the diagnosis of OA. The following discussion guides the provider through this examination. The main signs and symptoms of OA are pain, stiffness, and decreased function.

The pain tends to worsen with movement, activity, or extensive rest and decreases with rest. The pain is described as persistent and recurring with aching or tenderness with palpation of the joint. Upon examination, there may be crepitus, an audible crackling or grating sensation produced with the roughened articular or extraarticular surfaces approximate, usually occurring with motion, which may or may not be associated with the pain. Other symptoms include bony enlargement and malalignment, limited range of motion, joint deformity, and intraarticular joint effusion. Osteoarthritis symptoms usually worsen throughout the day, with increased stiffness with inactivity that will last approximately 5 to 10 minutes (Taruc-Uy & Lynch, 2013).

The weight-bearing joints, primarily the hip and knee, are the most commonly involved joints. The shoulder, lumbar and cervical spine, and the distal and proximal interphalangeal joints of the hand may be involved. Osteoarthritis is usually asymmetric. A patient may have severe, debilitating osteoarthritis of one joint and almost normal function of the contralateral side. Pain with range of motion and limitation of range of motion are common with the joints affected, but as with most conditions, each joint and each person will differ. In late stages of the disease, muscle atrophy around the affected joint will occur (Sinusas, 2012).

Pain with OA of the knee is most often felt around the knee and usually does not radiate. Loss of knee cartilage can lead to misalignment of the joint and possible leg length discrepancy. With OA of the medial knee compartment, a varus (bow-legged) deformity of the joint may occur. With progression of the disease, OA may occur in the lateral compartment of the knee with a resultant valgus or knock-knee deformity. With hip OA, pain is most commonly felt in the groin but may occur in the buttock and often down the anteromedial thigh to the knee. In addition, patients may complain of knee pain when the disease process is in the hip. With advanced OA, flexion deformity of the involved hip may develop. Patients often ambulate with an antalgic gait, with decreased weight-bearing on the involved side. As the disease progresses, a Trendelenburg gait may be evident (Doherty & Abhishek, 2019; Zhang, 2010).

With OA of the hand, gradual loss of joint range of motion can affect activities of daily living with it becoming more difficult for the patient to grasp small objects. With the progression of OA, the joints enlarge with the osteophyte formation that leads to deformity. These deformities are referred to as Heberden nodes when the distal interphalangeal joints are affected and Bouchard nodes when the proximal interphalangeal joints are involved. Lateral deformities of the joints may occur with the collateral ligaments becoming stretched, which can lead to the fingers overlapping and further functional disability (Haugen et al., 2011; Qin et al., 2017).

Generally, laboratory testing is not required to make the diagnosis of OA. Markers of inflammation, such as erythrocyte sedimentation rate and C-reactive protein level, are usually normal. If there is evidence of joint inflammation or synovitis, then immunologic tests, such as tests for antinuclear antibodies and rheumatoid factor, may be ordered. A measure of the patient's uric acid level is recommended, primarily if gout is suspected (Sinusas, 2012).

Plain radiography remains the mainstay with the clinical information for diagnosing OA. The Kellgren Lawrence grading system described by Kellgren and Lawrence in 1957 continues to be widely used in clinical practice to classify stages of OA and monitor progressions of the disease to enhance the plan of care. With this classification there are five grades, from 0 to 4, using the criteria of joint space narrowing and changes to bony structures. Grade 0 indicates that no radiographic features of osteoarthritis are present, and grade 4 is characterized by large osteophytes, marked joint space narrowing, severe sclerosis, and bony deformity (Braun & Gold, 2012; Kohn et al., 2016).

Studies are used more often when determining the pathology and progression of OA. MRI reveals the condition of the cartilage as it provides both morphologic and physiologic imaging techniques. A morphologic assessment of cartilage provides information about the tissue size and the integrity of the structure. MRI can determine image fissuring and focal or diffuse cartilage loss and can identify the presence of bone marrow lesions, visualization of the synovium, and periarticular inflammation (Braun & Gold, 2012; Guermazi et al., 2013).

The American College of Rheumatology (ACR) developed diagnostic guidelines for the clinical diagnosis of OA for the hip, knee, and hand. Using history, physical examination, and laboratory and radiographic findings, criteria include pain in the hip and two of the following: erythrocyte sedimentation rate <20 mm/hour, radiographic femoral or acetabular osteophytes, and radiographic joint space narrowing (superior, axial, or medial) (Altman et al., 1991).

For the knee, the following criteria are required using history, physical examination, and radiographic findings; they include pain in the knee and one of the following: patient over 50 years of age, less than 30 minutes of morning stiffness, and crepitus on active motion and osteophytes. With history, physical examination, and laboratory findings, criteria include pain in the knee and five of the following: patient over 50 years of age, less than 30 minutes of morning stiffness, crepitus on active motion, bony tenderness, bony enlargement, no palpable warmth of synovium, erythrocyte sedimentation rate (ESR) <40 mm/hour, rheumatoid factor (RF) <1:40, and synovial fluid signs of osteoarthritis (Altman et al., 1991).

Clinical classification criteria for OA of the hand include pain, aching, or stiffness in the hand and three of the following: hard tissue enlargement of two or more of the following joints: second and third interphalangeal or proximal interphalangeal joints and the first carpometacarpal joints of both hands, hard tissue enlargement of two or more distal interphalangeal joints, fewer than three swollen MCP joints, and deformity of at least one of the joints listed previously (Altman et al., 1991).

Rheumatoid Arthritis

The disease onset with rheumatoid arthritis (RA) is usually insidious, with predominant symptoms of pain, morning stiffness for more than 30 minutes, and swelling of multiple joints. Morning stiffness that lasts more than 1 hour indicates severe joint inflammation that rarely occurs in diseases other than RA. With early onset of RA, the typical joints involved include the metacarpophalangeal (MCP) and proximal interphalangeal (PIP) joints of the fingers, the interphalangeal joints of the thumbs, the wrists, and the metatarsophalangeal (MTP) joints of the toes. Elbows, shoulders, ankles, and knees are also commonly affected. With joint pain and swelling of the small joints, grip strength is decreased.

Involvement of the axial skeleton is commonly limited to the cervical spine that can result in serious neurologic compromise in patients with neurologic symptoms that include burning paresthesias and numbness. Patients complain of aching neck pain that is aggravated by cervical range of motion and often radiates into the occipital, retroorbital, or temporal areas. Chronic inflammation of the atlantoaxial joint can lead to laxity of the transverse ligament resulting in the dens no longer being positioned closely against the anterior arch of the atlas. As the dens drifts backward, it compresses the spinal cord during forward cervical flexion. Developing symptoms include a shocklike sensation and numbness down the upper extremities with forward cervical flexion.

With joint involvement, as the disease progresses, joint deformity can occur with subluxation. Common deformities in the fingers include ulnar deviation, swan-neck deformity, and boutonniere deformity. Extensor tendons slip to the ulnar aspect of the metacarpal head and thus cause the ulnar deviation. The swan-neck deformity (Fig. 16.3) occurs with hyperextension of the proximal interphalangeal joint and partial flexion of the distal interphalangeal joint. Boutonnière deformity (Fig. 16.4) is caused by flexion of the proximal interphalangeal joint with hyperextension of the distal interphalangeal joint.

Physical findings and symptoms of systemic and nonarticular manifestations with RA may include generalized aching, diffuse musculoskeletal pain, weight loss depression, deconditioning, and fatigue. A systematic review suggested that pain, sleep disturbance, cognitive, emotional, and physical function contribute to the fatigue. It remains unclear if depression is caused by negative cognitive perceptions, behavioral tendencies, or immune-mediated processes (Matteson & Davis, 2019).

Extraarticular involvement of RA is indicative of disease severity and is associated with increased morbidity and premature mortality. Successful management of the systemic manifestations of RA depends on the control of the underlying joint disease. Extraarticular manifestations (EAMs) mostly involve cutaneous cardiovascular and pulmonary systems. EAMs present a serious problem to the treating clinicians, as they are difficulty to diagnose yet need to be treated aggressively and need intense and frequent monitoring.

One of the most common cutaneous manifestations of RA is the development of nodules. Rheumatoid nodules occur in approximately one-fourth of patients with RA in both genders and vary in severity, size, and shape. These nodules are firm, obvious lumps that form subcutaneously and are generally located on or near the base of the arthritic joints. The typical locations for these nodules include the finger joints, elbows, forearms, knees, and the distal heels.

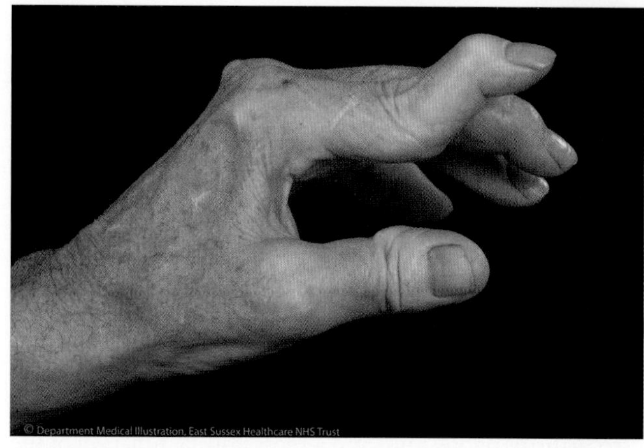

• **Fig. 16.3** Swan neck deformity of an index finger. (From Bulstrode, N. W., et al. [2022]. *Plastic surgery principles and practice.* Elsevier.)

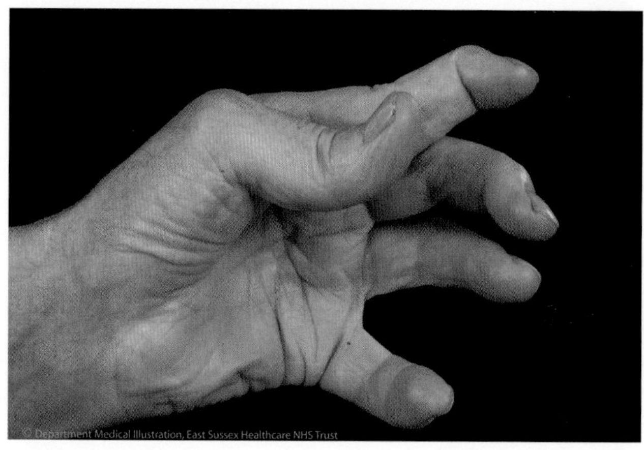

• **Fig 16.4** Boutonnière deformity of thumb. (From Bulstrode, N. W., et al. [2022]. *Plastic surgery principles and practice*. Elsevier.)

The leading cause of death among patients with RA is cardiovascular disease (CVD), for which these patients have a 50% higher risk than the general population (Marcucci et al., 2018). Additionally, a meta-analysis of studies of stroke and stroke subtypes in rheumatic diseases demonstrated a higher risk of cerebrovascular disease in RA patients, with persons less than 50 years of age having two times the risk in comparison to the general population (Wiseman et al., 2016).

Rheumatoid arthritis is also associated with several specific cardiac manifestations, which include pericarditis, myocardial disease, coronary vasculitis, and valvular involvement. A systematic review and meta-analysis of case-control studies that utilized an echocardiographic assessment of valvular and pericardial involvement in RA patients asymptomatic for cardiac disease revealed specific disease-related cardiac structure involvement. This asymptomatic heart involvement in RA is termed *silent rheumatoid heart disease* and has been significantly associated with an increased risk of heart failure (Wiseman et al., 2016).

Pulmonary involvement is another common extraarticular disease in RA. The prevalence of lung involvement in RA patients is approximately 50%. RA may affect all areas of the lung, including the airways, pleura, parenchyma, and vasculature, leading to significant morbidity and mortality. Lung disease is the second most common cause of death for those with RA, especially when these patients are susceptible to infection. Many of the respiratory manifestations associated with RA occur within the first 5 years of the diagnosed disease (Kelly et al., 2016).

The susceptibility to serious infection may be due to multiple predisposing factors that include disease activity, comorbidities, and the use of immunosuppressive drugs. The most common sites of serious infections involve the lower respiratory tract, skin, and soft tissues (Atzeni et al., 2017).

Studies support evidence that persons with RA are at an increased risk for osteoporosis for several reasons. Glucocorticoid medications prescribed for the treatment of RA have major effects on the metabolism of calcium, vitamin D, and bone that can lead to osteopenia, osteoporosis, and fractures. Persons with RA have twice the risk of hip and vertebral fractures, which is directly associated with low bone mineral density. In addition, pain and loss of joint function result in activity that further increases the risk of developing osteoporosis. The disease process of RA also directly affects bone loss, as studies indicated that the bone loss is most pronounced in areas immediately adjacent to the affected joints (National Institutes of Health [NIH], 2018).

The initial evaluation of patients with suspected RA must include a careful history and physical examination with laboratory tests that will identify characteristics associated with RA or that suggest an alternative differential diagnosis. This history includes personal and family medical history, and strict attention is paid to reported joint pain and edema and the presence, location, and duration of morning stiffness. The longer the symptoms have existed, the more likely there will be a diagnosis of RA.

Each joint should be palpated for tenderness and swelling and examined for signs of inflammation, nodules, and limited range of motion. The number and pattern of the joint involvement will indicate a typical pattern of RA as discussed previously.

In 2010, the American College of Rheumatology and European League Against Rheumatism collaborated and created new classification criteria for RA. These criteria were developed to assist with diagnosing RA earlier. The 2010 criteria do not include the presence of rheumatoid nodules or radiographic erosive changes, as these symptoms are less likely seen in early RA. Symmetric joint presentation is also not required in the 2010 criteria to allow for early asymmetric diagnosis (Wasserman, 2011). See the classification criteria for RA presented in Table 16.1 (from: https://www.aafp.org/pubs/afp/issues/2011/1201/p1245.html).

The laboratory tests that are most commonly recommended for the diagnosis of RA include assessments of the following: rheumatoid factor (RF), cyclic citrullinated peptide (CCP), erythrocyte sedimentation rate (ESR), C-reactive protein (CRP), and antinuclear antibody (ANA). RF is found in approximately 80% of patients with RA yet RF's sensitivity for the detection of RA is only 50%. Seventy to eighty percent of patients with established RA have serologic titers of anti-CCP antibody that are 95% specific for the disease. Determining the ESR and CRP levels in patients who are having symptoms suggestive of RA is also an important component of the laboratory prescription. The degree of elevation of both of these inflammatory markers most often mirrors the extent of RA pathology that is occurring. ANA measurement, complete blood cell (CBC) count, platelet count, serum uric acid measurement, and human leukocyte antigen (HLA) tissue testing assist with the differential diagnosis of RA, distinguishing it from other arthritic and immunologic pathologies. Because moderate hypochromic normocytic anemia is commonly seen, iron levels should be monitored (Katchamart et al., 2017).

Joint fluid should be assessed to measure the degree of inflammation while ruling out gout or septic arthritis. RA joint fluid tends to be more yellow to opalescent, with a higher white blood count and platelet count than osteoarthritic joint fluid. Arthrocentesis is a diagnostic tool that is needed to rule out septic arthritis, which may be a severe complication of RA.

Conventional radiography of the hands or feet in patients with undifferentiated inflammatory arthritis significantly supports the diagnosis of RA. Evidence recommends that radiographs of the hands should be performed in all persons who have clinical manifestations that suggest RA, whereas radiographs of the feet are recommended when radiography of the hands is normal (Katchamart et al., 2017).

In addition, the Leiden Early Arthritis Clinic in the Netherlands derived a clinical prediction rule for identifying RA among patients with undifferentiated arthritis (UA): the Leiden score. Furthermore, the rule guides follow-up and referral (van der Helm-van Mil et al., 2007).

Ghos et al. (2016) performed a group comparative longitudinal study model involving patients who had early symmetrical polyarthritis. It was concluded that the Leiden prediction rule is highly applicable to predict the progression of RA in undifferentiated arthritis patients.

Crystal-Associated Arthritis (Gout)

An acute gout flare is usually monoarthritic in the initial stages of the disease and peaks within hours, manifesting as a severely inflamed joint that is red, hot, edematous, and tender to the touch or movement. Gout attacks are usually self-limiting, with symptoms resolving within 2 weeks. However, ongoing joint damage occurs during the asymptomatic remission due to continuing monosodium urate (MSU) crystal deposition and inflammation (Ruoff & Edwards, 2016).

Attacks of arthritis caused by gout are very painful, leading to a decreased ability to perform activities of daily living. Diagnosis is usually based on the patient's clinical presentation and confirmed by findings of monosodium urate crystals in the synovial fluid. A good differential diagnosis of gout begins by taking a patient's medical history. Medications must be analyzed as well as the patient's diet and alcohol intake. Any involved joints must be examined for symptoms of inflammation: edema, erythema, increased temperature, and pain. Details of the flare are important for determining the severity of the pain, length of the attack, and joints affected. Untreated flares can last from hours to weeks and become chronic, which may lead to joint destruction. Uric acid–lowering drugs are effective to prevent further attacks and joint destruction, especially if started early in the course of the disease. Therefore an early and accurate diagnosis of gout is crucial (Gamala et al., 2018; Khanna et al., 2014).

Besides a diet rich in purines, increased adipose tissue is linked to hyperuricemia. Higher body mass index and weight gain are contributing factors to gout in men. Studies have evidenced a strong connection between obesity hyperuricemia and a higher risk of gout (Gancheva et al., 2019).

Some medications are associated with the development of the monosodium urate crystals because they affect the raising or lowering of serum urate concentrations. These drugs include thiazide and loop diuretics, low-dose aspirin, cyclosporine, levodopa, and uricosuric agents (Becker & Gaffo, 2019). The risk of incident gout was significantly associated with the use of beer or liquor, but not wine. Rates of gout among drinkers of similar amounts of alcohol per day were compared with those among nondrinkers. Drinking two or more beers daily increased the risk of gout by 2.5 compared with no beer intake. The risk of gout was also increased in males who reported drinking a similar amount of liquor per day, with the risk being lower than with beer (Becker & Neogi, 2019).

The diagnosis of gout based on hyperuricemia is a common misconception among providers who are nonrheumatologists. Although hyperuricemia is characteristic of gout, during gouty attacks it might drop to normal levels. Thus hyperuricemia is a weak marker for the differential diagnosis of gout.

The gold standard for the diagnosis of gout is the identification of monosodium urate (MSU) crystals in tissues. Involved joints need to be aspirated and the aspirated synovial fluid examined by polarized light microscopy. Samples should be examined as soon as possible, with the best determination arrived at within 6 hours. This is to avoid cellular dissolution and the disappearance of crystals. The synovial fluid is often opaque with low viscosity, and a leukocyte count that is often >10,000/mm^3. The diagnosis is confirmed with the presence of birefringent needle-shaped monosodium urate crystals. Additionally, the aspirated synovial fluid should undergo Gram stain and be cultured to rule out septic arthritis (Abhishek, 2017; Ragab et al., 2017).

Conventional radiography is the most widely used imaging in gouty arthritis diagnosis in clinical practice. It is widely available, inexpensive, fast, and acceptable by most patients. Musculoskeletal ultrasonography is another imaging method that may be utilized to evaluate gouty joints. This is a noninvasive technique that identifies where the crystals have been deposited in the joint. Monosodium urate crystals can be identified on ultrasound by hyperechoic irregular enhancement of the articular surface of the hyaline cartilage, called the double contour sign. The double contour sign suggests tophi within the joint or along tendons. Ultrasound features of the crystal deposition have high specificity and high positive predictive value but more limited sensitivity for early gout (Ogdie et al., 2016; Taylor & Law, 2019).

The newest modality to image monosodium urate crystal deposits is dual-energy CT (DECT) scan. The diagnostic findings are classified as positive if urate deposition is observed and as negative if no urate deposition is observed. Systematic review indicates that the pooled sensitivity and specificity of DECT for detecting gout were 0.87 and 0.84, respectively. DECT is advocated in cases where a definitive diagnosis cannot be made from signs, symptoms, and MSU analysis alone. It may additionally be a useful diagnostic imaging tool for patients who have difficulty undergoing joint aspiration (Gamala et al., 2018).

Factors to Consider in the Treatment of Arthritis

Osteoarthritis

Treatment choices fall into four main categories that include nonpharmacologic, pharmacologic, complementary and alternative, and surgical. Treatment should begin with the safest and most conservative interventions before proceeding to more invasive and expensive therapies. Treatment of OA must be patient centered and managed on an individual basis based on the degree of arthritis and disability and on any comorbidities that the patient may have. Currently recommended conservative treatments are weight loss, physical therapy/exercise, activity modification, drugs, braces/orthotics, and intraarticular injections

Activity modification includes the recommendation of low-impact exercises such as walking and the importance of physical activity for overall health. Low-impact aerobics activities that do not put stress on the joints include brisk walking, cycling swimming, water aerobics, light gardening, group exercise classes, and dancing. The combination of weight loss and moderate exercise promotes improvements in function, pain, and mobility in older adults with OA who are overweight or obese. Weight loss also leads to increased function in obese older adults.

The American College of Rheumatology advocates that exercise is one of the most effective nonpharmaceutical treatments to assist with reducing pain and improving movement in persons with osteoarthritis. Research has determined that for individuals with osteoarthritis, activities that combine strengthening and aerobic exercise reduce symptoms, improve joint motion and function, enhance coordination and balance, and control body weight. In addition, exercising has the potential to improve knee cartilage in patients at high risk of developing OA (Kraus et al., 2019).

Other factors to evaluate when interacting with patients with osteoarthritis are anxiety and depression. Several studies suggest that greater pain is associated with decreased coping, increased depression, reduced physical ability, and decreased quality of life (Parker et al., 2014).

When depression is diagnosed in addition to OA, there is a significant decrease in social interaction and increased physical limitation. Research indicates that the degree of OA pain is predictive of future fatigue, disability, and depressed mood. Persons with the comorbidity of anxiety and depression had increased provider visits, health care utilization, drug prescription, adverse surgical outcomes, and increased postsurgical pain. Higher levels of depressed mood are significantly associated with female gender. OA management strategies should include self-care, collaborative care, social/phone support, pharmacotherapy, music, educational videos about OA procedures, and yoga (Sharma et al., 2016).

Patients with OA frequently turn to complementary alternative medicine (CAM) for relief of the symptoms associated with the condition. The use of CAM among patients with OA is significantly higher than in the general population, with a reported prevalence of up to 90%. Thus the recommendation is that health care providers should include questions about the use of CAM with the routine assessment of patients with OA (Herman et al., 2004).

Dimethyl sulfoxide (DMSO) and methylsulfonylmethane (MSM) are two related nutritional supplements widely used for the symptomatic relief of OA. Brien et al. (2011) performed a meta-analysis of research concerning these two supplements in the treatment of OA of the knee. Evidence suggests that DMSO and MSM are not clinically effective in the reduction of pain during the treatment of OA. No definite conclusions could be drawn from the data, as the findings were mixed and dosing was not consistent.

The dietary supplements glucosamine and chondroitin sulfate are also popular in the general population of persons with OA. The glucosamine/chondroitin arthritis intervention trial (GAIT) evaluated the efficacy and safety of these supplements as a treatment for knee pain from OA. The results indicated that alone or in combination, pain was not decreased effectively in the overall group of patients with OA of the knee. The statistical analyses did suggest that the combination of glucosamine and chondroitin sulfate may be effective in the subgroup of patients with moderate-to-severe knee pain (Clegg et al., 2006).

Some herbal products are also used topically for OA. A 2013 study of the evidence on topical herbal products suggested that arnica gel and comfrey extract gel might be helpful. The research further concluded that capsicum extract gel most likely is not beneficial. The evidence on any other products was insufficient for conclusions to be reached (Cameron, 2013).

Rheumatoid Arthritis

Clinical evidence clearly indicates that joint damage with RA starts at the very beginning of the disease, therefore early diagnosis and treatment are critical to interrupt the disease process and improve long-term outcomes. Providers are met with a challenge to immediately diagnose RA and ideally refer the patient to a specialized arthritis clinic. Generally, treatment goals for a patient with RA are to significantly decrease pain and to maintain and improve mobility and function by minimizing stiffness, edema, and joint destruction. Therapy for RA has evolved from simple symptomatic treatment with antiinflammatories to prescribing pharmacologic agents that target the underlying pathophysiology with disease-modifying antirheumatic drugs (DMARDS). Therapy goals are targeted to have little or no evidence of the disease progression. The management of treatment must be highly individualized because the disease process is individually varied with patients often having different desired outcomes. A younger patient diagnosed early may want to have disease remission, whereas an older patient with progressed symptoms may want a decrease in painful symptoms (Burmester & Pope, 2017; McMahon, 2018).

Because fatigue is a common symptom of RA, inflamed joints should be rested, but it is important for the patient to stay physically active. Exercise and physical activity are most beneficial as a significant part of RA treatment. Home exercise should emphasize low-impact aerobics, muscle strengthening, and flexibility. These exercises can help prevent and reverse the loss of joint motion, contractions, and decreased muscle strength associated with RA (Gecht-Silver & Duncombe, 2018).

Referral for physical and occupational therapy is paramount for helping to relieve pain, decrease inflammation, and preserve joint integrity and function for patients with RA. Physical therapists and occupational therapists play a vital role in helping patients to improve and maintain function that may be limited due to RA.

Referral to a dietician is also recommended due to the weight loss and weight gain experienced by patients with RA. Although there is no definite correlation between diet and RA, studies have determined that the type of inflammation associated with RA may be modulated by certain foods.

Patient education is highly recommended to help patients with RA understand the disease process, treatment, possible outcomes, and the role of exercise and self-care that is most important to support patient management. Health education enhances the patient's knowledge of the illness with aims to modify health habits and lifestyle in order to be able to collaborate in therapy (Khoury et al., 2015).

The Arthritis Foundation offers programs on topics that include self-management skills, social support, biofeedback, and psychotherapy. These programs have been shown to reduce pain, depression, and disability in persons with arthritis and enable them to gain some control over their condition. The brochures available describe exercise benefits and types of exercises, how to start, and how to keep compliant. Patients are educated about the possible effects of not exercising.

The Arthritis Foundation Exercise Program (AFEP) is a group recreational program that is now supported by the Aquatics Exercise Association. The AFEP promotes physical activity as a strategy for self-managing RA symptoms and improving or maintaining mobility, strength, and physical function. The AFEP can be modified for patients who are sedentary with limited joint mobility but is also effective for persons who are relatively active with only mild joint impairment or other symptoms.

The Arthritis Foundation Exercise Program is held at recreation centers, senior centers, and other community facilities; patients meet in groups of 15 to 20 people for 1 hour twice weekly. A randomized, controlled trial of the AFEP funded by the Centers for Disease Control and Prevention confirmed these findings, particularly in persons who attend more than half of the class sessions (Callahan et al., 2018).

Crystal-Associated Arthritis (Gout)

The keystone treatment for gout is achieved by a number of approaches that include urate-lowering drug therapy, lifestyle modification, and other strategies for risk reduction. The British Society for Rheumatology/British Health Professionals in Rheumatology published guidelines for the management of gout in 2007. These were revised and updated in 2017 because of the availability of new pharmaceutical treatment options and increases in the incidence, prevalence, and severity of gout. The guidelines include key recommendations for the management of acute attacks, modification of lifestyle and risk factors, and the optimal use of urate-lowering therapies. The goals of intervention fall into two main categories: (1) to stop acute gouty attacks and prevent recurrent attacks; and (2) to correct the underlying hyperuricemia (Hui et al., 2017).

According to both the American College of Rheumatology (ACR) guidelines and the European League Against Rheumatism (EULAR) recommendations, the UA goal for urate-lowering therapy (ULT) is <6 mg/dL to facilitate faster dissolution of crystals for patients with severe gout until total crystal dissolution and resolution of gout occurs (Richette et al., 2017).

Ten percent of the uric acid produced in the body comes from foods. Patients must be educated in gout management recommendations for diet and exercise. The ACR used input from national and international medical experts and published key recommendations for gout management, which include increased intake of vegetables, decreased intake of purine-rich meat and seafood, and decreased alcohol consumption, especially beer, with no alcohol during an acute gout attack (Morelli, 2019).

The Academy of Nutrition and Dietetics recommends referral to a registered dietitian or nutritionist for education and the development of a gout-friendly diet that is nutritious (Gordon, 2019). Because risk factors for gout include adiposity and weight gain, weight loss in overweight patients is beneficial for decreasing the serum urate and gout symptoms in patients with diagnosed gout.

Neilson et al. (2017) performed a systematic review of longitudinal studies that reported weight loss in overweight/obese patients with gout. Findings reported the beneficial effects of weight loss on serum urate levels, achievement of the serum urate target, and a reduction in gout attacks. Maglio et al. (2017) assessed the long-term effect of bariatric surgery on the incidence of gout and hyperuricemia in participants of the Swedish Obese Subjects study. The study concluded that bariatric surgery prevents gout and hyperuricemia in obese subjects.

Treatment Options for the Older Adult With Arthritis

Pharmacologic Intervention

Osteoarthritis

Pharmacologic intervention for osteoarthritis is used primarily to help patients manage pain and maintain an active lifestyle. Acetaminophen is often recommended as the first drug of choice to treat mild or moderate osteoarthritic pain without symptoms of inflammation. When acetaminophen is ineffective or if the clinical symptoms are inflammatory, nonsteroidal antiinflammatory drugs (NSAIDs) are prescribed for the symptomatic treatment of pain with OA. Traditional NSAIDs generally cause more gastric symptoms than acetaminophen and thus present a limiting factor in the long-term use of these agents. The cyclooxygenase (COX)-2 inhibitors present an alternative when acetaminophen is ineffective for long-term intervention. The lowest effective dose is advised initially, increasing if the response is not significant (Ciccone, 2015; Lozada & Pace, 2019).

In addition, the analgesic tramadol has been prescribed for highly resistant OA pain. However, Zeng et al. (2019) performed an observational study of more than 88,000 patients diagnosed with OA. An initial prescription of tramadol was associated with a significantly higher rate of mortality over 1-year follow-up compared with commonly prescribed NSAIDs in patients 50 years of age and older.

The Agency for Healthcare Research and Quality (AHRQ) compared analgesics recommended for osteoarthritis. No analgesic reviewed was significantly more effective than another. The AHRQ comparison additionally stated that acetaminophen was only slightly inferior to NSAIDs in reducing osteoarthritic pain but was associated with a lower risk of gastrointestinal (GI) symptoms. The AHRQ report also noted that topical diclofenac had efficacy similar to that of oral NSAIDs in patients with localized OA (AHRQ, 2021).

Newer pharmacologic agents have emerged for mild to moderate OA that actually attempt to slow or reverse the pathologic changes in OA: disease-modifying osteoarthritic drugs (DMOADs). There are two general types of DMOADs: agents that work to improve the viscosity and function of synovial fluid (viscosupplementation) and drugs that act as precursors to the normal joint tissues (glucosamine and chondroitin sulfate).

With viscosupplementation, hyaluronan (hyaluronic acid) is injected into a joint affected by OA to help restore the normal viscosity of the synovial fluid, thus reducing joint stress and limiting the progression of articular destruction leading to decreased pain and increased function. Viscosupplementation typically requires three to five weekly injections of hyaluronan. A decrease in pain is often experienced within days after the injection with duration of relief being variable. Research indicates beneficial results for 6 months to 1 year after the series of injections (Bannuru et al., 2019; Ciccone, 2015; Henrotin et al., 2015).

Glucosamine and chondroitin are dietary supplements that may help protect articular cartilage and reverse joint degeneration associated with OA. These compounds are vital for the production of glycosaminoglycans, proteoglycans, and hyaluronic acid, essential components of articular cartilage and synovial fluid (Ciccone, 2015).

Glucosamine and chondroitin sulfate have been used for arthritic pain in Europe for a significant number of years and continue to be popular supplements worldwide (Lozada & Pace, 2019). However, the glucosamine/chondroitin arthritis intervention trial (GAIT) enrolled 662 patients with knee OA for a 24-month, double-blind, placebo-controlled study conducted in nine US states. Results of the trial indicated that there was limited benefit from glucosamine (500 mg TID), chondroitin sulfate (400 mg TID), or the combination of the two in patients with knee OA.

Overall, the supplements alone or in combination did not decrease pain significantly at 24 weeks, but in patients with moderate-to-severe pain at baseline, the pain response was significantly improved in those who received combined therapy in contrast to those who received the placebo (NCCIH, 2017; Sawitzke et al., 2017). Additionally, chondroprotective agents (matrix metalloproteinase [MMP] inhibitors and growth factors) are being tested as disease-modifying agents in the management of OA. MMP-13 is found in the cartilage of patients with OA but not in the cartilage of adults not diagnosed with OA (Gege et al., 2012). The researchers also examined the synthesis and biologic evaluation of an MMP-13 selective inhibitor that has demonstrated efficacy as a disease-modifying intraarticular injection for OA.

Rheumatoid Arthritis

Pharmacologic intervention for the treatment of RA has two primary goals: to decrease the joint inflammation and to slow the rate of the progression of the disease while minimizing pain, stiffness, inflammation, and complications of the disease. The general categories of medications that are utilized include a diverse group of agents known as disease-modifying antirheumatic drugs (DMARDs) and adjunctive agents such as corticosteroids, NSAIDs, corticosteroids, and analgesics. DMARDs interrupt the immune response associated with RA, whereas the adjunctive gents are used primarily to decrease joint inflammation but do not halt the progression of RA.

Early RA treatment is guided by two mutually inclusive concepts: early aggressive therapy and treat to target. Early and aggressive therapy with DMARDs is the gold standard of care, as these agents can both arrest the disease progression and promote remission before there is extensive damage to the affected joints. In addition, when prescribed with glucocorticoids and NSAIDs, DMARDs more often help improve the long-term physical outcomes of patients with RA and thus contribute to significant improvement in quality of life and function.

The target to be treated with RA is the disease activity measured by the following: tender joint count, swollen joint count, measure of sedimentation rate and C-reactive protein for inflammation, patient global assessment, and provider assessment (Aletaha & Smolen, 2018; Pisetsky, 2017; Smith & Brown, 2022; Walsh et al., 2017).

Many types of medications are available for the treatment of rheumatoid arthritis. As noted earlier, two prevailing concepts—early aggressive therapy and treat to target (T to T)—guide early RA treatment. Early aggressive therapy with T to T approaches is designed to decrease inflammation, prevent damage, and change the course of the disease process to limit late deformities (Combe et al., 2017). However, drug pharmacokinetics and pharmacodynamics in the older adult population are different and the drug side effects should be monitored closely. Furthermore, the incidence of different comorbid conditions has increased in this age group due to the high number of medications usually prescribed; therefore caution must be taken with close monitoring of side effects (Kobak & Bes, 2018).

DMARDs are typically classified into nonbiologic and biologic agents. These medications control synovitis and erosive changes during the active stages of RA. The advent of DMARDs for the treatment of RA significantly improved the potential for persons with RA. Traditional or conventional DMARDs, the nonbiologic DMARDs, include the following medications: hydroxychloroquine (HCQ), azathioprine (AZA), sulfasalazine, methotrexate, leflunomide, cyclosporine, gold salts, D-penicillamine, and minocycline. Biologic agents block the central proinflammatory cytokines active with RA and their effects. Biologic DMARDs include medications such as adalimumab, certolizumab, etanercept, golimumab, and infliximab (Ciccone, 2015; Cohen & Cannella, 2019; Pietsky, 2017; Smith & Brown, 2022; Smolen et al., 2017).

In 2008, the American College of Rheumatology (ACR) developed recommendations and algorithms for prescribing nonbiologic and biology DMARDs for patients diagnoses with RA (Singh et al., 2012). These recommendations were updated and published in April 2012 (Singh et al., 2015). The ACR recommends that before DMARDS are prescribed, patients should receive the pneumococcal, hepatitis, and influenza vaccinations as well as vaccinations for human papillomavirus and herpes zoster virus.

The most widely used nonbiologic DMARDs are methotrexate, sulfasalazine, leflunomide, and hydroxychloroquine. Methotrexate has become the cornerstone agent prescribed for patients newly diagnosed with RA and is the most widely used immunosuppressant for RA management due to its long-term efficacy (Aletaha & Smolen, 2018; Ciccone, 2015; Cohen & Cannella, 2019; McCormick, 2019; Moreland et al., 2012).

Methotrexate, originally a chemotherapy agent, given in much lower doses for RA, inhibits the metabolism of folic acid, a core substance necessary for the production of key immune system cells. It is taken weekly on the same day each week, as a pill, liquid, or injections. Symptoms most often improve 4 to 6 weeks after initiating treatment. Sulfasalazine is usually prescribed for RA and for arthritis associated with ankylosing spondylitis and inflammatory bowel disease. Leflunomide inhibits the production of certain inflammatory cells to reduce inflammation. Hydroxychloroquine was initially developed as a medication for malaria; later it was discovered that the agent also improved symptoms of arthritis (Ciccone, 2015; Cohen & Cannella, 2019; Goodman et al., 2010; Moreland et al., 2012).

Biologic DMARDs are the most recently approved drugs for RA and are usually used in combination with analgesics, antiinflammatories, and steroids to alter the clinical symptoms of RA. Some of these agents inhibit the action of tumor necrosis factor-alpha, which is a cytokine that that appears to be a key chemical mediator that promotes inflammation and joint erosion in RA. Therefore the progression of the disease process is delayed. Other DMARDs block the IL-1 protein that is present in excess in patients diagnosed with RA, thereby inhibiting inflammation and cartilage damage.

The TNF inhibitors that bind TNF, preventing its interaction with its receptors, include the following agents: etanercept, infliximab, adalimumab, certolizumab, and golimumab. Non-TNF biologic agents include rituximab, anakinra, abatacept, tocilizumab, sarilumab, tofacitinib, baricitinib, and upadacitinib. Biologic agents are expensive, and thus the consensus is that they should be used only after at least one nonbiologic DMARD, usually methotrexate, has been prescribed without significant success (Aletaha & Smolen, 2018; Singh et al., 2012; Smith & Brown, 2022; Smolen et al., 2017).

Pharmacologic therapy for the treatment of RA has significantly improved with research regarding the pathogenesis, optimal management, and optimal outcome measure of RA. The American College of Rheumatology (ACR) (Singh et al., 2015) and the European League Against Rheumatism (EULAR) (Smolen et al., 2017) both recommend drug therapy that targets remission of RA or low disease activity.

EULAR recommends combining biologic DMARDs and targeted synthetic DMARDs with methotrexate but does not advocate the use of biologic DMARD monotherapy. The ACR does not guard against the use of biologic DMARD monotherapy once methotrexate does not appear to have significant results. Furthermore, the ACR recommends combining conventional synthetic DMARDs with each other more strongly than does the EULAR. Randomized trials and indirect comparisons evidence that when combined with methotrexate, all biologic DMARDs and targeted synthetic DMARDs have similar efficacy. All drugs exhibit decreasing efficacy with increasing duration of the disease process or medicinal exposure. If methotrexate in combination with short-term glucocorticoids does not result in remission of the disease process, biologic DMARDs should be added, especially in patients with continuing high disease activity with the presence of autoantibodies (Aletaha & Smolen, 2018; Ciccone, 2015; Fleischmann et al., 2017; Pietsky, 2017; Smith & Brown, 2022).

Gout

Pharmacology strategies to treat the hyperuricemia associated with gout focus on limiting acute episodes triggered by urate crystal deposition, preventing recurrent attacks, and correcting the hyperuricemia. The American College of Rheumatology has established treatment guidelines and pharmacologic guidelines based on the acute and chronic presentation of the disease (Neogi, 2012).

Presently, the main pharmacologic treatment of hyperuricemia that causes gout is the use of allopurinol, a xanthine oxidase inhibitor; benzbromarone, which promotes the excretion of uric acid; and febuxostat, another xanthine oxidase inhibitor, when allopurinol is not effective or results in severe side effects. These medications have been approved to prevent or lessen future gout inflammatory attacks by slowing the rate at which the body synthesizes uric acid (Benn et al., 2018; Goodman & Fuller, 2021; Ragab et al., 2017). However, the US Food and Drug Administration (FDA) has recommended limiting the use of febuxostat due to more recent research that indicates an increased risk of death with febuxostat versus allopurinol (Gerriets & Jialai, 2019).

Acute episodes of gout are counteracted using NSAIDs, colchicine, or glucocorticoids, each of which act through different mechanisms. NSAIDs are effective in treating the pain and inflammation of an acute attack. NSAIDs are generally prescribed for patients without comorbid illnesses, but they are inappropriate for persons with renal impairment, congestive cardiac failure, and peptic ulcer disease, and with those treated with anticoagulants.

Additionally, high doses of NSAIDs can induce gastric toxicity. Glucocorticoids have many well-described antiinflammatory actions and may be given orally or as an intraarticular injection. However, these agents may interfere with blood pressure or glucose control. Colchicine has antiinflammatory effects but is less commonly prescribed presently because of its narrow therapeutic range and numerous side effects. Colchicine is recommended for patients who are unable to be treated with NSAIDs or corticosteroids (Gliozzi et al., 2015; Ragab et al., 2017).

The European League Against Rheumatism, in its most recent guidance on gout issued in 2016, advocated for the use of an exogenous uricase, pegloticase, for refractory gout (Richette et al., 2017). The presence of refractory gout indicates that the symptoms have not resolved with standard means of treatment and the disease has become chronic and unmanageable. Pegloticase has been approved by the FDA for the treatment of refractory gout. The enzyme uricase metabolizes urate into a more soluble compound, which is readily excreted by the kidney. Uricase is present in most mammalian species, but not in humans. However, some patients develop antipegloticase antibodies and thus pegloticase continues to be considered a last-resort intervention (Guttman et al., 2017).

Physical Rehabilitation

Research widely recommends physical activity as an essential component for patient management of the different types of arthritis. Physical activity can reduce pain, fatigue, and function limitation and thus improve patients' quality of life and level of independence. Because a significant number of persons diagnosed with arthritis have a higher risk for complications such as hypertension, cardiovascular diseases, and diabetes, being physically active is also important for secondary reasons (Arem et al., 2015; Egan, 2017; Leese et al., 2018; Wahid et al., 2016).

The role of the physical and occupational therapist in the management of RA is well established. Although RA is systemic, and OA is a localized joint condition, the general rehabilitation goals and outcomes for patients with RA and OA are similar. Physical and occupational therapists play an integral role in the nonpharmacologic management of RA and OA (Goodman et al., 2017; O'Sullivan et al., 2019).

Goals of rehabilitation for patients with arthritis include the following: relief of pain, improvement in range of motion (ROM), increased strength and endurance, prevention or modification of deformities, and provision of counseling and educational services. Heat, either superficial or deep, is an effective modality in addition to exercise. Thus rehabilitation includes exercises to prevent contractures, increase strength and flexibility, and increase the patient's cardiorespiratory/aerobic condition (Goodman et al., 2017; Nelson et al., 2014; O'Sullivan et al., 2019).

Modalities should not be used as an intervention without exercise (Cameron, 2013). Exercise programs should be prescribed by a physical therapist and modified for each patient's individual level of involvement, body build, previous activity level, and comorbidities. Physical and occupational therapists address exercise programs for hand involvement, education regarding joint protection and self-care, and instruction in use of assistive devices. These rehabilitative experts also recommend assistive devices and orthotics when needed and instruct patients on their use (Schur & Gibofsky, 2019; Smith & Brown, 2022).

Orthoses and Supportive Equipment

Orthotic devices are an essential part of rehabilitation management for patients with arthritis, particularly for patients with RA. Orthotics assist in decreasing pain and inflammation, improve function, reduce deformity, and correct biomechanical malalignment. Lower extremity orthoses are prescribed for patients with RA to assist in providing stability and proper alignment as well as to shift weight-bearing off of the affected extremity. Approximately 80% of patients diagnosed with RA have significant foot involvement. Many of these anatomic changes are accommodated by providing a deep, wide, soft leather shoe. A metatarsal pad is typically prescribed to remove weight from painful metatarsophalangeal (MTP) joints, and a rocker-bottom sole facilitates rolloff. Custom inserts can be fabricated to address hindfoot pronation (Goodman et al., 2017; O'Sullivan et al., 2019; Smith & Brown, 2022).

Knee orthoses may be used to improve the following problems: edema, pain, patellar misalignment, hyperextension, and collateral or cruciate ligament instability. Therapeutic shoes are recommended for the treatment of foot problems in patients diagnosed with RA, especially in patients with foot deformities or erosion in the foot joints (Bergstra et al., 2016; Marsman et al., 2013).

Tenten-Dlepenmaat et al. (2017) performed a literature search for studies investigating the effect of ready- or custom-made therapeutic shoes for patients with RA. The literature search was conducted up to January 2017. Within-group results indicated that therapeutic shoes are likely to be effective in patients with RA. Orlova and Karateev (2016) evaluated the clinical efficiency of orthotic intervention in the rehabilitation of patients with RA. They concluded that the 6-month application of knee, ankle, and wrist orthoses reduced pain and joint swelling and improved locomotor indicators, functional status, and quality of life in patients with RA. Thus orthotic intervention was recommended as part of a comprehensive rehabilitation program.

Assistive devices help keep joints in the best position for functioning, provide leverage, and extend functional motion. These may include zipper pulls, buttoning aids, Velcro fasteners, and long-handled shoehorns to assist with dressing. Several kitchen devices are available, including electric can openers, food processors, reachers, built-up handles, and grips. Tub bars and handrails provide additional stability and security to decrease fall potential. These and other devices are readily addressed by occupational therapists. Physical therapists are movement experts who can recommend the best assistive devices for gait and balance.

Surgical Intervention

A number of surgical interventions are available to help patients with arthritis to relieve pain, correct deformities, and improve function. These interventions may include myofascial techniques, excisions, reconstructions, arthrodesis, and joint replacements. When to perform the surgery is a complex decision; age, stage of disease, level of disability, location of the involved joints, and comorbidities must be considered (Smith & Brown, 2022).

Osteoarthritis in the hip and knees often leads to total joint arthroplasties (TJA) (Carr et al., 2012; Cross et al., 2014; de Achaval et al., 2015). With the aging population and the obesity epidemic, demands for TJA have increased significantly. It is predicted that by 2030, demands in the United States for primary TJA of the hip will grow by 174% and that for the knee will grow by 673% (See et al., 2018).

With advanced OA of the ankle, arthrodesis was the first-line treatment for decades due to the poor results of the first-generation total ankle replacements. The review of the literature by Barg et al. (2015) indicated that total ankle replacement with newer types of prosthesis has resulted, with mean success rates of up to 90% at 10 years post-op. Arthroscopic intervention is often the surgical intervention with mild to moderate OA of the ankle. Osti, Del Buono, and Malfulli (2016) reported the clinical and functional outcomes following arthroscopic management of anterior impingement with mild to moderate OA of the ankle in former soccer players. They concluded this was a safe, effective, and low-cost option that allows former athletes to return to ordinary daily activities and recreational sport activities. Additionally, TJA is most often the main surgical treatment for shoulder OA. It involves either a hemiarthroplasty or a total shoulder replacement (Craig et al., 2020; Orvets et al., 2018; Pandya et al., 2018; Simovitch et al., 2018).

Deformities of the hand or wrist usually lead to the loss of one's ability to grip, grasp, and pinch functionally. The surgical opportunities for RA of the hand and wrist include the following: synovectomy, tenosynovectomy, tendon realignment, reconstructive surgery, or arthroplasty, and arthrodesis.

Cervical spine instability often results in patients with RA due to the degeneration of ligaments and bone in the cervical spine area. Riches et al. (2016) assessed the patient-rated outcome measures (PROMs) related to hand and wrist surgery in patients with RA. Results indicated that highly significant improvements in both function and pain scores were reported across the cohort as a whole following hand surgery. Overall, patients reported improved outcomes in functional, stiffness, and pain domains.

Okura et al. (2018) also conducted a retrospective questionnaire survey to investigate the long-term outcomes of elbow, wrist, and hand surgery for RA. The original patient-reported outcome assessment tool revealed that elbow, wrist, and hand surgery provided long-lasting benefits in RA patients, with pain relief being the most favorable effect. Patients diagnosed with RA of the cervical spine who have refractory pain, neurologic compromise, or intrinsic spinal cord changes on magnetic resonance imaging (MRI) are most often candidates for surgical intervention.

Surgeries can be highly effective at restoring mobility and alleviating pain. Marques et al. (2018) performed a cross-sectional study that evaluated the results of cervical spine surgeries due to RA instability between January 2000 and 2012. They concluded that the procedures were relatively safe with a high rate of neurologic improvement. Rigid techniques appeared to lead to a more improved result when compared to wiring ones.

Metabolic Bone Disease

Approach to the Older Adult With Metabolic Bone Disease

Osteopenia and Osteoporosis

Osteoporosis has been clinically defined on the basis of bone mineral density (BMD) assessment. As defined by the World Health Organization (WHO) criteria, osteoporosis is the reduction in BMD of 2.5 standard deviations (SD) or more below the mean peak BMD of young adults when measured by dual-energy x-ray absorptiometry (DEXA). Osteopenia, low bone mass, is a milder decrease in BMD and is defined as a BMD value between 1.0 and 2.5 SD units below the mean value of young adults measured by DEXA (World Health Organization, 2004).

Osteoporosis is the most common bone disease worldwide with a progressive prevalence both in developed and developing countries. The bone disease is characterized by low bone mass and deterioration of bone tissue with changes in bone microarchitecture. Compromised bone strength and an increase in the risk of fractures often result due to the disease (Tabatabaei-Malazy et al., 2017). Fractures associated with osteoporosis, especially fractures of the hip and spine, are a significant cause of disability, mortality, and health care use. Osteoporosis is more prevalent among older adults and among women, with the prevalence projected to increase significantly over the new few decades as the number of older adults is expected to have an unprecedented increase in number (O'Donnell, 2018).

It is estimated that 10 million Americans have been diagnosed with osteoporosis, and approximately 80% are female. In addition, about 50% of women over the age of 50 will fracture a bone secondary to the disease, with this incidence equal to a combined risk of breast, uterine, and ovarian cancer (National Osteoporosis Foundation, n.d.). Adults age 80 and over have the highest prevalence of low bone mass. Caucasian and Asian women are more likely to develop osteoporosis, with African American and Hispanic women having the lowest prevalence (Looker & Frenk, 2015).

Etiology and Pathophysiology

Osteoporosis in older adults is caused by an imbalance of bone resorption in excess of bone formation. With aging, there is a decrease of osteoblastic activity that results in significantly less bone formation. Menopause then causes an increase in the osteoclastic activity, resulting in increases in bone reabsorption. Osteoporosis is classified as primary or secondary, depending on the related etiology. The cause of primary osteoporosis is unknown but is related to prolonged negative calcium balance, progressive estrogen or testosterone deficiency, smoking, low body mass index (BMI), or sedentary lifestyle. Secondary osteoporosis is often associated with prolonged pharmaceutical therapy with antiseizure medications, chemotherapy, proton pump inhibitors, selective serotonin reuptake inhibitors, and glucocorticoids.

The condition may also occur secondary to a number of conditions such as alcoholism, malnutrition, hyperthyroidism, and kidney disease (National Institute of Arthritis and Musculoskeletal and Skin Diseases, n.d.).

Osteoporosis is closely associated with inadequate calcium intake, but insufficient vitamin D contributes to osteoporosis by reducing the body's absorption of calcium. Vitamin D promotes calcium absorption in the gastrointestinal tract and maintains adequate serum calcium and phosphate concentration to facilitate normal mineralization of bone and to prevent hypocalcemic tetany. It is also needed for bone growth and bone remodeling by osteoblasts and osteoclasts. Together with calcium, vitamin D helps to protect older adults from osteoporosis (NIH Office of Dietary Supplements, n.d.).

In association, Cavalli (2016) screened 7305 persons of both sexes and analyzed the influence of factors associated with the development of osteoporosis. Additional important risk factors for developing osteoporosis were identified, including the following: family or personal history of osteoporotic fracture, RA, Crohn disease, ulcerative colitis, hypothyroidism, poor sun exposure, and oophorectomy before the age of 50.

Osteoporosis is a major cause of disability worldwide primarily due to its association with fractures. It is a serious disease associated with older adults that can impact their quality of life by increasing their susceptibility to fractures of the hip, spine, and wrist. Up to 50% of women and 20% of men are predicted to experience a fragility fracture at some point during their lifetime (Barton). According to US Medicare data, 65% of women between the ages of 65 and 85 who sustained a fracture were neither examined nor treated for osteoporosis within 6 months prior to the fracture (National Committee for Quality Assurance, n.d.).

Bone mass peaks between the ages of 25 and 35, and then the rate of bone resorption starts to exceed the rate of bone formation. Studies of bone microarchitecture have indicated that trabecular bone loss usually begins in the third decade of life, before gonadal sex steroid deficiency develops, whereas cortical loss typically begins in the sixth decade (Drake et al., 2015).

The most devastating fractures associated with osteoporosis are hip fractures. After sustaining a hip fracture, 50% of older adult patients fail to regain their prefracture mobility, with 25% ending up in long-term residential care and 25% dying within 12 months. Osteoporosis is a familial disease, and thus children of persons who have experienced an osteoporotic fracture are more likely to have low BMD themselves. Significant heritability has been evidenced in osteoporosis-related traits that include BMD, fracture risk, bone turnover rate, and bone geometry (Clark & Duncan, 2015).

Osteoporosis is a polygenic disorder, determined by the effects of several genes; some of these have modest effects on bone mass, whereas others suggest determinants of fracture risk. Genome-wide association studies (GWASs) have identified a number of promising genetic variants that are associated with osteoporosis and related traits.

The primary goals of GWASs are to discover new molecular and biologic pathways involved in the regulation of bone metabolism. The aim of these discoveries is to develop a a medicinal treatment for osteoporosis (Guo et al., 2019; Liu et al., 2019; Lovsin et al., 2018).

Chesi and colleagues (2019) investigated loci, DNA regions previously established to be associated with BMD in the GWAS. The study identified two genes, ING3 and EPDR1, which in turn revealed strong effects on human osteoblasts. They concluded that follow-up studies that investigate biologic pathways affected by these genes may identify targets for therapies to strengthen bone mineral density.

Paget Disease

Adult Paget disease of bone (PDB) is a noninflammatory, metabolic, skeletal condition that is characterized by localized abnormally rapid osteoclastic bone resorption with compensatory increased osteoblastic activity. It is a chronic, slowly progressive skeletal condition and is the second most common metabolic bone condition after osteoporosis. The new bone in those with PDB is structurally abnormal, dense, and fragile and may occur in one or more regions of the body. The condition primarily affects older adults, with persons under 40 years of age seldom diagnosed with the disease. The prevalence of the disease in the United States is estimated to be 1% to 2% of the general population. PDB is most prevalent in Great Britain, affecting 3% to 5% of the population, and in countries with a history of significant immigration from Britain (Abdulla et al., 2018; Kravets, 2018; Tuck et al., 2017).

Paget disease of bone occurs more frequently in men than in women of all ages over 55 years. The incidence has been reported to increase with age and was estimated to be 0.3 cases per 10,000 among women ages 55 to 59 and 0.5 cases per 10,00 among men of similar age. For persons 85 year so of age and older, this rate rose to 5.4 among women and 7.6 among men. Fortunately, the prevalence of PDB has become less common and less severe in the United Kingdom (Appelman-Dijkstra & Papapoulos, 2018; Michou & Orcel, 2016; Valenzuela & Pietschmann, 2017).

Britton et al. (2017) analyzed data from the database of the Paget's Disease Research Group of Western Australia that included 323 patients with PDB recruited between 1988 and 2013. The research established that in large cohort studies, PDB presented with a milder severity than in previous decades.

Etiology and Pathophysiology

The microstructure of bone in PDB is exceedingly abnormal. Under normal circumstances the process of bone remodeling involves resorption of bone by osteoclasts, which are multinucleated cells followed by new bone formation carried out by osteoblasts. During bone formation, some osteoblasts are trapped within the bone matrix where they differentiate into osteocytes, which play an important role in regulating osteoblast and osteoclast activity by producing a receptor activator of nuclear factor kappa B ligand (RANKL) and sclerostin (Setiawati & Rahardjo, 2018; Vallet & Ralston, 2016).

In PDB there is loss of the normal regulation of bone resorption and formation. There is an increased activity of osteoclasts that become large and numerous, with studies indicating that they can grow 10 to 100 times their normal number. These numerous enlarged osteoclasts have as many as 100 nuclei in contrast to 3 to 5 nuclei in normal osteoclasts. In response to the rapid bone resorption, bone formation becomes greatly accelerated, sixfold to sevenfold greater than normal (Kravets, 2018; Valenzuela & Pietschmann, 2017; Vallet & Ralston, 2016).

Paget disease of bone most often follows three stages. The first phase is osteolytic and is characterized by intense bone resorption and hypervascularization. The second phase is mixed osteoblastic and osteolytic, causing an increased production of new bone matrix by exceedingly numerous osteoblasts being recruited to resorption sites that occurs in parallel with continuing bone resorption by osteoclasts. However, normal lamellar bone is replaced in the form of woven bone that results in thickening of the cortex by endosteal and periosteal bone deposition with enlargement of the bones. The third phase of PDB is sclerotic, with bone resorption progressively diminishing, leaving a dense, sclerotic, disorganized bone that is weaker than normal. These phases may be present simultaneously at different skeletal sites (Cundy, 2017; Kravets 2018; Tuck et al., 2017; Winn et al., 2017). As a result, the bone becomes deformed and enlarged, and it is susceptible to fractures. The axial skeleton is often involved, and studies indicate that the bones most commonly affected include the pelvis (70%), femur (55%), lumbar spine (53%), skull (42%), and tibia (32%), but pagetic bone lesions can occur at any site of the skeleton (Appelman-Dijkstra & Papapoulos, 2018; Tuck et al., 2017; Valenzuela & Pietschmann, 2017).

The exact cause of Paget disease of bone is unknown, but overall the most likely pathogenesis is a combination of environmental factors that affect genetically predisposed people (Abdulla et al., 2018). Several hypotheses, not necessarily mutually exclusive, have been proposed to explain the pathology of Paget disease of bone with the dominant ones being genetic and environmental causes (Appelman-Dijkstra & Papapoulos, 2018; Cundy, 2017; Vallet & Ralston 2016; Visconti et al., 2017).

Prominent studies have supported a dominant environmental cause of the disorder to be a slow paramyxovirus family (e.g., measles virus, respiratory syncytial virus, canine distemper virus) of pagetic osteoclasts in genetically susceptible persons. Pagetic osteoclasts have been shown to contain intranuclear inclusion bodies that resemble paramyxovirus nucleocapsids (Appelman-Dijkstra & Papapoulos, 2018; Kravets 2018; Vallet & Ralston 2016; Visconti et al., 2017). However, a study of a large cohort of individuals diagnosed with PDB found no evidence that supported an association between the condition and a persistent infection with measles or other paramyxoviruses. This study supported the belief that paramyxoviruses and viral proteins can promote the formation of osteoclasts with features similar to those of pagetic osteoclasts, especially in association with genetic alterations (Appelman-Dijkstra & Papapoulos, 2018; Visconti et al., 2017).

Other environmental factors that may influence the development of Paget disease of bone have been identified based on decreasing incidence and severity of the disease. This has been attributed to better childhood nutrition with increased calcium and vitamin D intake, lower exposure to infections, and improved physical activity associated with a lower mechanical load on the skeleton and fewer skeletal injuries (Abdulla et al., 2018; Audet et al., 2017; Kravets, 2018; Vallet & Ralston 2016). Audet et al. (2017) investigated environmental factors through a questionnaire in 176 pagetic patients who lived in the same Canadian geographic area. PDB was significantly associated with wood-fired heating in childhood or adolescence, regardless of the form of PDB.

Genetics factors play an important role in PDB. Approximately 10% to 20% of individuals affected by Paget disease of bone have a family history of the disease. The inheritance of the condition follows an autosomal dominant pattern with incomplete penetrance. As many as 50% of patients with a family history of the disorder and 5% to 10% of patients with a sporadic form of the illness carry mutations in the SQSTM1 gene, which is responsible for encoding p62, a protein that plays a key role in regulating osteoclast function. Patients with SQSTM1 mutations are significantly associated with severe PDB, are diagnosed earlier, and have a high degree of penetrance with increasing age. PDB cases diagnosed without a reported family history are termed *sporadic*. The disease develops as a result of isolated de novo mutations, environmental triggers, or possibly incomplete penetrance that obscurs family history (Albagha, 2015; Britton et al., 2017; Tuck et al., 2017; Vallet & Ralston, 2016).

Steps for Diagnosing Metabolic Bone Disease

Osteopenia and Osteoporosis

The initial evaluation for diagnosing osteopenia/osteoporosis should begin with a history of clinical risk factors (CRFs) for fractures, including underlying medical conditions or medications that contribute to bone loss. The medical history may indicate symptoms of possibly correctable low bone density (gluten intolerance and celiac disease) or comorbidities that could influence intervention decisions.

An accurate measurement of body weight is important because low body weight (less than 127 pounds) and weight loss of 5% or more are associated with an increased risk of fracture. An accurate measurement of height is also recommended, as a height loss of 1.5 inches or more, or a loss of 0.75 inches compared to a previous measured height, is also indicative of a likelihood of vertebral fracture. Assessments of spinal points of tenderness, gait, posture, balance, and muscle strength are included in the exam (Lewiecki, 2019; Rosen & Drezner, 2019).

Basic biochemical and urine testing are advised. The following basic blood tests are recommended: CBC, calcium, phosphorus, alkaline phosphatase, 25-hydoxyvitamin D level, creatinine, thyroid-stimulating hormone (TSH) level, and liver enzymes. Tests for identifying secondary causes of osteoporosis include urinalysis and 24-hour urine for calcium tests that are helpful screening tools for identifying patients with common disorders of calcium metabolism. Knowledge of a patient's parathyroid hormone (PTH) level is essential for ruling out hyperparathyroidism and antigliadin, and antiendomysial antibody testing can help identify celiac disease (Bethel et al., 2019; Lewiecki et al., 2018; Rosen & Drezner, 2019).

Dual-energy x-ray absorptiometry (DEXA) is the gold standard for measuring bone mineral density (BMD) in clinical practice. The International Society for Clinical Densitometry (ISCD) recommends that BMD be measured ideally at L1 to L4, the total hip, and the femoral neck. Accuracy and precision of DEXA are excellent with recommendations of DXA measurements of the spine and hip because fractures at these sites have the greatest impact on patients' health and independent function. A strong correlation exists between mechanical strength and BMD measured by DXA biomechanical studies. In observational studies of patients who are not treated for low BMD, there is a highly significant relationship between fracture risk and BMD measured by DXA. In addition, there is a direct relationship between a decrease in fracture risk with medicinal intervention and increases in BMD by DXA (Choksi et al., 2018; Lewiecki 2019; Rosen & Drezner, 2019; Yuan et al., 2016; Bethel et al., 2019). In the United States, the majority of professional groups recommend BMD assessment in postmenopausal women 65 years of age and older and for all men older than 70 years regardless of risk factors (Camacho et al., 2016; Cosman et al., 2015; Curry et al., 2018; International Society for Clinical Densitometry, 2019; Jeremiah et al., 2015; Lewiecki et al., 2018; Link, 2016).

The combination of BMD scores and CRFs predicts fracture risk more accurately than BMD scores or CRFs alone. To assist providers in making a more successful quantitative assessment of fracture risk, a fracture risk assessment tool (FRAX) was developed. This is a computer-based algorithm that estimates the 10-year probability of hip fracture and major osteoporotic fracture. FRAX can be accessed online at http://www.shef.ac.uk/FRAX. FRAX was developed after an analysis of data from 12 large prospective observational studies that included approximately 60,000 untreated men and women internationally. Thus FRAX provides a quantitative estimation of fracture risk that is based on robust data from large populations with both genders and with ethnic and geographic diversity (Bethel et al., 2019; Choksi et al., 2018; Lewiecki, 2019; Link, 2016; Rosen & Drezner, 2019).

Other tests for diagnosing osteopenia/osteoporosis include quantitative ultrasound (QUS) and quantitative computed tomography (QCT). QUS emits sound waves in the ultrasonic range between 0.1 and 1.0 megahertz (MHz) and measures two parameters, the speed of sound (SOS) and broadband ultrasound attenuation (BUA). The calcaneus is the only validated skeletal site for the use of QUA in osteoporosis management. A higher bone density is indicated with a higher SOS and BUA. QUA is a low-cost portable screening, but it is not as accurate as DXA and thus cannot be used to monitor the response to treatment. If central DXA is not available, calcaneal QUS can be used to identify individuals who need pharmacologic intervention for low BMD (Bethel et al., 2019; Choksi et al., 2018; Lewiecki et al., 2018; Link, 2016).

Quantitative computed tomography measures BMD at the spine and provides a volumetric three-dimensional measurement offering details of the cortical and trabecular bone. QCT scanning of the spine is a significantly sensitive technique when repeated measurements are needed to detect small changes in BMD. However, QCT requires a higher radiation dose than DXA and is used less commonly than DXA. Medicare data indicate that approximately 5% of all BMD assessments are done with QCT scanning. QCT may be prescribed for testing more often in smaller, rural areas, as they often already have a CT scanner for trauma cases and may not be able to readily afford a DXA machine as well (Bethel et al., 2019; Choksi et al., 2018; Lewiecki, 2019; Link, 2016).

Bone turnover markers (BTMs) are laboratory tests of serum and urine that are usually available in clinical practice. BTMs reflect bone formation or bone resorption, which may be elevated in high-bone-turnover states that happens particularly in early postmenopausal osteoporosis. In clinical practice, BTMs can potentially predict fracture risk independent of BMD and may be useful for monitoring the metabolic effects of pharmacologic and nonpharmacologic therapy. Currently available serum markers of bone formation (osteoblast products) include the following: bone-specific alkaline phosphatase (BSAP), osteocalcin (OC), carboxyterminal propeptide of type I collagen (PICP) and aminoterminal propeptide of type I collagen (PINP). However, significant controversy exists regarding the use of these biochemical markers (Bethel et al., 2019; Lewiecki, 2019).

Plain radiography continues to be recommended to assess overall skeletal integrity. Radiographic findings can suggest the presence of bone loss but are not as accurate as BMD testing for diagnosing osteopenia/osteoporosis. In addition, bone biopsy is rarely used in clinical practice but may be helpful for excluding underlying pathologic conditions, such as multiple myeloma. Typically, an iliac crest biopsy is performed in a surgical area and may be performed when a therapeutic procedure such as kyphoplasty or vertebroplasty for fixation of a vertebral compression fracture is done (Choksi et al., 2018; Lewiecki et al., 2018; Link, 2016).

Paget Disease

Clinical Manifestations

Paget disease was originally described by Sir James Paget in 1877, a condition he referred to as osteitis deformans (Paget, 1877). Paget disease of bone (PBD) is often detected incidentally when an increased serum alkaline phosphatase level is noted on routine blood work or when a radiograph is obtained for an unrelated reason. The characteristic incidental nature of the diagnosis does not indicate that all patients are symptom-free, yet at least 20% to 25% are symptomatic when diagnosed.

Classical symptoms of PDB include bone pain, bone deformities, symptoms secondary to fractures, diminished hearing, symptoms resultant of nerve root compression, and headaches. Paget disease most commonly involves the axial skeleton, but any area can be affected. Predominately, the condition is polyostotic, involving multiple bones, but in approximately one-third of patients it is monostotic and involves only one bone (Singer, 2016).

Bone pain is the most common symptom reported and may be caused by the pagetic lesions or by complications of the condition such as arthritis or osteosarcoma. Pain is usually described as continuous and increasing at rest, especially noticed at night, and is alleviated by movement. This differs from pain caused by osteoarthritis associated with juxtaarticular Paget disease that is aggravated by movement.

In the later stages of the condition, a variety of deformities may occur, including kyphosis; shortened or bowed long bones; leonine facies, frontal bossing of the forehead; and dental abnormalities. Characteristic long bone deformities include anterior bowing of the tibia and anterolateral bowing of the femur. These deformities often lead to gait changes that result in joint and back pain. The increased stress on the adjacent joints caused by the deformities may produce symptomatic degenerative arthritis. Vertebral compression fractures or lumbar spinal stenosis may result, leading to neural impingement. Fractures are common in patients with PDB and may be traumatic, pathologic, complete, or incomplete. They are most often transverse and perpendicular to the bone cortex with the most common locations of the fractures being just inferior to the lesser trochanter of the femur and in the proximal one-third of the tibia. Because pagetic bone characteristically exhibits an increased vascularity, these fractures can lead to an acute blood loss.

Involvement of the bones of the skull may lead to osteoporosis circumscripta that causes an enlarged skull. Headaches described as a band tightening around the head, dizziness, or vertigo may then develop. Pagetic lesions of the temporal bone and the ossicles can cause hearing loss deafness. Other rare complications include anosmia, trigeminal neuralgia, and facial and bulbar palsy.

Clinical Assessment

Paget disease typically presents in a generally healthy older adult with elevated alkaline phosphatase, normal serum calcium, normal 25-hydroxy-viatmin D level, and no evidence of hepatobiliary disease (Kravets, 2018; Tan & Ralston, 2014). The diagnosis of Paget disease is most often confirmed by a thorough clinical evaluation, detailed patient history, and a variety of specialized tests that include blood tests, x-rays, and urine tests.

The most commonly used biochemical marker of Paget disease of bone is the serum alkaline phosphatase (ALP) level in the blood, which indicates osteoblast activity. An elevation of ALP may be the only evidence of the disease's presence when a patient is asymptomatic. Other possible causes of isolated raised ALP will need to be excluded, such as vitamin D deficiency, hyperparathyroidism, hyperthyroidism, renal osteodystrophy, and malignancy. Thus serum calcium, blood calcium levels, 24-hour urine calcium measurement, thyroid function tests, parathyroid hormone levels, and a 25-hydroxyvitamin D test may be indicated for differential diagnosis.

The diagnosis must confirm that the source of an elevated ALP is bone and not the liver by measuring the bone-specific ALP and obtaining liver function tests. Most patients with PDB have normal levels of calcium and phosphorus; however, patients who sustain fractures and suffer from limited mobility may develop hypercalcemia due to increased osteoclast activity. Also of interest, extremely active Paget disease is associated with increased bone formation that leads to elevated calcium needs that in turn may cause hypocalcemia. Hypocalcemia may then trigger secondary hyperparathyroidism. Bone metastases, including prostate cancer and myeloma, may be differentiated by blood tests, plain x-rays, and other imaging. If malignancy is diagnosed, a bone biopsy may be necessary to determine the presence of PDB (Kravets, 2018; Michou & Orcel, 2016; National Organization for Rare Disorders [NORD], n.d.; Shamus, n.d.; Tuck et al., 2017; Vallet & Ralston, 2016).

Plain radiographs of bones suspected to be involved by PDB are essential for determining the extent of deformity, detecting any potential fracture and lytic areas, and evaluating the adjacent joints. Radionuclide bone scans are screening tests used in addition to the plain radiographs, as they are very sensitive for detecting areas of increased bone cell activity, allowing the extent of disease to be determined. The three phases of PDB are evident with radiographs. The early lytic phase gives the characteristic blade-of-grass appearance that progresses through the bone at approximately 8 mm per year. The second phase shows a combined image of osteolysis and osteosclerosis, with the final phase reflected by primary sclerosis (Al Nofal et al., 2015; Kravets, 2018; Michou & Orcel, 2016; Tuck et al., 2017; Vallet & Ralston, 2016).

Factors to Consider in the Treatment of Metabolic Disease

Osteoporosis/Osteopenia

Intervention for the treatment of osteoporosis presents a challenge for the provider because patients with osteoporosis, unlike patients with cardiovascular diagnoses, may be completely asymptomatic until they experience a fracture (Ahn & Ham, 2016; Jaleel et al., 2018). Many studies show that fracture risk in osteoporotic patients may be reduced by 70% with bone-protective therapy. However, providers of osteoporosis treatment have struggled with suboptimal treatment adherence, which affects many other silent chronic diseases as well (Rossi et al., 2018).

Poor adherence with pharmacologic treatment for osteoporosis can reduce the therapeutic benefit. Research indicates that adherence has not improved satisfactorily despite the increase in treatment prescription, resulting in an increased risk of fractures and all-cause mortality (Jaleel et al., 2018). Adherence encompasses both compliance and persistence. Compliance is defined as the extent to which a patient follows the prescribed dosage of treatment, whereas persistence is the cumulative time duration from initiation to discontinuation of the drug (Park et al., 2017).

Health literacy is the degree to which patients have the ability to obtain, process, and understand basic health information and services needed to make appropriate health care decisions (Du et al., 2018). Patients with limited health literacy are less likely to obtain or be compliant with preventive care (Roh, 2018).

Roh et al. (2017) measured the health literacy of 116 patients with distal radius fracture and a diagnosis of osteoporosis. The results indicated that patients with inadequate health literacy, adverse drug events, or medical comorbidities have higher rates of nonadherence with treatment. Treatment satisfaction was associated with higher medication adherence among older adults. Osteoporosis and osteopenia are prevalent among the older adult population, making this population more susceptible to the development of mobility restrictions or severe disabilities that ultimately reduce their ability to remain independent. Studies project that the number of adults over the age of 50 with low bone mass will increase to 71.2 million people, a 29% increase from 2010. Although few older adults are illiterate, aging results in normal changes in cognition, vision, and hearing. Thus the provider should repeat essential information and provide brochures that have high-contrast print and larger font sizes (CDC, 2020).

Vitamin D Recommendations for Preventing Osteoporosis

A committee from the Institute of Medicine concluded that persons are at risk of vitamin D deficiency at levels ranging from 12 to 20 ng/mL. Practically all people are sufficient at levels ≥20 ng/mL. The committee stated that 50 is the serum 25(OD)D level that covers the needs of 97.5% of the population. Serum concentrations >50 ng/mL are associated with potential adverse effects (Institute of Medicine, Food and Nutrition Board). For practically all adults ages 19 through 50 and for men until age 71, 1000 milligrams will cover daily calcium needs. Women over 50 and both men and women 71 years of age and older need no more than 1200 milligrams per day to ensure they are meeting their daily needs for good bone health (Vieth, 2011).

Treatment Paget Disease

Treatment of Paget disease is not curative but can provide prolonged periods of remission. Literature generally supports treating the following patients diagnosed with PDB: all symptomatic patients, asymptomatic patients whose biochemical markers indicate an increase in bone remodeling, and patients with pagetic lesions located on weight-bearing regions or adjacent to joints.

Four main categories of treatment exist for persons diagnosed with Paget disease of bone: nonpharmacologic therapy, pharmacologic therapy using either bisphosphonates or calcitonins, pain management, and surgical intervention. Nonpharmacologic therapy primarily focuses on physical therapy as a means of improving muscle strength and will be discussed in the Physical Rehabilitation section. Please refer to the Pharmacologic Intervention and Surgical Intervention sections for further discussion. Good oral hygiene is important throughout treatment for PDB, and thus regular dental visits should be advised. Fall prevention is also important with treatment to decrease the risk of fractures. Weight control may reduce weight-bearing pain in the lower extremities. No special diet is evidenced for preventing or treating Paget disease. For overall bone health, a balanced diet rich in calcium and vitamin D is essential, as recommended by the Institute of Medicine of the National Academy of Sciences. Exercise and activity should be encouraged to help patients maintain healthy bones, good joint mobility, and independent activities of daily living (Alikhan, 2018; Bouchette & Boktor 2019; NIH, 2018; NORD, n.d.).

Treatment Options for the Older Adult With Metabolic Disease

Pharmacologic Treatment

The goals of pharmaceutical prescription with osteoporosis is to restore the balance of resorption and absorption of osteocytes. The FDA has approved many medications for the treatment of osteoporosis that fall into two basic categories: antiresorptive and anabolics. Antiresorptive drugs include bisphosphonates (alendronate, ibandronate, risedronate, zoledronic acid), denosumab, calcitonin, estrogen/estrogen-progestin, an estrogen agonist/antagonist (raloxifene), and a tissue-specific estrogen complex (estrogen/bazedoxifene). Teriparatide, a parathyroid hormone analog; abaloparatide, a parathyroid hormone-related protein analog; and romosozumab-aqqg, a sclerostin inhibitor; are the FDA-approved anabolic medicines available at this time. Romosozumab-aqqg, teriparatide and abaloparatide are the only drugs for osteoporosis that have a defined treatment length. The FDA recommends that treatment be limited to no more than 18 months or 2 years. Thus these drugs are prescribed for cases of severe osteoporosis that have not responded well to antiresorptive medications (Cosman et al., 2015; Rosen & Drezner, 2019).

The National Osteoporosis Foundation (NOF) developed recommendations for the initiation of drug therapy that are widely accepted and support the use of bisphosphonates to prevent fracture in patients diagnosed with osteoporosis (Cosman et al., 2015; Rosen & Drezner, 2019). There is an absence of high-quality drug comparison trials that determine the relative efficacy of the individual medications. Thus the choice of therapy should be determined based on efficacy, safety, cost, convenience, and other patient-related factors (Barrionuevo et al., 2019; Crandell et al., 2014; Cummings et al., 2017; Eastell et al., 2019; Shoback et al., 2020).

The pharmacologic treatment goal of PDB is to reduce osteoclast function. Other treatment is aimed at relieving symptoms and complications of the condition. Pharmacologic treatment with a bisphosphonate is recommend for most patients with active Paget disease who are at risk for progressive skeletal and extraskeletal complications. All modern bisphosphonates are nitrogenous and produce their effect by inhibiting farnesyl diphosphate synthase, thus causing apoptosis of osteoclasts.

Treatment with bisphosphonates is indicated for patients who experience symptoms caused by active bone lesions; for prophylaxis when biochemically active pagetic lesions are located in high-risk areas, such as weight-bearing bones or a site of potential nerve compression; when the alkaline phosphatase level is two to four times the normal limit; when surgery is planned that involves bone affected by Paget disease; and when hypercalcemia develops secondary to immobilization (Kravets, 2018). Currently, the US Food and Drug Administration (FDA) has approved six bisphosphonates for the treatment of Paget disease of bone. These include zoledronic acid (Reclast) and pamidronate disodium (Aredia), which are given intravenously, as well as Etidronate (Didronel), tiludronate (Skelid), Alendronate (Fosamax), and Risedronate (Actonel), which are given orally. Etidronate disodium and tiludronate disodium are less potent than alendronate and risedronate. Oral calcium and vitamin D supplements are recommended when these agents are prescribed to decrease hypocalcemia or vitamin D deficiency (Kravets, 2018; Muschitz et al., 2017; NORD, n.d.; Singer et al., 2014; Tuck, et al., 2017).

Subcutaneous injection of salmon calcitonin was the first drug therapy of choice for Paget disease. This agent has been shown to reduce elevated bone turnover by 50%. The use of calcitonins is limited mostly to patients who do not tolerate bisphosphonates. Miacalcin, an injection given daily or three times weekly, is the only calcitonin approved for Paget disease (Kravets, 2018; NORD, n.d.; Tuck et al., 2017). Denosumab is another alternative agent for treating Paget disease when bisphosphonates are not tolerated. This drug blocks the principal endogenous factor regulating osteoclast recruitment, RANKL, which is essential for the formation, function, and survival of osteoclasts. The recommended dosage is 60 mg via subcutaneous injection given every 6 months. Unfortunately, denosumab is much less effective than bisphosonates, and more studies are needed (Muschitz et al., 2017; Tuck et al., 2017; Vallet & Ralston, 2016).

Pain directly attributed to Paget disease is mostly relieved through bisphosphonate intervention. However, some pain may result from bone deformity, arthritic, or neurologic complications. Patients with mild to moderate pain may be managed with analgesic therapy that includes acetaminophen, nonsteroidal antiinflammatory drugs (NSAIDs), or the COX-2 inhibitors. These may be prescribed in addition to the main pagetic therapy chosen (Alikhan, 2018; NORD, n.d.; Vallet & Ralston, 2016).

Physical Rehabilitation

Osteoporosis and Osteopenia

Physical activity is one of the most effective age-related modifiable factors for maintaining and increasing BMD. Regular exercise with an emphasis on particular dosing can improve muscle strength, bone density, balance, and flexibility, ultimately decreasing the risk of falls and resulting fractures. Research has well established that the load of weight-bearing exercise is particularly valuable in maintaining bone mass and decreasing the risk of related fractures (Dohrn et al., 2016; Fornusek & Kilbreath, 2017; Howe et al., 2011; Kopiczho, 2019; Rosen & Drezner, 2019; Winters-Stone et al., 2013; Zhao et al., 2014). During physical activity, two types of mechanical stimuli interact to provide the mechanical stress required for bone density growth. Weight-bearing and resistive activities provide forces exerted by the joint force reaction and the ground force reaction. Increased bone density results from the mechanical adaptation of bone tissue to increasing loads produced by the attaching muscles secondary to these force reactions (Kemmeler et al., 2004; Kopiczho, 2019; Matsuo, 2009).

The 2014 Health Professional's Guide to Rehabilitation of the Patient With Osteoporosis (Cosman et al., 2015) offers concise recommendations for the treatment of osteoporosis for adults 50 years of age and older. Physical rehabilitation and exercise interventions that include moderate-intensity impact exercise maintain and increase BMD. Research has determined that physical therapy intervention for patients with osteoporosis or osteopenia should include the following: weight-bearing activity, flexibility and strengthening exercise, postural exercise, and balance exercise. It is evidenced that these exercises also decrease back pain associated with progressed osteoporosis and vertebral fractures. Rehabilitation intervention then includes education for the patient and safe home exercise. Physical and occupational therapists can also provide prescriptions for assistive devices and an evaluation of the home environment to decrease the risk factors for falls (Cosman et al., 2015; National Osteoporosis Foundation, n.d).

Paget Disease

Paget disease should be managed in an outpatient setting with physical, occupational, or speech therapy. Inpatient rehabilitation may be indicated for patients who have become deconditioned and are unable to perform activities of daily living independently or care for themselves at home. Physical therapy is important in the treatment process and the rehabilitation of persons diagnosed with Paget disease because it helps them to improve muscle strength, maintain joint range of motion and flexibility, increase endurance, and avoid deconditioning. Rehabilitation is essential after total joint replacement, fracture repair, laminectomy, or other major surgery associated with Paget disease. The pain associated with increased skeletal abnormalities leads to a loss of muscle strength, decreased range of motion, and reduced cardiovascular endurance, resulting in functional limitations such as slower walking and shorter distances. Exercise supervised by the physical therapist can help patients to maintain muscle strength, flexibility, and joint range of motion, and to increase endurance. Strengthening muscles can help minimize the skeletal complications association with Paget disease. Physical therapists can help patients to improve cardiovascular function and cardiac output, thus improving the patient's ability to perform activities of daily living. Recommendations may be made for orthotics and supportive devices (Chow, 2018; National Organization for Rare Disorders, n.d).

Orthoses and Supportive Equipment

Osteoporosis and Paget Disease

Long-term immobilization is not recommended for patients with osteoporosis, unless there are acute vertebral fractures or chronic pain, to prevent further muscle weakness, deconditioning, and decreased bone density due to the lack of weight-bearing activity (Cosman et al., 2015; Dohrn et al., 2016). In patients with vertebral fractures or chronic pain resulting from fractures, trunk orthoses may be required. These may include back braces, lumbosacral and dorsolumbosacral corsets, and posture training support devices (PTS) that assist with pain relief by decreasing the loads on the fracture site while aligning the vertebra (Cosman et al., 2015).

The goals of the utilization of orthoses may include any combination of limiting range of motion, improving posture, decreasing pain and fatigue, and improving function. For patient compliance with orthotic management of osteoporosis, a well-coordinated multidisciplinary team approach is indicated to professionally manage the care. Orthoses are commonly prescribed to treat and support patients with vertebral compression fractures (VCFs). They offer a low-risk and cost-effective treatment option for VCF; however, there is limited research that supports the use of orthoses in the treatment of VCFs. Thus physical therapy intervention must be included when orthoses are utilized. Spinal orthoses can be uncomfortable, leading to patient noncompliance, and they are associated with risk for pressure sores and decreased pulmonary capacity (Newman et al., 2015; Raiser & Alfano, 2019).

Deformity and abnormal biomechanics that result from Paget disease are often helped by orthotics. The literature is limited, but foot supports for leg discrepancies and spinal orthoses are often prescribed to decrease pain (Tan & Ralston, 2014; Tuck et al., 2017).

Surgical Intervention

Osteoporosis

Vertebral compression fractures (VCFs) are the most common fractures associated with osteoporosis. Fortunately, only 30% to 40% of these fractures are symptomatic, but the resulting neurologic deficits and pain most often severely limit a person's ability to perform ADLs and reduce one's quality of life (Anderson et al., 2013; Lou et al., 2018; Makris & Reid, 2017). Goals of treatment for VCFs include decreased pain and stabilization of the vertebrae. Research supports reserving surgery for patients with significant vertebral instability or neurologic compromise (Luo et al., 2016; Yuan et al., 2016). Vertebral augmentation surgeries such as percutaneous vertebroplasty (PVP) and balloon kyphoplasty (BKP) are minimally invasive techniques that are widely recommended for osteoporotic VCFs. Vertebroplasty is performed by percutaneously injecting radiopaque bone cement or other therapeutic material into the compression fracture or unstable painful vertebral body. Balloon kyphoplasty is an image-guided procedure in which a balloon is inserted into the vertebrae that then creates a cavity, which is filled with material (Anderson et al., 2013; Kochan et al., 2020). Luo et al. (2018) performed a review of all meta-analyses, evaluating trials of vertebral augmentation compared with nonoperative intervention for VCF. Their results indicated that current literature suggests that vertebral augmentation is more effective in improving pain outcomes compared with nonoperative intervention. Zhang et al. (2017) evaluated new-level fracture risk after PVP or BKP compared with conservative nonoperative treatment to determine if these procedures increase the risk for new vertebral compression fractures at untreated levels. A meta-analysis of comparative studies was performed, and results of their analysis did not reveal an increased risk of fracture.

Paget Disease

Orthopedic surgery may be a necessity for the correction of resulting deformities, joint replacement, prophylactic nailing to prevent probably fracture, and nerve compression. The bone activity associated with Paget disease should be controlled with drug therapy, especially bisphosphonates, prior to surgery to decrease vascularity and the risk of excessive blood loss. Pretreatment also reduces the potential for postoperative complications such as loosening of prostheses or rapid progression of the pagetic bone (Tan & Ralston, 2014; Tuck et al., 2017). Jorge-Mora et al. (2016) performed a systematic review of articles about patients with Paget disease of bone that affected the spine and were treated surgically over a span of 30 years. The main indications for surgery were neurologic symptoms and pain.

The Clinical Guideline for Diagnosis and Management of Paget Disease of Bone in Adults recommends total hip or knee arthroplasties for patients who additionally develop OA and in whom other medical treatment is not successful. The guideline additionally recommends fixation of fracture through the affected bone in PDB; however, the clinical outcomes in femoral neck and subtrochanteric fractures were poor. Osteotomy is evidenced intervention of the correction of bone deformity and improvement of pain in patients with PDB, with the benefit outweighing the risks involved in most cases (Ralston et al., 2019). Spinal surgery is considered for patients with PDB who have developed spinal stenosis and spinal cord compression with a successful decrease in symptoms (Jorge-Mora et al., 2016). Vertebroplasty has demonstrated good results with little complication in those who have mechanical pain with Paget disease (Jorge-Mora et al., 2016; Pedicelli et al., 2011).

Approach to the Older Adult With Fracture

Pathologic Fracture

Vertebral Compression Fracture

Vertebral compression fractures (VCFs) are the consequence of an axial/compressive load greater than that tolerated by the bony integrity, resulting in a fracture from the biomechanical failure of the bone (Hoyt et al., 2020; Patel et al., 2021; Urrutia et al., 2019). Vertebral compression fractures are defined as a loss of approximately 20% or at least 4 mm of anterior, middle, or posterior vertebral height. About 60% to 75% of VCFs occur in the thoracolumbar spine (T12–L2) followed by the lower lumbar region (L2 to L5) (Dewar, 2015; Hoyt et al., 2020; Patel et al., 2021).

These fractures typically occur in the anterior spinal column, which is composed of the anterior two-thirds of each of the following: the vertebral body, intervertebral disc, and longitudinal ligament (Donnally et al., 2020; Patel et al., 2021; Urrutia et al., 2019). Vertebral compression fractures are most often the result of osteoporosis in older adults and are directly correlated with aging as bone density progressively decreases.

The prevalence of VCF in postmenopausal women in the United States who are over 50 years of age is approximately 25% and 40% by the age of 80 with an annual incidence of approximately 10.7% for women and 5.7% for men (Goldstein et al., 2015; Hoyt et al., 2020). Fortunately, only 30% to 40% of these fractures are symptomatic, but the resulting neurologic deficits and pain most often severely limit a person's ability to perform ADLs and restrict one's quality of life (Anderson et al., 2013; Lou et al., 2018; Makris & Reid, 2017). For diagnostic and treatment strategies for VCFs, see the previous section on osteoporosis.

Hip Fracture

Hip fractures are a leading cause of disability and mortality in older adults, with greater than 95% of these fractures being caused by falling. More than 300,000 older adults are hospitalized for hip fractures each year, with 80% of these fractures occurring in older women (CDC, 2019). However, even though the risk of hip fracture is higher in older women, mortality rates due to hip fracture are higher in men (Gurger, 2019). The overall in-hospital mortality of this population with hip fracture is approximately 5%, with complications associated with the fracture event being the main causes of death.

Hip fractures can lead to systemic inflammatory response and lung injury, both of which increase the risk of respiratory infections and death during the postinjury recovery time (Gan et al., 2015). Even with advanced surgical methods and postoperative care, the 1-year mortality rate in older adults with hip fractures is between 20% and 30%. Gurger (2019) evaluated the risk factors that impact this 1-year mortality rate in the older adult with hip fractures after treatment with primary arthroplasty and proximal femoral nail (PFN). It was concluded that delayed surgery and postoperative complications may be the most important risk factors for this 1-year mortality rate. Katsoulis et al. (2017) investigated 122,808 participants from eight different cohorts in Europe and the Unites States for a mean of 12.6 years, which included 4273 accidental hip fractures with 27,999 resultant deaths. Hip fractures were positively associated with short- and long-term all-cause mortality in both males and females.

Tang et al. (2016) compared the physical condition and ability of 733 older adults before and after hip fractures. Functional recovery was measured by their ability to independently care for themselves with bathing, dressing, eating, and going to the restroom. The researchers concluded that fewer than 505 returned to a prefracture level of function regardless of their previous level of function and that for adults older than 85 years with comorbidities and dementia, the likelihood of returning to a high level of function was extremely low.

Stress Fracture

Stress fractures are caused by repeated loads whose intensities are less than that required to fracture a bone in a single incident. In the older adult population, this type of fracture most often occurs in persons with rheumatic diseases, osteoporosis, and knee arthroplasty. There are two categories of stress fracture: fatigue fracture and insufficiency fracture. Fatigue fracture results from an abnormal load upon healthy bone, and insufficiency fracture results from normal loading on abnormal bone. Knowing which category the fracture belongs to helps clinicians to predict the sites of injury and the diagnosis that will guide them to the correct treatment option. The majority of stress fractures with older adults are insufficiency fractures (Guler & Cerci, 2020; Matcuk et al., 2016). Stress fractures are most commonly diagnosed in the lower extremities, with the most frequent sites involving the metatarsal bones, calcaneus, proximal, and distal tibia. Bilateral involvement has been diagnosed in up to 16% of stress fracture cases (Guler & Cerci, 2020; Ozdemir & Yilmaz, 2016). Periprosthetic stress fractures around the knee can occur after total knee arthroplasty and can be diagnosed in the femur, tibia, and patella (Ozdemir & Yilmaz, 2016; Takai et al., 2018).

Traumatic Fracture

Falls and motor vehicle accidents are the most common means of injury among those in the older adult population. Older adult patients with traumatic injury have higher mortality rates than younger adults regardless of the mechanism involved. Those with an injury severity score greater than

15 most often die while in the hospital. Older adults are more susceptible to injury from minor causes and then have decreased potential to recover from any injury (Colwell & Moreira, 2021). Additionally, compared to younger adults with major trauma, older patients have longer hospital and ICU stays and are more likely to be discharged to a nursing home (Beck et al., 2018).

Gioffre-Glorio et al. (2018) studied 4554 patients 65 years and older who had sustained home injuries or car accidents from 2012 to 2016. The most common injuries were head injuries, followed by fractures of the upper and lower extremities. The highest prevalence of injury occurred in adults 75 to 84 years old. Hip fractures were most prevalent in the lower extremity, and the most frequent upper extremity fractures were to the wrist and proximal humerus. Rib fractures were most often associated with pneumothorax, hemothorax, or pulmonary contusions. Traumatic fractures occurred more in women in each year and in each older adult age group.

Bergh et al. (2020) reported on incidence of fracture locations of 23,917 persons who had sustained 27,169 fractures. The mean age of those who sustained the fracture was 57.9 years, and 64.5% occurred in women. Proximal femur fractures were most closely associated with older age, occurring 77.2% in patients 75 years of age and older. Other common fracture locations in females over 50 years were the distal radius, proximal femur, and proximal humerus. Zhu et al. (2020) performed a retrospective study to describe the epidemiologic characteristics of fracture in older adults in China during the COVID-19 pandemic; the study included 436 patients with 453 fractures. The majority of the fractures occurred at home (72.7%), with low-energy falls being the major means of injury.

Steps for Diagnosing Fractures

Signs and symptoms of stress fractures typically present with insidious onset but without a history of trauma or injury. Patients usually complain of pain with activity that is relieved with rest. The pain lasts progressively longer after the exercise or activity. Clinical diagnostic tests are limited. Point tenderness with palpation and the single leg hop test often reproduces pain. Fulcrum testing of the long bones also can elicit pain. Radiographic imaging initially includes plain radiography, which is readily available, inexpensive, and has low radiation exposure. If x-rays are negative but diagnosis is in question, magnetic resonance imaging (MRI) is recommended as a second-line imaging modality; it has a sensitivity of 100% and specificity of 100%.

A problem with MRI is the expense of the test and the lack of availability in all settings. Computer tomography (CT) is another modality used to image stress fractures, but it has a lower sensitivity than MRI. Laboratory tests are usually not needed but may assist the clinician in determining the mechanism of fracture if questioned: serum 25, D3 calcium, phosphate, parathyroid hormone, thyroid-stimulating hormone, alkaline phosphatase, albumin, and prealbumin may be considered (Barros et al., 2017; Denay, 2017; Matcuk et al., 2016; May & Marappa-Ganeshan, 2021; McInnis & Ramey, 2016; Miller et al., 2018).

Radiography is the gold-standard diagnostic modality for traumatic fracture in all age groups. Champagne et al. (2019) performed a systematic review and subgroup meta-analysis to assess the effectiveness of ultrasound (US) in the detection of upper and lower extremity bone fractures in adults compared to radiology, MRI, and CT scan in secondary and tertiary care centers. The results indicated that ultrasonography demonstrates good diagnostic detection of these fractures, especially in the foot and ankle.

Hip Fractures

The American College of Radiology (ACR) Appropriateness Criteria recommend initial imaging with conventional radiography. The guidelines were modified in 2019 to recommend for either CT or MRI as "usually appropriate" if radiographic results do not indicate fracture but a fracture is still suspected due to signs and symptoms (Ross et al., 2019). A 2019 meta-analysis of evidence researched CT scans for radiographic occult proximal hip fractures. Results showed a sensitivity of 94% and specificity of 100% with an added benefit of the speed of CT, particularly for persons with confusion at the time of injury (Kellock et al., 2019).

Wilson et al. (2020) performed a systematic review and meta-analysis to evaluate the diagnostic accuracy of limited MRI protocols for detecting radiographically occult proximal femoral fractures. Eleven studies with 938 patients and 247 proximal femoral fractures met the inclusions criteria. Evidence from the study indicated that limited MRI protocols can be used as the standard of care in patients with a suspected but radiographically occult hip fracture. A protocol composed of coronal T1-weighted and short tau inversion recovery (STIR) sequences is 100% sensitive.

Factors to Consider in the Treatment of Fracture

Research estimates that approximately 40% of falls in older adults are preventable. Polypharmacy, a chronic co-prescription of multiple medications, has been recognized as one of the most significant factors associated with falls with the older adult population. Thus it is suggested that medications in older patients should be revised on a regular basis with the number of medications kept to a minimum (Zaninotto et al., 2020).

Investigations indicate that cardiovascular agents, central nervous system drugs, analgesics, and endocrine medications particularly increase fall risk that can lead to fractures in older adults (Richardson et al., 2015; Zia et al., 2017). Older adults have both an increased rate of trauma and an increased potential to injury even from minimal forces. Low-risk stress fractures are treated with relative rest and weight-bearing restriction/activity modification until the patient is symptom-free, followed by gradual return to activity as tolerated. High-risk stress fractures include sites such as the tension-side femoral neck, patella, anterior tibia, medial malleolus, talus, tarsal navicular, proximal fifth metatarsal, and great toe sesamoids. These sites may require a period of non–weight bearing and may require surgical consultation given the high risk of suboptimal healing (Denay, 2017; Liem et al., 2013; McInnis & Ramey, 2016).

High-risk stress fractures most often do not respond to conservative management and often result in significant morbidity. Except for residual pain, low-risk stress fracture complications are generally few. High-risk stress fractures generally are more likely to progress toward nonunion and thus require surgical intervention (May & Marappa-Ganeshan, 2021; Miller & Best, 2016). In the more active older adult population, the incidence of stress fractures has been increasing. Studies indicate that stress injuries in older adults are associated with poor muscle strength. Risk factors include the footwear used, exercise surface, smiling, and alcohol consumption. Intrinsic risk factors include gender, age, race, fitness level, biomechanical factors, and previous history of stress fracture (Barros et al., 2017; Matcuk et al., 2016).

Treatment Options for the Older Adult With Fracture

Pharmacologic Intervention

A Cochrane review indicated that there is high-quality evidence that calcium combined with vitamin D results in small and significant decreases in the risk of hip fracture (16%), vertebral fracture (14%), and any nonvertebral fracture (11%). These studies recommend an intake of 800 IU/day of vitamin D and 1000 mg of calcium each day (Fares, 2018). Additionally, a meta-analysis reported that an increased intake of vegetables, but not fruits, was associated with a lower risk of hip fractures in older adults (Luo et al., 2016). Post fracture, patients may benefit from calcium and vitamin D supplements even though research does not indicate a clear benefit or faster healing (DeFroda et al., 2017). Medicinal recommendations in the treatment of postmenopausal osteoporosis to prevent fractures is discussed in the section on osteoporosis.

To address pain following surgery for fractures in older adults, NSAIDs are not recommended and clinicians are advised to offer the patient non-NSAIDs every 6 hours unless contraindicated. If pain continues, opioids can be prescribed, accompanied by a constipation prophylaxis. If non-NSAIDs and opioids do not relieve the pain, nerve blocks are often considered (Fischer et al., 2021). Guay et al. (2017) performed a Cochrane review that found moderate-quality evidence for decreasing pneumonia, time to mobility, and medication costs after single-shot blocks. High-quality evidence indicated that a regional block decreases pain with movement within 30 minutes after block intervention.

Physical Rehabilitation

Stress injuries are best managed by an interprofessional team that includes physical and occupational therapists and orthopedic nurses (Kiel & Kaiser, 2021). An interdisciplinary team identifies and addresses the surgical implications but also the complex analgesia, medical, cognitive, nutritional, social, and rehabilitation needs of these older adults, leading to improved outcomes (McDonough et al., 2021; Riemen & Hutchison, 2016; Terzis et al., 2021).

All guidelines recommend physical therapy assessment and mobilization on the first day following surgery. Not receiving a physical therapist intervention on the first postoperative day is a strong predictor for poor mobility upon discharge. An occupational therapist is also recommended to assess and educate patients about safe transfer techniques, hygiene tasks, and self-care (Riemen & Hutchison, 2016). After transfer from the acute care setting, patients with continued impairments and functional deficits after hip fracture need a physical therapy referral within 72 hours by a facility or home care physical therapist. It is recommended that referring clinicians provide for additional therapies if strength, balance, and functional deficits remain after 8 to 16 weeks (McDonough et al., 2021). Smith et al. (2015) performed a Cochrane review and found that older adults who are part of multidisciplinary care and rehabilitation models have significantly lower complications rates, decreased lengths of hospital stay and institutional placement, and better function and ambulation ability than prefracture.

Both high-low and high-risk stress fractures need a period of immobilization to allow the fracture to heal. There are two phases of rehabilitation. Phase 1 is active rest. During this time, aerobic fitness is advocated using no-impact activities like cycling, deep water walking, and swimming. If the patient is unable to ambulate without pain, temporary immobilization is indicated. Once the patient has been pain-free for 1 to 2 weeks, phase 2 may be initiated. This phase should include rehabilitation to strengthen the muscles of the injured extremity, improve proprioception, strengthen the core and pelvic girdle muscle, and progress the patient to pre-injury levels of activity. Both phases are best treated with physical therapy (Kiel & Kaiser, 2021; May & Marappa-Ganeshan, 2021).

Terzis et al. (2021) researched the effects of a rehabilitation program on the static balance, mobility, and strength of lower extremities in older adults who had fractured hips from a fall and received surgery as compared with nonoperated persons. The authors concluded that the intervention led to significant improvement in static balance, mobility, and strength of the loser extremities after hip fracture. Evidence-based rehabilitation should be prescribed for older adults who fall, with and without surgical intervention. Weight-bearing exercises and reducing home hazards have significant benefit in lowering the incidence of falls among older adults and thus reducing fracture occurrences. Prevention of fractures in older adults includes rehabilitation therapies, patient education, prevention of osteoporosis, and fall prevention, with special consideration given to reducing home hazards (Fares, 2018).

Casting and Orthoses

Ankle fractures in older adults that are stable under stress radiographs or axial loading are often treated with a stable orthosis or a special walker/boot that puts the foot in neutral and limits supination with weight bearing. Casts may be indicated initially for 3 to 5 days when severe soft tissue swelling is evident. The orthosis is normally worn for 6 weeks until the fracture is healed. Radiographs are most often obtained at 1 week after the injury to rule out secondary dislocation. Cast immobilization with off-loading is also recommended for older adults with poor bone quality (Rammelt, 2016).

Surgical Intervention

Most hip fractures are treated surgically, leading to better results for pain control and early mobilization to reduce the risks associated with prolonged bed rest and immobilization. Surgical intervention with open reduction followed by stabilization with internal fixation (ORIF) is indicated when there are pelvic fractures and proximal femur fractures that include the following: displaced or nondisplaced intracapsular femoral neck fractures, femoral head fracture-dislocations, intertrochanteric fractures, and subtrochanteric fractures (Kisner et al., 2018). For the older adult patient, the surgical intervention of choice for these types of fractures usually is a hemiarthroplasty (HA) or a total hip arthroplasty (THA) (Wang, F., et al., 2015; Tang et al., 2017).

The HA replaces the articular surface of the femoral head with the acetabular articular surface not surgically altered. With THA the articular surfaces of both joint components, the acetabulum and femur, are replaced (Kisner et al., 2018; Magee et al., 2016). Surgery should be performed within the first 24 hours after fracture to decrease the potential for perioperative complications such as pneumonia, pulmonary embolism, deep vein thrombosis, urinary trat infections, and pressure ulcers. When is surgery is delayed for more than 48 hours, statistics indicate that mortality risk increases significantly (Fischer et al., 2012; Klestil et al., 2018; Mears & Kates, 2015).

The American Academy of Orthopaedic Surgeons (AAOS, 2014) and the UK National Institute for Health and Care Excellence (NICE, 2017) recommend offering THA to older adults who meet certain criteria, with the anticipated functional benefits. These recommendations are for older adults who could ambulate independently prior to fracture, are not cognitively impaired, and are medically fit for both the anesthesia involved and the procedure. Three main surgical approaches are used with total hip replacement: the anterolateral, direct lateral, and posterolateral approaches (Kisner et al., 2018). The AAOS guideline for hip fractures presents moderate evidence that supports higher dislocation rates when a posterior approach is used in the treatment of displaced femoral neck fractures with hip arthroplasty (AAOS, 2014).

Heterotopic Ossificans

Approach to the Older Adult With Heterotopic Ossification

Heterotopic ossification (HO), also known as paraosteoarthropathy, myositis ossificans, and heterotopic calcification, refers to the abnormal formation of lamellar bone in nonosseous tissue, such as muscle, nerves, and connective tissue (Biz et al., 2015; Hoyt et al., 2020; Mujtaba et al., 2019; Sun & Hanyu-Deutmeyer, 2019).

The two major types of HO are acquired and genetic, with acquired being significantly more dominant. Acquired HO subdivides into three etiologic categories: neurogenic, orthopedic, and traumatic. Neurogenic HO is associated with traumatic brain injury (TBI), cerebral vascular accident (CVA), brain tumors, and spinal cord injury (SCI). Orthopedic HO results from arthroscopy, fracture fixation, joint dislocation, and joint arthroplasty. Finally, traumatic HO occurs with severe burns and high-velocity blast injuries (Cholok et al., 2019; Mujtaba et al., 2019; Sun & Hanyu-Deutmeyer, 2019). The pathophysiology of HO is uncertain, but theories suggest that failure to regulate the immune system or inflammatory response leads to the development of inciting cells; these then inappropriately activate mesenchymal stem cells that could differentiate into cartilage, bone, or tendon/ligament and become osteoblasts that lead to exaggerated ectopic bone proliferation (Cholok et al., 2019; Meyers et al., 2019; Mujtaba et al., 2019; Ohlmeier et al., 2019; Peterson et al., 2015). Heterotopic ossification may also be a result of rare hereditary conditions such as fibrodysplasia ossificans progressiva and progressive osseous hyperplasia (Hoyt, 2018).

Complications With Trauma

People who have heterotopic ossification associated with trauma can be classified into two broad categories: civilian patients and combat casualties, with distinct differences in prevalence and treatment. With civilian traumatic injuries, HO is diagnosed in approximately 11% to 20% of patients with traumatic brain or spinal cord injuries, in 20% of patients with forearm fractures, in 52% of patients with femoral shaft fractures, and in 60% of severe burn patients. The frequency of HO increases significantly, with combat casualties as high as 65% in post blast, extremity injured persons with amputations (Dey et al., 2017; Edwards et al., 2016). Chronic muscular trauma leads to traumatic myositis ossificans. The most common sites are the quadriceps femoris muscle and the brachialis muscles. The most common sites for traumatic neurogenic HO are the hips, extensor sides of elbows, shoulders, and knees (Sun & Hanyu-Deutmeyer, 2019). In patients with spinal cord injury, risk factors for HO include the severity of the injury and the level of the spinal cord injury. Injuries to the thoracic and cervical spine most often result in greater HO severity (Cholok et al., 2019).

Heterotopic ossification occurs in more than 60% of persons with extensive third-degree burns. HO associated with burns is frequently identified around joints and at sites with a large number of scleraxis-expressing cells (Dey et al., 2017; Peterson et al., 2013). The ectopic bone with severe burns often leads to nerve compression that results in pain, open or nonhealing wounds, and the restricted use of joints. For patients with burn injuries, HO is most often documented in the upper extremities, especially in the elbow (Dey et al., 2017; Orchard et al., 2014).

Complications With Surgical Procedures

In total joint arthroplasty, HO most commonly occurs with arthroplasty of the hips, knees, elbows, and shoulder (Sun & Hanyu-Deutmeyer, 2019). Heterotopic ossification is a recognized complication of total hip arthroplasties (Ohlmeier et al., 2019). The incidence of HO following total hip replacement (THR) and revision of THR has been reported to be as high as 26% to 41% (Meyers et al., 2019).

Ohlmeier et al. (2019) evaluated patients 6 months after total hip arthroplasty (THA) and evidenced HO in 21% of the participants. A meta-analysis from 2015 presented the average frequency of HO occurrence following THA at 30% (Zhu et al., 2015). Zheng et al. (2020) investigated the incidence in location of HO following hip arthroscopy. This retrospective study enrolled 327 patients who had hip arthroscopy intervention from January 2010 to December 2015. They concluded that HO is a minor complication of hip arthroscopy but can induce severe pain and functional impairment and usually forms in the arthroscopic portal or capsulotomy area.

Steps for Diagnosing Heterotopic Ossification

Patients with possible HO typically complain of inflammatory symptoms that include muscle pain, edema, erythema, and warmth in the area of the ectopic bone formation. Heterotopic ossification characteristically leads to progressive loss of range of motion when posttraumatic inflammation is usually no longer prevalent. With no intervention, joint ankylosis occurs (Lee et al., 2021). Early diagnosis of posttraumatic HO is imperative for timely intervention and prophylactic management of HO. Delaying the diagnosis of HO results in the progression of HO with the increased potential to lead to complications such as nerve impingement, joint contractures, pain, and limited range of motion (Dey et al., 2017). The early inflammatory phase signs and symptoms often mimic other pathologies that must be ruled out such as cellulitis, thrombophlebitis, osteomyelitis, or tumor. Additionally, deep vein thrombosis (DVT) and HO have been positively associated (Meyers, 2019).

Plain radiographs are typically the first imaging technique used to detect nongenetic HO with distinctive features that lead to the diagnosis of HO. No ossification is found by radiographs in the early phases of HO, as there are no calcific changes. This low-density mass may be the only sign of HO detected by CT (Meyers, 2019; Mujtaba et al., 2019; Weerakkody & Knipe, 2021).

Mature intramuscular HO appears as a well-developed and well-demarcated radio-dense mass with radiodensity most apparent in the periphery of the lesions reflecting a calcified outline or shell to the mass, which is termed *egg-shell calcification*. This represents a peripheral cortex with a well-defined cancellous bone interior and is detected by plain radiography and both contrast-enhanced and non-contrast CT (Dey et al., 2017; Meyers, 2019; Mujtaba et al., 2019). Magnetic resonance (MR) can also detect early lesions with HO due to the increased tissue vascularization and density. As the lesion is maturing, MR imaging results in nonspecific findings and mimics other pathologic processes. Once mature HO presents as cancellous fate outlined by hypointense cortical bone that is well detected by MR, no further imaging is considered necessary for diagnosis (Dey et al., 2017; Mujtaba et al., 2019).

The Brooker staging system is the most widely accepted classification system for the differential diagnosis of HO and includes four grades based on anteroposterior (AP) radiograph of the pelvis and hip. Grades 3 and 4 are considered clinically diagnostic (Biz et al., 2015; Lee et al., 2021; Ohlmeier et al., 2019; Weerakkody & Knipe, 2021). See the Brooker classification of HO in Fig.16.5.

Mujtaba et al. (2019) performed a literature review of HO and THR to develop guidelines for the prevention and management of patients with existing HO. Evidence included scintigraphy as the most sensitive method in diagnosing HO. Scintigraphy involves the administration of a radio-pharmaceutical followed by a series of scans that provide information about dynamic blood flow, blood accumulation, and the accumulation of the diagnostic medication in the bone. Scintigraphy was effective in identifying the maturity of HO, as there is a decrease in uptake of the radiopharmaceutical with more mature ectopic bone. Wang, Q. et al. (2018) evaluated ultrasonography for depicting HO progression. The study suggested that ultrasonography has potential for monitoring the development of HO and for providing a quantitative evaluation on HO when used with plain radiography.

With laboratory diagnostic studies, alkaline phosphatase is the most commonly ordered lab, but often is not elevated in the early stages of HO formation and may take up to 2 weeks to be elevated. Evidence indicates that serum alkaline phosphatase with levels greater than 250 is associated with HO in persons with a THA. The level of alkaline phosphatase does not correlate with the severity of the injury, however. Other inflammatory markers investigated include the erythrocyte sedimentation rate (ESR) and C-reactive protein. An ESR greater than 35 mm/hr usually indicates the development of HO (Mujtaba et al., 2019).

Factors to Consider in the Treatment of Heterotopic Ossification

Several studies have confirmed risk factors for developing HO, which include male gender, the presence of prior HO,

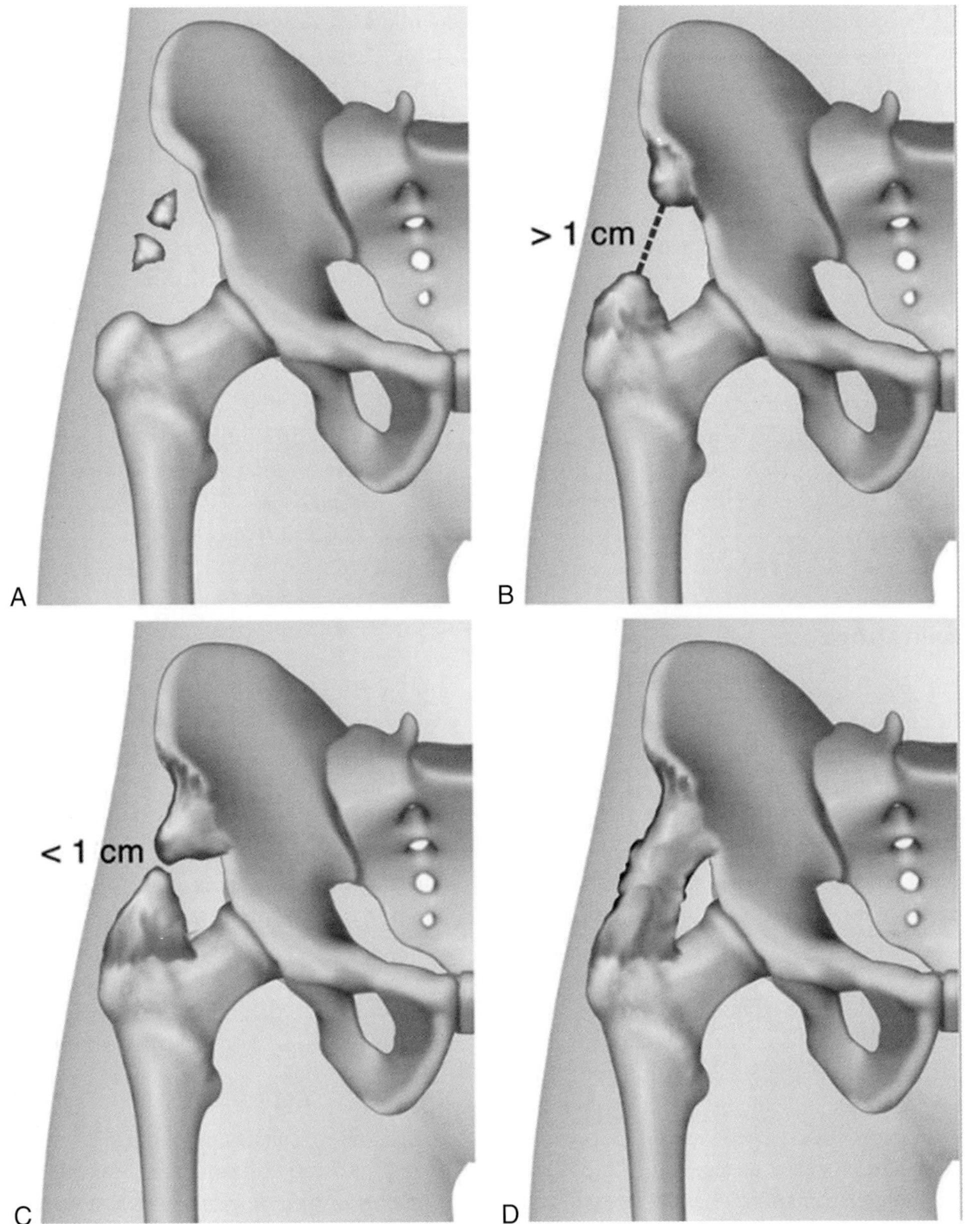

• **Fig. 16.5** Brooker classification of heterotopic ossification. (From Chas, S., et al. [2018]. Efficacy of prophylactic radiotherapy in the treatment of heterotopic ossification. *Cyclone, The Royal College of Radiologists*, 30, 6.)

and previous hip surgery. Some pathologies are also associated with a higher incidence of HO such as ankylosing spondylitis, hypertrophic osteoarthritis, diffuse idiopathic skeletal hyperostosis, Paget disease, Parkinson disease, and RA (Biz et al., 2015; Sun & Hanyu-Deutmeyer, 2019). Identifying patients with a high risk for developing HO is vital to the prophylaxis of HO. Routine prophylactic intervention is not recommended. Davis et al. (2016) assessed the influence of ethnicity on the incidence of HO after THA. They investigated the 6-month postoperative anteroposterior radiographs of 1449 primary THAs and retrospectively graded them for the presence of HO, using the Brooker classification. African American ethnicity was an independent risk factor for HO formation following THA, and prophylaxis treatment must be considered with this group.

Treatment Options for the Older Adult With Heterotopic Ossification

Pharmacologic Intervention

The most commonly prescribed medications for HO include antiinflammatory agents to decrease the prostaglandin synthesis that is necessary for osteogenic differentiation into the ectopic bone (Biz et al., 2015; Cholok et al., 2019; Meyers et al., 2019; Mujtaba et al., 2019). Numerous NSAIDs have demonstrated efficacy, yet postoperatively, the nonselective COX inhibitor, indomethacin, has become the gold standard, with dosing most often prescribed at 25 mg three times daily for up to 6 weeks after surgery (Lee et al., 2021; Meyers et al., 2019). More recently, COX-2 selective inhibitors are being prescribed more often due to the gastrointestinal effects of the nonselective NSAIDs (Biz et al., 2015; Meyers et al., 2019; Oni et al., 2014). Oni et al. (2014) examined the effect of the selective COX-2 inhibitor, celecoxib, on the rates of HO following THA. A control group of 108 patients did not receive celecoxib, and 106 patients did receive the medication. Celecoxib was associated with a significant reduction in the incidence of HO in patients after receiving THA. In agreement, Łęgosz et al. (2019) examined 117 articles concerning HO and THR; they concluded that NSAIDs and COX-2 inhibitors are commonly used for HO. This literature review also reported that numerous studies evidenced that treatment with bisphosphonates was ineffective.

Physical Rehabilitation

Historically, any passive range of motion (PROM) was considered contraindicated with HO, as PROM could lead to further ectopic bone development. An extensive review of the literature evidenced that active and PROM exercises, in addition to splinting, increase function with developing or diagnosed HO (Casavant & Hastings, 2006; Goodman et al., 2020; Sims et al., 2019). Following a thorough assessment, physical therapist intervention is determined based on the patient's phase of healing. During the first 2 weeks postsurgery or injury (the acute and edematous phase), intervention goals are to decrease edema and the potential for scar development and to reduce pain and thereby promote maximum participation in the rehabilitation program. Range-of-motion exercises are indicated depending on joint stability, with an emphasis on regular exercise to prevent muscle atrophy. From 2 to 6 weeks of recovery, the patient continues to be in the inflammatory phase. Unorganized scar tissue has developed that is soft and can be deformed, so range of motion can improve significantly. Progressive low-load exercise with static splinting is recommended for the best improvements. Functional activities must be encouraged throughout rehabilitation (Casavant & Hastings, 2006; Goodman et al., 2020).

The fibrotic phase begins during the sixth to twelfth week of recovery. Scar tissue is fully formed but continues to respond to progressive strengthening exercises and passive stretching. By 3 months after surgery or injury, the scar tissue is organized and fibrotic. The patient is weaned from splints and is encouraged to continue a regular strengthening program at home for up to 6 months after recovery (Casavant & Hastings, 2006; Goodman et al., 2020). Denormandie et al. (2018) reviewed resection of HO of the hip. They recommended beginning physical rehabilitation once the drains are removed, usually at 1 week after resection. The rehabilitation should progress as tolerated with a focus on function. Weight bearing should progress as tolerated depending on the patient's health and potential for femoral neck fracture. Sims et al. (2020) presented two case studies of patients with trauma injuries and the development of HO after aggressive rehabilitation. They concluded that range-of-motion exercise is indicated; however, progression should be made depending on the patient's complaints of extreme pain. They are also recommended increasing motion and strength with an emphasis on active and functional exercise during the inflammatory stage.

Radiation

Localized low-dose radiation is commonly prescribed and is most effective when administered in close proximity to the area of injury in combination with NSAIDs (Archdeacon et al., 2014; Biz et al., 2015; Cholok et al., 2019; Lee et al., 2012; Meyers et al., 2019; Mujtaba et al., 2019). External beam radiation therapy utilized for HO prophylaxis is usually prescribed to a dose of 7 to 8 single fraction, but studies have evidenced that several fractionation and dosing regimens are appropriate. The current standard verified by evidenced-based research continues to be to give the same dose of single fraction 7 to 8 Gy within 24 hours preoperatively or within 72 hours postoperatively (Lee et al., 2012; Łęgosz et al., 2019; Seegenschmiedt et al., 2001). The low radiation treatment dose is considered a safe treatment with minimal side effects. Potential side effects include fatigue, delayed wound healing, and joint edema. With such low radiation doses the chances of secondary cancer from the radiation treatment is very low (Lee et al., 2012; Łęgosz et al., 2019). Sheybani et al. (2014) analyzed records exceeding 3500 patients who had THR as an intervention. They concluded that there was no increase in malignancy risk after the radiation prophylaxis treatment.

Surgical Resection

Patients with persistent symptoms including decreasing range of motion and function after radiation and medicinal intervention have few management options other than surgical intervention. The main goal of surgical resection is to change the position of the affected joint due to the ectopic bone or to improve its range of motion. Surgical resection of the ectopic bone with nongenetic HO is usually performed by 6 months after the osseous maturation is complete. Evidence indicates that excision before 6 months may be associated with an enhanced risk of HO recurrence (Meyers et al., 2019; Pavey et al., 2015). No additional benefits have been evidenced with further delay of surgical management (Almangour et al., 2016; Chen et al., 2015; Meyers et al., 2019; Pavey et al., 2015).

Myositis and the Older Adult

Idiopathic inflammatory myopathies (IIMs), also known collectively as myositis, refer to a group of rare systemic autoimmune diseases that can affect both adults and children. The conditions are hallmarked by skeletal muscle inflammation and weakness. Despite the simple name, myositis encompasses more than simply autoimmune inflammation in muscle tissue. This inflammation also frequently affects other organs that may include the skin, joints, lungs, gastrointestinal tract, and heart, indicating the systemic nature of this disease (Barsotti et al., 2018; Lundberg et al., 2018; Meyer et al., 2019; Oddis & Aggarwal, 2018; Orlandi et al., 2016; Rider et al., 2018).

Autoimmune diseases develop as a result of chronic inflammation secondary to interactions between genes and the environment (Miller et al., 2018). Based on muscle symptoms, skin rash, and histopathologic features, the most recent classification of IIMs includes adult dermatomyositis, polymyositis (PM), inclusion body myositis (IBM), antisynthetase syndrome (ASS), and, since the early 2000s, autoimmune necrotizing myopathy (Barsotti et al., 2018; Lundberg et al., 2018; Miller et al., 2018; Orlandi et al., 2016). IBM is one of the most common inflammatory myopathies in patients older than the age of 50.

IBM is a progressive skeletal muscle disorder characterized by muscle inflammation, weakness, and atrophy. The symptoms and rate of progression vary significantly from person to person. Inclusion body myositis is a sporadic disorder that occurs more often in males with a male-to-female ration of 3:1. Its prevalence is estimated to be between 51 and 139 individuals per 1 million in the general population of those over 50. Despite growing awareness of this condition, research indicates that it remains underdiagnosed.

Inclusion body myositis is not more prevalent in any specific ethnic or racial group; however, it apparently occurs less often in person of African descent (NORD, n.d.). Research on the demographics and clinical history of patients with IBM is significantly limited, as each study involved a very small sample of patients. Paltiel et al. (2015) conducted a cross-sectional, self-reporting survey with 916 participants diagnosed with IBM in North America. The mean age was 70.4 with the mean time from first symptoms to diagnosis being 4.7 years. One-half of the participants reported that IBM was their initial diagnosis, with the majority reporting difficulty with ambulation and activities of daily living.

Pathogenesis

The underlying cause of IBM is complex, poorly understood, and believed to involve the interaction of genetic, immune-related, and environmental factors. Some individuals may have a genetic predisposition for developing IBM, but the condition typically is not inherited (National Institute of Health [NIH] Genetic and Rare Diseases [GARD], n.d.). Idiopathic inflammatory myopathies have an insidious onset leading to proximal muscle weakness and disability. Muscle tissue biopsy is characterized by the presence of inflammatory and degenerative features. Inflammatory features include endomysial inflammation, invasion of non-necrotic fibers by inflammatory cells, and upregulation of major histocompatibility complex (MHC) class I. The degenerative features include the formation of rimmed vacuoles, tubule filaments seen on electron microscopy, mitochondrial changes in muscle tissue, and the accumulation of many myotoxic proteins that are referred to as inclusions (Gang et al., 2014).

Research indicates that the two most popular theories for the pathogenesis of IBM are as follows: an autoimmune pathway and a degeneration pathway with aging considered an important factor that contributes to mitochondrial abnormalities. Autoimmunity has a key role in the pathogenesis of myositis, with autoantibodies identified in over 50% of diagnosed patients. These autoantibodies target both nuclear and cytoplasmic components of the cell, and they have conventionally been divided into two subsets: myositis-associated autoantibodies (MAAs) and myositis-specific autoantibodies (MSAs).

MAAs refer to autoantibodies that are also found in other conditions in which myositis can occur. MSAs are present in the majority of adult cases and are mostly mutually exclusive (Barsotti & Lundberg, 2018a, 2018b; Betteridge & McHugh, 2016; McHugh & Lundberg, 2018; Tansley, 2018). However, IBM has not responded to several of the conventional medicinal therapies normally used to treat autoimmune disorders, indicating that distinct factors account for its unmanageable nature. In particular, cytotoxic T cells found in the muscle of patients diagnosed with IBM are highly differentiated and their phenotype overlaps with those of T cells in T-cell large granular lymphocytic leukemia, a similarly refractory condition (NORD, n.d.).

In addition to the inflammatory process, studies have noted that some muscle tissue of individuals with IBM shows degenerative changes. Specifically, the muscle tissue of affected persons often contains subcellular compartments called vacuoles. Aberrant protein aggregates in IBM vacuolated muscle fibers are similar to features observed in brain tissue from persons with Alzheimer disease and Parkinson disease with Lewy bodies. The protein aggregation has been called inclusion bodies that give the disorder its name. This significant degenerative component supports the degenerative theory of IBM instead of an inflammatory one (Askanas et al., 2009; Gang et al., 2014; NORD n.d.).

Myositis and Diagnosis

Clinical Features

Dermatomyositis (DM) may occur at any age with the incidence higher in females. Weakness is typically experienced in the proximal upper and lower extremities and often in the cervical flexors. This can present acutely over days to weeks, or more slowly over a few months. Weakness of oropharyngeal and esophageal muscles occurs in up to 30% of patients and results in dysphagia. A characteristic rash is associated with dermatomyositis that may precede or accompany the progressive muscle weakness. This rash appears as a periorbital purplish discoloration (heliotrope rash), a papular erythematous rash over the knuckles (Gottron papules; Fig. 16.6), and an erythematous macular rash on the face,

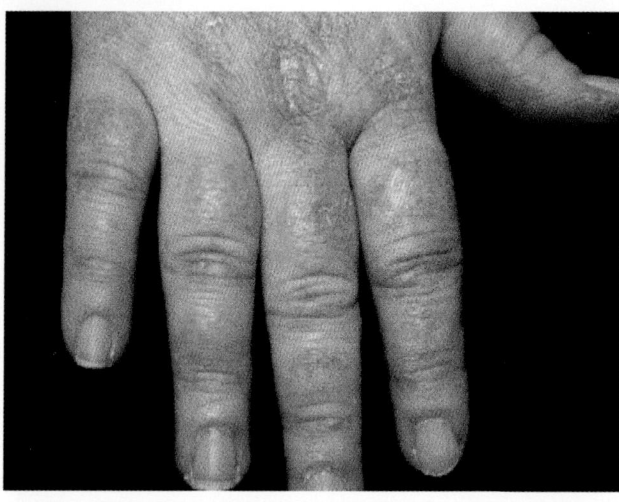

• **Fig. 16.6** Grotton papules. (From Jeffrey P. Callen, Robert L. Wortmann, *Dermatomyositis, Clinics in Dermatology*, 24:5, 2006, Pages 363–373.)

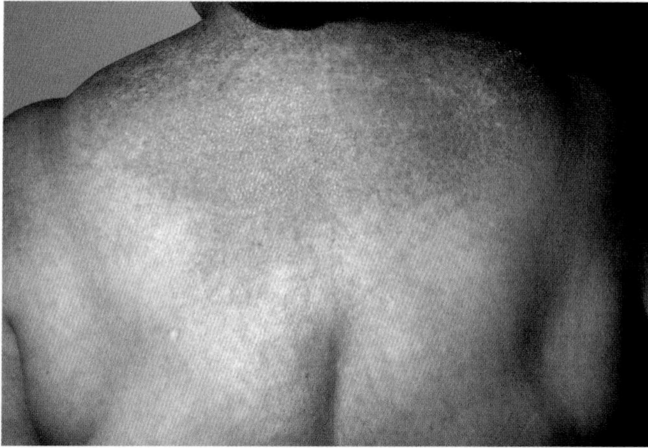

• **Fig. 16.7** Dermatomyositis, shawl sign. (From Micheletti, R. G., et al. [2023]. *Andrews' diseases of the skin clinical atlas* [2nd ed.]. Elsevier.))

neck, and anterior chest, shoulders, and upper back (shawl sign; Fig. 16.7).

Often the rash also develops on the extensor surfaces of elbows, knuckles, and knees (Gottron sign). There may be edema in the affected areas, and the rash may become more evident with sun exposure; subcutaneous calcification is often present. Adult patients with DM may experience weight loss or a low-grade temperature. Multiple systemic complications are associated with DM that include cardiac, pulmonary, gastrointestinal, and rheumatologic involvement. Systemic malignancies may also occur in adult-onset DM, and the condition is associated with infectious disorders such as HIV (Lundberg et al., 2018; Meyer et al., 2017; NIH, n.d.; Oldroyd et al., 2017).

Polymyositis (PM) is rarely diagnosed in persons younger than 20 with onset generally occurring between the ages of 30 and 60. These patients typically present with symmetrical weakness in a proximal distribution in the arms and legs. Patients also report muscle tenderness and myalgia, as well as problems with swallowing. Cardiac conduction system abnormalities and heart failure are associated with approximately 30% of these individuals, and there is an increased risk of malignancy. Up to 20% of all autoimmune myopathies are diagnosed as immune-mediated necrotizing myopathy (IMNM) in adults and children. The symptoms may first occur acutely or more insidiously with proximal upper and lower extremity weakness that progresses over time; facial muscle weakness is also reported. IMNM is also diagnosed with mixed connective tissue disease and scleroderma and as a paraneoplastic complication of lung cancer or gastrointestinal adenocarcinomas. Antisynthetase syndrome (ASS) is a particularly severe subtype of myositis and presents with inflammatory symmetrical polyarthritis of the small joints of the hands and feet. Constitutional symptoms include fevers, weight loss, Raynaud phenomenon, and skin changes known as mechanic's hands that are scaling, cracking, and fissuring with bleeding along the lateral and palmar aspects of the fingers (Lundberg et al., 2018; Meyer et al., 2017; NIH, n.d.; Oldroyd et al., 2017).

Inclusion body myositis typically presents with a slow onset of progressive, asymmetrical, proximal, and distal atrophy and weakness in adults over 50 years of age with males diagnosed more predominately. The primary muscles affected include the quadriceps femoris, wrist, and finger flexors, and ankle dorsiflexors. Approximately 35% to 50% of affected patients need a wheelchair for mobility within 14 years. Dysphagia occurs in approximately 60% of affected individuals and is often the presenting complaint, preceding the onset of extremity weakness by up to 7 years. Head drop and camptocormia may develop due to axial muscle involvement. Sarcoidosis has been associated with IBM as well as generalized sensory polyneuropathy. Muscle cramping, myalgia, or tenderness do not usually manifest with IBM. Patients with IBM usually remain ambulatory with use of an assistive device until 10 to 15 years post diagnosis when a wheelchair is usually needed (Lloyd, 2021; Lundberg et al., 2018; Muscular Dystrophy Association [MDA], 2019; NORD, n.d.; Oldroyd et al., 2017).

Diagnostic Evaluation

The diagnosis of myositis is based on clinical symptoms that include the subacute development of symmetrical muscle weakness and fatigue, which occurs prominently in proximal muscles, and laboratory results that indicate skeletal muscle inflammation. A precise medical history and physical examination are essential prerequisites for an accurate diagnosis of myositis. This includes symptom description, onset and progression, a discussion of risk factors, and a discussion of personal and family history.

As part of this history, it is recommended that the patient complete a questionnaire concerning ADLs and their health-related quality of life. The Health Assessment Questionnaire (HAQ) was historically the most common tool for measuring functional status in rheumatology. Wolfe et al. (2004) validated a revised version of the HAQ and determined that their HAQII was reliable when compared to the HAQ. The 36-item Short Form Survey (SF-36) is recommended for self-reported quality of life. Medicare uses it for routine monitoring and assessment of care outcomes in adult patients (Rider et al., 2009).

Rider et al. (2009) validated the Myositis Damage Index (MDI) in patients with juvenile and adult myositis to describe the degree and types of damage and then to develop predictors of damage. The study determined that the MDI has good content, construct, and predictive validity in cases of juvenile and adult myositis. This index is recommended for diagnosing myositis and then for future reevaluation of patients with diagnosed myositis, as anatomic, physiologic, and functional damage is common in myositis patients after a median of 5 years duration in adult-onset patients (Aggarwal et al., 2018; Rider et al., 2009).

Measurements of strength and related functional limitations are essential for the diagnosis of myositis conditions. Muscle strength is most commonly assessed with a manual muscle test (MMT), which has been validated for use as an outcome measure for those with myositis. MMT has adequate inter- and intrarater reliability and validity when performed by a trained examiner. Muscle strength may also be evaluated using dynamometry. Function can be assessed with task-oriented tasks that are reliable, valid, and easily performed, such as the Timed Up and Go, 10-meter walk test, and 30-second chair to stand test (Rider et al., 2009).

Laboratory tests include measuring muscle enzyme levels and identifying myositis antibodies in addition to the routine complete blood count. Muscle enzyme levels that include creatinine kinase (CK), aldolase, and transaminases are usually elevated, with CK having good sensitivity and specificity for the diagnosis of muscle disease. Transaminase elevation may suggest a diagnosis of liver involvement, but this is rare with myositis (Cassius et al., 2019; Meyer et al., 2017). Creatinine kinase activity is elevated in dermatomyositis, polymyositis, ASS, and IMNM.

With IBM, serum CKs are usually normal or only slightly elevated. However, serum CK levels do not correlate with the severity of clinical weakness manifested with any of the subsets of myositis (McGrath, Rider). Identifying MSA assists with diagnosing and characterizing the subtypes of myositis, guides additional workup and screening, predicts response to treatment, and indicates prognosis. The MSAs not only identify clinical subgroups of myositis but are also closely associated with distinct clinical phenotypes. The MSA phenotypes are additionally closely associated with the histopathology features of muscle biopsies (Barsotti & Lundberg, 2018a, 2018b; Cassius et al., 2019; Cruellas et al., 2013; Meyer et al., 2017; Moghadam-Kia et al., 2017).

Electrophysiologic tests recommended for diagnosing myositis conditions include electromyography (EMG) and nerve conduction tests. Nerve conduction studies can evidence any axonal sensory neuropathy. Characteristic EMG findings include the following: increased spontaneous activity, early recruitment, and low-amplitude, short-duration, polyphasic motor unit action potentials (McGrath, 2018).

Magnetic resonance imaging (MRI) of skeletal muscle can show edema that is associated with active inflammation. In addition, adding an MRI as a test with a muscle biopsy significantly decreased the false-negative rate of diagnosing myositis (Van De Vlekkert et al., 2015).

Muscle biopsy is recommended in the diagnostic workup of all patients with autoimmune myositis as this is the most accurate test for making the diagnosis and distinguishing it from other muscle disorders. The muscle selected to biopsy is ideally a muscle that is moderately weak but not severely weak. Severely weak muscle tissue tends to show nonspecific end-stage fibro-fatty changes. Muscle biopsy identifies the vacuoles and inclusion bodies associated with IBM. Histologically, IBM is characterized by endomysial inflammation consisting of CD8 T cells and macrophages invading the nonnecrotic muscle fibers. Additionally, muscle biopsy identifies the degree of atrophy (Moghadam-Kia et al., 2017). Skin biopsy is a good diagnostic test for skin symptoms related to dermatomyositis (Moghadam-Kia et al., 2017).

Screening for cancer is another important diagnostic tool. Cancer-associated myositis is diagnosed most frequently for patients with dermatomyositis; estimates indicate that as much as 20% to 30% of patients with dermatomyositis develop cancer. Patients with necrotizing myositis are also at a higher risk than the general population. Risk factors for cancer-associated myositis include a family or previous history of cancer and the presence of serum TIF1-maggam or NXP2 autoantibodies. In addition, patients who experience a rapid onset of disease and poor response to treatment are at a higher risk.

Myositis is also frequently associated with interstitial lung disease, which is a predominant cause of morbidity and mortality. Early detection should include the following basic screening procedures based on age and gender: mammogram for females over 30 years of age, pelvic exam and pap smear for all females, colonoscopy for patients over age of 50, prostate-specific antigen (PSA) blood test for males 50 years of age and older, chest x-ray, CBC annually, and skin cancer screening. Pulmonary function tests are additionally recommended, as they are minimally invasive method to follow progression and treatment responsiveness (Fayyaz et al., 2019; Hozumi et al., 2016; Li S., 2019; Moghadam-Kia et al., 2017; Yang et al., 2017).

Factors to Consider in the Treatment of Myositis

Pharmacologic management of myositis involves intervention for the remission of the condition, followed by maintenance of remission. Conventional interventions include glucocorticoids in combination with another or multiple immunosuppressive medications. Biologic therapies that target immunopathogenic pathways provide further treatment that is being increasingly utilized. When interstitial lung disease is a comorbidity, agents that modulate T-cell function and deplete B cells are also recommended (Barsotti et al., 2018; Oldroyd et al., 2017).

A multidisciplinary approach to treatment is recommended, which includes physical therapy, occupational therapy, and speech-swallowing therapy. Since the early 2000s, many studies have investigated the safety and effects of exercise in adults with myositis. The emerging evidence indicates that exercise is an effective intervention to optimize health and reduce disability in adult patients diagnosed with myositis. Intensive physical exercise reduces inflammation, decreases fatigue, and increases aerobic capacity and muscle strength (Alexanderson, 2018; Ihalainen et al., 2018; Munters et al., 2016; Oddis & Aggarwal, 2018; Pearson et al., 2017).

Treatment Options for the Older Adult With Myositis

Pharmacologic Intervention

Although there is an absence of clear data from randomized controlled trials of the efficacy of glucocorticoids in adults with myositis, treatment with glucocorticoids continues to be the first therapeutic pharmacologic choice for the initial management of nearly all patients diagnosed with myositis. Glucocorticoids reduces the muscular inflammation that leads to the associated improvement of muscular symptoms such as weakness.

Improvements generally occur in the first 6 months after the initiation of the treatment. The multitude of side effects of glucocorticoids is well evidenced; however, these effects may be minimized by managing the duration and dosing of these agents. Traditionally, glucocorticoids are started at a higher dose of 1 mg/kg/day; this is maintained for 2 to 4 weeks then is gradually decreased by 20% to 25% each month until 5 to 10 mg/day is reached. Lower dosages should be considered with the comorbidities that are common in the older adult such as diabetes mellitus, hypertension, or glaucoma. For patients with severe myositis symptom manifestations such as marked muscle weakness, severe dysphagia, or rapidly progressive interstitial lung disease, an intravenous methylprednisolone for 3 consecutive days followed by the high-dose oral glucocorticoid regimen previously discussed is recommended (Barsotti et al., 2018; Oddis & Aggarwal, 2018; Oldroyd et al., 2017).

Traditional treatment for muscular involvement includes the glucocorticoids and conventional immunosuppressive or immunomodulatory agents such as methotrexate, azathioprine, mycophenolate mofetil, tacrolimus, and intravenous immune globulin. Since 2005, several case reports, case series, open-label trials, and reports from registries have suggested a positive effect of treatment with biologics such as rituximab, tocilizumab, abatacept, etanercept, ajulemic acid, and infliximab (Barsotti et al., 2018; Oddis & Aggarwal, 2018; Olive et al., 2016; Orlandi et al., 2016).

Physical Rehabilitation

The aging process, regardless of pathology, is characterized by a significant reduction in muscle strength and muscle mass (Gonzalez-Gay et al., 2018; Li, X et al., 2017). Studies have established the health benefits of enhancing muscular fitness. Regular physical activity and exercise are associated with numerous physical and mental health benefits in men and women. Of particular importance concerning older adults is that exercise preserves bone mass, increases strength, and decreases fall risk (Dankel et al., 2016; Farinatti et al., 2013; Fernandez-Lezaun et al., 2017; Garber et al., 2011; Grgic et al., 2018; Mayhew & Cyrino, 2019). Many studies have established the effect of exercise rehabilitation on strength gains in those with muscle diseases, including myositis (Alexanderson, 2018; Harris-Love, 2005).

All patients diagnosed with myositis should be evaluated by a physical therapist with experience in neuromuscular disease to implement an individualized exercise program (Lloyd, 2021). Stretching and passive range-of-motion exercises are important for severely weak patients to prevent joint contractures. Physical therapy rehabilitation programs can also teach patients compensatory movements that reduce fall risk. Multiple studies with small sample sizes have indicated that many forms of aerobic exercise and moderate intensity strength training are beneficial for patients diagnosed with myositis (Alexanderson, 2018; Cronin et al., 2017; Habers & Takken, 2011; Munters et al., 2013). Tiffreau et al. (2017) compared a standardized, hospital-based rehabilitation program followed by home-based exercises with home-based physiotherapy in patients with myositis. Study participants were evaluated at inclusion, at the end of the rehabilitation program, and 6 and 12 months later. The program was well tolerated and had a positive effect on function and quality of life. Munters et al. (2016) performed a controlled pilot study to investigate the effects of a 12-week endurance exercise training program on the molecular profile of skeletal muscle in patients with established myositis compared to a control group of patients with myositis who did not exercise. The resulting data concluded that endurance exercise in this population activated an aerobic phenotype and promoted muscle growth while simultaneously suppressing the inflammatory response in the muscles. The muscle growth reversed the muscle atrophy process and suppressed the inflammatory response.

Occupational therapy is recommended for assistance with functional impairment from upper extremity weakness to improve the patient's ability to perform activities of daily living. Severe muscle weakness of finger and wrist flexors and reduced grip strength are prevalent symptoms of patients with myositis. Therefore individualized hand exercise is important in the treatment of myositis and should be initiated by an occupational therapist (Alexanderson, 2018; Lloyd et al., 2014). Patients with dysphagia should be referred to a speech-language pathologist. They are skilled to work not only with speech but with compensatory swallowing maneuvers to improve the swallowing safety for these patients and maintain better nutrition (Lloyd, 2021).

Orthoses and Supportive Treatment

Many patients with muscle weakness secondary to myositis benefit from assistive devises such as a walker or a cane. It is recommended that patients with foot and ankle weakness be evaluated for ankle foot orthoses (AFOs) that can improve safety by enhancing gait and knee stability and decreasing fall potential while increasing independence with gait. Furthermore, finger or wrist splints may be indicated for patients with upper extremity weakness (Hoenig & Cary, 2022; Lloyd, 2021). Home health intervention from physical and occupational therapists is important for assessing safety and needed equipment such as raised toilet seats and grab bars. A home environmental safety evaluation is recommended as well. These professionals are also able to assess for the need of a wheelchair for patients with progressed weakness.

Myofascial Pain Syndrome

Approach to the Older Adult With Myofascial Pain Syndrome

The prevalence of musculoskeletal pain increases with advancing age to 40% to 60%. Myofascial pain syndrome (MPS) is commonly diagnosed in older adults and causes chronic pain in several areas of the body (Bourgaize et al., 2018; Kim et al., 2016). Myofascial pain syndrome affects approximately 85% to 95% of persons with chronic pain (Anandkumar, 2018; Malanga et al., 2010) and is one of the main contributors to low back pain that is associated with poor quality of life, fatigue, limitations in activities of daily living, and disability (Chen et al., 2019; Malanga et al., 2010; Urits et al., 2019). Myofascial pain syndrome is also associated with other complaints, such as depression, mental stress, anxiety, and decreased quality of life (Shakouri et al., 2020). Myofascial trigger points (MTPs) are a primarily cause of myofascial pain syndrome, and two primary categories of MTPs have been identified. Active trigger points (TrPs) cause spontaneous local, and referred pain and latent TrPs cause pain only when activated with palpation or compression (Cerezo-Tellez et al., 2016; Donnelly, 2019; Kim et al., 2016; Niel-Asher, 2014).

Donnelly (2019) defined TrPs as extremely irritable areas in a taut band of a skeletal muscle; they are painful and involve compression stretch, overload, or contraction of the muscle, with the pain typically perceived distant from the TrP. This injury exacerbates acetylcholine release with increased motor end-plate activity that leads to the palpable trigger points within the peripheral muscle. Continual contraction leads to the release of vasoactive components and inflammatory factors that promote the localized muscle pain (Borg-Stein & Iaccarino, 2014; Bourgaize et al., 2018; Donnelly, 2019).

Research also supports that latent TrPs provide nociceptive input into the dorsal horn even though these TrPs are not spontaneously painful (Bourgaize et al., 2018; Goodman & Fuller, 2021). Due to OA being one of the primary reasons for disability with the older adult population, studies have determined that the myofascial pain in knee OA and the existence of associated myofascial TrPs could play a crucial role in pain and impairment in patients diagnosed with OA (Dor & Kalichman, 2017; Sanchez-Romero et al., 2019).

Cerezo-Terrez et al. (2016) carried out a cross-sectional descriptive from January 2012 to December 2014 that included three primary health care centers. The objective of the study was to assess the prevalence of active and latent MTPs in persons with chronic nonspecific neck pain. The results indicated that MPS is a common source of pain in patients who present with chronic nonspecific neck pain. Additionally, latent or active TrPs were identified in 93% of community-dwelling older adults with chronic low back pain who were involved in a university-based pain management program (Lisi et al., 2015).

Steps for Diagnosing Myofascial Pain Syndrome

Research has recognized myofascial pain as a clinical diagnosis even though there is a lack of consensual diagnostic criteria (Dommerholt et al., 2018; Fernandez-de-las-Penas & Dummerholt, 2018; Goodman & Fuller, 2021). Myofascial pain syndrome is primarily based on clinical findings. Thus patient history, physical exam, and diagnostic testing are important components to the accurate diagnosis and identification of patient pathophysiology. Most patients with MPS complain of local muscle pain and referred pain in specific patterns (Tantanatip & Chang, 2021; Ting et al., 2020). The referred pain is often associated with sensory symptoms such as paresthesia, dysesthesia, and local skin tenderness. The underlying problem(s) may involve a limited number of muscles or may be regional or more generalized (Goodman & Fuller, 2021). Myofascial pain syndrome and fibromyalgia (FM) are two of the most common forms of chronic musculoskeletal pain (Bourgaize et al., 2018). The muscles most commonly affected with MPS include muscles of the cervical and shoulder areas (trapezius, scalene, sternocleidomastoid) and the pelvic girdle. Clinically, MPS and FM present similarly, but there are significant differences that lead to the correct differential diagnosis and treatment.

Rivers et al. (2015) performed an international study of 214 pain specialists with the objective of determining the consensus of the clinical features and presentation of MPS. Seventy-six percent of the practitioners agreed that MPS is differentiated from other chronic musculoskeletal pain conditions. Determination of the diagnosis should include a combination of any three of the following signs: muscle stiffness/spasm, limited range of motion, symptoms that are aggravated with stress, or a palpable taut band/nodule. Additionally, it was emphasized that for the diagnosis of MPS the patient must present with the presence of pain for greater than 3 months with both local and regional pain manifestation. Mayoral del Moral et al. (2018) conducted a study to determine whether two independent physical therapist examiners could agree on a diagnosis of MPS. They examined 10 muscles bilaterally with the following measures: painfully restricted passive range of motion, muscle strength limited by pain, palpable taut band, area of spot tenderness, jump sing, local twitch response, pain referral reported, pressure pain threshold, matchstick test, and skin rolling test. The results determined that the interrater reliability between the two examiners showed significant agreement, suggesting that their clinical outcome measures with a good patient history of cause can be valid and reliable for a diagnosis of MPS.

Electromyography and ultrasound confirm the diagnosis. End-plate noise is usually found in TrPs with electromyography (Saxena et al., 2015; Bourgaize et al., 2018), and diagnostic ultrasound can identify TrPs as they are more hyperechoic compared to the surrounding muscles (Chang, K. V., et al., 2017, 2018; Kumbhare et al., 2016; Tantanatip & Chang, 2021). Shakouris et al. (2020) compared serum concentrations of important inflammatory biomarkers and oxidative stress between patients with MPS and healthy persons. Results of the case-controlled study indicated that patients with MPS had significantly higher concentrations of the inflammatory biomarkers hs-CRP, MDA, and PLA2 and lower concentrations of superoxide dismutase (SOD) compared with the healthy participants. Lab tests can also be helpful in identifying predisposing conditions such as vitamin deficiencies (C, B_1, B_6, B_{12}, folic acid), hypothyroidism, and hypoglycemia (Finely, 2019).

Treatment Options for the Older Adults With Myofascial Pain Syndrome

Pharmacologic Intervention

Medications often prescribed for symptoms of MPS include NSAIDs, tricyclic antidepressants, benzodiazepine receptor agonists (BZRAs), and muscle relaxants (Tantanatip & Chang, 2021; Wright, 2020). Wright performed a narrative review regarding the clinical use of BZRAs for treating chronic pain based on relevant publications through February 2020. The author concluded that best practice recommendations include limiting the duration of use to 2 to 4 weeks. Trigger points associated with MPS are reported to respond to injections with a local anesthetic such as lidocaine, steroid, or botulinum toxin. Typically, a regimen of multiple treatments spaced over several weeks is most successful (Hammi et al., 2021). The injections cause a temporary relaxation of the taut trigger point that results in improved perfusion with release of the actin-myosin chains, and thus lengthening of the muscle fibers occur with removal of the metabolic waste products (Hammi et al., 2021; Ricci & Ozcakar, 2019; Wong & Wong, 2012).

Physical Rehabilitation

Early physical rehabilitation is essential to decrease the sensitization of the TrPs because additional TrPs can develop with continued stress on the involved muscle fibers continuing to reduce daily function and quality of life (Kim et al., 2016). Inactivation of the trigger points is essential for decreasing the pain and symptoms that are exacerbated with MPS.

Myofascial pain syndrome is one of the most frequent underlying reasons for dysfunction seen by physical therapists (Takla, 2018). Treatment interventions reported by physical therapists include stretching, soft tissue mobilization, thermotherapy, laser, transcutaneous electrical stimulation, ultrasound, strengthening, and biofeedback (Anandkumar, 2018; Chen et al., 2015; Takla, 2018). A physical therapist's assessment will identify and address the underlying contributing cause(s) of the development of MPS based on common differential diagnostic techniques, and the therapist can provide posture training and education for eliminating the causes. Studies indicate that myofascial release therapy reduces pain and thus contributes to improved quality of sleep and enhanced quality of life (Arguisuelas et al., 2017; Arun, 2014). Dry needling has become a successful intervention for decreasing the associated trigger points and thereby decrease pain (Anandkumar, 2018; Ceballos-Laita et al., 2019; Chen et al., 2019).

Essential to the rehabilitation of the trigger points that lead to MPS is to determine the underlying cause of the myofascial trigger point (MTrPs). The exact mechanisms are not known, but evidence indicates that mechanical factors are associated with the development of MTrPs, with studies confirming that prolonged abnormal postures and ergonomic factors are often a direct cause (Fernandez-de-las-Penas et al., 2006; Tantanatip & Chang, 2021). Workspace modifications, such as the inclusion of an ergonomic chair, specialized keyboard, sit-stand workstation, and adjustable computer screen, may also help. Li, S et al. (2019) evaluated the current evidence with randomized controlled trials on the efficacy of acupuncture techniques for MPS that included 33 trials involving 1692 patients treated with acupuncture. The authors concluded that the evidence suggests that most acupuncture therapies, including acupuncture combined with other therapies, are effective for reducing pain and improving physical function for persons with MPS. A home program with self-exercise for myofascial release is supported in the literature to decrease the pain and restore the extensibility of the soft tissue (Kim et al., 2016).

Fibromyalgia

Approach to the Older Adult With Fibromyalgia

Fibromyalgia (FM) is a chronic pain condition that is characterized by widespread pain and affects approximately 2% to 5% of the general population (Jones, A et al., 2015; Serpas et al., 2022). The underlying component of FM, pain, reduces physical function among this population (Dailey et al., 2016; Torma et al., 2013).

Fibromyalgia is considered a syndrome that does not have a well-defined underlying pathologic disease. The primary reason for FM signs and symptoms is sensitization including, central sensitivity syndromes, recently identified as nociplastic pain (Maffei, 2020; Minerbi & Fitzcharles, 2021). Fibromyalgia is characterized by joint stiffness, chronic pain at multiple tender joints, and systemic symptoms that include cognitive dysfunction, sleep disturbances, anxiety, fatigue, and depressive disorders (Maffei, 2020; Wang, S. M., et al., 2015). There is limited research on fibromyalgia in the older adult population, and thus there is little evidence as to how FM affects the older adult population even though people in this age group often have pain, reduced mobility, and sleep disruption (Fitzcharles et al., 2013; Jacobson et al., 2015). Studies indicate that patients with FM age significantly earlier and faster than the general population (Martinez-Velilla et al., 2015). Additionally, older adults most often have higher medical comorbidities with an increased likelihood of adverse effects, drug interactions, and altered drug tolerance from pharmaceutical therapies for fibromyalgia.

These coexisting factors then increase the risk of falls, fractures, and other injuries with standard treatment for FM (Welsh et al., 2019). Jacobson et al. (2015) performed a longitudinal, observational study of 51 subjects with FM (55 to 95 years) and 81 control subjects (58 to 95 years) with serial history and exam data obtained over a 6-year period. The most common symptoms reported for those with FM were muscle pain, stiffness, and awakening tired and in pain. Compared with the control group, the group with FM had significantly more comorbidities of asthma, chronic fatigue, chronic obstructive pulmonary disease (COPD), depression, gastroesophageal reflux disease (GERD), irritable bowel syndrome, osteoarthritis, obstructive sleep apnea, and RA.

Steps for Diagnosing Fibromyalgia

There is controversy on the assessment and diagnosis of FM with studies indicating of 75% of people with fibromyalgia are not diagnosed (Arnold et al., 2011; Maffei, 2020). Hauser and Fitzcharles (2018) reported on the interdisciplinary, strongly evidence based guidelines recommended by Canada, Germany, and the European League Against Rheumatism (EULAR). According to this evidence, FM should be seen as a continuum disorder like other disorders such as diabetes, hypertension, and depression, not as a discrete disorder that can be present or absent at a particular point in time. The diagnosis of FM should be made after a complete history and physical examination. Currently, no specific diagnostic laboratory tests or biomarkers are available for the diagnosis of FM, and thus the diagnosis is clinically based (Fitzcharles et al. 2013).

Depression is evidenced to be the most common comorbidity with FM, and a systematic review concluded that there is a lifetime prevalence of approximately 63% (Kleykamp et al., 2021, Serpas et al., 2022). Furthermore, mood disorders, including depression, are estimated to be approximately three times higher in persons diagnosed with FM than in the general population (Loge-Hagen et al., 2019; Serpas et al., 2022). Thus these diagnoses must be assessed.

The preliminary American College of Rheumatology (ACR) 2016 criteria are presently used to validate a clinical diagnosis of FM (Wolfe et al., 2016). These standards do not suggest palpation of tender points, a method that has been used historically. As an alternative, patients are examined by the Fibromyalgia Impact Questionnaire, which can be accessed at https://www.rheumatology.org/I-Am-A/Rheumatologist/Research/Clinician-Researchers/Fibromyalgia-Impact-Questionnaire-FIQ (Wolfe et al., 2011). It presents a widespread pain index (WPI) that divides the body into 19 regions and scores the number of regions reported as painful; it also provides a symptom severity score that assesses the severity of fatigue, unrefreshing sleep, and cognitive symptoms. The widespread pain index and symptom severity scores are combined, with a maximum score of 31. A cutoff score of 12 to 13 is statistically significant for distinguishing those who fulfilled the ACR criteria from those who did not. The Symptom Severity Scale (SSS) and Extent of Somatic Symptoms (ESS) are other tools used to assess these symptoms (Maffei, 2020).

Based on the generalized pain criteria and clinical assessment, FM diagnostic criteria were updated in 2016 with the recommendation that the following conditions be present for the diagnosis of FM: (1) generalized pain, defined as pain exiting in at least four of five areas; (2) symptoms present at a similar level for at least 3 months; (3) a WPI >7 and an SSS >5 or a WPI of 4 to 6 and an SSS >9; and (4) a diagnosis of FM that is considered valid irrespective of other diagnoses (Serpas et al., 2022; Wolfe et al., 2016). All recent guidelines recommend that the diagnosis of fibromyalgia should be reviewed with each affected patient after the initial diagnosis so that the patient can participate in the decision making on therapeutic options. Evidence indicates that this approach reduces the patient anxiety that most often accompanies chronic pain and decreases the number of repeated diagnostic procedures that are unnecessary. Additionally, this process enhances the ability of the provider to prescribe the correct medications (Petzke et al., 2015; Wolfe et al., 2016).

Treatment Options for the Older Adult With Fibromyalgia

Pharmacologic Intervention

Pharmacologic interventions for patients diagnosed with FM are primarily directed to treat the symptoms. Research indicates that only 10% to 25% of persons treated with pharmacotherapy receive a 50% decrease in pain intensity (Maffei, 2020; Moore et al., 2013). A Cochrane review of the randomized controlled trials (RCTs) concerning which approved medications are strongly recommended for the treatment of FM by the FDA and EMA indicated that only 10% of the participants reported a clinically relevant decrease in pain symptoms. However, Espejo et al. (2018) determined that some medications appear to significantly improve the quality of life for individuals with FM. Very few medications have been approved by the US FDA for the treatment of FM, and thus these patients are often treated on an off-label basis (Calandre et al., 2015; Maffei, 2020).

The three medications approved for FM include two selective serotonin and norepinephrine reuptake inhibitors (SNRIs), duloxetine and milnacipran, and one anticonvulsant, pregabalin (Maffei, 2020; Serpas et al., 2022). The updated guidelines from systematic reviews by the German Pain Society concluded that amitriptyline and duloxetine are recommended for comorbid depressive disorders or generalized anxiety disorder and pregabalin is recommended for generalized anxiety disorder. Strong opioids were not recommended (Sommer et al., 2017). Due to the generalized symptoms of FM and the limited drugs approved, many patients are treated by combining different agents. Thorpe et al. (2018) performed a systemic review of double-blinded, randomized controlled trials conducted through September 2017; their objective was to assess the efficacy, safety, and tolerability of combination pharmacotherapy compared to monotherapy, placebo, or both, for the treatment of fibromyalgia pain in adults. These combinations include NSAIDs, antidepressants, opioids, and anticonvulsants. The authors concluded that there are very few high-quality clinical trials that evaluate the efficacy of specific drug combinations for treating FM. They surmised that determining if combination pharmacotherapy is effective for decreasing FM pain depends on the specific drugs prescribed. The authors recommended that when prescribing multimodal pharmacotherapy to closely monitor patients for risk of toxicity.

Rehabilitation

Guidelines for the treatment of FM from Canada, Israel, Germany, and EULAR agree that therapy should be tailored to each individual patient, and include the first-line role of nonpharmacologic therapies. They agreed with strong recommendations for the use of exercise and emphasized its effect on pain, physical function, and well-being. In addition, strong evidence supported the use of acupuncture and hydrotherapy to decrease pain and fatigue and improve quality of life. There was weak evidence on the effectiveness of meditative movement therapies or mindfulness-based stress reduction therapies. A survey of the European guidelines indicates that a multidisciplinary approach is necessary to determine the best intervention for persons with FM. In addition to pharmacologic intervention, evidence suggests including behavioral therapy, exercise, patient education, and pain management.

Multiple studies and systematic reviews support supervised, paced aerobic exercises that have positive effects on well-being and physical function while decreasing the pain and tender points associated with FM. A gradual increase in exercise intensity is encouraged. Winkelmann et al., (2017) coordinated 13 scientific societies and two patient self-help organizations to update the guidelines on treatment of fibromyalgia. Literature was searched for systematic reviews of randomized, controlled trials on physical and occupational therapy from 2010 through May 2016. The researchers concluded that low to moderate intensity endurance and strength training are strongly recommended. Chiropractic, laser therapy, magnetic field therapy, massage, and transcranial magnetic stimulation were not recommended. These systemic reviews also concluded that multimodal therapy with a combination of aerobic exercise and at least one psychological therapy session for a duration of at least 24 hours was strongly recommended for patients with severe forms of fibromyalgia (Schiltenwolf et al., 2017).

Polymyalgia Rheumatica

Approach to the Older Adult With Polymyalgia Rheumatica

Polymyalgia rheumatica (PMR) is a chronic auto-inflammatory rheumatic condition that affects persons over 50 years of age. Polymyalgia rheumatica is the second most common inflammatory rheumatic disease occurring in older adults after rheumatoid arthritis and is rarely diagnosed in individuals younger than 50 years (Camellino & Dejaco, 2018; Gonzalez-Gay et al., 2017; Milchert & Brzosko, 2017; Partington et al., 2018). Sixty-five to seventy-five percent of patients with PMR are female. The incidence of PMR increases with age, with the highest prevalence occurring in persons in their 70s. It is clinically characterized by pain and stiffness predominately in the cervical area, proximal shoulders, and pelvic girdles (Partington et al., 2017). It has been noted in the literature as secondary fibrositis, periarthrosis humeroscapularis, peri-extra-articular rheumatism, myalgic syndrome of the aged, pseudo-polyarthrite rhizomelic , and anarthritic rheumatoid disease. The condition is most common in Scandinavian countries, with a higher prevalence in northern European populations and individuals of Scandinavian descent (Gonzalez-Gay et al., 2017; Raheel et al., 2017).

The pathogenic mechanisms that cause PMR are not clearly defined. Because evidence concludes that PMR occurs almost exclusively in persons over 50 years of age, there may be age-related immune alterations in genetically predisposed individuals that lead to the development of the disease (Guggino et al., 2018). The actual genetics of PMR remain inconclusive; however, the higher incidence in those of Northern European heritage suggest a genetic role in the pathophysiology of the disease (Saad, 2020; Kreiner et al., 2017).

Immunogenetic studies have suggested an association between the condition and specific polymorphisms in genes related to immune regulation. There is a higher susceptibility in individuals who carry the HLA-DRB1*04 allele; however, the strength of this association varies with different populations. Interleukin and tumor necrosis factor-alpha gene polymorphisms are associated with the susceptibility to and severity of PMR (Guggino et al., 2018; Kreiner et al., 2017; Saad, 2020). Kreiner et al. (2017) measured gene expression in muscle biopsies from 8 patients diagnosed with PMR and 10 control participants. The study was the first to demonstrate changes in the gene expression in skeletal muscle in PMR. Several genes were identified that play a role in the pathophysiology of PMR.

A strong association has been established between PMR and giant cell arteritis (GCA), a systemic, granulomatous vasculitis that primarily affects the aorta and its branches (Crowson & Mattson, 2017; Guggino et al., 2018; Salvarani & Muratore, 2022). Approximately one-half of people with GCA have PMR, and approximately 10% of individuals diagnosed with PMR have GCA (Nesher & Breuer, 2016; Salvarani & Muratore, 2022). Ungprasert et al. (2017) performed a systematic review and meta-analysis of observational studies that compared the risk of coronary artery disease (CAD) and PMR. Results indicted a significantly increased risk of CAD among patients with PMR.

Even though evidence demonstrates that PMR causes severe pain and stiffness in the proximal muscle groups, no muscle biopsies and electromyographic findings have indicated inflammation in the muscle. The inflammation primarily occurs at the level of the synovium and bursae associated with the proximal joints. The synovitis of PMR is characterized by vascular proliferation and leukocyte infiltration, predominantly macrophages and T lymphocytes (Gonzalez-Gay et al., 2017; Guggino et al., 2017; Saad, 2020). Increased interstitial concentrations of pro-inflammatory cytokines have been detected by studies and may be important in the pathogenesis of the disease as well (Gonzalez-Gay et al., 2017; Guggino et al., 2017; Schinnerling et al., 2017). Several infections have been investigated as possible triggers to induce the monocyte and dendritic cell activation and production of pro-inflammatory cytokines that lead to PMR. However, the association is considered weak and the results inclusive (Guggino et al., 2017; Sobrero et al., 2018; Tshimologo et al., 2017).

Tshimologo et al. (2017) explored primary care PMR patient beliefs about the causes of their PMR. Seventy-two percent of the respondents claimed that statins were the most common group of drugs attributed to developing PMR symptoms. However, a literature review by Manzo (2019) concluded that PMR and statin-associated muscle symptoms (SAMS) are two completely different pathologic conditions, as SAMS is a myopathy and PMR has no muscular component involvement. However, the possibility that SAMS may cause an increase in the manifestation of PMR should be considered with discontinuation of the medication.

Steps for Diagnosing Polymyalgia Rheumatica

A thorough history is critical for diagnosing PMR, as all self-care activities of daily living that depend on the shoulder and pelvic girdles are significantly affected; these activities include dressing, toileting, getting in and out of a bathtub, and turning over in bed. These functional activities are affected so quickly that the patient will usually remember the exact day when PMR symptoms started (Manzo et al., 2021).

Bilateral shoulder or hip pain, stiffness, and muscle aches are the cardinal clinical features of PMR (Gonzalez-Gay et al., 2018; Helliwell et al., 2018; Milchert & Brzosko, 2017; Sobrero et al., 2018). Patients complain of pain and stiffness in the upper arms, cervical area, pelvic girdle, hips, and thighs. The onset of symptoms is usually rapid, developing over a few days and in some cases overnight. Symptoms are reported to be characteristically worse in the morning and improve progressively during the day, yet they are worse after rest or when the patient is inactive over a length of time. The morning stiffness usually lasts at least 30 minutes and typically for more than 45 to 60 minutes. The severe pain impacts the person's ability to perform activities of daily living, such as dressing, brushing one's hair, getting out of bed, or standing from sitting, thus leading to disability. Pain that increases at night is also typical and often awakens the patient, who then complains of having difficulties returning to sleep (Gonzalez-Gay et al., 2018; Helliwell et al., 2018; Milchert & Brzosko, 2017). These symptoms can also be associated with other nonspecific symptoms, such as low-grade fever, malaise, fatigue, poor appetite, and weight loss (Gonzalez-Gay et al., 2017; Jones & Birrell, 2016; Partington et al., 2018).

No gold-standard test exists for the differential diagnosis of PMR, thus in clinical practice the diagnosis of PMR continues to be based on the characteristic clinical manifestations, laboratory evidence of systemic inflammation, rapid response to low doses of glucocorticoids, and the exclusion of other disorders that may present with proximal pain and stiffness (Helliwell et al., 2018; Jones, GT et al., 2015; Muratore et al., 2018; Sobrero et al., 2018). Of utmost importance is a thorough assessment before starting treatment. The characteristic symptoms of PMR, such as proximal pain and stiffness, systemic symptoms, musculoskeletal manifestations, and evidence of inflammation, occur within a range of other conditions that can mimic PMR. These conditions need to be considered and excluded through careful history and examination (Jones et al., 2020; Muratore et al., 2018). Furthermore, patients in the typical age range for PMR often suffer with multimorbidity (Helliwell et al., 2018; Partington et al., 2018).

Comorbidity in patients with PMR is a significant issue for the clinical assessment and management of patients with PMR. Clinical guidelines recommend assessment for comorbidity in all patients suspected of having PMR (Chatzigeorgiou & Mackie, 2018; Dejaco et al., 2015). There is an increased prevalence of comorbid conditions with inflammatory rheumatic diseases in persons with PMR compared to the general population, and these can affect the outcomes of treatment (Baillet et al., 2016; Chatzigeorgiou & Mackie 2018).

For an accurate diagnosis of PMR, guidelines endorsed by the American College of Rheumatology (ACR) and the European League Against Rheumatism (EULAR) advise the exclusion of conditions that may cause similar symptoms (Dejaco et al., 2017; Partington et al., 2018). Ungprasert et al. (2017) performed a systematic review and meta-analysis of observational studies to compare the risk of coronary artery disease (CAD) in patients with PMR versus subjects without it. Published studies indexed in MEDLINE and EMBASE were searched through April 2016. The results demonstrated a significantly increased risk of CAD among patients with PMR.

Systematic reviews of studies investigated by radiologists and rheumatologists advocate the use of ultrasonography to help diagnose PMR because several intra- and extraarticular ultrasonographic results have been associated with PMR, including biceps tenosynovitis, bursitis, and synovitis. A meta-analysis evidenced the superior accuracy of diagnosing PMR with the use of ultrasonography due to its ability to detect subacromial bursitis versus other areas of inflammation. Unilateral subacromial bursitis had an 80% sensitivity and a 68% specificity, and bilateral subacromial bursitis had a 66% sensitivity and an 89% specificity (Mackie et al., 2015; Mahmood et al., 2020). Use of ultrasonographic criteria has been reported to increase the specificity of the EULAR/ACR classification system for PMR from 81.5% to 91.3% (Macchioni et al., 2014; Mahmood et al., 2020).

Laboratory tests may indicate inflammation consistent with PRM or assist with ruling out another diagnosis. The primary test recommended are the elevated erythrocyte sedimentation rate (ESR) and the C-reactive protein (CRP) level. With PMR, ESR will be elevated >30 or 40 mm/h and CRP will be >6 mg/dL, indicating an ongoing inflammatory condition. Other laboratory studies commonly see in PMR include normochromic anemia, thrombocytosis, and leukocytosis. Liver enzymes, particularly alkaline phosphatase, are often elevated (Gonzalez-Gay et al., 2018; Mahmood et al., 2020).

Factors to Consider in the Treatment of Polymyalgia Rheumatica

Untreated PMR is markedly disabling due to the combination of pain, extensive stiffness, and accompanying secondary signs and symptoms that can lead to significant disability (Goodman et al., 2020; Liew et al., 2018). It is recommended that a patient with PMR be evaluated for giant cell arteritis because this condition often is concurrent with PMR and causes irreversible blindness. Response to the gold-standard medication, glucocorticoids, is usually remarkable, thus if improvement of symptoms does not occur after1 week, the PMR diagnosis should be questioned and the patient should be reevaluated (Goodman et al., 2020; Gonzalez-Gay et al., 2017). In terms of prognosis, studies indicate that when PMR is promptly diagnosed and appropriate treatment has been initiated, there is an excellent prognosis. Mortality among persons with proper treatment is not significantly greater than that of the general population (Acharya & Musa, 2021). Longevity in persons with both PMR and giant-cell arteritis is also good unless severe aortitis is diagnosed. Complications associated with PMR include an increased risk of cardiovascular disease primarily due to premature atherosclerosis that results from the chronic inflammation (Acharya & Musa, 2021; Ungprasert et al., 2017). Persons with PMR also have a higher potential of developing inflammatory arthritis. Small joint synovitis, younger age group, and positive anti-CCP are associated with this development (Yates et al., 2019).

Treatment Options for the Older Adult With Polymyalgia Rheumatica

Pharmacologic Intervention

Oral glucocorticoids (GCs) are the mainstay of medicinal therapy for the treatment of polymyalgia rheumatica (Chino et al., 2019; Matteson et al., 2016). Usually, symptoms are significantly improved with a once-daily low dose of GCs as recommended by the EULAR and the ACR. An initial starting dose of prednisolone, between 12.5 mg to 25 mg daily continued for 2 to 4 weeks, is the recommendation. Patients generally experience a quick improvement in symptoms, usually within 24 to 72 hours with most patients responding within a week after the onset of glucocorticoid therapy. Once the dose has been tapered off to 10 gm per day, the daily dose can be decreased by 1 mg each month until discontinuation of the prednisolone therapy (Dejaco et al., 2015; Gonzalez-Gay et al., 2017; Liew et al., 2018; Mori & Koga, 2016; Yates et al., 2017). Of utmost importance for the prescribing provider, GC adverse events are common, occurring in up to 65% of diagnosed patients. The most common side effects include weight gain, swelling, mental disturbances, and gastrointestinal problems. Thus regular monitoring of blood pressure, weight, and fasting glucose is essential, as well as assessment for osteoporosis (Camellino & Dejaco, 2018).

However, approximately 50% of patient with PMR experience a relapse while being treated. When relapse symptoms are consistent with PMR indicators, then an increase of 10% to 20% of the glucocorticoids is recommended (Dejaco et al., 2015; Koster & Warrington, 2015; Mahmood et al., 2020). If steroids were successfully discontinued before relapse, recommendations are to restart induction therapy at the lowest effective dosage and then again taper as tolerated (Mahmood et al., 2020; Weyand & Goronzy, 2014). When there are severe symptoms with relapse, a single dose of intramuscular methylprednisolone at 120 mg has been advocated to help with the induction of the glucocorticoids (Dasgupta et al., 2010; Mahmood et al., 2020). After two relapses, steroid-sparing medications such as methotrexate, azathioprine, a TNF inhibitor, or an interleukin 6 (IL-6) may be prescribed (Gonzalez-Gay et al., 2017; Mahmood et al., 2020).

Physical Rehabilitation

There is no recent evidence that reports on physical rehabilitation intervention for patients with PMR. The Italian Society of Rheumatology clinical practice guidelines for the management of polymyalgia rheumatica indicate strong evidence in support of an individualized exercise program for patients with PMR aimed at maintaining muscular mass and function, and decreasing fall risk, especially in older adults on long-term GCs and for frail individuals (Ughi et al., 2020).

The 2015 EULAR and ACR panel agreed with these recommendations (Dejaco et al., 2017). Physical therapy for nonpharmaceutical treatments for diagnoses associated with chronic inflammation of joints and connective tissue, and bone disorders is well documented (Kisner et al., 2018). Because PMR is an inflammatory response that often involves bursitis and tenosynovitis, physical rehabilitation can evaluate and treat patients with PMR using this pathogenesis as the foundation of the plan of care. Physical therapy is valuable with this population as a means to decrease the potential of early functional impairment and severe disability with a combination of modalities, functional activities, and exercise (Goodman & Fuller, 2021; Muratore et al., 2018). Physical therapists are valuable patient educators for home programs and client education about preserving bone and muscle. Isono et al. (2018) reported a case of PMR that developed during hospitalization at another hospital. They concluded that history taking by physical and occupational therapists is paramount in the symptomatic diagnoses of inpatients suspected of having PMR.

Orthoses and Supportive Equipment

There is no evidence that reports on orthoses and supportive equipment for persons diagnosed with PMR. Please refer to other sections of this chapter that discuss inflammatory diagnoses.

Soft Tissue Injuries

Approach to the Older Adult With Soft Tissue Injuries

Research concerning soft tissue injuries and older adults is limited. Muscle strength, endurance, work capacity, and muscle power progressively decline with aging, with significant decreases after 50 years of age for women and men. Aging is also associated with decreases in muscle mass and muscle quality, along with increases in adipose tissue (Baker, 2017; Boros & Freemont, 2017; Haraldstad et al., 2017; Hiol et al., 2021; McCarthy & Hannafin, 2014).

Changes in tendons with aging include reduced blood flow and the gradual loss of normal tendon homeostasis components due to increased and repetitive mechanical load (Boros & Freemont, 2017; McCarthy & Hannafin, 2014). With aging, there is an increased incidence of tendinopathy with impaired healing ability, primarily due to the impaired ability of the tenocytes to respond because of injury and comorbidities (Birch et al., 2017; Loiselle, 2017).

Metabolic changes that occur during aging are significant contributing factors to these decreases. There is a decrease in muscle protein that leads to a decrease in muscle repair capacity with aging. Strength declines 10% to 15% per decade, and decrease accelerates to 25% to 40% per decade (Siparsky et al., 2014). Concurrent with these changes is an increase in susceptibility to soft tissue maladaptation with activities of daily living (Baker, 2017; Rader et al., 2016; Thorpe et al., 2021). Recovery time for these injuries increases significantly with aging, and research indicates that with soft tissue injuries, older adults/workers/athletes develop more chronic disability and require more care that is more costly than it is for younger populations (Baker, 2017; Minetto et al., 2020; Siparsky et al., 2014). Most research performed with ligaments has been done on the anterior cruciate ligament (ACL). The ACL degenerates with increasing age, with collagen fiber disorientation being the most prevalent change that occurs earliest (Hasegawa et al., 2012; McCarthy & Hannafin, 2014). Aging also leads to ligament decreased metabolism, numbers of mechanoreceptors that cause poor proprioception, and increased apoptosis of cells (Boros & Freemont, 2017; McCarthy & Hannafin, 2014).

Strains

A strain is an injury to a muscle or tendon. Muscle strain injuries are prevalent in the aging population, and they commonly result from physical/mechanical stresses. With aging, activities of daily living often result in skeletal-muscle-strain injury that is then associated with losses in muscle performance and increases in tissue edema, inflammation, degeneration, pain, discomfort, and soreness (Baker, 2017).

Lee et al. (2018) explored the incidence, characteristics, complications, and socioeconomic impacts association with falls in community-dwelling older adults utilizing a questionnaire-based survey with a sample population of 2012 older adults. The low back was most commonly injured, followed by the wrist, hip, and elbow with sprains and strains being the most frequent (67.3%) types of injuries among outpatient participants.

Little et al. (2013) evaluated the 12-month incidence of exercise-related injuries to community-dwelling older adults in a study that included 167 participants. A questionnaire was developed and issued to the participants, who documented self-reported injuries. The most common type of injury was acute muscle strain (32%), followed by strain due to overuse (23%) and sprains (23%). Seventy percent of the injuries required medical treatment, with 75% of these persons visiting medical offices.

Sprains

A sprain is a stretch (plastic deformation), partial rupture, or complete rupture of at least one ligament. Consecutively, the ankles, knees, and wrists are most often involved. Ankle injury is one of the most common reasons that patients access primary care settings and emergency departments. Once these ankle injuries have been examined, ankle sprains are found to constitute a large percentage of the final diagnoses. Ankle sprains are extremely prevalent and have a significant risk of recurrence. Thus residual ankle instability results for many patients, making them more prone to recurrent chronic lesions. This often leads to decreased physical activity, posttraumatic ankle osteoarthritis, and a more sedentary lifestyle (Correia et al., 2021; Doherty et al., 2017; Ferkel et al., 2020; Petersen, J et al., 2013).

Research indicates that a history of lateral ankle sprain (LAS) and aging will increase the potential for disrupted sensorimotor action potentials to the lower extremity postural muscles through the peripheral and central nervous systems. Older adults compensate for this decreased corticospinal excitability of the postural muscles by depending on the hip musculature strategies (Baudry et al., 2015; Terada et al., 2015).

Terada et al. (2015) examined postural control during a single-leg balance task in older adults with and without a history of LAS. The results of the research indicated that older adults with an ankle sprain history exhibited altered postural control and had more rigid postural control than older adults without injury and thus had a greater potential for falls. Briet et al. (2016) studied the correlation between pain self-efficacy or symptoms of depression and ankle-specific limitations and pain intensity in patients diagnosed with lateral ankle sprain. Self-efficacy and older age were statistically significant for more ankle-specific symptoms and limitations 3 weeks after injury.

Tendinopathy

Aging causes tendon degeneration with changes to the tendon structure and composition that influence the mechanical function of tendons (Lange et al., 2019; Li, Y., et al., 2019). The incidence of tendon diseases related to aging, including tendinopathy, is increasing, with older adults suffering more severe injury (Li, Y., et al., 2019). Tendons are fibrous connective tissue whose primary function is to transmit muscular forces to the bones on which they attach, allowing joint movement. Therefore tendons constantly experience mechanical loading in varying degrees (Lang et al., 2019; McCarthy & Hannafin, 2014; Zhang & Wang, 2015; Zhou et al., 2014).

Aging reduces the number of tendon cells and reduces their activity, thereby decreasing the ability of the injured tendon to repair itself and contributing to a steady decline in the ability of tendons to repair injuries as people age. These age-related changes decrease the mechanical properties, structure, and strength of tendons, increasing their susceptibility to injury that reduces quality of life (Lang et al., 2019; Li, Y., 2019; Zhang & Wang, 2015). Additionally, with increases in age there is decreased blood supply to tendons, with a noted presence of lipids, cartilaginous metaplasia, and osseous metaplasia (Birch et al., 2016; Li, Y., et al., 2019). Research indicates that aging is a predisposing factor for developing tendinopathy, with tendon tissue injuries occurring more frequently with aging (Albers et al., 2016; Lang et al., 2019; McCarthy & Hannafin, 2014).

Slane et al. (2017) evaluated the effects of aging on healthy Achilles tendons using shear wave elastography. The results indicated that aging alters spatial variations in Achilles tendon elasticity, thus increasing injury potential.

Steps for Diagnosing Soft Tissue Injuries

Sprains

A correct diagnosis of sprains is of utmost importance for determining treatment and acceptable rehabilitation. The diagnosis of a sprain depends primarily on the medical history and physical examination. Sprain injuries are classified as grade I, II, or III, varying from mild to severe based on the degree of damage and the number of ligaments affected. Lateral ankle sprains are diagnosed significantly more often; they are the result of a combination of inversion and adduction of the foot in supination, most often damage the anterior talofibular and calcaneofibular ligament (lateral ligament complex), and are the most frequent ankle sprains. Eversion sprains that affect the medial ligament compartment occur significantly less frequently (Feger et al., 2015; Oliveira et al., 2016; Petersen, W et al., 2013). Most patients complain of pain, develop edema, and demonstrate functional limitations (Feger et al., 2015; Oliveira et al., 2016).

Recovery after an acute ankle sprain injury requires protection of the ankle ligaments for stability, reducing edema and tenderness, and exercises to regain range of motion and strength (Feger et al., 2015).

Treatment Options for the Older Adult With Soft Tissue Injuries

Pharmacologic Intervention

Doherty et al. (2017) provided a systematic overview of the systematic reviews that evaluated treatment strategies for acute ankle sprains and chronic ankle instability. They concluded that there is strong evidence for the use of NSAIDs along with exercise therapy.

Jones et al. (2020) searched medical databases up to January 2020 for studies that compared NSAIDs with paracetamol, opioids, complementary or alternative medicines, or combinations of these. The main results indicated that there is no difference between NSAIDs and paracetamol in terms of their effect on pain after 1 to 2 hours, or after 2 to 3 days, with low-certainty evidence indicating no difference after a week or more. The use of NSAIDs may result in small increases in gastrointestinal adverse complaints. Moderate-certainty evidence suggested that there is no difference between NSAIDs and opioids in terms of their effect on pain at 1 hour or 4 or 7 days. NSAIDs lead to fewer gastrointestinal and neurologic adverse effects compared with opioids. There was little to no difference between NSAIDs and paracetamol combined with opioids in terms of their effect on pain, edema, return to function, or unwanted side effects. However, this evidence was of low certainty. The authors found no studies comparing NSAIDs with complementary or alternative medicines.

Physical Rehabilitation

Moderate exercise has beneficial effects on tendons. Long-term exercise increases tendon-tissue mass, collagen content, cross-sectional area, load to failure, ultimate tensile strength, and weight-to-length ratio (Zhang & Wang, 2015). Research shows that early movement is beneficial for decreasing the symptoms associated with lateral ankle sprains (Petersen et al., 2013). Physical therapy intervention with progressive exercise is evidenced not only to improve function but to prevent the recurrence of ankle sprains

(Correia et al., 2021; Petersen et al., 2013). There is moderate evidence that supports exercise and manual therapy techniques to address pain, edema, and improved function (Doherty et al., 2017).

Orthoses

Peterson et al. (2013) performed a systematic literature review regarding evidence for the treatment and prevention of lateral ankle sprains. Several options were analyzed for external ankle protection, including the use of bandages, tape, lace-up braces, and semirigid ankle orthoses. There was good evidence from high-level randomized trials that braces are effective for the prevention of future ankle sprains.

Surgical Intervention

The initial treatment of chronic ankle instability includes functional and prophylactic physical rehabilitation. Surgical intervention becomes a choice only if rehabilitation fails to restore structural and functional ankle stability. Multiple surgical techniques have been utilized through the decades as surgical interventions advanced for ankle ligament reconstruction surgery. Anatomic and nonanatomic procedures, allograft, suture tape augmentation, and arthroscopic techniques are available as surgical choices. Ferkel et al. (2020) described these various techniques and reported that the gold standard remains the open anatomic Brostrom repair with the Gould augmentation, which can be used to address issues regarding early range of motion and limited immobilization.

Lohrer et al. (2016) performed a systematic review from 1945 until September 2014 analyzing the results of operative treatment for midportion Achilles tendinopathy with the intention of providing evidence-based recommendations for the best surgical intervention. Two different operative techniques and their combinations were identified, which included open procedures and minimally invasive surgeries. Preoperatively, all patients received conservative treatment for at least 3 months that included immobilization, eccentric exercise, stretching, cryotherapy, ultrasound therapy, laser therapy, orthotics, extracorporeal shock wave therapy, sclerosing injections, and antiinflammatory medication. The open procedure group (542 patients) included longitudinal tenotomies with debridement of the affected area of the tendon with or without tendon augmentation and gastrocnemius lengthening or recession. The minimally invasive group (172 patients) included percutaneous longitudinal tenotomies, endoscopic debridement, and minimally invasive gastrocnemius lengthening or recession. Statistically, no difference was determined between the two groups in terms of success rates and patient satisfaction. Studies involving the open techniques indicated there were more complications than the studies on minimally invasive techniques. In their systematic review, the authors recommended the minimally invasive surgery as the primary operative choice due to its lower complication rate.

Key Points

- The older adult patient is at risk for a number of musculoskeletal injuries.
- Osteoarthritis is the most common musculoskeletal issue in the older adult population.
- An interdisciplinary approach to managing older adult patients leads to the best possible rehabilitation.
- Multiple modalities (surgery, physical therapy, occupational therapy, etc.) can be used to treat the older adult patient.

More information about tools and Interprofessional Education Collaborative (IPEC) competencies mentioned in this chapter can be found in Appendix 1: Tools and Appendix 2: IPEC Competencies.

References

Abdulla, O., Naqvi, M. J., Shamshuddin, S., Bukhari, M., & Procoter, R. (2018). Prevalence of Paget's disease of bone in Lancaster: Time for an update. *Rheumatology*, *57*, 931–932. https://doi.org/10.1093/rheumatology/kex505.

Aberg, A. C., & Ehrenberg, A. (2017). Inpatient geriatric care in Sweden-Important factors from an inter-disciplinary team perspective. *Archives of Gerontology and Geriatrics*, *72*, 113–120. https://doi.org/10.1016/j.archger.2017.06.002.

Abhishek, A. (2017). Managing gout flares in the elderly: Practical considerations. *Drugs Aging*, *34*, 873–880.

Acharya, S., & Musa, R. (2021, January). Polymyalgia rheumatica: *StatPearls [Internet]*. StatPearls Publishing. PMID: 30725959.

Agency for Healthcare Research & Quality Analgesics for Osteoarthritis (AHRQ). (2021, October 24).: An Update of the 2006 Comparative Effectiveness Review. https://effectivehealthcare.ahrq.gov/topics/osteoarthritis-pain/research

Ahn, Y. H., & Ham, O. K. (2016). Factors associated with medication adherence among medical-aid beneficiaries with hypertension. *Western Journal of Nursing Research*, *38*(10), 1298–1312. https://doi.org/10.1177/0193945916651824.

Albagha, O. M. (2015). Genetics of Paget's disease of bone. *BoneKey Reports*, *4*, 756. https://doi.org/10.1038/bonekey.2015.125.

Albers, I. S., Zwerver, J., Diercks, R. L., Dekker, J. H., & Van den Akker-Scheek, I. (2016). Incidence and prevalence of lower extremity tendinopathy in a Dutch general practice population:

A cross-sectional study. *BMC Musculoskeletal Disorders, 17,* 16. https://doi.org/10.1186/s12891-016-0885-2.

Aletaha, D., Neogi, T., Silman, A., Funovits, J., Felson, D. T., Bingham, C., et al. (2010). 2010 Rheumatoid arthritis classification criteria: An American College of Rheumatology/European League Against Rheumatism collaborative initiative. *Arthritis & Rheumatology, 62*(9), 2569–2581. https://doi.org/10.1002/art.27584.

Aletaha, D., & Smolen, J. S. (2018). Diagnosis and management of rheumatoid arthritis: A review. *Journal of the American Medical Association, 320*(13), 1360–1372. siuL10.1001/jama.2018.13103.

Alexanderson, H. (2018). Exercise in myositis. *Current Treatment Options in Rheumatology, 4*(4), 289–298. https://doi.org/10.1007/s40674-018-0113-3.

Alikhan, M. M. (2018). Paget disease. *Medscape* https://emedicine.medscape.com/article/334607-overview.

Almangour, W., Schnitzler, A., Salga, M., Debaud, C., et al. (2016). Recurrence of heterotopic ossification after removal in patients with traumatic brain injury: A systematic review. *Annals of Physical and Rehabilitation Medicine, 59*(4), 263–269. https://doi.org/10.1016/j.rehab.2016.03.009.

Al Nofal, A. A., Altayar, O., Ben Khadra, K., et al. (2015). Bone markers in Paget's disease of the bone: A systemic review and meta-analysis. *Osteoporosis International, 26,* 1875–1891.

Alpizar-Rodriguez, D., & Finckh, A. (2017). Environmental factors and hormones in the development of rheumatoid arthritis. *Seminars in Immunopathology, 39,* 461–468. https://doi.org/10.1007/s00281-017-0624-2.

Altman, R., Alarcón, G., Appelrouth, D., Bloch, D., Borenstein, D., Brandt, K., Brown, C., Cooke, T. D., Daniel, W., Feldman, D., Greenwald, R., Hochberg, M., Howell, D., Ike, R., Kapila, P., Kaplan, D., Koopman, W., Marino, C., McDonald, E., & Wolfe, F. (1991). The American College of Rheumatology criteria for the classification and reporting of osteoarthritis of the hip. *Arthritis & Rheumatology, 34*(5), 505–514. https://doi.org/10.1002/art.1780340502.

American Academy of Family Physicians Clinical Preventive Services Recommendations. (2017). *Summary of recommendations for clinical preventive services.* https://www.aafp.org/dam/AAFP/documents/patient_care/clinical_recommendations/cps-recommendations.pdf

American Academy of Orthopaedic Surgeons (AAOS) Management of Hip Fractures in the Elderly. (2014, September 5). *Evidence-based clinical practice guideline.* https://www.aaos.org/globalassets/quality-and-practice-resources/hip-fractures-in-the-elderly/hip-fractures-elderly-clinical-practice-guideline-4-24-19--2.pdf

American Association of Colleges of Nursing (AACN). (2016). *Adult-gerontology.* acute/primary care NP competencies. https://cdn.ymaws.com/www.nonpf.org/resource/resmgr/files/np_competencies_2.pdf

American College of Rheumatology (ACR). (2020). *Exercise and arthritis.* https://www.rheumatology.org/I-Am-A/Patient-Caregiver/Diseases-Conditions/Living-Well-with-Rheumatic-Disease/Exercise-and-Arthritis

American Physical Therapy Association (APTA). (2019). *Evidence-based community programs.* https://www.apta.org/uploadedFiles/APTAorg/Practice_and_Patient_Care/Patient_Care/Arthritis/ArthritisFoundationExerciseProgram.pdf

Anandkumar, S. (2018). Effect of dry needling on myofascial pain syndrome of the quadratus femoris: A case report. *Physiotherapy Theory and Practice, 34*(2), 157–164. https://doi.org/10.1080/09593985.2017.1376021.

Anderson, P. A., Froyshteter, A. B., & Tontz, W. L. (2013). Meta-analysis of vertebral augmentation compared with conservative treatment for osteoporotic spinal fractures. *Journal of bone and mineral research: The Official Journal of the American Society for Bone and Mineral Research, 28*(2), 372–382. https://doi.org/10.1002/jbmr.1762.

Appelman-Dijkstra, N. M., & Papapoulos, S. E. (2018). Paget's disease of bone. *Best Practice & Research Clinical Endocrinology & Metabolism, 32,* 657–668. https://doi.org/10.1016/j.beem.2018.05.005.

Archdeacon, M., d'Heurle, A., Nemeth, N., & Budde, B. (2014). Is preoperative radiation therapy as effective as postoperative radiation therapy for heterotopic ossification prevention in acetabular fractures. *Clinical Orthopaedics and Related Research, 472*(11), 3389–3394. https://doi.org/10.1007/s11999-014-3670-2.

Arem, H., Moore, S. C., Hartge, P., et al. (2015). Leisure time physical activity and mortality: A detailed pooled analysis of the doe-response relationship. *Journal of the American Medical Association, 175,* 959–967.

Arguisuelask, M., Lisonk, J., Sanchez-Zuriagak, D., Martinez-Hurtadok, I., & Domenech-Fernandezk, J. (2017). Effects of myofascial release in nonspecific chronic low back pain: A randomized clinical trial. *Spine, 1*(42), 1 627–634. https://doi.org/10.1097/BRS.0000000000001897.

Arliani, G. G., Astur, D. C., Yamada, R. K., Yamada, A. F., Miyashita, G. K., Mandelbaum, B., et al. (2014). Early osteoarthritis and reduced quality of life after retirement in former professional soccer players. *Clinics, 69,* 589–594.

Arnett, D. K., Blumenthal, R. S., Albert, M. A., Buroker, A. B., Goldberger, Z. D., Hahn, E. J., & Ziaeian, B. (2019). 2019 ACC/AHA Guideline on the primary prevention of cardiovascular disease: Executive summary: A report of the American College of Cardiology/American Heart Association Task Force on Clinical Practice Guidelines. *Journal of the American College of Cardiology, 74*(10), 1376–1414. https://doi.org/10.1016/j.jacc.2019.03.009.

Arnold, L. M., Clauw, D. J., McCarberg, B. H., & FibroCollaborative, (2011). Improving the recognition and diagnosis of fibromyalgia. *Mayo Clinic Proceedings, 8,* 457–464. https://doi.org/10.4065/mcp.2010.0738.

Arthritis Foundation. (2019a). *Gout.* https://www.arthritis.org/diseases/gout

Arthritis Foundation. (2019b). *Nutrition guidelines for people with rheumatoid arthritis.* https://www.arthritis.org/living-with-arthritis/arthritis-diet/anti-inflammatory/rheumatoid-arthritis-diet.php

Arthritis Foundation. (2019c). *Rheumatoid arthritis self-care.* https://www.arthritis.org/about-arthritis/types/rheumatoid-arthritis/self-care.php

Arthritis Foundation. (2019d). *Self-help arthritis devices.* https://www.arthritis.org/health-wellness/healthy-living/managing-pain/joint-protection/self-help-arthritis-devices

Arthritis Foundation. (2019e). *Supplement and herb guide for arthritis symptoms.* https://www.arthritis.org/health-wellness/treatment/complementary-therapies/supplements-and-vitamins/supplement-and-herb-guide-for-arthritis-symptoms

Arun, B. (2014). Effects of myofascial release therapy on pain related disability, quality of sleep and depression in older adults with chronic low back pain. *International Journal of Physiotherapy and Research, 2*(1), 318–323. ISSN 2321-1822 www.ijmhr.org/ijpr.html.

Askanas, V., Engel, W., & Nogalska, A. (2009). Inclusion body myositis: A degenerative muscle disease associated with intra-muscle fiber multi-protein aggregates, proteasome inhibition, endoplasmic reticulum stress and decreased lysosomal degradation. *Brain Pathology, 19*, 493–506. https://doi.org/10.111/j.1750-3639.2009.00290.x.

Audet, M. C., Jean, S., Beaudoin, C., Guay-Belanger, S., Dumont, J., Brown, J., & Michou, L. (2017). Environmental factors associated with familial or non-familial forms of Paget's disease of bone. *Joint Bone Spine, 84*(6), 719–723. https://doi.org/10.1016/j.jbspin.2016.11.010.

Atzeni, F., Masala, I., di Franco, M., & Sarzi-Puttini, P. (2017). Infections in rheumatoid arthritis. *Current Opinion in Rheumatology, 29*(4), 323–330. https://doi.org/10.1097/BOR.0000000000000389.

Azeez, M., Clancy, C., O'Dwyer, T., Lahiff, C., et al. (2020). Benefits of exercise in patients with rheumatoid arthritis: A randomized controlled trial of a patient-specific exercise programme. *Clinical Rheumatology, 39*, 1783–1792. https://doi.org/10.1077/s10067-020-04937-4.

Baillet, A., Gosses, L., Carmoa, L., et al. (2016). Points to consider for reporting, screening for and preventing selected comorbidities in chronic inflammatory rheumatic diseases in daily practice: A EULAR initiative. *Annals of the Rheumatic Diseases, 75*, 965–973.

Baker, B. A. (2017). An old problem: Aging and skeletal-muscle = strain injury. *Journal of Sport Rehabilitation, 26*, 180–188. https://doi.org/10.1123/jsr.2016.0075.

Bannuru, R. R., Osani, M. C., Vaysbrot, E. E., Arden, N. K., et al. (2019). OARSI guidelines for the non-surgical management of knee, hip, and polyarticular osteoarthritis. *Osteoarthritis and Cartilage, 27*(11), 1578–1589. https://doi.org/10.1016/j.joca.2019.06.011.

Bannuru, R. R., Schmid, C., Kent, D. M., et al. (2015). Comparative effectiveness of pharmacologic interventions for knee osteoarthritis: A systematic review and network meta-analysis. *Annals of Internal Medicine, 162*, 46–54. https://doi.org/10.7326/M14-1231.

Barbour, K. E., Helmick, C. G., Boring, M., & Brady, T. J. (2017). Vital signs: Prevalence of doctor-diagnosed arthritis and arthritis-attributable activity limitation—United States, 2013–2015. *Morbidity and Mortality Weekly Report, 66*, 246–253. https://doi.org/10.15585/mmwr.mm6609e1.

Barg, A., Wimmer, M. D., Wiewiordki, M., Wirtz, D. C., Pagenstert, G. I., & Valderrabano, V. (2015). Total ankle replacement—Indications, implant designs, and results. *Deutsches Ärzteblatt International, 111*, 177–184. https://doi.org/10.3238./Arztebl.2015.0177.

Barnes, S.N. (2017). *2012 Updated recommendations for treating rheumatoid arthritis*. Content last reviewed March 2017. Agency for Healthcare Research and Quality. https://www.ahrq.gov/chain/practice-tools/practice-guidelines/2012-updated-recommendations-for-treating-rheumatoid-arthritis.html

Barrionuevo, P., Kappor, E., Alahdab, A. N., Benkhadra, K., Almasri, J., et al. (2019). Efficacy of pharmacological therapies for the prevention of fractures in postmenopausal women: A network meta-analysis. *Journal of Clinical Endocrinology & Metabolism, 104*(5), 1623–1630.

Barros, A., Karmali, S., Rosa, B., & Goncalves, R. (2017). Stress fracturs in older athletes: A case report and literature review. *Clinical Case Reports, 5*(6), 849–854. https://doi.org/10.1002/ccr3.954.

Barsotti, S., Cioffi, E., Tripoli, A., Tavoni, A., d'Ascanio, A., Mosca, M., & Neri, R. (2018). The use of rituximab in idiopathic inflammatory myopathies: Description of a monocentric cohort and review of the literature. *Reumatismo, 70*(2), 78–84.

Barsotti, S., & Lundberg, I. E. (2018a). Current treatment for myositis. *Current Treatment Options in Rheumatology, 4*(4), 299–315. https://doi.org/10.1007/s40674-018-0106-2.

Barsotti, S., & Lundberg, I. E. (2018b). Myositis an evolving spectrum of disease. *Immunological Medicine, 41*(2), 46–54. https://doi.org/10.1080/13497413.2018.1481571.

Barton, D., Griffin, D., & Carmouche, J. (2019). Orthopedic surgeons' views on the osteoporosis care gap and potential solutions: Survey results. *Journal of Orthopaedic Surgery and Research, 14*(72). https://doi.org/10.1186/s13018-019-1103-3.

Baudry, S., Collignon, S., & Duchateau, J. (2015). Influence of age and posture on spinal and corticospinal excitability. *Experimental Gerontology, 69*, 62–69. https://doi.org/10.1016/j.exger.2015.06.006.

Beaudreuil, J. (2017). Orthoses for osteoarthritis: A narrative review. *Annals of Physical and Rehabilitation Medicine, 60*(2), 102–106. doi.org/10.1016/.rehab.2016.10.005.

Beck, B., Cameron, P., Lowthian, J., Fitzgerald, M., et al. (2018). Major trauma in older persons. *BJS Open, 2*(5), 310–318. https://doi.org/10.1002/bjs5080.

Becker, M.A., & Gaffo, A.L. (2019). Clinical manifestations and diagnosis of gout. In N. Dalbeth (Ed.), *UpToDate*. https://www-uptodate-com.libproxy.txstate.edu/contents/clinical-manifestations-and-diagnosis-of-gout?search=medications%20causing%20gout&source=search_result&selectedTitle=1~150&usage_type=default&display_rank=1

Becker, M.A., & Neogi, T. (2019). Lifestyle modification and other strategies to reduce the risk of gout flares and progression of gout. In N. Dalbeth (Ed.), *UpToDate*. https://www-uptodate-com.libproxy.txstate.edu/contents/lifestyle-modification-and-other-strategies-to-reduce-the-risk-of-gout-flares-and-progression-of-gout?sectionName=ALCOHOL&search=medications%20causing%20gout&topicRef=1667&anchor=H1015801285&source=see_link#H1015801285

Benn, C., Dua, P., Gurrell, R., et al. (2018). Physiology of hyperuricemia and urate-lowering treatments. *Frontier Medicine, 5*, 160. https://doi.org/10.3389/fmed.2018.00160. article.

Bergh, C., Wennergran, D., Moller, M., & Brisby, H. (2020). Fracture incidence in adults in relation to age and gender: A study of 27,169 fractures in the Swedish Fracture Register in a well-defined catchment area. *PLoS One, 15*(12), e0244291. https://doi.org/10.1371/journal.pone.0244291.

Bergstra, S. A., Markusse, I. M., Ronday, H. K., et al. (2016). Erosions in the foot at baseline are predictive of orthopaedic shoe use after 10 years of treat to target therapy in patients with recent onset rheumatoid arthritis. *Clinical Rheumatology, 35*(8), 2101–2107. https://doi.org/10.1007/s10067-015-3145-1.

Bethel, M., Carbone, L., Lohr, K., Machua, W., & Diamond, H. (Eds.). (2019). Osteoporosis workup. *Medscape*. https://emedicine.medscape.com/article/330598-workup#c7

Betteridge, A., & McHugh, N. (2016). Myositis-specific autoantibodies: An important tool to support diagnosis of myositis. *Journal of Internal Medicine, 280*, 8–23. https://doi.org/10.111/joim.12451.

Beydoun, H. A., el-Amin, R., McNeal, M., Perry, C., & Archer, D. F. (2013). Reproductive history and postmenopausal rheumatoid arthritis among women 60 years or older: Third National Health and Nutrition Examination Survey. *Menopause, 20*(9), 930–935.

Birch, H. L., Peffers, M. J., & Clegg, P. D. (2016). Influence of ageing on tendon homeostasis. *Advances in Experimental Medicine and Biology, 920*, 247–260. https://doi.org/10.1007/978-3-319-33943-6_24.

Birch, H. L., Peffers, M. J., & Clegg, P. D. (2017). Influence of ageing on tendon homeostasis. *Advances in Experimental Medicine and Biology, 920*, 247–260. https://doi.org/10.1007/978-3-319-33943-6_24

Biz, C., Pavan, D., Frizziero, A., Baban, A., & Iacobellis, C. (2015). Heterotopic ossification following hip arthroplasty: A comparative radiographic study about its development with the use of three different kinds of implants. *Journal of Orthopaedic Surgery and Research*, *10*, 176. https://doi.org/10.1186/s13018-015-0317-2.

Blalock, D., Miller, A., Tilley, M., & Wang, J. (2015). Joint instability and osteoarthritis. *Clinical Medicine Insights. Arthritis and Musculoskeletal Disorders*, *8*, 15–23. https://doi.org/10.4137/CMAMD.S22147.

Bohannon, R. W. (1997). Comfortable and maximum walking speed of adults aged 20–79 years: Reference values and determinants. *Age and Ageing*, *26*(1), 15–19. https://doi.org/10.1093/ageing/26.1.15. PMID: 9143432.

Borg-Stein, J., & Iaccarino, M. A. (2014). Myofascial pain syndrome treatments. *Physical Medicine and Rehabilitation Clinics of North America*, *25*(2), 357–374. https://doi.org/10.1016/j.pmr.2014.01.012.

Boros, K., & Freemont, T. (2017). Physiology of ageing of the musculoskeletal system. *Best Practice & Research Clinical Rheumatology*, *31*(2), 203–217. https://doi.org/10.1016/j.berh.2017.09.003.

Bouchette, P., & Boktor, S. W. (2019, January). Paget disease: *StatPearls [Internet]*. StatPearls Publishing. https://www.ncbi.nlm.nih.gov/books/NBK430805/.

Bourgaize, C., Newton, G., Kumbhare, D., & Srbely, J. (2018). A comparison of the clinical manifestation and pathophysiology of myofascial pain syndrome and fibromyalgia: Implications for differential diagnosis and management. *Journal of the Canadian Chiropractic Association (JCCA)*, *62*(1), 26–41. PMID: 30270926.

Braun, H. J., & Gold, G. E. (2012). Diagnosis of osteoarthritis: Imaging. *Bone*, *51*(2), 278–288. https://doi.org/10.1016/j.bone.2011.11.019.

Brien, S., Prescott, P., & Lewith, G. (2011). Meta-analysis of the related nutritional supplements dimethyl sulfoxide and methylsulfonylmethane in the treatment of osteoarthritis of the knee. *Evidence-based complementary and alternative medicine: eCAM*, *2011*, 528403. https://doi.org/10.1093/ecam/nep045.

Briet, J., Houwert, R., Hageman, M., Hietbrink, F., et al. (2016). Factors associated with pain intensity and physical limitations after ankle sprains. *Injury*, *47*(11), 2565–2569. https://doi.org/10.1016/j.injury.2016.09.016.

Britton, C., Brown, S., Ward, L., Rea, S., Ratajczak, T., & Watsh, J. (2017). The changing presentation of Paget's disease of bone in australia, a high prevalence region. *Calcified Tissue International*, *101*, 564–569. https://doi.org/10.1007/s00223-017-0312-1.

Brooks, A. J., Koithan, M. S., Lopez, A. M., Klatt, M., Lee, J. K., Goldblatt, E., & Lebensohn, P. (2019). Incorporating integrative healthcare into interprofessional education: What do primary care training programs need? *Journal of Interprofessional Education & Practice*, *14*, 6–12. https://doi.org/10.1016/j.xjep.2018.10.006.

Brouwer, R. W., Jakma, T. S. C., Verhagen, A. P., et al. (2005). Braces and orthoses for treating osteoarthritis of the knee. *Cochrane Database of Systematic Reviews*, CD004020. https://doi.org/10.1002/14651858.CD004004020.pub2.

Buhr, G., Dixon, C., Dillard, J., Nickolopoulos, E., Bowlby, L., Canupp, H., & McConnell, E. (2019). Geriatric resource teams: Equipping primary care practices to meet the complex care needs of older adults. *Geriatrics (Basel)*, *4*(4), 59. https://doi.org/10.3390/geriatrics4040059.

Bullock, J., Rizvi, S., Saleh, A., Ahmed, S., et al. (2018). Rheumatoid arthritis: A brief overview of the treatment. *Medical Principles and Practice*, *27*(6), 501–507. https://doi.org/10.1159/000493390.

Burmester, G., & Pope, J. (2017). Novel treatment strategies in rheumatoid arthritis. *The Lancet*, *389*, 2338–2348. www.thelancet.com.

Burn, E., Edwards, C., Murray, D., Silman, A., et al. (2019). Lifetime risk of knee and hip replacement following a diagnosis of RA: Findings from a cohort of 13,961 patients from England. *Rheumatology*, *58*(11), 1950–1954. https://doi.org/10.1093/rheumatology/kez143.

Calandre, E., Rico-Villademoros, F., & Slim, M. (2015). An update on pharmacotherapy for the treatment of fibromyalgia. *Expert Opinion on Pharmacotherapy*, *16*(19), 1347–1368. https://doi.org/10.1517/14656566.2015.1047343.

Callahan, L. F., Mielenz, T., Freburger, J., et al. (2008). A randomized controlled trial of the People with Arthritis Can Exercise Program: Symptoms, function, physical activity, and psychosocial outcomes. *Arthritis & Rheumatology*, *59*(1), 92–101.

Camacho, P., Petak, S., Binkley, N., et al. (2016). American Association of Clinical Endocrinologists and American College of Endocrinology clinical Practice Guidelines for the Diagnosis and Treatment of Postmenopausal Osteoporosis–2016. *Endocrine Practice*, *22*(Suppl. 4). https://journals.aace.com/doi/pdf/10.4158/EP161435.GL.

Camellino, D., & Dejaco, C. (2018). Update on treatment of polymyalgia rheumatica. *Reumatismo*, *70*(1), 59–66.

Cameron, M. H. (2013). Physical agents in clinical practice: Chapter 2: *Physical agents in rehabilitation: From research to practice* (4th ed.). Elsevier.

Cameron, M., & Chrubasik, S. (2013). Topical herbal therapies for treating osteoarthritis. *Cochrane Database of Systematic Reviews*, *5*(5), CD010538. https://doi.org/10.1002/14651858.CD010538. 3.

Carr, A. J., Robertsson, O., Graves, S., Price, A. J., et al. (2012). Knee replacement. *The Lancet*, *379*(9823), 1331–1340. https://doi.org/10.1016/S0140-6736(11)60752-6.

Casavant, A. M., & Hastings, H. (2006). Heterotopic ossification about the elbow: Aa therapist's guide to evaluation and management. *Journal of Hand Therapy*, *19*(2), 255–266. https://doi.org/10.1197/j.jht.2006.02.009.

Cassius, C., Le Buanec, H., Bouaziz, J. D., & Amode, R. (2019). Biomarkers in Adult Dermatomyositis: Tools to Help the Diagnosis and Predict the Clinical Outcome. *Journal of immunology research*, *2019*, 9141420. https://doi.org/10.1155/2019/9141420.

Cavalli, L., Guazzini, A., Cianferotti, L., Parri, S., et al. (2016). Prevalence of osteoporosis in the Italian population and main risk actors: Results of *BoneTour* campaign. *BMC Musculoskeletal Disorders*, *17*(1), 396. https://doi.org/10.1186/s12891-016-1248-8.

Ceballos-Laita, L., Jimenez-del-Barrio, S., Marin-Zurdo, J., Moreno-Calvo, A., et al. (2019). Effects of dry needling in HIP muscles in patients with HIP osteoarthritis: A randomized controlled trial. *Musculoskeletal Science and Practice*, *43*, 76–82. https://doi.org/10.1016/j.msksp.2019.07.006.

Centers for Disease Control and Prevention (CDC). (2019a). *Arthritis disabilities and limitations*. https://www.cdc.gov/arthritis/data_statistics/disabilities-limitations.htm

Centers for Disease Control and Prevention (CDC). (2019b). *Arthritis-related statistics*. https://www.cdc.gov/arthritis/data_statistics/national-statistics.html

Centers for Disease Control and Prevention (CDC). (2020). *Health literacy*. https://www.cdc.gov/healthliteracy/developmaterials/audiences/olderadults/understanding-challenges.html

Centers for Disease Control and Prevention (CDC). (2021). *Home and recreational safety.* https://www.cdc.gov/homeandrecreationalsafety/falls/adulthipfx.html

Cerezo-Tellez, E., Torres-Lacomba, M., Mayoral-del Moral, O., et al. (2016). Prevalence of myofascial pain syndrome in chronic non-specific neck pain: A population-based cross-sectional descriptive study. *Pain Medicine, 17,* 2369–2377. https://doi.org/10.1093/pm/pnw114.

Chaleshgar-Kordasiabi, M., Enjezab, B., Akhlaghi, M., & Sabzmakan, I. (2018). Barriers and reinforcing factors to self-management behavior in rheumatoid arthritis patients: A qualitative study. *Musculoskeletal Care, 16*(2), 241–250. https://doi.org/10.1002/msc.1221.

Champagne, N., Eadie, L., Regan, L., & Wilson, P. (2019). The effectiveness of ultrasound in the detection of fractures in adults with suspected upper or lower limb injury: A systematic review and subgroup meta-analysis. *BMC Emergency Medicine, 19,* 17–32. https://doi.org/10.1186/s12873-019-0226-5.

Chang, K., Yang, S. M., Kim, S. H., Han, K. H., Park, S. J., & Shin, J. I. (2014). Smoking and rheumatoid arthritis. *International Journal of Molecular Sciences, 15*(12), 22279–22295. https://doi.org/10.3390/ijms151222279.

Chang, K. V., Wu, W. T., Han, D. S., & Ozcaker, L. (2017). Static and dynamic shoulder imaging to predict initial effectiveness and recurrence after ultrasound-guided subacromial corticosteroid injections. *Archives of Physical Medicine and Rehabilitation, 98*(10), 1984–1994. https://doi.org/10.1016/j.apmr.2017.01.022.

Chang, K. V., Wu, W. T., Lew, H., & Ozcaker, L. (2018). Ultrasound imaging and guided injection for the lateral and posterior hip. *American Journal of Physical Medicine and Rehabilitation, 97*(4), 285–291. https://doi.org/10.1097/PHM>0000000000000895.

Chapman, L. S., Redmond, A. C., Landorf, K. B., Rome, K., et al. (2019). Foot orthoses for people with rheumatoid arthritis: A survey of prescription habits among podiatrists. *Journal of Foot and Ankle Research, 12*(7). https://doi.org/10.1186/s13047-019-0314-5.

Chatzigeorgiou, C., & Mackie, S. L. (2018). Comorbidity in polymyalgia rheumatica. *Reumatismo, 70*(1), 35–43.

Chen, S., Yu, S. Y., Yan, H., et al. (2015). The time point in surgical excision of heterotopic ossification of post-traumatic stiff elbow: Recommendation for early excision followed by early exercise. *Journal of Shoulder and Elbow Surgery, 24*(8). https://doi.org/10.1016/j.jse.2015.05.044. 11065–0071.

Chen, Y., Li, X., Xu, J., Chen, J., et al. (2019). Acupuncture for lumbar myofascial pain: Protocol for a systematic review of randomized controlled trials. *Medicine, 98,* 26. https://doi.org/10.1097/MD.0000000000016271.

Chesi, A., Wagley, Y., Johnson, M., Manduchi, E., Su, C., et al. (2019, March 19). Genome-scale Capture C promoter interactions implicate effector genes at GWAS loci for bone mineral density. *Nature Communications* https://doi.org/10.1038/s41467-019-09302-x.

Cheung, T., & McInnes, I. (2017). Future therapeutic targets in rheumatoid arthritis? *Seminars in Immunopathology, 39,* 487–500. https://doi.org/10.1007/s00281-017-0623-3.

Chidi-Ogbolu, N., & Baar, K. (2019). Effect of estrogen on musculoskeletal performance and injury risk. *Frontiers in Physiology, 9,* 1834. https://doi.org/10.3389/fphys.2018.01834.

Chino, K., Kondo, T., Sakai, R., Saito, S., Okada, Y., et al. (2019). Tocilizumab monotherapy for polymyalgia rheumatica: A prospective, single center, open-label study. *International Journal of Rheumatic Diseases, 22*(12). https://doi.org.libproxy.txstate.edu/10.1111/1756-185X.13723.

Choksi, P., Jepsen, K., & Clines, G. (2018). The challenges of diagnosing osteoporosis and the limitations of currently available tools. *Clinical Diabetes and Endocrinology, 4,* 12. https://doi.org/10.1186/s40842-018-0062-7. article.

Cholok, D., Chung, M., Ranganathan, K., Ucer, S., et al. (2019). Heterotopic ossification and the elucidation of pathologic differentiation. *Bone, 109,* 12–21. https://doi.org/10.1016/j.bone.2017.09.019.

Chow, D.C. (2018). Campagnoio, D.I. Ed Rehabilitation for Paget disease. *Medscape.* https://emedicine.medscape.com/article/311688-overview#a2

Ciccone, C. (2015). *Pharmacology in rehabilitation* (5th ed.). Pharmacological Management of Rheumatoid Arthritis and Osteoarthritis. F.A. Davis Company.

Clark, G., & Duncan, E. (2015). The genetics of osteoporosis. *British Medical Bulletin, 113*(1), 73–81. https://doi.org/10.1093/bmb/ldu042.

Clegg, D., Reda, D., Harris, C., Klein, M., et al. (2006). Glucosamine, chondroitin sulfate, and the two in combination for painful knee osteoarthritis. *New England Journal of Medicine, 354,* 795–808. https://doi.org/10.1056/NEJMoa052771.

Cohen, S., & Cannella, A. (2019). Patient education: Disease-modifying antirheumatic drugs (DMARDs) in rheumatoid arthritis (Beyond the Basics). In D. E. Furst (Ed.), *UpToDate.* https://www.uptodate.com/contents/disease-modifying-antirheumatic-drugs-dmards-in-rheumatoid-arthritis-beyond-the-basics?search=disease-modifying-antirheumatic-drugs-dmards-beyond-the-basics&source=search_result&selectedTitle=1~150&usage_type=default&display_rank=1

Colon, C., Molina-Vicenty, I., Frontera-Rodriquez, M., et al. (2018). Muscle and bone mass loss in the elderly population: Advances in diagnosis and treatment. *Journal of Biomedicine (Syd), 3,* 40–49. https://doi.org/10.7150/jbm.23390.

Colwell, C., & Moreira, M. (2021). Geriatric trauma: Initial evaluation and management. In J. Grayzel (Ed.), *UpToDate.* https://www.uptodate.com/contents/geriatric-trauma-initial-evaluation-and-management

Combe, B., Landewe, R., Daien, C. I., Hus, C., Aletaha, D., et al. (2017). 2016 update of the EULAR recommendations for the management of early arthritis. *Annals of the Rheumatic Diseases, 76*(6), 948–959.

Coombs, L. A., Max, W., Kolevska, T., Tonner, C., & Stephens, C. (2019). Nurse practitioners and physician assistants: an under-estimated workforce for older adults with cancer. *Journal of the American Geriatrics Society, 67,* 1489–1494. https://doi.org/10.1111/jgs.15931.

Correia, F., Molinos, M., Neves, C., Janela, D., et al. (2021). Digital rehabilitation for acute ankle sprains: Prospective longitudinal cohort study. *JMIR Rehabilitation and Assistive Technologies, 8*(3), e31247. https://doi.org/10.2196/31247. PMID: 34499038.

Cortiella-Masdeu, A., Sopena, E., Gomez, P., Florensa, J., Qanneta, R., & Moltó, E. (2016). Evaluation of the activity of a functional and interdisciplinary (social and healthcare) geriatric unit (FISHGU) for hospitalized patients at an acute hospital. *International Journal of Integrated Care, 16*(6), 1. http:libproxy.txstate.edu/login?url=http://search.ebscohost.comlogin.aspx?direct=true&db=edb&AN=120725036&site=eds-live&scope=site.

Cosman, F., de Beur, S. J., LeBoff, M. S., et al. (2015). Erratum to: Clinician's guide to prevention and treatment of osteoporosis. *Osteoporosis International, 26,* 2045–2047. https://doi.org/10.1007/s00198-015-3037-x.

Costenbader, K. H., Feskanich, D., Mandl, L. A., & Karlson, E. W. (2006). Smoking intensity, duration, and cessation, and the risk of rheumatoid arthritis in women. *American Journal of Medicine, 119*(6), e1–e9. https://doi.org/10.1016/j.amjmed.2005.09.053.

Craig, R. S., Goodier, H., Singh, J. A., Hopewell, S., & Rees, J. L. (2020). Shoulder replacement surgery for osteoarthritis and rotator cuff tear arthropathy. *Cochrane Database of Systematic Reviews, 2020*(4). https://doi.org/10.1002/14651858.CD012879.pub2. Art. No.: CD012879.

Crandall, C. J., Newberry, S. J., Diamant, A., Lim, Y. W., Gellad, W. F., Booth, M. J., Motala, A., & Shekelle, P. G. (2014). Comparative effectiveness of pharmacologic treatments to prevent fractures: An updated systematic review. *Annals of Internal Medicine, 161*(10), 7–11. https://doi.org/10.7326/M14-0317.

Cronin, O., Keohane, D. M., Molloy, M. G., & Shanahan, F. (2017). The effect of exercise interventions on inflammatory biomarkers in healthy physically active subjects: A systematic review. *QJM, 110*(10), 629–637. https://doi.org/10.1093/qimed/hcx091.

Cross, M., Smith, E., Hoy, D., Nolte, S., Ackerman, I., Fransen, M., … March, L. (2014). The global burden of hip and knee osteoarthritis: Estimates from the global burden of disease 2010 study. *Annals of the Rheumatic Diseases, 73*(7), 1323–1330. https://doi.orb.libproxy.txstate.edu/10.1136/annrheumdis-2013-201763.

Crowson, C., & Matteson, E. (2017). Contemporary prevalence estimates for giant cell arteritis and polymyalgia rheumatica, 2015. *Seminars in Arthritis and Rheumatism, 47*(2), 253–256. https://doi.org/10.1016/j.semarthrit.2017.04.001.

Cruellas, M. G., Viana, V., Levy-Neto, M., Souza, F. H., & Shinjo, S. K. (2013). Myositis-specific and myositis-associated autoantibody profiles and their clinical associations in a large series of patients with polymyositis and dermatomyositis. *Clinics (Sao Paulo, Brazil), 68*(7), 909–914. https://doi.org/10.6061/clinics/2013(07)04.

Cudejko, T., van der Esch, M., Schrijvers, J., Richards, R., et al. (2018). The immediate effect of a soft knee brace on dynamic knee instability I persons with knee osteoarthritis. *Rheumatology (Oxford), 57*(10), 1735–1742. https://doi.org/10.1093/rheumatology/key162.

Cummings, S. R., Cosman, F., Lewiecki, E. M., Schousboe, J. T., Bauer, D. C., et al. (2017). Goal-directed treatment for osteoporosis: A progress report from the ASBMR-NOF working group on goal-directed treatment for osteoporosis. *Journal of Bone and Mineral Research, 32*(1), 3. https://doi.org.libproxy.txstate.edu/10.1002/jbmr.3039.

Cundy, T. (2017). Treating Paget's disease—Why and how much? *Journal of Bone and Mineral Research, 32*(6), 1163–1164. https://doi.org/10.1002/jbmr.3156.

Cundy, T. (2018). Paget's disease of bone. *Metabolism, 80*, 5–14. https://doi.org/10.1016/j.metabol.2017.06.010.

Curry, S. J., Krist, A. H., Owens, D. K., et al. (2018). Screening for osteoporosis to prevent fractures: US Preventive Services Task Force Recommendation Statement. *Journal of the American Medical Association, 319*(24), 2521.

Cymet, T. C., & Sinkov, V. (2006). Does long-distance running cause osteoarthritis? *Journal of the American Osteopathic Association, 106*, 342–345.

Daily, D. L., Law, L. A., Vance, C. G., et al. (2016). Perceived function and physical performance are associated with pain and fatigue in women with fibromyalgia. *Arthritis Research & Therapy, 18*(1), 68. https://doi.org/10.1186/s13075-016-0954-9.

Dalbeth, N., Phipps-Green, A., Frampton, C., Neogi, T., Taylor, W. J., & Merriman, T. R. (2018). Relationship between serum urate concentration and clinically evident incident gout: An individual participant data analysis. *Annals of the Rheumatic Diseases, 77*(7), 1048.

Dalen, C. I., Hua, C., Combe, B., & Landewe, R. (2017). Non-pharmacological and pharmacological interventions in patients with early arthritis: A systematic literature review informing the 2016 update of EULAR recommendations for the management of early arthritis. *RMD Open, 3*(1), e000404. https://doi.org/10.1136/rmdopen-2016-000404/ecollection 2017.

Dankel, S. J., Loenneke, J. P., & Loprinzi, P. D. (2016). Dose-dependent association between muscle-strengthening activities and all-cause mortality: Prospective cohort study among a national sample of adults in the USA. *Archives of Cardiovascular Diseases, 109*(11), 626–633.

Das, S., & Padhan, P. (2017). An overview of the extraarticular involvement in rheumatoid arthritis and its management. *Journal of Pharmacology & Pharmacotherapeutics, 8*(3), 81–86. https://doi.org/10.4103/jpp.JPP_194_16.

Dasgupta, B., Borg, F., Hassan, N., et al. (2010). BSR and BHPR guidelines for the management of polymyalgia rheumatica. *Rheumatology (Oxford), 49*(1), 189–190. https://doi.org/10.1093/rheumatology.kep303a.

Davis, G., Patel, R., Tan, T., Alijanipour, P., Naik, T., & Parivzi, J. (2016). Ethnic differences in heterotopic ossification following total hip arthroplasty. *Bone & Joint Journal, 98-B(, 6*, 761–766. https://doi.org/10.1302/0301-620X.98B6.36050.

de Achaval, S., Kallen, M. A., Amick, B., Landon, G., Siff, S., Edelstein, D., Ahzng, H., & Suarez-& Almazor, M. E. (2015). Patients' expectations about total knee arthroplasty outcomes. *Health Expectations, 19*(2), 299–308. https://doi.org.libproxy.txstate.edu/10.1111/hex.12350.

Defillo-Draiby, J.C., Page, J.S. (2016). Fibromyalgia syndrome, a geriatric challenge. *Rhode Island Medical Journal Archives*, December webpage. www.RIMED.Org.

DeFroda, S. F., Cameron, K. L., Posner, M., Kriz, P. K., et al. (2017). Bone stress injuries in the military: Diagnosis, management, and prevention. *American Journal of Orthopedics, 46*(4), 176–183. PMID: 28856344.

Dejaco, C., Duftner, C., Buttgereit, F., et al. (2017). The spectrum of giant cell arteritis ad polymyalgia rheumatica: Revisiting the concept of the disease. *Rheumatology, 66*, 506–515. https://doi.org/10.1093/rheumatology/kew273.

Dejaco, C., Singh, Y., Perel, P., et al. (2015). Recommendations for the management of polymyalgia rheumatica: A European League Against Rheumatish/American College of Rheumatology Collaborative Initiative. *Arthritis & Rheumatology, 67*, 259080.

De l'Escalopier, N., Anract, P., & Biau, D. (2016). Surgical treatment for osteoarthritis. *Annals of Physical and Rehabilitation Medicine, 59*(3), 227–233. https://doi.org/10.1016/j.rehab.2016.04.003.

Denay, K. (2017). Stress fractures. *Current Sports Medicine Reports, 16*(1), 7–8. https://doi.org/10.1249/JSR.0000000000000320.

Denormandie, P., de l'Escalopier, N., Gatin, L., Grelier, A., & Genet, F. (2018). Resection of neurogenic heterotopic ossification (NHO) of the hip. *Orthopaedics & Traumatology: Surgery & Research, 104*, S121–S127. https://doi.org/10.1016/j.otsr.2017.04.015.

Dewar, C. (2015). Diagnosis and treatment of vertebral compression fractures. *Radiolic Technology, 86*(3), 301–320. quiz 321–323. PMID:25739109.

Dey, D., Wheatley, B., Cholok, D., Agarwal, S., et al. (2017). The traumatic bone: Trauma-induced heterotopic ossification. *Translational Research, 186*, 95–111. https://doi.org/10.1016/j.trsl.2017.06.004.

Di Giuseppe, D., Discacciati, A., Orsini, N., & Wolk, A. (2014). Cigarette smoking and risk of rheumatoid arthritis: A dose-response meta-analysis. *Arthritis Research & Therapy, 16*(2), R61. https://doi.org/10.1186/ar4498.

Divisato, G., Scotto di Carlo, F., Petrillo, N., Esposito, T., & Gianfrancesco, F. (2018). ZNF687 mutations are frequently found in pagetic patients from South Italy: Implication in the pathogenesis of Paget's disease of bone. *Clinical Genetics, 93*(6), 1240–1244. https://doi.org/10.1111/cge.13247.

Doghramji, P. (2018). Long-term treatment of gout: New opportunities for improved outcomes. *Clinician Reviews*. https://www.pce-consortium.org/documents/Gout.pdf

Doherty, C., Bleakly, C., Delahunt, E., & Holden, S. (2017). Treatment and prevention of acute and recurrent ankle sprain: An overview of systematic review with meta-analysis. *British Joournal of Sports Medicine, 51*(2), 113–125. https://doi.org/10.1136/bjsports-2016-096178.

Doherty, M., & Abhishek, A. (2019). Clinical manifestations and diagnosis of osteoarthritis. In D. Hunter (Ed.), *UpToDate*. https://www-uptodate-com.libproxy.txstate.edu/contents/clinical-manifestations-and-diagnosis-of-osteoarthritis?search=Osteoarthritis%20and%20hip%20and%20knee%20pain&source=search_result&selectedTitle=6~150&usage_type=default&display_rank=5

Dohrn, I. M., Stahle, A., & Roaldsen, K. S. (2016). "You have to keep moving, be active": Perceptions and experiences of habitual physical activity in older women with osteoporosis. *Physical Therapy, 96*(3), 361–370. https://doi.org/10.2522/ptj.20150131.

Dommerholt, J., Finnegan, M., Hooks, T., & Chou, L. W. (2018). A critical overview of the current myofascial pain literature—July 2018. *Journal of Bodywork & Movement Therapies, 22*, 673–684. https://doi.org/10.1016/j.jbmt.2018.06.005.

Dong, H., Xu, Y., Zhang, X., & Tian, S. (2017). Visceral adiposity index is strongly associated with hyperuricemia independently of metabolic health and obesity phenotypes. *Scientific Reports, 7*(1), 8822. https://doi.org/10.1038/s41598-017-09455-z.

Donnally, C. J., III, DiPompeo, C. M., & Varacallo, M. (2020). Vertebral compression fractures: *StatPearls [Internet]*. StatPearls Publishing. https://www.ncbi.nlm.nih.gov/books/NBK448171/.

Donnelly, J. (Ed.), (2019). *Travell, Simons & Simons' myofascial pain and dysfunction: The trigger point manual* (3rd ed.). Wolters Kluwer.

Dor, A., & Kalichman, K. (2017). A myofascial component of pain in knee osteoarthritis. *Journal of Bodywork and Movement Therapies, 21*(3), 642–647. https://doi.org/10.1016/j.jbmt.2017.03.025.

Dore, A. L., Golightly, Y., Mercer, V., Shi, X., Renner, J., Jordan, J., & Nelson, A. (2014). Lower-extremity osteoarthritis and the risk of falls in a community-based longitudinal study of adults with and without osteoarthritis. *Arthritis Care and Research, 67*(5), 633–639. https://doi.org/10.1002/acr.22499.

Drake, M., Clarke, B., & Lewiechi, M. (2015). The pathophysiology and treatment of osteoporosis. *Clinical Therapeutics, 37*(8), 1837–1850. https://doi.org/10.1016/j.clinthera.2015.06.006.

Dreant, N., & Poumellec, M. A. (2019). Total thumb carpometacarpal joint arthroplasty: A Retrospective functional study of 28 MOOVIS prostheses. *Hand (NY), 14*(1), 59–65. https://doi.org/10.1177/1558944718797341.

Du, S., Zhou, Y., Fu, C., et al. (2018). Health literacy and health outcomes in hypertension: An integrative review. *International Journal of Nursing Sciences, 5*(3), 301–309. https://doi.org/10.1016/j.ijnss.2018.06.001.

Duivenvoorden, T., Brouser, R. W., van Raaij, T. M., et al. (2015). Braces and orthoses for treating osteoarthritis of the knee. *Cochrane Database of Systematic Reviews, 2015*(3), CDOO4020. https://doi.org/10.1002/14651858. CD004020.pub3.

Durcan, L., Grainger, R., Keen, H., Raylor, W., & Dalbeth, N. (2016). Imaging as a potential outcome measure in gout studies: A systematic literature review. *Seminars in Arthritis and Rheumatism, 45*(5), 570–579. https://doi.org/10.1016/j.semarthrit.2015.09.008.

Eastell, R., Rosen, C. J., Black, D. M., Cheung, A. M., Murad, M. H., & Shoback, D. (2019). Pharmacological management of osteoporosis in postmenopausal women: An Endocrine Society clinical practice guideline. *Journal of Clinical Endocrinology & Metabolism, 104*(5), 1595. https://doi.org/10.1210/jc.2019-00221.

Edwards, D., Kuhn, K., Potter, B., & Forsberg, J. (2016). Heterotopic ossification: A review of current understanding, treatment, and future. *Journal of Orthopaedic Trauma, 30*, S27–S30. https://doi.org/10.1097/BOT.0000000000000666.

Egan, B. M. (2017). Physical activity and hypertension. *Hypertension, 69*, 383. https://doi.org/10.1161/HYPERTENSIONAHA.117.09012.

Elherik, F. K., Dolan, S., Antrum, J., Unglaub, F., et al. (2017). Functional and patient-reported outcomes of the Swanson metacarpophalangeal arthroplasty in the rheumatoid hand. *Archives of Orthopaedic and Trauma Surgery, 137*(5), 725–731. https://doi.org/10.1007/s00402-017-2675-1.

Ellis, G., & Sevdalis, N. (2019). Understanding and improving multidisciplinary team working in geriatric medicine. *Age and Ageing, 48*(4), 498–505. https://doi.org/10.1093/ageing/afz021.

Espejo, J. A., Garcia-Escudero, M., & Oltra, E. (2018). Unraveling the molecular determinants of manual therapy: An approach to integrative therapeutics for the treatment of fibromyalgia and chronic fatigue syndrome/myalgic encephalomyelitis. *International Journal of Molecular Sciences, 19*(9). https://doi.org/10.3390/ijms19092673.

Fares, A. (2018). Pharmacological and non-pharmacological means for prevention of fractures among elderly. *International Journal of Preventive Medicine, 9*, 78–86. https://doi.org/10.4103/ijpvm.IJPVM_114_18.

Farkhutdinova, L. M. (2019). About the basics of comprehensive geriatric assessment. *Arhiv Vnutrennej Mediciny*(4), 245. https://doi.org/10.20514/2226-6704-2019-9-4-245-252.

Farinatti, P. T., Geraldes, A. A. R., Bottaro, M. F., et al. (2013). Effects of different resistance training frequencies on the muscle strength and functional performance of active women older than 60 years. *Journal of Strength and Conditioning Research, 27*(8), 2225–2234.

Farrokhi, S., Voycheck, C. A., Klatt, B. A., Gustafson, J. A., Tashman, S., & Fitzgerald, G. K. (2014). Altered tibiofemoral joint contact mechanics and kinematics in patients with knee osteoarthritis and episodic complaints of joint instability. *Clinical Biomechanics (Bristol, Avon), 29*(6), 629–635. https://doi.org/10.1016/j.clinbiomech.2014.04.014.

Fayyaz, B., Rehman, H. J., & Uqdah, H. (2019). Cancer-associated myositis: An elusive entity. *Journal of Community Hospital Internal Medicine Perspectives, 9*(1), 45–49. https://doi.org/10.1080/20009666.2019.1571880.

Feger, M., Goetschius, J., Love, H., Saliba, S., et al. (2015). Electrical stimulation as a treatment intervention to improve function, edema or pain following acute lateral ankle sprains: A systematic review. *Physical Therapy in Sport, 16*(4), 361–369. https://doi.org/10.1016/j.ptsp.2015.01.001.

Fenton, S., Sandoo, A., Metsios, G., Duda, J., et al. (2018). Sitting time is negatively related to microvascular endothelium-dependent function in rheumatoid arthritis. *Microvascular Research, 117*, 57–60.

Ferkel, E., Nguyen, S., & Kwong, C. (2020). Chronic lateral ankle instability: Surgical management. *Clinics in Sports Medicine, 39*, 829–843. https://doi.org/10.1016/j.csm.2020.07.004.

Fernandez-de-Las-Penas, C., Alonso-Blance, C., Cuadrado, M. L., Gervin, R. D., & Pareja, J. A. (2006). Myofascial trigger points and their relationship to headache clinical parameters in chronic tension-type headache. *Headache, 46*(8), 1264–1272. https://doi.org/10.1111/j.15264610.2006.00440.x.

Fernandez-de-Las-Penas, C., & Dummerholt, J. (2018). International consensus on diagnostic criteria and clinical considerations of myofascial trigger points: A Delphi study. *Pain Medicine, 19*(1), 142–150. https://doi.org/10.1093/pm/pnx207.

Fernandez-Lezaun, E., Schumann, M., Makinen, T., et al. (2017). Effects of resistance training frequency on cardiorespiratory fitness in older men and women during intervention and follow-up. *Experimental Gerontology, 95*, 44–53.

Finely, J. E. (2019). Physical medicine and rehabilitation for myofascial pain workup. *Medscape* https://emedicine.medscape.com/article/313007-workup.

Fischer, H., Maleitzke, T., Eder, C., Ahmad, S., Stockle, U., & Braun, K. F. (2021). Management of proximal femur fractures in the elderly: Current concepts and treatment options. *European Journal of Mecical Research, 26*, 86–101. https://doi.org/10.1186/s40001-021-00556-0.

Fitzcharles, M. A., Shir, Y., Ablin, J. N., et al. (2013). Classification and clinical diagnosis of fibromyalgia syndrome: Recommendations of recent evidenced-based interdisciplinary guidelines. *Evidence-Based Complementary and Alternative Medicine, 2014*, 528952.

Fitzcharles, M.A., Ste-Marie, P.A., Shir, Y., & Lussier, D. (2014). *Drugs Aging, 31*, 711–719. https://doi.org/10.1007/s40266-014-0210-4

Fleischmann, R., Schiff, M., van der Heijde, D., et al. (2017). Baricitinib, methotrexate, or combination in patients with rheumatoid arthritis and no or limited prior disease-modifying antirheumatic drug treatment. *Arthritis & Rheumatology, 69*(3), 506–517. https://doi.org/10.1002/art.39953.

Fornusek, C. P., & Kilbreath, S. L. (2017). Exercise for improving bone health in women treated for stage I-III breast cancer: A systematic review and meta-analyses. *Journal of Cancer Survivorship, 11*, 525–541. https://doi.org/10.1007/s11764-017-0622-.

Frecklington, M., Dalbeth, N., McNair, P., Gow, P., et al. (2018). Footwear interventions for foot pain, function, impairment and disability for people with foot and ankle arthritis: A literature review. *Seminars in Arthritis and Rheumatism, 47*, 814–824. https://doi.org/0.1016/j.semarthrit.2017.10.017.

Freeman, J. (2018). RA surgery: How successful is surgery in treating rheumatoid arthritis? *Rheumatoid Arthritis*: Rheumatoid Arthritis Support Network. https://www.rheumatoidarthritis.org/treatment/surgery/

Fritz, S., & Lusardi, M. (2009). White paper: "Walking speed: The sixth vital sign.". *Journal of Geriatric Physical Therapy, 32*(2), 2–5.

Gallagher, K., Godwin, J., Hendry, G., Steultjens, M., & Woodburn, J. (2018). A protocol for a randomized controlled trial of prefabricated versus customized foot orthoses for people with rheumatoid arthritis: The FOCOS RA trial [Foot Orthoses-customized v Off-the-Shelf in Rheumatoid Arthritis]. *Journal of Foot and Ankle Research, 11*(24). https://doi.org/10.1186/s13047-018-0272-3.

Gamala, M., Linn-Rasker, S. P., Nix, M., Heggelman, B., Laar, J., et al. (2018). Gouty arthritis: Decision-making following dual-energy CR scan in clinical practice, a retrospective analysis. *Clinical Rheumatology, 37*, 1879–1884. https://doi.org/10.1007/s10067-018-3980-y.

Gan, L., Zhong, J., Zhang, R., Sun, T., et al. (2015). The immediate intramedullary nailing surgery increased the mitochondrial DNA release that aggravated systemic inflammatory response and lung injury induced by elderly hip fracture. *Mediators of Inflammation, 2015* https://doi.org/10.1155/2015/587378. article ID 587378.

Gancheva, R., Koundurdjiev, A., Ivanova, M., Kundurzhiev, T., & Kolarov, Z. (2019). Obesity, echocardiographic changes and Framingham risk score in the spectrum of gout: A cross-sectional study. *Archives of Rheumatology, 34*(2), 176–185. https://doi.org/10.5606/ArchRheumatol.2019.7062.

Gang, Q., Bettencourt, C., Machado, P., Hanna, M. G., & Houlden, H. (2014). Sporadic inclusion body myositis: The genetic contributions to the pathogenesis. *Orphanet Journal of Rare Diseases, 9*, 88. https://doi.org/10.1186/1750-1172-9-88.

Garber, C. E., Blissmer, B., Deschenes, M. R., et al. (2011). American College of Sports Medicine position stand. Quantity and quality of exercise for developing and maintaining cardiorespiratory, musculoskeletal, and neuromotor fitness in apparently healthy adults: Guidance for prescribing exercise. *Medicine & Science in Sports & Exercise, 43*(7), 1334–1359. https://doi.org/10.1249/MSS.0b013e318213f3fb.

Gecht-Silver, M., & Duncombe, A. (2018). Patient education: Arthritis and exercise (beyond the basics). In Z. Isaac (Ed.), *UpToDate*. https://www.uptodate.com/contents/arthritis-and-exercise-beyond-the-basics?topicRef=513&source=see_link

Gege, C., Bao, B., Boer, J., et al. (2012). Discovery and evaluation of a non-Zn chelating, selective matrix metalloproteinase 13 (MMP-13 inhibitor for potential intra-articular treatment of osteoarthritis. *Journal of Medicinal Chemistry, 55*(2), 709–716. ISSN: 1520-4804.

Gellis, Z. D., Kim, E., Hadley, D., Packel, L., Poon, C., Forciea, M. A., & Johnson, J. (2019). Evaluation of interprofessional health care team communication simulation in geriatric palliative care. *Gerontology & Geriatrics Education, 40*(1), 30–42. https://doi.org/10.1080/02701960.2018.1505617.

Gerriets, V., & Jialai, I. (Updated 2019, December15). Gebuxostat. In *StatPearls* [Internet]. StatPearls Publishing. https://www.ncbi.nlm.nih.gov/books/NBK544239/

George, C., & Minter, D.A. (Updated 2019, June 4). Hyperuricemia. In *StatPearls* [Internet]. StatPearls Publishing. https://www.ncbi.nlm.nih.gov/books/NBK459218/

Ghosh, K., Chatterjee, A., Ghosh, S., Chakraborty, S., Chattopadhyay, P., Bhattacharya, A., & Pal, M. (2016). Validation of Leiden score in predicting progression of rheumatoid arthritis in undifferentiated arthritis in Indian population. *Annals of Medical and Health Sciences Research, 6*(4), 205–210. https://doi.org/10.4103/amhsr.amhsr_339_15.

Gibson, K.S., Woodburn, J., Porter, D., & Telfer, S. Functionally optimized orthoses for early rheumatoid arthritis foot disease: A study of mechanisms and patient experience. *Arthritis Care Research*, 66(10), 1456–1464. https://doi.org/10.1002/acr.22060

Gioffre-Glorio, M., Murabito, L., Visalli, C., Pergolizzi, F., & Fama, F. (2018). Trauma in elderly patients: A study of prevalence, comorbidities and gender differences. *Il Giornale di Chirurgia [Journal of Surgery], 39*(1), 35–40. https://doi.org/10.11138/gchir/2018.39.1.035.

Giuliante, M. M., Greenberg, S. A., McDonald, M. V., Squires, A., Moore, R., & Cortes, T. A. (2018). Geriatric interdisciplinary team training 2.0: A collaborative team-based approach to delivering care. *Journal of Interprofessional Care, 32*(5), 629–633. https://doi.org/10.1080/13561820.2018.1457630.

Gliozzi, M., Malara, N., Muscoli, , & Mollace, V. (2015). The treatment of hyperuricemia. *International Journal of Cardiology, 213*, 23–27. https://doi.org/10.1016/j.ijcard.2015.08.087.

Glyn-Jones, S., Palmar, A. J. R., Agricola, R., Price, A. J., Vincent, T. L., Weinans, H., & Carr, A. J. (2015). Osteoarthritis. *The Lancet, 386*, 376–387. http://doi.org/10.1016/ S0140-6736(14)60802-3.

Goldstein, C., Chutkan, N., Choma, T., & Orr, R. (2015). Management of the elderly with vertebral compression fractures. *Neurosurgery, 77*(4), S33–S45. https://doi.org/10.1227/NEU.0000000000000947.

Gomes Carreira, A. C., Jones, A., & Natour, J. (2010). Assessment of the effectiveness of a functional splint for osteoarthritis of the trapeziometacarpal joint on the dominant hand: A randomized controlled study. *Journal of Rehabilitation Medicine, 42*(5), 469–474. https://doi.org/10.2340/16501977-0542.

Gonzalez-Gay, M., Matteson, E., & Castaneda, S. (2017). Polymyalgia rheumatica. *The Lancet, 390*, 1700–1712. https://doi.org/10.1016/s0140-6736(1)31825-1.

Gonzalez-Gay, M., Pina, T., Prieto-Pena, D., Calderon-Goercke, M., et al. (2018). Drug therapies for polymyalgia rheumatica: A pharmacotherapeutic update. *Expert Opinion on Pharmacotherapy, 19*(1), 1235–1244. https://doi.org/10.1080/14656566.2018.1501360.

Goodman, C. C., & Fuller, K. S. (2021). Soft tissue, joint, and bone disorders: *Pathology: Implications for the physical therapist* (5th ed.). Elsevier.

Goodman, S. M., Mehta, B., Mirza, S. Z., et al. (2020). Patients' perspectives of outcomes after total knee and total hip arthroplasty: A nominal group study. *BMC Rheumatology, 4*, 3. https://doi.org/10.1186/s41927-019-0101-8.

Gordon, B. (2019). *Gout*. Academy of Nutrition and Dietetics eat right. https://www.eatright.org/health/wellness/healthy-aging/gout

Grgic, J., Schoenfeld, B. J., Davies, T. B., et al. (2018). Effect of resistance training frequency on gains in muscular strength: A systematic review and meta-analysis. *Sport Medicine, 48*(5), 1207–1220. https://doi.org/10.1007/s40279-018-0872-x.

Grotle, M., Hagen, K. B., & Natvig, B. (2008). Obesity ad osteoarthritis in knee, hip, and/or hand: An epidemiological study in the general population with 10 years follow-up. *BMC Musculoskeletal Disorders, 9*, 132–137.

Guay, F., Parker, M., Griffiths, R., & Kopp, S. (2017). Peripheral nerve blocks for hip fractures. *Cochrane Database of Systematic Reviews, 5*(5), CD001159. https://doi.org/10.1002/14651858.CD001159.pub2.

Guermazi, A., Roemer, F. W., & Genant, H. K. (2013). Role of imaging in osteoarthritis: Diagnosis, prognosis, and follow-up. *Medicographia, 35*, 164–171.

Guggino, G., Ferrante, A., Macaluso, F., et al. (2018). Pathogenesis of polymyalgia rheumatica. *Reumatismo, 70*(1), 10–17.

Guidelines for the initial evaluation of the adult patient with acute musculoskeletal symptoms, (1996). American College of Rheumatology Ad Hoc Committee on Clinical Guidelines. *Arthritis & Rheumatology, 39*(1), 1–8.

Guler, O., & Cerci, M. (2020). A comparative overview of metatarsal stress fractures in premenopausal and postmenopausal women: Our single-centre experience with eighty-one patients. *International Orthopedics, 44*(11), 2407–2412. https://doi.org/10.1007/s00264-020-04528-7.

Guo, L., Han, J., Guo, H., Lv, D., & Wang, Y. (2019). Pathway and network analysis of genes related to osteoporosis. *Molecular Medicine Reports, 20*(2), 985–994. https://doi.org/10.3892/mmr.2019.10353.

Guttmann, A., Krasnokutshy, S., Pillinger, M., & Berhanu, A. (2017). Pegloticase in gout treatment—Safety issues, latest evidence and clinical considerations. *Therapeutic Advances in Drug Safety, 8*(12), 379–388. https://doi.org/10.1177/2042098617727714.

Gurger, M. (2019). Factors impacting 1-year mortality after hip fractures in elderly patients: A retrospective clinical study. *Nigerian Journal of Clinical Practice, 22*(5), 648–651. https://doi.org/10.4103/njcp_327_18.

Habers, G. E. A., & Takken, T. (2011). Safety and efficacy of exercise training in patients with idiopathic inflammatory myopathy—A systematic *review*. *Rheumatology, 50*(11), 2113–2124. https://doi.org/10.1093/rheumatology/ker292.

Halle, A. D., Kaloostian, C., & Stevens, G. D. (2019). Occupational therapy student learning on interprofessional teams in geriatric primary care. *American Journal of Occupational Therapy, 73*(5). https://doi.org/10.5014/ajot.2019.037143. 7305185050p7305185051-7305185050p7305185010.

Hammi, C., Schroeder, J. D., & Yeung, B. (2021). Trigger point injection: *StatPearls [Internet]*. StatPearls Publishing. https:///www.ncbi.nlm.nih.gov/books/NBK542196.

Hanaoka, B. Y., Ithurburn, M. P., Rigsbee, C. A., et al. (2019). Chronic inflammation in rheumatoid arthritis and mediators of skeletal muscle pathology and physical impairment: A review. *Arthritis Care & Research, 71*(2), 173–177. https://doi.org/10.002/scr.23775.

Hanse, M., & Kjaer, M. (2014). Influence of sex and estrogen on musculotendinous protein turnover at rest and after exercise. *Exercise and Sport Sciences Reviews, 42*(4), 183–192.

Haraldstad, K., Rohde, G., Stea, T., Seiler, H., et al. (2017). Changes in health-related quality of life in elderly men after 12 weeks of strength training. *European Review of Aging and Physical Activity, 14*, 8–14. https://doi.org/10.1186/s11556-017-0177-3.

Harris-Love, M. O. (2005). Safety and efficacy of submaximal eccentric strength training for a subject with polymyositis. *Arthritis & Rheumatology, 53*(3), 471–474. https://doi.org/10.1022/art.21185.

Hasegawa, A., Otsuki, S., Pauli, C., Miyaki, S., et al. (2012). Anterior cruciate ligament changes in the human knee joint in aging and osteoarthritis. *Arthritis & Rheumatology, 64*(3), 696–704. https://doi.org/10.1002/art.334417.

Haugen, I. K., Englund, M., Aliabadi, P., Niu, J., Clancy, M., Kvien, T. K., & Felson, D. T. (2011). Prevalence, incidence and progression of hand osteoarthritis in the general population: The Framingham osteoarthritis study. *Annals of the Rheumatic Diseases, 70*(9), 1581–1586. https://doi.org/10.1136/ard.2011.150078.

Hawley, S., Cordtz, R., Dreyer, L., et al. (2018). Association between NICE guidance on biologic therapies with rates of hip and knee replacement among rheumatoid arthritis patients in England and Wales: An interrupted time-series analysis. *Seminars in Arthritis and Rheumatism, 47*(5), 605–610. https://doi.org/10.1016/j.semarthrit.2017.09.006.

Helliwell, T., Muller, S., Hider, S., et al. (2018). Challenges of diagnosing and managing polymyalgia rheumatica: A multi-method study in UK general practice. *British Journal of General Practice, 68*(676), e783–e793. https://doi.org/10.3399/bjgp18X699557.

Henrotin, Y., Raman, R., Richette, P., et al. (2015). Consensus statement on Viscosupplementation with hyaluronic acid for the management of osteoarthritis. *Seminars in Arthritis and Rheumatism, 45*(2), 140–149. https://doi.org/10.1016/j.semarthrit.2015.04.011.

Herman, C. J., Allen, P., Hunt, W. C., Prasad, A., & Brady, T. J. (2004). Use of complementary therapies among primary care clinic patients with arthritis. *Preventing Chronic Disease, 1*(4), A12.

Hiol, A., von Hurst, P., Conlon, A., Mugridge, O., & Beck, K. (2021). Body composition associations with muscle strength in older adults living in Auckland, New Zealand. *PLoS ONE, 16*(5), e0250439. https://doi.org/10.1371/journal.pone.0250439.

Hoenig, H., & Cary, M. (2022). Overview of geriatric rehabilitation: Program components and settings for rehabilitation. Schmader, K.E. Ed. *UpToDate*. https://www-uptodate-com.libproxy.txstate.edu/contents/overview-of-geriatric-rehabilitation-program-components-and-settings-for-rehabilitation?sectionName=Orthoses&search=management%20of%20inclusion%20body%20myositis&topicRef=5164&anchor=H1174941&source=see_link#H1174941

Holden, M. A., Callaghan, M., Felson, D., Birrell, F., et al. (2021). Clinical and cost-effectiveness of bracing in symptomatic knee osteoarthritis management: Protocol for a muticentre, primary care, randomised parallel-group, superiority trial. *BMJ Open, 11*, e048196. https://doi.org/10.1136/bmjopen-2020-048196.

Hootman, J. M., Helmick, C. G., Barbour, K. E., Theis, K. A., & Boring, M. A. (2016). Updated projected prevalence of self-reported doctor-diagnosed arthritis and arthritis-attributable activity limitation among US adults, 2015–2040. *Arthritis & Rheumatology, 68*(7), 1582–1587. https://doi.org/10.1002/art.39692. PMID: 27015600.

Hootman, J. M., Helmick, C. G., & Brady, T. J. (2012). A public health approach to addressing arthritis in older adults: The most common cause of disability. *American Journal of Public Health, 102*(3), 426–433. https://doi.org/10.2105/AJPH.2011.300423.

Horton, S. C., Walsh, C. A., & Emery, P. (2011). Established rheumatoid arthritis: Rational for best practice: Physicians' perspective of how to realise tight control in clinical practice. *Best Practice & Research: Clinical Rheumatology, 25*(4), 509–521. https://doi.org/10.1016/j.erh.2011.10.012.

Howe, T. E., Shea, B., Dawson, L. J., Downie, F., Murray, A. H., Ross, C., Harbour, R. T., Caldwell, L. M., & Creed, G. (2011). Exercise for preventing and treating osteoporosis in postmenopausal women. *Cochrane Database of Systematic Reviews, 7*, CD000333. https://doi.org/10.1002/14651858.CD000333.pub2.

Hoyt, B., Pavey, G., Potter, B., & Forsberg, J. (2018). Heterotopic ossification and lessons learned from fifteen years at war: A review of therapy, novel research, and future directions for military and civilian orthopedic trauma. *Bone, 109*, 3–11. https://doi.org/10.1016/j.bone.2018.02.0098756-3282/.

Hoyt, D., Urits, I., Orhurrhu, V., Orhurhu, M., et al. (2020). Current concepts in the management of vertebral compression fractures. *Current Pain and Headache Reports, 24*(16). https://doi.org/10.1007/s11916-020-00849-9.

Hozumi, H., Fujisawa, T., Nakashima, R., Johkoh, T., et al. (2016). Comprehensive assessment of myositis-specific autoantibodies in polymyositis/dermatomyositis-associated interstitial lung disease. *Respiratory Medicine, 121*, 91–99. https://doi.org/10.1016/j.rmed.2016.10.019.

Huded, J. M., Dresden, S. M., Gravenor, S. J., Rowe, T., & Lindquist, L. A. (2015). Screening for fall risks in the emergency department: A novel nursing-driven program. *Western Journal of Emergency Medicine: Integrating Emergency Care with Population Health, 16*(7), 1043–1046. https://doi.org/10.5811/westjem.2015.10.26097.

Hug, K. T., Alton, T. B., & Gee, A. O. (2015). Classifications in brief: Brooker classification of heterotopic ossification after total hip arthroplasty. *Clinical Orthopaedics and Related Research, 473*(6), 2154–2157. https://doi.org/10.1007/s11999-014-4076-x.

Hui, M., Carr, A., Cameron, S., Davenport, G., Doherty, M., et al. (2017). The British Society for Rheumatology guideline for the management of gout. *Rheumatology, 56*, 1056–1059. https://doi.org/10.1093/rheumatology/kex150.

Hurkmans, E., van der, Giesen, F., Vlieland, T., et al. (2009). Dynamic exercise programs (aerobic capacity and/or muscle strength training) in patients with rheumatoid arthritis. *Cochrane Database of Systematic Reviews, 2009*(4), CD006853. https://doi.org/10.1002/14651858.CD006853.pub2.

Ihalainen, J. K., Schumann, M., Eklund, D., et al. (2018). Combined aerobic and resistance training decreases inflammation markers in healthy men. *Scandinavian Journal of Medicine & Science in Sports, 28*(1), 40–47. https://doi.org/10.1111/sms.12906.

Institute of Medicine of the National Academies. (2019). *Dietary reference intakes for calcium and vitamin D*. http://www.nationalacademies.org/hmd/~/media/Files/Report%20Files/2010/Dietary-Reference-Intakes-for-Calcium-and-Vitamin-D/Vitamin%20D%20and%20Calcium%202010%20Report%20Brief.pdf on September 20, 2019.

International Society for Clinical Densitometry. (2019). *ISCCK official positions–Adult*. https://iscd.app.box.com/s/5r713cfzvf4gr28q7zdccg2i7169fv86

Ishikawa, H., Abe, A., Kojima, T., et al. (2018, April 16). Overall benefits provided by orthopedic surgical intervention in patients with rheumatoid arthritis. *Modern Rheumatology, 29*(2), 335–343. https://doi.org/10.1080/14397595.2018.1457468.

Isono, H., Ito, Y., & Takamura, N. (2018). Development of polymyalgia rheumatica during hospitalization and diagnosis based on history taking by physical and occupational therapists. *Journal of General and Family Medicine, 20*, 28–30. https://doi.org/10.1002/jgf2.221.

Iundusi, R., Scialdoni, A., Arduini, M., Battisti, D., et al. (2013). Stress fractures in the elderly: Different pathogenetic feature compared with young patients. *Aging Clinical and Experimental Research, 25*(Suppl. 1), S89–S91. https://doi.org/10.1007/s40520-013-0105-y.

Jacobson, S. A., Simpson, R. G., Lubahn, C., Hu, C., et al. (2015). Characterization of fibromyalgia symptoms in patients 55 to 95 years old: A longitudinal study showing symptom persistence with suboptimal treatment. *Aging Clinical and Experimental Research, 27*(1f), 75–82. https://doi.org/10.1007/s40520-014-0238-7.

Jaleel, A., Saag, K., & Danila, M. (2018). Improving drug adherence in osteoporosis: An update on more recent studies. *Therapeutic Advances in Musculoskeletal Disease, 10*(7), 141–149. https://doi.org/10.1177/1759720X81785539.

Jensen, L. K. (2008). Hip osteoarthritis: Influence of work with heavy lifting, climbing stairs or ladders, or combining kneeling/squatting with heavy lifting. *Occupational & Environmental Medicine, 65*(1), 6–19. https://doi.org/10.1136/oem.2006.032409. Epub 2007 Jul 18. PMID: 17634246.

Jeremiah, M., Unwin, B., Greenawald, M., & Casiano, V. (2015). Diagnosis and management of osteoporosis. *American Family Physician, 92*(4), 261–268.

Jill, M. H., Scott, M. D., Stephanie, J. G., Theresa, R., & Lee, A. L. (2015). Screening for fall risks in the emergency department: A novel nursing-driven program. *Western Journal of Emergency Medicine*(7), 1043. https://doi.org/10.5811westjem.2015.10.26097.

Jones, A., Palmer, A. J. R., Agricola, R., Price, A. J., Vincent, T. L., Weinans, H., & Carr, A. J. (2015). Osteoarthritis. *The Lancet, 386*, 376–387. www.thelancet.com.

Jones, G. T., Atzeni, F., Beasley, M., et al. (2015). The prevalence of fibromyalgia in the general population: A comparison of the American College of Rheumatology 1990, 2010, and modified 2010 classification criteria. *Arthritis & Rheumatology, 67*(2), 568–575. https://doi.org/10.1002/art.38905.

Jones, O., & Birrell, F. (2016). Diagnosis and management of polymyalgia rheumatica. *The Practitioner, 260*(1799), 13–16.

Jones, P., Lamdin, R., & Dalziel, S. R. (2020). Oral non-steroidal anti-inflammatory drugs versus other oral analgesic agents for acute soft tissue injury. *Cochrane Database of Systematic Reviews, Issue 8* https://doi.org/10.1002/14651858.CD007789.pub3. Art. No. CD007789.

Jorge-Mora, A., Amhaz-Escanlar, S., Lois-Iglesias, A., Leborans-Elris, S., & Pino-Minguez, J. (2016). Surgical treatment in spine Paget's disease: A systematic review. *European Journal of Orthopaedic Surgery and Traumatology, 26*, 27–30. https://doi.org/10.1007/s00590-015-1659-5.

Katchamart, W., Narongroeknawin, P., Chevaisrakuo, P., Dechanuwong, P., et al. (2017). Evidence-based recommendations for the diagnosis and management of rheumatoid arthritis for non-rheumatologists: Integrating systematic literature research and expert opinion of the Thai Rheumatism Association. *International Journal of Rheumatic Disease, 20*, 1142–1165.

Kato, E., Sawada, T., Tahara, K., Hayashi, H., Nishino, J., Matsui, T., & Tohma, S. (2017). The age at onset of rheumatoid arthritis is increasing in Japan: A nationwide database study. *International Journal of Rheumatic Disease, 20*(7). https://doi.org/10.1111/1756-185X.12998.

Katsoulis, M., Benetou, T., Karapetyan, D., Feskanich, F., et al. (2017). Excess mortality after hip fracture in elderly persons from Europe and the USA: The CHANCES project. *Journal of Internal Medicine, 281*(3), 300–310. https://doi.org/10.1111/joim.12586.

Kazak, A. E., Nash, J. M., Hiroto, K., & Kaslow, N. J. (2017). Psychologists in patient-centered medical homes (PCMHs): Roles, evidence, opportunities, and challenges. *American Psychologist, 72*(1), 1–12. https://doi.org/10.1037/a0040382.

Kellock, T. T., Khurana, B., & Mandell, J. C. (2019). Diagnostic performance of CT for occult proximal femoral fractures: A systematic review and meta-analysis. *American Journal of Roentgenology, 213*(6), 1324–1330. https://doi.org/10.221/AJR.19.215010.

Kelly, C., Iqbal, K., Iman-Gutierrez, L., Evans, P., & Manchegowda, K. (2016). Lung involvement in inflammatory rheumatic diseases. *Best Practice & Research Clinical Rheumatology, 30*(5), 870–888. https://doi.org/10.1016/j.berh.2016.10.004.

Kemmler, W., Weineck, J., Kalender, W. A., & Engelke, K. (2004). The effect of habitual physical activity, non-athletic exercise, muscle strength, and VO2max on bone mineral density is rather low in early postmenopausal osteopenic women. *Journal of Musculoskeletal & Neuronal Interactions, 4*(3), 325–334.

Khanna, P., Gladue, H., Singh, M., FitzGerald, J., Bae, S., et al. (2014). Treatment of acute gout: A systematic review. *Seminars in Arthritis and Rheumatism, 44*, 31–38. https://doi.org/10.1016/j.semarthrit.2014.02.003.

Khoury, V., Kourilovitch, M., & Massardo, L. (2015). Education for patients with rheumatoid arthritis in Latin America and the Caribbean. *Clinical rheumatology, 34*(Suppl. 1), S45–S49. https://doi.org/10.1007/s10067-015-3014-y.

Kiel, J., & Kaiser, K. (Updated 2021, August 4). Stress reaction and fractures. In *StatPearls* [Internet]. StatPearls Publishing. https://www.ncbi.nlm.nih.gov/books/NBK507835

Kim, M., Lee, M., Ki, Y., Oh, S., et al. (2016). Myofascial pain syndrome in the elderly and self-exercise: A single-blind, randomized, controlled trial. *Journal of Alternative and Complementary Medicine, 22*(3), 244–251. https://doi.org/10.1089/acm.2015.0205.

Kisner, C., Colby, L., & Borstad, J. (2018). Overview of common orthopedic surgeries and postoperative management: *Therapeutic exercise: Foundations and techniques* (7th ed.). F.A. Davis Company.

Klestil, T., Order, C., Stotter, C., Winkler, B., et al. (2018). Impact of timing of surgery in elderly hip fracture patients: A systematic review and meta-analysis. *Scitific Reports, 8*(1), 13993. https://doi.org/10.1038/s41598-018-32098-7.

Kleykamp, B. A., Ferguson, M. C., McNicol, E., et al. (2021). The prevalence of psychiatric and chronic pain comorbidities in fibromyalgia: An ACTION systematic review. *Seminars in Arthritis and Rheumatism, 51*(1), 166–174. https://doi.org/10.1016/j.semarthrit.2020.10.006.

Kobak, S., & Bes, C. (2018). An autumn tale: Geriatric rheumatoid arthritis. *Therapeutic Advances in Musculoskeletal Disease, 10*(1), 3–11. https://doi.org/10.1177/1759720X17740075.

Kochan, J.P. (Ed.). (2020). Percutaneous vertebroplasty and kyphoplasty. *Medscape*. https://emedicine.medscape.com/article/1835633-overview

Kohn, M. D., Sassoon, A. A., & Fernando, N. D. (2016). Classifications in brief: Kellgren-Lawrence classification of osteoarthritis. *Clinical Orthopaedics and Related Research, 474*(8), 1886–1893. https://doi.org/10.1007/s11999-016-4732-4.

Kolasinski, S. L., Neogi, T., Hochberg, M. C., Oatis, C., et al. (2020). 2019 American College of Rheumatology/Arthritis Foundation guideline for the management of osteoarthritis of the hand, hip, and knee. *Arthritis & Rheumatology, 272*(2), 220–233. https://doi.org/10.1002/art.41142.

Kopiczko, A. (2019). Bone mineral density in old age: The influence of age at menarche, menopause status and habitual past and present physical activity. *Archives of Medical Science, 16*(3), 657–665. https://doi.org/10.5114/aoms.2019.81314.

Koster, M. J., & Warrington, K. J. (2015). Latest advances in the diagnosis and treatment of polymyalgia rheumatica. *Practical Pain Management, 15*(9). https://www.practicalpainmanagement.com/pain/myofascial/inflammatory-arthritis/latest-advances-diagnosis-treatment-polymyalgia-rheumatica.

Küçükdevecii, A. A. (2019). Nonpharmacological treatment in established arthritis. *Best Practice & Research. Clinical Rheumatology, 33*(5), 101482. https://doi.org/10.1016/j.berh.2019.101482.

Kumari, R., & Saharawat, S. (2020). Effect of usage and compliance of hand splints on activities of daily living in patients with rheumatoid arthritis: A review. *International Journal of Health Sciences and Research, 10*(2), 223–227. ISSN: 2249-9517.

Kuo, C. F., Grainge, M., Mallen, C., Zhang, W., & Doherty, M. (2016). Comorbidities in patients with gout prior to and following diagnosis: Case-control study. *Annals of the Rheumatic Diseases, 75*, 210–217. https://doi.org/10.1136/annrheumdis-2014-206410.

Kraus, V. B., Sprow, K., Powel, K. C., Buchner, D., Boodgood, B., Piercy, K., & Kraus, W. E. (2019). Effects of physical activity in knee and hip osteoarthritis: A systematic umbrella review. *Medicine & Science in Sports & Exercise, 51*(6), 324–1339. https://doi.org.libproxy.txstate.edu/10.1249/MSS.0000000000001944.

Kwak, J. M., Koh, K. H., & Jeon, I. H. (2019). Total elbow arthroplasty. *Clinical Outcomes, Complications, and Revision Surgery, 11*(4), 369–379. https://doi.org/10.4055/cios.2019.22.4369.

Kravets, I. (2018). Paget's disease of bone: Diagnosis and treatment. *American Journal of Medicine, 131*, 1298–1303. https://doi.org/10.1016/j.amjmed.2018.04.028.

Kreiner, F., Borup, R., Nielsen, F., Schjerling, P., & Galbo, H. (2017). Gene expression profiling in patients with polymyalgia rheumatica before and after symptom-abolishing glucocorticoid treatment. *BMC Musculoskeletal Disorders, 18*, 341–360. https://doi.org/10.1186/s12891-017-1705-z.

Kumbhare, D., Elzibak, A., & Noseworthy, M. (2016). Assessment of myofascial trigger points using ultrasound. *American Journal of Physical Medicine and Rehabilitation, 95*(1), 72–80. https://doi.org/10.1097/PHM.0000000000000376.

Lange, E., Kucharski, D., Svedlund, S., Svensson, K., et al. (2019). Effects of aerobic and resistance exercise in older adults with rheumatoid arthritis: A randomized controlled trial. *Arthritis Care & Research, 71*(1), 61–70. https://doi.org/10.1002/acr.23589.

Larson, C., O'Brien, B., & Rennke, S. (2016). GeriWard Falls: An interprofessional team-based curriculum on falls in the hospitalized older adult. *Mededportal: The Journal of Teaching and Learning Resources, 12* https://doi.org/10.15766/mep_2374-8265.10410. 10410–10410.

Laurent, M., Dedeyne, L., Dupont, J., Mellaerts, B., Dejaeger, M., & Gielen, E. (2019). Age-related bone loss and sarcopenia in men. *Maturitas, 122*, 51–56. https://doi.org/10.1016/j.maturitas.

Lee, A., Maani, V., & Amin, P. (2021). *Radiation therapy for heterotopic ossification prophylaxis*. StatPearls Publishing. https://www.ncbi.nlm.nih.gov/books/NBK493155/.

Lee, L., Hillier, L. M., McKinnon Wilson, J., Gregg, S., Fathi, K., Sturdy Smith, C., & Smith, M. (2018). Effect of primary care-based memory clinics on referrals to and wait-time for specialized geriatric services. *Journal of the American Geriatrics Society, 66*(3), 631–632. https://doi.org/10.1111/jgs.15169.

Lee, Y., Kim, S., Chang, M., Nam, E., et al. (2018). Complications and socioeconomic costs associated with falls in the elderly population. *Annals of Rehabilitative Medicine, 42*(1), 120–129. https://doi.org/10.5535/arm.2018.42.1.120.

Leese, J., Macdonald, G., Tran, B., et al. (2018). Using physical activity trackers in arthritis self-management: A qualitative study of patient and rehabilitation professional perspectives. *Arthritis Care & Research, 71*(2), 227–236. https://doi-org.libproxy.txstate.edu/10.1002/acr.23780.

Łęgosz, P., Otworowski, M., Sibilska, A., et al. (2019). Heterotopic ossification: A challenging complication of total hip arthroplasty: Risk factors, diagnosis, prophylaxis, and treatment. *BioMed Research International*, 2019. https://doi.org/10.1155/2019/3860142.

Lewiecki, E. M. (2018). Osteoporosis: Clinical evaluation. In K. R. Feingold, B. Anawalt, & A. Boyce (Eds.), *Endotext [Internet]*. MDText.com. https://www.ncbi.nlm.nih.gov/books/NBK279049/.

Lewiecki, E.M. (2019). Osteoporotic fracture risk assessment. In J. E. Mulder (Ed.), *UpToDate*. https://www-uptodate-com.libproxy.txstate.edu/contents/osteoporotic-fracture-risk-assessment?sectionName=Fracture%20risk%20assessment%20tool&search=osteoporosis&topicRef=2035&anchor=H4&source=see_link#H4

Li, R., Tian, C., Postlethwaite, A., et al. (2017). Rheumatoid arthritis and periodontal disease: What are the similarities and differences? *International Journal of Rheumatic Diseases, 20*, 1887–1901. https://doi.org.libproxy.txstate.edu/10.1111/1756-185X.13240.

Li, S., Ge, Y., Yang, H., Wang, T., et al. (2019). The spectrum and clinical significance of myositis-specific autoantibodies in Chinese patients with idiopathic inflammatory myopathies. *Clinical Rheumatology, 38*(8), 2171–2179. https://doi.org/10.1007/s10067-019-04503-7.

Li, X., Wang, R., Xing, X., Shi, X., et al. (2017). Acupuncture for myofascial pain syndrome: A network meta-analysis of 33 randomized controlled trials. *Pain Physician, 20*(6), E883–E902. PMID: 28934793.

Li, Y., Dai, G., Shi, L., Lin, Y., et al. (2019). The potential roles of tendon stem/progenitor cells in tendon aging. *Current Stem Cell Research & Therapy, 14*(00). https://doi.org/10.1274/1574888X13666181017112233.

Liem, B. C., Trunswell, H. J., & Harrast, M. (2013). Rehabilitation and return to running after lower limb stress fractures. *Current Sports Medicine Reports, 12*(3), 200–217. https://doi.org/10.1249/JSR.0b013e3182913cbe.

Liew, D. F., Owen, C. E., & Buchanan, R. R. (2018). Prescribing for polymyalgia rheumatica. *Australian Prescriber, 41*(1), 14–19. https://doi.org/10.18773/austprescr.2018.001.

Link, T. M. (2016). Radiology of osteoporosis. *Canadian Association of Radiologists Journal, 67*(1), 28–40. https://doi.org/10.1016/j.carj.2015.02.002.

Lisi, A., Gallagher, R., Rodriguez, E., & Rossi, M. (2015). Deconstructing chronic low back pain in the older adult-step by step evidence and expert-based recommendations for evaluation and treatment. *Pain Medicine, 16*(7), 1282–1289. https://doi.org/10.1111/pme.12821.

Little, R., Paterson, D., Humphreys, D., & Stathokostas, L. (2013). A 12-month incidence of exercise-related injuries in previously sedentary community-dwelling older adults following an exercise intervention. *BMJ Open, E*, e002831. https://doi.org/10.1136/bmjopen-2013-002831.

Litwic, A., Edwards, M. H., Dennison, E. M., & Cooper, C. (2013). Epidemiology and burden of osteoarthritis. *British Medical Bulletin, 105*, 185–199. https://doi.org/10.1093/bmb/lds038.

Liu, J., Liu, A., Luo, J., Gong, L., et al. (2019). Influence of vertebral bone mineral density on total dispersion volume of bone cement in vertebroplasty. *Medicine, 98*(12), e14941. https://doi.org/10.1097/MD.0000000000014941.

Liu, U. J., Zhang, L., Papsian, C. J., & Deng, H. W. (2014). Genome-wide association studies of osteoporosis: A 2013 update. *Journal of Bone Metabolism, 21*(2), 99–116. https://doi.org/10.11005/jbm.2014.21.2.99.

Lloyd, T.E. (2021). Management of inclusion body myositis. *UpToDate*. https://www.uptodate.com/contents/management-of-inclusion-body-myositis/print

Lloyd, T. E., Mammen, A. L., Amato, A. A., Weiss, M. D., Needham, M., & Greenberg, S. A. (2014). Evaluation and construction of diagnostic criteria for inclusion body myositis. *Neurology, 83*(5), 426–433. https://doi.org/10.1212/WNL.0000000000000642.

Lo, C. W. T., Tsang, W. W. N., Yan, C. H., Lord, S. R., Hill, K. D., & Wong, A. Y. L. (2019). Risk factors for falls in patients with total hip arthroplasty and total knee arthroplasty: A systematic review and meta-analysis. *Osteoarthritis and Cartilage, 27*(7), 979–993. https://doi.org/10.1016/j.joca.2019.04.006.

Loge-Hagen, J. S., Saele, A., Juhl, C., et al. (2019). Prevalence of depressive disorder among patients with fibromyalgia: Systematic review and meta-analysis. *Journal of Affective Disorders, 245*, 1098–1105. https://doi.org/10.1016/j.jad.2018.12.001.

Lohrer, H., David, S., & Nauck, T. (2016). Surgical treatment for Achilles tendinopathy—A systematic review. *BMC Musculskelet Disord, 17*, 207–217. https://doi.org/10.1186/s12891-016-1061-4.

Loiselle, A. (2017). Tendon homeostasis, tendinopathy, and healing. *MSR T32 Musculoskeletal Basic Science Course* https://www.urmc.rochester.edu/MediaLibraries/URMCMedia/musculoskeletal-research/documents/Loiselle_CMSR-course-2017.pdf.

Looker, A., & Frenk, S. (2015). Percentage of adults Aged 65 and over with osteoporosis or low bone mass at the femur neck or lumbar spine: United States, 2005–2010. *National Center for Health Statistics* https://www.cdc.gov/nchs/data/hestat/osteoporsis/osteoporosis2005_2010.pdf on September 18, 2019.

Lou, W., Cui, C., Pourtaheri, S., & Garfin, S. (2018). Efficacy of cerebral augmentation for vertebral compression fractures: A review of meta-analyses. *Spine Surgery and Related Research, 2*(3), 163–168. https://doi.org/10.22603/ssrr.2017-0089.

Lourenzi, F., Jones, A., Pereira, D., et al. (2017). Effectiveness of an overall progressive resistance strength program for improving the functional capacity of patients with rheumatoid arthritis: A randomized controlled trial. *Clinical Rehabilitation, 31*(11), 1482–1491. https://doi.org/10.1177/0269215517698732.

Lovsin, N., Zupan, J., & Marc, J. (2018). Genetic effects on bone health. *Current Opinion in Clinical Nutrition and Metabolic Care, 21*(4), 233–239. https://doi.org/10.1097/MCO.0000000000000482.

Lozada, C., & Pace, S., & Diamond, H. (Eds.). (2019). Osteoarthritis treatment & management. *Medscape*. https://emedicine.medscape.com/article/330487-treatment#d9

Lundberg, I., Visser, M., & Werth, V. (2018). Classification of myositis. *Rheumatology, 14*, 269–278. https://doi.org/10.1038/nrrheum.2018.41.

Luo, S. Y., Li, Y., Luo, H., Xh, Y., et al. (2016). Increased intake of vegetables; but not fruits, may be associated with reduced risk of hip fracture: A meta-analysis. *Scientific Reports, 6*, 19783. https://doi.org/10.1038/srep19783.

Macchioni, P., Boiardi, L., Catanoso, M., Pazzola, G., & Salvarani, C. (2014). Performance of the new 2012 EULAR/ACR classification criteria for polymyalgia rheumatica: Comparison with the previous criteria in a single-study. *Annals of the Rheumatic Diseases, 73*(6), 1190–1193. https://doi.org/10.1136/rheumatology.kep286.

Mackie, S. L., Koduri, G., Hill, C. L., et al. (2015). Accuracy of musculoskeletal imaging for the diagnosis of polymyalgia rheumatica: Systematic review. *RMD Open, 1*(1), e000100. https://doi.org/10.1136/rmdopen-2015-00010021.

Maffei, M. E. (2020). Fibromyalgia: Recent advances in diagnosis, classification, pharmacology and alternative remedies. *International Journal of Molecular Sciences, 21*, 7877–7904. https://doi.org/10.3390/IJMS21217877.

Magee, D., Zachazewski, J., Quillen, W., & Manske, R. (2016). Pathology and intervention in musculoskeletal rehabilitation. *Management of osteoarthritis and rheumatoid arthritis*. Saunders.

Maglio, C., Peltonen, M., Neovius, M., Jacobson, P., Jacobsson, L., & Carlsson, L. M. (2017). Effects of bariatric surgery on gout incidence in the Swedish Obese Subjects study: A non-randomized, prospective, controlled intervention trial. *Annals of the Rheumatic Diseases, 76*(4), 688–693. https://doi.org/10.1136/annrheumdis-2016-209958. Epub 2016 Oct 8. PMID: 28076240.

Mahmood, S., Nelson, E., Padniewski, J., & Nasr, R. (2020). Polymyalgia rheumatica: An updated review. *Cleveland Clinic Journal of Medicine, 87*(9), 549–556. https://doi.org/10.3949/ccjm.87a.20008.

Makris, U. E., & Reid, M. C. (2017). Back pain and spinal stenosis. In J. B. Halter, J. G. Ouslander, & S. Studenski (Eds.), *Hazzard's geriatric medicine and gerontology* (7th ed.). McGraw-Hill Education.

Malanga, G. A., & Cruz Colon, E. J. (2010). Myofascial low back pain: A review. *Physical Medicine and Rehabilitation Clinics of North America, 21*(4), 711–724.

Mange, D., & Bougault, C. (2015). What understanding tendon cell differentiation can teach us about pathological tendon ossification. *Histology and Histopathology, 30*(8), 901–910. https://doi.org/10.14670/HH-11-614.

Mann, G. S., & Mologhianu, G. (2014). Osteoarthritis pathogenesis—A complex process that involves the entire joint. *Journal of Medicine and Life, 7*(1), 37–41.

Manzo, C. (2019). If something looks like an apple, is it necessary an apple? Reflections on so-called "statin-induced polymyalgia rheumatica.". *Reumatologia, 57*(3), 163–166. https://doi.org/10.5114/reum.2019.86427.

Manzo, C., Castagna, A., & Betul, S. (2021). Not just pain and morning stiffness duration in the daily experience of patients with polymyalgia rheumatica. Does the rheumatologist listen to all patient-reported outcomes? *Reumatologia, 59*(3), 200–202. https://doi.org/10.5114/reum.2021.106221.

Marcucci, E., Bartoloni, E., Alunno, A., Leone, M. C., Cararo, G., Luccioli, F., Valentini, V., Valentini, E., La Paglia, G. M. C., et al. (2018). Extra-articular rheumatoid arthritis. *Reumatismo, 70*(4), 212–224. https://doi.org/10.4081/reumatismo.2018.1106.

Marques, P. M., Cacho-Rodrigues, P., Ribeiro-Silva, M., et al. (2015). Surgical management of cervical spine instability in rheumatoid arthritis patients. *Acta Reumatologica Portuguesa, 40*(1), 34–39.

Marsh, M., & Newman, S. (2021). Trends and developments in hip and knee arthroplasty technology. *Journal of Rehabilitation and Assistive Technologies Engineering* https://doi.org/10.1177/2055668320952043. Feb 8; 8:2055668320952043.

Marsman, A. F., Dahmen, R., Roorda, L. D., et al. (2013). Foot-related health care use in patients with rheumatoid arthritis in an outpatient secondary care center for rheumatology and rehabilitation in the Netherlands: A cohort study with a maximum of fifteen years of followup. *Arthritis Care Research, 65*(2), 220–226. https://doi.org/10.1002/acr.21787.

Martinez-Velilla, N., Fernández-Sola, J., Santaeugenia, S., & Mas, M. A. (2015). Geriatric frailty applied to fibromyalgia patients. *Rheumatology International, 35*, 193–194. https://doi.org/10.1007/s00296-014-3048-5.

Matcuk, G., Mahanty, S., Skalski, M., Patel, D., et al. (2016). Stress fractures: Pathophysiology, clinical presentation, imaging features, and treatment options. *Emergency Radiology, 23*, 365–375. https://doi.org/10.1007/s10140-016-1390-5.

Matsuo, K. (2009). Cross-talk among bone cells. *Current Opinion in Nephrology and Hypertension, 18*(4), 292–297. https://doi.org/10.1097/mnh.0b013e32832b75f1.

Matteson, E., & Davis, J. (2019). Overview of the systemic and non-articular manifestations of rheumatoid arthritis. In J. R. O'Dell (Ed.), *UpToDate*. https://www-uptodate-com.libproxy.txstate.edu/contents/overview-of-the-systemic-and-nonarticular-manifestations-of-rheumatoid-arthritis?search=rheumatoid%20arthritis%20diagnosis&topicRef=7502&source=see_link

Matteson, E. L., Buttgereit, F., Dejaco, C., & Dasgupta, B. (2016). Glucocorticoids for management of polymyalgia rheumatica and giant cell arteritis. *Rheumatic Disease Clinics of North America, 42*(1), 75–90. https://doi.org/10.1016/j.rdc.2015.08.009.

May, T., & Marappa-Ganeshan, R. (Updated 2021, August 11). Stress fractures. In *StatPearls* [Internet]. StatPearls Publishing. https://www.ncbi.nim.nih.gov/books/NBK554538/

Mayoral del Moral, O., Lacomba, M., Russell, J., Mendez, S., & Sanchez, B. (2018). *Pain Medicine*, 19, 2039–2050. https://doi.org/10.1093/pm/pnx315

McAlindon, R. E., Bannuru, R. R., Sullivan, M. C., Arden, N. K., et al. (2014). OARSI guidelines for the non-surgical management of knee osteoarthritis. *Osteoarthritis Cartilage, 22*(3), 363–388. https://doi.org/10.1016/j.joca.2014.

McBain, H., Shipley, M., & Newman, S. (2018). Clinician and patient views about self-management support in arthritis: A cross-sectional UK survey. *Arthritis Care Research, 70*(11), 1607–1613. https://doi.org/10.1002/acr.23540.

McCarthy, M., & Hannafin, J. (2014). The mature athlete. *Sports Health, 6*(1), 41–48. https://doi.org/10.1177/1941738113485691.

McCormick, N. (2019). Which patient with rheumatoid arthritis will start biologics, how soon, and shy—Much to learn from a universal coverage setting. *Journal of the American*

Medical Association, *2*(12), e1917065. https://doi.org/10.1001/jamanetworkopen.2019.17065.

McDonough, C., Harris-Hayes, M., Kristensen, M., Overgaard, J., et al. (2021). Physical therapy management of older adults with hip fractures. *Journal of Orthopaedic & Sports Physical Therapy*, *51*(2), CPG1–CPG81. https://doi.org/10.2519/jospt.2021.0301.

McGrath, E. R., Doughty, C. T., & Amato, A. A. (2018 Octt). Autoimmune Myopathies: Updates on Evaluation and Treatment. *Neurotherapeutics*, *15*(4), 976–994. https://doi.org/10.1007/s13311-018-00676-2. PMID: 30341597; PMCID: PMC6277300.

McHugh, N., & Tansley, S. (2018). Autoantibodies in myositis. *Nature Reviews Rheumatology*, *14*, 290–303. https://doi.org/10.1038/nrrheum.2018.56.

McInnes, I. B., & Schett, G. (2007). Cytokines in the pathogenesis of rheumatoid arthritis. *Nature Reviews Immunology*, *7*(6), 429–442. Review.

McInnis, K. C., & Ramey, L. N. (2016). High risk stress fractures: Diagnosis and management. *Archives of Physical Medicine and Rehabilitation*, *8*(3 Suppl), S113–S124. https://doi.org/10.1016/j.pmrj.2015.09.019.

McMahon, M. (2018). Optimizing treatment strategies in the management of rheumatoid arthritis: Novel therapies for improved patient outcomes. *Journal of Managed Care Medicine*, *21*(4), 74–78. www.namcp.org.

Mears, S. C., & Kates, S. (2015). A guide to improving the care of patients with fragility fractures, edition 2. *Geriatric Orthopaedic Surgery & Rehabilitation*, *6*(2), 58–120. https://doi.org/10.1177/2150458515572697.

Menendez-Buetes, L. R., & Fernandez, S. (2017). Paget's disease of bone: Approach to its historical origins. Reumatología. *Clinica*, *13*, 66–72.

Metsios, G. S., & Kitas, G. D. (2018). Physical activity, exercise, and rheumatoid arthritis: Effectiveness, mechanisms and implementation. *Best Practice & Research Clinical Rheumatology*, *32*(5), 669–682. https://doi.org/10.1016/j.berh.2019.03.013.

Metsios, G. S., Moe, R. H., van der Esch, M., et al. (2019). The effects of exercise on cardiovascular disease risk factors and cardiovascular physiology in rheumatoid arthritis. *Rheumatology International*, *40*(3), 347–357. https://doi.org/10.1007/s00296-019-04483-6.

Meyer, A., Scirè, C. A., Talarico, R., et al. (2019). Idiopathic inflammatory myopathies: State of the art on clinical practice guidelines. *Rheumatic & Musculoskeletal Diseases Open*, *4*, e000784. https://doi.org/10.1136/rmdopen-2018-000784.

Meyer, A., Lannes, B., Goetz, J., Echaniz-Laguna, A., et al. (2017). Inflammatory myopathies: A new landscape. *Joint, Bone, Spine*, *85*, 23–33. https://doi.org/10.1016/j.jbspin.2017.03.005.

Meyers, C., Lisiecki, J., Miller, S., Levin, A., Fayad, L., Ding, C., & James, A. W. (2019). Heterotopic ossification: A comprehensive review. *Journal of Bone and Mineral Research Plus*, *3*(4), e10172. https://doi.org/10.1002/jbm4.10172.

Michael, J. W., Schlüter-Brust, K. U., & Eysel, P. (2010). The epidemiology, etiology, diagnosis, and treatment of osteoarthritis of the knee. *Deutsches Arzteblatt International*, *107*(9), 152–162. https://doi.org/10.3238/arztebl.2010.0152.

Michou, L., & Orcel, P. (2016). The changing countenance of Paget's disease of bone. *Joint Bone Spine*, *83*, 650–655. https://doi.org/10.1016/j.jbspin.2016.02.011.

Milchert, M., & Brzosko, M. (2017). Diagnosis of polymyalgia rheumatica usually means a favorable outcome for your patient. *Indian Journal of Medical Research*, *145*, 593–600. https://doi.org/10.4103/ijmr.IJMR_298_17.

Miller, F., Lamb, J., Schmidt, J., & Nagaraju, K. (2018). Risk factors and disease mechanisms in myositis. *Nature Reviews Rheumatology*, *14*, 255–268.

Miller, T. L., & Best, T. M. (2016). Taking a holistic approach to managing difficult stress fractures. *Journal of Orthopaedic Surgery and Research*, *11*(1), 98. https://doi.org/10.1186/s13018-016-0431-9.

Minerbi, A., & Fitzcharles, M. A. (2021). Fibromyalgia in older individuals. *Drugs & Aging*, *38*, 735–749. https://doi.org/10.1007/s40266-021-00879.

Minetto, M. A., Giannini, A., McConnell, R., Busso, C., Torre, G., & Massazza, G. (2020). Common musculoskeletal disorders in the elderly: The star triad. *Journal of Clinical Medicine*, *9*(4), 1216–1233. https://doi.org/10.3390/jcm9041216.

Mirmiran, R., Bush, T., Cerra, M., Grambart, S., et al. (2018). Joint clinical consensus statement of the American College of Foot and Ankle Surgeons and the American Association of Nurse Practitioners: Etiology, diagnosis, and treatment consensus for gouty arthritis of the foot and ankle. *Journal of Foot & Ankle Surgery*, *57*, 1207–1217. https://doi.org/10.1053/j.jfas.2018.08.018.

Moghadam-Kia, S., Aggarwal, R., & Oddis, C. (2018). Myositis in clinical practice—Relevance of new antibodies. *Best Practice & Research Clinical Rheumatology*, *32*, 887–901. https://doi.org/10.1016/j.berh.2019.03.0121521-6942.

Moghadam-Kia, S., Oddis, C. V., & Aggarwal, R. (2017). Modern therapies for idiopathic inflammatory myopathies (IIMs): Role of biologics. *Clinical Reviews in allergy & immunology*, *52*(1), 81–87. https://doi.org/10.1007/s12016-016-8530-2.

Moreland, L., O'Dell, J. R., Cofield, S., et al. (2012). A randomized comparative effectiveness study of oral triple therapy versus etanercept plus methotrexate in early, aggressive rheumatoid arthritis. *Arthritis & Rheumatology*, *64*(9), 2824–2835. https://www.ncbi.nlm.nih.gov/pmc/articles/PMC4036119/#!po=2.63158 on January 8, 2020.

Morelli, J. (2019). *Gout treatment guidelines by the American College of Rheumatology*. Arthritis Foundation. https://www.arthritis.org/about-arthritis/types/gout/articles/gout-treatments-guidelines.php.

Mori, S., & Koga, Y. (2016). Glucocorticoid-resistant polymyalgia rheumatica: Pretreatment characteristics and tocilizumab therapy. *Clinical Rheumatology*, *35*, 1367–1375. https://doi.org/10.1007/s10067-014-2650-y.

Mueller, R. B., Reshiti, N., Kaegi, T., Finckh, A., Haile, S. R., Schulze-Koops, H., Schiff, M., Spaeth, M., von Kempis, J., & SCQM Physicians, (2017). Does addition of glucocorticoids to the initial therapy influence the later course of the disease in patients with early RA? Results from the Swiss prospective observational registry (SCQM). *Clinical Rheumatology*, *36*(1), 59–66.

Mujtaba, B., Taher, A., Fiala, M., Nassar, S., et al. (2019). Heterotopic ossification: Radiological and pathological review. *Radiology Oncology*, *53*(3), 275–284. https://doi.org/10.2478/fapm-2019-0039.

Munters, L., Loell, I., Ossipova, E., et al. (2016). Endurance exercise improves molecular pathways of aerobic metabolism in patients with myositis. *Arthritis & Rheumatology*, *68*(7), 1738–1750. https://doi.org/10.1002/art.39624.

Munters, L. A., Dastmalchi, M., Andgren, V., et al. (2013). Improvement in health and possible reduction in disease activity using endurance exercise in patients with established polymyositis and dermatomyositis: A multicenter randomized controlled trial with a 1-year open extension follow-up. *Arthritis Care and Research*, *65*, 1959–1968. Doi.org/10.1002/acr.22068.

Muratore, F., Pazzola, G., Pipitone, N., & Salvarani, C. (2016). Recent advances in the diagnosis and treatment of polymyalgia rheumatica. *Expert Review of Clinical Immunology, 12*(10), 1037–1045. https://doi.org/10.1080.1744666S.2016.1178572.

Muratore, F., Salvarani, C., & Macchioni, P. (2018). Contribution of the new 2012 EULAR/ACR classification criteria for the diagnosis of polymyalgia rheumatica. *Reumatismo, 70*(1), 18–22.

Muschitz, C., Feichtinger, X., Haschika, J., & Kocijan, R. (2017). Diagnosis and treatment of Paget's disease of bone: A clinical practice guideline. *Wien Med Wochenschr, 167*, 18–24. https://doi.org/10.1007/s10354-016-0502-x.

Muscular Dystrophy Association (MDA). (2019, October 26). *Inclusion-body myositis (IBM)*. https://www.mda.org/disease/inclusion-body-myositis/signs-and-symptoms

Musumeci, G., Aiello, F. C., Szychlinska, M. A., Di Rosa, M., Castrogiovanni, P., & Mobasheri, A. (2015). Osteoarthritis in the XXIst century: Risk factors and behaviors that influence disease onset and progression. *International Journal of Molecular Sciences, 16*(3), 6093–6112. https://doi.org/10.3390/ijms16036093.

Mayhew, J. L., & Cyrino, E. S. (2019). Effect of resistance training with different frequencies and subsequent detraining on muscle mass and appendicular lean soft tissue, IGF-1, and testosterone in older women. *European Journal of Sport Science, 19*(2), 199–207. https://doi.org/10.1080/17461391.2018.1496145.

National Center for Complementary and Integrative Health (NCCIH). (2017). *Glucosamine/chondroitin arthritis intervention trial (GAIT)*. https://nccih.nih.gov/research/results/gait.

National Commission on Certification of Physician Assistants (NCCPA). (2018). *2018 Statistical profile of recently certified physician assistants*. https://www.nccpa.net/wp-content/uploads/2020/11/2018StatisticalProfileofRecentlyCertifiedPAs.pdf.

National Committee for Quality Assurance (NCQA). Osteoporosis *testing and management in older women (OTO, OMW)*. https://www.ncqa.org/hedis/measures/osteoporosis-testing-and-management-in-older-women.

National Institute for Health and Care Excellence (NICE). (2017). Hip fracture: Management. *In Clinical Guidelines. June 22, 2011*. https://www.nice.org.uk/guidance/cg124/resources/hip-fracture-management-pdf-35109449902789.

National Institute of Arthritis and Musculoskeletal and Skin Diseases. *Osteoporosis*. https://www.niams.nih.gov/health-topics/osteoporosis#tab-causes

National Institute of Health Genetic and Rare Diseases Information Center (NIH-GARD). *Inclusion body myositis*. https://rarediseases.info.nih.gov/diseases/3896/inclusion-body-myositis

National Institute of Health Osteoporosis and Related Bone Diseases National Resource Center. *Bone mass measurement: What the numbers mean*. https://www.bones.nih.gov/health-info/bone/bone-health/bone-mass-measure

National Institutes of Health National Institute on Aging. *Osteoarthritis*. https://www.nia.nih.gov/health/osteoarthritis on August 17, 2021.

National Institutes of Health Neurological Disorders and Stroke. *Inflammatory myopathies fact sheet*. https://www.ninds.nih.gov/health-information/patient-caregiver-education/fact-sheets/inflammatory-myopathies-fact-sheet.

National Institutes of Health Office of Dietary Supplements. *Vitamin D, fact sheet for health professionals*. https://ods.od.nih.gov/factsheets/VitaminD-HealthProfessional

National Institutes of Health Osteoporosis and Related Bone Diseases National Resource Center. (2018). *What people with rheumatoid arthritis need to know about osteoporosis. NIH Publication No. 18-7904*. https://www.bones.nih.gov/health-info/bone/osteoporosis/conditions-behaviors/osteoporosis-ra#resources

National Institutes of Health Osteoporosis and Related Bone Diseases National Resource Center. (2019). *Information for people newly diagnosed with Paget's disease of bone*. https://www.bones.nih.gov/health-info/bone/pagets/overview#h

National Organization for Rare Disorders (NORD). (n.d., a). *Rare disease database Paget's disease*. https://rarediseases.org/rare-diseases/pagets-disease/

National Organization for Rare Disorders (NORD). (n.d., b). *Rare disease database sporadic inclusion body myositis*. https://rarediseases.org/rare-diseases/sporadic-inclusion-body-myositis/

National Osteoporosis Foundation. (n.d., a). *Exercise to stay healthy*. https://www.nof.org/preventing-fractures/exercise-to-stay-healthy/

National Osteoporosis Foundation. (n.d., b). *What women need to know*. https://www.nof.org/preventing-fractures/general-facts/what-women-need-to-know.

Nielsen, S. M., Bartels, E. M., Henriksen, M., Wæhrens, E. E., Gudbergsen, H., Bliddal, H., Astrup, A., Knop, F. K., Carmona, L., Taylor, W. J., Singh, J. A., Perez-Ruiz, F., Kristensen, L. E., & Christensen, R. (2017). Weight loss for overweight and obese individuals with gout: A systematic review of longitudinal studies. *Annals of the Rheumatic Diseases, 76*(11), 1870–1882. https://doi.org/10.1136/annrheumdis-2017-211472. Epub 2017 Sep 2. PMID: 28866649; PMCID: PMC5705854.

Nelson, A., Allen, K., Golightly, Y., Goode, A., & Jordan, J. (2014). A systematic review of recommendations and guidelines for the management of osteoarthritis: The Chronic Osteoarthritis Management Initiative of the U.S. Bone and Joint Initiative. *Seminars in Arthritis and Rheumatism, 43*(6), 701–712. https://doi.org/10.1016/j.semarthrit.2013.1.012.

Neogi, T. (2012). Clinical significance of bone changes in osteoarthritis. *Therapeutic Advances in Musculoskeletal Disease, 4*(4), 259–267. https://doi.org/10.1177/1759720X12437354.

Neogi, T., Th, T. L., Jansen, A., et al. (2015). 2015 Gout classification criteria: An America College of Rheumatology/European League Against Rheumatism Collaborative Initiative. *Arthritis & Rheumatology, 67*(10), 2557–2568. https://doi.org/10.1002/art.39254.

Nesher, G., & Breuer, G. S. (2016). Giant cell Arteritis and polymyalgia rheumatica: 2016 Update. *Rambam Maimonides Medical Journal, 7*(4), e0035. https://doi.org/10.5041/RMMJ.10262.

Newman, M., Lowe, C. M., & Barker, K. (2015). Spinal orthoses for vertebral osteoporosis and osteoporotic vertebral fracture: A systematic review. *Archives of Physical Medicine and Rehabilitation, 97*(6), 1013–1025. https://doi.org/10.1016/j.apmr.2015.10.108.

Nguyen, C., Lefevre-Colau, M. M., Poiraudeau, S., & Rannou, F. (2016). Rehabilitation (exercise and strength training) and osteoarthritis: A critical narrative review. *Annals of Physical and Rehabilitation Medicine, 59*(3), 190–195. https://doi.org/10.1016/j.rehab:2016.02.010.

Niel-Asher, S. (2014). *The concise book of trigger points: A professional and self-help manual* (3rd ed.). North Atlantic Books.

Nielsen, S. M., Bartels, E. M., Henriksen, M., Waehrens, E. E., et al. (2017). Weight loss for overweight and obese individuals with gout: A systematic review of longitudinal studies. *Annals of the Rheumatic Diseases, 76*(11), 1870.

NIH Osteoporosis and Related Bone Diseases National Resource Center. (2018). *What people with rheumatoid arthritis need to know about osteoporosis*. https://www.bones.nih.gov/health-info/bone/osteoporosis/conditions-behaviors/osteoporosis-ra#:~:text=The%20 link%20between%20rheumatoid%20arthritis%20and%20osteoporosis,-Studies%20have%20found&text=In%20addition%2C%20pain%20and%20loss,direct%20result%20of%20the%20disease

Oddis, C., & Aggarwal, R. (2018). Treatment in myositis. *Nature Reviews Rheumatology, 14*, 279–290. https://doi.org/10.1038nrrheum.2018.42.

O'Donnell, S. (2018). Screening, prevention and management of osteoporosis among Canadian adults. Dépistage, prévention et prise en charge de l'ostéoporose chez les adultes canadiens Osteoporosis Surveillance Expert Working Group. *Health Promotion and Chronic Disease Prevention in Canada: Research, Policy and Practice, 38*(12), 445–454. https://doi.org/10.24095/hpcdp.38.12.02.

Ogdie, A., Taylor, W., Neogi, T., Fransen, J., Jansen, T., et al. (2016). Performance of ultrasound in the diagnosis of gout in a multicenter study: Comparison with monosodium urate monohydrate crystal analysis as the gold standard. *Arthritis &. Rheumatology, 69*(2), 429–438. https://doi.org/10.1002/art.39959.

Ohlmeier, M., Krenn, V., Thiesen, D. M., Sandiford, N. A., Gehrke, T., & Citak, M. (2019). Heterotopic ossification in orthopaedic and trauma surgery: A histopathological ossification score. *Scientific Reports, 9*, 18401. https://doi.org/10.1038/s41598-019-54986-2.

Okabayashi, R., Ishikawa, H., Abe, A., et al. (2021). Twenty years' follow-up of radiocarpal arthrodesis for rheumatoid wrists. *Modern Rheumatology, 31*(2), 312–318. https://doi.org/10.1080/14397595.2020.1782565.

Okura, C., Ishikawa, H., Abe, A., et al. (2018). Long-term patient reported outcomes of elbow, wrist, and hand surgery for rheumatoid arthritis. *International Journal of Rheumatic Diseases, 21*(9), 1701–1708. https://doi.org.libproxy.txstate.edu/10.1111/1756-185x.13340.

Oldroyd, A., Lilleker, J., & Chinoy, H. (2017). Idiopathic inflammatory myopathies—A guide to subtypes, diagnostic approach and treatment. *Clinical Medicine, 17*(4), 322–328.

Oliveira, J., Vardasca, R., Pimenta, M., Gabriel, J., & Torres, J. (2016). Use of infrared thermography for the diagnosis and grading of sprained ankle injuries. *Infrared Physics & Technology, 76*, 530–541. https://doi.org/10.1016/infrared.2016.04.014.

Oni, J. K., Pinero, J. R., Saltzman, B. M., & Jaffe, F. F. (2014). Effect of a selective COX-2 inhibitor, celecoxib, on heterotopic ossification after total hip arthroplasty: A case-controlled study. *Hip International, 24*(3), 256–262. https://doi.org/10.5301/hipint.5000109.

Orchard, G., Paratz, J., Blot, S., & Roberts, J. (2014). Risk factors in hospitalized patients with burn injuries for developing heterotopic ossification—A retrospective analysis. *Journal of Burn Care & Research, 36*(4), 465–470. https://doi.org/10.1097/BCR/0000000000000123.

Orlandi, M., Barsotti, S., Cioffi, E., Tenti, S., Toscano, C., Baldini, C., & Neri, R. (2016). The year in review 2016: Idiopathic inflammatory myopathies. *Experimental Rheumatology, 34f*, 966–974.

Orlova, E. V., & Karateev, D. E. (2016). Efficiency of orthotic intervention in the rehabilitation of patients with rheumatoid arthritis. *Sovremennaâ Revmatologiâ, 10*(3), 11–22. https://doi.org/10.14412/1996-7012-2016-3-11-22.

Orvets, N., Chamberlain, A., Patterson, B. M., Chalmers, P. N., Gosselin, M., Salazar, D., Aleem, A. W., & Keener, J. D. (2018). Total shoulder arthroplasty in patients with a B2 glenoid addressed with corrective reaming. *Journal of Shoulder and Elbow Surgery, 27*(6), S58–S64. https://doi.org/10.1016/j.jse.2018.01.003.

Osteoporosis. (2020, May 5). *Physiopedia*. https://www.physio-pedia.com/index.php?title=Osteoporosis&oldid=236815.

Osti, L., Del Buono, A., & Malfulli, N. (2016). Arthroscopic debridement of the ankle for a mild to moderate osteoarthritis: A midterm follow-up study in former professional soccer players. *Journal of Orthopaedic Surgery and Research, 11*, 37. https://doi.org/10.1186/s13018-016-0368-z.

O'Sullivan, S., Schmitz, S., & Fulk, G. (2019). Arthritis. Chapter 23: *Physical rehabilitation* (7th ed.). F A Davis.

Ozdemir, G., & Yilmaz, A. (2016). Bilateral periprosthetic tibial stress fracture after total knee arthroplasty: A case report. *International Journal of Surgery Case Reports, 24*, 175–178. https://doi.org/10.1016/j.ijscr.2016.04.023.

Paget, J. (1877). On a form of chronic inflammation of bones (osteitis deformans). *Medico-Chirurgical Transactions, 60*, 37–64.

Paget's disease. (2019, November 24). *Physiopedia*. https://www.physio-pedia.com/index.php?title=Paget%27s_Disease&oldid=226286

Paget's disease. (2012). In E. Shamus (Ed.), *Quick answers: Physiotherapy*. McGraw-Hill. http://accessphysiotherapy.mhmedical.com/content.aspx?bookid=855§ionid=49734768.

Paltiel, D., Ingvarsson, E., Lee, D., Leff, R., et al. (2015). Demographic and clinical features of inclusion body myositis in North America. *Muscle Nerve, 52*(4), 527–533. https://doi.org/10.1022/mus.24562.

Pandya, J., Johnson, T., & Low, A. K. (2018). Shoulder replacement for osteoarthritis: A review of surgical management. *Maturitas, 108*, 71–76. https://doi.org/10.1016/j.maturitas.2017.11.013.

Park, J., Park, E., Koo, D., et al. (2017). Compliance and persistence with oral bisphosphonates for the treatment of osteoporosis in female patients with rheumatoid arthritis. *BMC Musculoskeletal Disorders, 18*, 152. https://doi.org/10.1186/s12891-017-1514-4.

Parker, L., Moran, G. M., Roberts, L. M., Calvert, M., & McCahon, D. (2014). The burden of common chronic disease on health-related quality of life in an elderly community-dwelling population in the UK. *Family Practice, 31*(5), 557–563. https://doi.org.libproxy.txstate.edu/10.1093/fampra/cmu035.

Partington, R., Helliwell, T., Muller, S., et al. (2018). Comorbidities in polymyalgia rheumatica: A systematic review. *Arthritis Research & Therapy, 20*, 258–268. https://doi.org/10.1186/s13075-018-1757-y.

Patel, A., Petrone, B., & Carter, K. (2021). Percutaneous vertebroplasty and kyphoplasty: *StatPearls [Internet]*. StatPearls Publishing. https://www.ncbi.nlm.nih.gov/books/NBK525963/.

Pavey, G. J., Polfer, E. M., Nappo, K. E., Tintle, S. M., et al. (2015). What risk factors predict recurrence of heterotopic ossification after excision in combat-related amputations. *Clinical Orthopaedics and Related Research, 473*(9), 2814–2824. https://doi.org/10.1007/s11999-015-4266-1.

Pearson, M. J., Mungovan, S. F., & Smart, N. A. (2018). Effect of aerobic and resistance training on inflammatory markers in heart failure patients: Systematic review and meta-analysis. *Heart Trail Review, 23*(2), 209–223. https://doi.org/10.1007/s10741-018-9677-0.

Pedicelli, A., Papacci, F., Leone, A., et al. (2011). Vertebroplasty for symptomatic monostotic Paget disease [published correction appears in *Journal of Vascular and Interventional Radiology, 22*(5), 738. De Simone, Costantino [corrected to De Simone, Celestino]. *Journal of Vascular and Interventional Radiology, 22*(3), 400–403. https://doi.org/10.1016/j.jvir.2010.11.031.

Pérez, L. M., Enfedaque-Montes, M. B., Cesari, M., Soto-Bagaria, L., Gual, N., Burbano, M. P., & Inzitari, M. (2019). A community program of integrated care for frail older adults. *Journal of Nutrition, Health & Aging, 23*(8), 710–716.

Peterson, J., Eboda, O., Brownley, R., Cilwa, E., et al. (2015). Effects of aging on osteogenic response and heterotopic ossification following burn injury in mice. *Stem Cells and Development, 24*(2), 205–213. https://doi.org/10.1089/scd.2014.0291.

Peterson, J., Okagbare, P., De La Rosa, S., Cilwa, K., et al. (2013). Early detection of burn induced heterotopic ossification using transcutaneous raman spectroscopy. *Bone, 54*(1), 28–34. https://doi.org/10.1016/j.bone.2013.02.002.

Petersen, W., Rembitzki, I. V., Koppenburg, A. G., Ellermann, E., et al. (2013). Treatment of acute ankle ligament injuries: A systematic review. *Archives of Orthopaedic and Trauma Surgery, 133*(8), 1129–1141. https://doi.org/10.1007/s00402-013-1742-5.

Petzke, F., Bruckle, W., Eidmann, U., Heldmann, P., et al. (2017). General treatment principles, coordination of care and patient education in fibromyalgia syndrome. *Der Schmerz, 31*, 246–254. https://doi.org.libproxy.txstate.edu/10.10007/s00482-017-0201-6.

Pikwer, M., Bergstrom, U., Nilsson, J. A., Jacobsson, L., & Turesson, C. (2012). Early menopause is an independent predictor of rheumatoid arthritis. *Annals of the Rheumatic Diseases, 71*(3), 378–381.

Pils, K. (2016). Aspects of physical medicine and rehabilitation in geriatrics. *Wiener Medizinische Wochenschrift (1946), 166*(1–2), 44–47. https://doi.org/10.1007/s10354-015-0420-3.

Pisetsky, D. (2017). Advances in the treatment of rheumatoid arthritis: Cost and challenges. *North Carolina Medical Journal, 78*(5), 337–340. https://doi.org/10.18043/ncm.78.5.337.

Pretzer-Aboff, I., & Prettyman, A. (2015). Implementation of an integrative Hohlistic healthcare model for people living with Parkinson's disease. *Gerontologist, 55*(Suppl. 1), S146–S153.

Qato, D. M., Wilder, J., Schumm, L. P., Gillet, V., & Alexander, G. C. (2016). Changes in prescription and over-the-counter medication and dietary supplement use among older adults in the United States, 2005 vs 2011. *Journal of the American Medical Association Internal Medicine, 176*(4), 473–482. https://doi.org/10.1001/jamainternmed.2015.8581. PMID: 26998708; PMCID: PMC5024734.

Qin, J., Barbour, K. E., Murphy, L. B., Nelson, A. E., Schwartz, T. A., Helmick, C. G., Allen, K. D., Renner, J. B., Baker, N. A., & Jordan, J. M. (2017). Lifetime risk of symptomatic hand O\osteoarthritis: The Johnston County osteoarthritis project. *Arthritis & Rheumatology, 69*(6), 1204–1212. https://doi.org/10.1002/art.40097.

Rader, E. P., Layner, K., Triscuit, A. M., Chetlin, R. D., Ensey, J., & Baker, B. A. (2016). Age-dependent muscle adaptation after chronic stretch-shortening contraction in rats. *Aging and Disease, 7*(1), 1–13. https://doi.org/10.14336/AD.2015.0920.

Ragab, G., Elshahaly, M., & Bardin, T. (2017). Gout: An old disease in new perspective—A review. *Journal of Advanced Research, 8*(5), 495–511. https://doi.org/10.1016/j.jare.2017.04.008.

Raheel, S., Crowson, C., Matteson, E., et al. (2017). Epidemiology of polymyalgia rheumatica 2000–2014 and examination of incidence and survival trends over 45 years: A population-based study. *Arthritis Care & Research, 69*(8), 1282–1285.

Raiser, S. N., & Alfano, A. P. (2019). Orthoses for osteoporosis: *Atlas of orthoses & assistive devices* (pp. 115–125) (5th ed.). Elsevier.

Ralston, S. H., Corral-Gudino, L., Cooper, C., Francis, R., Fraser, W. D., et al. (2019). Diagnosis and management of Paget's disease of bone in adults: A clinical guideline. *Journal of Bone and Mineral Research, 34*(4). https://doi.org/10.1002/jbmr.3657.

Rammelt, S. (2016). Management of ankle fractures in the elderly. *EFFORT Open Reviews, 1*(5), 239–246. https://doi.org/10.1302/2058-5241.1.000023.

Rannou, F., & Poiraudeau, S. (2010). Non-pharmacological approaches for the treatment of osteoarthritis. *Best Practice & Research: Clinical Rheumatology, 24*(1), 93–106. https://doi.org/10.1016/j.berh.2009.08.013.

Reckrey, J. M., Soriano, T. A., Hernandez, C. R., DeCherrie, L. V., Chavez, S., Zhang, M., & Ornstein, K. (2015). The team approach to home-based primary care: Restructuring care to meet individual, program, and system needs. *Journal of the American Geriatrics Society, 63*(2), 358–364. https://doi.org/10.1111/jgs.13196.

Reilly, J. M., Aranda, M. P., Segal-Gidan, F., Halle, A., Han, P. P., Harris, P., & Cousineau, M. R. (2014). Assessment of student interprofessional education (IPE) training for team-based geriatric home care: Does IPE training change students' knowledge and attitudes? *Home Health Care Services Quarterly, 33*(4), 177–193. https://doi.org/10.1080/01621424.2014.968502.

Reina-Bueno, M., del Carmen Vazquez-Bautista, M., Perez-Barcia, S., et al. (2019). Effectiveness of custom-made foot orthoses in patients with rheumatoid arthritis: A randomized controlled trial. *Clinical Rehabilitation, 33*(4), 661–669. https://doi.org/10.1177/0269215518819118.

Rheumatoid Arthritis (2019, September 28). *Physiopedia.* https://www.physio-pedia.com/index.php?title=Rheumatoid_Arthritis&oldid=223690.

Ricci, V., & Ozcakar, L. (2019). Ultrasound imaging of the upper trapezius muscle for safer myofascial trigger point injections: A case report. *Physician and Sportsmedicine, 47*(3), 247–248. https://doi.org/10.1080/00913847.2019.1589105.

Richardson, K., Bennett, K., & Kenny, R. A. (2015). Polypharmacy including falls risk-increasing medications and subsequent falls in community-dwelling middle-aged and older adults. *Age and Ageing, 44*(1), 90–96. https://doi.org/10.1093/ageing/afu141.

Riches, P., Elherik, F., Dolan, S., Unglaub, F., & Breusch, S. (2016). Patient rated outcomes study into the surgical interventions available for the rheumatoid hand and wrist. *Archives of Orthopaedic and Trauma Surgery, 136*(4), 563–570. https://doi.org/10.1007/s00402-016-2412-1.

Richette, P., Doherty, M., Pascual, E., et al. (2017). 2016 updated EULAR evidence-based recommendations for the management of gout. *Annals of the Rheumatic Diseases, 76*(1), 29–42.

Rider, L., Aggarwal, R., Machado, M., et al. (2018). Update on outcome assessment in myositis. *Nature Reviews Rheumatology, 14*(5), 303–318. https://doi.org/10.1038/nrrheum.2018.33.

Rider, L., Lachenbruch, P., Monroe, J., Ravelli, A., et al. (2009). Damage extent and predictors in adult and juvenile dermatomyositis and polymyositis using the myositis damage index. *Arthritis & Rheumatology, 60*(11). 3425–3425.

Riemen, A., & Hutchison, J. (2016). The multidisciplinary management of hip fractures in older patients. *Orthopaedic Trauma, 30*(2), 117–122. https://doi.org/10.1016/j.mpoth.2016.03.006.

Riskowski, J., Dufour, A. B., & Hannan, M. T. (2011). Arthritis, foot pain, and shoe wear: Current musculoskeletal research on feet. *Current Opinion in Rheumatology, 23*(2), 48–155. https://doi.org/10.1097/BOR.0b013e3283422cf5.

Ritchie, C., Andersen, R., Eng, J., Garrigues, S. K., Intinarelli, G., Kao, H., & Barnes, D. E. (2016). Implementation of an interdisciplinary, team-based complex care support health care model at an academic medical center: Impact on health care utilization and quality of life. *PloS One, 11*(2), e0148096. https://doi.org/10.1371journal.pone.0148096.

Rivers, W. E., Garrigues, D., Graciosa, J., et al. (2015). Signs and symptoms of myofascial pain: An international survey of pain management providers and proposed preliminary set of diagnostic criteria. *Pain Medicine, 16*(9), 1794–1805. https://doi.org/10.1111/pme.12780.

Roh, Y. H., Hoh, J. H., Gong, H. S., et al. (2018). Comparative adherence to weekly oral and quarterly intravenous bisphosphonates among patients with limited heath literacy who sustained distal radius fractures. *Journal of Bone and Mineral Metabolism, 36*, 589. htps://doi.org/10.1007/s00774-017-0867-y.

Roh, Y. H., Koh, J. H., Noh, J. F., Gong, H. S., & Baek, G. H. (2017). Effect of health literacy on adherence to osteoporosis treatment among patients with distal radius fracture. *Archives of Osteoporosis, 12*(1), 42. https://doi.org/10.1007s/11657-017-0337-0.

Roll, S. C., & Hardison, M. E. (2017). Effectiveness of occupational therapy interventions for adults with musculoskeletal conditions of the forearm, wrist, and hand: A systematic review. *American Journal of Occupational Therapy, 71*(1). https://doi.org/10.5014/ajot.2017.023234. 7101180010p1-7101180010p12.

Roman-Blas, J. A., Castañeda, S., Largo, R., & Herrero-Beaumont, G. (2009). Osteoarthritis associated with estrogen deficiency. *Arthritis Research & Therapy, 11*(5), 241. https://doi.org/10.1186/ar2791.

Roos, E., & Dahlber, L. (2005). Positive effects of moderate exercise on glycosaminoglycan content in knee cartilage: A four-moth, randomized, controlled trial in patients at risk of osteoarthritis. *Arthritis & Rheumatology, 52*(11), 2005. https://doi.org/10.1002/art.21415.

Rosen, H., & Drezner, M. (2019). Clinical manifestations, diagnosis, and evaluation of osteoporosis in postmenopausal women. In J. E. Mulder (Ed.), *UpToDate*. https://www-uptodate-com.libproxy.txstate.edu/contents/clinical-manifestations-diagnosis-and-evaluation-of-osteoporosis-in-postmenopausalwomen?search=osteoporosis&topicRef=2064&source=see_link.

Ross, A. B., Lee, K. S., Chang, E. Y., et al. (2019). Expert panel on musculoskeletal imaging. ACR appropriateness criteria acute hip pain: Suspected fracture. *Journal of the American College of Radiology, 16*(Suppl. 5), S18–S25. https://doi.org/10.1016/j.jacr.2019.02.028.

Rossi, L., Copes, R., Osto, L., et al. (2018). Factors related with osteoporosis treatment in postmenopausal women. *Medicine, 97*, 28. https://doi.org/10.1097/MC.0000000000011524.

Roszyk, E., & Puszczewicz, M. (2017). Role of human microbiome and selected bacterial infections in the pathogenesis of rheumatoid arthritis. *Reumatologia, 55*(5), 242–250. https://doi.org/10.5114/reum.2017.71641.

Ruoff, G., & Edwards, L. (2016). Overview of serum uric acid treatment targets in gout: Why less than 6 mg/dL? *Postgraduate Medicine, 128*(7), 706–715. https://doi-org.libproxy.txstate.edu/10.1080/00325481.2016.1221732.

Saad, E. R. (2020). Polymyalgia rheumatica. *Medscape* https://emedicine.medscape.com/article/330815-overview.

Sadura-Sieklucka, T., Sokolowska, B., Prusinowska, A., Trzaska, A., et al. (2018). Benefits of wrist splinting in patients with rheumatoid arthritis. *Reumatologia, 56*(6), 362–367. https://doi.org/10.5114/reum.2018.80713.

Salvarani, C., & Muratore, F. (2022). Clinical manifestations and diagnosis of polymyalgia rheumatica. *UpToDate*. https://www.uptodate.com/contents/clinical-manifestations-and-diagnosis-of-polymyalgia-rheumatica.

Salzmann, G. M., Preiss, S., Zenobi-Wong, M., Harder, L. P., Maier, D., & Dvorák, J. (2017). Osteoarthritis in football. *Cartilage, 8*(2), 162–172. https://doi.org/10.1177/1947603516648186.

Sanchez, C., Pesesse, L., Gabay, O., et al. (2012). Regulation of subchondral bone osteoblast metabolism by cyclic compression. *Arthritis & Rheumatology, 64*, 1193–1203.

Sanchez-Romero, E., Pecos-Martin, D., Calvo-Lobo, C., Garcia-Jimenez, D., et al. (2019). Clinical features and myofascial pain syndrome in older adults with knee osteoarthritis by sex and age distribution: A cross-sectional study. *The Knee, 26*, 165–173. https://doi.org/10.1016/j.knee.2018.09.011.

Sawitzke, A. D., Shi, H., Finco, M. F., et al. (2010). Clinical efficacy and safety of glucosamine, chondroitin sulphate, their combination, celecoxib or placebo taken to treat osteoarthritis of the knee: 2-year results from GAIT. *Annals of the Rheumatic Diseases, 69*(8), 1459–1464. https://doi.org/10.1135/ard.2009.12009.

Saxena, A., Chansoria, M., Tomar, G., & Kumar, A. (2015). Myofascial pain syndrome: An overview. *Journal of Pain & Palliative Care Pharmacotherapy, 29*(1), 16–21. https://doi.org/10.3109/15360288.2014.997853.

Schiltenwolf, M., Eidmann, U., Kollner, V., Kuhn, T., et al. (2017). Multimodal therapy of fibromyalgia syndrome. *Der Schmerz, 31*, 285–288. https://doi.org.libproxy.txstate.edu/10.107/s00482-017-0205-2.

Schinnerling, K., Aguillon, J. C., Catalan, D., & Soto, L. (2017). The role of interleukin-6 signaling and its therapeutic blockage in skewing the T cell balance in rheumatoid arthritis. *Clinical and Experimental Immunology, 189*, 12–20.

Schur, P. H., & Gibofsky, A. (2019). Nonpharmacologic therapies and preventive measures for patients with rheumatoid arthritis. In J. R. O'Dell (Ed.). *UpToDate*. https://www-uptodate-com.libproxy.txstate.edu/contents/nonpharmacologic-therapies-and-preventive-measures-for-patients-with-rheumatoid-arthritis?search=exercise%20and%20rheumatoid%20arthritis&source=search_result&selectedTitle=1-150&usage_type=default&display_rank=1.

See, M. T. A., Kowitlawakul, Y., Tan, A. J. Q., & Liaw, S. Y. (2018). Expectations and experiences of patients with osteoarthritis undergoing total joint arthroplasty: An integrative review. *International Journal of Nursing Practice, 24*(2), e12621. https://doi.org/10.1111/ijn.12621.

Seegenschmiedt, M., Makoski, H., & Mickem, O. (2001). Radiation prophylaxis for heterotopic ossification about the hip joint-a multicenter study. *International Journal of Radiation Oncology, Biology, Physics, 51*(3), 756–765.

Senara, S. H., Wahed, W. A. Y., & Mabrouk, D. E. (2019). Importance of patient education in management of patients with rheumatoid arthritis: An intervention study. *Egyptian Rheumatology and Rehabilitation, 46*(1), 42–47. https://doi.org/10.4103/err.err_31_18.

Seror, R., Henry, J., Guston, G., Augin, H. J., Boutron-Ruault, M. C., & Mariette, X. (2019). Passive smoking in childhood increases the risk of developing rheumatoid arthritis. *Rheumatology, 58*, 1154–1162. https://doi.org/10.1093/rheumatology/key219.

Serpas, D. G., Zettel-Watson, L., & Cherry, B. J. (2022). Pain intensity and physical performance among individuals with fibromyalgia in mid-to-late life: The influence of depressive symptoms. *Journal of Health Psychology, 27*(7), 1723–1737. https://doi.org/10.1177/13591053211009286.

Setiawati, R. & Rahardjo, P. (2018). *Bone development and growth, osteogenesis and bone regeneration, Haishen Yang, IntechOpen*. https://doi.org/10.5772/intechopen.82452. https://www.intechopen.com/books/osteogenesis-and-bone-regeneration/bone-development-and-growth.

Shakoor, N., & Loeser, R. (2008). Osteoarthritis: 20 clinical pearls. *Journal of Musculoskeletal Medicine, 25*, 476–480.

Shakouris, S., Dolatkhah, N., Omidbakhsh, S., Pishgahi, A., & Hashemian, M. (2020). Serum inflammatory and oxidative stress biomarkers levels are associated with pain intensity, pressure pain threshold, and quality of life in myofascial pain syndrome. *BMC Research Notes, 13*, 520. https://doi.org/10.1186/s13104-020-05352-3.

Shao, J. H., Yu, K. H., & Chen, S. H. (2021). Effectiveness of a self-management program for joint protection and physical activity in patients with rheumatoid arthritis: A randomized controlled trial. *International Journal of Nursing Studies, 111*, 103752. https://doi.org/10.1016/j.ijnurstu.2020.103752.

Sharma, A., Kudesia, P., Shi, Q., & Gandhi, R. (2016). Anxiety and depression in patients with osteoarthritis: Impact and management challenges. *Open Access Rheumatology: Research and Reviews, 8*, 103–113. https://doi.org/10.2147/OARRR.S93516.

Sheybani, A., Tennapel, M., Lack, W., et al. (2014). Risk of radiation-induced malignancy with heterotopic ossification prophylaxis: A case-control analysis. *International Journal of Radiation Oncology, Biology, Physics, 89*(3), 584–589.

Shoback, D., Rosen, C. J., Black, D. M., Cheung, A. M., Murad, M. H., & Eastell, R. (2020). Pharmacological management of osteoporosis in postmenopausal women: An Endocrine Society guideline update. *Journal of Clinical Endocrinology & Metabolism, 105*(3), 587–594. https://doi.org.libproxy.txstate.edu/10.1210/clinem/dgaa048.

Shortridge, A., Steinheider, B., Ciro, C., Randall, K., Costner-Lark, A., & Loving, G. (2016). Simulating interprofessional geriatric patient care using telehealth: A team-based learning activity. *Mededportal: The Journal of Teaching and Learning Resources, 12* https://doi.org/10.15766/mep_2374-8265.10415. 10415–10415.

Siegel, P., Tencza, M., Apocada, B., & Poole, J. (2017). Effectiveness of occupational therapy interventions for adults with rheumatoid arthritis: A systematic review. *American Journal of Occupational Therapy, 71*, 7101180050. https://doi.org/10.5014/ajot.2017.023176.

Silva, P. G., de Carbalho Silva, F., de Rocha Correa Rocha Fernandes, A., & Natour, J. (2020). Effectiveness of nighttime orthoses in controlling pain for women with hand osteoarthritis: A randomized controlled trial. *American Journal of Occupational Therapy, 74*(3). https://doi.org/10.5014/ajot.2020.033621.

Simovitch, R., Flurin, P. H., Wright, T., Zuckerman, J. D., & Roche, C. P. (2018). Quantifying success after total shoulder arthroplasty: The minimal clinically important difference. *Journal of Shoulder and Elbow Surgery, 27*, 298–305. https://doi.org/10.1016/j.jse.2017.09.013.

Sims, J. A., Yoon, Y. C., & Baek, S. H. (2020). Heterotrophic ossification after aggressive rehabilitation in patients with trauma: A case report. *Journal of the Korean Fracture Society, 33*(1), 32–37. https://doi.org/10.12671/jkfs.2020.33.1.32.

Sims Gould, J., Tong, C., Ly, J., Vazirian, S., Windt, A., & Khan, K. (2019). Process evaluation of team-based care in people aged > 65 years with type 2 diabetes mellitus. *BMJ Open, 9*(8), e029965. https://doi.org/10.1136bmjopen-2019-029965.

Singer, F. (2016). Bone quality in Paget's disease of bone. *Current Osteoporosis Reports, 14*, 39–42. https://doi.org/10.1007/s11914-016-0303-6.

Singer, F., Bone, H., Hosking, D., Lyles, K., Murad, M., Reid, I., & Siris, E. (2014). Paget's disease of bone: An Endocrine Society clinical practice guideline. *Journal of Clinical Endocrinology & Metabolism, 99*(12), 4408–4422. https://doi.org/10.1210/jc.2014-2910.

Singh, H. A., Furst, D. E., Bharat, A., et al. (2012). 2012 Update of the 2008 American College of Rheumatology recommendations for the use of disease-modifying antirheumatic drugs and biologic agents in the treatment of rheumatoid arthritis. *Arthritis Care & Research, 64*(5), 625–639. https://doi.org/10.1002/acr.21641.

Singh, J., Yu, S., Chen, L., & Cleveland, J. (2019). Rates of total Joint replacement in the United States: Future projections to 2020–2040 using the National Inpatient Sample. *Journal of Rheumatology* https://doi.org/10.3899/jrheum.170990. Jrheum.170990.

Singh, J. A., Saag, K. G., Bridges, L., et al. (2015). 2015 American College of Rheumatology Guideline for the treatment of rheumatoid arthritis. *Arthritis Care & Research, special article* https://doi.org/10.1002/acr.22783.

Sinusas, K. (2012). Osteoarthritis: Diagnosis and treatment [published correction appears in *American Family Physician*, 2012 November 15, *86*(10), 893]. *American Family Physician, 85*(1), 49–56.

Siparsky, P., Kirkendall, D., & Garrett, W. (2014). Muscle changes in aging: Understanding sarcopenia. *Sports Health, 6*(1), 36–40. https://doi.org/10.1177/1941738113502296.

Siqueira, U. S., Valente, L. G., Mello, M. T., et al. (2017). Effectiveness of aquatic exercises in women with rheumatoid arthritis: A randomized, controlled, 16-week intervention-the HydRA trial. *American Journal of Physical Medicine and Rehabilitation, 96*(3), 167–175. https://doi.org/10.1097/PHM.0000000000000564.

Slane, L., Martin, J., DeWall, R., Thelen, D., & Lee, K. (2017). Quantitative ultrasound mapping of regional variations in shear wave speeds of the aging Achilles tendon. *European Radiology, 27*, 474–482. https://doi.org/10.1007/s00330-016-4409-0.

Śliwiński, Z., & Żak, M. (2019). [Physiotherapy in geriatrics—Its significance in overall treatment management]. *Wiadomosci Lekarskie (Warsaw, Poland: 1960), 72*(9 cz 1), 1667–1670. http:libproxy.txstate.edu/login?url=http://search.ebscohost.comlogin.aspx?direct=true&db=mdc&AN=31586980&site=eds-live&scope=site.

Smith, G. I., Yoshino, J., Reeds, D. N., Bradley, D., Burrows, R. E., Heisey, H. D., & Mittendorfer, B. (2014). Testosterone and progesterone, but not estradiol, stimulate muscle protein synthesis in postmenopausal women. *Journal of Clinical Endocrinology and Metabolism, 99*(1), 256–265. https://doi.org/10.1210/jc.2013-2835.

Smith, H.R., Brown, A., & Diamond, H.S. (Eds.). (2022). Rheumatoid arthritis treatment & management. *Medscape*. https://emedicine.medscape.com/article/331715-treatment#d13

Smolen, J. S., Aletaha, D., & McInnes, J. B. (2016). Rheumatoid arthritis. *The Lancet, 388*, 2023–2038. https://doi.org/10.1016/S0140-6736(16)30173-8.

Smolen, J. S., Landewe, R., Bijlsma, J., et al. (2017). EULAR recommendations for the management of rheumatoid arthritis with synthetic and biological disease-modifying antirheumatic drugs: 2016 update. *Annals of the Rheumatic Diseases, 76*(6), 960–977.

Sobrero, A., Manzo, C., & Stimamiglio, A. (2018). The role of the general practitioner and the out-of-hospital public rheumatologist in the diagnosis and follow-up of patients with polymyalgia rheumatica. *Reumatismo, 70*(1), 44–50.

Solai, L. K., Kumar, K., Mulvaney, E., Rosen, D., Rodakowski, J., Fabian, T., & Sewell, D. (2019). Geriatric mental healthcare training: A mini-fellowship approach to interprofessional assessment and management of geriatric mental health issues. *American Journal of Geriatric Psychiatry* https://doi.org/10.1016/j.jagp.2019.04.018.

Sommer, C., Alten, R., Bar, K. J., Bernateck, M., et al. (2017). Drug therapy of fibromyalgia syndrome. *Der Schmerz, 31*, 274–284. https://doi.org.libproxy.txstate.edu/10.1007/s00482-017-0207-0.

Sowers, M. F., McConnell, D., Jannausch, M., Buyutur, A. G., Hochberg, M., & Jamadar, D. (2006). Estradiol and its metabolites and their association with knee osteoarthritis. *Arthritis & Rheumatology, 54*(8), 2481–2487. https://doi.org/10.1002/art.22005.

Sözen, T., Özışık, L., & Başaran, N. Ç. (2017). An overview and management of osteoporosis. *European Journal of Rheumatology, 4*(1), 46–56. https://doi.org/10.5152/eurjrheum.2016.048.

Spahn, G., Grosser, V., Schiltenwolf, M., Schroter, F., & Grifka, J. (2015). Football as risk factor for a non-injury-related knee osteoarthritis – results from a systematic review and meta-analysis [in German]. *Sportverletz Sportschaden, 29*, 27–39. https://doi.org/10.1055/s-0034-1385731.

Sperber, N. R., Bruening, R. A., Choate, A., Mahanna, E., Wang, V., Powell, B. J., & Hastings, S. N. (2019). Implementing a mandated program across a regional health care system: A rapid qualitative assessment to evaluate early implementation strategies. *Quality Management in Health Care, 28*(3), 147–154. https://doi.org/10.1097QMH.0000000000000221.

Strelzow, J., Frank, T., Chan, K., Athwal, G., et al. (2019). Management of rheumatoid arthritis of the elbow with a convertible total elbow arthroplasty. *Journal of Shoulder and Elbow Surgery, 28*(11), 2205–2214. https://doi.org/10.1016/j.jse.2019.07.029.

Sugiyama, D., Nishimura, K., Tamaki, K., Tsuji, G., Nakazawa, T., Morninobu, A., & Kumagai, S. (2010). Impact of smoking as a risk factor for developing rheumatoid arthritis: A meta-analysis of observational studies. *Annals of the Rheumatic Diseases, 69*(1), 70–78. https://doi.org/10.1136/ard.2008.096487.

Sullivan, M. F., & Kirkpatrick, J. N. (2020). Palliative cardiovascular care: The right patient at the right time. *Clinical Cardiology, 43*(2), 205–212. https://doi.org/10.1002/clc.23307.

Sun, E., & Hanyu-Deutmeyer, A. A. (2019). Heterotopic ossification. [Updated 2019 June 4]: *StatPearls [Internet]*. StatPearls Publishing. file:///C:/Users/McDowell/Dropbox/chapter%20in%20text/Heterotopic%20Ossification%20-%20StatPearls%20-%20NCBI%20Bookshelf.html.

Tabatabaei-Malazy, O., Salari, P., Khashayar, P., & Larijani, B. (2017). New horizons in treatment of osteoporosis. *DARU Journal of Pharmaceutical Sciences, 25*(2). https://doi.org/10.1186/s40199-017-0167-z.

Taii, T., Matsumoto, T., Tanaka, S., Nakamura, I., et al. (2018). Wrist arthrodesis in rheumatoid arthritis using an LCP metaphyseal locking plate versus an AO wrist fusion plate. *International Journal of Rheumatology, 2018* https://doi.org/10.1155/2018/4719634. article ID 4719634.

Takai, H., Kii, S., Murayma, M., Nakene, N., & Takahashi, T. (2018). Ipsilateral stress fracture of the proximal fibula after total knee arthroplasty in a patient with severe valgus knee deformity on a background of Rheumatoid arthritis. *International Journal of Surgery Case Reports, 45*, 17–21. https://doi.org/10.1016/j.ijscr.2018.02.042.

Takla, M. (2018). Low-frequency high-intensity versus medium-frequency low-intensity combined therapy in the management of active myofascial trigger points: A randomized controlled trial. *Physiotherapy Research International, 23*, e1737–e1746. https://doi.org/10.1002/pri.1737.

Tan, A., & Ralston, S. H. (2014). Clinical presentation of Paget's disease: Evaluation of a contemporary cohort and symptomatic review. *Calcified Tissue International, 95*, 385–392.

Tang, V., Sudore, R., Stijacic, I., Cenzer, W., et al. (2017). Rates of recovery to pre-fracture function in older persons with hip fracture: An observational study. *Journal of General Internal Medicine, 32*(2), 153–158. https://doi.org/10.1007/s11606-016-3848-2.

Tang, X., Wang, D., Liu, Y., Chen, J., et al. (2020). The comparison between total hip arthroplasty and hemiarthroplasty in patients with femoral neck fractures: A systematic review and meta-analysis based on 25 randomized controlled trials. *Journal of Orthopaedic Surgery and Research, 15*(1), 596. https://doi.org/10.1186/s13018-020-02122-6.

Tantanatip, A., & Chang, K. V. (2021). Myofascial pain syndrome: *StatPearls [Internet]*. StatPearls Publishing. https://www.ncbinlm.nih.gov/books/NBK499882/.

Taruc-Uy, R., & Lynch, S. (2013). Diagnosis and treatment of osteoarthritis. *Primary Care: Clinics in Office Practice, 40*(4), 821–836.

Taylor, P., & Law, S. (2019). When the first visit to the rheumatologist is established rheumatoid arthritis. *Best Practice & Research Clinical Rheumatology, 33*(5), 101479. https://doi.org/10.1016/j.berh.2019.101479.

Tenten-Diepenmaat, M., Dekker, J., Heymans, M., Roorda, L., et al. (2019). Systematic review on the comparative effectiveness of foot orthoses in patients with rheumatoid arthritis. *Foot and Ankle Research, 12*(32). https://doi.org/10.1186/s130047-019-0338x.

Tenten-Diepenmaat, M., van der Leeden, M., Vlieland, T., Roorda, L., & Dekker, J. (2018). The effectiveness of therapeutic shoes in patients with rheumatoid arthritis: A systematic review and meta-analysis. *Rheumatology International, 38*(5), 749–762. https://doi.org/10.1007/s00296-018-4014-4.

Terada, M., Kosik, K., Johnson, N., & Gribble, P. (2015). Altered postural control variability in older-aged individuals with a history of lateral ankle sprain. *Gait & Posture, 60*, 88–92. https://doi.org/10.1016/j.gaitpost.2017.11.009.

Terroso, M., Rosa, N., Marguew, A. T., & Simoes, R. (2014). Physical consequences of falls in the elderly: A literature review from 1995 to 2010. *European Review of Aging and Physical Activity, 11*, 51–59. https://doi.org/10.1007/s11556-013-0134-8.

Terzis, N., Salonikidis, K., Apostolara, P., Roussos, N., et al. (2021). Can the exercise-based and occupational therapy improve the posture, strength, and mobility in elderly Greek subjects with hip fracture? A non-randomized control trial. *Journal of Frailty, Sarcopenia and Falls, 6*(2), 57–65. https://doi.org/10.22540/JFSF-06-057.

Theis, K. A., Murphy, L., Hootman, J. M., & Wilkie, R. (2013). Social participation restriction among US adults with arthritis: A population-based study using the International Classification of Functioning, Disability, and Health. *Arthritis Care & Research, 65*(7), 1059–1069.

Thorpe, D., Gannotti, M., Peterson, M., Want, C. H., & Freburger, J. (2021). Musculoskeletal diagnoses, comorbidities, and physical and occupational therapy use among older adults with and without cerebral palsy. *Disability and Health Journal, 4*(4), 101109. https://doi.org/10.1016/j.dhjo.2021.101109.

Thorpe, J., Shum, B., Moore, R. A., et al. (2018). Combination pharmacotherapy for the treatment of fibromyalgia in adults. *Cochrane Database of Systematic Reviews, 2*(2), CD010585. https://doi.org/10.1002/14651858.CD010585.pub2.

Tiffreau, V., Rannou, F., Kopciuch, F., Hachulla, E., Mouthon, L., Thoumie, P., Sibilia, J., Drumez, E., & Thevenon, A. (2017). Postrehabilitation functional improvements in patients with inflammatory myopathies: The results of a randomized controlled trial. *Archives of Physical Medicine and Rehabilitation, 98*(2), 227–234. https://doi.org/10.1016/j.apmr.2016.09.125.

Tijsen, L. M. J., Derksen, E. W. C., Achterberg, W. P., & Buijck, B. I. (2019). Challenging rehabilitation environment for older patients. *Clinical Interventions in Aging, 14*, 1451–1460. https://doi.org/10.2147/CIA.S207863.

Ting, K., Huh, A., & Roldan, C. (2020). Review of trigger point therapy for the treatment of myofascial pain syndromes. *Journal of Anesthesiology and Pain Therapy, 1*(3), 22–29. https://www.anesthesioljournal.com/articles/review-of-trigger-point-therapy-for-the-treatment-of-myofascial-pain-syndromes.pdf.

Toprak, C. Ş., Duruöz, M. T., & Gündüz, O. H. (2018). Static and dynamic balance disorders in patients with rheumatoid arthritis and relationships with lower extremity function and deformities: A prospective controlled study. *Archives of Rheumatology, 33*(3), 328–334. https://doi.org/10.5606/ArchRheumatol.2018.6720.

Torma, L. M., Houck, G. M., Wagnild, G. M., et al. (2013). Growing old with fibromyalgia: Factors that predict physical function. *Nursing Research, 62*(1), 16–24. https://doi.org/10.1097/NNR.0b013e318273b853.

Traistaru, M. R., Alexandru, D. O., Kamal, D., Rogoveanu, O. C., et al. (2019). Importance of rehabilitation in primary knee osteoarthritis. *Current Health Sciences Journal, 45*(2), 148–155. https://doi.org/10.12865/CHSJ.45.02.04.

Tran, G., Smith, T. O., Grice, A., Kingbury, S., McCrory, P., & Conaghan, P. G. (2016). Does sports participation (including level of performance and previous injury) increase risk of osteoarthritis? A systematic review and meta-analysis. *British Journal of Sports Medicine, 50*, 1459–1466. https://doi.org/10.1136/bjsports-2016-09614.

Tshimologo, M., Saunders, B., Muller, S., et al. (2017). Patients' views on the causes of their polymyalgia rheumatica: A content analysis of data from the PMR cohort study. *BMJ Open, 7*, e014301.

Tuck, S., Layfield, R., Walker, J., Mekkayil, B., & Francis, R. (2017). Adult Paget's disease of Bone: A review. *Rheumatology, 56*, 2050–2059. https://doi.org/10.1093/rheumatology/kew430.

Ughi, N., Sebastiana, G. D., Gerli, R., Salvarani, C., Parisi, S., et al. (2020). The Italian Society of Rheumatology clinical practice guidelines for the management of polymyalgia rheumatica. *Reumatismo, 72*(1), 1–15. https://doi.org/10.4081/Reumatismo.2020.1268. PMID: 32292016.

Ungprasert, P., Koster, M., Warrington, K., & Matteson, E. (2017). Polymyalgia rheumatica and risk of coronary artery disease: A systematic review and meta-analysis of observational studies. *Rheumatology International, 37*, 143–149. https://doi.org/10.1007/s00296-016-3557-5.

Urits, I., Burshtein, A., Sharma, M., et al. (2019). Low back pain, a comprehensive review: Pathophysiology, diagnosis, and treatment. *Current Pain and Headache Reports, 23*(3), 23. https://doi.org/10.1007/s11916-019-0757-1.

Urrutia, J., Besa, P., & Piza, C. (2019). Incidental identification of vertebral compression fractures in patients over 60 years old using computed tomography scans showing the entire thoracolumbar spine. *Archives of Orthopaedic and Trauma Surgery, 139*(11), 1497–1503. https://doi.org/10.1007/s00402-019-03177-9. Epub.

Valenzuela, E., & Pietschmann, P. (2017). Epidemiology and pathology of Paget's disease of bone—A review. *Wein Med Wochenschr, 167*, 2–8. https://doi.org/10.1007/s10354-016-0496-4.

Vallet, M., & Ralston, S. (2016). Biology and treatment of Paget's disease of bone. *Journal of Cellular Biochemistry, 117*, 289–299. https://doi.org/10.1002/jcb.25291.

Van der Helm-van Mil, A. H., le Cessie, S., van Dongen, H., et al. (2007). A prediction rule for disease outcome in patients with recent-onset undifferentiated arthritis. *Arthritis & Rheumatology, 56*(2), 433–440.

Van De Vlekkert, J., Maas, M., Hoogendijk, J., De Visser, M., & Man Schaik, I. (2015). Combining MRI and muscle biopsy improves diagnostic accuracy in subacute-onset idiopathic inflammatory myopathy. *Muscle & Nerve, 51*(2), 253–258. Doi.org/10.1022/mus.24307.

Venables, P., & Chir, M. (2019a). Diagnosis and differential diagnosis of rheumatoid arthritis. In J. R. O'Dell (Ed.), *UpToDate*. https://www-uptodate-com.libproxy.txstate.edu/contents/diagnosis-and-differential-diagnosis-of-rheumatoid-arthritis?search=rheumatoid%20arthritis%20diagnosis&source=search_result&selectedTitle=1~150&usage_type=default&display_rank=1

Venables, P., & Chir, M. (2019b). Patient education: Rheumatoid arthritis treatment (beyond the basics). In J. R. O'Dell (Ed.), *UpToDate*. https://www.uptodate.com/contents/rheumatoid-arthritis-treatment-beyond-the-basics

Verhoeven, F., Tordi, N., Prati, C., et al. (2016). Physical activity in patients with rheumatoid arthritis. *Joint Bone Spine, 83*(3), 265–270. https://doi.org/10.1016/j.jbspin.2015.10.002.

Vieth, R. (2011). Why the minimum desirable serum 25-hydroxyvitamin D level should be 75 nmol/L (30 ng/ml). *Best Practice & Research Clinical Endocrinology & Metabolism, 25*(4), 681–691. https://doi.org/10.1016/j.beem.2011.06.009. PMID: 21872808.

Visconti, M. R., Usategui-Martin, R., & Ralston, S. (2017). Antibody response to paramyxoviruses in Paget's disease of bone. *Calcified Tissue International, 101*(2), 141–147. https://doi.org/10.1007/s00223-017-0265-4.

Vos, T., Flaxman, A. D., Naghavi, M., Lozano, R., Michaud, C., Ezzati, M., et al. (2012). Years lived with disability (YLDs) for 1160 sequelae of 289 diseases and injuries 1990–2012: A systematic analysis for the global burden of disease study 2010. *The Lancet, 380*, 2163–2196.

Wabe, N., Wojciechowski, J., Wechalekar, M., et al. (2017). Disease activity trajectories in early rheumatoid arthritis following intensive DMARD therapy over 3 years: Association with persistence to therapy. *International Journal of Rheumatic Diseases, 20*, 1447–1456.

Wahid, A., Manek, N., Nichols, M., et al. (2016). Quantifying the association between physical activity and cardiovascular disease and diabetes: A systematic review and meta-analysis. *Journal of American Heart Association* https://ahajournals.org/doi/pdf/10.1161/JAHA.115.002495.

Walsh, A. M., Wechalekar, M. D., Guo, Y., Yin, X., Weedon, H., et al. (2017). Triple DMARD treatment in early rheumatoid arthritis modulates synovial T cell activation and plasmablast/plasma cell differentiation pathways. *PLoS One, 12*(9), e0183928. https://doi.org/10.1371/journal.pone.0183928.

Wang, F., Zhang, H., Ahang, Z., Ma, C., & Feng, X. (2015). Comparison of bipolar hemiarthroplasty and total hip arthroplasty for displaced femoral neck fractures in the healthy elderly: A meta-analysis. *BMC Musculoskeletal Disorders, 16*, 229. https://doi.org/10.1186/s12891-015-0696-x.

Wang, S. M., Han, C., Lee, S. J., Patkar, A. A., Masand, P. C., & Pae, C. U. (2015). Fibromyalgia diagnosis: A review of the past, present, and future. . *Expert Review of Neurotherapeutics, 15*(6), 667–679. https://doi.org/10.1586/14737175.2015.1046841.

Wang, Q., Zhang, P., Pengdong, L., Song, X., et al. (2018). Ultrasonography monitoring of trauma-induced heterotopic ossification: Guidance for rehabilitation procedures. *Frontiers in Neurology, 9*, 771. https://doi.org/10.3389/fneur.2018.0771.

Wang, V., Allen, K., Van Houtven, C. H., Coffman, C., Sperber, N., Mahanna, E. P., & Hastings, S. N. (2018). Supporting teams to optimize function and independence in Veterans: A multi-study program and mixed methods protocol. *Implementation Science: IS*, *13*(1). https://doi.org/10.1186/s13012-018-0748-3. 58–58.

Wasserman, A. (2011). Diagnosis and management of rheumatoid arthritis. *American Family Physician*, *84*(11), 1245–1252.

Weerakkody, Y., & Knipe, H. (2021). Heterotopic ossification. Reference article, *Radiopaedia.org*. https://radiopaedia.org/articles/19159.

Wei, J., Gross, D., Lane, N. E., Lu, N., Wang, M., Zeng, C., Yang, T., Leit, G., Choi, H. K., & Zhang, Y. (2019). Risk factor heterogeneity for medial and lateral compartment knee osteoarthritis: Analysis of two prospective cohorts. *Osteoarthritis and Cartilage*, *27*, 603–610.

Wellsandt, E., & Golightly, Y. (2018). Exercise in the management of knee and hip osteoarthritis. *Current Opinion in Rheumatology*, *30*(2), 151–159. https://doi.org/10.1097/BOR.0000000000000478.

Welsh, V. K., Clarson, L. E., Mallen, C. D., & McBeth, J. (2019). Multisite pain and self-reported falls in older people: Systematic review and meta-analysis. *Arthritis Research & Therapy*, *21*, 67. https://doi.org/10.1186s13075-019-1847-5.

Wen, A., Mac, C., Arndt, R., Katze, A. R., Richardson, K., Deutsch, M., & Masakia, K. (2019). An interprofessional team simulation exercise about a complex geriatric patient. *Gerontology & Geriatrics Education*, *40*(1), 16–29. https://doi.org/10.1080/02701960.2018.1554568.

Weyand, C. M., & Goronzy, J. J. (2014). Clinical Practice. Giant-cell arteritis and polymyalgia rheumatica. *New England Journal of Medicine*, *37*(1), 50–57. https://doi.org/10.1056/NEJMcp1214825.

Williams, L. A. (2019). The history, symptoms, causes, risk factors, types, diagnosis, treatments, and prevention of gout, part 2. *International Journal of Pharmaceutical Compounding*, *23*(1), 14–21.

Williams, N. H., Roberts, J. L., Din, N. U., Totton, N., Charles, J. M., Hawkes, C. A., … Wilkinson, C. (2016). Fracture in the elderly multidisciplinary rehabilitation (FEMuR): A phase II randomised feasibility study of a multidisciplinary. *BMJ Open*, *6*(10), e012422. https://doi.org/10.1136/bmjopen-2016-012422.

Wilson, M. P., Nobbee, D., Murad, M. H., Dhillon, S., et al. (2020). Diagnostic accuracy of limited MRI protocols for detecting radiographically occult hip fractures: A systematic review and meta-analysis. *American Journal of Roentgenology*, *215*, 559–567. https://doi.org/10.2214/AJR.19.22676.

Winkelmann, A., Bork, H., Dexl, C., Heldman, P., et al. (2017). Physiotherapy, occupational therapy and physical therapy in fibromyalgia syndrome: Updated guidelines 2017 and overview of systematic review articles. *Schmerz*, *31*(3), 255–265f. https://doi.org/10.1007/s00482-017-0203-4.

Winn, N., Lalam, R., & Cassar-Pullicina, V. (2017). Imaging of Paget's disease of bone. *Wien Med Wochenschr*, *167*, 9–17. https://doi.org/10.1007/s10354-016-0517-3.

Winters-Stone, K. M., Dobek, J., Nail, L. M., Bennett, J. A., Leo, M. C., et al. (2013). Impact = resistance training improves bone health and body composition in prematurely menopausal breast cancer survivors: A randomized controlled trial. *Osteoporosis International*, *24*(5), 1637–1646. https://doi.org/10.1007/s00198-012-2143-2.

Wiseman, S. J., Ralston, S. H., & Wardlaw, J. M. (2016). Cerebrovascular disease in rheumatic disease. A systematic review-analysis. *Stroke*, *47*(4), 943–950. https://doi.org//jrheum.081180/jrheum.081180/jrheum.08118010.1161/STROKEAHA.115.012052.

Wolfe, F. (2009). Fibromyalgia wars. *Journal of Rheumatology*, *36*(4), 671–678. https://doi.org/10.3899/jrheum.081180.

Wolfe, F., Clauw, D. J., Fitzcharles, M. A., et al. (2011). Fibromyalgia criteria and severity scales for clinical and epidemiological studies: A modification of the ACR preliminary diagnostic criteria for fibromyalgia. *Journal of Rheumatology*, *38*(6), 1113–1122.

Wolfe, F., Clauw, D. J., Fitzcharles, M. A., et al. (2016). Revisions to the 2010/2011 fibromyalgia diagnostic criteria. *Seminars in Arthritis and Rheumatism*, *46*(3), 319–329. https://doi.org/10.1016/j.semarthrit.2016.08.012.

Wolfe, F., Michaud, K., & Pincus, T. (2004). Development and validation of the Health Assessment Questionnaire II. *Arthritis & Rheumatology*, *50*(10), 3296–3305. https://doi.org/10.1002/art.20549.

Wojdasiewicz, P., Poniatowski, Ł. A., & Szukiewicz, D. (2014). The role of inflammatory and anti-inflammatory cytokines in the pathogenesis of osteoarthritis. *Mediators of Inflammation*, *2014*, 561459. https://doi.org/10.1155/2014/561459.

Wong, C. S., & Wong, S. H. (2012). A new look at trigger point injections. *Anesthesiology Research and Practice*, 492452. https://doi.org/10.1155/2012/492452.

World Health Organization (WHO). (2004). *WHO scientific group on the assessment of osteoporosis at primary health care level*. https://www.who.int/chp/topics/Osteoporosis.pdf.

World Health Organization (WHO). (2020, November). *Physical activity*. https://www.who.int/news-room/fact-sheets/detail/physical-activity.

Wright, S. L. (2020). Limited utility for benzodiazepines in chronic pain management: A narrative review. *Advances in Therapy*, *37*(3), 2604–2619. https://doi.org/10.1007/s12325-020-01354-6.

Yang, H., Peng, Q., Yin, L., Li, S., Shi, J., Zhang, Y., & Wang, G. (2017). Identification of multiple cancer-associated myositis-specific autoantibodies in idiopathic inflammatory myopathies: A large longitudinal cohort study. *Arthritis Research & Therapy*, *19*(1), 259. https://doi.org/10.1186/s13075-017-1469-8.

Yates, M., Kotecha, J., Watts, R. A., Luben, R., et al. (2019). Incidence of inflammatory polyarthritis in polymyalgia rheumatica: A population-based cohort study. *Annals of the Rheumatic Diseases*, *78*(5), 704–705. https://doi.org/10.1136/annrheumdis-2018-214386.

Yates, M., Watts, R. A., Swords, F., & MacGregor, A. J. (2017). Glucocorticoid withdrawal in polymyalgia rheumatica: The theory versus the practice. *Clinical and Experimental Rheumatology*, *35*(1), 1–2.

Yuan, W. H., Hsu, H. C., & Lai, K. L. (2016). Vertebroplasty and balloon kyphoplasty versus conservative treatment for osteoporotic vertebral compression fractures: A meta-analysis. *Medicine*, *95*(31), e4491. https://doi.org/10.1097/MD.0000000000004491.

Zaccardelli, A., Friedlander, M., Ford, J., & Sparks, J. (2019). Potential of lifestyle changes for reducing the risk of developing rheumatoid arthritis: Is an ounce of prevention worth a pound of cure. *Clinical Therapeutics*, *41*(7), 1323–1345. https://doi.org/10.1016/j.clinthera.2019.04.021.

Zaninotto, P., Huang, Y., Gessa, G., Abell, J., Lassale, C., & Steptoe, A. (2020). Polypharmacy is a risk factor for hospital admission due to a fall: Evidence from the English longitudinal study of ageing. *BMC Public Health*, *20*, 1804–1811. https://doi.org/10.1186/s12889-020-09920-x.

Zeng, C., Dubreuil, M., LaRochelle, M. R., et al. (2019). Association of tramadol with all-cause mortality among patients with osteoarthritis. *Journal of the American Medical Association, 321*(10), 969–982.

Zhang, H., Xu, C., Zhang, T., Gao, Z., & Zhang, T. (2017). Does percutaneous vertebroplasty or balloon kyphoplasty for osteoporotic vertebral compression fractures increase the incidence of new vertebral fractures? A meta-analysis. *Pain Physician, 20*(1), E13–E28.

Zhang, J., & Wang, J. (2015). Moderate Exercise Mitigates the Detrimental Effects of Aging on Tendon Stem Cells. *PLoS One, 10*(6), e0130454. https://doi.org/10.1371/journal.pone.0130454.

Zhang, W., Doherty, M., Peat, B., Bierma-Aeinstra, M. A., Arden, N. K., et al. (2010). EULAR evidence-based recommendations for the diagnosis of knee osteoarthritis. *Annals of the Rheumatic Diseases, 69*(3), 483–489.

Zhao, R., Zhao, M., & Zhang, L. (2014). Efficiency of jumping exercises in improving bone mineral density among premenopausal women: A meta-analysis. *Sports Medicine, 44*, 1392–1402. https://doi.org/10.1007/s40279-014-0220-8.

Zheng, L., Hwang, J. M., Hwang, D. S., Kang, C., et al. (2020). Incidence and location of heterotopic ossification following hip arthroscopy. *BMC Musculoskeletal Disorders, 21*, 132–136. https://doi.org/10.1186/s12891-020-3150-7.

Zhou, B., Zhou, Y., & Tang, K. (2014). An overview of structure, mechanical properties, and treatment for age-related tendinopathy. *Journal of Nutrition, Health & Aging, 18*(4), 441–448. https://doi.org/10.1007/s12603-014-0026-2. PMID: 24676328.

Zhu, Y., Chen, W., Xi, X., Yin, Y., et al. (2020). Epidemiologic characteristics of traumatic fracture in elderly patients during the outbreak of coronavirus disease 2019 in China. *International Orthopaedics, 44*(8), 1565–1570. https://doi.org/10.1007/s00264-020-04575-0.

Zhu, Y., Zhang, F., Chen, W., Zhang, Q., et al. (2015). Incidence and risk factors for heterotopic ossification after total hip arthroplasty: A meta-analysis. *Archives of Orthopaedic and Trauma Surgery, 135*(9), 1307–1314. https://doi.org/10.1007/s00402.-015-2277-8.

Zia, A., Kamanaruzzaman, S. B., & Tan, M. P. (2017). The consumption of two or more fall risk-increasing drugs rather than polypharmacy is associated with falls. *Geriatrics & Gerontology International, 17*(3), 463–470. https://doi.org/10.1111/ggi.12741.

Zimmerman, S., Greene, A., Sloane, P. D., Mitchell, M., Giuliani, C., Nyrop, K., & Walsh, E. (2017). Preventing falls in assisted living: Results of a quality improvement pilot study. *Geriatric Nursing, 38*(3), 185–191. https://doi.org/10.1016/j.gerinurse.2016.09.003. Epub 2016 Oct 21.

17

Cancer

HEIDI YULICO, RN, MS, SINCERE SIMONE MCMILAN, DNP, MS, BSN, AND SOO JUNG KIM, MSN, ANP, AGPCNP-BC

OBJECTIVES

Student Learning Objectives

After completing this chapter, the student should be able to do the following:

1. Discuss the prevalence of cancer in older adults, state the most common types of cancers, and discuss current screening recommendations and guidelines.
2. Discuss treatment modalities and potential treatment-related side effects/complications, and describe the clinician's role in identifying and managing these symptoms.
3. Discuss the implications of conducting a comprehensive geriatric assessment (CGA) pre- and posttreatment to identify fit versus frail patients and recognize the role CGA can play in treatment decision making.
4. Discuss some of the psychosocial and ethical considerations of treating cancer in the older adult.
5. Discuss the importance of effective communication and coordination of care among care providers throughout a patient's cancer journey.

Practitioner Objectives

After completing this chapter, the practitioner should be able to do the following:

1. Appropriately recognize signs of and screen for cancer in older adults.
2. Perform comprehensive geriatric assessments and generate appropriate referrals based on assessment findings.
3. Provide support for the patient and the patient's family and caregivers to assist them in managing treatment-related side effects.
4. Coordinate care and facilitate effective communication with the interdisciplinary oncology team.

Cancer Prevalence

The population in the United States is aging, and with increased life expectancy, the prevalence of cancer in aging individuals is also increasing (Fig. 17.1). The 10 leading cancer diagnoses in older adults age 85 and older are like that of the general population with the exception of stomach cancer in men and ovarian and urinary bladder cancer in women (see Table 17.1 for leading sites of new cancer cases and deaths in patients aged 85 and older in the United States).

Statistics show cancer is a leading cause of death globally (Siegel et al., 2019), and in the United States the highest cancer-related mortality occurs in 65- to 74-year-olds (Fig. 17.2). In the United States , more than half of all cancers and >70% of all cancer-related mortalities are among those who are 65 and older. However, despite changing demographics, older adults are often underrepresented in clinical trials. As a result, there is less evidence-based information available to guide the clinician in the treatment and care of aging individuals with cancer (Korc-Grodzicki & Tew, 2017).

Interprofessional Collaboration

The care of an older adult with cancer necessitates a team-based approach to care. The oncology interprofessional team may consist of physicians, nurse practitioners (NPs), physician assistants (PAs), nurses, case managers, social workers, rehabilitation medicine specialists, nutritionists, and pharmacists (Box 17.1). Each member of the team shares her or his expertise to develop a comprehensive, personalized care plan for the patient. Clear communication among providers, patients, and caregivers is essential to prevent fragmented care, to maintain the focus on patient's wishes and values, and to provide the best outcome for the older adult cancer patient.

Cancer Screening, Presentation and Management for the Older Adult

Cancer screening is the act of looking for cancer before it causes symptoms. PAs and NPs can play a critical role in the primary and secondary prevention of cancer, beginning with risk assessment and screening for older patients. By partnering with patients and their caregivers, modifiable health risk behaviors can be addressed such as tobacco use, obesity, physical inactivity, and poor nutrition. At the same time, there is opportunity to promote self-management strategies as listed in Box 17.2 that emphasize wellness, which is a cornerstone of practice (Cancer Prevention Overview, 2019).

Although screening can have positive benefits for patients, clinicians should be aware that there are risks associated with screening, including false-positive (being diagnosed with a disease you do not have) or false-negative results (not being diagnosed with a disease you do have). Both of these scenarios can have a negative psychological impact on patients and their caregivers. The burden of screening should also be carefully weighed with the patient and the patient's family or

HEALTHY PEOPLE BOX 2030 BOX 17.1

Healthy People 2030 lists the following objectives relating to cancer with the goal of improving quality of life and overall health:

- Reduce new cases of cancer and cancer-related illness, disability, and death.
- Promote evidence-based cancer screening and prevention strategies for lung, breast, cervical, and colorectal cancer to reduce cancer deaths.
- Improve care and survivorship for people with cancer.
- Increase the proportion of people who discuss interventions to prevent cancer with their care providers.

care partners, especially if there is a limited life expectancy or the risks of screening outweigh the benefits (i.e., finding the cancer may not improve the person's health or help the person live longer) (American Geriatrics Society [AGS] Choosing Wisely Workgroup, 2014). If a clinician suspects that a patient may have cancer and screenings or diagnostic procedures are recommended, it is important that patients be routinely assessed for signs of depression, adjustment disorders, caregiver strain, and cognitive impairment during this initial process. The development of these syndromes could potentially impact the patient's ability to cope or participate in self-management strategies, and this may ultimately impair the patient's ability to follow treatment regimens for cancer-directed therapies.

From 2012 to 2014, according to the most recent data available for adults over 70 years of age, the highest prevalence of cancers among men were prostate (8.2%), lung (6.1%), and colorectal (3.4%). Among women, cancers with the highest prevalence were breast (6.8%), lung (4.8%), and colorectal (3.4%) (Siegel et al., 2019). This section discusses the recommended screening guidelines and typical presentation of these cancers in older adults.

Prostate Cancer

Screening

Ways to Screen for Prostate Cancer

Digital Rectal Exam

A digital rectal exam (DRE) is a test that checks the lower rectum and pelvis for cancer (National Cancer Institute, 2019). The use of a DRE in cancer screening has been debated. Although it may still be used in practice by some clinicians, it has been suggested that a DRE not be conducted for prostate cancer screening either alone or in combination with a prostate specific antigen (PSA) screening as no controlled studies have shown a reduction in the morbidity or mortality of prostate cancer when detected by DRE at any age (Burke & Laramie, 2004). If a DRE is performed, no special patient preparation is needed but the clinician should be aware that if a patient has hemorrhoids or anal fissures, a DRE may cause irritation and patients should be informed of this prior to the examination. The goal of the exam is for the provider to assess the size of the prostate and feel for any asymmetry, soft spots, induration, or nodularity. The provider should also examine the wall of the lower colon/rectum during a DRE (National Cancer Institute, 2019).

Prostate Specific Antigen Test

Prostate specific antigen (PSA) is a protein made by the prostate. The PSA test is a blood test that measures the level of PSA in the blood. Patients do not need to fast for this test, but it is recommended that men abstain from ejaculation for 3 days prior to the test (Grossman et al., 2018). There is debate over the value of the PSA test for detecting prostate cancer. Although a PSA test itself cannot diagnose cancer, a high PSA level has been linked to an increased chance of having prostate cancer. Some medications such as Lipitor (atorvastatin),

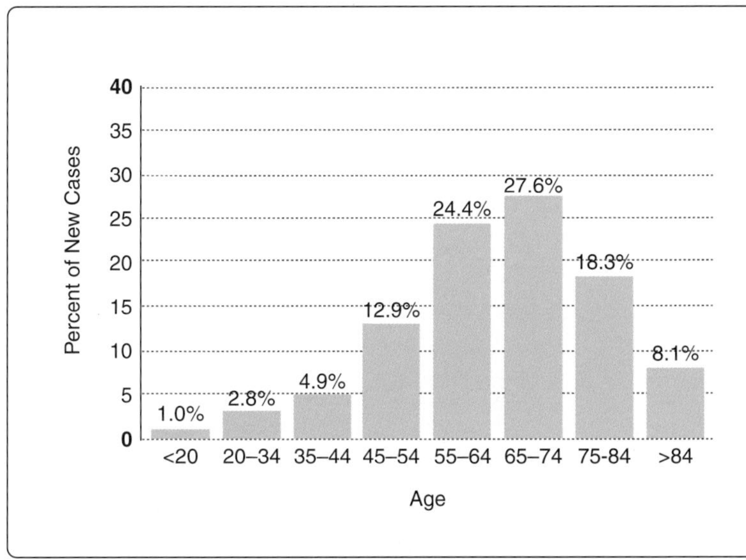

Cancer of any site is most frequently diagnosed among people ages 65–74.

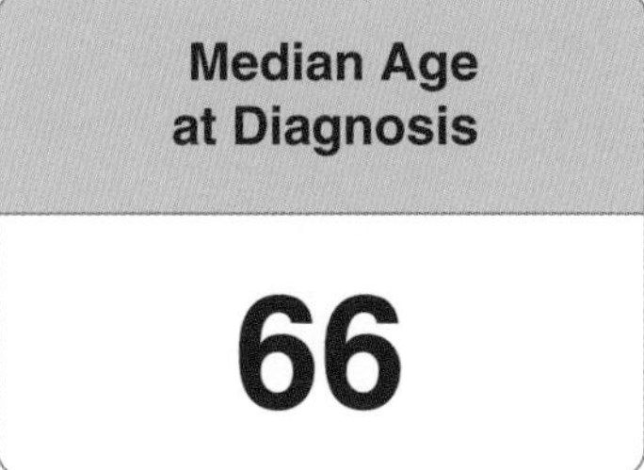

The Surveillance, Epidemiology, and End Results (SEER) 21 2012–2016, all races, both sexes.

• **Fig. 17.1** Percent of New Cases by Age Group: Cancer of Any Site (From the National Cancer Institute. [2019]. Cancer stat facts: Cancer of any site. https://seer.cancer.gov/statfacts/html/all.html.)

TABLE 17.1 Leading Site of New Cancer Cases and Deaths, Ages 85 Years and Older, United States

Incidence							
	Estimated Cases, 2019				Estimated Cases, 2019		
Males	**No.**	**%**	**Rate, 2011–2015**	**Females**	**No.**	**%**	**Rate, 2011–2015**
1. Lung & bronchus	9,800	16%	450.6	1. Breast	14,800	19%	332.8
2. Prostate	7,960	13%	366.0	2. Colon & rectum	11,200	14%	252.0
3. Urinary bladder	7,870	13%	361.7	3. Lung & bronchus	10,870	14%	244.4
4. Colon & rectum	6,640	11%	305.2	4. Pancreas	4,150	5%	93.4
5. Melanoma of the skin	4,000	6%	183.9	5. Non-Hodgkin lymphoma	3,710	5%	83.5
6. Non-Hodgkin lymphoma	3,090	5%	142.1	6. Urinary bladder	3,360	4%	75.5
7. Leukemia	2,740	4%	126.0	7. Leukemia	3,000	4%	67.6
8. Pancreas	2,270	4%	104.1	8. Melanoma of the skin	2,510	3%	56.5
9. Kidney & renal pelvis	1,730	3%	79.6	9. Uterine corpus	2,310	3%	51.9
10. Stomach	1,390	2%	63.8	10. Ovary	1,900	2%	42.7
All sites	**61,830**				**78,860**		

Mortality							
	Estimated Deaths, 2019				Estimated Deaths, 2019		
Males	**No.**	**%**	**Rate, 2012–2016**	**Females**	**No.**	**%**	**Rate, 2012–2016**
1. Prostate	9,860	20%	452.9	1. Lung & bronchus	10,200	19%	247.8
2. Lung & bronchus	9,700	20%	445.6	2. Breast	7,150	13%	173.7
3. Colon & rectum	4,380	9%	201.1	3. Colon & rectum	6,740	12%	163.7
4. Urinary bladder	3,410	7%	156.9	4. Pancreas	4,210	8%	102.2
5. Leukemia	2,590	5%	119.2	5. Leukemia	2,630	5%	63.8
6. Pancreas	2,530	5%	116.4	6. Non-Hodgkin lymphoma	2,570	5%	62.4
7. Non-Hodgkin lymphoma	2,160	4%	99.4	7. Ovary	2,060	4%	50.1
8. Liver & intrahepatic bile duct	1,230	3%	56.6	8. Urinary bladder	1,680	3%	40.7
9. Kidney & renal pelvis	1,200	2%	55.1	9. Liver & intrahepatic bile duct	1,380	3%	33.4
10. Esophagus	1,120	2%	51.4	10. Uterine corpus	1,330	2%	32.4
All sites	**49,040**			**All sites**	**54,210**		

Rates are per 100,000 population.
From DeSantis, C. E., Miller, K. D., Dale, W., Mohile, S. G., Cohen, H. J., Leach, C. R., Goding Sauer, A., Jemal, A., & Siegel, R. L. (2019). Cancer statistics for adults aged 85 years and older, *CA: A Cancer Journal for Clinicians, 69*(6), 452–467.

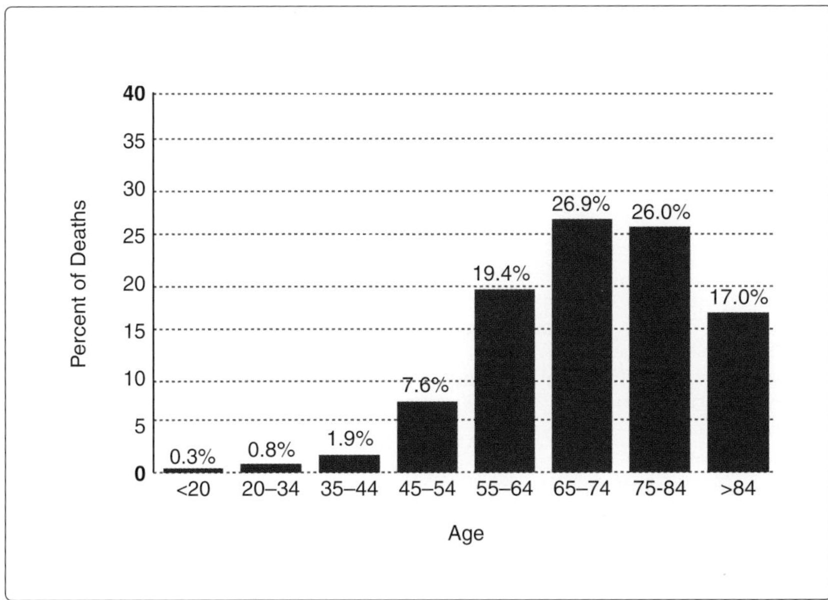

The percent of cancer of any site deaths is highest among people ages 65–74.

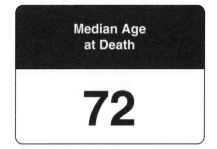

US 2012–2016, all races, both sexes.

• **Fig. 17.2** Percent of Deaths by Age Group: Cancer of Any Site (From the National Cancer Institute. [2019]. Cancer stat facts: Cancer of any site. https://seer.cancer.gov/statfacts/html/all.html.)

Zocor (simvastatin), and nonsteroidal antiinflammatory drugs (NSAIDS) such as aspirin, ibuprofen, and naproxen or conditions such as prostatitis can cause a PSA reading to be inaccurate.

If no prostate cancer is found through screening, the time between future screenings depends on the results of the PSA blood test. Men who choose to be tested who have a PSA of less than 2.5 ng/mL may only need to be retested every 2 years. Screening should be done yearly for men whose PSA level is 2.5 ng/mL or higher (American Cancer Society, 2019a).

According to the American Cancer Society, men who are age 50 or older, at average risk of prostate cancer, and expected to live at least 10 more years should have a chance to make an informed decision with their health care provider about whether to be screened for prostate cancer (Grossman et al., 2018). Men age 45 at high risk of developing prostate cancer, including African Americans and men who have a first-degree relative such as a father or brother diagnosed with prostate cancer when they were younger than age 65, and men age 40 at even higher risk such as those with more than one first-degree relative who had prostate cancer at an early age should also be given an opportunity to discuss the benefits of screening with their health care provider. The decision for or against screening should be made after the patient and provider discuss uncertainties, risks, and potential benefits of prostate cancer screening.

The US Preventative Services Task Force (USPSTF) recommends against PSA-based screening for prostate cancer in men 70 years and older (Grossman et al., 2018). One potential harm of PSA-based screening is overdiagnosis, which is the identification of asymptomatic cancer that would never cause a person symptoms or contribute to one's death. Treatment of these men can result in harms such as

• BOX 17.1 Brief description of the roles of several members of the interdisciplinary team:

Case managers: Professionals, usually registered nurses, who facilitate appropriate services referrals, which can include home care, skilled care, or rehabilitative care. Case managers explore a patient's social supports and educate patients and caregivers regarding safe disposition and long-term care planning.

Social workers: Professionals who help patients and caregivers navigate through challenging psychosocial situations. Social workers provide information on community resources, can evaluate social supports as well as patient and caregiver coping mechanisms, and can provide supportive psychotherapy to improve overall well-being.

Pharmacists: Professionals with expertise in the management of medications. Pharmacists can evaluate medication regimens for safety and efficacy. They provide medication safety education to patients and their caregivers and can prevent medication errors through medication reconciliation and prescription refill monitoring.

Rehabilitation medicine practitioners: Professionals such as physical and occupational therapists who help patients to maintain their functional independence in the community. Physical therapists focus on mobility, activities of daily living such as safe ambulation, balance, and fall prevention through gait assessment, whereas occupational therapists focus on upper body strength, instrumental activities of daily living, tasking, sequencing, and cognitive cueing.

Nutritionists: Professionals who partner with the care team to manage/optimize patient nutritional status.

CASE STUDY (FRAIL PATENT)

History of Present Illness

An 80-year-old female presents with a past medical history significant for hypertension, hyperlipidemia, right thigh Merkel cell carcinoma status postresection and radiation therapy in 2011, right thigh sarcoma status postresection and radiation therapy in 2017 and reexcision in 2018, right renal cell papillary carcinoma status post partial nephrectomy in 2013, and right upper lobe minimally invasive lung cancer status post right video-assisted thoracoscopic surgery and right upper lobe wedge resection. More recently, the patient was found to have a new left upper lobe cT1 N0 M0 adenocarcinoma. Due to her poor lung function, she was started on definitive stereotactic body radiation therapy (SBRT). The patient completed radiation therapy successfully. She continues follow-up with several providers including her medical oncologist, radiation oncologist, and surgical oncologist where she has routine follow-up laboratory tests and imaging. Given her age and multiple comorbidities, the patient was referred to geriatric medicine for an evaluation with the goal of maximizing her independence and coordinating her overall medical management. At this visit, the patient expresses experiencing occasional short-term memory loss (for example, misplacing items), depressed mood, functional decline with a history of falls, and fatigue. A comprehensive geriatric assessment is performed during the visit.

Clinical Data

Blood pressure: 120/52; pulse: 62 beats per minute, regular; respiration: 16 breaths per minute, no signs of acute respiratory distress; oxygen saturation: 98% on room air. Temperature 36.3°C orally; weight: 49.1 kilograms; body mass index 20.7.

Comorbidities

The patient's blood pressure has been stable within JNC8 recommended guidelines for her age; a recent lipid profile was normal. Her cancer treatment and surveillance are as per the preceding history of present illness.

Cognition

The patient has subjective complaints of short-term memory loss, including occasionally misplacing items, but notes she was able to remember where she placed them later. She expresses feeling overwhelmed caring for her husband who is disabled while simultaneously managing the stress of undergoing cancer treatment. A Mini Mental State Exam (MMSE) is performed, and the patient scores within the normal range of 29/30 (a score of <26 would be concerning for cognitive dysfunction). The patient scores 7/15 on the Geriatric Depression Scale (GDS) (suggestive of depression/adjustment disorder). Her distress score on the distress thermometer is 7/10 (a score >5 is suggestive of increased distress). The patient had prior neuroimaging via brain magnetic resonance imaging (MRI) within the past 2 months that was without acute intracranial abnormality.

Function

The patient has had several falls; the most recent was a few months ago at home when she lost her balance and tripped. She denies any injuries. A timed up and go test (TUG) is greater than 20 seconds (scores of >12 seconds suggest a higher risk for falls). The patient is not orthostatic on exam.

She has a walker but uses it only outside for long distances. She has a fear of falling and has cut down on her usual activities because she is afraid to go anywhere on her own.

Nutrition

The patient scores 6/14 on the Mini Nutritional Assessment (MNA) (indicative of malnutrition). She has had unintentional weight loss of greater than 10 pounds over the past several months. She has also been skipping meals due to the demands of caring for her husband.

Medications

The patient is on more than nine medications, which is indicative of polypharmacy.

Social Support

She reports that she is socially isolated as she has few friends, and those that she does have are not physically well themselves. She has no children or living relatives nearby.

Assessment and Plan

The patient has a history of multiple malignancies without evidence of recurrent disease on follow-up imaging, including CT scans, and has overall stable symptomatology from a cancer perspective. She continues on active surveillance and follows up with the oncology team closely.

On the spectrum of frailty, the patient is frail based upon her geriatric assessment.

Memory Loss

The patient's current score on the MMSE is not suggestive of an underlying cognitive disorder; however, because the MMSE is a screening tool it will be repeated at a subsequent follow-up visit for comparison. Laboratory tests to rule out reversible causes of memory loss are ordered, including a test for thyroid stimulating hormone (TSH), folate, and vitamin B_{12} levels; all are normal. She has no signs of active infection. The patient is referred to occupational therapy for cognitive rehabilitation. She is encouraged to use organizational strategies such as a note pad for daily tasks and a calendar for appointment reminders.

Depressed Mood/Adjustment Disorder/Distress

Given the patient's high level of distress and her GDS score, which suggests depression, emotional support is provided on this visit and suicidal ideation is assessed, which the patient denies. She declines treatment with pharmacotherapy (i.e., a selective serotonin-reuptake inhibitor [SSRI] such as sertraline) but is open to referral toa psychologist for supportive psychotherapy.

Social Support

The patient is referred to social work to explore supports and connect the patient and her husband to resources in the community, including cancer survivorship support groups, meals on wheels services, and home care services.

Gait Instability With a History of Falls, Deconditioning

The patient is educated on fall precaution measures and home safety modifications. She is encouraged to use a walker at all times. The patient is referred for home visiting nurse services to evaluate her home for safety and to start home physical and occupational therapy.

Nutrition

Nutrition counseling is provided, and the patient is encouraged to eat small, frequent meals and is counseled not to skip meals. The use of nutritional supplements is discussed, and the patient

Continued

CASE STUDY (FRAIL PATENT)—cont'd

is encouraged not to use these supplements as long-term meal replacements. Fortunately, the patient's husband has a home health aide, and the patient is encouraged to delegate meal preparation tasks to home health aide.

Medications

Medications are reviewed and no inappropriate polypharmacy is identified. Although the patient is on more than five medications, each of the medications is for the control of her comorbid conditions, including the multiple cancers. No new medications have been added over the past 6 months, and the patient is not on any potentially inappropriate medications for older adults. She is able to maintain responsibility for her own medication management and has an appropriate system for organizing, administering, and refilling her medications.

Coordination of Care

The provider communicates with patient's care team including her medical and surgical oncologists. The patient is encouraged to follow up with her primary care doctor for management of her primary care needs near her home.

Follow-up

The patient presents for a follow-up visit 3 months after the initial visit. She has completed in-home physical and occupational therapy and has not had any additional falls since the last assessment. She now has a home health aide who accompanies her to medical appointments. She has started going to beading class, which she enjoys, and notes improved mood and energy levels. She finds visits with the psychologist in person and on the phone extremely helpful. She is no longer skipping meals, and her weight and body mass index have been stable.

• BOX 17.2 Self-Management Strategies

- Stress reduction
- Improving sleep
- Setting priorities and goals
- Maintaining adequate nutrition
- Effective communication with family, caregivers, and medical team
- Appropriate exercise
- Advance care planning/decision making
- Complementary therapies
- Establishing and maintaining healthy relationships

erectile dysfunction and urinary incontinence, while providing them with no benefit. Overdiagnosis rates would be expected to increase with age and to be highest in men 70 years and older because older men have high risk of death from competing causes (Grossman et al., 2018). The USPSTF recommendation statement in the *Journal of the American Medical Association* states that there is inadequate evidence to assess whether the benefits for African American men and men with a family history of prostate cancer ages 55 to 69 years is different than the benefits for the average-risk population (Grossman et al., 2018). According to this recommendation statement, there is also inadequate evidence to assess whether there are benefits to starting screening in these high-risk groups before age 55 years (Grossman et al., 2018). Table 17.2 summarizes the potential benefits and harms of prostate cancer screening.

Presentation

Prostate cancer typically presents as an abnormal mass or enlargement of the prostate gland with or without elevation in the PSA level. Serum PSA levels increase in men with prostate cancer, and levels greater than 4 ng/dl are considered abnormal. Transrectal ultrasonography of the prostate may also be used to provide additional information following an abnormal DRE or elevated PSA and can be used in the staging of a carcinoma and to guide biopsy (Burke & Laramie, 2004). Prostate cancer is diagnosed with biopsy of the prostate gland. In the geriatric population, vague symptoms such as weight loss, urinary difficulties, constipation, bone pain, or fractures related to metastatic disease may also be the initial presenting signs of prostate cancer.

Management

The patient should be referred to an oncologist to determine treatment, as options vary depending on the extent of disease, the risk of recurrence, and the patient's characteristics such as age, comorbidity, and personal preferences. Older patients with multiple comorbid conditions with low-risk, localized cancer may opt for active surveillance rather than immediate treatment. The 2019 National Comprehensive Cancer Network (NCCN) guideline should be used to direct treatment plans. This guideline has helped to minimize overtreatment of low-risk disease over the years. For advanced disease, androgen deprivation therapy (ADT), chemotherapy, bone-directed therapy (such as zoledronic acid or denosumab), radiation, or a combination of these treatments with or without prostatectomy may be used. Newer forms of hormone therapy, such as abiraterone and enzalutamide, can also be used to treat advanced prostate cancer that is no longer responding to traditional hormone therapy (Siegel et al., 2019). Nurse practitioners and physician assistants caring for patients with prostate cancer should stay abreast of current evidence-based best practices concerning screening, treatment, and surveillance.

Breast Cancer

Screening

According to the USPSTF (2016), women ages 50 to 74 at average risk for breast cancer are recommended to undergo biennial screening mammography (U.S. Preventive Services Task Force, 2016). A screening mammogram can be used

TABLE 17.2 Potential Benefits and Harms of Prostate Cancer Screening

Potential Benefits of Prostate Cancer Screening	Potential Harms of Prostate Cancer Screening
• Screening offers a potential benefit of reducing the chance of death from prostate cancer in some men • Finds prostate cancers that may be at high risk of spreading; this may lower the chance of death from prostate cancer in some men • Some men prefer to know if they have prostate cancer	• False-positive results • Potential for additional testing and prostate biopsy • Overdiagnosis • Overtreatment • Treatment related complications such as incontinence and erectile dysfunction

From Grossman, D. C., Curry, S. J., Owens, D. K., Bibbins-Domingo, K., Caughey, A. B., Davidson, K. W., ... & Krist, A. H. (2018). Screening for prostate cancer: US Preventive Services Task Force recommendation statement. *Journal of the American Medical Association, 319*(18), 1901–1913.

to check for breast cancer in women who have no signs or symptoms of the disease (Center for Disease Control, 2018). A mammogram is an x-ray picture of the breast usually involving two or more x-ray images of each breast. Screening mammograms can also find tiny deposits of calcium called calcifications that sometimes can be a marker of underlying cancer development. For women age 75 or older with average risk, current evidence is insufficient to assess the balance of benefits and harms of screening mammography (U.S. Preventive Services Task Force, 2016).

Women who are at high-risk for developing breast cancer have different screening recommendations. According to the American Cancer Society, women at high-risk include those who have a lifetime risk of breast cancer of about 20% to 25% or greater according to risk assessment tools based mainly on family history (American Cancer Society, 2019b). Additionally, women who have a known BRCA1 gene mutation based on genetic testing; have a first-degree relative such as a parent, sibling, or child with a BRCA1 or BRCA2 gene mutation and have not had genetic testing themselves; women who had radiation therapy to the chest when they were between the ages of 10 and 30 years or have Li-Fraumeni syndrome, Cowden syndrome, or Bannayan-Riley-Ruvalcaba syndrome; or women who have a first-degree relatives with one of these syndromes would also be considered at high-risk (American Cancer Society, 2019b). Research has not shown a clear benefit of regular clinical breast exams done by a health professional or self-breast exams done by the patient. Although there is little evidence that these tests help find breast cancer early when women also get screening mammograms, there may be benefits to women being familiar with how their breasts normally look and feel so they can report any changes to a health care provider immediately (American Cancer Society, 2019b).

It is important to note that men can also be affected by breast cancer. Because men have less breast tissue than women, there are no recommendations for routine mammography in men. Additionally, male breast cancer is rare, making up 1% of all breast cancers diagnosed in the United States (National Breast Cancer Foundation, 2019). Screening is usually recommended only for men with a strong family history of breast cancer or genetic mutations of the type noted previously. The National Comprehensive Cancer Network recommends that men at higher risk for breast cancer be screened starting at age 35. NPs and PAs should note that men who have a BRCA gene mutation may also benefit from prostate cancer screening (National Breast Cancer Foundation, 2019).

Presentation

Breast cancer presents as an abnormality on mammography but can also present as any of the following: painful mass, painless mass, discoloration of breast tissue, dimpling of the breast tissue, or abnormal drainage from the nipple. A diagnosis of breast cancer requires a biopsy of the lesion and a determination of tumor estrogen/progesterone receptor (ER/PR) status and HER2 status. The presentation of breast cancer is similar in adult and geriatric patients (Shachar et al., 2017).

Management

The patient should be referred to an oncologist and surgeon who will review NCCN guidelines to determine treatment options. The most common treatment among women with early-stage (1 or 2) breast cancer is breast-conserving surgery (BCS) with adjuvant radiation. For patients with stage 3 disease, treatment would consist of mastectomy with adjuvant chemotherapy. Patients with metastatic (stage 4) disease most often receive radiation or chemotherapy alone versus no treatment based on their frailty score and comorbid conditions. These patients may, however, receive hormonal therapy. Most patients with hormone receptor-positive tumors receive hormonal therapy. Patients with metastatic triple-negative breast cancer may also receive immunotherapy drugs with chemotherapy (Siegel et al., 2019).

The NP or PA caring for breast cancer survivors should stay up to date on appropriate follow-up guidelines. In the United States, after curative breast cancer treatment patients should have a physical examination every 3 to 6 months in the first 3 years after primary treatment, then every 6 to 12 months for the next 2 years, and annually thereafter (Spronk et al., 2017). Mammograms are generally recommended annually on the intact breast for women who have received a unilateral mastectomy and annually on both breasts for women who have had lumpectomies (Spronk et al., 2017).

NPs and PAs should communicate with the patient's oncology team to determine if these recommendations are appropriate for the individual patient, as guidelines can change based on the patient's presentation and needs. In addition to physical assessment, it is important for practitioners to remember to monitor and assess for potential psychological impacts related to surviving cancer (Spronk et al., 2017). Practitioners should assess the patient's nutrition, weight, and physical activity level; monitor for signs of depression/anxiety; and check for any potential side effects of treatment such as pain, lymphedema, infection, fatigue, or cognitive change.

Lung Cancer

Screening

Although lung cancer is one of the most commonly seen cancers among both male and female patients, there was no proven screening test for lung cancer until 2010 when The National Lung Screening Trial (NLST) results were reported (Chudgar et al., 2015). The NLST was a randomized, multicenter study that compared low-dose helical computed tomography (CT) with chest radiography in the screening of older current and former heavy smokers ages 55 to 74 for early detection of lung cancer (National Lung Screening Trial Research Team, 2011). The NLST demonstrated that low-dose CT (LDCT) screening reduced mortality in a high-risk population based on age and smoking history compared with screening by radiograph. LDCT screening is significantly more sensitive than chest radiograph for identifying small, asymptomatic lung cancers. It is recommended that patients ages 55 to 80 years who have a 30 pack-year smoking history (patients who have smoked an amount that is equal to at least 1 pack a day for 30 years) or who currently smoke or have quit within the past 15 years have this test done once a year if scans are normal. Patients can stop getting screened at age 80, once they have gone 15 years or longer without smoking or if there is a limited life expectancy. It is important to be aware that CT screening can have false-positive findings, which may lead to additional testing such as serial imaging or invasive procedures (Wood et al., 2012). All patients who currently smoke or have a history of smoking should be advised of the risks and benefits of screening for lung cancer. Clinicians should also counsel all patients who smoke to quit and counsel against the initiation of smoking for those who do not.

Another environmental exposure that puts patients at risk for the development of lung cancer is radon. Radon is a radioactive gas that comes from the natural breakdown of uranium in soil, rock, and water (American Cancer Society, 2015). Prolonged radon exposure, exposures in homes above 4 picocuries per liter (pCi/L) (the remediation level EPA recommends), exposures among those who smoke or have smoked, and exposures through high-risk jobs such as mining puts patients at particularly high risk for developing lung cancer. Radon exposure is the second most common cause of lung cancer in the United States (American Cancer Society, 2015). According to the Environmental Protection Agency (EPA), any home can have a radon problem regardless of its age, sealant, or if the home does or does not have a basement. The EPA estimates that 1 in 15 homes in the United States has elevated levels of radon (above 4 picocuries per liter (pCi/L). Therefore all patients should be counseled to have their homes tested and treated for radon.

Presentation

Lung cancer presents as an abnormality on chest imaging such as x-ray, CT scan, or MRI and is diagnosed with biopsy of the lesion and classified as either small-cell lung cancer (SCLS) or non-small-cell lung cancer (NSCLC) for the purposes of treatment. Lung cancer can also present as persistent cough, hemoptysis, unintentional weight loss, shortness of breath, or fatigue. These symptoms can be similar in adult and geriatric patients (Sinha et al., 2017).

Management

Patients should be referred to an oncologist and surgeon who will review NCCN guidelines to determine the treatment plan. Most patients with SCLC with receive chemotherapy. Patients with stage 1 and 2 NSCLC will undergo surgery with partial wedge resection, lobectomy, or complete pneumonectomy. Patients with stage 3 NSCLC will undergo chemotherapy or radiation with fewer undergoing surgery. NSCLC can also be treated with targeted and immunotherapy drugs such as angiogenesis inhibitors, epidermal growth factor inhibitors, and anaplastic lymphoma kinase inhibitors (Siegel et al., 2019).

Colorectal Cancer (CRC)

Screening

The USPSTF recommends screening for colorectal cancer (CRC) starting at age 50 and continuing until age 75. The decision to screen for CRC in adults aged 76 to 85 years is recommended on an individual basis (Bibbins-Domingo et al., 2016). For patients in this age group, clinicians should take into account the patient's overall health and prior screening history when deciding if CRC screening is appropriate. Screening in this age group should be considered for patients who have never been screened for colorectal cancer, who are healthy enough to undergo treatment if colorectal cancer is detected, and who do not have comorbid conditions that would significantly limit their life expectancy (Bibbins-Domingo et al., 2016). The USPSTF does not recommend routine screening for CRC in adults 86 years and older. Risk factors for the development of CRC include aging, family history, male sex, and black race (Bibbins-Domingo et al., 2016). There are many screening tests available to detect early-stage colorectal cancer, including stool-based tests, direct visualization tests, and serology tests.

Stool-Based Tests

- *Fecal immunochemical test:* Because blood vessels in larger colorectal polyps or cancers are often fragile and easily damaged by the passage of stool, a fecal immunochemical test (FIT) test detects occult blood in the stool. This test reacts to part of the human hemoglobin protein, which is found in red blood cells. One benefit of this test it that it can be done at home. Patients are asked to place a small amount of stool on a special card (or in a tube), which is then sent for processing. No drug or dietary restrictions are required for this test. Clinicians should be aware that blood in the stool can also have noncancerous causes. If a noncancerous cause of bleeding, such as hemorrhoids, were present at the time of testing, this could yield a false-positive result. If the test is positive, a colonoscopy will be needed for further investigation. This test must be done every year.
- *Guaiac-based fecal occult blood test:* The guaiac-based fecal occult blood test also detects occult blood in the stool but in a different way than a FIT. The test allows the patient to check more than one stool sample at home. Patients are given a special kit that must be returned to their provider's office or a designated laboratory. Like the FIT, this test is done yearly. If the test results are positive, a colonoscopy will be needed to find the reason for the bleeding. Medications such as aspirin and nonsteroidal antiinflammatory drugs can affect the test results, and patients are usually asked to stop these medications for 7 days before testing. However, patients who are on aspirin for cardiac or neurologic protective reasons or are on anticoagulation for causes such as deep vein thrombosis or pulmonary embolism would need approval from their cardiologist, neurologist, or hematologist prior to stopping these medications. Of note, vitamin C in doses greater than 250 mg daily can affect the chemicals in the test and give false-negative results. Patients should be counseled that vitamin C from either supplements, fruits, or juices should be avoided for 3 days before testing. Additionally, it is recommended that foods such as red meat not be consumed for 3 days before testing due to the risk of altered test results. Advanced practice providers (APPs) should note that fecal occult blood testing done during a digital rectal exam in the office, which only checks one stool sample, is not sufficient for proper screening.
- *Stool DNA test:* A stool DNA test (also known as a multitargeted stool DNA test, or MT-sDNA) looks for cells in the stool with DNA mutations, which can be shed by certain genes in cancer or polyp cells. Cologuard is the only test currently available that checks for both DNA changes and blood in the stool (Bibbins-Domingo et al., 2016). Patients receive a kit in the mail to use to collect their stool sample at home. The sample is then returned as per kit instructions. This test is done every 3 years. Because the test is still new, not all insurances may cover the cost. If DNA changes or blood are found, a colonoscopy is required.

Stool-based tests can miss many polyps and some cancers, so it is important to discuss the options with patients when deciding which test to recommend or order. Patients should be informed that an abnormal stool-based test would warrant investigation with a colonoscopy.

Direct Visualization Tests

Colonoscopy and Flexible Sigmoidoscopy

A colonoscopy can find and remove small clumps of cells on the inner lining of the colon called polyps. A colonoscopy is the only screening method that not only detects cancer at its earliest stages but can also prevent it. The pre-procedure preparation that a patient must complete prior to a colonoscopy must be considered when deciding whether to order or proceed with colonoscopy. The pre-procedure preparation may be especially challenging for some older individuals. It usually requires the patient to fast or only consume clear liquids starting the day before the test and also complete a "bowel prep" to clear the colon so the provider performing the test can have better visualization. This bowel prep usually requires patients to take oral laxatives over a specific period of time. Patients who are very frail may have difficulty completing this prep, especially if there are limitations in their mobility to and from the bathroom. Patients with cognitive impairment may not understand the pre-procedure preparation instructions or may forget to complete the preparation in its entirety, which would affect the clinical significance of the colonoscopy. Patients who cannot maintain adequate hydration are at risk for dehydration and electrolyte imbalance. Patients who are older, frailer, or at high risk for falls may need special arrangements prior to completing a bowel prep.

Clinicians should ensure that patients have adequate social supports if there is any concern for safety while completing the pre-procedure preparation. Blood thinners are usually held prior to colonoscopies, but the specific time frame for stopping these medications should be discussed on an individualized basis. Diabetic patients may need to have their oral medications or insulin doses adjusted while not eating or on a clear liquid diet. Sedation is necessary to complete a colonoscopy, which can have its own risk for patients with known or undiagnosed cognitive impairment including post-procedure delirium, which is an acute change in mental status. Patients are asked to have someone drive them home, which should be considered beforehand if they live alone or have few social supports. Colonoscopies carry a small risk of bleeding, bowel tears, or infection. Colonoscopies are currently recommended every 10 years, starting at age 50.

A flexible sigmoidoscopy is similar to a colonoscopy, but a shorter tube is used to examine the lower part of the colon. A sigmoidoscope can look at the inside of the rectum and part of the colon to detect and possibly remove any abnormalities. The sigmoidoscope allows the clinician to see the entire rectum but less than half of the colon. If a flexible sigmoidoscopy is abnormal, a standard colonoscopy will be needed. This test is recommended every 5 years but is not widely used as a screening test for colorectal cancer in the United States.

Virtual Colonoscopy

A virtual colonoscopy or CT colonography uses CT scan technology to create two-dimensional and three-dimensional images of the colon. This test does not require sedation but requires the same preparation as a colonoscopy. Virtual colonoscopies can sometimes miss small or flat polyps, and if the procedure detects a polyp, the patient will then have to undergo a standard colonoscopy. This test can have false-positive test results and exposes patients to a small amount of radiation. In addition, because the test is still new, not all insurances may cover its cost.

Presentation

Colorectal cancer (CRC) typically presents as an abnormal polyp on flexible sigmoidoscopy or colonoscopy but can also present as abnormal rectal bleeding, a positive Guaiac-based fecal occult blood test, or a positive stool DNA test. Most colorectal cancers evolve from premalignant adenomas, and the estimated time of progression from polyp to cancer is 5 to 10 years. Removal of these lesions prevents the development of cancer (Burke & Laramie, 2004). In the geriatric patient, atypical symptoms such as anemia, weight loss, changes in bowel pattern, new onset diarrhea, or constipation can also indicate a new cancer in the colon.

As of 2017 the death rate has dropped from its peak for colorectal cancer by 53% among males (since 1980) and by 57% among females (since 1969) (Siegel et al., 2020). Colon cancer when caught and treated early can have a generally favorable outcome; however, disease can recur. Follow-up after colon cancer treatment with curative intent aims to detect recurrences in a timely manner (Duineveld et al., 2016). In a retrospective study of consecutive patients with colon cancer who were treated in two hospitals in the Netherlands, researchers found that from a total of 446 patients who were been treated for colon carcinoma with curative intent, 74 developed recurrent disease (17%) (Duineveld et al., 2016). In 43 of those 74 patients, recurrent disease was detected during a scheduled follow-up visit, and 41 out of 43 patients were asymptomatic. When symptoms were present, the most prevalent symptoms were abdominal pain, altered defecation, and weight loss (Duineveld et al., 2016).

It is suggested that patients with resected stage 2 or 3 CRC posttreatment have an encounter with a clinician every 3 to 6 months for the first 3 years and every 6 months during years 4 and 5. Although most recurrences develop within the first 3 years, recurrence beyond 3 years is not uncommon, particularly in patients treated for locally advanced rectal cancer (Moy et al., 2016). This underscores the importance of NP and PA follow-up for patients diagnosed with and treated for colon cancer. NPs and PAs should routinely obtain comprehensive histories on patients with CRC aimed at highlighting symptoms that could suggest cancer recurrence. These should include an assessment of recent weight loss, changes in appetite, abdominal pain/distention, changes in stool patterns including changes in fecal color, consistency, and assessment for the presence of blood per rectum. A comprehensive physical examination should also be performed. It is also recommended that a rectal examination be completed for patients who have undergone low anterior resection or transanal excision for rectal cancer (Moy et al., 2016). NPs and PAs should discuss this with the patient's oncologist or gastrointestinal surgeon, as the specialist may prefer to do the rectal examination.

Serum carcinoembryonic antigen (CEA) levels are suggested at each follow-up visit in patients with colon or rectal cancer for at least the first 2 to 3 years after primary resection, even if preoperative CEA levels were normal. The NP or PA should coordinate with the patient's cancer team to determine if this level should be followed in the primary care or oncology clinic. If CEA monitoring is undertaken, an elevated CEA should be confirmed by retesting, particularly if the values are between 5 and 10 ng/mL (Moy et al., 2016). It is suggested that all patients with colon or rectal cancer undergo a complete colonoscopy either before surgical resection or within a few months after resection to exclude synchronous polyps and cancer. A repeat colonoscopy 1 year after primary resection of colon or rectal cancer is suggested to exclude new lesions, and if normal, subsequent follow-up intervals of 3 to 5 years are recommended depending on the results of the prior colonoscopy (Moy et al., 2016).

Patients who have undergone low anterior resection for rectal cancer and who have not received radiation therapy are suggested to undergo flexible proctosigmoidoscopy every 6 months for 2 to 5 years. This recommendation is controversial, however, and consensus-based guidelines from the National Comprehensive Cancer Network (NCCN) no longer recommend surveillance proctosigmoidoscopy in this population (Moy et al., 2016). For patients with colon or rectal cancer, it is suggested that annual surveillance CT scans of the chest and abdomen be performed for at least 3 years if the patient would be eligible for aggressive therapy, including curative-intent surgery. For patients with rectal cancer, it is suggested that an annual pelvic CT be done if pelvic radiation therapy was not administered (Moy et al., 2016). NPs and PAs should be aware that the following tests are not suggested for routine surveillance: fecal occult blood testing, liver function tests, complete blood count, chest radiograph, or positron emission tomography (PET) scanning (Moy et al., 2016). These tests may be warranted for other reasons and should be discussed with the patient's oncology team. NPs and PAs should remain vigilant about staying current on the most up-to-date surveillance guidelines for patients with CRC, including patients with CRC of different stages or metastatic disease.

Management

The patient should be referred to an oncologist and surgeon who will review NCCN guidelines to determine the treatment plan. Treatment of older CRC patients presents different challenges than treatment of younger patients due to the high number of comorbid conditions and potential psychosocial issues older patients may have, which may impact patient's tolerability of the treatment. More than 70% of CRC cases are diagnosed at an early stage (1 to 3) and are treated with surgical resection. Surgery is usually well tolerated in older patients, especially with the advances in laparoscopic resections. Excellent survival can be achieved in patients with complete resection. Older patients who are not surgical candidates may be referred for other treatment options such as colonic stenting (in a palliative setting), systemic chemotherapy, radiofrequency ablation (of liver metastases), or radiation therapy. Systemic chemotherapy can be used in the neoadjuvant or adjuvant setting and include fluoropyrimidines, oxaliplatin plus a fluoropyrimidine, or irinotecan plus 5-fluoracil. In the past 2 decades, several classes of biologic agents have been approved for the treatment of metastatic CRC. They are vascular endothelial growth factor therapies (bevacizumab, aflibercept, ramucirumab), epidermal growth factor receptor-targeted agents (cetuximab and panitumumab), and multikinase inhibitors (regorafenib). These agents can be used in combination with cytotoxic chemotherapy or as a single agent (Hubbard, 2016).

Additional Cancers

Genitourinary Cancer (GU)

Screening

For asymptomatic adults the USPSTF concludes that the current evidence is insufficient to assess the balance of benefits and harms of screening for bladder cancer (USPSTF, 2016). Risk factors for bladder cancer include cigarette smoking, prolonged exposure to urinary foreign bodies and infections, exposure to aminobiphenyl, or other occupational or environmental exposures from coal and products used in rubber or textile industries. Worksites reported to be associated with an increased risk of bladder cancer include dry cleaners, paper manufactures, rope and twine makers, and apparel factories (Burke & Laramie, 2004).

Presentation

Bladder cancer (BC) is the fifth most commonly diagnosed cancer in the United States, and the median age of patients' diagnosed with BC is 73. Bladder cancer can present as new onset hematuria or red blood cells noted on urinalysis. Use of cystoscopies and bladder washing with cytologic examinations have proven useful in the surveillance of patients who have been previously treated for bladder cancer but has not proven effective as a screening measure (Burke & Laramie, 2004). In the older adult patient, vague symptoms of weight loss, dysuria, hematuria, or abdominal pain can also be presenting symptoms of bladder cancer. Bladder cancer is diagnosed with positive biopsy of the bladder lesion.

Management

The patient should be referred to an oncologist and surgeon who will review NCCN guidelines to determine the treatment plan. The patient's level of fitness according to a comprehensive geriatric assessment (CGA) must also be determined prior to initiating treatment, as management of BC in older adults is complicated by their functional status and numerous other comorbidities that afflict them. A fit BC patient will be able to undergo a complete transurethral resection of the bladder tumor (TURBT) and intravesical bacillus Calmette-Guerin (BCG) therapy. High risk-frail patients who are unfit for general anesthesia can be offered BCG alone as a low-risk local procedure. Muscle invasive bladder cancer (MIBC) is defined as cancer that has invaded the muscularis propria of the bladder wall and involves multimodality therapy that includes radical cystectomy, chemotherapy (cisplatin, gemcitabine, methotrexate, vinblastine, or doxorubicin), or chemoradiation. Due to significant toxicities, the patient must be carefully screened with CGA prior to initiating treatment to determine tolerability (Kanesvaran, 2017).

Melanoma/Skin Cancer

Screening

Skin cancer, primarily melanoma, is a leading cause of morbidity and mortality in the United States. The USPSTF has found insufficient evidence to recommend for or against using visual examinations by clinicians to screen adults for skin cancer; however, encouraging patients to be aware of changes in their skin that could be indicative of cancer may be an important tool in early detection. The recommended frequency of skin self-exams may be patient specific, but preferably they should occur once a month. According to the American Cancer Society, patients should be aware of their normal pattern of moles, freckles, and blemishes.

Presentation

In older adults, differentiating normal versus age-related skin changes versus skin cancer can be challenging. Skin cancer is classified as basal call, squamous cell, or melanoma. All present as abnormal lesions on the skin or dermis tissue and are diagnosed with a positive biopsy.

Management

The patient should be referred to an oncologist and surgeon who will review NCCN guidelines to determine a treatment plan. For people who are at increased risk for skin cancer, such as people with reduced immunity, people who have had skin cancer before, and people with a strong family history of skin cancer, regular skin exams are important.

Blood Malignancies: Acute Myeloid Leukemia (AML) and Myelodysplastic Syndrome (MDS)

Screening and Presentation

Leukemias may be identified during routine blood tests or a chest x-ray, or a CT scan may reveal swollen lymph nodes or signs of infection. Currently, there are no standardized leukemia screening methods that are recommended for regular testing in the general population (Moffitt Cancer Center, 2020). Although there is no routine leukemia screening test, people with certain risk factors, such as a prior exposure to benzene or a family history of leukemia, should be vigilant in monitoring for possible symptoms, including fatigue, fever, night sweats, unexplained weight loss, bone pain, and anemia.

Management

The patient should be referred to a hematologist-oncologist who will review NCCN guidelines to determine a treatment plan.

AML in older adult patients tends to have a more aggressive biology, and performing CGA prior to selecting a treatment plan is extremely important to determine the patient's tolerability to proposed treatment. Optimal treatment of older adult patients with AML includes standard induction therapy of intensive chemotherapy with traditional chemotherapy (cytarabine for 7 days and an anthracycline or anthracenedione mitoxantrone for 3 days). Patients who are frail and unable to tolerate intensive therapy can be offered lower-intensity therapy with hypomethylating agents such as azacitidine or decitabine. Fit patients can also be considered for allogeneic hematopoietic stem cell transplantation (HSCT) but must have good social support and functional status to complete treatment.

Myelodysplastic syndrome (MDS) in the older adult patient is characterized by ineffective hematopoiesis and cytopenias. Treatment for MDS should be adapted to risk and the patient's fitness. Supportive care, such as transfusions, hematopoietic growth factors, and antibiotics, to control symptoms of cytopenias remains the primary therapy for frail patients. Fit older adult patients can be treated with hypomethylating agents such as azacitidine and decitabine. Lenalidomide may also benefit patients with low-risk MDS and can be considered in patients who are transfusion dependent. The only curative therapy for MDS is an allogeneic HSCT, but this option should be considered only in patients with good functional status and social support (Huang & Rao, 2017).

Head and Neck Cancers

Screening

NPs and PAs should be aware that patients who routinely drink alcohol, currently use tobacco products, or have used tobacco products in the past are at risk for head and neck cancer (Screening PDQ, 2020). Additional risk factors can include sun exposure, radiation exposure, inhalation of asbestos, wood or nickel dust, and poor oral hygiene. Although these are some risk factors, all patients should be assessed for head and neck cancer. A clinician should assess the nose, mouth, and throat of their patients for abnormalities and palpate for masses in the neck. General health screenings should be encouraged at least yearly and as needed and as directed by the clinician. Clinicians should recommend that patients receive regular dental checkups as part of the assessment for head and neck cancer. The human papillomavirus (HPV), a common sexually transmitted disease, has been associated with the development of some head and neck cancers, particularly in the upper throat and back of the tongue. Risk factors for HPV-related head and neck cancers include certain sexual behaviors and smoking marijuana.

Presentation

Warning signs of head and neck cancer can include frequent nose bleeds, ongoing nasal congestion, a persistent sore throat or changes in one's voice including hoarseness, a growth or nonhealing sore in the mouth or throat, constant earaches, bloody phlegm or saliva for several days, a lump in the neck lasting more than 2 weeks, changes in skin or a mole, and problems swallowing (Cleveland Clinic, 2020). Head and neck cancers (HNC) usually present as squamous cell carcinomas within the paranasal sinuses, nasal cavity, oral cavity, pharynx, and larynx (Fig. 17.3) (Maggiore et al., 2017).

Management

The patient should be referred to an oncologist and surgeon who will review NCCN guidelines to determine a treatment plan. The majority of HNC patients present with locally advanced disease, which often requires multimodality

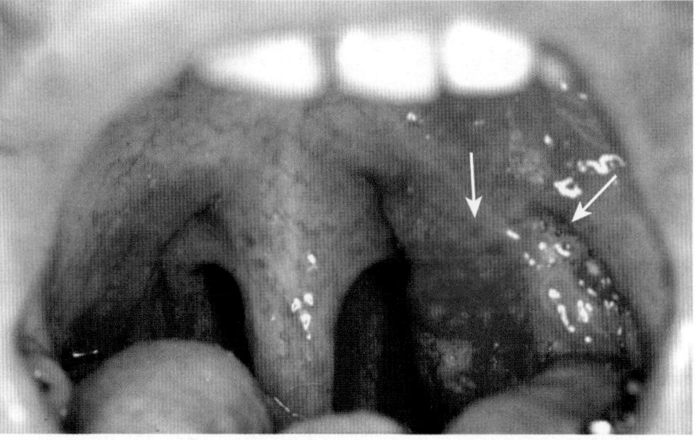

• **Fig. 17.3** Squamous Cell Carcinoma (From Richardson, M. A. et al. (2010). *Cummings otolaryngology head and neck surgery* (5th edition). Mosby, 1358-1374, Figure 100-8.)

therapy such as resection and concurrent chemoradiation. These treatments can lead to significant acute and late-term toxicities that can impact the patient's quality of life and survival. Patients must be carefully screened with CGA prior to determining and initiating therapy. Surgical resection is the recommendation for early stage HNC, but radiation monotherapy may be preferable in patients with early-stage disease or those with poor functional status or multiple comorbidities. For patients with recurrent or metastatic HNC, chemotherapy is the recommended treatment (Maggiore et al., 2017).

Role of a Comprehensive Geriatric Assessment (CGA) in Cancer Treatment

Aging is accompanied by changes in several areas, including physical, functional, cognitive, and socioeconomic domains. Comorbidity among older adults is more common, as is the incidence of geriatric syndromes that may include gait imbalance, delirium, and malnutrition. Additionally, cancer treatment may worsen geriatric syndromes and comorbidities, further complicating anticancer therapy.

The aging process is unique and varies among individuals. It is influenced by factors such as genetics, environment, and the patient's lifestyle. It is important to assess functional age, which can be different from the patient's chronologic age, when planning cancer treatment for older cancer patients. Additionally, there is high prevalence of frailty and prefrailty in older patients with cancer, with average estimates of approximately 42% and 43%, respectively. In addition to cancer itself, the treatments offered can be stressors that challenge the patient's physiologic reserve, increasing risk for the development of frailty.

The International Society of Geriatric Oncology (SIOG) recommends that oncologists include a geriatric assessment as part of their evaluation, as it provides a comprehensive medical, functional, and psychosocial evaluation of the older cancer patient to aid in treatment decision making. However, in practice settings where time and resources may be limited, it may be more feasible to select a brief frailty screening tool. Thereafter, in those who are identified as vulnerable or frail, the clinician can offer CGA and refer the patient to a geriatric clinic for further evaluation if available. Regardless of the tool selected, the key is to evaluate a patient's level of fitness as she or he is being considered for cancer treatment to guide treatment planning and to optimize care.

Fit Versus Frail

It is also important to recognize that some older adults may be as fit as younger adults, others may have slight declines in physiological reserve, and some may be frail. It is important to identify those who are fit, because they are more likely to benefit from standard therapy. Fit older adults generally have fewer comorbidities, are functionally independent, and may or may not have geriatric syndromes. Conversely, frail patients have more comorbidities, functional dependencies, and geriatric syndromes, and they are more likely to experience adverse outcomes and treatment-related toxicities. Frail patients may not experience lasting benefits from treatment due to these factors, which put them at increased risk of morbidity and mortality. Screening for frailty allows the clinician to assess the patients functional age and level of fitness when considering the goals of care and treatment options. Several frailty screening tools are available, including the CGA, the electronic Rapid Fitness Assessment (eRFA), the Fried Frailty Criteria, Balducci Frailty Criteria, and the Canadian Study of Health and Aging Clinical Frailty Scale.

The *Comprehensive Geriatric Assessment (CGA)* is an intensive multidimensional diagnostic evaluation of the older adult, which includes an evaluation of cognition, functional status, nutritional status, social support, psychological and emotional status, polypharmacy, and comorbidities (Fig. 17.4). The CGA is a collection of validated tools that can be used as a method for evaluating older adults. The CGA provides objective data that clinicians can use to risk stratify the older cancer patient and aid in treatment planning and follow-up. It provides a comprehensive overview of the older adult's level of fitness and reveals areas that may impact an older adult's tolerance to cancer therapy. A major value of the CGA is the results, which lead to actionable interventions by the interdisciplinary team that may improve outcomes (Box 17.3). For example, in patients with dependencies in activities of daily living (ADLs) and instrumental activities of daily living (IADLs), referrals for home services may be indicated to support patients through cancer treatment. CGAs have been associated with improved outcomes in the older cancer patient population, and its use is supported by national and international medical organizations prior to initiating cancer treatment and at appropriate follow-up points throughout the patient's treatment course, which may include during and after treatment, with a change of treatments, or as determined appropriate by the clinician (Balducci & Extermann, 2000; Chen et al., 2014; Clegg et al., 2014; Exterman & Hurria, 2007; Fried et al., 2001; Hurria and Balducci, 2009; Korc-Grodzicki & Tew, 2017; Korc-Grodzicki et al., 2015; Rockwood et al., 2005; Shahrokni et al., 2017a, 2017b).

It is important to perform CGAs (Fig. 17.3), as they may lead to the detection of impairments that are potentially reversible and may improve patient outcomes. When a CGA is performed, clinicians may wonder what interventions to implement based on the results obtained. Multicenter studies have found that geriatric assessments identify older cancer patients at heightened risk for chemotherapy-related toxicity and mortality. A study by McCorkle and colleagues found that when geriatric nurse practitioners performed geriatric assessments and incorporated interventions based on impairments identified in older adults with cancer, it led to a survival advantage. A study by Goodwin and colleagues showed that breast cancer patients who had received geriatric assessments and interventions based on the findings were much more likely to return to their baseline functioning. These studies highlight the value of

COMPREHENSIVE GERIATRIC ASSESSMENT				
Name:		Date of birth:		Gender:
Physical Health				
Chronic disorder				
Vision	Adequate Inadequate	Eyeglasses: Y N		Needs evaluation
Hearing	Adequate Inadequate	Hearing aids: Y N		
Mobility	Ambulatory: Y N	Assistive device:		
	Falls: Y N			Needs evaluation
Nutrition	Albumin:	TLC:	HCT:	
	Weight:	Weight loss or gain: Y N		Needs evaluation
Incontinence	Y N	Treatment:	Y N	Needs evaluation
Medications	Total number:	Reviewed & revised:	Y N	
	Adverse effects/allergy:			
Screening	Cholesterol:	TSH:	B12:	Folate:
	Colonoscopy: Date:		N/A	
	Mammogram: Date:		N/A	
	Osteoporosis: Date:		N/A	
	Pap smear: Date:		N/A	
	PSA: Date:		N/A	
Immunization	Influenza: Date:			
	Pneumonia: Date:			
	Tetanus: Date:		Booster:	
Counselling	Diet	Exercise Calcium	Vitamin D	
	Smoking	Alcohol Driving	Injury prevention	
Mental Health				
Dementia	Y N	MMSE score: Date:	Cause (if known):	
Depression	Y N	GDS score: Date:	Treatment:	Y N
Functional Status				
ADL	Bathing: I D	Dressing: I D		Toileting: I D
	Transferring: I D	Feeding: I D		Continence: Y N

• **Fig. 17.4** Comprehensive Geriatric Assessment (From Varcarolis's Canadian Psychiatric Mental Health Nursing, ed3, Elsevier, 2023.)

geriatric assessment–guided treatment processes in the care of older adults with cancer (Mohile et al., 2015). In addition to the patient's cancer status and prognosis, the results of the CGA should be considered in discussions with patients, families, and caregivers; these conversations should cover the potential risks and benefits of treatment, being mindful of patients' goals and preferences. The results of the CGA can be useful for primary care providers, oncologists, supportive care professionals, and symptom management specialists. A comprehensive approach to care is recommended,

BOX 17.3 Geriatric Assessment Guided Interventions

Functional Impairment

- Consider referral to physical or occupational therapy.
- Consider referral to home visiting nurse services.
- Consider referral to social work or case management.

At Risk for Malnutrition, Malnourishment, or Weight Loss

- Consider nutritional counseling to optimize nutrition.
- Consider nutritional supplements (i.e., Ensure, Glucerna, Boost).
- Identify community resources (i.e., home-delivered meals, federal resources such as Supplemental Nutrition Assistance Program [SNAP]).
- Discuss the use of feeding tubes and intravenous nutrition with the cancer care team, patient, and family in keeping with patient's stated care goals.

Depression, Distress, Anxiety

- Treat anxiety and depression with consideration of pharmacotherapy, if appropriate (i.e., selective serotonin-reuptake inhibitors [SSRIs]).
- Consider referral for supportive psychotherapy with a psychologist or social worker.
- Consider referral to a psychiatrist for the diagnosis, treatment, and prevention of mental, emotional, and behavioral disorders including substance use disorders.
- Refer to mental health resources available in community, such as support groups.

Cognitive Impairment

- Evaluate and treat reversible causes of memory loss (including but not limited to infection, electrolyte imbalance, vitamin deficiency, thyroid disorder).
- Consider referral to home visiting nurse services for home safety evaluation.
- Consider referral to social work or case management for identification of community resources.
- Identify social supports (i.e., caregiver). Connect patient/caregiver to community resources.
- Consider referral to a memory disorders clinic or neurocognitive clinic.

Poor Social Support

- Identify caregiver in the community.
- Evaluate for areas of financial strain.
- Connect patient/caregiver to community resources.
- Consider referral to social work or case management.

Polypharmacy

- Review patient's medication with consideration of Beers criteria for potentially inappropriate medications.
- Consider de-prescribing (cutting down medications that can be safely omitted).
- Consider asking a pharmacist for a medication review.
- Utilize Internet tracking systems that monitor for overprescribing.

as several factors play a key role in the health of aging individuals with cancer, such as functional status, psychosocial health, and the environment (Hurria & Balducci, 2009; Korc-Grodzicki & Tew, 2017).

Psychological Effects of Cancer on the Older Adult

In addition to the increased prevalence of cancer in aging individuals, it is also projected that by 2026 there will be greater than 20 million cancer survivors in the United States. Studies are emerging that suggest there may be a greater prevalence of depression and anxiety in older cancer survivors compared to those with no cancer history. It is essential that clinicians address the psychosocial components of aging and cancer in older patients to help them maintain a quality of life that is acceptable to them. Screening for depression and distress and initiating appropriate interventions should be incorporated in the care plan for current older adult cancer patients and cancer survivors (American Cancer Society, 2020). Some common tools used to screen for emotional distress are the Geriatric Depression Scale (GDS), the Distress Thermometer, the Patient Health Questionnaire-2 (PHQ-2), and the Patient Health Questionnaire-9 (PHQ-9). The GDS is used to assess for depression in older adults. There are two forms of the GDS, a long form that has 30 questions and a short form that has 15 questions. The GDS questions have high correlation with depressive symptoms, and the short form can be completed in approximately 5 to 7 minutes. When using the GDS short form, scores of 0 to 4 are considered normal, depending on age, education, and complaints. Scores of 5 to 8 indicate mild depression, scores from 9 to 11 indicate moderate depression, and scores between 12 and 15 indicate severe depression. Distress can be defined as a mix of anxiety and depressive symptoms. Some level of distress among cancer patients may be expected, but up to a third of cancer patients experience significant distress that can be debilitating and have negative effects on coping. The distress thermometer can identify patient concerns in practical, family, emotional, spiritual, and physical areas. The purpose of the distress thermometer is to make it easier for patients to talk to their doctors about the emotional effects caused by the diagnosis, symptoms, and treatment of cancer. Distress using this tool is measured from 0 to 10, where 0 is no distress and 10 is significant distress. The PHQ-2 and PHQ-9 are tools used to screen for depression. The PHQ-2 can be used as a quick screening tool that, if answered positively, should prompt the clinician to complete the PHQ-9. These tools can be used to diagnose depression, measure the severity of symptoms, and assess a patient's response to treatment (Hurria & Balducci, 2009; Korc-Grodzicki and Tew, 2017).

Treatment Modalities

Radiation

Radiation therapy, or radiotherapy, is a type of cancer treatment that uses high doses of radiation to kill cancer cells and shrink tumors. High-dose radiation kills cancer cells or slows their growth by damaging the cell's DNA, causing the cancer cells to stop dividing or die. It is important to educate patients so that they understand that radiation therapy does not kill cancer cells right away. It takes days or weeks of treatment before DNA is damaged enough for cancer cells to die. Then, cancer cells keep dying for weeks or months after radiation therapy ends. There are two main types of radiation therapy, external beam radiation and internal radiation. External beam radiation is the most common type of radiation therapy used for cancer treatment. High-energy rays or beams are directed from outside the body into the tumor. With internal radiation, also known as brachytherapy, a radioactive implant is put inside the body in or near the tumor. Depending on the cancer type and treatment plans, a temporary or a permanent implant may be used. Brachytherapy allows a higher dose of radiation in a smaller area than might be possible with external radiation.

The type of radiation used depends on cancer type, tumor size and location, and the patient's general health and medical history. Age modifies the efficacy and toxicity profile of radiation treatment for many disease sites, because age itself modifies influential tumor and patient factors (Smith & Smith, 2014). It is also important to take into consideration not only the patient's cancer but other comorbidities. If a patient's life expectancy is short, the potential gains in overall and cancer-free survival that may be attributed to radiation treatment will be diminished (this is not meant to minimize the potential role of palliative radiation). For older patients, the clinician must empirically weigh the trajectory and risks for noncancer morbidity and mortality, including impacts on overall health and function, to provide patients with a holistic view of their entire health spectrum and overall needs.

It is essential that clinicians caring for patients with cancer or a history of cancer be aware of the late and long-term effects of radiation treatment (Fig. 17.5). Late and long-term side effects of cancer treatment are not the same. Late side effects are side effects of cancer treatment that become apparent after treatment has ended and can appear months or years posttreatment. For example, for a patient who has undergone chemotherapy, a late side effect of treatment could be the development of osteoporosis or a second primary cancer. Long-term side effects can be caused by the cancer itself or the treatment of cancer and may continue for months or years. For example, peripheral neuropathy is a long-term side effect of chemotherapy. Long-term side effects usually begin during treatment and may persist after treatment ends.

Chemotherapy

Age should not be the only factor considered when developing a treatment plan for an older adult. Older adults can often benefit from systemic therapy the same as younger patients. A systematic review of 345 cooperative group trials found no evidence of poorer survival or increased treatment-related mortality with experimental treatments in older patients when compared with younger patients, despite concerns about an increased risk of toxicity (Kumar et al., 2007). If the decision to give chemotherapy is made, it is important to understand why chemotherapy is being given. Is it being given for palliation of symptoms or with a curative intent? The need for maintaining dose and dose intensity can be very different depending on the setting.

Older adults may have a decreased tolerance to chemotherapy in general, with an increased incidence of various toxicities. Some side effects are rather drug specific, such as cardiac failure with anthracyclines or neuropathy with taxanes/cisplatin (International Society of Geriatric Oncology [SIOG], 2020).

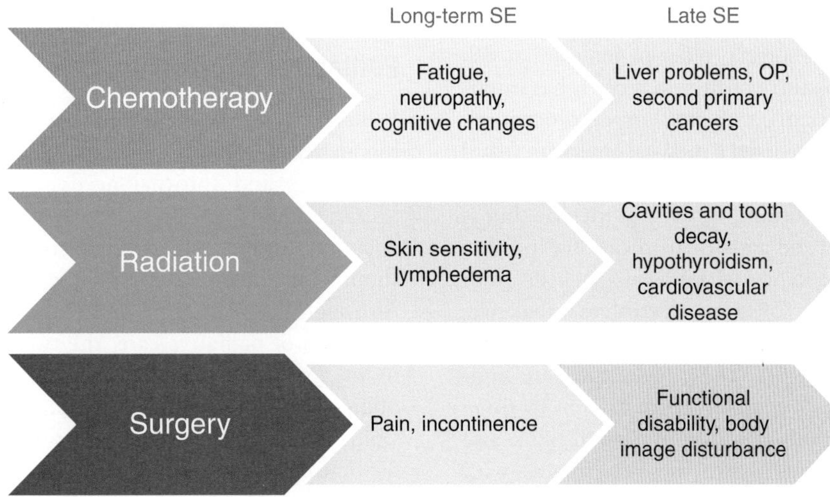

• **Fig. 17.5** Longer Term and Late Side Effects of Cancer Treatment (Created by Sincere McMillan.)

Chemotherapy toxicity tools such as that offered by the Cancer & Aging Research Group (CARG) and the Chemotherapy Risk Assessment Scale for High-Age Patients (CRASH) tool can help clinicians identify patients at risk for chemotherapy toxicity. It is important to be aware of the pharmacologic and clinical data for specific chemotherapy drugs. The most current information can be found on the National Cancer Institute website, which lists A–Z cancer drugs (www.cancer.gov). For most classical chemotherapeutic drugs, there may be some data available on age-related pharmacokinetics and dosing. However, it should be stated that dose adaptation based on age-related pharmacologic changes is an unvalidated approach, as clinical trials prospectively testing the efficacy and toxicity of age-related dose adaptation versus standard dosing are lacking. A geriatric assessment is currently the best way to obtain a broad view on the general health of the patient and is advised in all cancer patients > 70 years of age. If a patient is deemed to be at a higher risk of toxicity with standard dose therapy, there may be good alternatives to chemotherapy that can be discussed further with the patient's oncologist.

Surgery

Surgical approaches to cancer care for older adults can be considered for a curative intent or to palliate symptoms. Patients may benefit from a comprehensive assessment prior to any planned surgical intervention to better understand their overall fitness level. Fit older adults may be able to tolerate surgery with better outcomes than their frailer counterparts. It is always important to take into consideration the normal age-related physiologic changes that may impact surgical outcomes. Surgical interventions can cause physical deconditioning in even the fittest patient, and patients and their families should be aware that reconditioning often takes longer than deconditioning. This requires a frank, honest, and open discussion with patients and families before surgery, during which the postoperative recuperation expectations and the timeline are outlined; this discussion will take into consideration not so much the patient's age, but the patient's comorbidities and overall underlying health status. In addition to the physical toll of surgery, older patients are at risk for delirium, an acute cognitive change that often has multifactorial components and can occur after surgical procedures.

Delirium should be considered a medical emergency, and the multidisciplinary team should be involved to address the patient's risk factors for delirium, which can include, but is not limited to, anesthesia and narcotic medication exposure, blood loss, hypoxia, substance withdrawal (such as from benzodiazepine or alcohol), infection, electrolyte imbalance, and uncontrolled pain. Delirium prevention techniques are preferred as first-line strategies. These techniques are nonpharmacologic and include frequent reorientation to time, place, person, and situation; exposure to natural light; and early mobility. Providers can discuss these techniques with family members in advance of surgical procedures so they are familiar with nonpharmacologic management strategies.

Once patients are discharged from the hospital, often their recovery continues either at home or in a skilled facility. After surgery, follow-up with the primary care provider can be as important as follow-up with the surgeon. Identification of who will be responsible for medication reconciliation and assessment of the status of comorbid conditions (i.e., controlled or uncontrolled) is an important aspect of postoperative care of the older patient with cancer.

Immunotherapy

Immunotherapy for the treatment of cancer is a viable treatment option for many patients. Immunotherapy uses certain parts of a patient's immune system to fight disease (American Society of Clinical Oncology [ASCO], 2020). One example of immunotherapy is called chimeric antigen receptor (CAR)T cell therapy in which immune cells are removed from a patient, armed with new proteins that allow them to recognize cancer, and then given back to the patient in large numbers. These cells then persist in the body, essentially becoming "living drugs" (LaRussa, 2015). Bone marrow transplantation for blood cancers such as leukemia takes a donor's healthy blood-forming cells and puts them into the patient's bloodstream, where they begin to grow and make healthy red blood cells, white blood cells, and platelets. Immunotherapy can lead to side effects and toxicities that are distinct from those associated with traditional chemotherapeutic agents. These side effects can become life threatening if not anticipated and managed appropriately. The knowledge about the efficacy and toxicity of immunotherapy in older adults with cancer is limited, as most of the studies have involved a low number of older patients. Geriatric assessment for older adults receiving immunotherapies may be useful to gauge fitness for more intense therapies, such as combined immunotherapy, chemoimmunotherapy, or chemotherapy/radiation plus immunotherapy strategies. Geriatric assessments allow for a tailored approach to treatment, which becomes especially important in the care of the heterogeneous older adult population (see Table 17.3).

Palliative/ Supportive Care

Palliative care is interdisciplinary and focuses on improving patients' quality of life by addressing their physical, emotional, and spiritual needs. Some clinicians, as well as patients and families, may have misconceptions about what constitutes palliative or supportive care. Clinicians should understand that palliative care is not hospice care. Although hospice care is sometimes considered within the spectrum of palliative care, the two terms are not synonymous. Palliative care specialists work collaboratively with oncology care teams to help patients maintain the best possible quality of life while also providing caregiver support, facilitating communication among members of the health care team, and assisting with discussions focusing on goals of care.

TABLE 17.3 Cancer Treatment Symptom Management at a Glance

Treatment Side Effects	Clinician Interventions
Chemotherapy	
Fatigue	TUG, ADL, IADL, referral to PT/OT, encourage rest breaks as needed
Weight loss	MNA, diet log, nutritionist referral, consider use of nutritional supplements, address nausea/vomiting
Cognitive impairment	Mini-Cog, MoCA, MMSE, GDS, CAM, neuropsychiatry referral, cognitive rehabilitation, promote safe independence, address actual and potential safety concerns
Neuropathy	Monofilament screening, podiatry, occupational therapy
Radiation	
Skin sensitivity	Encourage use of emollients, avoid direct exposure to sunlight, monitor for signs of infection, avoid injury, monitor for signs of bruising, dermatology referral
Lymphedema	Monitor for signs of infection, encourage stretching, use of compression garments, lymphedema therapy
Surgery	
Pain	Ongoing pain assessment, nonopioids for mild pain, stepwise approach to opioid use: start with low doses and titrate up, consider use of adjuvants, integrative approaches, monitor for psychosocial distress
Functional impairment	TUG, ADL, IADL, referral to PT/OT, referral for home care
Altered body image	Explore the patients concerns, use effective communication strategies such as empathy, cognitive behavioral therapy, stress-reduction techniques, support groups

ADL, Activities of daily living; CAM, confusion assessment method; GDS, Geriatric Depression Scale; IADL, instrumental activities of daily living; MMSE, Mini Mental State Examination; MNA, Mini-Nutrition Assessment; MoCA, Montreal Cognitive Assessment; OT, occupational therapy; PT, physical therapy; TUG, Timed Up and Go Test.

CASE STUDY (FIT PATIENT)

Mr. L. is an 85-year-old male with a medical history significant for mild hypertension, hyperlipidemia, and arthritis. He has newly diagnosed, locally advanced rectal adenocarcinoma. Due to o the geriatric clinic for CGA prior to initiating treatment and to determine if he can tolerate standard treatment versus palliative treatment.

He presents to the geriatric clinic with his 80-year-old wife, who is in good health, and one of his daughters. The APP collects the following complete health history, physical exam results, and CGA.

History of Present Illness

Mr. L was in his usual state of health until 2 months ago when he started having occasional blood with bowel movements and more frequent bowel movements. He has a history of hemorrhoids, so he attributed the bleeding to the hemorrhoids. More recently he noticed more fatigue and shortness of breath at his biweekly exercise class, and mild anemia was noted on recent blood work. He underwent further evaluation; a colonoscopy revealed two rectal masses and a biopsy was consistent with intramuscular adenocarcinoma and a tubular adenoma. He denies unintentional weight loss, nausea, vomiting, fever, or pain and continues to have a good appetite.

Past Medical History

Mild hypertension, hyperlipidemia, arthritis.

Past Surgical History

Left knee replacement 10 years ago, tonsillectomy as a child.

Family History

Mother died at age 90 of cerebrovascular accident (CVA), father died age 95 of pneumonia, one brother A&W at 82, one sister A&W at 86 with history of breast cancer.

Social History

Retired accountant with a master's degree in accounting. Lives with wife in single-level private home in an independent 55+ community. Has two daughters and one son who live close by and are involved in his care.

Alcohol

Two glasses of wine a week, no tobacco or drug use.

Continued

CASE STUDY (FRAIL PATENT)—cont'd

Medications

Lisinopril 20 mg po daily, HCTZ 25 mg po daily, Lipitor 40 mg po daily, Tylenol 1000 mg po prn joint pain, multivitamin 1 a day.

Allergies

None.

Review of System

See HPI for pertinent positives and negatives; also complains of pain and stiffness in knees in the morning.

Vitals

BP: 124/65 P: 68 RR: 17 breaths/min O2Sat: 98% RA Weight 163 pounds, BMI 28.

Physical Exam

General: Well groomed, well nourished, not in distress
Skin: + seborrheic keratosis on the back
HEENT: PERRLA
Nodes: No palpable peripheral adenopathy
Pulmonary: Clear to A&P, no wheezing
Heart: RRR, no murmur
Abdomen: NABS, soft, nontender
Extremities: Trace edema to feet bilat
Neuro: No focal neurologic deficit, stable gait, A&Ox3

Geriatric Assessment

Comorbidities: His blood pressure has been stable within JNC8 recommended guidelines for his age; a recent lipid profile was normal.

Cognitive Function

Patient has good cognitive function as evident on normal score on MOCA exam (28/30). Patient scores 2/15 on the Geriatric Depression Scale (GDS), which is within normal range (negative for depression). His distress score on the distress thermometer is 4/10 (no distress).

Functional Capacity

Independent in all ADLs and IADLs. No recent falls. TUG <10 sec.

Nutrition

Patient scores 12/14 on the Mini Nutritional Assessment (MNA) (indicative of normal nutritional status).

Medications

No inappropriate polypharmacy.

Social Support

Well supported by wife and family.

On the spectrum of frailty, patient is fit based on geriatric assessment and should tolerate standard treatment with support of the medical team and family.

Coordination of Care

The provider communicated with the patient's care team, including his medical and surgical oncologists. The patient was encouraged to continue follow-up with his primary care doctor for management of his primary care needs near his home.

2-Week Follow-up

The patient returned to the geriatric clinic after meeting with the oncologist to discuss a treatment plan. The oncologist recommended standard treatment with neoadjuvant fluorouracil/leucovorin/oxaliplatin (FLOX) chemotherapy followed by a laparoscopic partial colectomy with anastomosis, with curative intent.

The NP in the geriatric clinic looked up the chemotherapies in the online Memorial Sloan Kettering Geriatric Plan (https://libguides.mskcc.org/GeriatricPlan) and found the following potential complications related to this treatment:

Fluorouracil: Diarrhea, nail changes, hand and foot syndrome, increased tearing of eyes, confusion/disorientation with high doses)
Leucovorin: GI upset, seizures, syncope, nausea/vomiting, urticaria
Oxaliplatin: Diarrhea, peripheral neuropathy, ataxia, hypomagnesemia, hypocalcemia, sensitivities to cold foods/fluids, lip numbness

Recommendations

- The NP counseled the patient and family about monitoring for and treatment of diarrhea. Discussed dietary modifications and encouraged small but frequent high-calorie, high-protein meal options while in treatment and for after surgery.
- Encouraged maintaining adequate hydration with at least six glasses of water a day, more when diarrhea is present.
- Discussed the importance of continuing with twice-weekly exercise program to maintain strength.
- Encouraged the patient to check blood pressure and monitor for any persistent high or low readings.
- Informed the patient that he should follow-up with the primary care physician for medication adjustment if changes in blood pressure occur.
- Notified the patient that he should monitor for any gait troubles related to dizziness, weakness, or neuropathy of feet.
- Referred the patient to a support group for colorectal patients.
- Explained that the patient must return to the clinic after completing chemotherapy and prior to surgery.

3-Month Follow-up

The patient has completed chemotherapy. He has managed diarrhea with dietary modifications and Imodium as needed. He has lost 5 pounds, discontinued HCTZ, and reduced his dose of lisinopril to 10 mg po daily due to persistent lower blood pressure. His blood pressure today is 120/68 P 64. MOCA remained the same at 28/30. Distress level and depression screening scores have stayed the same, but MNA scores have gone down to 10/14 due to poor appetite and weight loss.

Continued

CASE STUDY (FRAIL PATENT)—cont'd

A complete H&P was preformed, and the patient was cleared for upcoming surgery. He was also referred to an outpatient and inpatient nutritionist to assist with his diet.

4-Month Follow-up

The patient presents to the geriatric clinic s/p complete resection of the tumor with a new colostomy. He is now NED with plans to return to OR in a few months for take down of the ostomy. Inpatient stay was significant for postoperative delirium on days 1 through 3, ileus, and hypotension. He was followed by the geriatric inpatient team while admitted, but due to the prolonged hospital stay related to the ileus he became dependent on a walker, lost an additional 5 pounds, and was discharged to a rehabilitation facility to regain strength. He stayed at the rehab facility for 2 weeks and was discharged home using a cane only. He presents to the clinic today with his wife, ambulating with a cane, and is now back to his preoperative weight. CGA is preformed and reveals that MOCA has declined to 24/30 and his TUG is >20 with one fall in the rehab center. He is dependent in some ADLs and IADLs using a cane for ambulation. The patient scores 2/15 on the Geriatric Depression Scale (GDS) (no depression). His distress score on the distress thermometer is 4/10 (no distress). The patient scores 10/14 on the Mini Nutritional Assessment (MNA) (indicating that he is at risk for malnutrition).

Lab work is WNL and blood pressure is 122/68 on lisinopril 10 mg po daily only. His physical exam is significant for new ostomy, functioning well with pink stoma. In general, the patient has successfully completed cancer treatment. He is referred to occupational therapy for cognitive training and assistance with improving IADLs and to outpatient physical therapy for gait training and conditioning. He will return to his primary care provider for general care and continued follow-up of blood pressure and cognition.

Cases Wrap-up

The cases discussed in this chapter demonstrate the importance of using the CGA prior to initiating and throughout cancer treatment to identify the vulnerabilities an older cancer patient may have. These vulnerabilities could lead to frailty, which can significantly impact the patient's overall biopsychosocial status and ultimately his or her quality of life. Frailty is a dynamic process, and performing geriatric assessments can reveal deficits that would not be found on routine care alone. This can lead to interventions that can impact clinical outcomes as illustrated in the cases presented here.

Cancer treatment is made more complex in the geriatric patient due to diminished functional reserve, comorbidities, and altered physical, physiologic, and psychosocial capacity. Often subtle alterations in health or functional status can signal the onset of toxicities or complications that can result in serious consequences. Using a pocket guide, such as *The Geriatric Plan: The MSKCC Ambulatory Nurses Guide to Assist Older Adults Though Cancer Treatment*, can help the care provider screen for and identify the most common and significant symptoms associated with cancer treatment and make suggestions on how to intervene to minimize severity, reduce distress, improve the patient's quality of life, and maintain care of the patient in the ambulatory clinic (Carrow et al., n.d.).

• BOX 17.4 Resources

- National Comprehensive Cancer Network (NCCN) Older Adult Oncology Guidelines
- *The Geriatric Plan: The MSKCC Ambulatory Nurses Guide to Assist Older Adults Though Cancer Treatment*: A handbook for nursing clinicians to provide a systematic framework to address needs of older cancer patients the in ambulatory care setting. (Carrow, M., Derby, S., Frierson, L., Gooch, M., Mulligan-Stoiber, A. M., Ricci, J., Roth, J., & Yulico, H. [n.d.]. *The Memorial Sloan Kettering Cancer Center GERIATRIC PLAN©*. https://libguides.mskcc.org/GeriatricPlan.)
- ConsultGeri: A clinical website for The Hartford Institute for Geriatric Nursing. Includes e-learning resources and webinars
- National Cancer Institute, www.cancer.gov
- Oncology Nursing Society, www.ONS.org
- American Society of Clinical Oncology (ASCO), www.ASCO.org

Conclusion

Caring for the older adult with cancer can be challenging and rewarding for NP and PA clinicians. The prevalence of cancer in older adults make it likely that NPs and PAs working not just in oncology but in different specialties and settings will be caring for older adults who either have or have had a malignancy during their lifetime. Awareness of the presentation of cancer in older adults, the treatment regimen options, the possible long-term side effects and interactions of comorbidities and medications with cancer treatment regimens require NPs and PAs to maintain proficiency in knowledge about cancer prevention, presentation, and treatment. Box 17.4 provides a list of resources to assist PAs and NPs in the care of older adults with cancer.

Key Points

- Nurse practitioners and physician assistants play an important role in caring for older adults before, during, and after a cancer diagnosis.
- NPs and PAs can use the comprehensive geriatric assessment (CGA) to help risk stratify patients prior to cancer treatment.
- Cancer treatment must be tailored to the patient and take into account the patient's physical, mental, and psychosocial function.

More information about tools and Interprofessional Education Collaborative (IPEC) competencies mentioned in this chapter can be found in Appendix 1: Tools and Appendix 2: IPEC Competencies.

References

American Cancer Society. (2015). *Radon and cancer*. https://www.cancer.org/cancer/cancer-causes/radiation-exposure/radon.html.

American Cancer Society. (2019a). *American Cancer Society recommendations for prostate cancer early detection*. https://www.cancer.org/cancer/prostate-cancer/detection-diagnosis-staging/acs-recommendations.html.

American Cancer Society. (2019b). *American Cancer Society recommendations for the early detection of breast cancer*. https://www.cancer.org/cancer/breast-cancer/screening-tests-and-early-detection/american-cancer-society-recommendations-for-the-early-detection-of-breast-cancer.html.

American Cancer Society. (2020). *Emotional, mental health, and mood changes*. https://www.cancer.org/treatment/treatments-and-side-effects/physical-side-effects/emotional-mood-changes.html.

American Geriatrics Society (AGS). Choosing wisely Workgroup. (2014). American Geriatrics Society identifies another five things that healthcare providers and patients should question. *Journal of the American Geriatrics Society, 62*(5), 950–960.

American Society of Clinical Oncology (ASCO). (2019). *Digital rectal exam (DRE)*. https://www.cancer.net/navigating-cancer-care/diagnosing-cancer/tests-and-procedures/digital-rectal-exam-dre.

American Society of Clinical Oncology (ASCO). (2020, May 13). *Understanding immunotherapy*. https://www.cancer.net/navigating-cancer-care/how-cancer-treated/immunotherapy-and-vaccines/understanding-immunotherapy.

Balducci, L., & Extermann, M. (2000). Management of the frail person with advanced cancer. *Critical Reviews in Oncology/Hematology, 33*(2), 143–148.

Bibbins-Domingo, K., Grossman, D. C., Curry, S. J., Davidson, K. W., Epling, J. W., García, F. A., … & Kurth, A. E. (2016). Screening for colorectal cancer: US Preventive Services Task Force recommendation statement. *Journal of the American Medical Association, 315*(23), 2564–2575.

Burke, M. M., & Laramie, J. A. (2004). *Primary care of the older adult: A multidisciplinary approach*. Elsevier Health Sciences.

Carrow, M., Derby, S., Frierson, L., Gooch, M., Mulligan-Stoiber, A.M., Ricci, J., Roth, J., & Yulico, H. (n.d.). *The Memorial Sloan Kettering Cancer Center GERIATRIC PLAN©*. https://libguides.mskcc.org/GeriatricPlan.

Center for Disease Control and Prevention. (2018). *What is breast cancer screening?* https://www.cdc.gov/cancer/breast/basic_info/screening.htm.

Chen, X., Mao, G., & Leng, S. X. (2014). Frailty syndrome: An overview. *Clinical Interventions in Aging, 9*, 433–441.

Chudgar, N. P., Bucciarelli, P. R., Jeffries, E. M., Rizk, N. P., Park, B. J., Adusumilli, P. S., & Jones, D. R. (2015). Results of the national lung cancer screening trial: Where are we now? *Thoracic Surgery Clinics, 25*(2), 145–153.

Cleveland Clinic. (2020). *Head & neck cancer FAQS: Throat cancer*. https://my.clevelandclinic.org/health/diseases/17041-head--neck-cancer-frequently-asked-questions.

DeSantis, C. E., Miller, K. D., Dale, W., Mohile, S. G., Cohen, H. J., Leach, C. R., Goding Sauer, A., Jemal, A., & Siegel, R. L. (2019). Cancer statistics for adults aged 85 years and older, 2019. *CA: A Cancer Journal for Clinicians, 69*(6), 452–467.

Duineveld, L. A., van Asselt, K. M., Bemelman, W. A., Smits, A. B., Tanis, P. J., van Weert, H. C., & Wind, J. (2016). Symptomatic and asymptomatic colon cancer recurrence: A multicenter cohort study. *Annals of Family Medicine, 14*(3), 215–220.

Extermann, M., & Hurria, A. (2007). Comprehensive geriatric assessment for older patients with cancer. *Journal of Clinical Oncology, 25*(14), 1824–1831.

Fried, L. P., Tangen, C. M., Walston, J., Newman, A. B., Hirsch, C., Gottdiener, J., & McBurnie, M. A. (2001). Frailty in older adults: Evidence for a phenotype. *The Journals of Gerontology Series A: Biological Sciences and Medical Sciences, 56*(3), M146–M157.

Grossman, D. C., Curry, S. J., Owens, D. K., Bibbins-Domingo, K., Caughey, A. B., Davidson, K. W., … & Krist, A. H. (2018). Screening for prostate cancer: US Preventive Services Task Force recommendation statement. *Journal of the American Medical Association, 319*(18), 1901–1913.

Huang, L., & Rao, A. (2017). Acute myeloid leukemia and myelodysplastic syndrome. In B. Korc-Grodzicki & W. Tew (Eds.), *Handbook of geriatric oncology practical guide to caring for the older cancer patient* (pp. 233–240). Springer.

Hurria, A., & Balducci, L. (2009). *Geriatric oncology: Treatment, assessment and management*. Springer Science & Business Media.

International Society of Geriatric Oncology (SIOG). (2020). *Chemotherapy in senior adults*. http://siog.org/content/chemotherapy-senior-adults.

Kanesvaran, R. (2017). Bladder and renal cancer. In B. Korc-Grodzicki & W. Tew (Eds.), *Handbook of geriatric oncology practical guide to caring for the older cancer patient* (pp. 208–215). Springer.

Korc-Grodzicki, B., Holmes, H. M., & Shahrokni, A. (2015). Geriatric assessment for oncologists. *Cancer Biology & Medicine, 12*(4), 261.

Korc-Grodzicki, B., & Tew, W. P. (Eds.). (2017). *Handbook of geriatric oncology*. Springer.

Kumar, A., Soares, H. P., Balducci, L., & Djulbegovic, B. (2007). Treatment tolerance and efficacy in geriatric oncology: A systematic review of phase III randomized trials conducted by five National Cancer Institute–sponsored cooperative groups. *Journal of Clinical Oncology, 25*(10), 1272–1276.

LaRussa, A. (2015). *Chimeric antigen receptor (CAR) T-cell therapy*. https://www.lls.org/treatment/types-of-treatment/immunotherapy/chimeric-antigen-receptor-car-t-cell-therapy.

Lu, D., Andersson, T. M., Fall, K., Hultman, C. M., Czene, K., Valdimarsdóttir, U., & Fang, F. (2016). Clinical diagnosis of mental disorders immediately before and after cancer diagnosis: A nationwide matched cohort study in Sweden. *JAMA Oncology, 2*(9), 1188–1196.

Maggiore, R., VanderWalde, N., & Crawley, M. (2017). Head and neck cancers in older adults. In B. Korc-Grodzicki & W. Tew (Eds.), *Handbook of geriatric oncology practical guide to caring for the older cancer patient* (pp. 233–240). Springer.

Moffitt Cancer Center. (2020). *Leukemia screening*. https://moffitt.org/cancers/leukemia/diagnosis/screening/.

Mohile, S. G., Velarde, C., Hurria, A., Magnuson, A., Lowenstein, L., Pandya, C., … & Dale, W. (2015). Geriatric assessment-guided care processes for older adults: A Delphi consensus of geriatric oncology experts. *Journal of the National Comprehensive Cancer Network, 13*(9), 1120–1130.

Moy, B., Jacobson, B.C., & Goldberg, R.M. (2016). Surveillance after colorectal cancer resection. *UpToDate*. http://www. uptodate. com/contents/surveillance-after-colorectal-cancer-resection.

National Breast Cancer Foundation. (2019). *Male breast cancer*. https://www.nationalbreastcancer.org/male-breast-cancer

National Cancer Institute. (2019). *Cancer stat facts: Cancer of any site*. https://seer.cancer.gov/statfacts/html/all.html.

National Lung Screening Trial Research Team. (2011). The national lung screening trial: Overview and study design. *Radiology, 258*(1), 243–253.

Rockwood, K., Song, X., MacKnight, C., Bergman, H., Hogan, D. B., McDowell, I., & Mitnitski, A. (2005). A global clinical measure of fitness and frailty in elderly people. *Canadian Medical Association Journal, 173*(5), 489–495.

Screening PDQ. (2019). Cancer prevention overview (PDQ®): *PDQ Cancer Information Summaries [Internet]*. National Cancer Institute (US).

Screening PDQ. (2020). Oral cavity, pharyngeal, and laryngeal cancer prevention (PDQ®): *PDQ Cancer Information Summaries [Internet]*. National Cancer Institute (US).

Shachar, S., Jolly, T., Walde, V., & Muss, H. (2017). Breast cancer. In B. Korc-Grodzicki & W. Tew (Eds.), *Handbook of geriatric oncology practical guide to caring for the older cancer patient* (pp. 133–144). Springer.

Shahrokni, A., Kim, S. J., Bosl, G. J., & Korc-Grodzicki, B. (2017a). How we care for an older patient with cancer. *Journal of Oncology Practice, 13*(2), 95–102.

Shahrokni, A., Tin, A., Downey, R. J., Strong, V., Mahmoudzadeh, S., Boparai, M. K., ... & Korc-Grodzicki, B. (2017b). Electronic rapid fitness assessment: A novel tool for preoperative evaluation of the geriatric oncology patient. *Journal of the National Comprehensive Cancer Network, 15*(2), 172–179.

Siegel, R. L., Miller, K. D., & Jemal, A. (2019). Cancer statistics, 2019. *CA: A Cancer Journal for Clinicians, 69*(1), 7–34.

Siegel, R. L., Miller, K. D., & Jemal, A. (2020). Cancer statistics, 2020. *CA: A Cancer Journal for Clinicians, 70*(1), 7–30.

Sinha, S., Alexander, M., & Gajra, A. (2017). Lung cancer. In B. Korc-Grodzicki & W. Tew (Eds.), *Handbook of geriatric oncology practical guide to caring for the older cancer patient* (pp. 161–167). Springer.

Smith, G. L., & Smith, B. D. (2014). Radiation treatment in older patients: A framework for clinical decision making. *Journal of Clinical Oncology, 32*(24), 2669.

Spronk, I., Korevaar, J. C., Schellevis, F. G., Albreht, T., & Burgers, J. S. (2017). Evidence-based recommendations on care for breast cancer survivors for primary care providers: A review of evidence-based breast cancer guidelines. *BMJ Open, 7*(12), e015118.

US Department of Health and Human Services (USPSTF) Office of Disease Prevention and Health Promotion. (2020). *Healthy people 2030*. https://health.gov/healthypeople.

US Preventive Services Task Force. (2016). *Final recommendation statement breast cancer screening*. https://www.uspreventiveservicestaskforce.org/Page/Document/RecommendationStatementFinal/breast-cancer-screening1.

US Preventative Services Task Force. (2018). *Final recommendation statement: Prostate cancer: Screening*. https://www.uspreventiveservicestaskforce.org/Page/Document/RecommendationStatementFinal/prostate-cancer-screening1.

Wood, D. E., Eapen, G. A., Ettinger, D. S., Hou, L., Jackman, D., Kazerooni, E., ... & Massion, P. P. (2012). Lung cancer screening. *Journal of the National Comprehensive Cancer Network, 10*(2), 240–265.

18

Mental Health/Behavioral Health

JENNIFER COX, MSW, LICSW

OBJECTIVES

Student Learning Objectives

After completing this chapter, the student should be able to do the following:

1. Describe the qualities unique to behavioral health presentations in the older adult.
2. Summarize the approach to assessment and diagnosis of behavioral health conditions in the older adult.
3. Appraise the unique aspects of the presentation and management of common behavioral health conditions in the older adult.

Practitioner Objectives

After completing this chapter, the practitioner should be able to do the following:

1. Carefully evaluate older adults presenting with behavioral health symptoms, and effectively differentiate psychiatric symptoms from medical or neurologic symptoms.
2. Determine when referral to a geriatric behavioral health specialist is required, and describe the roles and functions of varied allied behavioral health professionals, including psychologists, social workers, and case managers.
3. Develop practice approaches based on accurate assessment, current scientific evidence, and informed clinical judgment for the older adult client with mental health conditions.

Introduction

For clinicians who want to provide the highest quality care to older adults, skillfully navigating the evaluation and treatment of mental health concerns in later life is a priority and a necessity, but it is also a formidable challenge. It is not unusual to see a well-meaning practitioner bypass a patient completely and interview an older patient's adult child to conduct a behavioral health assessment, which is discriminatory and inappropriate. However, conducting assessments and failing to recognize the unique features and contributing factors of advanced age on mental health can lead to grossly inaccurate differential diagnoses. Cognitive decline and medical comorbidity, including medication interactions and side effects, are more likely to be contributing factors to a psychiatric presentation in older adults than they are in a general adult population.

Common medical problems that would be more consistent with psychiatric or psychological disorders in younger populations, such as thyroid dysfunction, vitamin deficiencies, sensory deficits, and vascular problems, all can manifest symptoms in older adults. Complicating the assessment picture, older adults are more likely to report mental health problems as physical problems or fail to report distressing psychiatric symptoms at all (Speer & Schneider, 2006).

The complex interplay between medical and psychiatric conditions in the context of generational beliefs about mental health concerns and the overall stigma toward behavioral health in this population demands a careful and thorough assessment that includes patients and collateral contacts when available. Evidence suggests that older adults, and in particular African American older adults are disproportionately harmed by negative perceptions (stigma) of asking for help with mental health concerns and, as a result, can avoid seeking help or admitting they have a concern (Conner et al, 2011). Providers, caregivers, and older adults themselves may have been slow to realize the importance of treating and managing mental health concerns in older adults, but this oversight is thankfully changing. Healthy People 2020 (HP2020), an initiative that provides science-based, 10-year national objectives for improving the health of all Americans, has listed the behavioral health of seniors as one out of three emerging issues in the area mental health and mental disorders (Office of Disease Prevention and Health Promotion, 2020). Consequently, this chapter explores best practices for the assessment and treatment of behavioral health concerns for the older adult patient, emphasizing the importance of an integrated approach with care providers, patients, and their caregivers.

Interprofessional Care

Older adult mental health includes a wide range of conditions, is often complex and complicated by other coexisting medical conditions, and can be difficult to assess, treat, and manage. Expecting primary care providers, much less acute care providers, to carry out this task in isolation is unfair and unrealistic. Thus, an integrated, interdisciplinary team approach to managing behavioral health concerns in older adults is needed and helpful for improved patient care and outcomes in older adult patients. Since the early 2000s, the American Geriatrics Society has held the position that interdisciplinary care offers the best way to provide high-quality care to older adults with complex needs (Mion et al., 2006).

Who should be included in the care team for patients with behavioral health concerns? Whenever possible, a psychiatrist serves as an ideal care partner, and, in the best-case scenario, this psychiatrist is well versed in the care and management of geriatric concerns. In addition, due to polypharmacy's central position in the care of older adults and the need to manage and monitor psychiatric medications, a geriatric psychiatrist would be an ideal consultant. Unfortunately, the field currently experiences a crisis-level shortage of these physician specialists. In the absence of a geriatric specialist, adult psychiatry remains an important asset to the interdisciplinary team.

A pharmacist also contributes significantly to the behavioral health interdisciplinary team, especially when a patient has a long medication list, is prescribed high-risk medications such as antipsychotics or benzodiazepines, or has cognitive or neurologic disorders. Care providers of hospitalized patients often have access to pharmacists to consult on their care, a luxury less available in outpatient settings. When psychiatry or geriatric psychiatry remains an unavailable resource, primary care providers must manage the medications of older adults with mental health concerns. In those cases, consulting with a pharmacist can be extremely valuable.

Physician assistants and nurse practitioners also play a critical role in caring for older adults with behavioral health concerns. The American Academy of Physician Assistants (AAPA, 2020) listed this approach in its vision statement: "PAs transforming health through patient-centered, team-based medical practice." Finally, the American Association of Nurse Practitioners (AANP, 2020) also endorses and advocates an integrated, interdisciplinary path.

In behavioral health care, nonmedical professionals can be an equally important part of an interdisciplinary care team. Psychologists, who provide assessment, cognitive testing, and psychotherapy, and licensed mental health professionals, who offer psychotherapy and behavioral therapy, are key players in behavioral health care. Nonpharmacologic interventions can be as effective as, and sometimes even more effective than, medication interventions for common behavioral health concerns such as depression and anxiety, without the concomitant risks or challenges of medication therapy. For this reason, psychological and behavioral interventions always should be considered an appropriate first-choice intervention for behavioral health concerns in older adult patients.

Case managers are an absolutely essential part of a successful interdisciplinary approach. They can be nurse case managers, social work case managers, or others trained in this capacity. These valuable professionals ensure communication between medical and behavioral health providers, facilitate care planning meetings with or without patients and families present, conduct thorough histories involving collateral contacts and other caregivers, and answer questions while providing a point of contact for patients and families. It does not benefit patients and providers to have many different content experts managing patient care if they are not sharing information and coordinating their efforts. A case manager is the best hub in the wheel of integrated behavioral health care.

Many sources, including clinical studies, confirm the importance and benefits of an interdisciplinary team approach. For instance, the American Psychological Association (APA) has addressed the need to include psychology into the care of older adults (Keita, 2011). The association views interdisciplinary teams as central to the new health care system. In fact, the APA's Integrated Health Care for an Aging Population Initiative "focuses on efforts to promote psychologists' involvement and contributions to the expanding model of health care" (Keita, 2011; also see American Psychological Association, 2008). In addition, Tanaka (2003) mentions a study with elder care that included an intervention team of a geriatrician, a nurse, and a social worker. Together, they listed the patient's issues, developed a care plan, and coordinated the plan's implementation. This research recommends interdisciplinary teams for inpatients and outpatients as well as the provision of psychosocial counseling, patient and family education, discharge planning, and posthospital care. Although the study showed no effects on survival, this approach "significantly reduced functional decline during hospitalization and improved mental health in patients" (Tanaka, 2003). Another study focused on implementing an innovative integrated service delivery for seniors in France (De Stampa et al., 2014). Using qualitative data (focus groups with case managers), the researchers concluded that this approach aids in the reduction of service fragmentation, which, in turn, increases the quality of care provided to seniors with complex needs.

Indeed, the interdisciplinary team approach offers the best way to cover the complex interplay between the older adult patients' medical and psychiatric conditions such as those covered in this chapter: depression, anxiety, suicidality, chronic and major mental illness, and substance abuse. In turn, this more comprehensive way of assessing and treating older adult patients allows practitioners to provide higher-quality care to older adults. As their quality of life improves, so does that of their caregivers and families.

Assessment

Careful assessment is the most important aspect of the successful evaluation of, and intervention for, behavioral health concerns in the older adult patient. It is absolutely essential for the health care provider to conduct a thorough medical assessment in conjunction with, and ideally before, every behavioral health assessment. Specifically, a clinician will want to review the following laboratory results before the first behavioral health interview: complete blood count (CBC) with differential, comprehensive metabolic panel, urinalysis, B_{12}, folate, thyroid stimulating hormone (TSH), and syphilis screening to rule out medical conditions potentially underlying behavioral changes. Of particular

CASE STUDY

Elizabeth, an 86-year-old single Caucasian woman, has lived alone and independently in an apartment for the past 10 years. She had retired from her job as a music director at her church 20 years prior. She never married nor had children. When she turned 75, she moved several states to be closer to her only living relative, her older sister Jeanne. Jeanne passed away 5 years later. Elizabeth has lived alone, with limited social and community supports, ever since. She has multiple chronic medical conditions, including chronic hypertension, chronic obstructive pulmonary disease (COPD), an essential tremor, and an implanted pacemaker. She recently received the diagnosis of mild cognitive impairment and early stage Alzheimer's disease.

Elizabeth came to her current primary care provider (PCP) with a prescription for lorazepam, prescribed by her former physician, for 30 1-mg tabs to be used as needed monthly. Because Elizabeth had been on this medication for several years, her new provider continued to prescribe it. As time went on, Elizabeth began running out of lorazepam before the end of the month and calling the office to request three to four extra pills until she could refill her prescription. Her primary care provider, who had been reluctant to continue the lorazepam prescription in the first place, initially complied but, after the first few requests, began to refuse. In addition, she told Elizabeth that she would stop prescribing the medication altogether and would place her on a taper regimen. Upon hearing this, Elizabeth became extremely upset and called the primary care office several times, alternately crying and arguing. Her PCP asked her to come in for an office visit to discuss the situation.

In the office, Elizabeth explained that lately she felt like she needed the lorazepam more because the stresses of managing her life independently overwhelmed her. She tearfully reported that memory lapses and mistakes with her finances were occurring more frequently. She also noted unsteadiness and increasing worries about falling. As she had no social supports, she feared that she would "die on the floor and no one would know." The PCP referred Elizabeth to the behavioral health clinician for an evaluation of anxiety and depression as well as to the Visiting Nurses Association (VNA) for an in-home safety assessment and case management services.

The behavioral health clinician evaluated Elizabeth and found scores on validated instruments indicating diagnoses of depression and anxiety, both exacerbated by her declining cognitive ability. The VNA caseworker determined that an assisted living environment would be a safer choice for Elizabeth than living alone and helped Elizabeth apply for a subsidized apartment. Elizabeth also received referrals to an individual therapist to work with her weekly. She became involved in the social activities and groups offered at the assisted living facility. After consulting with Elizabeth's individual therapist, her primary care provider tapered her off the lorazepam over 16 weeks and initiated escitalopram (Lexapro) to better control her anxiety and eliminate the risks of benzodiazepines. Six months later, Elizabeth's mood and anxiety were much improved, demonstrating the benefits of the collaborative, interdisciplinary approach.

importance in this sequence is the urinalysis, because urinary tract infections (UTIs) in older women and older men are a common cause of behavioral change, including psychiatric symptoms such as hallucinations, sudden changes in sleep and appetite, and a new onset or worsening of preexisting confusion and agitation (Gbinigie et al., 2018). Additionally, evaluating labs carefully for signs of infection and screening for recent anesthesia, falls, or other medical events distinguishes sudden behavior changes that could be psychiatric in nature from delirium, which can cause altered mental status that looks like psychosis but is, in fact, a medical emergency.

Finally, patients need to be carefully questioned for recent medication changes, particularly with respect to benzodiazepine use, and their medication compliance assessed. Sudden withdrawal or overuse from benzodiazepines can cause mood, behavior, and mental status changes. Older adults are far more likely than younger cohorts to react to medication changes, withdrawal, or interactions with altered mental status and behavioral changes (Hauviller et al., 2016). It is essential that clinicians be knowledgeable about medications that can alter behavior or cause other adverse side effects in older adults (Tables 18.1 to 18.3) (Lindsey, 2009). Practitioners must keep in mind that older adults can be a vulnerable population and that their medications can be managed—and in some cases misappropriated—by others. In addition, they may not be either in control of or aware of inaccuracies in medication compliance. Primary care and urgent care practitioners cannot be expected to conduct investigations into every case they encounter. However, by keeping these issues in mind, they help determine what information is needed and whether it is necessary to follow up with additional collateral sources or refer clients to social work or case management to get more information on their living and family situation.

Once a medical evaluation has been reviewed, but before initiating the behavioral health interview, a practitioner must consider whether any sensory impairment is present that may prevent the patient from participating fully in the interview. This point sounds obvious but frequently is overlooked. Hearing impairment compromises the quality of a patient's ability to participate in or understand a behavioral health assessment. Many older adults who grow accustomed to not being able to hear well enough to participate in meaningful conversation will not alert interviewers to their hearing deficit. These patients have developed a "disengaged" method of coping with their hearing impairment in order to avoid fatigue, embarrassment, or frustration with their limitations in unfamiliar social situations (Heffernan et al., 2016). One must be careful to ensure that the examination area has as little background noise as possible such as that found in busy emergency departments or other acute care settings. It is important to ensure that the patient can see the practitioner's face, in case he or she uses lip reading or visual cues to supplement comprehension when hearing is impaired. Due to these common mistakes, older adults are at times judged to have cognitive impairment when they simply cannot hear well enough to answer questions or participate in a conversation fully. To conduct more accurate assessments in these types of contexts, it is wise for the clinician to invest in an inexpensive "pocket talker" (a small device that amplifies the clinician's voice into headphones worn by the patient) or another amplifying device.)

TABLE 18.1 Anxiolytic Medications and Recommended Dosing for Use in Older Adults

Generic (Brand) Name	Initial Dosage	Maximum Daily Dosage	Major Adverse Effects
Benzodiazepines			
Alprazolam (Xanax)	0.125 mg to 0.25 mg twice per day	0.25 mg to 2 mg twice per day	Incoordination, cognitive impairment, depression, drowsiness, fatigue, irritability, light headedness, sedation, appetite changes, weight loss or gain, constipation, dry mouth, difficulty urinating, dysarthria
Lorazepam (Ativan)	0.25 mg to 0.5 mg twice per day	0.5 mg to 4 mg twice per day	Sedation and respiratory depression
Oxazepam (Serax)	10 mg twice per day	10 mg to 30 mg twice per day	Edema, drowsiness, ataxia, dizziness, memory impairment, headache, paradoxical excitement, incontinence, blood dyscrasia, jaundice, dysarthria, tremor, diplopia, syncope (rare)
Temazepam (Restoril)	7.5 mg at night	7.5 mg to 5 mg at night	Confusion, dizziness, drowsiness, fatigue, anxiety, headache, lethargy, hangover, euphoria, vertigo, diarrhea, dysarthria, weakness, blurred vision, diaphoresis
Hypnotic Agents			
Eszopiclone (Lunesta)	1 mg to 2 mg at bedtime	1 mg to 2 mg at bedtime	Headache, unpleasant taste
Gabapentin (Neurontin)	100 mg at bedtime	100 mg to 300 mg/3600 mg[a] at bedtime	Somnolence, dizziness, ataxia, fatigue, peripheral edema, diarrhea, tremor, weakness, nystagmus, diplopia
Mirtazapine (Remeron)	7.5 mg at bedtime	7.5 mg to 45 mg at bedtime	Somnolence, increased appetite with weight gain, increased serum cholesterol, constipation, dry mouth
Nortriptyline (Pamelor)	10 mg to 25 mg at bedtime	10 mg to 100 mg at bedtime	Orthostasis, hypertension, myocardial infarction, ataxia, extrapyramidal symptoms, seizures, glucose dysregulation, syndrome of inappropriate antidiuretic hormone, sexual dysfunction, dry mouth, anorexia, constipation, nausea, vomiting, diarrhea, weight gain (or loss), urinary retention, impotence, blood dyscrasia, increased levels in liver function test values, paresthesia, mydriasis
Trazodone (Desyrel)	25 mg at bedtime	25 mg to 200 mg at bedtime	Orthostasis, ventricular irritability, sedation, dizziness, gait instability, mild cognitive impairment, seizures, weight gain, priapism, headache, dry mouth, edema, nausea, diarrhea
Zaleplon (Sonata)	5 mg at bedtime	5 mg to 10 mg at bedtime	Few common adverse effects. *Less common effects*: Chest pain, edema, amnesia, dizziness, hallucinations, light headedness, incoordination, anorexia, dyspepsia, nausea, constipation, dry mouth, tremor, weakness, arthralgia
Zolpidem (Ambien)	5 mg at night	5 mg to 10 mg at night	Few common adverse effects. *Less common effects*: Palpitations, headache, dizziness, light headedness, amnesia, nausea, diarrhea, dry mouth, constipation

[a]For insomnia, the recommended dosage of gabapentin is up to 300 mg per day; for essential tremor, restless leg syndrome, and neuropathic pain, the recommended dosage is up to 3600 mg per day.

From Jacobson, S. A., Pies, R. W., & Katz, I. R. (2007). *Clinical manual of geriatric psychopharmacology*. American Psychiatric Publishing, Inc.; Lindsey, P. (2009). Psychotropic medication use among older adults: What all nurses need to know. *Journal of Geriatric Nursing, 35*(9), 28–38. https://doi.org:10.3928/00989134-20090731-01; Smith, J. C. (2005). *Relaxation, meditation, and mindfulness: A mental health practitioner's guide to new and traditional approaches*. Springer Publishing Co.

TABLE 18.2 Antidepressant Medications and Recommended Dosing for Use in Older Adults

Generic (Brand) Name	Initial Dosage	Maintenance Dosage	Major Adverse Effects
Selective Serotonin Reuptake Inhibitors (SSRIs)			
Citalopram (Celexa)	10 mg to 20 mg per day	10 mg to 40 mg per day	Nausea, vomiting, dry mouth, headache, somnolence, insomnia, increased sweating, tremor, diarrhea, sexual dysfunction
Escitalopram (Lexapro)	10 mg per day	5 mg to 20 mg per day	Suicidal behavior, fever, insomnia, dizziness, somnolence, paresthesia, light headedness, migraine, tremor, vertigo, abnormal dreams, irritability, fatigue, lethargy, palpitations, hypertension, flushing, chest pain, nausea, diarrhea, constipation, indigestion, vomiting, dry mouth, heartburn, flatulence, gastroesophageal reflux, ejaculation disorder, urinary frequency
Fluoxetine (Prozac)	10 mg per day	5 mg to 40 mg per day	Nausea, vomiting, diarrhea, insomnia, nervousness, restlessness, agitation, anxiety, light headedness, drowsiness, fatigue, headache, tremor, initial weight loss, possible long-term weight gain, hyponatremia, syndrome of inappropriate antidiuretic hormone (SIADH), increased risk of bleeding (upper gastrointestinal and intraoperative) with co-administration of nonsteroidal antiinflammatory drugs, aspirin, and warfarin (Coumadin)
Paroxetine (Paxil, Paxil CR)	10 mg per day	5 mg to 40 mg per day	Headache, somnolence, dizziness, insomnia, dry mouth, constipation, diarrhea, ejaculatory disturbances, weakness, diaphoresis
Sertraline (Zoloft)	12.5 mg to 25 mg per day	25 mg to 200 mg per day	Insomnia, somnolence, dizziness, headache, fatigue, dry mouth, diarrhea, nausea, ejaculatory disturbances
Non-SSRIs			
Bupropion (Wellbutrin, Wellbutrin SR, Wellbutrin XL)	37.5 mg to 75 mg per day; SR: 75 mg to 100 mg every morning; XL: 150 mg every morning	150 mg in two to three divided dosages; SR: 100 mg twice per day; XL: 150 mg per day	Dizziness, anxiety, agitation, dry mouth, insomnia, headache, nausea, constipation or diarrhea, tremor
Duloxetine (Cymbalta)	20 mg per day	20 mg to 60 mg per day	Nausea, dry mouth, constipation, poor appetite, diarrhea, headache, insomnia, somnolence, fatigue, diaphoresis, dizziness
Mirtazapine (Remeron, Remeron SolTab)	7.5 mg at bedtime	7.5 mg to 45 mg at bedtime	Somnolence, increased appetite with weight gain, increased serum cholesterol, constipation, dry mouth
Venlafaxine (Effexor, Effexor XR)	25 mg twice per day; XR: 37.5 mg per day	150 mg per day in divided dosages; XR: 150 mg per day	Headache, somnolence, dizziness, insomnia, nervousness, nausea, dry mouth, constipation, anorexia, abnormal ejaculation/orgasm, weakness, diaphoresis
Tricyclic Antidepressant Drugs			
Desipramine (Norpramin)	25 mg per day	100 mg per day	Serotonin syndrome, anticoagulant effect with warfarin, cardiotoxicity, orthostasis, hypotension, hypertension, anticholinergic effects, tremor, agitation, insomnia
Nortriptyline (Pamelor)	10 mg to 25 mg per day	50 mg per day	Orthostasis, hypertension, myocardial infarction, ataxia, extrapyramidal symptoms, seizures, glucose dysregulation, SIADH, sexual dysfunction, dry mouth, anorexia, constipation, nausea, vomiting, diarrhea, weight gain/loss, urinary retention, impotence, blood dyscrasia, increased levels in liver function test values, paresthesia, mydriasis

From Jacobson, S. A., Pies, R. W., & Katz, I. R. (2007). *Clinical manual of geriatric psychopharmacology*. American Psychiatric Publishing, Inc.; Lindsey, P. (2009). Psychotropic medication use among older adults: What all nurses need to know. *Journal of Geriatric Nursing, 35*(9), 28–38. https://doi.org:10.3928/00989134-20090731-01; Morgan, B. D., White, D. M., & Wallace, A. X. (2005). Substance abuse in older adults. *Geropsychiatric and Mental Health Nursing*, 193-212; Norman, M. A., Whooley, M. E., & Lee, K. (2004). Depression and other mental health issues. *Current Geriatric Diagnosis and Treatment*, 100-113.

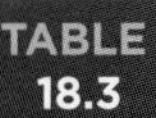

TABLE 18.3 Antipsychotic Medications and Recommended Dosing for Use in Older Adults

Generic (Brand) Name	Initial Dosage	Maintenance Dosage	Major Adverse Effects
Typical Antipsychotic Agent			
Haloperidol (Haldol)	0.25 mg to 0.5 mg per day	0.25 mg to 4 mg per day	Extrapyramidal symptoms, tardive dyskinesia, neuroleptic malignant syndrome
Atypical Antipsychotic Agents			
Aripiprazole (Abilify)	5 mg per day	2.5 mg to 15 mg per day	Headache, agitation, anxiety, insomnia, somnolence, akathisia, light headedness, weight gain, nausea, dyspepsia, constipation, vomiting
Clozapine (Clozaril)	6.25 mg to 12.5 mg per day	6.25 mg to 400 mg per day (slow titration)	Agranulocytosis, neuroleptic malignant syndrome, deep venous thrombosis and pulmonary embolism, glucose dysregulation, weight gain, increased serum creatine kinase, increased serum lipids (including triglycerides), seizures, tachycardia, confusion, sedation, dizziness, salivary pooling
Olanzapine (Zyprexa)	2.5 mg per day	2.5 mg to 15 mg per day	Orthostatic hypotension, sedation, weight gain, glycemic dyscontrol, elevation of serum lipids (triglycerides), anticholinergic effects (e.g., constipation), nausea, dizziness (not orthostatic), tremor, insomnia, overactivation, akathisia, neuroleptic malignant syndrome, tardive dyskinesia
Quetiapine (Seroquel)	25 mg at bedtime	50 mg to 400 mg at bedtime	Sedation, orthostatic hypotension, dizziness, agitation, insomnia, headache, neuroleptic malignant syndrome
Risperidone (Risperdal)	0.25 mg to 0.5 mg at bedtime	0.25 mg to 3 mg at bedtime	Hypotension (especially orthostatic), tachycardia, dysrhythmias, electrocardiogram changes, syncope, sedation, headache, dizziness, restlessness, akathisia, anxiety, extrapyramidal symptoms, tardive dyskinesia, neuroleptic malignant syndrome
Ziprasidone (Geodon)	20 mg twice per day with food	20 mg to 80 mg twice per day with food	Extrapyramidal symptoms, somnolence, headache, dizziness, nausea, akathisia

From Edlund, B. J. (2007). Pharmacotherapy in older adults: a clinician's challenge. *Journal of gerontological nursing*, *33*(7), 3; Jacobson, S. A., Pies, R. W., & Katz, I. R. (2007). *Clinical manual of geriatric psychopharmacology*. American Psychiatric Publishing, Inc.; Lindsey, P. (2009). Psychotropic medication use among older adults: What all nurses need to know. *Journal of Geriatric Nursing, 35*(9), 28–38. https://doi.org:10.3928/00989134-20090731-01; Norman, M. A., Whooley, M. E., & Lee, K. (2004). Depression and other mental health issues. *Current Geriatric Diagnosis and Treatment*, 100-113.

A comprehensive mental status examination performed by a clinician includes an assessment of the following: appearance, behavior, speech, mood, affect, thought process (are the patient's thoughts logical, organized, goal directed, and related?), thought content (does the patient have any bizarre or unusual thoughts, such as believing he has special powers or that someone is controlling his thoughts?), insight, and judgment (Box 18.1). A thorough evaluation of a client's mental status should include subjective symptoms, such as the patient's evaluation of his mood, and objective assessments made by the clinician, such as whether or not the patient's motor activity is normal or whether the patient's speech is normal, slowed, or pressured. Conducting an assessment for an older adult should not differ much from performing

• BOX 18.1 Mental Status Exam Components

1. General observations
   a. Appearance
   b. Speech
   c. Behavior
   d. Cooperativeness
2. Thinking
   a. Thought process
   b. Thought content
   c. Perceptions
3. Emotion
   a. Mood
   b. Affect
   c. Suicidal or homicidal ideation
4. Cognition
   a. Orientation/attention
   b. Memory
   c. Insight
   d. Judgement

similar assessments on any adult beyond taking extra care to ensure the patient can see and hear clearly. However, in an assessment of an older adult, conducting a cognitive evaluation has more significance than similar assessments of younger patients. Ideally, a cognitive assessment—and the same cognitive assessment each time with the same mental status screening tool—would be performed concurrently by the same clinician at least quarterly for older adults with behavioral health concerns. Standardized assessments tools commonly employed include the Mini Mental Status Exam (MMSE) (Heart and Stroke, n.d.), the Montreal Cognitive Assessment (MoCA) (US Department of Veterans Affairs, n.d.), or the Mini-Cog (Mini-Cog, n.d.). (See the appendix for copies.) The MoCA or Mini-Cog are good options in the public domain (the MMSE, by contrast, is subject to a licensing agreement). In addition, practitioners often employ an unofficial Mental Status Exam (MSE) (Psychiatry Database, n.d.). The MSE provides a systematic way of describing a patient's mental state at the time of assessment, including recorded subjective and objective observations. If a patient is seen in an acute setting, getting a general sense of the patient's cognitive baseline will help differentiate symptoms of psychiatric disturbance from cognitive impairment. In the outpatient or chronic care setting, an assessment will give helpful information to compare over time and observe changes, if any, in a client's cognition (Wray et al., 2012).

The question of whether to obtain collateral reports in behavioral health assessment always is difficult. It is unreasonable to assume that a patient is an unreliable reporter simply because of his or her age. Many adults in their 80s and 90s remain cognitively intact and are reliable historians. On the other hand, especially in settings where a patient is not well known to the practitioner and no cognitive evaluation baseline is available, one must ensure that he or she collects the most accurate information possible. Therefore it is recommended that the practitioner always request that a patient give permission to speak to a collateral contact when performing the assessment. One particularly helpful strategy, with the patient's permission, is to invite the patient's collateral contact into the interview and propose that the collateral, without interruption or participating in the interview itself, note his or her answers to the questions being asked of the patient. Reviewing these answers separately with the clinician at the conclusion of the interview offers an unobtrusive and timesaving way to determine congruence in the two reports. In situations where the collateral cannot be invited into the interview, obtaining permission to call that person on the telephone or otherwise interview him or her separately is the respectful way to ensure the fullest picture. The patient interview takes place first, and then the meeting with the identified contact occurs afterward.

In the event that two largely different reports are received, which is not uncommon when cognitive impairment is present, the practitioner's work becomes complicated and requires additional investigation to determine the full story. It is worth noting that older adults suffering from cognitive impairment often do not mean to mislead or misrepresent their situation to medical providers, and often they are not aware that the information they are providing is not or is no longer accurate. Older adults suffering from short-term memory loss related to moderate Alzheimer disease may give factually accurate details about their lives, abilities, and routines, but their information may be several years or more out of date and no longer currently relevant. This is important because if patients represent themselves as being able to drive or organize their own appointments independently, for example, a practitioner pressed for time may take their word that they are able to follow up on and arrange a behavioral health service independently, when this is in fact outside the scope of their current ability. In those situations, the interdisciplinary approach is extremely helpful. To begin, for the generalist acute or primary care practitioner pressed for time, the assistance of social workers, case managers, or nurses often can provide a clearer sense of a patient's "big picture." They can assist with interviewing collateral contacts, reaching out to the staff in residential care settings, or reviewing medical records from referral sources. In cases where mental health and cognitive issues are both present, time spent on these efforts is invaluable to ensure that the recommended intervention is appropriate, achievable, and realistic for that individual's current condition and ability.

When evaluating an older patient's current behavioral health needs, evaluation of his or her psychiatric history is equally important. Although advances in technology and the standardization of the inventories and scales certainly have changed the face of diagnostics, one must keep in mind that widespread mental health treatment, diagnosis, and visibility is a relatively recent phenomenon (Edelstein et al., 2008). In other words, it is still common to interview older adults who speak in euphemisms about their own or family members' mental health conditions or who reference mental health conditions that would be described and treated differently in modern clinical settings. As the current cohort of middle-aged and young adults age, this may fade as a clinical consideration.

For example, in interviews of older people with behavioral health concerns, patients have shared that either they or someone they know have had a "nervous breakdown" in the past. Clinical experience shows that an older adult's use of the term "nervous breakdown" is extremely vague. It describes any number of psychiatric conditions, ranging from an episode of relatively moderate depression in the context of environmental stress to a manic episode to, at the extreme end, a description of psychosis. Similarly, different standards of care can give younger clinicians an inaccurate sense of the severity of a patient's psychiatric history. A patient reporting that she spent 6 weeks in a psychiatric hospital for depression in 1964 might impress the medical professional with the severity of her depression, but the average length of stay in a psychiatric hospital presently is a tiny fraction of what it was in the not-so-distant past. Patients who today would be discharged within a week, or never admitted to an inpatient facility at all, may have spent long periods in a residential psychiatric setting in the past.

Further, the ever-changing climate of health care funding has fundamentally altered the way in which patients initially interact with and receive services from the modern mental health care system. Since the 1960s, psychiatric care has shifted from a primarily inpatient-based treatment modality to a variety of outpatient treatment options. A recent report from the National Association of State Mental Health Directors notes,

> [I]n 2014 state mental health systems provided services to 7.3 million individuals but only 493,517 (6.8 percent) of those individuals received inpatient psychiatric services during the year (2 percent received inpatient psychiatric services in state psychiatric hospitals and 4.8 percent in other psychiatric inpatient settings). (Lutterman et al., 2017)

Therefore a client's psychiatric history must be evaluated carefully, with the clinician collecting various data points and perspectives, if possible.

The APA formulated 21 guidelines for psychological practice with older adults, which emphasize the need to understand cognitive and functional changes associated with aging as well as the need for a comprehensive understanding of the medical context of behaviors and the wide variety of settings in which many older adults live (American Psychological Association, 2014). Medical practitioners may want to review these guidelines to familiarize themselves with best practices endorsed by the professional association of psychologists. Of note, guideline 18 states, "In working with older adults, psychologists are encouraged to understand the importance of interfacing with other disciplines, and to make referrals to other disciplines and/or to work with them in collaborative teams and across a range of sites, as appropriate" (American Psychological Association, 2014). This emphasis by the APA on interdisciplinary practice illustrates the importance of this issue for all providers. The APA guidelines do not recommend specific tools for the behavioral health assessments of older adults. Rather, they encourage psychologists (and other providers) to be familiar with current research on the impact of patient age on assessment and to integrate data from other spheres, such as medicine, social services, and caregivers, into their own assessment protocols (American Psychological Association, 2014).

Depression

Depression is not, and never has been, a normal part of the aging process. The Healthy People 2020 initiative underscores the importance of addressing depression in all age groups. One of the Mental Health and Mental Disorders objectives addresses this topic: "Increase the proportion of primary care physician office visits where adults 19 years and older are screened for depression" (Office of Disease Prevention and Health Promotion, 2020). With regard to depression, several issues are idiosyncratic to the older age group, requiring proper assessment and treatment. These factors include ageism, perceived stigma about mental health care, multiple health problems, and the tendency for older adults to be more prone to medication side effects (Levine, 2018).

The *Diagnostic and Statistical Manual of Mental Disorders*, Fifth Edition (DSM-5), provides eight criteria for the diagnosis of clinical depression and further specifies that to be diagnosed with depression, the patient must experience five or more symptoms during the same 2-week period. At least one of the symptoms should be either (1) depressed mood or (2) loss of interest or pleasure. The DSM-5 has a list of criteria for diagnosing depression (American Psychiatric Association, 2013).

Dysthymia, a related but different disorder, is described as persistent depression in which a patient has been experiencing symptoms of and met diagnostic criteria for clinical depression continuously for more than 2 years (American Psychiatric Association, 2013). In some cases, when patients report an extended or even lifelong history of depression, they could more accurately be diagnosed with dysthymia, although in practice settings this degree of specificity is generally not common.

Is depression more prevalent in older adults than in younger age groups? The evidence is mixed. Some research demonstrates that old age is actually a happy period in people's lives on average, compared to reports of happiness at other ages. Von Humbolt and Leal (2015) identified three contributing factors to a higher sense of happiness and well-being in later life. They argued that, because older adults have developed steady and stable social relationships, often have achieved a degree of economic stability/sense of occupational accomplishment, and have developeexistential meaning and spiritual activities, they often self-report a high quality of life. Similarly, Blanchflower and Oswald (2008) described happiness throughout the adult life span as a U-shaped curve, reaching a low point in middle age and steadily rising into old age. Rates of depression as reported

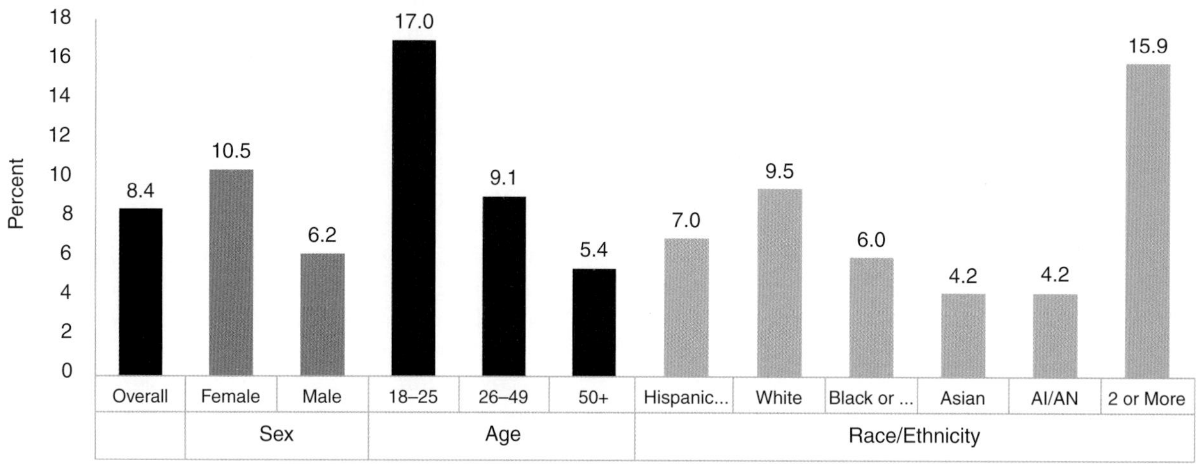

• **Fig. 18.1** Past Year Prevalence of Depressive Episodes Among US Adults (2020). (From National Institute of Mental Health. [2022]. Major depression. https://www.nimh.nih.gov/health/statistics/major-depression.shtml#part_155029.)

by the National Institute of Mental Health appear to indicate that the prevalence of depressive episodes is lowest in the 50+ age cohort (Fig. 18.1).

That said, other evidence indicates that older adults, especially those in long-term care facilities, are more likely to be clinically depressed, with a prevalence of 8% to 15% for the former and 30% for the latter (Chang et al., 2006). Therefore the identification of and screening for depression are especially critical in acute and chronic care medical settings. Additional research suggests that, even if depression in later life actually occurs less commonly than at younger ages, the consequences of depression in older age are more serious and result in greater risk to patients. These might include increased risks for mortality, suicide, reduced social functioning, and self-neglect (Blazer, 2003).

How does one interpret these seeming contradictions? The answer is not immediately clear. To begin, simply assessing whether a given adult is "happy" does not necessarily imply that the opposite condition is depression. In addition, the existence of these contrary conclusions may signify the need for more research into this topic for a more expansive understanding. What remains clear, however, is that depression in older adults is a serious concern. As the previously noted statistics demonstrate, this diagnosis remains a larger problem in the subgroup of older adults with significant medical problems or who are living in long-term care settings. Despite the lack of agreement on prevalence, the evidence supports the fact that depression in older adults is treatable and outcomes are good when patients are referred to treatment (Fiske et al., 2009).

In any case, this exploration includes the research pointing to increased happiness in old age to make a larger point: depression in the older adult population is not a normal outcome of being old. Because of bias against older adults or anxiety about getting old themselves, clinicians sometimes allow their beliefs about what it must be like to be old to lead them to make assumptions that older people are, by definition, unhappy, and therefore undercount the significance of depression as a clinical concern. As discussed, research demonstrates that this is not necessarily true (Blanchflower & Oswald, 2008; Taylor, 2011). Despite the fact that many older adults experience some decline in health or mobility or some social losses, clinical depression does not constitute the default response to the normal changes occurring in this stage of life. Furthermore, depression in an older adult can effectively be treated with a wide range of interventions, including medication and various modalities of psychotherapy (Fiske et al., 2009). Therefore it is important to screen all older adults for depression and to provide appropriate treatment if evidence of depression is present.

Several helpful, brief screening tools for depression have been developed for adult populations (Box 18.2). The Geriatric Depression Scale (GDS), developed by Yesavage et al., has been tested extensively with older adults and has been found to have excellent specificity and sensitivity against diagnostic criteria for depression when used across a wide

• BOX 18.2 Screening Tools for Depression

Beck Depression Inventory (BDI) (Beck et al., 1961)
Patient Health Questionnaire (PDQ) (Spitzer et al., 2003)
Major Depression Inventory (MDI) (Cuijpers et al., 2007)
Center for Epidemiologic studies Depression Scale (CES-D) (Radloff, 1977)
Hamilton Depression Rating Scale (HDRS) (Hamilton, 1980)
Zung self rated Depression Scale (Zung, 1965)
Geriatric Depression Scale (GDS) (Greenberg, 2019)
Cornell Scale for Depression in Dementia (CSDD) (Alexopolous et al., 1988)

See reference list for more information on sources.

variety of clinical settings (Greenberg, 2019). The GDS is available in the public domain in both a long and short form. The short form (15 items) has been demonstrated to be as effective in screening for depression as the longer version and is therefore adequate for use in most settings. It has become the most commonly used instrument for evaluating depression in older adults. A second, less common screening tool, the Brief Carroll Depression Rating Scale (BCDRS), has been shown in some research to have even a slightly higher sensitivity and better predictive value for depression in older adults (Koenig et al., 1988), but, in most contemporary clinical settings, the GDS is the standard tool. Consequently, this tool also has been translated into many languages and utilized with older populations from various cultural and ethnic backgrounds. Research into the applicability and validity of the scale with non-English-speaking populations has demonstrated its appropriateness in translation as well as in the original form (Lai, 2000).

Once an assessment has been completed, accessing appropriate treatment for depression is the next step. The integrated behavioral health model, in particular, works very well to help connect patients with a behavioral health clinician. Primary care providers, including nurse practitioners and physician assistants, can use a brief assessment such as the GDS short form to screen clients for depression during routine visits and then immediately can refer those who screen positive for depression to in-house behavioral health services. This could include psychiatrists, psychologists, and licensed mental health professionals. Indeed, as mentioned previously, the American Psychological Association released a "Blueprint for Change" in 2008, explicitly endorsing a model of integrated medical and behavioral health care for older adults based in the primary care setting (American Psychological Association, 2008).

Fortunately, nonmedication treatment interventions for depression have been found to be useful in geriatric populations. In particular, psychotherapy interventions—including behavioral therapy, cognitive behavioral therapy, brief psychodynamic therapy, problem-solving therapy, life review, and validation therapy—have been found to be effective in treating late-life depression (Fiske et al., 2009). The efficacy of nonmedication interventions in this population is welcome news, because all older adults remain at risk of complications from polypharmacy. Prescribing medications for older adults can be complicated by compromised physical health and differences in drug metabolization due to age or the risk of potential negative side effects less common in younger age groups. (For more details about nonmedication interventions, please see this chapter's Anxiety section.)

Although social isolation can contribute to depression in all age groups, this factor is a problem with particular prevalence and relevance in the older adult population. Some studies indicate that social isolation is the largest risk factor for depression in older adults (Cacioppo & Cacioppo, 2018) and therefore is of the utmost concern for those crafting policy and interventions for aging populations. Determining whether a patient is lonely or socially isolated is crucial to determining whether that individual is at risk for or suffering from depression. In addition to using the DSM-5 to identify social isolation in older adults (Cuncic, 2020), other diagnostic tools include the Mini Social Phobia Inventory and the Liebowitz Social Anxiety Scale (Cuncic, 2020). Events and conditions common to the life stage contribute to the increasing social isolation of many older adults. These include decreasing mobility and the death of family and lifelong friends, along with children and extended family moving and living far away.

Many places in the United States have taken seriously the necessity and importance of reducing the inappropriate institutionalization of older adults in nursing homes for financial and quality of life reasons. However, the emergence of programs that provide care in the older adult's homes (the "aging in place" model) has not offered an adequate solution to the problems of loneliness and isolation that many older adults experience as their community dwindles and their ability to get around independently wanes. An accurate identification of social isolation therefore helps a practitioner make preventive recommendations if depression is not present. Again, the interdisciplinary approach is critical. Identifying socially isolated older adults and referring them to caseworkers or community agencies who could work on relieving the problem can provide an easy and highly effective way to prevent depression from developing in this vulnerable population, whether the individual is institutionalized or at home.

Finally, a challenge in assessing and treating depression in older adults is a significant overlap in symptoms of depression with those of advancing dementia. These include the following:

- Changes in appetite, particularly loss of appetite
- Sleep/wake cycle dysregulation, including over- or under-sleeping and terminal or intermittent insomnia
- Apathy, withdrawal from familiar social activities and supports
- Lack of attention to hygiene
- Changes in motivation to attend to housekeeping and activities of daily living
- Increased confusion and diminished cognitive performance

If these symptoms are mistaken for depression when they actually result from cognitive decline, or vice versa, significantly inappropriate treatment can result. A misdiagnosis can end up either with a prescription for superfluous antidepressants and inappropriate safety planning in the former case or the failure to effectively address a treatable, reversible problem in the latter.

Differentiating the 4Ds—cognitive *d*ecline, *d*epression, *d*ementia, and *d*elirium—is challenging for all clinicians (Table 18.4). Several diagnostic clues can be used to guide the differential diagnosis of depression versus cognitive decline or dementia. For instance, if the patient or caregiver reports that these symptoms have developed gradually, over months or even years, the etiology may be more related to cognitive decline than clinical depression. Symptoms that develop more acutely, over a period of weeks, may be more indicative of depression. Patients suffering from depression tend to be more self-aware of impairments in memory, problem solving, and cognition and bring these to the attention of providers, recognizing them as concerns. Patients experiencing cognitive changes tend to be less self-aware and often fail to recognize these impairments themselves, pushing back on them when pointed out by caregivers or providers. A quick diagnostic experiment easily performed in a routine appointment is to ask the patient some basic memory or problem-solving questions. A patient who confabulates or reacts angrily to the cognitive challenge remains more likely to be experiencing cognitive decline than depression.

Even to the skilled interviewer, despite these general rules of thumb, depression can masquerade as early or moderate dementia and vice versa. As a result, a simple depression screening tool in the primary care or acute care setting does not always provide information enough to determine the full picture. Nonetheless, brief screening and identifying depressive symptoms are vital first steps in assessment. Interventions, including first-line antidepressant therapy and a recommendation for behavioral intervention, should be initiated at that time. However, at the 8- to 12-week follow-up, if no improvement is seen or worsening symptoms are in evidence, best practice recommends taking the next step of referring the patient to a more specialized clinician, a geriatric psychiatrist or neuropsychologist, who can complete a full and careful clinical screening to obtain an accurate diagnosis.

Selective serotonin reuptake inhibitors (SSRIs) are the most appropriate initial treatment for depression when brief screening methods indicate a clinical concern. Common SSRIs include fluoxetine (Prozac), sertraline (Zoloft), citalopram (Celexa), escitalopram (Effexor), and paroxetine (Paxil). SSRIs generally are considered to be well tolerated in all age groups, but some specific concerns apply when prescribing them for older adults (Herron & Mitchell, 2018). There is a high incidence of polypharmacy in the older adult population, and drug interactions are an important consideration. Citalopram and escitalopram have the least likelihood of drug interactions (Herron & Mitchell, 2018) and therefore would be good choices when a patient already takes many other medications. Fluoxetine and paroxetine are more associated with drug interactions so may be more appropriate choices when a patient is not on many other medications.

When prescribing antidepressant medications, hyponatremia and a prolonged QT interval are two specific considerations to keep in mind. Almost all SSRIs are associated with a rare but potentially dangerous side effect of hyponatremia in the geriatric population. Increased risk comes with older age, female gender, and a history of hyponatremia. When SSRIs are prescribed to a patient already taking a diuretic, ongoing monitoring for hyponatremia is wise.

TABLE 18.4 Features of Depression, Delirium, and Dementia

Features	Depression	Delirium	Dementia
Onset	Weeks to months (rapid)	Hours to days (acute)	Months to years (slow, indefinite)
Duration	Short	Variable	Long/lifetime
Mood	Consistent	Labile	Fluctuation
Disabilities	Recognizes	New disabilities appear (acute)	May conceal deficits
Answers	"Don't know"	May be incoherent (acute)	Offers response but not correct, but may be close to correct
MMSE	Performance fluctuates	Acute fluctuations	Fairly stable with downward trajectory over time
Progression	Resolves with treatment	Resolves with treatment	Ongoing

MMSE, Mini mental status exam (http://www.nernc.org/psychMunse.asp).
From Insel, K. C., & Badger, T. A. (2002). Deciphering the 4 D's: Cognitive decline, delirium, depression, and dementia—a review. *Journal of Advanced Nursing, 38*(4), 360–368.

With regard to a prolonged QT interval, almost all psychotropic medications can result in prolongation, but citalopram and escitalopram in particular are associated with this concern. Therefore particular care should be used when prescribing these medications to cardiac patients (Herron & Mitchell, 2018). An initial baseline ECG and a follow-up ECG a few weeks after the initiation of therapy are useful in determining whether this effect is present.

Some evidence suggests that older adult populations take longer to achieve positive results with antidepressant treatment (Herron & Mitchell, 2018). So although evaluating results after 4 weeks may be sufficient for younger patients, in the case of older adults, waiting 6 to even 12 weeks may be more appropriate. If no significant improvement can be shown after the initiation of SSRI therapy, venlafaxine (Effexor) or mirtazapine (Remeron) should be considered. Venlafaxine has side effects of hypertension and increased risk of hyponatremia (Frank, 2014), which may be problematic in certain older adults, and mirtazapine can result in increased appetite and sedation. These qualities, however, may make the medication an attractive choice for patients for whom decreased appetite and insomnia are prominent features of depression.

A referral to a geriatric behavioral specialist is indicated, as mentioned, when a patient does not report an improvement after treatment with an antidepressant or if the symptoms worsen or there is an increase in behavioral agitation. Psychiatrists, psychologists, neuropsychologists, and licensed clinical social workers are among those who can conduct a more in-depth behavioral health screening and determine the best and most appropriate interventions. For patients who have failed first-line trials of antidepressant medication or patients with significant polypharmacy or many adverse medication reactions, a geriatric psychiatrist is the most appropriate referral. For more specificity in differentiating depression from dementia or other neurocognitive disorders, a geriatric psychiatrist or neuropsychologist would be the best choice. For clients who have complicated trauma histories or extensive mental health issues, a referral to a psychologist or licensed clinical social worker is appropriate, either with or without a psychiatrist referral, for a comprehensive behavioral health intervention.

Electroconvulsive therapy (ECT), although considered by some to be an outdated treatment, remains a clinically appropriate and sometimes lifesaving intervention for older adults with severe depression that fails to respond to medication interventions, especially those with psychotic features, catatonia, or failure to thrive (Snyder et al., 2017). ECT has been shown to be safe, well tolerated, and highly effective in geriatric populations with severe or life-threatening depression symptoms. Positive response rates range from 47% to 80% (Snyder et al., 2017). In all populations, ECT is associated with the risk of short-term memory loss. Research suggests this risk is perhaps more pronounced in older populations, but ECT is still clinically appropriate in cases of severe depression. In cases where ECT may be beneficial, a referral to a psychiatrist is the most appropriate initial intervention. The psychiatrist must be the one to coordinate and supervise the treatment. In sum, when properly diagnosed, depression in the older adult population can be adequately treated, simultaneously contributing to one's quality of life and care.

Anxiety

Anxiety and depression together are the most common mental health conditions encountered by medical professionals in the primary and acute care settings. Anxiety significant enough to register as a diagnosable behavioral health concern affects 10% to 20% of all older adults (Bassil et al., 2011). Anxiety is often comorbid with depression across all age groups, including the geriatric population. Like depression, anxiety significantly reduces quality of life but is responsive to treatment interventions, careful assessment, and prompt referrals. All of these result in good clinical outcomes. Stresses and challenges that accompany aging are all good reasons to be anxious. These include increasing health concerns, fear of falling, fear of becoming debilitated or of losing independence and autonomy, and memory problems. Many older adults dread losing their dignity, suffering extensively before dying, or running out of financial resources. Simultaneously, many also lose social supports that they may have relied on at earlier stages in their lives. Given this reality, it is not surprising that many older adults experience at least intermittent anxiety. Anxiety that persists for longer than 6 months or interferes with a patient's ability to function, however, can and should be treated. Symptoms of an anxiety disorder are as follows:

- Excessive worry or fear
- Withdrawal from normal or routine social situations
- Preoccupation with health and safety
- Racing heart, shallow breathing, chest pain, trembling, nausea, and sweating in the absence of a medical explanation
- Sleep disturbance
- Memory problems (Bassil et al., 2011)

More than with depression, older patients suffering from anxiety may not recognize their symptoms as anxiety or as out of the realm of normal. Some may have suffered from anxiety for most of their adult lives, and therefore the way they feel is normal for them. Wetherell et al. (2011) underscored this point in their discussion of general anxiety disorder (GAD) among older adults. They found that the condition often has persisted for 20 to 30 years. In addition, some seniors may not realize that their symptoms result from anxiety and, instead, may attribute them to their medical problems, not realizing that excessive concern and fixation on medical problems is itself a separate problem (Balsamo et al., 2018). Finally, as people age and their neuroplasticity declines, thinking can become increasingly concrete and rigid. One downstream effect of this cognitive rigidity is an inability to solve problems effectively or evaluate various possible outcomes, causing people to become more fearful and less able to manage their normal worries and concerns. Finally, insinuating that a patient is anxious when he or she is seeking excessive reassurance around medical concerns can seem dismissive or alienate patients. Consequently, helping older adults recognize their anxiety symptoms as a distinct and treatable condition sometimes can be a delicate challenge.

Thus anxiety, along with depression and other mental health issues, can be difficult to diagnose in the older adult patient. Often a great deal of overlap exists between the physical and cognitive symptoms of anxiety and those of other physical and medical conditions, as well as cognitive decline. Furthermore, because older persons frequently experience sleep disruption, insomnia is a less reliable symptom of anxiety than for younger populations (Balsamo et al., 2018). Another factor in diagnostic difficulty is what Lenze and Wetherell (2011, p. 301) have labeled the medical community's "treatment gap": "anxiety disorders in older adults [that] are rarely detected and essentially never correctly diagnosed." This results in a "de facto treatment algorithm" for older adults, which includes doing nothing, resorting to drug therapy, or treating solely with antidepressants. To address this gap in care the researchers have proposed the use of evidence-based psychotherapy, combined treatments, or collaborative care (i.e., an interdisciplinary team approach) (Lenze & Wetherell, 2011).

Tools that aim to evaluate anxiety specifically in geriatric populations have been developed and include the Geriatric Anxiety Inventory (GAI) (American Psychological Association, 2020), the Adult Manifest Anxiety Scale–elderly version (AMAS-E) (Roberts et al., 2016), and the Geriatric Anxiety Scale (GAS). If a primary or acute care setting does not have one of these validated tools available, a good place to start is simply to ask patients if they feel like they worry too much, worry more than most people, find it difficult to stop worrying, or if worrying interferes with their daily activities (Box 18.3). An affirmative response to any of these questions is enough to consider initiating treatment with an SSRI or to refer the patient to a behavioral health provider. Anxiety is slightly more challenging to treat with medication than is depression. In addition, some common medications used to treat anxiety effectively in young and middle-aged adults have significant drawbacks when used in older adult populations. (Refer back to Tables 18.1 to 18.3.) Although medication is absolutely an appropriate intervention for the older patient presenting with anxiety symptoms, practitioners often inappropriately prescribe anxiety medications, specifically benzodiazepines, despite treatment guidelines recommending against their use. One study indicated that despite older adults' elevated risk for negative side effects and poor outcomes of benzodiazepine therapy, nearly one in ten women over age 65 is prescribed a benzodiazepine, and over a third of those prescriptions are long term (Markota et al., 2016).

As drug therapy, benzodiazepines can be effective in relieving acute anxiety, but they also put older people at increased risk for memory impairment, gait disturbance, and falls. They are also particularly dangerous if mis- or overused and therefore are not ideal for patients who may have mild or moderate cognitive impairment and manage their own medications. When prescribed, they should be used with caution and only for short periods of time (1 or 2 weeks) to avoid these risks as well as the danger of dependence. In an overview of antianxiety medications in older adults, pharmacist M. D. Coggins (2017) wrote that benzodiazepines for "severe or debilitating" anxiety can be considered, but best practice would be to prescribe them for no longer than 4 to 6 weeks. In the same article, he noted that "a key to optimizing benzodiazepines is to ensure patients are not started on these medications if at all possible" (Coggins, 2017, p. 9).

Buspirone or SSRIs are considered the best choices to treat anxiety in older adults as they have fewer risks than benzodiazepines. Specifically, escitalopram (Lexapro) and sertraline (Zoloft) are generally well tolerated and have been shown to have beneficial effects in reducing anxiety symptoms in this population (Crocco et al., 2017). Current prescribing guidelines suggest starting at a very low dose, typically half the starting dose of a young adult, and increasing to therapeutic levels over 4 to 6 weeks to avoid increasing anxiety levels with the initiation of treatment.

Research also supports the idea that cognitive therapy and other behavioral interventions may actually be more effective than medication in managing anxiety in all populations, including older adults. For this reason, a recommendation to pursue cognitive behavioral therapy, either instead of or concurrently with medication interventions, remains a best practice (Fiske et al., 2009). Behavioral interventions, such as therapy with a psychologist or other licensed mental health professional, have no side effects or risk of drug interactions and may provide as much or more benefit to relieve acute anxiety. The question then arises, how do practitioners engage older patients with therapy? Many in this generation are uncomfortable sharing their problems with peers, let alone with a trained therapist whom they do not know very well. Several additional factors directly related to aging can affect the therapeutic environment. These include needing more time to process information, sensory deficits such as hearing loss, the stigma attached to therapy, and, at times, lack of transportation (Brenes et al., 2010). Like their younger cohorts, seniors have different personality types as well as likes and dislikes. As such, what works for one person may not work for another. Offering a variety of therapeutic methods increases the likelihood of older patients participating in therapy.

• BOX 18.3 Screening Questions to Assess Anxiety

1. Do you often feel nervous or anxious?
2. Do you feel like you worry too much or can't stop yourself from worrying?
3. Do you feel afraid, like something terrible might happen?
4. Do you think you worry more than you should or more than other people do?
5. Do you have anxious, nervous feelings most days of the week?

Normalizing anxiety, or any behavioral health concern, is an effective technique to help older adults consider a referral to a behavioral health provider. Mentioning that many older adults worry about things a great deal, or that many worriers find talking about it either in a group or individually helpful, can ease the stigma associated with mental health care somewhat, especially in a population where that stigma remains particularly strong. Group therapy in particular provides an effective intervention for anxiety. It helps to normalize the experience of anxiety and gives older adults needed peer support as well as psychoeducation and support from the group leader. Unfortunately, group therapy for older people is not always easy to find or utilize. Often, local area access points for the older adult, senior centers and visiting nurse agencies, may have that information available. Community geriatric social workers also serve as an invaluable resource for such referrals.

Other interventions, such as mindfulness training, are known to be effective in the older adult population. Some studies have found that mindfulness-based stress reduction (MBSR) training for older adults has the potential to relieve anxiety symptoms and to improve cognitive functioning (Lenze et al., 2014). Much research exists on the efficacy of introducing exercise interventions as a treatment for depressive and anxiety disorders, but little focuses specifically on the subgroups of older adults. Biblio and telephone therapy (BTT), a cognitive-behavioral treatment program for late-life anxiety disorders, has been used successfully to treat late-life anxiety. In BTT, written materials (bibliotherapy) were paired with telephone contact (Brenes et al., 2010). These two approaches allowed the sessions to be conducted in clients' homes, an especially needed technique during difficult times such as the COVID-19 global pandemic in 2020. Wetherell et al. (2011) have recommended acceptance and commitment therapy (ACT), a type of individual psychotherapy. This evidence-based treatment highlights the importance of acceptance as a process that facilitates psychological flexibility and provides a buffer against ineffectual coping. Worry and depression decreased with ACT. Their results point to the efficacy of treating older patients with ACT and other forms of one-on-one therapy (Wetherell et al., 2011).

In general, more research into all of these areas would benefit the field in order to continue improving the delivery of care to older adults experiencing anxiety.

Suicidality

In addition to depression and anxiety, suicide is a significant concern in every age category. Older adults are no exception. In fact, suicide rates in older adults are high and climbing. Of all demographics, older men have the highest rates of suicide completion and are at the highest risk for suicide in the United States and in almost all industrialized countries (Szanto et al., 2002). Many older adults suffering from depression, plagued by multiple medical problems, and experiencing loss of loved ones to death, come to view suicide as a way to end their suffering or relieve the burden on their caregivers. Screening for suicidality is important in the older population, especially because evidence demonstrates that appropriate mental health intervention can reduce suicide rates. A simple and easy way to do this is by asking a few key questions (Box 18.4).

• BOX 18.4 Brief Screening Questions for Suicide Risk Assessment

1. Have you had thoughts, either specific or general, about killing yourself?
2. Have you recently wished you were dead?
3. Do you feel like your family would be better off if you were dead?
4. Have you ever tried in the past to kill yourself?
5. If you were going to kill yourself, how might you do so?

Screening for depression in acute care and primary care settings always should be accompanied by a suicide risk assessment if a positive result is found on the depression screening. Even without a depression screen, however, many emergency departments and other acute care settings now have universal screening protocols for all patient visits, in light of research demonstrating that many individuals who go on to complete suicide have emergency department encounters within a week prior. However, subsequent research suggests that even with the presence and use of these protocols, suicide risk screening is less common in older adults than in younger cohorts. One large study across eight emergency departments in seven states found that despite a universal protocol for suicide risk screening, screening rates decreased with age, to a low of 68% of screenings completed on patients >85 years of age (Betz et al., 2016). Although at least part of this disparity likely can be explained by the decreased ability of older adult patients to participate in the screening (due to altered mental status or advanced cognitive impairment), this cannot account for all of it. At least part of the explanation also can be an inaccurate perception that older adults are unlikely, or less likely, to attempt suicide or a failure on the part of clinicians to consider depression or suicidality in older adult populations.

Underscreening for depression and suicidality in the older adult population is particularly concerning in light of the fact that the reality of suicide in this populations runs contrary to the perception. Furthermore, emerging evidence suggests that the suicide rate among the rapidly aging baby boom cohort, born approximately 1946 to 1964, is higher than that of previous age cohorts (Phillips, 2014). It also appears that older adults are more likely to plan suicides in advance, less likely to ask for help, and more likely to complete attempted suicides than are younger individuals. (Phillips, 2014). This combination of factors makes clear the importance of improving suicide screening in older adults yet also highlights the challenges of doing so.

As of this writing, more research needs to be done into the most effective ways to screen for and prevent suicides in older adults, particularly in light of the advancing aging of the baby boom generation. Currently, no validated suicide screening tools specific to older adult populations are available. Nonetheless, standard adult suicide risk assessments, such as the Columbia Suicide Risk Screening, have been found to be reliable in older adult populations. More research and the development of age-specific screening tools would be welcomed by clinicians in the field.

A persistent myth about suicide assessment is that asking patients directly if they are thinking about suicide can make them more likely to attempt suicide by putting the idea in their minds. This is quite untrue. The best way to evaluate whether someone is at risk of attempting suicide is to ask them if they have considered it. Several excellent, brief screening tools are available in the public domain such as the Ask Suicide-screening Questions (ASQ) toolkit provided by the National Institute of Mental health (National Institute of Mental Health, n.d.). Used mostly in primary care settings, the Patient Health Questionnaire (PHQ) offers another public-domain tool. This assessment has a two- and a nine-question version (PHQ-2 and PHQ-9). Both have been validated in adult populations for identifying at-risk patients. Another alternative is the Columbia Suicide Severity Rating Scale (C-SSRS), a more extensive screening tool popularly used in hospital settings, which comes in several versions (See the appendix for examples of all these tools.) Any positive response indicating suicidal ideation should be followed up carefully and immediately with further intervention.

One thing to keep in mind, however, when holding these conversations with older patients is that many more older adults have thoughts of death and dying than are actively suicidal or plan to act on an impulse to take their lives. Thinking about dying is quite normal in old age, particularly in the "old-old" subgroup, ages 85 and older. Death becomes a somewhat regular occurrence in the life of the majority of older adults, as their friends, family, and members of their community die around them. For many seniors, the fear of dying recedes. In fact, many older adults will openly say that they are ready to die or that they no longer are upset by or afraid of death. Therefore a practitioner must keep in mind the importance of neither over- nor underreacting when discussing death, dying, and suicidality with older adults. Instead, they must listen carefully for red flags that would indicate a patient is contemplating taking action to end his or her life, such as the following:

- A previous history of suicide attempts or family history of suicide
- Expressing hopelessness, helplessness, and lack of future orientation
- Asking direct questions about what kinds or combinations of medications would be lethal or other medical questions about death
- Describing a plan to hurt themselves
- Trying to say goodbye or thanking you for what you've done for them
- Precipitants or triggering events, significant losses, or new, frightening diagnoses
- Evidence of psychotic symptoms, especially command hallucinations

Practitioners who suspect a patient is thinking about harming him- or herself must ask pointed questions to determine the patient's plan, means, and intent. Have these patients thought about how they would kill themselves? If so, do they have the means easily accessible to them, especially firearms? Most important, do they intend to act on these thoughts? Although it is common for older people to think about dying and even occasionally have passive suicidal thoughts, if patients indicate that they have a well thought out plan, easily accessible means, or intend to harm themselves, this constitutes a behavioral health emergency. This patient should not be left alone. The medical staff member must ensure he or she gets safely to a setting where further behavioral health examination can occur. As with the other challenges facing this aging population, a proper diagnosis will save lives.

Chronic and Major Mental Illness

Caring for older adults who have a lifetime history of chronic, major mental illness such as schizophrenia and other thought disorders, bipolar disease, and personality disorders is an emerging challenge in the field. Improvements in medical care and community and living environments for the chronically mentally ill has resulted in this population living longer, but with more complex presentations than ever before. Medical providers encounter patients who have been on psychiatric medications for sometimes 50 years or more; who may still be taking older, less common medications that today's prescribers are less familiar with; or for whom medications have stopped working. Geriatric psychiatry is a highly specialized field with, unfortunately, a serious shortage of prescribers and other clinical professionals. Therefore the management and care of the older, chronically mentally ill adult often is left to general psychiatrists and primary care medical providers.

For a variety of reasons, the lack of clarity with regard to diagnosis is a huge barrier to effective care in this population. Inaccurate and inappropriate diagnoses often are written down at some point in time and follow patients from chart to chart, facility to facility, and provider to provider without investigation or update. This concern is especially an acute problem for clients who have few social supports and are living in nursing homes, group homes, or other residential settings. For example, the number of patients referred with diagnoses of bipolar disorder, but who are not on mood-stabilizing drugs, have no evidence of a history of mania, and for whom no one knows where the diagnosis originated is believed to be surprisingly and dismayingly high. Although a specific percentage is unknown, many researchers credit the overdiagnosis of schizophrenia and underdiagnosis of bipolar disorder in the United States until the 1980s as a primary reason for many older patients' records carrying forward the inaccurate diagnoses without substantiation (Umapathy et al., 2000). These historical deficits in mental health diagnosis and care, combined with the additional challenges presented by patients of advanced age, complicate vague, inaccurate, and unsupported diagnoses. Many "schizophrenic" older adults, upon further investigation, have no evidence of a lifetime psychotic disease or instead have bipolar disease, depression, personality disorder, or substance use disorder. Each is a specific mental health condition with distinct features, diagnostic criteria, and different treatment plans. The DSM-5 contains the gold-standard diagnoses for the characteristics of mental health disorders. Contributing to the stigma that negatively affects this population is the acceptance of a casual, unsupported diagnosis. It seems impossible to emphasize enough the importance of a careful and thorough assessment.

The initial diagnosis of schizophrenia, bipolar disease, schizoaffective disorder, or other thought disorders often are unlikely to be made late in the life course. A patient presenting with symptoms of one of these disorders for the first time after age 60, or reporting a history of being diagnosed with one of these disorders after age 60, is a diagnostic clue that their diagnosis may be inaccurate. Although not common in the general population, there are rare cases of a first episode of mania in late life or a brief psychotic disorder in later life (Singh, et al., 2015). Nonetheless, most of those late-life diagnoses are inaccurate. One of the strongest indicators that a patient's psychiatric symptoms are related to a major mental illness is a diagnosis before age 30. This consideration underscores the need for the medical and psychiatric history. In addition, many older adults experience psychotic symptoms or mania as a result of other neurocognitive disorders. The emergence of these symptoms late in life is an indication that a referral to neurology may be more appropriate than a referral to psychiatry.

Another rule of thumb for assessment is that patients manifesting visual hallucinations (VHs) are more likely to experience these due to organic causes (such as brain lesions or Parkinson disease) than patients experiencing auditory hallucinations (AHs). Auditory hallucinations, on the other hand, classically are associated with psychotic diseases. True visual hallucinations in schizophrenic and schizoaffective patients are relatively uncommon. These guidelines, by no means, are accurate in every case but can be used to generalize when assessing mental illness in older patients, especially because the risk of neurologic disease is elevated.

More than anything else, assessment and care for this specialized subpopulation of older adults with chronic major mental health history takes time. The pressure to see and treat patients quickly and meet productivity targets in medicine is an unavoidable, unfortunate reality of our current medical system. These patients, however, cannot appropriately be cared for without allowing extra time to collect as extensive a history as possible from the patient, collateral contacts, or, ideally, both. For instance, consider the patient with a diagnosis of schizophrenia, sent for evaluation from a nursing home, who has recently been eating and drinking poorly, has lost a great deal of weight, and is listless, apathetic, and withdrawn. After ruling out a medical explanation for the symptoms, a complete behavioral health investigation would include seeking answers to a number of questions. For example, where and when did the patient receive a diagnosis of schizophrenia, and has it been a lifelong concern? What clinical correlates confirmed it? Has this patient ever been psychiatrically hospitalized? How many times and for how long? What psychotic features have been observed, such as paranoia, delusions, or hallucinations? Are they historically present even when the patient is medication adherent? Is the patient refusing food and drink because of fears that he is being poisoned or because he is depressed and is passively suicidal? Has she ever made a suicidal statement, gesture, or attempt? What medications have been trialed and with what result? Is the patient refusing medications, or is he observed when he takes them? Is it possible she has stopped taking them and is hiding them from the nursing home staff? What procedure does the facility follow to ensure medication compliance? Has the patient ever tried an injectable medication or required medication over objection? What does this patient's baseline look like when he is feeling the most well? How is this patient's cognition, currently and at baseline?

Carefully collecting the answers to these questions, potentially to be provided to a psychiatrist and considered when making treatment decisions, provides the foundation of individualized, effective treatment, as opposed to generic, ineffective treatment. Unearthing many decades of psychiatric history from a mentally ill older adult cannot be done quickly and sometimes requires multiple sources of information, but it is the only way to provide the quality of care these patients deserve. Such investigations, lengthy and detailed as they are, highlight again the importance of a collaborative care model in practicing geriatric medicine. It is unlikely and unrealistic to expect that the primary or urgent care practitioner can reliably conduct these investigations, but a nurse case manager, social worker, or similar professional can. Regular interdisciplinary collaboration can paint a detailed picture resulting in the best and most appropriate care.

In addition to the challenges of assessment and diagnosis, a clear association has been made between chronic mental illness and chronic medical illness. Extensive evidence supports the hypothesis that patients who suffer from major mental illness are extremely likely to have comorbid medical problems as they age and are more likely to have chronic medical problems than their non–mentally ill counterparts. Some research even suggests that good mental health is actually a protective factor against developing chronic and acute health conditions as people age (Keyes, 2005). Part of this result likely stems from social and environmental factors and stigma. Mentally ill adults are more likely to live in poverty and less likely to have health insurance, may receive inadequate screening and treatment for health problems, or may neglect their physical heath as a result of symptoms of their mental illness (de Hert et al., 2011). Compliance with treatment plans may be compromised as well, especially for patients who live either alone or in living environments with inadequate support or supervision. Therefore caring for the chronically mentally ill older adult almost always requires a collaborative, integrated approach. In the best-case scenario, primary care providers in either chronic or acute settings always would refer these clients to a case manager, social worker, or integrated behavioral health provider in order to provide wraparound environmental and social support to improve medical outcomes.

The patient, unless legally determined otherwise, is always the expert and the authority on his or her health and should be treated as such. That said, the best care can be provided when trust and rapport develop with the patient such that he or she gives the medical provider permission to speak with collateral contacts who can shed additional light on his or her daily functioning, ability to manage his or her medications, treatment compliance, and so on. People with chronic mental illness vary widely in terms of their highest level of functioning, ranging from extremely capable on some occasions to nearly incapacitated on others. Collateral contacts may give the practitioner a more accurate sense of what the patient's level of functioning is at its low point, which the patient may not be able to accurately assess. This guides medical personnel's treatment and prescribing decisions, taking into account how the patient manages when he or she is not doing well. For example, when prescribing medications that require careful daily adherence and management to prevent negative outcomes, enlisting a visiting nurse service may be the best option, rather than relying on patient self-management.

Understanding a patient's relationship to medical providers, and attempting to repair it if needed, is probably one of the most effective strategies one can use to improve a patient's ability to manage his or her medical problems and follow a recommended treatment plan. A practitioner must remember that a trauma-informed, person-centered approach to mental health care (Box 18.5), although becoming more standard now, was not at all common even a few decades ago. Mentally ill older adults are likely to have had traumatic experiences with medical professionals and may be appropriately quite distrustful or afraid of doctors and other providers, nurses, medications, and treatments. The only effective strategy to make gains here is, again, taking time to build a relationship with patients and to understand their concerns about treatment plans or providers. The lived experiences and perspectives of mentally ill patients, especially those with severe mental illness, have historically been ignored, and these patients have often been mistreated by the larger medical system. It should therefore be no surprise that they might reject or ignore efforts to care for them. Providing quality care and treatment for this population is challenging and requires persistence and patience on the part of the medical providers who care for them.

Some chronic major mental illnesses have specific considerations as people age. As a general rule, long periods of nontreatment tend to make symptoms of mental illness worse and more treatment resistant. This is particularly true of psychosis. As a result, some people with chronic psychotic diseases who have been treatment nonadherent for long periods of time may not respond as well to treatment with antipsychotic drugs as will younger people with fewer episodes of prolonged psychosis. Many older adults with lifelong psychotic diseases may have residual symptoms, even when medication adherent, that cannot be treated with medication and only can be addressed by controlling the patient's environment or simply must be accepted as baseline. Long periods of psychosis also damage brain function, and as a result people with psychotic diseases are at significantly higher risk for dementia (Almeida et al., 2019). For individuals with these psychotic disorders, cognitive screening should be part of routine encounters with medical providers to monitor for cognitive decline. Managing comorbid psychotic disease and dementia is difficult. Almost all antipsychotic medications have black-box warnings for use in patients with dementia. Consequently, patients who have begun to experience cognitive decline or dementing processes should be referred to a psychiatrist, preferably a geriatric psychiatrist, for medication management.

Patients who have been taking antipsychotic medications for long periods of time, particularly first-generation antipsychotics, such as chlorpromazine (Thorazine), fluphenazine (Prolixin), haloperidol (Haldol), thioridazine (Mellaril), and trifluoperazine (Stelazine), are at risk of developing, or may have already developed, tardive dyskinesia (TD). This condition causes involuntary movements of the face, body, and limbs. The risk for developing TD increases the longer a patient has been taking these medicines. Patients on these drugs should be monitored at least once a year for involuntary movement using the Abnormal Involuntary Movement Scale (AIMS). The goal of regular screening for TD is to prevent it, because the condition can be irreversible once it occurs. The Food and Drug Administration (FDA) has approved two medications for the treatment of TD: valbenazine (Ingrezza) and deutetrabenazine (Austedo). Unfortunately, both have only limited efficacy. Suspicions about TD development

• BOX 18.5 What Is Trauma-Informed Care?

Trauma-informed care is essentially a philosophy of care provision that emphasizes the role of trauma in forming the reactions and behaviors of people who have suffered from it. It takes into account person-specific environmental and emotional triggers, then it seeks to provide care that is respectful of these triggers and avoids them to the extent possible.

Trauma-informed care is based on the understanding that many patients have suffered traumatic experiences and that the care provider is sensitive to and respectful of this possibility whether or not the provider knows about the trauma or is specifically addressing it. As a result of this understanding, providers treat all patients *as if* they have a trauma history and seek to create a care experience that takes this potential for previous adverse experiences into account.

warrant a swift consultation with psychiatry to consider medication changes. Of note, the first-generation antipsychotics work very well for some older adult patients. In those cases, the benefit of using these medications outweighs the risks of movement disorders. However, for the majority, the older medications should be changed. Newer antipsychotics, sometimes called atypical antipsychotics such as aripiprazole (Abilify), clozapine (Clozaril), ziprasidone (Geodon), risperidone (Risperdal), quetiapine (Seroquel), and olanzapine (Zyprexa), are less likely to cause extrapyramidal symptoms.

Although newer atypical antipsychotics can be helpful, switching to them does not insulate patients from TD and other negative side effects. Several of the atypical antipsychotics, in particular clozapine and olanzapine, have been shown to increase blood sugar and promote weight gain. Both side effects may make managing comorbid diabetes more difficult. All antipsychotics increase the risk of QT interval prolongation, creating a risk for life-threatening arrhythmia. Thioridazine and ziprasidone carry the highest risk of this complication and therefore should be used with caution in cardiac patients. Clozapine is known to cause neutropenia and agranulocytosis in some patients and requires at least monthly blood draws to monitor. All of the medications in this class have been shown to increase the risk of stroke, cardiac events, and sudden death in patients with dementia (Gareri et al., 2014). Thus, medication changes and management must be undertaken seriously and done with much care.

Bipolar disease also presents unique challenges in older adults. Many people diagnosed with bipolar illness as young adults have been very well managed on lithium for long periods of time—sometimes 30 years or longer. As they age, however, lithium sometimes becomes problematic. First, there is an elevated risk of lithium toxicity, drug interactions, and decreased renal function. Lithium dosing and monitoring must be managed extremely carefully as patients age (D'Souza et al., 2011). Interestingly, despite these concerns, some evidence shows that lithium actually has neuroprotective properties and reduces the risk of dementia (Shulman, 2010). More practically, little research has been conducted on other mood-stabilizing alternatives to lithium in this population because lithium is and has long been the first-line treatment choice for bipolar disorder (Shulman, 2010). As with most clinical considerations with older adults, consideration of the risk/benefit balance (and careful monitoring, of course) should guide treatment decisions.

Keeping a risk/benefit framework in mind, clozapine is a medication that older adults with chronic and serious mental illnesses may be taking. Practitioners rarely choose it as a first-line treatment because of its significant potential for adverse side effects. These include potentially fatal agranulocytosis, leukopenia, weight gain, and metabolic abnormalities. Rigid guidelines are in place for initiating clozapine therapy, including verification by the pharmacist of initial white blood count (WBC) of at least 3500, an absolute neutrophil count (ANC) of at least 2000 mm, and weekly monitoring of WBC and ANC for at least 6 months (Citrome & Volavka, 2002). Because of these prescribing and monitoring difficulties, it has been sometimes referred to as a "last resort" medication for patients with psychotic diseases. Risks aside, however, clozapine's effectiveness is undeniable, especially as it sometimes is the only effective medication for certain patients with schizophrenia, schizoaffective disorder, or other psychotic illnesses. Careful monitoring can mitigate its adverse consequences. For patients who have been well managed on clozapine, a practitioner must keep in mind that if a patient becomes medication noncompliant, clozapine cannot be restarted at the patient's previous maintenance dose. A break in treatment for more than 2 days requires that it be restarted carefully and titrated back up slowly to the previous therapeutic dose. Failing to do this can result in severe adverse consequences, including death. Ongoing management of this medication demands careful attention and close monitoring.

Manifestations of neurocognitive disorders (including all types of dementia, Parkinson disease, Huntington disease, amyotrophic lateral sclerosis, and others) constitute another category of concern with older adults and psychiatric symptoms. Much research indicates that patients who have preexisting chronic mental illnesses have a higher likelihood of developing these neurologic conditions. Untangling the etiology of psychiatric symptoms in patients with comorbid neurologic diseases is extremely difficult and sometimes impossible. Even in nondemented older people without neurologic disease, social isolation, sensory deficits (including hearing and vision loss), or polypharmacy may result in psychosis (Targum, 2001). Regardless of the etiology, the psychiatric symptoms resulting from these conditions sometimes require psychiatric intervention and management with similar medications to those that would be used in solely psychiatric illnesses.

In general, atypical antipsychotics are the preferred medications for managing psychosis in older people regardless of etiology, but their use should be conservative. Patients should be tapered off these medications once the desired benefit has been achieved. Current recommendations for targeting psychotic symptoms are to begin with very low doses and increase only until the target symptoms are reduced, then lower the dose every 3 months to ensure the treatment is still necessary (O'Connor, 2006). Research indicates that psychotic symptoms in older adults as a result of neurologic, sensory, or other organic problems do not generally require sustained treatment with antipsychotics. In fact, most states have regulations requiring that older patients in residential settings who are prescribed antipsychotic medications demonstrate attempts to reduce these medications within 6 months. These regulations exist because of the very real adverse effects of these medications on older patients. As previously mentioned, most antipsychotics have a "black box" warning for older patients with dementia. In practical terms, despite these negatives, these are the strategies in the current toolbox available to clinicians who need to treat these symptoms to relieve patient suffering and manage symptoms of psychosis. Therefore when necessary, they should be used cautiously and sparingly, and then discontinued as soon as possible.

A final note about the use of antipsychotic medication for psychiatric symptoms is that some specific cautions apply for patients with Parkinson disease. Haloperidol (Haldol) is contraindicated for use in Parkinson's disease, because it can dramatically worsen symptoms and can even precipitate death. Clozapine has been shown to have the most benefits without worsening Parkinson symptoms, but due to safety issues this medication is rarely and reluctantly prescribed. Most often, quetiapine, risperidone, and olanzapine are used. Newer medications such as pimavanserin (Nuplazid) are being developed specifically for use in Parkinson patients. Because common antipsychotic treatments can worsen parkinsonian symptoms, greater caution and monitoring are required when managing care for these patients (Yuan et al., 2017).

Patients suffering from psychotic disorders, such as schizophrenia and schizoaffective and mood disorders with psychotic symptoms, may not always be capable of making informed decisions about their health care because of their mental illness. These patients differ from those who suffer from cognitive impairment in the sense that their conditions are considered to be reversible—that is, with appropriate treatment they may regain the ability to appropriately manage their care. All states have legal ways to substitute judgment for these patients without having to petition for guardianship, as one would in the case of an irreversible cognitive impairment. These situations usually require a psychiatrist to begin the process of obtaining legal permission to administer medication or pursue other needed medical interventions. Some states have encouraged the creation of psychiatric advance directives, documents patients sign when they are well. The directive covers the times when patients may be unable to make decisions by outlining what care and treatment they want when impaired by their mental illness. These are not yet commonly used and are not offered in all states. When available, they are a useful tool that patients can use to specify what treatments they wish to be given to them during a psychiatric crisis.

Personality Disorders

In some ways, grouping personality disorders with chronic and severe mental illness seems strange, because personality disorders fall into a gray area of psychiatric practice. They more accurately can be understood not as illnesses, but as maladaptive variants of common character traits that significantly impair functioning over time. That said, however, there are people for whom characterological problems are so severe as to dramatically impact their functioning and ability to form and maintain relationships with other people across the life span. As they age, a common and unfortunate consequence is that they tend to have very few social supports, often having become estranged from or abandoned by their friends and family. This often results in these patients needing more time, attention, and energy from professionals, including paid caregivers and medical professionals. They can be difficult to manage. Some familiarity with the characteristics of personality-disordered individuals can be helpful for clinical staff; these can be found in the DSM-5. Unfortunately, the current understanding of the prognosis of entrenched personality disorder in late life is limited. Few personality disorders are considered responsive to treatment, and anecdotally some clinicians believe that narcissistic personality disorder can actually be made worse by attempting insight-oriented therapy or other behavioral health treatment interventions. Thus when caring for older personality-disordered patients, management, rather than treatment, is often the goal.

Cluster A personality disorders often also are referred to as the odd, eccentric cluster. These include paranoid, schizoid, and schizotypal personality disorders. Common features to this cluster are poor social skills and social withdrawal. These personality disorders are relatively rare (meaning all three disorders combined constitute less than 1% to 3% of the population) and all share patterns of disordered thinking, but they do not generally experience florid psychosis. For these patients, no interventions have been shown to be effective. Treatment with psychotropic medications is not indicated. Nonetheless, understanding that their social deficits, suspiciousness, and discomfort interacting with people are fixed and unlikely to change can help providers be more empathic when working with them, respect their limitations, and not challenge their disordered thoughts (as long as it is not necessary to do so for safety). Determining who carries a cluster A personality disorder diagnosis can be challenging, as these diagnoses are rarely recorded in medical charts or documentation. Generally, clients who seem avoidant, suspicious, eccentric, isolated or have bizarre beliefs and behaviors, without a history of a major mental illness or thought disorder, could be in this population. The key to working successfully with these patients is to be sensitive to their limitations and mindful that their interpersonal deficits are unlikely to improve. Respecting their limits and fixed beliefs is the best way to build trust and rapport.

Cluster B personality disorders sometimes also are referred to as the dramatic, emotional cluster. These are the most common types of personality disorder, affecting together an estimated 4% to 5% of the general population, and about 80% of all personality-disordered people. They include narcissistic, borderline, histrionic, and antisocial personality disorders. Managing these patients can be a challenge. They share a difficulty with both impulse control and emotional regulation and, in general, lack insight into the ways their behaviors affect others. They can often be perceived as sabotaging themselves by seeming to manufacture crises, ignore health advice, or act in ways that undermine their self-care and safety. In contrast to patients with cluster A disorders who tend to be socially isolated by choice, patients with cluster B disorders often become estranged from most or all of their social supports due to their behavior. Nonetheless, they continue to actively, and sometimes problematically, seek out social and emotional support.

The conventional wisdom used to be that there were no effective treatments for personality disorders and that people afflicted with them could never change. However, this idea has been challenged, particularly with regard to borderline personality disorder (BPD), for which several different treatment protocols have been developed with some success. Treatment for BPD in older age, however, has not been extensively studied. Antisocial and narcissistic personality disorders rarely respond to treatment, and research on effective, evidence-based interventions is scant. For patients with cluster B personality disorders, who can present as high-need, high-contact patients in frequent crisis, good professional boundaries are essential. High-quality, respectful care always should be provided with the understanding that these patients have little insight into how their behavior affects other people and therefore must be managed carefully to ensure they can maintain positive, long-term relationships with health care providers.

The final group, cluster C, is sometimes called the anxious, fearful cluster. This includes avoidant, dependent, and perfectionistic personality disorders. Like cluster A personality disorders, these are fairly uncommon, together accounting for perhaps 1% to 2% of the general population and maybe 10% of all people with personality disorders. These disorders share pathologic levels of anxiety that do not respond to any interventions and can present as requiring unusual and unsustainable levels of reassurance or contact with health care providers. As with many other personality disorders, there is little evidence demonstrating that these character profiles can be meaningfully changed. Therefore, again, maintaining firm, calm professional boundaries is essential. An interdisciplinary team approach benefits all patients who present with a suspected or previously diagnosed personality disorder (and who typically require frequent contact with health care professionals) because this approach can help prevent provider burnout by sharing the task of sometimes quite difficult patient management.

Older patients with a chronic, major mental illness such as schizophrenia and other thought disorders, bipolar disease, and personality disorders require extra care and concern because not enough is known about this cohort and these diagnoses. An interdisciplinary team approach with patients in each category provides the best option for assessment and treatment.

Substance Abuse

In a manner similar to younger populations, substance use disorders (SUD) with older adults complicates the context. Historically, there has been a perception that older adults do not have high rates of SUD. This belief possibly evolved as a result of the low proportion of older adults in substance abuse treatment settings or a failure to adequately screen and identify substance abuse disorders. Current epidemiologic evidence suggests that substance use disorders are underdiagnosed in the older adult population and are increasing as the baby boom generation enters older adulthood (Kuerbis et al., 2014). Multiple studies indicate that the greater use of both alcohol and nonprescribed illicit drugs in older age is increasing. The Healthy People 2020 initiative included this concern in its Mental Health and Mental Disorders objectives: "Increase the proportion of persons with co-occurring substance abuse and mental disorders who receive treatment for both disorders" (Office of Disease Prevention and Health Promotion, 2020). In light of these findings, a pressing need exists to develop more effective identification and treatment protocols for SUD in the older adult population.

SUDs have many faces. Alcohol use disorders (AUD) are the most common form of SUD with older patients (Kuerbis et al., 2014). Alcohol, legal and widely available, enjoys a high societal tolerance for its use. Many older adults have consumed alcohol their entire adult lives and do not consider it a concern, much less a "substance" they are or could be abusing. Excluding alcohol and considering only illicit drug use, marijuana is the most commonly used drug in the older adult population (Lloyd & Striley, 2018). As efforts to legalize medical and recreational marijuana make it more accessible to the general population in many states, the prevalence of its use can be expected to continue to increase. Beyond marijuana, the abuse of and dependence on opioid medications will continue to pose a high public health risk in all population age groups, including the older population. Older adults who are naïve about addiction remain at risk of developing opioid dependence from medications prescribed for new or deteriorating medical conditions. Furthermore, a downstream effect of the opiate crisis affecting all strata of American society is that adults already grappling with opiate dependence are aging into this group. Opiate dependence is emerging as a particularly difficult problem to address in rural populations (Grantmakers in Aging, 2017). Finally, as discussed earlier in this chapter, benzodiazepine use, abuse, and dependence are significant concerns in older adult populations, especially considering their increased vulnerability to adverse consequences when using these medications (Singh & Sarkar, 2016). Use and abuse of other illegal drugs, such as methamphetamine, cocaine, stimulants, and others, likely will exist in this population segment, but current research does not support significant concerns about them with seniors.

Turning first to consider the issue of alcohol use disorders (AUDs), one notes that all age populations have a high prevalence of AUD and SUD. Screening for these in the primary and acute care settings is important at any age, followed by referral to and availability of effective and appropriate treatment. There are, however, some age-cohort-specific issues to consider when identifying and treating AUD in older adults. Prominent among these are denial and fear of stigma. Research indicates older adults are more likely to have negative views of people who suffer from AUD and are less likely to identify as such or ask for help from health care providers (Dibartolo & Jarosinski, 2017). Additionally, the long-term effects of alcohol dependence, such as confusion, memory issues, gait disturbance, and vascular problems, may not raise red flags in medical settings but may be ascribed to aging itself (National Institute on Aging, 2017). Clinical correlates for alcohol use, abuse, or dependence may be misidentified as medical complications of advanced age, older adults may not be specifically screened for AUD, and older patients are relatively unlikely to identify the problem themselves, leaving AUD underrecognized, undiagnosed, and therefore not treated.

One reason older adults may not self-identify as having an AUD is that they genuinely do not realize that their drinking is unusual or problematic. It is well known to clinicians that as people age, their ability to metabolize alcohol changes, but this is not common knowledge in the patient population. When blood alcohol concentration is measured after drinking, older adults have higher readings than younger adults after consuming the same quantity. Consequently, adults drinking the same quantity as they always have can be at risk for significantly different consequences than when they were younger (National Institute on Aging, 2017). Because older adults may not understand this consideration of drinking in later life, they also may not realize they are at higher risk of problematic intoxication, balance problems and falls, and drug interactions or dependence.

Tools specific to screening for AUD in older adults have not been extensively developed or researched (Dibartolo & Jarosinski, 2017). Therefore screening tools validated for adults age 18+ are likely to be the best available choices for providers to incorporate into their practice. The two most common brief assessment tools by far are the AUDIT-C (National Institute on Drug Abuse, n.d.) and the CAGE-AID (National HIV Curriculum, n.d.). Both are three- or four-question screening tools in the public domain that have been extensively tested and validated for use with adult populations. The Centers for Medicare and Medicaid Services (CMS) have adopted the AUDIT-C as the validated screening tool of choice in hospitals for this purpose. In the absence of tools specific to older adults, either is a good choice to use when screening for AUD. The CAGE-AID has been adapted to include screening for drug use in addition to alcohol use. Given the increased risks of consuming alcohol at older ages, it makes sense for providers to counsel their patients and provide this information at routine patient encounters, even in the absence of a positive result for problem drinking. Older adults may be willing to moderate or reevaluate their drinking habits in response to education from medical providers.

Older adult patients should be provided the same treatment options for AUD, when available, as all adults. Community-based resources such as Alcoholics Anonymous (AA) or other peer-based support models, intensive outpatient programs, or individual substance abuse counseling are good choices for patients who are not alcohol dependent. A detox protocol is indicated for patients who are drinking at levels high enough to meet criteria for alcohol dependence. The criteria for diagnosing alcohol dependence can be found in the DSM-5. Although alcohol detox can be managed on either an inpatient or an outpatient basis, a benzodiazepine taper following a clinical regimen such as the CIWA-Ar is most frequently used (University of Maryland School of Medicine, n.d.). Health care providers must remember that complications of alcohol withdrawal such as confusion, hypertensive crisis, delirium tremens, and others are more common at older ages (Kraemer & Conigliaro, 1999). Therefore inpatient detox may be a safer and more appropriate choice for patients ages 65 and older.

Little research has been conducted on marijuana use by older adults beyond simply noting that use in older adult cohorts is prevalent and apparently increasing (Lloyd & Striley, 2018). Any existing age-specific research on marijuana abuse and treatment appears to be more focused on adolescents and young adults. That said, a small amount of research indicates that in older adult populations there may be some potential for drug-drug interactions in people using marijuana across all delivery methods. The recommendation is therefore to monitor the condition and lab results of older adults using marijuana, medically or recreationally, especially those with chronic kidney or liver conditions (Alsherbiny & Li, 2018).

Addressing opiate abuse and dependence in the older adult population is twofold: clinicians must provide appropriate care for adults with a history of opiate dependence at younger ages who age into the older adult population and for patients developing a problem with opiate dependence as a result of medications prescribed for chronic conditions and pain. Given the emphasis on reducing prescriptions for opiate medication at the policy and clinical levels, many patients find themselves in crisis when long-term opiate prescriptions are reduced or stopped. Providers often find managing these situations stressful.

A complete discussion of the opioid crisis, the management of chronic pain patients, and opioid dependence is outside the scope of this chapter, but with regard to opioid abuse and dependence in the older adult population, there are some key points to consider. First, practitioners must remember that many older patients who have become dependent on opioid medications do not realize it. They have been taking medications as prescribed, have never obtained "street" or illegal drugs, and only realize their dependence when prescriptions are reduced or eliminated. Unfortunately, many older adults who have been prescribed long-term opiate medications will require a detox protocol when reducing or eliminating these prescriptions. These patients must be treated sensitively and sympathetically, as their problem is iatrogenic. Opiate detox, like detox from alcohol, can be done in both inpatient and outpatient settings. Unfortunately, inpatient settings for treatment and recovery of opiate dependence rarely are designed for or appropriate for older adults.

In a similar way, benzodiazepine abuse and dependence often are not recognized by older patients or their caregivers and families. Despite the known risks and negative outcomes associated with the use of these medications in older adults, rates of their prescription are higher in this age group than with any other age (Coggins, 2017). As with opioid medications, patients may not realize these medications are problematic until they recognize that they are using them more frequently, running out before their prescription refills, and experiencing withdrawal symptoms when they do not have access to these medications. Withdrawal from benzodiazepines can be potentially life threatening and, as with alcohol, may be best managed in inpatient settings for older patients with other medical problems.

A major barrier to appropriate substance abuse treatment for older adults is the unfortunate lack of age-specific treatment options. Older adults may feel out of place or uncomfortable in substance abuse treatment programs designed for and populated by younger adults. Often these programs are not designed to support older adults with their more complicated medical profiles or support needs. Older adults are less likely to have legal problems or abuse "street" drugs like heroin, methamphetamine, and cocaine. They are more likely to be abusing or dependent on prescribed drugs, and group treatment may feel like an extremely unfamiliar and uncomfortable treatment modality, especially when they have little in common with the younger participants. There is a significant lack of research and resources targeting substance abuse treatment and recovery specifically for older adults. Much work is needed to address these emerging challenges in this vulnerable population.

Key Points

- The assessment and diagnosis of behavioral health concerns in older adults are challenging issues. An accurate differential diagnosis remains essential to providing appropriate care. The appropriate assessment of older adults to accurately diagnose and treat new or chronic mental health concerns takes significant time and effort to complete.
- Polypharmacy, metabolic changes in later life, and comorbid medical conditions make the management of psychotropic medications in this population challenging, and it requires careful ongoing monitoring.
- Research into best practices for mental health treatment specific to this age cohort is lacking. More work needs to be done to identify effective interventions for older adults, specifically with regard to substance abuse.
- An integrated approach is essential to providing high-quality, coordinated care.

More information about tools and Interprofessional Education Collaborative (IPEC) competencies mentioned in this chapter can be found in Appendix 1: Tools and Appendix 2: IPEC Competencies.

References

Almeida, O., Ford, A., Hankey, G., Yeap, B., Golledge, J., & Flicker, L. (2019). Risk of dementia associated with psychotic disorders in later life: The health in men study (HIMS). *Psychological Medicine, 49*(2), 232–242. https://doi.org/10.1017/S003329171800065X.

Alexopoulos, G. S., Abrams, R. C., Young, R. C., & Shamoian, C. A. (1988). Cornell scale for depression in dementia. *Biological psychiatry, 23*(3), 271–284.

Alsherbiny, M., & Li, C. (2018). Medicinal cannabis—Potential drug interactions. *Medicines, 6*(1), 3. https://doi.org/10.3390/medicines6010003.

American Academy of Physician Assistants (AAPA). (n.d.). *Vision statement*, About section. https://www.aapa.org/about/.

American Association of Nurse Practitioners. (2020). *Team-based care*. https://www.aanp.org/advocacy/advocacy-resource/position-statements/team-based-care.

American Psychiatric Association. (2013). *Diagnostic and statistical manual of mental disorders* (5th ed.). https://doi.org/10.1176/appi.books.9780890425596.

American Psychological Association, & Presidential Task Force on Integrated Care for an Aging Population. (2008). *Blueprint for change: Achieving integrated health care for an aging population*. American Psychological Association. https://www.apa.org/pi/aging/programs/integrated/integrated-healthcare-report.pdf.

American Psychological Association. (2014, January). Guidelines for psychological practice with older adults. *American Psychologist, 69*(1), 34–65. https://doi.org/10.1037/a0035063.

American Psychological Association. (2020, June). *Geriatric anxiety inventory (GAI)*. https://www.apa.org/pi/about/publications/caregivers/practice-settings/assessment/tools/geriatric-anxiety.

Balsamo, M., Cataldi, F., Carlucci, L., & Fairfield, B. (2018). Assessment of anxiety in older adults: A review of self-report measures. *Clinical Interventions in Aging, 13*, 573–593. https://doi.org/10.2147/CIA.S114100.

Basil, N., Ghandour, A., & Grossberg, G. (2011). How anxiety presents differently in older adults. *Current Psychiatry, 10*(3), 65–72.

Beck, A. T., Ward, C., Mendelson, M., Mock, J., & Erbaugh, J. J. A. G. P. (1961). Beck depression inventory (BDI). *Arch gen psychiatry, 4*(6), 561–571.

Betz, M. E., Arias, S. A., Segal, D. L., Miller, I., Camargo, C. A., Jr., & Boudreaux, E. D. (2016). Screening for suicidal thoughts and behaviors among older patients visiting the emergency department. *Journal of the American Geriatric Society, 64*(10), e72–e77. https://doi.org/10.1111/jgs.14529.

Blanchflower, D. G., & Oswald, A. J. (2008). Is well-being U-shaped over the life cycle. *Social Science & Medicine, 66*(8), 1733–1749. https://doi.org/10.1016/j.socscimed.2008.01.030.

Blazer, D. G. (2003). Depression in late life: Review and commentary. *The Journals of Gerontology. Series A, Biological Sciences and Medical*

Sciences, 58(3), 249–265. https://doi.org/10.1093/gerona/58.3.m249.

Borson, S. (n.d.). Standardized Mini-Cog© Instrument [Measurement Instrument]. http://mini-cog.com/wp-content/uploads/2018/03/Standardized-English-Mini-Cog-1-19-16-EN_v1-low-1.pdf.

Brenes, G. A., McCall, W. V., Williamson, J. D., & Stanley, M. A. (2010). Feasibility and acceptability of bibliotherapy and telephone sessions for the treatment of late-life anxiety disorders. *Clinical Gerontologist, 33*(1), 62–68.

Cacioppo, J. T., & Cacioppo, S. (2018). The growing problem of loneliness. *Lancet, 391*(10119), 426. https://doi.org/10.1016/S0140-6736(18)30142-9.

Chang, Y. Y., Gou, D. W., & Hwang, C. C. (2006). Depression in the elderly. *Long-Term Care Magazine, 10*, 207–215.

Citrome, L., & Volavka, J. (2002). Optimal dosing of atypical antipsychotics in adults: A review of the current evidence. *Harvard Review of Psychiatry, 10*(5), 280–291. https://doi.org/10.1080/10673220216279.

Coggins, M. D. (2017). Medication monitor: Antianxiety medications. *Today's Geriatric Medicine, 10*(2), 9.

Conner, K. O., Copeland, V. C., Grote, N. K., Koeske, G., Rosen, D., Reynolds, C. F., & Brown, C. (2010). Mental health treatment seeking among older adults with depression: The impact of stigma and race. *American Journal of Geriatric Psychiatry, 18*(6), 531–543. https://doi.org/10.1097/JGP.0b013e3181cc0366.

Crocco, E. A., Jaramillo, S., Cruz-Ortiz, C., & Camfield, K. (2017). Pharmacological management of anxiety disorders in the elderly. *Current Treatment Options in Psychiatry, 4*(1), 33–46. https://doi.org/10.1007/s40501-017-0102-4.

Cuijpers, P., Dekker, J., Noteboom, A., Smits, N., & Peen, J. (2007). Sensitivity and specificity of the Major Depression Inventory in outpatients. *BMC Psychiatry, 7*(1), 1–6.

Cuncic, A. (2020). *Symptoms and diagnosis of social anxiety*. Very Well Health website. https://www.verywellmind.com/social-anxiety-disorder-symptoms-and-diagnosis-4157219.

de Hert, M., Correll, C. U., Bobes, J., Cetkovich-Bakmas, M., Cohen, D., Asai, I., Detraux, J., Gautam, S., Möller, H. J., Ndetei, D. M., Newcomer, J. W., Uwakwe, R., & Leucht, S. (2011). Physical illness in patients with severe mental disorders. I. Prevalence, impact of medications and disparities in health care. *World Psychiatry: Official Journal of the World Psychiatric Association (WPA), 10*(1), 52–77. https://doi.org/10.1002/j.2051-5545.2011.tb00014.x.

de Stampa, M., Vedel, I., Trouvé, H., Ankri, J., Saint Jean, O., & Somme, D. (2014). Multidisciplinary teams of case managers in the implementation of an innovative integrated services delivery for the elderly in France. *BMC Health Services Research, 14*, 159. https://doi.org/10.1186/1472-6963-14-159.

Dibartolo, M. C., & Jarosinski, J. M. (2017). Alcohol use disorder in older adults: Challenges in assessment and treatment. *Issues in Mental Health Nursing, 38*(1), 25–32. https://doi.org/10.1080/01612840.2016.1257076.

D'Souza, R., Rajj, T. K., Mulsant, B. H., & Pollock, B. G. (2011). Use of lithium in the treatment of bipolar disorder in late life. *Current Psychiatry Reports, 13*(6), 488–492. https://doi.org/10.1007/s11920-011-0228-9.

Edelstein, B., Woodhead, E. L., Segal, D. L., Heisel, M. J., Emily, H., Bower, E. H., Lowery, A. J., & Stoner, S. A. (2008). Older adult psychological assessment: Current instrument status and related considerations. *Clinical Gerontologist, 31*(3). https://uccs.edu/Documents/dsegal/Older-adult-psychological-assessment-CG-2008.pdf.

Edlund, B. J. (2007). Pharmacotherapy in older adults: a clinician's challenge. *Journal of gerontological nursing, 33*(7), 3.

Fiske, A., Wetherell, J. L., & Gatz, M. (2009). Depression in older adults. *Annual Review of Clinical Psychology, 5*, 363–389. https://doi.org/10.1146/annurev.clinpsy.032408.153621.

Frank, C. (2014). Pharmacologic treatment of depression in the elderly. *Canadian Family Physician [Medecin de Famille Canadien], 60*(2), 121–126.

Gareri, P., Segura-Garcia, C., Manfredi, V. G., Bruni, A., Ciambrone, P., Cerminara, G., De Sarro, G., & De Fazio, P. (2014). Use of atypical antipsychotics in the elderly: A clinical review. *Clinical Interventions in Aging, 9*, 1363–1373. https://doi.org/10.2147/CIA.S63942.

Gbinigie, O. A., Ordóñez-Mena, J. M., Fanshawe, T. R., Plüddemann, A., & Heneghan, C. (2018). Diagnostic value of symptoms and signs for identifying urinary tract infection in older adult outpatients: Systematic review and meta-analysis. *Journal of Infection, 77*(5), 379–390. https://doi.org/10.1016/j.jinf.2018.06.012.

Grantmakers in Aging. (2017). *Heartache, pain and hope: Rural communities, older people, and the opioid crisis: An introduction for funders*. https://www.giaging.org/documents/170823_GIA_Rural_Opioid_Paper_FINAL_for_web.pdf.

Greenberg, S. (2019). The Geriatric Depression Scale (GDS). *Try This: Best Practices in Nursing Care to Older Adults, 4* https://hign.org/sites/default/files/2020-06/Try%20This%20General%20Assessment%204.pdf.

Hauviller, L., Eyvrard, F., Garnault, V., Rousseau, V., Molinier, L., Montastruc, J. L., & Bagheri, H. (2016). Hospital re-admission associated with adverse drug reactions in patients over the age of 65 years. *European Journal of Clinical Pharmacology, 72*(5), 631–639. https://doi.org/10.1007/s00228-016-2022-4.

Heart & Stroke Foundation of Canada. (n.d.). Mini Mental Status Exam (MMSE). https://www.heartandstroke.ca/-/media/pdf-files/canada/clinical-update/allen-huang-cognitive-screening-toolkit.ashx?la=en&hash=631B35521724C28268D0C2130D07A401E33CDBB0.

Heffernan, E., Coulson, N. S., Henshaw, H., Barry, J. G., & Ferguson, M. A. (2016). Understanding the psychosocial experiences of adults with mild-moderate hearing loss: An application of Leventhal's self-regulatory model. *International Journal of Audiology, 55*(Suppl. 3), S3–S12. https://doi.org/10.3109/14992027.2015.1117663.

Herron, J., & Mitchell, A. (2018). Depression and antidepressant prescribing in the elderly. *Prescriber: Journal of Prescribing and Medicines Management, 29*(3), 12–17. https://doi.org/10.1002/psb.1654.

Insel, K. C., & Badger, T. A. (2002). Deciphering the 4 D's: Cognitive decline, delirium, depression and dementia—A review. *Journal of Advanced Nursing, 38*(4), 360–368. https://doi.org/10.1046/j.1365-2648.2002.02196.x.

Jacobson, S. A., Pies, R. W., & Katz, I. R. (2007). *Clinical manual of geriatric psychopharmacology*. American Psychiatric Publishing, Inc.

Keita, G.P. (2011). Advancing health and well-being. *In the Public Interest blog* (American Psychological Association), *42* (10). https://www.apa.org/monitor/2011/11/itpi

Keyes, C. L. M. (2005). Chronic physical conditions and aging: Is mental health a potential protective factor? *Ageing International, 30*(1), 88–104. https://doi.org/10.1007/BF02681008.

Koenig, H. G., Meador, K. G., Cohen, H. J., & Blazer, D. G. (1988). Self-rated depression scales and screening for major depression in the older hospitalized patient with medical illness. *Journal of the American Geriatrics Society*, *36*(8), 699–706. https://doi.org/10.1111/j.1532-5415.1988.tb07171.xs.

Kraemer, K. L., Conigliaro, J., & Saitz, R. (1999). Managing alcohol withdrawal in the elderly. *Drugs & Aging*, *14*(6), 409–425. https://doi.org/10.2165/00002512-199914060-00002.

Kroenke, K., Spitzer, R. L., & Williams, J. B. W. (2003). The Patient Health Questionnaire-2: Validity of a Two-Item Depression Screener. *Medical Care*, *41*(11), 1284–1292. http://www.jstor.org/stable/3768417.

Kuerbis, A., Sacco, P., Blazer, D. G., & Moore, A. (2014). Substance abuse among older adults. *Clinics in Geriatric Medicine*, *30*(3), 629–654. https://doi.org/10.1016/j.cger.2014.04.008.

Lai, D. W. (2000). Measuring depression in Canada's elderly Chinese population: Use of a community screening instrument. *Canadian Journal of Psychiatry [Revue Canadienne de Psychiatrie]*, *45*(3), 279–284. https://doi.org/10.1177/070674370004500308.

Lenze, E. J., Hickman, S., Hershey, T., Wendelton, L., Ly, K., Dixon, D., Doré, P., & Wetherell, J. L. (2014). Mindfulness-based stress reduction for older adults with worry symptoms and co-occurring cognitive dysfunction. *International Journal of Geriatric Psychiatry*, *29*(10), 991–1000. https://doi.org/10.1002/gps.4086.

Lenze, E. J., & Wetherell, J. L. (2011). Anxiety disorders: New developments in old age. *American Journal of Geriatric Psychiatry*, *19*(4), 301–304.

Levine, D. (2018, June 15). Why mental illness is so hard to spot in seniors. *U.S. News & World Report*. https://health.usnews.com/health-care/patient-advice/articles/2018-06-15/why-mental-illness-is-so-hard-to-spot-in-seniors.

Lindsey, P. (2009). Psychotropic medication use among older adults: What all nurses need to know. *Journal of Geriatric Nursing*, *35*(9), 28–38. https://doi.org/10.3928/00989134-20090731-01.

Lloyd, S. L., & Striley, C. W. (2018). Marijuana use among adults 50 years or older in the 21st century. *Gerontology & Geriatric Medicine*, *4* https://doi.org/10.1177/2333721418781668. 2333721418781668.

Lutterman, T., Shaw, R., Fisher, W., & Manderscheid, R. (2017). *Trend in psychiatric inpatient capacity, United States and each state, 1970 to 2014*. National Association of State Mental Health Directors. https://www.nasmhpd.org/sites/default/files/TACPaper.2.Psychiatric-Inpatient-Capacity_508C.pdf.

Markota, M., Rummans, T. A., Bostwick, J. M., & Lapid, M. I. (2016). Benzodiazepine use in older adults: Dangers, management, and alternative therapies. *Mayo Clinic Proceedings*, *91*(11), 1632–1639. https://doi.org/10.1016/j.mayocp.2016.07.024.

Maryland Department of Health. (n.d.). *Abnormal involuntary movement scale (AIMS)*. https://mmcp.health.maryland.gov/pap/docs/Abnormal%20Involuntary%20Movement%20Scale.pdf.

Mini-Cog©. (n.d.). Standardized Mini-Cog© Instrument. https://mini-cog.com/mini-cog-instrument/standardized-mini-cog-instrument/

Mion, L., Odegard, P. S., Resnick, B., Segal-Galan, F., & Geriatrics Interdisciplinary Advisory Group, American Geriatrics Society. (2006). Interdisciplinary care for older adults with complex needs: American Geriatrics Society position statement. *Journal of the American Geriatrics Society*, *54*(5), 849–852. https://doi.org/10.1111/j.1532-5415.2006.00707.x.

Morgan, B. D., White, D. M., & Wallace, A. X. (2005). Substance abuse in older adults. *Geropsychiatric and mental health nursing*, 193–212.

National HIV Curriculum. (n.d.). *CAGE-AID questionnaire*. https://www.hiv.uw.edu/page/substance-use/cage-aid.

National Institute of Mental Health. (n.d.). *Ask suicide-screening questions (ASQ) toolkit*. https://www.nimh.nih.gov/research/research-conducted-at-nimh/asq-toolkit-materials/index.shtml.

National Institute on Aging. (2017, May). *Facts about aging and alcohol*. US Department of Health and Human Services, National Institutes of Health. https://www.nia.nih.gov/health/facts-about-aging-and-alcohol.

National Institute on Drug Abuse. (n.d.). *Instrument: AUDIT-C questionnaire*. https://cde.drugabuse.gov/instrument/f229c68a-67ce-9a58-e040-bb89ad432be4.

Norman, M. A., Whooley, M. E., & Lee, K. (2004). Depression and other mental health issues. *Current geriatric diagnosis and treatment*, 100–113.

O'Connor, D. (2006). Psychotic symptoms in the elderly—Assessment and management. *Australian Family Physician*, *35*(3), 106–108. https://www.racgp.org.au/afpbackissues/2006/200603/200603oconnor.pdf.

Office of Disease Prevention and Health Promotion (ODPHDP). (2020). *Healthy People 2020 Initiative: Topics & objectives*. https://www.healthypeople.gov/2020/topics-objectives.

Phillips, J. (2014). A changing epidemiology of suicide? The influence of birth cohorts on suicide rates in the United States. *Social Science & Medicine*, *114*, 151–160. https://doi.org/10.1016/j.socscimed.2014.05.038.

Psychiatry DataBase. (n.d.). *Mental status exam (MSE)*. https://www.psychdb.com/teaching/mental-status-exam-mse.

Radloff, L. S. (1977). The Center for Epidemiology Studies Scale for Depression: A Self-Report depression scale for research in the general population. *Appl Psychol M.*, *3*, 383–401.

Roberts, M., Fletcher, R., & Merrick, P. (2016). Evaluation of the factor structure of the Adult Manifest Anxiety Scale--Elderly version (AMAS-E) in community dwelling older adult New Zealanders. *New Zealand Journal of Psychology* https://www.thefreelibrary.com/Evaluation+of+the+factor+structure+of+the+Adult+Manifest+Anxiety...-a0486712409.

Schottenfeld, L., Petersen, D., Peikes, D., Ricciardi, R., Burak, H., McNellis, R., & Genevro, J. (2016). *Creating patient-centered team-based primary care*. Agency for Healthcare Research and Quality, U.S. Department of Health and Human Services.

Shulman, K. I. (2010). Lithium for older adults with bipolar disorder: Should it still be considered a first line agent? *Drugs & Aging*, *27*(8), 607–615. https://doi.org/10.2165/11537700-000000000-00000.

Singh, P., Pandey, N., & Tiwari, S. (2015). Late life mania: A brief review. *Journal of Geriatric Mental Health*, *2*(2), 68–73. https://doi.org/10.4103/2348-9995.174269.

Singh, S., & Sarkar, S. (2016). Benzodiazepine abuse among the elderly. *Journal of Geriatric Mental Health*, *3*(2), 123–130. https://doi.org/10.4103/2348-9995.195605.

Smith, J. C. (2005). *Relaxation, meditation, and mindfulness: A mental health practitioner's guide to new and traditional approaches*. Springer Publishing Co.

Snyder, A., Venkatachalam, V., & Pandurangi, A. (2017). Electroconvulsive therapy in geriatric patients: A literature review and program report from Virginia Commonwealth University, Richmond, Virginia, USA. *Journal of Geriatric Mental Health*, *4*(2), 115–122. https://doi.org/10.4103/jgmh.jgmh_9_17.

Speer, D. C., & Schneider, M. G. (2006). Mental health needs of older adults and primary care: Opportunity for interdisciplinary geriatric team practice. *Clinical Psychology*, *10*(1), 85–101. https://doi.org/10.1093/clipsy.10.1.85.

Suicide Prevention Lifeline. (n.d.). *Columbia suicide severity rating scale*. https://suicidepreventionlifeline.org/wp-content/uploads/2016/

09/Suicide-Risk-Assessment-C-SSRS-Lifeline-Version2014.pdf#:~:text=Risk%20Assessment%20%28Lifeline%20crisis%20center%20version%29%20Columbia-Suicide%20Severity,public%20health%20initiative%20involving%20the%20assessment%20of%20suicidality

Szanto, K., Gildengers, A., Mulsant, B. H., Brown, G., Alexopolous, G. S., & Reynolds, C. F., 3rd (2002). Identification of suicidal ideation and prevention of suicidal behavior in the elderly. *Drugs & Aging, 19*(1), 11–24. https://doi.org/10.2165/00002512-200219010-00002.

Tanaka, M. (2003). Multidisciplinary team approach for elderly patients. *Geriatrics and Gerontology, 3*(2), 69–72.

Targum, S. D. (2001). Treating psychotic symptoms in elderly patients. *Primary Care Companion to the Journal of Clinical Psychiatry, 3*(4), 156–163. https://doi.org/10.4088/pcc.v03n0402.

Taylor, S. (2011, December 10). Happiness in old age: Why are those over 70s so happy? *Psychology Today* https://www.psychologytoday.com/us/blog/out-the-darkness/201112/happiness-in-old-age-why-are-those-over-70s-so-happy.

Umapathy, C., Mulsant, B. H., & Pollock, B. G. (2000). Bipolar disorder in the elderly. *Psychiatric Annals, 30*(7), 473–480. https://doi.org/10.3928/0048-5713-20000701-08.

University of Maryland School of Medicine. (n.d.). *Clinical institute withdrawal assessment of alcohol scale, revised (CIWA-Ar)*. https://umem.org/files/uploads/1104212257_CIWA-Ar.pdf.

US Department of Veterans Affairs. (n.d.). *Montreal cognitive assessment (MoCA)*. https://www.parkinsons.va.gov/resources/MOCA-Test-English.pdf.

von Humboldt, S., & Leal, I. (2015). The old and the oldest-old: Do they have different perspectives on adjustment to aging? *International Journal of Gerontology, 9*(3), 150–160. https://doi.org/10.1016/j.ijge.2015.04.002.

Wetherell, J. L., Afari, N., Ayers, C. R., Stoddard, J. A., Ruberg, J., Sorrell, J. T., Liu, L., Petkus, A. J., Thorp, S. R., Kraft, A., & Patterson, T. L. (2011). Acceptance and commitment therapy for generalized anxiety disorder in older adults: A preliminary report. *Behavior Therapy, 42*(1), 127–134.

Wray, L. O., Mavandadi, S., Klaus, J. R., Tew, J. D., Jr., Oslin, D. W., & Sweet, R. A. (2012). The association between mental health and cognitive screening scores in older veterans. *American Journal of Geriatric Psychiatry: Official Journal of the American Association for Geriatric Psychiatry, 20*(3), 215–227. https://doi.org/10.1097/JGP.0b013e3182410cdb.

Yuan, M., Sperry, L., Malhado-Chang, N., Duffy, A., Wheelock, V., Farias, S., O'Connor, K., Olichney, J., Shalaie, K., & Zhang, L. (2017). Atypical antipsychotic therapy in Parkinson's disease psychosis: A retrospective study. *Brain and Behavior, 7*(6), e00639. https://doi.org/10.1002/brb3.639.

Zung, W. W. (1965). A self-rating depression scale. *Archives of General Psychiatry, 12*(1), 63–70.

19 Home Care

KRIS T. PYLES SWEET, DMSC, PA-C AND KATHY KEMLE, MS, PA-C, DFAAPA

OBJECTIVES

Student Learning Objectives

After completing this chapter, the student should be able to do the following:

1. Describe the changes in the health care system that have led to the proliferation of medical home visits.
2. Identify the unique approach to home care of those with serious or chronic illnesses.
3. Identify the reimbursement mechanisms of home care.

Practitioner Objectives

After completing this chapter, the practitioner should be able to do the following:

1. Apply evidence-based medicine to promote optimal outcomes for patients and caregivers in the home care setting while maintaining appropriate cost-effective allocation of resources.
2. Develop plans of care in collaboration with other health care professionals, patients, and caregivers that affect the patient's overall health and well-being, including behavioral health, family health and relationships, functional impairments, environmental adaptations, medication management, and health promotion.
3. Recognize and manage ethical issues that may arise in the home care setting, such as changing living arrangements, identifying appropriate decision makers, handling conflicts, and maintaining professional boundaries.

Introduction

Home care or house call practice refers to the provision of medical services in the home by a physician, nurse practitioner (NP), or physician assistant (PA) and is a growing component of care, especially in those with serious medical illnesses such as frail older adults. Usually, the patients have significant mobility impairment and cannot easily access an office. This chapter provides an overview of the history of house calls or home visits in the United States and how care is provided through home-based primary care for older adults.

Interprofessional Collaboration

Because house call patients have a complex set of medical, psychological, and social needs, there is a great need for interprofessional collaboration among practitioners from a number of disciplines, including nurses' aides, pharmacists, nurses, nurse practitioners, physician assistants, physical therapists, occupational therapists, speech therapists, and social workers. It is imperative that all understand their own roles and those of their colleagues. They must work together to promote interventions that are safe, timely, efficient, effective, and equitable for everyone.

Aides provide assistance with activities of daily living and are rich sources of information about the needs and abilities of the patient and family. They are instrumental to preserving mobility and preventing pressure wounds. Pharmacists can review medications and advise on combinations that may be ineffective or dangerous. Nurses provide a detailed review of the patient and the home environment, assess wellness, check on medication compliance, and offer other care. Nurse practitioners and physician assistants diagnose and manage illness, as they do in other settings. Physical therapists evaluate and treat musculoskeletal disorders and educate patients and others on the safe and appropriate use of assistance devices. Occupational therapists assist with splints and review the home environment for safety issues. Speech therapists help to evaluate for dysphagia and make suggestions about the food consistencies most appropriate for the patient's swallowing ability. Social workers can help patients and families identify and receive the benefits for which they are eligible and they may also help with advance directives.

History of Medical Home Visits

Medical home visits are those that occur in the patient's home for medical evaluation and management as part of ongoing care, episodic acute care, or postacute convalescence. They may be performed by physicians, but nurse practitioners and physician assistants occupy a growing niche in the provision of this model of care (Leff et al., 2015). A small number/percentage of providers today provide medical home visits or work in house call practices, but this can be expected to grow as population demand and technology combine to create an environment where home care becomes more necessary and accessible for older adults.

Prior to World War II, house calls were the usual mode of care, as physicians enjoyed better transportation than their

CASE STUDY 19.1

An 89-year-old man is referred to a home visit program after two falls at his home within 3 weeks of each other. He suffered minor injuries and has curtailed his usual daily activities to try to avoid any further falls. His initial lab work included a urinary analysis (UA), a complete blood count (CBC), an electrolyte panel, a test for renal and hepatic values, and normal HgbA1C. The CT brain scan done at the urgent care center is negative for pathology, but the referring provider is worried about his blood pressure (BP) of 168/98 and starts hydrochlorothiazide. The patient describes each fall as associated with arising from a chair and feeling slightly lightheaded. He is arising more slowly and is using a cane, which used to belong to his wife.

The evaluation reveals severe orthostatic hypotension with a standing BP of 92/64 and 120/80 supine. The patient's pulse remains in the 60s. He has poor balance, loss of proprioception, and mild cognitive impairment. His medications are metoprolol, 50 mg daily; hydrochlorothiazide, 25 mg daily; donepezil, 10 mg daily; saw palmetto; flaxseed oil; aspirin, 81 mg daily; acetaminophen, 500 mg q 4 hours PRN pain; and metformin 500 mg BID.

Further labs obtained reveal a serum B_{12} level of 101 (low), a vitamin D level of 10 (low), and a TSH level of 4.2 (normal).

Next Steps

The first step is for the practitioner to address medications that could be causing or contributing to the patient's condition. Metoprolol should be decreased because it is probably contributing to his decreased heart rate and may be causing cognitive impairment. He is also orthostatic, which may be causing some of his falls. Close monitoring of blood pressure and stopping the hydrochlorothiazide should be done next. Then, if bradycardia persists, the practitioner should consider stopping the donepezil. The patient's B_{12} deficiency may be related to his metformin and he may have hypoglycemia at times as a contributor. The practitioner should discontinue the metformin, as HgBA1C is normal, and monitor blood sugars. Two additional medication supplements should be ordered, 5000 micrograms of B_{12} orally, once daily, and D3 4000 units, once daily.

An order is placed for physical and occupational therapy to assess and arrange for the proper assistive device and to assess the patient's home for hazards. He is advised to begin an exercise and strengthening program including tai chi along with the physical therapy. Discussion and arrangements are made for the patient to receive a rapid alert device that he can use to summon help.

Two weeks later, the patient's BP is 110/70, and he has not fallen. At 1 month, he is gaining in strength and balance. Repeat mental status testing reveals a return to normal baseline cognition with a Mini-Mental State Examination (MMSE) score of 29 and a clock-drawing test. Six months later, he has not fallen and has resumed participating in local senior activities.

TABLE 19.1 House Call Competencies

Patient Care	Medical Knowledge	Interpersonal Skills	Professionalism
History and physical	Falls	End-of-life decisions	Medical ethics
Physical diagnosis	Functional assessment	Interdisciplinary teams	Understand shared humanity
Observational skills	Indicators of frailty	PA is guest in home	See patients as people experiencing illness
Medical, social environmental hazards	Effects of functional decline	Provide medical and Emotional support	
	Overall mortality		
	Determination of decision-making capacity		

From Hayashi, J., & Christmas, C. (2009). House calls and the ACGME competencies. *Teaching and Learning in Medicine, 21*(2):140–147. https://doi.org/10.1080/10401330902791115.

patients. Hospitals and other advanced care institutions were less accessible, and diagnostic tools were easily carried in the traditional "doctor's black bag." By 2001, less than 10% of US physicians made home visits, averaging five per week (DeCherrie, 2018). Perceived barriers that led to this decline include lack of opportunity, excessive costs with insufficient reimbursement under the fee-for-service payment system, inadequate time with the patient, concern about potential liability, excessive travel time and costs involved, and a general lack of training for health care providers on the management of complex diseases in the home. (See Table 19.1.) The rise of the hospital during the latter half of the 20th century as the center of the medical delivery system and the increasing concentration of technology that was housed at hospitals also served to further remove care from the home. Fragmented care led to poor control of chronic diseases, placing further strain on the system and on providers.

Why Did Home Care Return?

In 1996, there were only 984,000 home visits billed to the Center for Medicare and Medicaid Services (CMS) (Schuchman et al., 2018); however, by 2016, this trend

TABLE 19.2 Common Disorders in Homebound Elderly Persons

Often Multifactorial With Clusters Medical/Psychosocial Interactions	
Cardiac disease	Hypertension Coronary artery disease Congestive heart failure
Pulmonary	Chronic obstructive pulmonary disease (COPD) Pulmonary hypertension
Diabetes mellitus	Complications
Musculo-skeletal disorders	Osteoarthritis Spinal arthritis
Neurological	Stroke Dementia
Constitutional	Obesity Low body weight Generalized weakness
Chronic kidney disease	
Psychological	Schizophrenia Paranoid disorders Depression Substance abuse
Neoplasms	

From Oiu, W., Dean, M., Liu, T., George, L., et al. (2010). Physical and mental health of the homebound elderly: An overlooked population. *Journal of the American Geriatrics Society, 58*(12): 2433–2438.

had dramatically reversed, with 2.2 million house calls and 3.2 million visits in assisted living facilities (ALFs). The return of home visits was spurred by a number of factors, including the ever-growing population of individuals with functional impairments and multiple serious chronic illnesses (older adults and disabled younger individuals) (see Table 19.2 and Box 19.1 for common diagnoses of homebound patients enrolled in home-based primary care practices); the de-institutionalization of persons via the Federal Rebalancing program, which has realigned funding to move patients from institutions into home-based care; the ongoing fragmentation of families leading to a decline in social supports, as well as the availability of family members to provide transportation to appointments; and a change from a fee-for-service to more value-based system of reimbursement. The improved technology of portable electronic medical records and the availability of point-of-care testing (including handheld ultrasound, diagnostic studies, and the emergence of smartphones) has further stimulated this increase and can be expected to continue to do so. Liability concerns have proven to be unfounded with only two cases reported, one of which was dismissed (Schuchman et al., 2018).

• BOX 19.1 Common Disorders in Younger Homebound Individuals

- Depression/cognitive impairment
- Substance abuse
- Obesity
- Tobacco abuse
- Asthma
- Developmental disabilities

The Center for Medicare and Medicaid Services has encouraged more home visits by allowing more liberal patient qualifiers such as poor medication adherence, excessive emergency room or hospital use, frequent missed appointments, and a need to assess the home environment for safety. Poor medication adherence is defined as failure to comply with appropriate prescription use resulting in harm by an exacerbation of the disease process or medication side effects. Previously, qualifications required difficulty accessing appointments, which was defined as requiring the assistance of at least one person to allow for access to the office setting. It did not include the strict housebound requirement needed for home health agency services, which is defined as only leaving the home for occasional medical appointments/testing and attending religious services, as well as a "considerable and taxing effort" to leave the home (Center for Medicare Advocacy, 2013). In addition, providers had to document the reason a home visit was being done in lieu of an office visit on every medical record note, but as of January 2019, this last was no longer required.

The strongest incentive for growth in home care and house call practices has been the recognition of the immense benefits of home-based primary care for patients, providers, and the health care system. For patients, these are extensive and include improved function, hospital and emergency center avoidance with subsequently fewer nosocomial infections, less hospital-induced delirium and disability from disuse, and fewer iatrogenic disorders (Box 19.2). Home visits offer more person-centered care with improved satisfaction, better quality of life, better psychosocial support, improved symptom management, a more thorough assessment and management of geriatric syndromes, as well as the evaluation of hidden diagnoses. Problems may be identified and treatment initiated earlier, allowing patients to avoid more serious complications.

For caregivers, the benefits include improved emotional and social supports, education in care provision and expectations for their care recipient, improved rapport with the provider, and improved satisfaction with their caregiver role (Box 19.3).

Providers enjoy enhanced assessment of the patient and the patient's environment, better rapport (which often provides for a more relaxed and productive discussion of difficult subjects and decreases potential liability), less burnout, greater provider satisfaction, and excellent training opportunities for students of the health professions (Table 19.3). However, these providers also face stressors unique or more common to their practice, such as complex patients with

• BOX 19.2 Benefits of Home-Based Care for Patients

- Improved function
- Hospital and EC avoidance
  - Fewer nosocomial infections, iatrogenic complications
  - Less hospital-based disability and delirium
- Hidden diagnoses uncovered and treated
- Person centered care/higher satisfaction/improved quality of life
- Symptoms addressed
- Geriatric syndromes addressed
- Psychosocial support
- Earlier intervention to decrease adverse effects

• BOX 19.3 Benefits of Home-Based Primary Care for Caregivers

- Emotional/social support
- Education
- Rapport with provider
- Improved satisfaction with role

TABLE 19.3 Benefits of Home-Based Primary Care for Providers and the Health Care System

Providers	System
Enhanced assessment of patient/environment	Decreased overall costs
Improved rapport Difficult subject discussion Decreased potential liability	Fewer hospital admissions
Training opportunities	Fewer readmissions
	Decreased length of stay
	Decreased LTC stays
	Fewer EC visits
	Lower prescription drug costs

significant mental health issues, more complex patients with limited availability of diagnostic equipment, insect infestation, and concerns for personal safety (O'Brien, 2019).

Modern Home Care/House Call Practice

A key advantage of home care is being able to assess the patient as well as the patient's environment, which allows the provider to have more insight about how to better care for an older adult. Assessing transfer skills from couch to chair or mobility from one room to the next is helpful for determining a patient's ability to ambulate and function within her or his living environment. This information alone can aid in an accurate assessment of activities of daily living (ADLs). This, in turn, can help the practitioner to determine the correct durable medical equipment (DME) for the patient's needs within the environment. It also provides an opportunity to directly assess potential fall risks (Box 19.4). Because most falls occur while transferring and in areas frequented by patients, including the bathroom, this is a wonderful chance to evaluate the environment and common risks.

• BOX 19.4 Home Safety Fall Risks

- Lack of appropriate height/safety furnishings
- Unsecured throw rugs
- Poor lighting
- Inappropriate footwear
- Improper or broken assistive devices
- Clutter especially in "command centers"[a]
- Stairs with high risers
- Lack of handrails in bathroom
- Inappropriately low toilet seats
- Lack of handrails on stairs
- Inaccessible baths/showers
- Excessive height of kitchen counters

[a]Command centers are areas within a home where persons spend most of their time; they are frequently very cluttered.

Home care also provides the opportunity for the practitioner to observe interpersonal relationships never seen in the office. For example, one can see the caregiver directly providing hygienic care and transferring the loved one, and the health care provider can also inspect the refrigerator and kitchen for adequate and illness-appropriate foods. The provider then can determine if there is a need for and facilitate development of a support system for the homebound older adult based on observations and interactions witnessed over time in the person's home. In-home assessments can overcome environmental obstacles for family members to assist and alleviate potential problems while incorporating their values. One may also note if family members are willing or able to give care to an older adult. Many times these issues can be hidden in the office setting.

Caring for a complex patient outside of the office can prove difficult, but understanding the skills needed is crucial to a good outcome. Understanding components of a comprehensive assessment of systems as well as a review of the patient's medical and family history will aid in developing a complete picture. The nuances of specific exams, such as those required by neurology or orthopedics specialists, performed in the home setting can assist the practitioner in focusing on functional decline. In the neurologic and musculoskeletal examinations, paying attention to gait, observing the patient navigating in the home, and noting his or her ability to get in and out of bed or up from a favorite chair, as well as returning safely to it, are all essential to help the patient avoid falls. To perform the service well, a home care provider, similar to other primary care providers, must have a comprehensive knowledge of diseases and conditions that affect the older adult population. The ability to diagnose and manage common acute and chronic conditions leads to better care by avoiding potentially high-cost, high-risk environments such as the hospital or emergency room.

Polypharmacy is a common issue in older adults and can potentially be deadly. It is imperative that the PA or NP working in home care understand medication, its use, and interactions. A distinct advantage offered by a home care provider is the opportunity to see all of the medications that a patient has in the home, not just those the patient reports or brings to a medical appointment. In the home setting, a provider can see more fully what over-the-counter (OTC) products, including vitamins, supplements, and herbals, that a patient might be using, while assessing medication compliance. This is essential because OTC medications may interact with the patient's prescriptions or may actually precipitate symptoms, and they often go unreported in the office, hospital, or other traditional medical care setting. Knowledge of de-prescribing (discussed more fully in Chapter 7) can be advantageous in order to pinpoint a particular side effect or duplication of actions.

Functional decline and impairment are concerns for older adults and are usually the precipitators for the initiation of house call medicine. A myriad of medical disorders can result in functional decline and may trigger ancillary services providers, such as physical, occupational, and speech therapists, to become involved in the patient's care. Decline can affect other body systems, resulting in skin breakdown, wounds, falls, and overall frailty. Frailty is the number one cause of mortality in the United States for older adults.

Engaging the caregiver or family member, an essential part of house call medicine, requires a different set of skills than that needed in the office setting. It is imperative for the provider to understand the family dynamics within the home. Identifying which family members or others who reside in the same home as the patient and are, or are not, involved in the older adult patient's care is an important aspect of providing house call medicine. The caregiver's own limitations may affect his or her ability to care for the patient. For example, it is common for a small frail woman to care for a larger but less able spouse. The inability to move him safely can lead to injuries for the wife and complications for the patient as she struggles to provide his needed hygienic care. Awareness of community resources that will encourage family members/caregivers to care for themselves can make a difference in how they approach depression, stress, and burnout, which can easily result in premature long-term care placement or even abuse via neglect. This may include homemaker services, nursing assistants, and education in safe and effective care by home health nurses, as well as physical occupational, speech, and other therapists.

Stand-alone house call or home care practices are growing in both urban and rural areas to meet the needs of older adults and others with disabling conditions that limit their access to traditional office-based practices. A house call practice may also be an extension of an existing office or clinic-based practice. An often overlooked benefit for a mixed office and house call practice is improved efficiency in the office, as complex stretcher-bound patients require more staff time and decreased room turnover within the office. It also provides a way to retain patients within a practice that may also provide care for a spouse, child, or other family member of the home care patient.

Home-Based Primary Care Models

An appreciation of the benefits of home care for older adults led CMS to fund demonstration projects for new models of home-based care, as studies demonstrated substantial value in lowered costs coupled with high patient and caregiver satisfaction. Much of the savings were realized by avoiding unnecessary hospitalizations and by coordination of services. For example, Mary Naylor's program using nurse practitioners to provide comprehensive discharge planning along with home visits decreased health care costs by 50%, primarily by reducing 90- and 180-day readmissions. A study by Nabagiez et al. (2013), in a program that employed PAs in a home visit service postoperatively, demonstrated a 25% readmission rate in patients undergoing cardiac surgery with a 44% reduction in infection-related hospitalizations. The most common intervention was an adjustment of medications (90%) especially diuretics, antibiotics, and hypoglycemic agents, with other interventions being imaging studies (7%) and wound care (2%) (Nabagiez, 2013). A follow-up study looking at costs showed a savings of $937,500 over 2 years with a cost of $25,399. or a savings of $39 for each $1 spent (Nabagiez et al., 2016). The Veterans Administration Home Based Primary Care (VA HBPC) program, staffed by an interdisciplinary team of medical providers, mental health professionals, and others depending on the site, showed a 60% reduction in hospital days with the highest patient and caregiver satisfaction scores of any VA program (Schuchman, 2018).

In 2012, Independence at Home, a Center for Medicare and Medicaid Services demonstration project, was funded for 3 years, with participants eligible to receive 80% of shared savings after a minimum savings of 5 % was achieved. Programs were required to maintain established quality measures, which included follow-up within 48 hours of a hospitalization or emergency department (ED) visit, medication reconciliation, and yearly documentation of an advanced directive preference. This program produced a high level of satisfaction for both patients and caregivers. A mechanism for providing accessibility to care 24/7 was needed, and most programs had telephonic means to do this, usually staffed by nurses with backup available from a physician, physician assistant, or nurse practitioner. Each program enrolled 10,000 beneficiaries with two or more chronic conditions, two or more activities of daily living (ADL) deficiencies, and who had received hospital or postacute services in the prior year. Initial results were very promising, with successful programs saving $2000 per patient per year, mainly via reductions in hospitalizations, 30-day readmissions, and emergency room visits (Schuchman et al., 2018). Quality measure improvements were seen in posthospitalization follow-up within 48 hours of discharge, medication reconciliation, and advance care preference documentation. The most successful program was staffed entirely by nurse practitioners (Yao et al., 2017).

In May of 2019, an early follow-up report on the program did not show significant savings, perhaps because the study was underpowered to detect a difference in overall costs and there was an increase in the use of home health care agencies, which drove costs higher. Other concerns felt to contribute to these disappointing results included measuring effects, difficulty identifying the comparison groups, identifying savings compared with what group, the ability for the beneficiaries to elect to enter or disenroll from the program at any time, and difficulty identifying other programs utilizing incentive payments. Continuing positive reports include no difference in overall mortality, a tendency toward decreased expenditures in the last 3 months of life in program participants, and very high satisfaction in patients and their caregivers (Kimmey et al., 2019).

As of 2018, reimbursement for home-based primary care was 100% more than the 1997 rate (Schuchman et al., 2018). The VA has a hospital at home (HAH) program, and managed care corporations such as Optum Care Landmark and Clover Health have developed their own systems.

Home-Based Primary Care Programs

Staffing

Most programs include an interdisciplinary team with nurses, social workers, other allied health professionals, physicians, nurse practitioners, and physician assistants. Staff mixtures vary widely based on the program's mission and level/type of funding. Outside the VA program, no studies on optimal staffing have been published, so each program must determine its needs based on its own parameters. Many programs have multiple missions and even business plans incorporated into their structures.

Providers must have a combination of primary care, geriatrics, and palliative care skill sets to meet the needs of older adults in home-based care or house call program. They must be able to elicit and align patient goals with care, provide support for patient and caregiver access to needed services, assess and intervene in geriatric syndromes, and manage symptoms throughout the life span. Additionally, the home-based care or house call provider must learn to be comfortable in a setting where control lies with the patient or family and caregiver rather than in a health care environment, which favors control by the health care team. This is also an opportunity for the provider to assure the patient and caregivers that she or he respects their wishes regarding cleanliness, so providers should ask if they should remove their shoes, wear shoe covers or masks, and the like. Providers should place their home care bag on a clean surface or disposable garbage bag away from possible contamination by children or pets. They should wash their hands as they would for any encounter and before entering the bag for equipment, or they should use a hand sanitizer. Home visits truly represent patient-centered care and maximize self-empowerment by allowing dignity of choice.

Equipment: The House Call Black Bag

The bag must be organized so that "clean" and "used" supplies are stored separately. The bag and supplies should be cleaned with a hospital-grade disinfectant before and after visits. It should be placed in a clean plastic bag in the vehicle, out of sight and locked to prevent theft.

One should also carry an adequate supply of clean zippered plastic bags, plastic garbage bags, a sharps container, and disposable underpads. Personal protective equipment (gowns, gloves, masks, eye protection) should also be readily available. If the home environment is possibly contaminated, decisions regarding the equipment to take should be made prior to the visit and changes made as deemed appropriate.

Single-use items such as paper towels, disinfectant wipes, and dressing supplies should be placed in plastic bags and into the garbage with instructions to the patient to avoid opening them. Reusable items such as pulse oximeters, blood pressure cuffs, thermometers, oto-ophthalmoscopes, and ultrasound transducers should be cleaned with disinfectant wipes prior to returning them to the bag. All of the equipment should be thoroughly cleaned upon returning to the operational base.

The basic house call bag includes a pulse oximeter, sphygmomanometer with multiple cuff sizes, digital thermometer (oral or otoscopic), digital scales, stethoscope, oto-ophthalmoscope, vinyl gloves, hand sanitizer, disposable measuring tape, flashlight, batteries, biohazard bag, and possibly a vaginal speculum. Many providers also carry lab testing supplies with hemoccult cards, urine sample containers, bacterial culture swabs, and phlebotomy supplies. Items needed for minor procedures like bandage scissors, toenail clippers, small forceps, K-Y jelly, scalpels, suture kits, silver nitrate sticks, and ear curettes may also be useful. A wound care bag with saline, sterile gauze, Kerlix, Opsite, hydrogel ointment, elastic bandages, and abdominal pads is often recommended (Yang, 2019). Smartphones and Internet capability allow for more rapid management of unusual cases.

The "advanced" bag might include a portable ECG machine and a point-of-care ultrasound, which is useful for cardiac, lung, and anterior jugular views for jugular venous distension, bladder volume, and possibly deep vein thrombosis (DVT) assessment (Bonnel et al., 2019). Portable transducers allow for visualization of structures on phones or laptops/tablets. Challenges to use of ultrasound in the home include habitus and positioning challenges that lead to nondiagnostic studies, excessive gain (obscuring the image due to changes in tissue attenuation of the ultrasound beam) in study images, and differences in screen sizes (laptop versus smartphone); however, the authors concluded that home health ultrasound (HHUS) could decrease delays between data acquisition and clinical decision making (Bonnel et al., 2019). This is an evolving technology, so its full benefits and limitations have yet to be determined. It is now being used in evaluation of the pneumonia associated with the COVID 19 pandemic, so it may be used more often in the future.

Because of the severity of medical conditions managed in home-based care, mortality rates are high, so providers need to be skilled in end-of-life care or maintain close contacts with a community hospice. A 2017 study (Soones et al., 2017) found homebound status to be an independent risk factor for death, with half of community-dwelling Medicare beneficiaries being homebound in the year prior to their death, probably due to limited geographic mobility as a marker for frailty, which is overall the *most* common cause of death by percentage. Although there is no breakdown of the cause of mortality in homebound persons, as of 2017, heart disease was the most common in adults from 65 to 85 years old. Stroke was the fourth leading cause for both younger older adults and for the oldest old, those 85 and older. Alzheimer disease or other forms of dementia ranked number 5 in those over age 65 and number 3 in the over-85 group (Heron, 2019). Most patients enrolled in home-based primary care die at home (70%) versus the national average of about 33%, perhaps because their goals of care remain the primary focus and determinant of where care is rendered (Schuchman, 2018). However, many community dwellers may wish to pursue a palliative approach but are not yet eligible for hospice services. Because the prognosis in many terminal disorders can be difficult to predict and hospice requires an expected life expectancy of 6 months or less, some patients (especially those with uncertain diagnoses such as an ill-defined neoplasm) may not qualify for hospice. Patients may be referred to hospice for a trial if they do not decline, but they may be removed and reenrolled at another time. There is no penalty charged to health care providers for too-early referrals, but the hospice may be fined for an excess of patients who do not decline in the usual manner.

Home-based primary care programs are moving into palliative medicine, an area of workforce shortage, highlighting the need for NPs and PAs to be skilled in symptom and complex disease management. They can thus provide symptom relief for physical, psychological, and spiritual concerns.

Safety Concerns

Common concerns for home care providers include visiting in high-crime areas, the potential for weather-related issues, and traffic accidents. It should be remembered that crime can occur anywhere but that these concerns can be partially alleviated by visiting during daylight hours, using teams, training clinicians in defined de-escalation techniques, and providing an emergency panic button via a mobile application. Actually, more house call providers have been injured by environmental hazards and animals than as a result of crime. Further, it should be emphasized to all potential clients that team members do not carry drugs. Providers should remain attuned to the weather and avoid potentially dangerous storms. Traffic accidents can be monitored via mobile applications.

Infection Control

The increase in transmissible diseases, including the coronavirus, has placed a new emphasis on assuring the sanitary practice of home care medicine. Providers should be aware of the possible prevalence of infectious disease within their home community and take steps to mitigate transmission of potentially lethal pathogens to their clients. This begins in the preappointment phase during which time staff should ask about the history of tuberculosis and other diseases among household members so that they can inform the visiting clinician about needed precautionary equipment. Providers who are ill should avoid visiting until they are well. There should be clear policies regarding bedbugs and other illness vectors.

Characteristics of Staff

Physicians making home visits are concentrated in internal medicine, family medicine, and geriatrics, and they tend to bill for more office visits, certification/recertification for home health agencies, and other medical services in addition to house calls. In 2013 internists made 1,077,953 visits, family practice and general practice doctors together accounted for about 1 million, and geriatricians made 186,608. There was little change in the number of visits by these clinicians between 2012 and 2013 (Yao et al., 2017), whereas there has been a steady rise in the number of house call visits by NPs since 2008 (Fig. 19.1).

Nurse practitioners are in the vanguard of home care clinicians, providing the majority of nonpodiatry visits in residences and domiciliary facilities. One may speculate this may have to do with nursing roots and their experience in home health care. In 2013, approximately 3000 NPs made more than 1.1 million visits to Medicare fee-for-service beneficiaries, representing about 20% of all medical home care visits and providers. About 10% of the NPs who participated in home visits made more than 1000 visits yearly and tended to serve a larger geographic area than physicians working in home care (Yao et al., 2017). States that allow for greater autonomy have shown the largest growth in the participation of NPs in home care, but significant barriers remain (Box 19.5).

Physician assistants are much less involved in home visits, reflecting their strong ties to physicians and heavier concentration in surgical specialties. However, they too recorded an increase from 2012 to 2013 from 268,066 visits to 311,007 (Yao et al., 2017). PAs face more regulatory challenges than NPs in that some federal and state regulations limit their role as "dependent practitioners," whereas NPs are considered licensed independent practitioners in some areas. Changes in legislation/regulations recognize

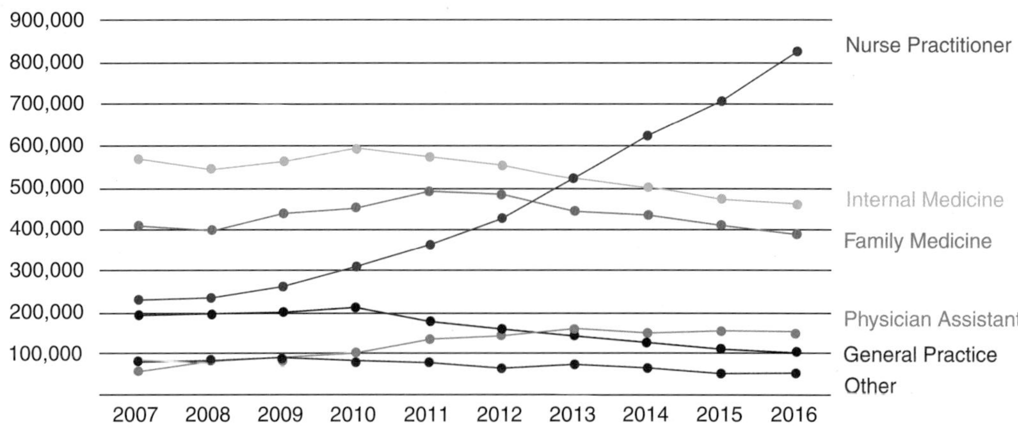

• **Fig. 19.1** House Call Visits by Provider Type. (From Kingan, M. J. Clinical news: Nurse practitioners bring back the house call. *Today's Geriatric Medicine, 11*[5], 6.)

• BOX 19.5 Barriers and Limitations of Home-Based Care

- Reduced access to high-tech diagnostic tests such as CT scans
- Limitations of community resources
- Low volume/high acuity of patients limits ability to cover costs.
- Fee for service/outdated care codes do not reflect complexity of case
- Lack of trained providers
- Regulatory and legislative barriers
- Fear of liability

the contributions of physician assistants in optimal team practice, but both types of providers face ongoing obstacles to their ability to provide care to their fullest scope of practice.

Rehabilitation specialists, particularly occupational therapists and physical therapists, are limited in their capacity to maximize function because of restrictions within traditional Medicare or even within managed care resulting from the expense associated with their services. Their utilization is also more targeted to episodic care or to the evaluation and management of a specific problem, such as fall reduction. Most HBCP rely on home health agency affiliations for this care.

Although many patients have high mental health and community resource needs, few house call programs can afford a social worker, so many partner with other agencies for these services. Pharmacists can assist with polypharmacy and in reducing complex medication lists, but like social workers, they cannot bill for their services, so most programs rely on community or hospital-based pharmacists where needed. Another means of accessing mental health and pharmacy expertise is via telehealth, a heavily relied upon and growing part of home care delivery.

The ability to order home health services, especially skilled nursing, as well as durable medical equipment is an indispensable component for the patient and family. There are specific codes and language involved in ordering them, so the clinician must be aware of needed documentation in the patient note to provide payment for these items. The practitioner should also be certain to respond promptly to requests from equipment and home health suppliers for information, so as to avoid unnecessary delays in the provision of needed devices and time constraints instituted by Medicare and other insurances.

Durable Medical Equipment

Durable medical equipment (DME) is any equipment used to augment the mobility and safety of the patient, inside and outside of the home. These items include, but are not limited to, a walker, a cane, a nebulizer, or a hospital bed; they may be covered by Medicare with limitations. Certain criteria for all DME orders need to include the name of beneficiary, the specific item ordered, the provider's National Provider Identification (NPI) number, the provider's signature, and the date of order (Medicare Learning Network, 2013). Practitioners need to be aware that Medicare defers to local agencies, known as Medicare local determination contractors, regarding criteria and the necessity of items being ordered to determine eligibility for payment (Mamuya et al., 2018).

Documentation of the need for DME is a critical step to secure much needed equipment for patients seen through house call practices. See Box 19.6 for examples of wording that can be used to request specific equipment commonly ordered for patients being cared for at home.

• BOX 19.6 Suggested Verbiage for Durable Medical Equipment

Face-to-Face Notes

All require diagnosis, height, and weight

Trapeze Bar

The patient is bed confined and needs a trapeze bar to sit up because of respiratory condition, to change body position for other medical reasons, or to get in and out of bed

Automatic Bath Lift

Has an inability to transfer to the bathtub or shower independently using assistive device (including but not limited to care, walker, bathtub rails)
Requires maximum assistance by the caregiver to transfer to the bathtub or shower
Has bathtub or shower that meets the manufacturer's recommended depth, width, and height for safe bath lift installation and operation

Toilet Grab Bars

The patient has decreased functional mobility and is unable to safely self-toilet or self-bathe without assistive equipment

Raised Toilet Seat

The patient has a medical condition that limits ability to ambulate to bathroom safely

Low Air Loss Mattress

Group 1 If patient is completely immobile; otherwise he or she must be partially immobile or have any single pressure wound on the trunk or pelvis and demonstrate one of the following conditions: impaired nutritional status, incontinence, altered sensory perception, or compromised circulatory status
Group 2 If patient has a stage II pressure wound on the trunk or pelvis, has been on a comprehensive sore treatment program including the use of a group 1 support surface for at least one month, has sores that have worsened or remained the same over the past month; also covered if patient has large or multiple stage III or IV wounds on the trunk or pelvis, or if he or she has had a recent myocutaneous flap or skin graft for a pressure sore on the trunk or pelvis and has been on a group 2 or 3 support surface

Power Wheelchair

Also needs right upper extremity (rue) and left upper extremity (lue) strength
The patient has a mobility limitation that significantly impairs his or her ability to participate in bathing, feeding, toileting, grooming, or dressing in customary locations in the home, which can be improved through the use of a powered wheelchair
The patient's mobility limitation cannot be sufficiently resolved by the use of a cane or walker
The patient's home has adequate access between rooms, maneuvering space, and surfaces for the use of the wheelchair
A cane or walker cannot meet this patient's mobility needs because
State primary reason
State secondary reason
The patient has not expressed an unwillingness to use the power wheelchair in the home
A manual wheelchair cannot meet the patient's needs due to the following:
State reason
A scooter cannot meet the patient's mobility needs due to the following:
The home is too small to accommodate a scooter
Patient is unable to transfer safely on/off without difficulty
Patient is unable to use handlebars on scooter
Patient is unable to maintain postural stability while on a scooter

Power Scooter

Requires RUE and LUE strength
The patient has a mobility limitation that significantly impairs his or her ability to participate in feeding, bathing, toileting, dressing, or grooming in the customary locations in the home, which can be improved with the use of a power scooter
The patient's mobility limitation cannot be sufficiently resolved through the use of a cane or walker
The patient's home has adequate access between rooms, maneuvering space, and surface for the use of the scooter
The patient has not expressed an unwillingness to use the power scooter that is provided in the home
The patient can safely self-propel the wheelchair or has a caregiver who is able to provide assistance
The patient has the physical and mental ability to safely operate the scooter in the home
A cane or walker cannot meet the patient's mobility needs due to the following:
State primary reason
State secondary reason
A manual wheelchair cannot meet the patient's mobility needs due to the following:
State primary reason
The patient is able to transfer on and off the scooter, maintain postural stability while in the scooter, and operate the handlebar tiller on the scooter

Reclining Wheelchair

Requires RUE and LUE strength
The patient cannot independently traverse from wheelchair to bed
The patient cannot weight shift independently
The patient has history of stage II pressure wounds
The patient is wheelchair bound
The patient has a mobility limitation that significantly impairs his or her ability to participate in feeding, bathing, toileting, dressing, or grooming in the customary locations in the home, which can be improved with the use of a manual wheelchair
The patient's mobility limitation cannot be sufficiently resolved by the use of a cane or walker.
The patient's home has adequate access between rooms, maneuvering space, and surface for the use of the wheelchair
The patient has not expressed an unwillingness to use the manual wheelchair in the home
The patient can safely self-propel the wheelchair or has a caregiver who is able to provide assistance
The patient requires a light weight wheelchair because the patient requires the reduced weight to self-propel

(Continued)

• BOX 19.6 Suggested Verbiage for Durable Medical Equipment—cont'd

Cane

The patient has a mobility limitation that significantly impairs his or her ability to participate in feeding, bathing, toileting, dressing, or grooming in the customary locations in the home, which can be improved with the use of a cane

A cane is medically necessary to prevent falling and improve ambulation

The patient is able to safely use the cane

Hospital Bed

The patient needs a semielectric hospital bed with a therapeutic mattress

The patient needs the head of the bed to be elevated to > 30 degrees most of the time due to the following:
State primary reason

The patient requires frequent changes in body position or has an immediate need for a change in body position
If wounds are an issue, describe wounds
Patient has multiple stage II, large stage III/stage IV wounds
Location, size, stage

Hoyer Lift

Patient's caregiver is expressing increased difficulty transferring the patient in and out of bed to wheelchair/chair; the patient would be bed confined without the use of a lift; will request a Hoyer lift to aid in transfer safety

Light-Weight Manual Wheelchair

Requires RUE and LUE strength

The patient has a mobility limitation that significantly impairs his or her ability to participate in feeding, bathing, toileting, dressing, or grooming in the customary locations in the home, which can be improved with the use of a manual wheelchair

The patient's mobility impairment cannot be sufficiently resolved with the use of a cane or walker

The patient's home has adequate access between rooms, maneuvering space, and surface for the use of the wheelchair

The patient has not expressed an unwillingness to use the manual wheelchair that is provided in the home

The patient can safely self-propel the wheelchair or has a caregiver who is able to provide assistance

The patient requires a light-weight wheelchair because he or she needs the reduced weight to self-propel

Rollator Walker

The patient has a mobility limitation that significantly impairs his or her ability in a mobility-related activity of daily living in the home

The patient is able to safely use the walker

The functional mobility deficit can be sufficiently resolved with the use of a walker

Seat Chair Lift

The patient has severe arthritis of the knees

The patient does not have a neuromuscular disease

The patient is completely incapable of standing from a regular armchair or any chair in his or her home

Once standing, the patient is able to ambulate

All appropriate therapeutic modalities to enable the patient to transfer from a chair to a standing position have been tried and failed

Nebulizer

Dx. J 44.9. Chronic obstructive pulmonary disease (COPD)

Nebulizer with tubing, filters, mouthpiece for administration of albuterol .083% vial every 4 hours and as needed for wheezing or asthma

Incontinence Supplies

Dx. R32. Incontinence

Knee Orthosis

The patient has lower-extremity weakness and had a trial of physical therapy; however, the patient continues to need the additional support for his or her joints to assist in transfers and decrease the potential for falls

The patient currently takes pain medication; the expectation is that the need for these would decrease with the use of a knee orthosis

Lumbar Orthosis

The lumbar orthosis is expected to reduce pain by restricting trunk movement

Due to the patient's diagnosis, he or she will benefit from supporting weakened spinal muscles or spinal deformities

Blood Pressure Machine

The patient requires an automated blood pressure machine, as he or she has a diagnosis of hypertension and must monitor blood pressure (BP) at home

An automated blood pressure machine is required, as the patient does not have a caregiver knowledgeable enough to take BP manually

Enteral Needs and Supplies

Dx. G 93.1. Gastrostomy tube present
R13.19. Dysphagia

Missions of Home-Based Primary Care (HBPC)

Missions are often based on the population served such as longitudinal primary care for home limited vulnerable patients, improved end-of-life care for the terminally ill, episodic visits for acute care patients to augment traditional primary care, patients in need of improved transitions of care, patients who need care for a particular disease like amyotrophic lateral sclerosis (ALS), home ventilator patients, and others; other missions are oriented toward those who dislike office-based care and are frequent users of the acute care system. Many HBPC practices have more than one mission or target population. Nearly all limit their services to a specific geographic area or to a limited population. Some programs assume all primary care, whereas others serve as complements to the patient's primary provider by offering enhanced or acute medical visits and assistance, social services, education for the patient and caregiver, or value-added technology, such as telehealth capability.

Business Plans of Home-Based Primary Care

There are several different business plans under which home-based primary care practices operate. These may be fee-for-service plans funded by Medicare, Medicaid, other insurers, or via private pay. They may be arranged via risk-sharing/value-based contracts or a combination of all of these. Many also incorporate philanthropic grants and may be partially supported by educational institutions.

Private pay models include so-called concierge practices, which typically enroll patients via a yearly fee, which provides 24/7 access to a physician or other clinician. The patient may also pay a fee for visits, on a sliding scale based on the day of the week or the time of day. In general, the concierge clinician cannot bill Medicare or Medicaid for this practice, so this option is generally limited to wealthier clients. Most limit their patient panels to a few thousand and report higher satisfaction with their work and private lives than do other physicians. On a charitable basis, many also see nonpanel patients who cannot afford their fees.

One of the more recent developments is direct primary care, in which a physician provides services on a per-member per-month basis with discounted fees for procedures, tests, and even pharmaceuticals. These providers do not file insurance, which reduces their overhead by allowing them to avoid hiring administrative personnel to file insurance claims. Monthly fees are typically much less than insurance and vary based on the cost of living in the geographic area. Usually the practice begins as a group of home visit clinicians, and as their panels increase, they transition to a small office practice. Practitioners enjoy the freedom to spend more time with each patient and focus on maintaining their health.

There are now a number of HBPC practices who partner with health plans and share risk for large numbers of lives; one example is Landmark Health, which covers 14 health plans in 13 states. They share the savings with their partners after quality metrics are met. They report a 30% to 40% reduction in hospital admissions with high patient satisfaction. Medicare Advantage plans like Optum Care and Clover Health provide 24/7 care via phone or video app (Berresford, 2020).

Other examples of this type of program are offered at Mount Sinai, Johns Hopkins, and Cleveland Clinic, all of which send paramedics to homes when the physician is unable to make an acute call. They communicate with the physician via skype regarding vital signs, medication review, and other aspects of the physical exam (Berresford, 2020).

The Future of Home-Based Care

There is a growing recognition that many serious illnesses can be safely managed in the home environment and indeed may have superior outcomes over those in the hospital. The home has other benefits for patients, such as fewer nosocomial infections, fewer iatrogenic outcomes (especially delirium), and less hospital-associated disability, which occurs when patients are confined to bed for prolonged periods. Although it is less well measured, there is probably also a component of psychological support from being at home, which aids in recovery.

Examples of illnesses that may require hospitalization but are often safely treated at home include pneumonia and deep venous thrombosis. The availability of home intravenous infusions for long-term antibiotics or other drugs has expanded our ability to provide hospital at home (HAH) services and can be expected to grow. The increase in cases of coronavirus with its contagious and potentially lethal nature has led to more use of telemedicine and telemonitoring to prevent close contacts of ill patients within hospitals. At the time of this writing there is not much known about the effectiveness of this practice.

There has been wide adoption of home care in other countries with single-payer systems, like the UK, which also has a long history of physician-led home visits. Countries that have embraced the use of physician associates in home care include Germany, Australia, and others. Early studies show excellent acceptance by patients and caregivers and no measured differences in the quality of care in patients seen for routine appointments. There is little or no evidence of a difference in quality between general practitioners and physician associates in acute care visits, nor in practice utilization patterns, probably because they have not yet been sufficiently studied (van den Berg et al., 2010).

Another government demonstration project, Primary Care First, which was slated to begin in January 2020 but was delayed, is believed to hold promise for further savings (Berresford, 2020). The project is only available in certain regions, primarily in the coastal states, and as of this writing the deadline to apply has passed. It emphasizes the doctor-patient relationship and care coordination to reduce overall costs and to target practices at multiple levels of readiness to assume risk. There are two options for providers. One provides for experienced primary care practices to assume responsibility for those Medicare patients who lack a primary care provider. The practice assumes financial risk for the patients in exchange for a reduced administrative burden and performance-based payments. The second option targets programs that include hospice and palliative medicine services and is designed for populations with serious illnesses (SIPs), incentivizing the practices to provide patient-centered care and to avoid high-cost areas of care, such as the emergency center and hospital. Nurse practitioners and physician assistants who are certified in internal or general medicine, family medicine, geriatric medicine, and hospice/palliative medicine are included as providers who are eligible to participate.

Increasing use of telehealth will allow for further expansion of services. Patient portals are increasingly being used to improve communication between patients and providers; however, little is known about their effectiveness in

CASE STUDY 19.2

A 69-year-old Hispanic male who was status post a recent cerebral vascular accident (CVA) with left-sided weakness was referred to a house call service upon discharge from rehabilitation. His medical history included seizures and neuropathy on the left side as residual effects of his last CVA, as well as muscle weakness, hypertension, hyperlipidemia, and acid reflux. There was no history of tobacco or alcohol use. The patient's family history was positive for hypertension (mother and brother) and CVA (father). His wife is now a fulltime caretaker because the patient is not able to turn over by himself.

Medication included gabapentin, levetiracetam, losartan, atorvastatin, and cyclobenzaprine. Hypertension had been diagnosed many years prior, but no specific date was available. The patient's first CVA was in 2014, but he was able to regain full-function status. Although this subsequent CVA was more painful and damaging, the patient's family expected him to recover fully. The most recent CVA left the patient with left-sided weakness and slight paralysis, but he was in stable condition with a good prognosis given the diligence of care provided by his wife.

Home health visits along with physical and speech therapy were ordered by the discharging provider and carried out in the home. The speech therapist ordered a swallow study that revealed negative issues with mastication and swallowing, and the patient was discharged from therapy fairly soon after returning home. The physical therapist visited in the patient's home for several months with good results, and physical therapy was then discontinued. Home health nursing services continued weekly to reduce any chance for readmission to hospital (Siclovan, 2018). Improvement continued while the patient's wife aided in-home exercises given by a therapist.

Progress was maintained, and the patient's wife was interested in discontinuing all in-home treatment. Because the patient recovered from the first CVA, the wife fully expected him to have the same results. The wife was informed of the benefit of continued house calls and other in-home services, and the patient was referred to a community primary care provider.

Several months later, the wife called the house call office requesting refills of medication. She explained she was unable to get her husband to an appointment due to her own physical disabilities and could not afford alternative transportation. An appointment was scheduled for immediate follow-up.

After his discharge from the house call service, the patient had another stroke. His wife took him to the ED without ongoing follow-up care. The patient was immediately added back to the house call service schedule for further care. The patient was found to be in worsening functional decline with increased difficulty swallowing. Home health, speech therapy, and physical therapy were ordered immediately; however, it soon became apparent that recovery was unlikely, and with the help of counseling by the house call provider, the wife decided to pursue hospice at home. The patient continued to be followed by both the house call service and hospice until his death at home. His wife expressed appreciation for the assistance of both teams, which allowed her to keep the patient at home, as had been his goal.

home-based primary care. One study conducted in 2014 found that VA-based HBPC recipients had limited knowledge of the portal, limited computer and Internet access, and high satisfaction with the value of surrogates acting as intermediaries, but they also had a desire to learn more about patient portal use, indicating a willingness to engage (Mishuris, 2014). This suggests that further growth in computer use and Internet access may be beneficial for the current cohort of patients. This may be particularly important for rural residents, who remained 78% less likely to receive home-based services than their metropolitan counterparts in 2014 (Yao et al., 2017). As younger generations who have more familiarity with telehealth age into disease and disability, it is likely that better acceptance will follow.

Summary

Home-based primary care holds great promise for patients and caregivers, health care providers, and the health care system to assure high-quality care at a lower cost for individuals with serious medical illnesses. Nurse practitioners and physician assistants are playing an increasing role in expanding access to care through home care and house call practices. The growing availability of the home-based medical practice is an absolutely essential component to addressing patient and family care needs in our currently overstressed medical care delivery system.

Key Points

- Home-based primary care is cost-effective, high-quality care that is being recognized as essential for the value-based system of care, emphasizing outcomes over volume of care delivered.
- The inherent advantages of team-based care are readily apparent in the house call practice.
- Patients and caregivers report high satisfaction with house call services.
- The house call practice is a viable option for NPs and PAs who have strong interpersonal skills and enjoy developing relationships with their patients.

More information about tools and the Interprofessional Education Collaborative (IPEC) competencies mentioned in this chapter can be found in Appendix 1: Tools and Appendix 2: IPEC Competencies.

References

Berresford, L. (2020, January 3). House calls for homebound patients: Has their time come. *Medscape Medical News.*

Bonnel, A., Baston, C., Wallace, P., Panebianco, N., & Kinosian, B. (2019). Using point of care ultrasound on home visits: The Home-Oriented Ultrasound Examination (HOUSE). *Journal of the American Geriatrics Society, 67*(12), 2662–2663. https://doi.org/10.1111/jgs.16188.

Center for Medicare Advocacy. (2013, November 7). *New CMS proposed homebound policy would leave medicare beneficiaries without coverage.* https://www.medicareadvocacy.org/new-cms-proposed-homebound-policy-will-leave-medicare-beneficiaries-without-coverage/

Hayashi, J., & Christmas, C. (2009). House calls and the ACGME competencies. *Teaching and Learning in Medicine, 21*(2), 140–147. https://doi.org/10.1080/10401330902791115.

Heron, M. (2019). Deaths: Leading causes for 2017. *National Vital Statistics Reports, 68*(6).

Kimmey, L., Anderson, M., Cheh, V., LI, E., et al. (2019, May). *Evaluation of the IAH demonstration: An examination of the first four years.* Mathematica Policy Research.

Leff, B., Weston, C. M., Garrigues, S., Patel, K., & Ritchie, C. (2015). Home based primary care practice in the United States: Current state and quality improvement approaches. *Journal of the American Geriatrics Society, 63*(5), 963–969.

Mamuya, W., Hoover, Jr., R.D., Brennan, S.V., & Gurk, P.J. (2018). *Face-to-face and written order requirements for certain types of DME.* https://www.cgsmedicare.com/pdf/f2f_wo_requirements_high-costdme.pdf.

Medicare Learning Network. (2013, May 31). *Detailed written orders and face-to-face encounters.* https://www.cms.gov/Research-Statistics-Data-and-Systems/Monitoring-Programs/Medicare-FFS-Compliance-Programs/Medical-Review/Downloads/DetailedWrittenOrdersandFacetoFaceEncounters.pdf.

Mishuris, R., Stewart, M., Fix, G., Marcello, T., et al. (2014). Barriers to patient portal access among veterans receiving home-based primary care: A qualitative study. *Health Expectations, 18,* 2296–2305.

Nabagiez, J., Shariff, M., Khan, M., Molly, W., & McGinn, J. T., Jr. (2013). Physician assistant home visit program to reduce hospital readmissions. *Journal of Thoracic and Cardiovascular Surgery, 145*(1), 225–231. 232–233.

Nabagiez, J. P., Shariff, M. A., Molloy, W. J., Demissie, S., & McGinn, J. T., Jr. (2016). Cost analysis of physican assistant home visit program to reduce readmissions after cardiac surgery. *Annals of Thoracic Surgery, 102*(3), 696–702. https://doi.org/10.1016/j.athoracsur.2016.03.077.

O'Brien, K., Bradley, S., Ramirez-Zohfeld, V., & Lindquist, L. (2019). Stressors facing home-based primary care providers. *Geriatrics, 4,* 17.

Oiu, W., Dean, M., Liu, T., George, L., et al. (2010). Physical and mental health of the homebound elderly: An overlooked population. *Journal of the American Geriatrics Society, 58*(12), 2433–2438.

Schuchman, M., Fain, M., & Cornwell, T. (2018). The resurgence of home-based primary care models in the United States. *Geriatrics (Basel), 3*(3), pii: E41.

Van den Berg, N., Meinke, C., Matzuke, M., & Heynann, R. (2010). Delegation of GP home visits to qualified practice assistants: Assessment of economic effects in an ambulatory healthcare center. *BMC Health Services Research, 10,* 155.

Yao, N., Rose, K., Le Baron, V., Camacho, F., & Boling, P. (2017). Increasing role of nurse practitioners in house call programs. *Journal of the American Geriatrics Society, 65,* 847–852.

20 Acute Care

TRACY MCCLINTON, DNP, AGACNP-BC, APRN, EBP-C

OBJECTIVES

Student Learning Objectives

After completing this chapter, the student should be able to do the following:

- Identify symptoms of acute coronary syndrome as related to myocardial infarction or ischemia.
- Distinguish myocardial ischemia from myocardial infarction, ST segment elevation (STEMI), or non-ST segment elevation (NSTEMI).
- Recommend appropriate treatment measures for myocardial infarction and myocardial ischemia for the geriatric patient.
- Identify the symptoms of stroke and transient ischemic stroke.
- Prioritize the necessary immediate management of stroke.
- Evaluate the risks and benefits of treatment when managing geriatric patients who experience strokes.
- Identify symptoms of bowel obstruction in the geriatric patient.
- Assess the need for the invasive and noninvasive management of bowel obstruction.
- Consider the quality of life of the geriatric patient if considering laparotomy.
- Understand the impact of hip fracture in the geriatric patient.
- Prioritize the goals of treatment when managing the patient with hip fracture.
- Recall the importance of the interprofessional team in managing the geriatric patient with hip fracture.
- Review possible causes of transverse myelitis.
- Understand the presentation of symptoms associated with transverse myelitis.
- Recall the appropriate treatment for managing transverse myelitis.
- Recognize the clinical signs of sepsis.
- Understand the impact of sepsis on the mortality rate in the geriatric population.
- Recall the treatment in managing sepsis and the underlying source.
- Summarize the STEDI (Stopping Elderly Accidents, Deaths, and Injuries) Initiative
- Understand the importance of a comprehensive geriatric assessment (CGA).
- Explain why geriatric patients may present differently than other patients who experience trauma.

Practitioner Objectives

After completing this chapter, the practitioner should be able to do the following:

- Understand the various presentations of acute coronary syndrome as related to myocardial ischemia versus myocardial infarction, ST segment elevation (STEMI), or non-ST segment elevation (NSTEMI).
- Differentiate ECG changes, coronary involvement, and the anatomic location of various myocardial infarctions.
- Recall the risks and benefits of treatment measures for the geriatric patient experiencing acute coronary syndrome (ACS).
- Recognize the signs of stroke and transient ischemic stroke.
- Understand the application of the Glasgow Coma Scale when performing a neurologic examination.
- Determine the appropriate diagnostic imaging to correctly diagnose various types of strokes.
- Recall the importance of the FAST ultrasound in geriatric patients presenting with symptoms of bowel obstruction.
- Distinguish the need for invasive and noninvasive management of bowel obstruction.
- Recognize the need for surgery consultation when appropriate.
- Correctly diagnose hip fracture upon physical examination.
- Identify potential complications the geriatric patient may encounter.
- Specify consultations needed during the geriatric patient's hospitalization post hip fracture.
- Recognize the presentation of transverse myelitis.
- Recall the importance of serologic testing in diagnosing and managing transverse myelitis.
- Summarize the goals of treatment in transverse myelitis.
- Differentiate between sepsis and systemic inflammatory response syndrome.
- Recognize specific diagnostic tests for analyzing and managing sepsis.
- Identify the primary treatment for managing sepsis.
- Discuss the impact of trauma on the geriatric patient's quality of life.
- Understand the importance of the STEADI (Stopping Elderly Accidents, Deaths, and Injuries) initiative when addressing trauma prevention related to falls.
- Prioritize the need for the primary survey and assessment of geriatric patients who experience trauma.

Introduction

CASE STUDY 20.1

Mr. N. C. is a 75-year-old male who presents to the emergency department with complaints of intermittent chest pain, left arm pain, diaphoresis, and shortness of breath. He rates the chest pain an 8 out of 10 on the pain scale and describes it as dull and radiating. He is morbidly obese, has a 30-pack per year smoking history, and suffered a non-ST segment elevation (NSTEMI) 1 year ago. Despite instructions from his cardiologist, Mr. N.C. continues to smoke and has been noncompliant with his diet, antihypertensives, and statins. How should this patient's care be managed during his hospital stay?

Myocardial Infarction

Definitions

Acute coronary syndrome (ACS): Myocardial ischemia (unstable angina) or myocardial infarction (with or without ST elevation; NSTEMI or STEMI).

Coronary artery bypass graft (CABG): Surgical coronary revascularization of the coronary arteries by use of bypass grafting, which may be indicated for patients with recurrent ischemia, STEMI, severe heart failure, cardiogenic shock, or who do not respond to percutaneous coronary intervention (Garatti et al., 2018).

Coronary computed tomographic angiography (CCTA): A diagnostic noninvasive tool used to detect coronary artery disease, allowing visualization of the coronary anatomy involving the lumen of the arteries and its walls to identify stenosis and occlusion, which cause ischemia of the myocardium (DeFilippo & Capasso, 2016).

GI cocktail: Maalox or Mylanta, viscous lidocaine, and Donnatal.

Killip classification: A prognostic classification based on the presence and severity of patients with STEMI (Ferri, 2021).

Non-ST elevated myocardial infraction (NSTEMI); A cardiac event involving partial blockage of a coronary artery with evidence of myocyte necrosis and with no ST segment elevation on the ECG.

Patient activation measure (PAM): A validated assessment tool that evaluates how engaged patients are in their health care (Humphries et al., 2021).

Q wave: Signifies current or previous myocardial infarction (Barkley, 2021; Hobson et al., 2018).

Stable angina: The presence of predictable substernal chest discomfort or pain due to inadequate oxygen to the myocardium, which may be exercise induced or induced by anxiety and resolves in minutes. It is reproduced by the same activities and generally resolves with rest or pharmacologic treatment (Joshi & de Lemos, 2021).

ST-elevated myocardial infarction (STEMI): Acute cardiac injury signifying ischemia and identifiable on the ECG with an elevated "ST" segment requiring opening of the blocked coronary artery (Barkley, 2021).

ST-segment: Depression may signify ischemia or infarction; elevation may indicate myocardial infarction, pericarditis, or left ventricular aneurysm (Barkley, 2021; Hobson et al., 2018).

Unstable angina (UA): The presence of unpredictable substernal chest discomfort or pain without myocardial necrosis, which occurs between stable angina and acute myocardial infarction (Sandoval et al., 2018). The presence varies and usually indicates coronary artery disease.

Myocardial infarction (MI) is one of the five leading causes of hospitalizations and is related to an 80% mortality rate among individuals ages 65 and older (Barkley, 2021; Centers for Disease Control and Prevention [CDC], 2021). One-third of adult patients with MIs present with an ST-segment elevated myocardial infarction (STEMI). Patients with non-ST-segment elevated myocardial infarctions (NSTEMI) generally have more comorbidities overall than those with STEMIs (Huedebert et al., 2020). Patients generally present with symptoms of acute coronary syndrome (ACS) and require management of unstable angina (UA), STEMI, and NSTEMI. ACS related to NSTEMI accounts for approximately 546,000 events (Noe et al., 2020). Of the approximate 1.2 million individuals in the United States who are hospitalized with ACS, two-thirds are diagnosed with NSTEMI; individuals ages 65 years and older account for more than half of those admissions, and almost half are women (Lange & Mukherjee, 2020).

The incidence of NSTEMIs continues to rise due to diabetes, hypertension, and obesity in the aging population. This increased incidence of NSTEMI poses increased risks of STEMIs in the future in addition to the risk of long-term mortality (Huedebert et al., 2020). Chronic inflammation is a major contributor to ACS/MI in the older adult due to peripheral vascular disease, rheumatoid arthritis, psoriasis, infection, or a chronic inflammatory disorder (Lange & Mukherjee, 2020).

Prevention of diabetes mellitus, hypertension, and hypercholesterolemia is key to decreasing the risks and burdens of chronic inflammation that result in MI. A healthy diet and exercise, including healthy behaviors such as smoking cessation, are always key in the prevention of cardiovascular disease, which leads to MI. Interventions to the aforementioned inflammatory disease processes, respectively, include intensive glycemic control, hypertension treatment, and treatment with HMG-CoA reductase inhibitor also known as *statins*. Contrary to past recommendations, the US Preventive Services Task Force (USPSTF) recommends against the initiation of low-dose aspirin in adults 60 years of age or older for the primary prevention of heart disease (Mora et al., 2022).

Interprofessional Collaboration

Interprofessional collaboration is key to the management of diseases in the aging population and in health care systems to improve patient outcomes and decrease mortality. The nurse practitioner (NP) and physician assistant (PA) must collaborate with individuals in multiple disciplines to provide evidence-based care to the geriatric patient, whose condition may rapidly change. This includes the physician who may be deemed the collaborating physician or supervising provider. Other professionals include, but are not limited to, the nurse, respiratory therapist, doctor of pharmacy, nutritionist, physical therapist, and case manager. It is important that the NP and PA communicate their roles and responsibilities clearly to the patients, families, and others working within the patient care team (Interprofessional Education & Collaboration [IPEC], 2016). Engaging with other professionals helps the NP and PA to formulate a cohesive patient care plan for each individual and additionally meets the needs of diverse geriatric patients across the continuum of care. Integrating the knowledge and experience of other health care professionals while providing timely, instructive feedback to other team members will improve the team's cohesiveness, patient safety, and health care outcomes. Maintaining a climate of mutual respect and shared values for each team member builds a rapport that will benefit the patient and the team (IPEC, 2016).

The scope of the acute care nurse practitioner is developed by formal education and includes the abilities to independently perform comprehensive health assessments, order and interpret diagnostic tests, perform skills and procedures, formulate differential and primary diagnoses, plan and delegate care, and evaluate the outcomes of interventions (American Association of Colleges of Nursing [AACN], 2021). The NP's scope in acute care is broad, although privileges are set by the hospital or facility setting. This also holds true to the PA's privileges. The process of granting clinical privileges ensures the provider has the skills necessary to perform duties specific to the patient population (AAPA, 2022). PAs also have diverse medical knowledge, which includes, but is not limited to, performing history and physical examinations, consultation, discharge; formulating diagnoses; developing, implementing, and managing treatment plans; ordering and interpreting diagnostics; and more. Specialty privileges and scope of practice for the PA are dependent on the privileges granted by the institution (AAPA, 2022).

In the diagnosis of myocardial infarction, the acute care nurse practitioner and the physician assistant have equal responsibility in diagnosis and treatment of the geriatric population in the acute care setting, based on their hospital privileges. For the sake of this chapter, the discussion will include the scope, understanding that privileges may vary by state, hospital, or facility. Other professionals caring for the geriatric patient who has sustained an MI include registered nurses who generally provide nursing care. Nursing care includes, but is not limited to, completing physical examinations of the patients with scheduled assessments; administering medications as ordered; initiating electrocardiograms (ECGs); monitoring continuous ECGs when necessary; drawing basic and serial laboratory diagnostics to monitor cardiac markers and electrolytes; and monitoring respiratory status, urinary output, and hemodynamic parameters. Respiratory therapists also have a role in caring for geriatric patients who have sustained an MI. Their role includes, but is not limited to, monitoring and managing the patient's oxygen and airway, which may also include providing aerosol treatments, intubation, and ventilator management. Pharmacists, nutritionists, physical therapists, and case managers also have roles in managing the care of the cardiac patient. These responsibilities include, but are not limited to, delivering and managing medications specific to patients' weight and allergies for their plans of care; determining proper diet and calorie counts individualized for each patient; determining patients' ambulatory abilities, limitations, and exercises necessary to perform activities of daily living during their hospital stay and prior to discharge; and determining the proper disposition of patients and the means they will use to care for themselves upon discharge, including issues regarding medication, transportation, and shelter.

It is important for the acute care nurse practitioner/physician assistant to understand that cardiovascular changes within the older adult consist of more fibrous and rigid heart valves with calcium deposits and stiffening of cardiac vessels and ventricles and a decrease in the number of cells in the sinus and sinoatrial nodes causing a decrease in conduction. Other physiologic changes that impact the aging patient include a decrease in the average and maximal rate. The heart of geriatric patients generally does not tolerate tachyarrhythmias well due to reduced ventricular compliance; it therefore takes longer for the heart to return to its resting heart rate when stressed (Barkley, 2021).

Upon history and physical examination, the acute care provider should note that chest discomfort may or may not be severe and has one of the following features: occurs with or without exertion and lasts greater than 10 minutes; is of recent onset of less than 2 weeks; or has a crescendo increasing pattern in severity, frequency, or length (Giugliano et al., 2018). Older adult patients with neuropathies may lack pain due to diabetes; 15% of patients sustaining an MI have no pain (Barkley, 2021). Additionally, geriatric individuals may experience symptoms such as confusion, increased fatigue, malaise, and weakness. As the origin of pain from MI in women is more commonly related to gastrointestinal (GI) symptoms, treatment with a GI cocktail will help to quickly resolve GI symptoms and rule out MI.

Chest discomfort is usually located in the substernal region and radiates to the left arm, shoulder, jaw, or neck. Although patients with stable angina may exhibit an unremarkable physical examination, in addition to pain not relieved by nitroglycerin, physical findings of patients experiencing an MI or large area of ischemia may include nausea, vomiting, diaphoresis; pale, cool skin; tachycardia; a third or fourth heart sound; basilar rales; dyspnea; feeling of impending doom; and, sometimes, hypotension (Barkley, 2021; Giugliano et al., 2018).

Upon physical examination, the acute care provider may observe that patients suffering from STEMI exhibit the Levine sign, with a clenched fist held over the sternum

• BOX 20.1 Killip Classification

The Killip classification is an independent predictor of all-cause 30-day mortality:

1. Killip class I includes individuals with no clinical signs of HF. Mortality rate is 6%.
2. Killip class II includes individuals with rales or crackles in the lungs, S3 gallop, and elevated jugular venous pressure. Mortality rate is 17%.
3. Killip class III describes individuals with frank acute pulmonary edema. Mortality rate is 38%.
4. Killip class IV describes individuals in cardiogenic shock or hypotension (measured as systolic blood pressure <90 mm Hg) and evidence of peripheral vasoconstriction (oliguria, cyanosis, or sweating). Mortality rate is 67%.

From Ferri, F. F. (2021). *Ferri's clinical advisor 2022*. Elsevier.

(Mohammadian et al., 2022). Although a hypertensive response is generally seen initially in STEMIs, patients may also be normotensive after infarction and may return to an elevated blood pressure 3 to 6 months post infarction. Elevated temperature secondary to the cytokine release of necrosing tissue may begin within 4 to 8 hours of STEMI and may reach 101° to 102° Fahrenheit (Mirvis & Goldberger, 2021). The patient may also exhibit tachypnea and generally a normal jugular venous pulse when the left ventricle is involved. Palpation of the precordium may also be normal with palpation of the carotid arterial pulse indicating a slow pulse (fewer than 60 beats per minute), suggesting reduced stroke volume or a sharp, brief upstroke in patients with mitral regurgitation (Mirvis & Goldberger, 2021). Although moist rales and some diffuse wheezing may be auscultated in lung fields, based on the Killip classification (Box 20.1), class I patients on the New York Heart Association (NYHA) functional classification suffering from MI may not have rales, whereas patients in classes II through IV present with rales. A patient's NYHA classification can be a predicator in physical examination findings. Note that upon cardiac examination, patients sustaining STEMI may exhibit pericardial friction rubs. Delayed onset and pericarditis, known as post-MI (Dressler) syndrome, can present as late as 3 months after infarction (Mirvis & Goldberger, 2021). Additionally, the geriatric patient may present with confusion or disorientation.

A diagnosis of STEMI and NSTEMI consists of ECG, cardiac biochemical markers (also known as cardiac biomarkers or cardiac enzymes) and stress testing (nuclear or treadmill). An ECG should be obtained and interpreted within 10 minutes of the patient's arrival, regardless of the setting. Coronary computed tomographic angiography (CCTA) may improve the accuracy of the diagnosis. Patients who present with chest pain and are at high risk of MI should be evaluated carefully and admitted through a critical pathway such as a chest pain unit or coronary care unit. Note that geriatric patients may present with vague symptoms rather than classic chest pain, including fatigue, nausea, vomiting, dyspnea, or midepigastric or postprandial pain (Fihn et al., 2012). ECG changes and monitoring of cardiac markers are important for diagnosing MI in patients presenting with chest pain; for patients with a negative ECG and negative cardiac markers with chest pain, further diagnostics should include a stress test or CCTA (Di Carli et al., 2018).

Although the ECG of geriatric individuals may not meet typical criteria for MI, ECG changes may include other ST or T-wave changes, such as ST-segment depression or T-wave inversion (Table 20.1) (Barkley, 2021, Goldberger & Mirvis, 2021; Tintinalli, 2020). Increased age is a risk factor for individuals >75 years of age, who account for 33% of all cases of ACS, including noncardiac chest pain (considered as a fourth type of chest pain). For this reason, a more thorough workup should be performed on these patients. Patients older than 75 years who experienced stable symptoms of coronary artery disease are shown to have a positive stress test associated with risk of cardiovascular death or MI (Lowenstern et al., 2020).

A hallmark of injury is an ST-segment elevation greater than 1 mm above baseline, whereas infarction may produce a pathologic Q wave more than 1 mm wide (0.04 s) or >25% the height of the QRS complex (Barkley 2021, Mirvis & Goldberger, 2021). Severe myocarditis can mimic ECG patterns of acute MI, such as Q waves or ST-segment elevations. Note that there can be variability of ECG patterns that are associated with acute myocardial ischemia. A non-Q-wave infarct can potentially develop into a Q-wave infarct (Fig. 20.1) (Mirvis et al., 2020). Based on ST-segment criteria for acute myocardial infarction (AMI), ECG changes are detected as associated with anatomic locations, as noted in Table 20.1.

For patients presenting with chest pain, negative serial ECGs, and positive biochemical markers, a diagnosis of NSTEMI should be made (Antman & Loscalzo, 2018). Unstable angina and NSTEMI acute coronary syndrome are characterized by the absence of ST elevation or ST segment depression and are also indicative of ischemia (see Fig. 1 in Lang & Mukherjee, 2020). Serial cardiac biochemical markers, also known as serum cardiac enzymes, should be initiated immediately upon evaluation of the patient presenting with chest pain. These markers include cardiac-specific troponin T (cTnT), cardiac-specific troponin I (cTnI), creatine phosphokinase (CK), and its myocardial band (MB) isoenzyme (CK-MB) measurements (Antman & Loscalzo, 2018). As cTnT and cTnI may increase many times higher above the upper reference limits, they are the preferred biochemical markers in hospitals and may remain elevated post STEMI for 7 to 10 days. It is not cost effective to monitor serial cTnI or cTnT and CK-MB in every patient. Troponins, cTnI and cTnT, rise more quickly, every 3 hours versus every 6 hours, respectively (Antman & Loscalzo, 2018; Barkley, 2021). Elevations of total CK and isoenzymes, total human lactate dehydrogenase isoenzyme (also known as LD), and the human heart LD_1 are nonspecific markers indicative of tissue damage. However, the latter two will not increase until approximately 8 to

TABLE 20.1 EKG Criteria for Myocardial Infarction

Anatomic Location of Infarct	Electrocardiogram Changes	Coronary Artery Involvement
Inferior	ST-segment elevations Leads II, III, and aVF	Diaphragmatic involving the right coronary artery (80–90%) or left circumflex artery
Inferolateral	ST-segment elevations Leads II, III, aVF, V5, and V6	Left circumflex artery
Anterior (Rosen & Tininalli)	ST-segment elevations V1–V4	Left anterior descending artery
Anterolateral (Ferri, Tintinalli, Barkley, 2021)	ST-segment elevations V1–V6, I, aVL	Left anterior descending artery or left circumflex artery
Lateral (Ferri, Rosen, Barkley, 2021, Tininalli)	ST-segment elevations I, aVL, V5, V6	Left circumflex artery
Anteroseptal (Barkley 2021, Tintinalli)	ST-segment elevations V1, V2, V3	Left anterior descending Artery
Posterior (Barkley 2021, Ferri, Tintinalli)	Reciprocal changes in V1, V2, and/or V3. Tall R waves: and ST depression without T-wave inversion may be seen	Right coronary artery or left circumflex artery
Right ventricular (Barkley 2021, Rosen)	V_4R to V_6R	Right coronary artery

Data from Ferri, F. F. (2021). *Ferri's clinical advisor 2022*. Elsevier; Barkley, T. W. (2021). *Practice considerations for adult-gerontology acute care nurse practitioners* (3rd ed.). Barkley and Associates, Inc. https://www.npcourses.com/ebook/practice-considerations-agacnp-3rd-edition/; Walls, R. M., Hockberger, R. S., Gausche-Hill, M., Bakes, K. M., Thomas, J., & Brady, W. (2018b). Acute coronary syndrome. In *Rosen's emergency medicine: Concepts and clinical practice* (9th ed., pp. 891–928). Elsevier.

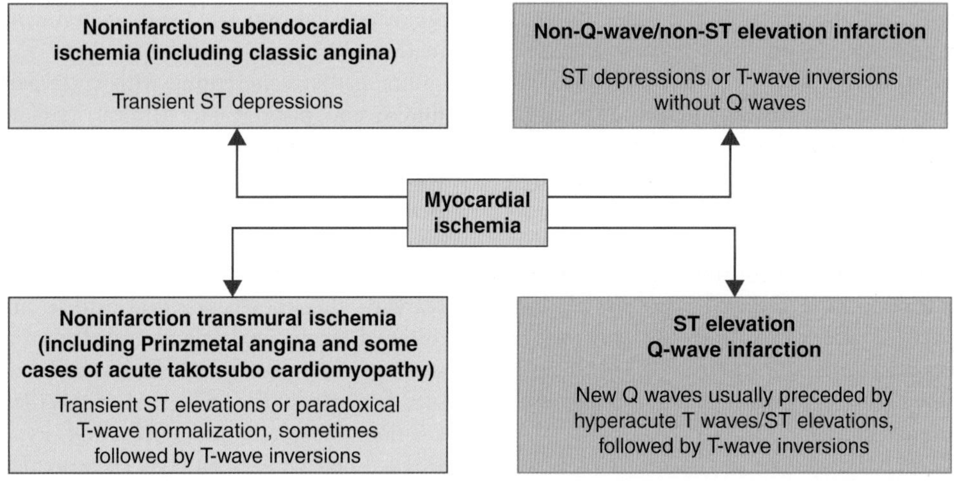

• **Fig. 20.1** Variable EKG Patterns of Myocardial Infarction. (From Goldberger AL, Goldberger ZD, Shvilkin A. *Goldberger's Clinical Electrocardiography: A Simplified Approach*. 9th ed. Philadelphia:Elsevier; 2017.)

10 days and peak at 72 hours on average (Barkley, 2021). Due to variability in the rising of biochemical markers—for instance, myoglobin rising within 1 to 2 hours and CK-MB rising within 4 to 12 hours—serial enzyme testing is warranted every 6 to 8 hours (Barkley, 2021).

Additionally, elevated levels of B-type natriuretic peptide (BNP) and high-sensitivity C-reactive protein (hs-CRP) are indicators of future cardiac complications. Other laboratory monitors for the patient suffering from a suspected MI include a complete metabolic count (CBC), a basic metabolic panel (BMP) or comprehensive metabolic panel (CMP), a lipoprotein profile, prothrombin time (PT), and partial thromboplastin time (PTT).

If the ECG reveals normal findings with persistent chest pain, increased risk factors and other symptoms necessitate a repeat ECG. Imaging studies to differentiate MI from aortic dissection pulmonary embolism or other intrathoracic causes of chest pain should include a high-quality portable chest x-ray, transthoracic echocardiography, and a contrast chest computed tomography scan (Ferri, 2021). For patients with STEMI, the thrombolysis in myocardial infarction (TIMI) can be used to determine the 30-day mortality rate (Fig. 20.2). The TIMI grading ranges from 0 to 3. Grade 0 indicates complete occlusion; grade 1 indicates some perfusion of contrast beyond the infarct obstruction; grade 2 indicates full perfusion of the entire infarct vessel; and grade 3 indicates full perfusion of the infarcted vessel with normal flow (Antman & Loscalzo, 2018; Mirvis & Goldberger, 2021, Fig. 2). As the TIMI risk score increases, the mortality rate increases (Ferri, 2021). This is important for the geriatric patient, as age increases the risk of mortality. In research by Ferri, (2021), the TIMI risk score showed a greater than 40-fold graded increase in mortality, with scoring ranging from 0 to >8. The variables are divided into three categories: historic, exam, and presentation:

Historic
- Age 65 to 74 (2 points), >75 (3 points)
- Diabetes/hypertension or angina (1 point)

Exam
- SBP <100 mm Hg (3 points)
- Heart rate >100 bpm (2 points)
- Killip 2 to 4 (2 points)
- Weight <67 kg (1 point)

Presentation
- Anterior ST elevation or left bundle branch block (LBBB) (1 point)
- Time to reperfusion >4 hour (1 point) (Ferri, 2021; Golla & Satya, 2022)

Treatment

Emergency management of acute coronary syndrome for patients who may be suffering an MI with or without percutaneous coronary intervention (PCI) includes chewable aspirin 162 to 325 mg, sublingual nitroglycerin 91 every 5 minutes up to three doses, ticagrelor or clopidogrel, and supplemental oxygen titrating to maintain a saturation of 92% or greater and for management of dyspnea (Fig. 20.3A). Continuous cardiac and hemodynamic monitoring should be initiated, and at least 24-hour observation is necessary for the geriatric patient to rule out STEMI and to direct a further treatment plan (Barkley, 2021).

In addition, treatment of discomfort from a NSTEMI or STEMI should include intravenous (IV) morphine, in small increments in the geriatric patient so as not to oversedate or cause a vagotonic effect that could result in bradycardia or heart block in patients who suffer inferior infarctions (Antman & Loscalzo, 2018). Intravenous beta-blockers may also control pain by diminishing myocardial oxygen demand and ultimately decreasing ischemia. However, all intravenous medications may affect the geriatric patient drastically and must be initiated with caution.

Treatment measures of ACS in individuals who are at low risk of a subsequent ischemic event and who do not benefit from fibrinolytic therapy or PCI should include an immediate antianginal (sublingual nitroglycerin immediately) and an antiischemic (oral within 24 hours, beta-blocker, or diltiazem or verapamil), a statin (prior to discharge), an antiplatelet (aspirin immediately and ticagrelor or clopidogrel or prasugrel), and an anticoagulant (Lange & Mukherjee, 2020). Treatment measures of ACS in individuals who are at high risk of a subsequent ischemic event and who do not benefit from fibrinolytic therapy should include an antianginal (sublingual nitroglycerin immediately and an oral within 24 hours, beta-blocker, or diltiazem or verapamil), a statin (prior to discharge), and an antiplatelet (aspirin immediately and clopidogrel, prasugrel, or ticagrelor), an anticoagulant, and invasive management (Lange & Mukherjee, 2020).

However, note that ticagrelor is a reversible inhibitor of the platelet P_2Y_{12} (Andreotti et al., 2015, Madhaven et al., 2018). This is important when considering the risk of bleeding when treating the geriatric population. The Prospective Randomized Platelet Inhibition and Patient Outcomes (PLATO) randomized trial of 18,624 patients greater than 75 years of age showed that ticagrelor reduced the number of 1-year cardiovascular deaths, including those associated with MI (Andreotti et al., 2015; Husted et al., 2012; Madhaven et al., 2018). In addition, life-threatening bleeding was not increased with ticagrelor compared with clopidogrel. Major bleeding related to non-CABG was more frequent.

Patients with STEMI in the anterior location, heart failure (HF), or ejection fraction (EF) less than or equal to 40% should receive an angiotensin-converting enzyme (ACE) inhibitor within the first 24 hours (Heidenreich et al., 2022). However, for patients with STEMI who are already receiving an ACE inhibitor or beta-blocker and who have an EF less than or equal to 40%, with symptomatic HF, diabetes mellitus, and no contraindications, aldosterone antagonist should be administered (Heidenreich et al., 2022). Beta-blockers should be avoided in patients with decompensated heart failure, evidence of low output state, increased risk of cardiogenic shock, active asthma, or reactive airway disease; and diltiazem or verapamil should be avoided in patients with significant left ventricular dysfunction; both medications should be avoided in patients who have a PR interval >0.24 (Fihn et al., 2012; Lange & Mukherjee, 2020).

Treatment measures for STEMI include fibrinolytic therapy, if no contraindications are present, or PCI (also known as coronary angioplasty), initiated within 120 minutes of the patient's presentation (see Fig. 20.4) (Antman & Loscalzo, 2018). Primary PCI, referred to as angioplasty or stenting, should be initiated when there is a high risk of bleeding or when cardiogenic shock is present. PCI is superior to fibrinolytic therapy and is the preferred standard of care, as it generally results in more favorable outcomes (Ferri, 2021). STEMI treated with rapid reperfusion with primary PCI within 120 minutes has been shown to reduce mortality by

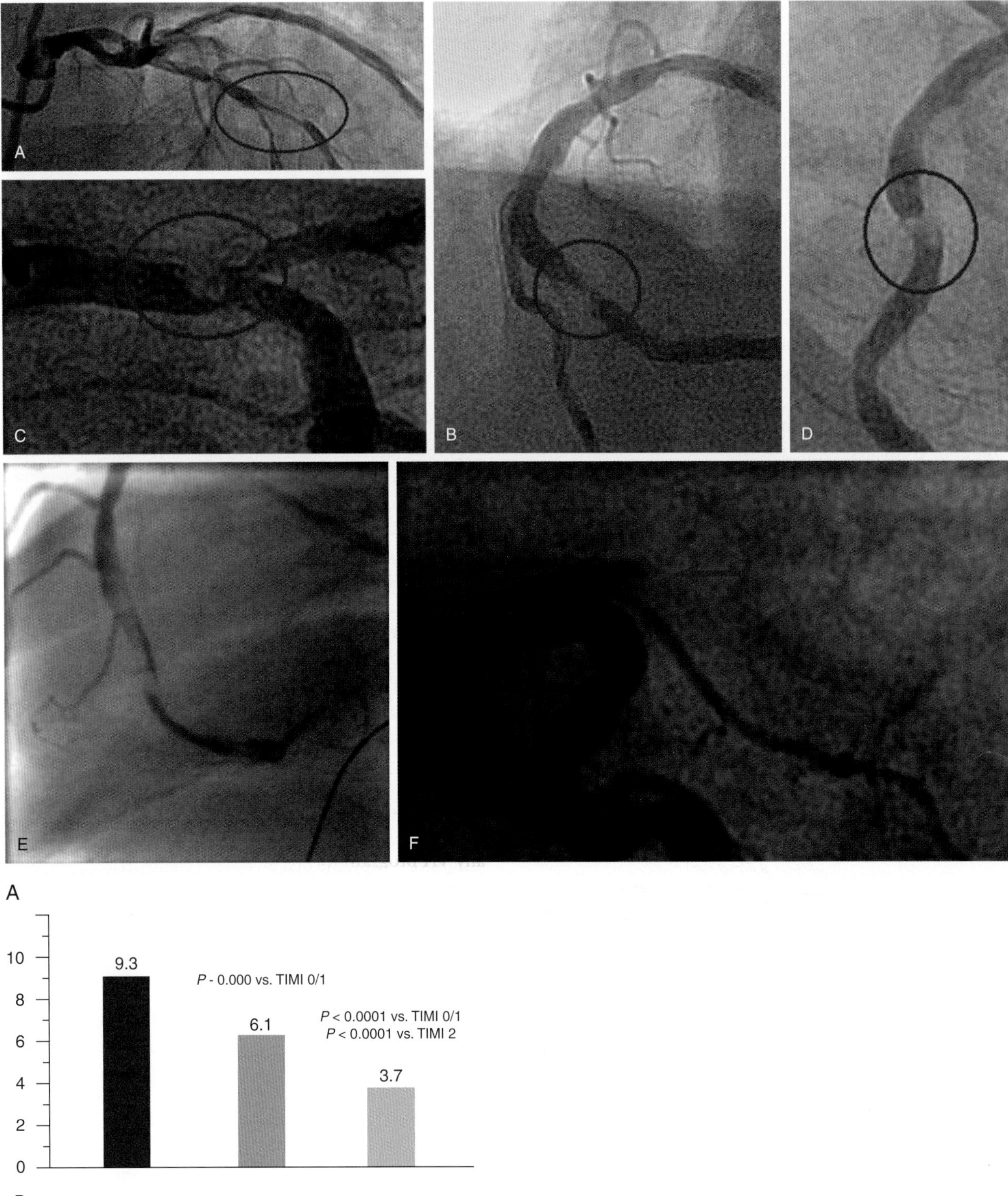

• **Fig. 20.2** Thrombolysis in Myocardial Infarction Grading. (A) Grades of thrombus as defined by the classic thrombolysis in myocardial infarction (TIMI) thrombus grading. A, Grade 0: No thrombus present. The marked plaque *(red circle)* exhibits smooth and clear borders without haziness located in the middle segment of the left anterior descending artery. B, Grade 1: Suspected thrombus in the plaque occupying the middle-distal right coronary artery *(red circle)*. C, Grade 2: Eccentric plaque and associated thrombus located in the distal left main coronary artery *(red circle)*. D, Grade 3: Thrombus in the middle segment of the right coronary artery *(red circle)*. E, Grade 4: Represented by heavy layers of thrombus almost completely obstructing distal flow. F, Grade 5: Total thrombotic occlusion of the proximal left anterior descending artery in a patient with an acute anterior wall myocardial infarction *(red arrow)*. (From Topaz, O., & Topaz, A. [2018]. Thrombus classifications: Critical tools for diagnostic and interventional cardiovascular procedures. In O. Topaz [Ed.], *Cardiovascular thrombus: From pathology and clinical presentations to imaging, pharmacotherapy and interventions* [pp. 175–187]. Elsevier.) (B) As the TIMI risk score increases, the mortality rate increases. (From Ferri, F. F. [2021]. *Ferri's clinical advisor 2022*. Elsevier.)

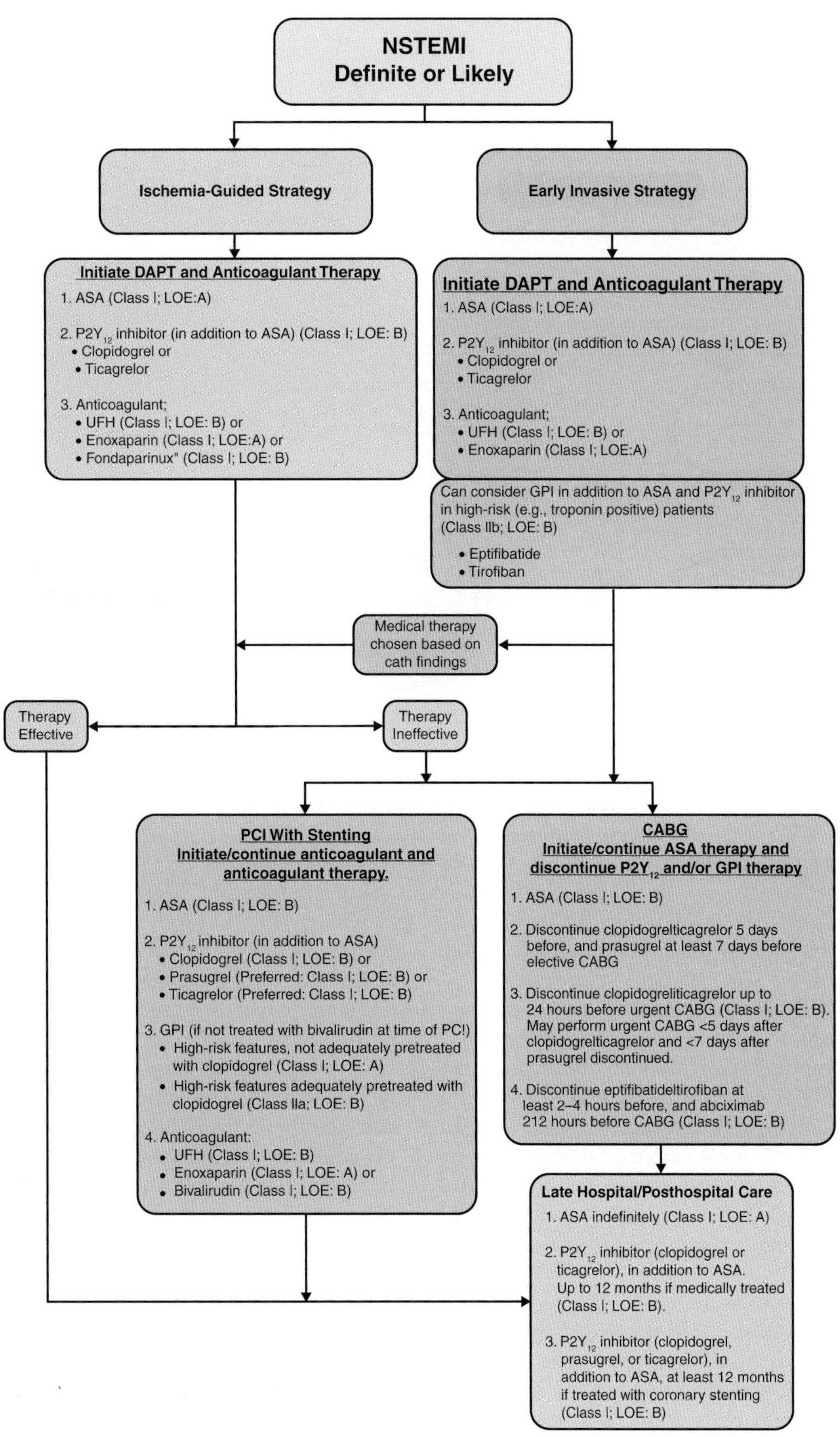

NSTEMI
Definite or Likely
Ischemia-Guided Strategy
Early Invasive Strategy
Initiate DAPT and Anticoagulant Therapy
1. ASA (Class I; LOE:A)
2. P2Y12 inhibitor (in addition to ASA) (Class I; LOE: B)
• Clopidogrel or
• Ticagrelor
3. Anticoagulant;
• UFH (Class I; LOE: B) or
• Enoxaparin (Class I; LOE:A) or
• Fondaparinux" (Class I; LOE: B)
Initiate DAPT and Anticoagulant Therapy
1. ASA (Class I; LOE:A)
2. P2Y12 inhibitor (in addition to ASA) (Class I; LOE: B)
• Clopidogrel or
• Ticagrelor
3. Anticoagulant;
• UFH (Class I; LOE: B) or
• Enoxaparin (Class I; LOE:A)
Can consider GPI in addition to ASA and P2Y12 inhibitor in high-risk (e.g., troponin positive) patients (Class IIb; LOE: B)
• Eptifibatide
• Tirofiban
Medical therapy chosen based on cath findings
Therapy Effective
Therapy Ineffective
PCI With Stenting
Initiate/continue anticoagulant and anticoagulant therapy.
1. ASA (Class I; LOE: B)
2. P2Y12 inhibitor (in addition to ASA)
• Clopidogrel (Class I; LOE: B) or
• Prasugrel (Preferred: Class I; LOE: B) or
• Ticagrelor (Preferred: Class I; LOE: B)
3. GPI (if not treated with bivalirudin at time of PC!)
• High-risk features, not adequately pretreated with clopidogrel (Class I; LOE: A)
• High-risk features adequately pretreated with clopidogrel (Class IIa; LOE: B)
4. Anticoagulant:
• UFH (Class I; LOE: B)
• Enoxaparin (Class I; LOE: A) or
• Bivalirudin (Class I; LOE: B)
CABG
Initiate/continue ASA therapy and discontinue P2Y12 and/or GPI therapy
1. ASA (Class I; LOE: B)
2. Discontinue clopidogrelticagrelor 5 days before, and prasugrel at least 7 days before elective CABG
3. Discontinue clopidogreliticagrelor up to 24 hours before urgent CABG (Class I; LOE: B). May perform urgent CABG <5 days after clopidogrelticagrelor and <7 days after prasugrel discontinued.
4. Discontinue eptifibatideltirofiban at least 2–4 hours before, and abciximab 212 hours before CABG (Class I; LOE: B)
Late Hospital/Posthospital Care
1. ASA indefinitely (Class I; LOE: A)
2. P2Y12 inhibitor (clopidogrel or ticagrelor), in addition to ASA. Up to 12 months if medically treated (Class I; LOE: B).
3. P2Y12 inhibitor (clopidogrel, prasugrel, or ticagrelor), in addition to ASA, at least 12 months if treated with coronary stenting (Class I; LOE: B)

• **Fig. 20.3** Non-ST Elevation-Acute Coronary Syndrome. (From Cohen, M., & Visveswaran, G. [2020]. Defining and managing patients with non-ST-elevation myocardial infarction: Sorting through type 1 vs other types. *Clinical Cardiology, 43,* 242–250. https://doi.org/10.1002/clc.23308.)

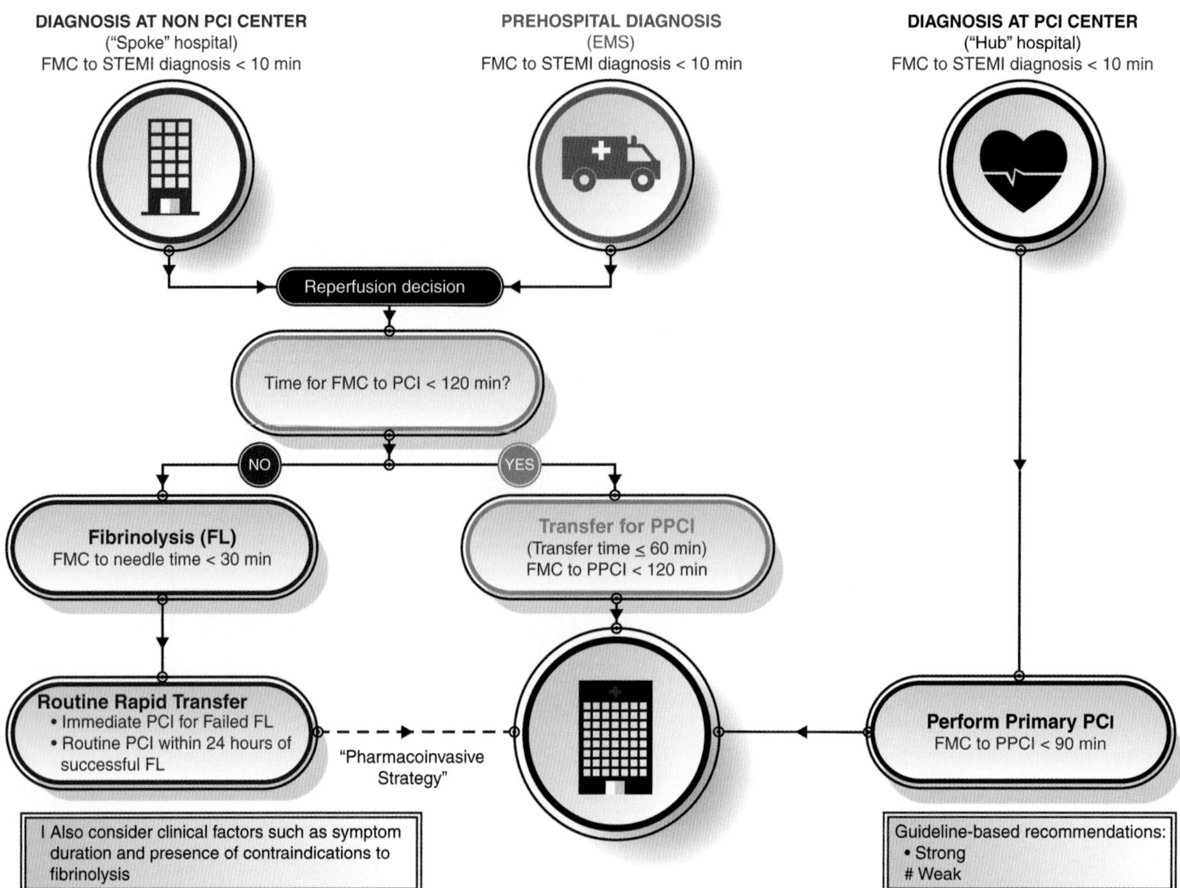

• **Fig. 20.4** ST-Elevation Myocardial Infarction (STEMI) Reperfusion Strategies. *EMS*, Emergency medical services; *FL*, fibrinolysis; *FMC*, first medical contact; *PCI*, percutaneous coronary intervention; *PPCI*, primary percutaneous coronary intervention. (From Wong, G. C., et al. [2019]. 2019 Canadian Cardiovascular Society/Canadian Association of Interventional Cardiology guidelines on the acute management of ST-elevation myocardial infarction: Focused update on regionalization and reperfusion. *Canadian Journal of Cardiology, 35*[2], 107–132.)

2% compared with fibrinolytic therapy alone (Bhatt et al., 2022).

For patients presenting to a non-PCI-capable hospital (see Fig. 20.4), it is vital that an immediate assessment is completed that captures the (1) time from symptom onset, (2) risk of STEMI-related complications, (3) bleeding risk with fibrinolysis, (4) presence of severe heart failure or shock, and (5) time required to transfer the patient to a PCI-capable facility with the decision about fibrinolytic therapy having been made (which should be done within 30 minutes of the patient's presentation) (Ferri, 2021).

Patients over the age of 70 are nearly twice as likely to experience hemorrhagic stroke with the use of fibrinolytics, more so with the use of a tissue plasminogen activator (tPA) or reteplase (rPA) than with the use of streptokinase (Antman & Loscalzo, 2018; Box 20.2). Fibrinolytic therapy includes thrombolytic agents such as tissue plasma activator or alteplase (tPA), reteplase (r-PA), Tenecteplase (TNK-t-PA), and streptokinase (Table 20.3; Ferri, 2021). Tenecteplase, also known as TNKase, is another fibrinolytic therapy that can be initiated (Table 20.2). However, in patients ages 75 years and greater, an invasive approach is preferrable due to the increased risk of complications associated with bleeding (Lange & Mukherjee, 2020).

Limiting the size of the infarct is vital in all patients suffering from MI. The most important intervention is timely reperfusion, regardless of whether patients receive fibrinolytic therapy. The limitation of factors that increase oxygen consumption should be the priority, including reducing physical and emotional stressors, avoiding adrenergic agonists whenever possible, and promptly treating tachyarrhythmias. Management of infections and fever, accompanied by tachycardia. should be considered (Mirvis & Goldberger, 2021).

Definite contraindications to fibrinolytic therapy include a drug allergy to fibrinolytics, a history of cerebrovascular hemorrhage, an ischemic stroke within the previous 3 months (exception to acute ischemic stroke within 4.5 hours), uncontrolled hypertension (reliable arterial pressure systolic >180 mm Hg and/or diastolic >110 mm Hg) at any time during acute presentation, suspicion of aortic dissection, suspicion or known active bleeding or bleeding diathesis (except menses), surgery to the cranium or spine within 2 months, and extensive closed head trauma or facial trauma within the previous 2 months (Antman & Loscalzo, 2018;

Ferri, 2021). Relative contraindications to fibrinolytic therapy can be determined by establishing a risk-to-benefit ratio and include current use of anticoagulants, an international normalized ratio (INR) greater than or equal to 2, invasive or surgical procedures in the previous 2 weeks, cardiopulmonary resuscitation lasting greater than 10 minutes, known bleeding within the previous 2 to 4 weeks, pregnancy, active peptic ulcer, and a history of severe, poorly controlled hypertension (Antman & Loscalzo, 2018; Ferri, 2021). The most frequent complication to fibrinolytic therapy is hemorrhage, with hemorrhagic stroke as the most serious. The risk of these complications increases with age, and the risk of hemorrhagic stroke nearly doubles in patients greater than 70 years of age (Antman & Loscalzo, 2018). For geriatric patients, the risk-to-benefit ratio should always be considered prior to the initiation of therapy.

Patients who sustain STEMI and do not respond to fibrinolytic therapy and do not reperfuse or who reocclude after therapy should be transferred to a PCI-capable hospital where cardiac catheterization and coronary angiography should be performed (Antman & Loscalzo, 2018; Ferri, 2021). Patients who fail reperfusion have persistent chest pain and ST-segment elevation >90 minutes and require a *rescue* PCI. Those who develop recurrent ischemia post reperfusion and demonstrate a re-elevated ST-segment or chest pain should be considered for an *urgent* PCI (Antman & Loscalzo, 2018).

Coronary artery bypass graft (CABG) is revascularization of the coronary arteries, which improves heart function and survival. It is indicated for patients with recurrent ischemia, coronary anatomy that does not allow PCI, or for patients with STEMI who have severe heart failure or who experience cardiogenic shock. It improves heart function and survival (Dellinger & Parrillo, 2019).

In patients undergoing CABG, close glucose monitoring with an insulin infusion should be administered to maintain a serum glucose of <180 mg/dl to reduce the risk of sternal wound infection (American College of Cardiology [ACC]/American Heart Association [AHA]/Society for Cardiovascular Angiography & Interventions [SCAI], 2022). Antiplatelets should be discontinued prior to surgery with

• BOX 20.2 Contraindications to Intravenous Tissue Plasminogen Activator

Absolute Contraindications

- Initial head CT suggests time of onset is inaccurate
- Suggestion of intracranial hemorrhage on pretreatment imaging
- Subarachnoid hemorrhage
- Intracranial neoplasm or arteriovenous malformation
- Active internal bleeding
- Uncontrolled hypertension greater than 185/110 mm Hg despite antihypertensive treatment
- Current bacterial endocarditis
- Head trauma, intracranial/intraspinal surgery, or myocardial infarction within 3 months
- Known bleeding diathesis
  - INR >1.7 or PT >15 s
  - Platelets <100,000 mm^3
  - Heparin within 48 hours if PTT is elevated
  - PTT outside of the normal range
  - Dose of nonwarfarin oral anticoagulant within the previous 12 hours

Relative Contraindications

- Minor or rapidly resolving deficits
- Seizure
- Major surgery in the previous 2 weeks
- GI or urinary hemorrhage in the previous 3 weeks
- Puncture at noncompressible site within 7 days (including lumbar puncture)

CT, Computed tomography; *GI*, gastrointestinal; *INR*, international normalized ratio; *PT*, prothrombin time; *PTT*, partial thromboplastin time.

TABLE 20.2 Fibrinolytic Agents and Their Specificity

Fibrinolytic Agent	Dose	Fibrin Specificity	Fibrinogen Depletion	Antigenic	Patency Rate (90-min Timi 2 OR 3 Flow)
Fibrin Specific					
Tenecteplase (TNK)	Single IV weight-based bolus	++++	Minimal	No	85%
Reteplase (r-PA)	10 units + 10-unit IV boluses given 30 min apart	++	Moderate	No	84%
Alteplase (t-PA)	90-min weight-based infusion	++	Mild	No	73%–84%
Non-Fibrin Specific					
Streptokinase	1.5 million units IV given over 30–60 min	No	Marked	Yes	60%–68%

From Levine, G. N., Parekh, M., Litvak, P., Martini, S., & Kent, T. (2023). Ischemic stroke. In *Cardiology secrets* (6th ed., pp. 482–492). Elsevier.

TABLE 20.3 Modified Fisher Scale for Subarachnoid Hemorrhage

Grade	Subarachnoid Blood	Intraventricular Blood	Risk of Symptomatic Vasospasm
1	Minimal	None	24%
2	Minimal	Present	33%
3	Diffuse	None	33%
4	Diffuse	Present	40%

Data from Long, B., Robertson, J., & Koyfman, A. (2019). Emergency medicine evaluation and management of small bowel obstruction: Evidence-based recommendations. *Journal of Emergency Medicine*, *56*(2), 166–176. https://doi.org/10.1016/j.jemermed.2018.10.024; Maung, A. A., Johnson, D. C., Piper, G. L., Barbosa, R. R., Rowell, S. E., Bokhari, F., Collins, J. N., Gordon, J. R., Ra, J. H., & Kerwin, A. J. (2012). Evaluation and management of small-bowel obstruction. *Journal of Trauma and Acute Care Surgery*, *73*(5), 362–369. https://doi.org/10.1097/ta.0b013e31827019de

aspirin continued until the time of surgery; ticagrelor and clopidogrel discontinued at least 24 hours before surgery; short-acting glycoprotein IIb/IIIa inhibitor (eptifibatide and tirofiban) discontinued 4 hours prior; abciximab discontinued 12 hours prior; and P2Y12 receptor inhibitors clopidogrel discontinued 5 days prior, ticagrelor discontinued 3 days prior, and prasugrel discontinued 7 days prior to CABG to reduce the risk of major bleeding (ACC/AHA/SCAI, 2022). Beta-blockers before CABG, if no contraindications, may be beneficial to reduce the incidence of atrial fibrillation postoperatively and may reduce in-hospital 30-day mortality rates.

Patients suffering from ACS should be admitted to a coronary care unit where continuous cardiac monitoring and hemodynamic monitoring, when appropriate, can be administered. Patients who have sustained a STEMI should be monitored on bed rest for the first 6 to 12 hours at minimum. Patients considered at low risk after a STEMI may be transferred from the coronary care unit within 24 hours. However, when no complications are indicated, post-STEMI patients should be encouraged to sit in a chair within the first 24 hours (Antman & Loscalzo, 2018).

Diet should consist of NPO, also known as "nothing by mouth." or clear liquids with the first 4 to 12 hours after STEMI due to the risk of emesis and aspiration. Consulting with a dietitian can be helpful for managing diets, which should consist of small portions with 30% or less of the calories coming from fat and a cholesterol count of 300 mg/d or less (Antman & Loscalzo, 2018). Patients with diabetes mellitus should receive special restrictions.

Post ischemic events, patients should be considered for additional diagnostic testing such as an exercise or nuclear stress test to assess for ischemia for those who have not had a coronary angiography. Exercise testing after STEMI, with a baseline ECG 48 hours prior, may be performed to assess (1) functional capacity and the ability to perform activities of daily living, (2) the efficacy of medical therapy, and (3) the risk of subsequent cardiac events (Wenger & Engberding, 2017). Early post-MI exercise testing may be performed using the traditional submaximal exercise test, 3 to 5 days (as long as no complications are present) of symptom-limited exercise, to take place in 5 days or later.

Left ventricular (LV) function should be assessed and echocardiography completed to rule out the presence of thrombus (Golla & Satya, 2022). Patients with LV function less than 40% and who may be eligible for implantable defibrillators should have LV function reevaluated within 90 days or within 42 days if revascularization was not performed. For patients who sustained STEMI, cardiac rehabilitation is recommended (Golla & Satya, 2022).

Discharge medications for all patients who sustained an ACS should include antithrombotic therapy (81 mg aspirin indefinitely, ticagrelor, or clopidogrel), a statin or lipid-lowering agent, a beta-blocker (except when contraindicated in HF), an ACE inhibitor or angiotensin receptor blocker (ARB) (except when contraindicated), an aldosterone inhibitor, and, for those with a history or high risk for gastrointestinal bleeding, a proton pump inhibitor (Golla & Satya, 2022; Pollack et al., 2020). In many cases, dual antiplatelet therapy is indicated (Pollack et al., 2020). Dual antiplatelet therapy is foundational for the secondary prevention of ACS and against stent thrombosis, but it may be less effective in reducing atrial fibrillation (Pollack, 2020). For patients treated for NSTEMI who also have atrial fibrillation, "triple" antithrombotic therapy consisting of aspirin, a $P2Y_{12}$, and an oral anticoagulant should be considered (Lopes et al., 2019). In the AUGUSTUS clinical trial, patients with atrial fibrillation and recent PCI or ACS were treated with a $P2Y_{12}$ antagonist and an antithrombotic regimen, which included apixaban, without aspirin, resulting in less bleeding. In addition, there were fewer hospitalizations with no significance in the incidence of ischemic events of the vitamin K antagonist, aspirin, or both (Lopes et al., 2019).

Special Considerations for the Older Adult Who Suffers from STEMI

Geriatric patients pose unique risk factors, clinical influences, and treatment considerations (Fig. 20.5). This may contribute to a poor prognosis when treating older adults for STEMI as opposed to treating younger patients and

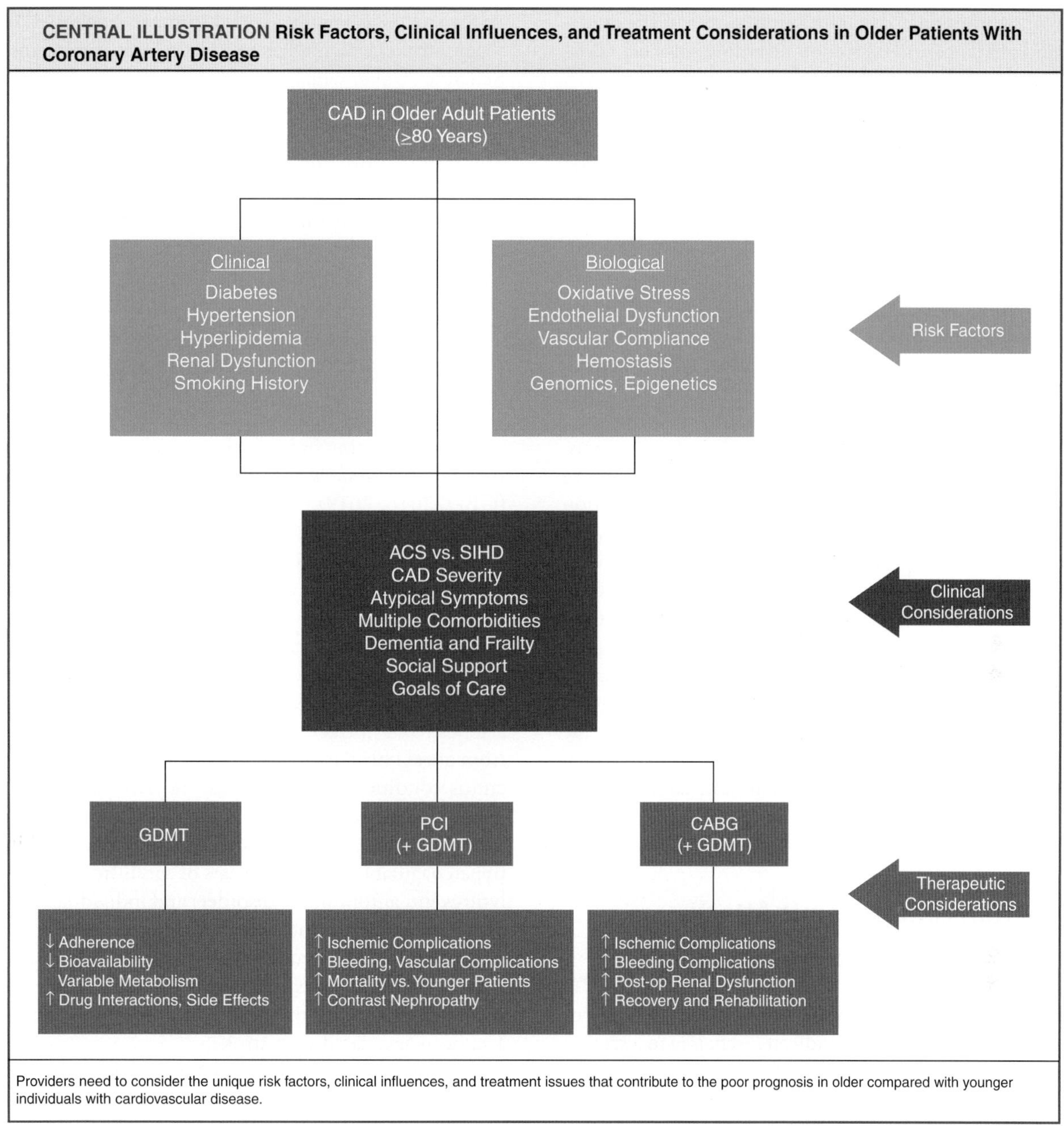

• **Fig. 20.5** Treatment Considerations for Older Patients With Myocardial Infarction. *ACS*, Acute coronary syndrome; *CABG*, coronary artery bypass graft; *CAC*, coronary artery calcium; *CAD*, coronary artery disease; *DES*, drug-eluting stent(s); *GDMT*, guideline-directed medical therapy; *MACE*, major adverse cardiovascular event(s); *MI*, myocardial infarction; *NSTEACS*, non–ST-segment elevation acute coronary syndrome; *PCI*, percutaneous coronary intervention; *SIHD*, stable ischemic heart disease; *STEMI ST*, ST segment elevation myocardial infarction. (From Madhavan M., Gersh B., Alexander K., et al. [2018]. Coronary artery disease in patients ≥80 years of age. *Journal of the American College of Cardiology, 71*[18], 2015–2040. https://doi.org/10.1016/j.jacc.2017.12.068.)

leads to a growing high-risk population regarding adverse events (Madhavan et al., 2018). Older patients are at risk of challenges related to cardiovascular, pathologic, and age-related changes and polypharmacy. When managing the geriatric patient, it is important for providers to consider the bleeding complications, decreased bioavailability, renal dysfunction, and increased recovery and rehabilitation time that may occur (Madhavan et al., 2018). Clinical considerations include multiple comorbidities, possible dementia, frailty, social support, and goals of care regarding outcome and disposition (Madhavan ct al., 2018).

Prevention

Posthospitalization planning should include systems to prevent readmission; exercise-based cardiac rehabilitation or secondary prevention programs; a detailed evidence-based plan that promotes medication adherence, timely follow-up, appropriate dietary and physical activity guidelines; and guidance and education regarding smoking cessation (Wenger & Engberding, 2017).

Patient education is the key to preventing reoccurrence of ACS. Readmissions post hospital discharge after PCI, the most common revascularization treatment, occur at rates of between 4.7% and 15.6% (Kwok et al., 2017). Older individuals are more likely to experience readmission (Kwok et al., 2017). In addition, Medicare and Medicaid 30-day readmissions for acute AMI do not meet the terms for reimbursement according to the Centers for Medicare and Medicaid Services (CMS) Hospital Readmissions Reduction Program (HRRP) (Centers for Medicare and Medicaid Services, 2021). Evidence supports patient engagement as a key indicator that influences patient outcomes post myocardial infarction (Peters & Keeley, 2017). For these reasons, patient education regarding the importance of adherence post discharge is vital. Utilization of the Patient Activation Measure (PAM) tool revealed that patients who were more engaged in their care, based on their higher scores, were more likely to adhere to treatment plans and make healthier lifestyle choices after an acute MI and less likely to sustain unplanned readmissions (Humphries et al., 2021). Engaging patients in self-management activities is vital in the progression of everyone's health-related quality of life (HRQOL) (Newland et al., 2020). Evidence supports the belief that the higher the patient's engagement in his or her care—which involves the patient's knowledge, skill, and confidence in managing his or her health—the more likely the patient's HRQOL outcome will improve (Newland et al., 2020).

Stroke/Transient Ischemic Attack

Definitions

Cerebrovascular attack (CVA): Also known as *stroke* or acute *ischemic stroke (AIS);* indicates ischemia to a section of the brain due to a blockage of blood flow that manifests with focal neurologic signs and requires emergent mechanical or pharmacologic intervention.

Endovascular thrombectomy (EVT): Mechanical extraction of a thrombus post ischemic stroke.

Transient ischemic attack (TIA): Temporary ischemia to a section of the brain that manifests with focal neurologic signs and resolves within minutes or hours without treatment.

CASE STUDY 20.2

Mrs. V. A. is a 76-year-old female with a history of type 2 diabetes, dyslipidemia, hypertension, and peripheral vascular disease. She presents to the emergency department with her husband, who reports of slurred speech, left-sided weakness, left-sided facial droop, and tingling, which started 2 hours prior to arrival. Her home medications consist of an 85 mg aspirin, metformin 500 mg, and losartan 25 mg po daily. How would you manage this patient?

Strokes are generally divided into two categories: hemorrhagic stroke, which refers to a bleed in the brain, and acute ischemic stroke, which refers to a disruption in the blood supply to an area of the brain. Transient ischemic strokes (TIAs) are referred to as ischemic strokes or "mini strokes." This chapter primarily discusses ischemic strokes unless otherwise indicated. Globally, cerebrovascular attack (CVA), or stroke, remains the third-leading cause of death. Stroke incidence increased by 70% from 1990 to 2019, and the prevalence of stroke increased by 85% with an increase in deaths and disability-adjusted life-years (DALYs) by 43% and 32% respectively (Global Burden of Disease [GBD], 2016, 2019). The aging population and ongoing increase in risk factors contribute to an accumulation of risk for the geriatric population. There was a 225% increase in the stroke prevalence rate for individuals ages 70 years and younger. Ischemic stroke showed an incidence of 62.4% of all strokes (GBD, 2016, 2019).

Chronic comorbidities such as cardiovascular disease and diabetes further increase the risk of stroke and transient ischemic attacks (TIAs) in the aging population. Risk factors such as obesity, hypertension, hyperlipidemia, and smoking further increase the risk of stroke. Other causes of CVA include, but are not limited to, atherosclerotic disease (of the aorta, carotid arteries, vertebral arteries, basilar arteries, and intracranial atherosclerosis), cardiac emboli from atrial fibrillation, MI, congestive cardiomyopathy, vasculitis conditions such as lupus, moyamoya disease, severe anemia, sickle cell disease, and platelet and hypercoagulable disorders; susceptible individuals include those at risk for a hypercoagulable state (>55 years of age/history of thrombolytic event, autoimmune disorder) and individuals with cancer (Barkley, 2021). Individuals diagnosed with COVID-19 are at risk for a hypercoagulable state, in addition to those with cancer and individuals who use birth control. Drug use, such as the use of cocaine or methamphetamine, has also been associated with stroke.

Symptom recognition of CVA or TIA is vital to improve outcomes for the patient, including reducing the chances of death and disability. For these reasons, patient and public education on how to identify stroke should be taught by health care professionals during routine visits when dealing with high-risk populations. One of the most common methods used to help patients recognize the symptoms of CVA is the FAST mnemonic, which indicates Facial drooping, Arm weakness, Speech difficulties, and Time to call 9-1-1 (American Stroke Association [ASA], 2021). However, some educational programs have used the BE-FAST mnemonic, where "B" is for balance and "E" is for eyes (Aroor et al., 2017). The use of the BE-FAST mnemonic additionally allows one to recognize symptoms in patients who may exhibit gait imbalance, leg weakness, visual impairment (visual loss, diplopia, or blurring), headache, or dizziness but who may not meet the FAST mnemonic criteria (Aroor et al., 2017).

Health care providers should be knowledgeable and competent in performing a thorough neurologic assessment, in addition to a comprehensive physical examination, health history, and review of systems. A thorough assessment is crucial when examining the patient at risk of a CVA or TIA. Prehospital stroke scales used in the diagnosis of intracranial large-vessel occlusion include the Cincinnati Prehospital Stroke Scale (CPSS), Conveniently Grasped Field Assessment Stroke Triage (CG-FAST), FAST-PLUS (Face-Arm-Speech-Time plus severe arm or leg motor deficit) test, Gaze-Face-Arm-Speech-Time (G-FAST), Prehospital Acute Stroke Severity (PASS), Los Angeles Motor Scale (LAMS), and Rapid Arterial oCclusion Evaluation (RACE) (Dippel et al., 2021). The CG-FAST, G-FAST, and RACE have shown acceptable to good accuracy and similar accuracy to the National Institutes of Health Stroke Scale (NIHSS) (Dippel et al., 2021). Many of the prehospital stroke scales can be used from a mobile app.

Obvious signs of stroke include hemiplegia, facial droop, slurred speech, unilateral weakness, numbing, or tingling, in addition to the aforementioned signs. Hemiplegia is generally a sign of stroke, where facial tingling, slurred speech, dizziness, headache and gait disturbance, or any focal neurologic deficit that peaks in minutes and lasts less than 24 hours is diagnosed as a TIA (Foschi et al., 2022). However, patients with any ischemic brain lesion on imaging are considered to have experienced a minor ischemic stroke (MIS) or TIA and usually have mild nondebilitating symptoms (Amarenco, 2020). Other symptoms of stroke upon further assessment include expressive aphasia, disruption in the ability to verbally express or communicate, and receptive aphasia, the inability to comprehend verbal communication. Additionally, stroke symptoms may include memory loss, confusion, loss of gross motor ability, visual hallucinations, visual disturbances, and other forms of sensory loss (Barkley, 2021).

Utilization of the NIHSS is recommended for the neurologic assessment for CVA in the emergency department or hospital setting (Dippel et al., 2021; Powers et al., 2019. When patients present with symptoms of stroke, the stroke team or medical emergency team should be notified immediately.

Interprofessional Collaboration in Acute Management of Stroke and Transient Ischemic Attack

The acute care nurse practitioner or physician assistant responding to patients who exhibit signs of stroke should complete a neurologic examination, order appropriate imaging and diagnostics, and consult with the neurologist for ongoing management if stroke or MIS/TIA is diagnosed. Interprofessional collaboration with the nursing staff, neurologists, physical therapist, and case manager are vital for acute management and preparation for discharge. The neurologist can assist with management of the patient during the acute management and upon discharge during patient follow-up. The role of physical therapist is important to identify and prepare the patient for any limitations regarding activities of daily living and fall prevention. Case management is key to assist in proper discharge placement, when helping to decide if a patient should be discharged home with physical therapy visits, to a rehabilitation clinic, or to long-term assisted living. Interprofessional collaboration is an important factor to achieving best outcomes for the patient who has sustained a stroke or TIA.

Upon completion of a thorough neurologic assessment, the acute care nurse practitioner or physician assistant should consider any physiologic possibilities that could mimic stroke or TIA. Vital signs should be checked immediately, as should the patient's oxygen saturation and blood glucose level. Symptoms of hypoxemia, hypoglycemia, and hyperglycemia resemble those of stroke or TIA, so the provider should consider these possibilities if the patient appears confused and exhibits aphasia or visual disturbances. A noncontrast computed tomography (CT) of the head should be ordered and simultaneously the patient should be transferred to a higher level of care. This includes a critical or intensive care unit or neurologic intensive care unit, if available, where the patient should be given hourly neurologic assessments.

Although an ischemic stroke may not be visualized by a noncontrast CT, excluding intracranial hemorrhage or tumors it may detect any contraindications to thrombolytics (Powers et al., 2019). The diagnostic evaluation of acute ischemic stroke (AIS) should be confirmed by a neurology expert such as a neurologist or neuroradiologist prior to administering thrombolytics. Consultations can be initiated onsite or via a telemedicine neurologic consult. Although magnetic resonance imaging (MRI) is often seen as the gold standard for diagnosing stroke shortly after ischemic stroke, CT is the only imaging tool that is readily available and that is required prior to diagnosing stroke (Aben et al., 2020; Powers et al., 2019). Because stroke can be diagnosed by CT alone, thrombolytic administration should not be delayed while waiting to administer further diagnostics (Powers et al., 2019). A computed tomographic angiography (CTA) can be completed at the same time to identify large vessel occlusion.

However, considerations of the geriatric patient should be taken into account when deciding to add a CTA, which requires intravenous contrast dye. Use of contrast dye could affect kidney function and further cause contrast-induced nephrology (CIN) or acute kidney injury (AKI). See the Special Considerations for the Older Adult Experiencing Stroke/Transient Ischemic Attack section.

Treatment

Patients who screen positive for CVA should be transported to a stroke center or hospital with the capability to deliver acute stroke care. Geriatric patients who are medically eligible and who are less than age 80 should receive intravenous (IV) alteplase within 4.5 hours of symptom onset, even if there is a consideration for endovascular thrombectomy (EVT) due to large vessel occlusion (Powers et al., 2019).

Reperfusion treatment of IV alteplase of 0.9 mg/kg, with a maximum dose of 90 mg over 60 minutes with an initial bolus of 10% given over 1 minute, should be initiated as quickly as possible (Powers et al., 2019). Blood pressure should be lowered safely to less than 185/110 mm Hg prior to reperfusion therapy with a blood glucose level greater than 50 mm/dl. Patients taking antiplatelet monotherapy prior to stroke may be administered IV alteplase granted the benefit outweighs the risk. Patients who received low-molecular-weight heparin within the previous 48 hours should not receive IV alteplase, nor should patients taking anticoagulants, thrombin inhibitors, or direct factor Xa inhibitors. For these patients, a direct factor Xa activity assay, an ecarin clotting time (ECT), and a coagulation panel, including an international normalize ratio (INR), should be monitored. For patients with AIS and platelets <100,000/mm^3, INR>1.7, aPTT>40 s, or PT>15 s, IV alteplase is contraindicated, as the safety and efficacy are unknown (Powers et al. 2019). If IV alteplase is initiated in patients who are not on anticoagulants and previous findings are noted on the laboratory results, therapy should be discontinued. Antiplatelet agents that inhibit the glycoprotein IIb/IIIa receptor are also contraindicated with IV alteplase. Other contraindications to IV alteplase include, but are not limited to, aortic arch dissection, suggestions of subarachnoid hemorrhage or intracranial hemorrhage, intracranial neoplasm, active internal bleeding, uncontrolled hypertension greater than 185/110, head trauma, bacterial endocarditis, known bleeding diathesis, dose of nonwarfarin oral anticoagulant within the previous 12 hours, seizure, major surgery within the previous 2 weeks, gastrointestinal or urinary hemorrhage in the previous 3 weeks, and lumbar puncture or puncture at a noncompressible site within the previous 7 days (see Table 20.3) (Levine et al., 2023; Powers, et al., 2019).

Upon any indication of neurologic decline during reperfusion therapy, IV alteplase should be discontinued to obtain a head CT and until intracranial hemorrhage is ruled out. Follow-up CT or MRI should be obtained within 24 hours of alteplase initiation, and placement of central lines, indwelling Foley catheters, nasogastric tubes, or any other invasive procedures should be avoided.

Vital signs and neurologic assessments should be monitored closely. Continuous electrocardiogram and oxygen saturation monitoring should be present with airway management being a priority. Blood pressure should be monitored every 15 minutes upon the initiation of alteplase for the first 2 hours, every 30 minutes for 6 hours, then every hour for 16 hours. When administering IV antihypertensives, blood pressure should be monitored every 15 minutes. Any temperature greater than or equal to 38°C should be investigated to determine the source and treated with antipyretics, in addition to treatment of the underlying cause. In patients with AIS, blood glucose should be kept in a range of 140 to 180 mg/dL. Monitoring glucose levels every 6 hours with use of a sliding scale is appropriate for patients who are not receiving oral intake. Once patients begin to receive oral intake, blood glucose can be monitored before meals and at bedtime with supplemental subcutaneous regular insulin per sliding scale, per the facility's protocol.

In patients who sustained acute ischemic strokes due to large vessel occlusion, EVT is considered the standard of care when symptom onset is within 6 hours. EVT is also considered the standard of care for stroke patients who present beyond 6 hours with favorable perfusion imaging (Powers et al., 2019). Patients 80 years and older with fewer comorbidities have demonstrated better outcomes after EVT (Mehta et al., 2021). In patients who undergo mechanical thrombectomy, with or without reperfusion, blood pressure should be maintained at less than 180/110 mm Hg.

Special Considerations for the Older Adult Experiencing Stroke/Transient Ischemic Attack

Patients with end-stage renal disease who receive hemodialysis (HD) are at increased risk of stroke (Mark et al., 2021). Older adults on HD should receive IV alteplase. However, older adults with a history of diabetic hemorrhagic retinopathy, the risk of vison loss should be weighed against the risk on not receiving alteplase and worsening, permanent neurologic deficits. For older patients with preexisting disabilities, the decision to receive alteplase should consider the quality of life and the risk for higher mortality associated with reperfusion therapy. Older adults who sustained an AIS within the previous 3 months are not eligible for IV alteplase. As other diagnoses can mimic stroke, such as hypoglycemia, hyperglycemia, and neurologic symptoms related to infections (urinary tract infections, pneumonia), the proper diagnosis and management of stroke are the keys to decreasing morbidity and mortality.

As previously mentioned, when contemplating a CTA for geriatric patients, renal function and the risk of AKI should be considered. Geriatric patients with normal renal function are at risk of AKI with the use of contrast dye with CTA. Because geriatric patients may have decreased kidney function and are at higher risk of developing CIN and AKI, hydration with isotonic saline should be considered. Other preventive measures against CIN and AKI include the use of sodium bicarbonate and acetylcysteine. Evidence shows that there is no significant difference in the prevention of kidney damage when using the previous pharmacologic interventions over isotonic saline (Weisbord et. al, 2018).

It is always necessary for acute care providers of older adults to consider the impact of procedures and pharmacologic therapy, including the risk of hemorrhage with fibrinolytics (Madhavan et al., 2018). Special considerations should be made when managing the patient with stroke to ensure that the benefits of therapy outweigh the risks.

Hemorrhagic Stroke

Intracranial hemorrhage (ICH) and subarachnoid hemorrhage (SAH) account for approximately 13% to 17% of all strokes, with ICH more common than SAH (Barkley, 2021; Benjamin et al., 2017). Risk factors of hemorrhagic stroke include uncontrolled hypertension, anticoagulants, illicit drug use, alcoholism due to injury to the cerebral vessels, and hematologic disorders such as thrombocytopenia and factors VIII and XI deficiencies (Barkley, 2021).

Symptoms of hemorrhagic strokes vary depending on the location and severity. Symptoms include, but are not limited to, nausea, vomiting, headache, vertigo, impaired gait, impaired vision, aphasia, pinpoint pupils, irregular eye movements, quadriplegia, facial weakness, gaze palsies, and coma (Camargo et al., 2017). Noncontrast head CT remains the diagnostic choice for ICH. For SAH; the use of the modified Fischer scale can be utilized to indicate the severity of the hemorrhage by findings indicated on the noncontrast CT (see Table 20.3) (Winn et al., 2022). Acute laboratory tests include a coagulation panel as indicated in AIS and an extensive history, a physical and neurologic examination, and imaging to investigate causes and prevent transformation of ischemic infarction (Camargo et al., 2017). If the CT of the head is negative for a SAH but symptoms suggest otherwise, a lumbar puncture must be performed. Treatment of hemorrhagic strokes includes supportive care in the intensive care unit. The neurology surgery consult may consider possible evacuation of any hematomas, clipping, or placement of an external ventricular drain (EVD), which is dependent on the location of the hemorrhage.

Systolic blood pressure should be maintained at less than or equal to 140 mm Hg. Intravenous antihypertensives may be needed to manage blood pressure. However, nitroglycerin and nitroprusside cause cerebral vasodilation and should be avoided (Barkley, 2021). Any coagulopathy should be corrected by reversing anticoagulants specific to the patient's medication profile and coagulation panel. The health care professional should monitor the patient's coagulation panel, PT, PTT, and INR every 3 to 6 hours.

In the event that an EVD is placed, intracranial pressure (ICP) should be monitored closely with a goal of less than 20 mm Hg. Cerebral perfusion (mean arterial pressure minus the ICP) should be maintained at greater than 60 or 50 to 70 mm Hg (Barkley, 2021). Hourly neurologic checks should be performed utilizing the Glasgow Coma Scale (GCS). The GCS gives a numeric score of the lowest at 3 and the highest at 15, revealing the patient's overall responsiveness (Magee & Manske, 2021; Table 20.4). A goal of <9 with strict bed rest and minimal stimulation should be maintained. In patients who have experienced a hemorrhagic, stroke stool softeners should be initiated to avoid constipation and defecation strain, which could further extend a brain hemorrhage. Patients experiencing ICH or SAH should be placed in seizure precautions. Prophylactic antiepileptic medications remain controversial (Barkley, 2021). Supportive care for the patient who has suffered SAH is vital to decrease the risk of vasospasm.

Prevention

Decreasing risks to reduce recurrent stroke is key. Risk factors include hypertension, diabetes, smoking, hyperlipidemia, obstructive sleep apnea, alcohol use, and a lack of physical activity (Oza et al., 2017). Adherence to antithrombotic therapy is also key to reducing the reoccurrence of ischemic stroke and TIA. Patient education that consists of detailed information regarding taking the necessary steps to reduce the risks of stroke is essential. Monitoring and managing blood pressure and glucose levels are important steps in addition to taking medications as prescribed and maintaining a healthy diet. Smoking cessation is necessary for those who use tobacco products or who vape, as use of these products increase the risk of stroke. Patients who exhibit signs or who are at risk of obstructive sleep apnea should have a sleep study performed during their hospital stay or immediately upon discharge to identify possible obstructive sleep apnea, which is also a risk factor for stroke. Limiting or eliminating alcohol consumption is also necessary for the patient recovering from stroke to decrease the patient's risk of recurrence. Providers should encourage physical exercise of 120 to 150 minutes per week, such as brisk walking or jogging, when possible (Oza et al., 2017).

As patients aim to lead a healthy lifestyle post stroke and to prevent stroke reoccurrence, it is vital that health care providers encourage patients to adhere to their medication regimen. Patients who suffered with ischemic stroke or TIA should be discharged on aspirin, a combination of aspirin and extended-release dipyridamole, or clopidogrel. Prasugrel is contraindicated in patients with a history of stroke or TIA (Kass & Goldsmith, 2022).

Bowel Obstruction

Definitions

Adhesions: Bands of scar tissue formed in the bowel post-surgery (Baiu & Hawn, 2018).

Bilious vomiting: Nausea and dark green bile vomitus caused by an obstruction inside the bowel.

Bowel obstruction: Blockage of the intestinal flow that may be mechanical, functional, or in the form of a lesion, due to the lack of peristalsis.

FAST ultrasound: The focused-abdominal-sonography in trauma evaluation considered the standard of care in adults with traumatic injury or with suspected peritoneal injury or dysfunction. The FAST views the right upper

CASE STUDY 20.3

Ms. C. I. is an 88-year-old female who was admitted to the observational unit in your hospital less than 6 hours prior with diffuse abdominal pain accompanied by nausea and bilious vomiting. She has been diagnosed with dehydration and fever secondary to a gastrointestinal virus contracted from her grandchild. You are called to manage her worsening abdominal pain and upon your physical examination you are unable to detect bowel sounds. The patient also reports worsening constipation over the past 48 hours. How should you manage this patient?

TABLE 20.4 Glasgow Coma Scale

				Time 1()	Time 2()
Eyes	Open	Spontaneously	4	____	____
		To verbal command	3		
		To pain	2		
		No response	1		
Best motor response	To verbal command	Obeys	6	____	____
	To painful stimulus	Localizes pain	5		
		Flexion—withdrawal	4		
		Flexion—abnormal (decorticate rigidity)	3		
		Extension (decerebrate rigidity)	2		
		No response	1		
Best verbal response		Oriented and converses	5	____	____
		Disoriented and converses	4		
		Inappropriate words	3		
		Incomprehensible sounds	2		
		No response	1		
Total			3–15	____	____

From Magee, D. J., & Manske, R. (2021). Head and face. In *Orthopedic physical assessment* (pp. 73–163). Saunders Elsevier.

quadrant, left upper quadrant, suprapubic, and pericardium and can further detect intraperitoneal and pericardial fluid (Fornari & Lawson, 2021).

Obstipation: When fluid and air cannot advance in the colon, causing the lack of flatulence or bowel movements (Baiu & Hawn, 2018).

There are approximately 350,000 cases of small bowel obstructions (SBOs) annually in the United Sates with 65% occurring secondary to adhesions, 10% from hernias, with neoplasms and Crohn's disease accounting for 5% each (Reddy & Cappell, 2017). A bowel obstruction is a medical emergency and should be diagnosed and managed as soon as possible as 35% of bowel obstructions can lead to death if untreated for more than 36 hours (Federle & Lau, 2018; Reddy & Cappell, 2017).

SBOs can be categorized as follows: partial or complete; simple or closed; by severity of low grade to high grade; and by position of high, proximal, occurring in the jejunum or low, distal occurring in the ileum (Federle & Lau, 2018). Complications of SBO include bowel strangulation, infarction, perforation, peritonitis, gangrenous bowel, and sepsis. The mortality rate of untreated strangulated bowel (also known as ischemic bowel) is 100% (Federle & Lau, 2018).

Gastrointestinal discomfort is a cardinal sign of bowel obstruction. The patient with bowel obstruction may present with diffuse abdominal pain, constipation, obstipation, nausea, bilious vomiting, or fever, and may have hypoactive to no bowel sounds. Absent or decreased bowel sounds indicate decreased peristalsis, which may indicate a bowel obstruction. Other indicators include the absence of flatus or bowel movements. Upon physical examination, high-pitched bowel sound may be heard initially with tenderness upon palpation and tympany upon percussion (Reddy & Cappell, 2017). However, bowel sounds are not always indicative of the severity of bowel obstruction. Patients with bowel obstruction may also appear with signs of sepsis and dehydration.

Performing a FAST ultrasound may be helpful in assessing for markers of obstruction (Long et al., 2019). However, a CT of the abdomen and pelvis is most appropriate for a definitive diagnosis (ten Broek et al., 2018). Suspected acute SBO should be diagnosed with a CT of the abdomen and pelvis with IV contrast, as patient presentation, physical examination, and laboratory findings alone are not sufficient in diagnosis of SBO. Although laboratory findings may reveal leukocytosis, with hematocrit, blood urea nitrogen (BUN), and creatinine indicative of volume depletion, a CT of the abdomen with IV contrast is preferred (Price, 2020). Although a CT of the abdomen and pelvis without IV contrast may be appropriate, contrast will aid in the distinction between a partial and complete SBO (Chang et al., 2020).

In patients who are not vomiting, enteral contrast may be ingested 1 to 4 hours prior to an abdominal CT via nasogastric (NG) tube or orally. Failure of contrast to reach the cecum in 24 to 36 hours is indicative of bowel obstruction requiring surgery exploration (ten Broek et al., 2018). Contrast that reaches the cecum predicts nonsurgical resolution of the SBO (Barkley, 2021, Jacobs, 2022; Reddy & Cappell, 2017). However, CT of the abdomen with IV contrast remains the ideal choice for quickly diagnosing SBO in all patients (Long & Koyfman, 2019).

Special Considerations of the Older Adult Experiencing Bowel Obstruction

Because those in the geriatric population generally have more comorbidities of diabetes, cardiovascular disease, and kidney disease, these patients may experience poorer outcomes if surgery is delayed greater than 24 hours (Karmanos et al., 2016). The quality of life and frailty of the geriatric patient should be taken into strong consideration, particularly if considering laparotomy (ten Broek et al., 2018. The risk of delayed healing postsurgery and the impact on quality of life should be discussed with the geriatric patient in preparation for recovery, physical therapy, and disposition upon discharge. The acute care provider should communicate to the geriatric patient possible and expected outcomes. This includes pain management, sepsis, the possibility of prolonged ventilator support, physical therapy, and rehabilitation.

Treatment

A surgery consult should be initiated for management of a bowel obstruction, and the patient should be admitted to a higher level of care for close monitoring. An NG tube should be placed to decompress distention proximal to the obstruction and to control emesis and prevent aspiration (Smith et al., 2021). Although many bowel obstructions may be resolved with conservative management via placement of an NG tube, IV fluids, bowel rest with no oral intake, intravenous antiemetics, bed rest, and discontinuation of any medications that inhibit GI motility are priorities. With SBOs, surgical intervention is often necessary (Long et al., 2019; Price, 2020). Level I recommendations have strong evidence indicating that hemodynamic instability in SBOs warrants surgical intervention (Table 20.5) (Long et al., 2019; Maung et al., 2012).

Patients managed without surgical intervention should be monitored closely for worsening or resolving bowel obstructions, indicating serial abdominal radiography every 8 to 12 hours (Reddy & Cappell, 2017). Worsening symptoms may be indicative of ischemia, necrosis, or perforation. With resolving bowel obstructions, patients' symptoms will often show improvement, including decreased abdominal pain, distention, passage of flatus, and increased bowel movements (Reddy & Cappell, 2017).

SBOs are more common than large bowel obstructions (LBOs) and generally more frequently require surgical intervention (Smith et al., 2021). Up to 90% of patients who sustain an SBO without peritonitis may be successfully managed nonoperatively (Catena et al., 2016; Reddy & Cappell, 2017). Evidence indicates that patients 80 years of age and older who experience emergent exploratory laparotomies have an increased risk of mortality. Laparoscopic treatment is further classified as a level 2 recommendation (see Table 20.5), indicating it is not highly recommended for the geriatric patient (Long et al., 2019; ten Broek et al., 2018). When operative treatment is required, laparoscopy may be beneficial for special cases of acute simple bowel obstruction (ten Broek et al., 2018).

Surgical intervention requires adequate bowel preparation. In older adults who are at risk of fluid and electrolyte abnormalities, polyethylene glycol-electrolyte lavage (PEG-ELS) solution should be used for bowel preparation. The use of PEG-ELS is especially important given the population of geriatric patients who have electrolyte imbalances, renal insufficiency, end-stage liver disease, and heart failure, whereas the use of hyperosmotic laxative regimens may cause electrolyte shifts and are renally excreted (A-Rahim & Falchuk, 2021). Surgical preparation with preoperative broad-spectrum antibiotics should be initiated, which may include tazobactam-piperacillin, 3.375 grams IV every 6 hours, ticarcillin-clavulanate, 3.1 grams IV every 6 hours, or a carbapenem, and it may depend on the preference of the surgery consult (Price, 2020).

TABLE 20.5 Criteria for the Diagnosis of Idiopathic Acute Transverse Myelitis Eastern Association for the Surgery of Trauma Practice Management Guideline for Managing Small Bowel Obstruction

Recommendation	Level
1. Patients with generalized peritonitis or other evidence of clinical deterioration (fever, leukocytosis, tachycardia, acidosis, continuous pain) should undergo timely surgical exploration.	1
2. Patients with no evidence of clinical deterioration can safely undergo nonoperative management initially.	1
3. CT findings consistent with bowel ischemia require a low threshold for operative intervention.	2
4. Laparoscopic treatment of SBO is a viable option compared with laparotomy in selected cases.	2
5. Water-soluble contrast should be considered for patients with partial SBO that has not resolved in 48 h.	2

SBO, Small bowel obstruction.
From Lim, P. A. C. (2020). Transverse myelitis. *Essentials of Physical Medicine and Rehabilitation*, 952–959. https://doi.org/10.1016/B978-0-323-54947-9.00162-0

Interprofessional Collaboration in Managing the Geriatric Patient With Bowel Obstruction

Collaboration with the surgeon and the interprofessional team remains the standard of care when managing geriatric patients postoperatively and in the acute care setting. The geriatric patient remains at risk due to physiologic and anatomic changes. Challenges the geriatric patient may face include postoperative complications such as delirium, ventilator-associated pneumonia, infection, and pain, which may delay ambulation and recovery. Close collaboration with the interprofessional team should be maintained regarding appropriate medications, prevention of polypharmacy, pain management, adequate nutrition, safe ambulation postoperatively, and appropriate disposition—all of which require an interprofessional team approach.

The geriatric patient should receive nothing by mouth until further indicated by the surgeon. Patient's will often return from surgery with a nasogastric tube, and removal of the NGT should be left to the surgeon's discretion. The nutritionist should be consulted to provide support in management of the patient's nutrition. Physical therapists and occupational therapists should be consulted to assist the patient with activities of daily living and ambulation when appropriate in preparation for discharge.

Hip Fracture

Definitions

Delirium: Acute onset of confusion characterized by a change in cognition (Nguyen & Lui, 2020).

Hip fracture: Fracture of the proximal part of the femur (Dove & Jenkins, 2022).

Intermittent pneumatic compression (IPC): An intermittent inflating calf compression device used in prophylaxis deep vein thrombosis (DVT) postoperatively or during hospitalization when ambulation is limited or not feasible (Morris & Roberts, 2022).

CASE STUDY 20.4

Ms. J. R. is an 81-year-old who presented to the emergency department with left-sided hip pain after sustaining a fall when walking her dog. She was found on the sidewalk by a neighbor and has been admitted to the hospital for a fractured left hip. As the provider managing her care for the night shift, how would you proceed to ensure this patient receives optimal care during her hospital stay?

Hip fracture is one of the leading causes of hospitalizations in the geriatric population ages 65 and older, with the mean age being greater than 80 years (Dove et al., 2022; Ferris, 2022). According to the Centers for Disease Control and Prevention, more than 300,000 geriatric patients experience hip fractures, and chances increase as adults age, with an estimated global cost of $130,000 billion by 2050 (CDC, 2016; Nguyen et al., 2020). Caucasian females have a greater incidence of osteoporosis than other groups, which places them more at risk for hip fracture.

In the acute care setting, obvious signs of hip fracture include an acute onset of pain after falling with bruising and swelling around the hip and limited weight-bearing. An externally rotated hip upon physical examination as well as limited range of motion are indications of a hip fracture. Although most hip fractures can be diagnosed using anteroposterior and lateral radiographs, MRI can detect occult fractures not detected on radiographs (Ross et al., 2019). Fall prevention is vital in the outpatient and inpatient settings, as approximately 95% of hip fractures are secondary to falls (CDC, 2016).

Potential complications in the geriatric patient further decrease quality of life and mortality while increasing the cost of hospitalization. These complications include, but are not limited to, cardiovascular adverse events such as DVTs, pulmonary emboli, myocardial infarctions, congestive heart failure, and CVAs. Other complications of hip fracture include infections such as pneumonia, urinary tract infections, surgical wound infections, and pressure ulcers. Depression, social isolation, and functional decline are also complications of hip fractures that contribute to increased mortality (Nguyen & Lui, 2020).

Treatment

The goals of treatment for the geriatric patient who sustained a hip fracture are to minimize pain, restore mobility with complete weight-bearing ambulation, decrease mortality, and improve quality of life (Elsevier, 2022). Consultation of an orthopedic surgeon should be initiated, and a neurosurgeon should be consulted if there is suspected neurologic injury, particularly injury to the sciatic nerve, upon physical examination. Although most hip fractures are treated surgically with a goal of surgical fixation within 24 to 48 hours, for patients with severe dementia, with multiple or significant comorbidities, or who were nonambulatory prior to injury, nonoperative management may be the treatment of choice (Dove & Jenkins, 2022). Treatment of hip fracture in the geriatric patient is dependent on the location and severity of the fracture, in addition to comorbidities and other factors that may impact the patient's outcome.

Patients should be placed in fall precautions, with management of pain and deep vein thrombosis prophylaxis. DVT prophylaxis is important for the prevention of thrombi post injury and immobility. IPC prophylaxis in addition to low-molecular-weight heparin (LMWH) or aspirin is recommended (Anderson et al., 2019). Laboratory testing should include a complete blood count, a comprehensive metabolic panel, a coagulation panel, and a type and screen. Other diagnostics include a chest radiograph, an ECG, and a urinalysis (Dove & Jenkins, 2022). Prior to surgery, broad-spectrum antibiotics should be initiated with isotonic IV fluids for hydration.

Postoperatively patients generally remain in the acute care setting approximately 2 to 5 days after hip surgery (Halter et al., 2017). Adequate pain management is vital to ensure early ambulation, with minimal sedating affects, to minimize deconditioning, falls, and postoperative complications. Pain can be managed with IV morphine, being sure to decrease the dosage as necessary for pain control, as geriatric patients are more at risk of adverse reactions to narcotics and sedating medications. For this reason, it is important to remember to "start low and go slow." Beginning with low doses of medications known to cause sedation, respiratory depression, or hypotension decreases the risks for adverse effects concerning the geriatric patient. Utilizing the interdisciplinary team approach will help to improve patient outcomes, decrease the hospital length of stay, and prevent subsequent falls.

Interprofessional Collaboration in Managing the Geriatric Patient With Hip Fracture

As with managing the care of all patients admitted to an inpatient setting, an extensive interprofessional team should be consulted to decrease all risks of morbidity and mortality in the geriatric patient who has sustained a hip fracture. In addition to the adult gerontology acute care nurse practitioner or physician assistant, orthopedic surgeon, and the registered nurse, the interdisciplinary team should also consist of the respiratory therapist, the occupational therapist, the physical therapist, the dietician, and the social worker or case manager. The occupational therapist (OT) and physical therapist (PT) will work closely with the patient postoperatively to help the patient ambulate and perform activities of daily living while understanding the perceived functional ability versus the actual functional ability. Providing extensive education is also an important role of OT and PT, as they provide therapeutic strategies to prevent future falls (Riemen & Hutchinson, 2016).

The case manager also plays a vital role in preparing for the older adult's disposition and in assisting the patient, interdisciplinary team, and caregiver in deciding whether to discharge the patient home or if a rehabilitation or skilled facility is more appropriate (Halter et al., 2017). Rehabilitation should also be coordinated in communication with the patient, the interprofessional team, and any support system the patient may have; the intent is to achieve optimal recovery and to meet the patient's goals to obtain and maintain a reasonable quality of life. All parties must be aware of the expectation of acute intensive physical therapy, which requires approximately 3 hours per day (Halter et al., 2017). Individuals who are not able to comply with such rigorous therapy should be considered for a more long-term approach, based on the patient's physical capabilities and the availability of resources.

The acute care provider should educate the patient and family to continue DVT prophylaxis for approximately 30 days postoperatively. Additionally, patients should be educated on the possible limitations with ambulation that may last up to 1 year postoperatively and may require the use of a medical device (Halter et al., 2017). Patients older than 85 years are more likely to require long-term care and have poorer outcomes regarding lower extremity baseline function (Halter et al., 2017).

Transverse Myelitis

Definitions

Autonomic dysfunction: A dysfunction in the autonomous nervous system that may result in a lack of functional control; it includes orthostatic hypotension, drooling, bladder dysfunction, gastrointestinal dysfunction, and excessive sweating (Xu & Lu, 2019).

Multiple sclerosis: A neurodegenerative autoimmune disease that affects the central nervous system and can progress to irreversible disability (Adam et al., 2021).

Neurogenic bladder: Atypical function of the bladder caused by brain or spinal cord injury or disease that can lead to upper urinary tract damage (Lee, 2021).

Neuromyelitis optica spectrum of disorders (NMOSD): A rare antibody-mediated demyelinating disease of the nervous system that results in extensive spinal cord involvement leading to inflammation (myelitis), optic neuritis, and possible episodes of hiccoughs and intractable vomiting (Huda et al., 2019; Monreno-Escobar et al., 2021).

Transverse myelitis: A rare inflammatory process in a transverse region of the spinal cord; it leads sensory and motor changes that can result in the rapid onset of paraplegia (Sudhakar et al., 2022).

CASE STUDY 20.5

Mrs. Z is a 65-year-old patient who presents to the emergency department with her spouse and complaints of bilateral paraplegia of acute onset upon awakening. Her spouse reports she was recently treated for shingles and has been running a fever along with bowel and bladder incontinence, which she had never experienced before. She further complains of lower back pain. What are your differential diagnoses, and how do you plan to manage this patient?

Transverse myelitis (TM) ranges from 1.3 to 8 cases per 1 million and increases to 24.6 cases per 1 million when multiple sclerosis (MS) or neuromyelitis optic spectrum disorders (NMOSD) are included (Moreno-Escobar et al., 2021). MS often presents with transverse myelitis in patients of African or Asian descent; however, MS is a rare cause of myelitis in Caucasians (Hauser, 2022). Neuromyelitis optica is a severe myelopathy that is associated with optic neuritis and may precede or succeed myelitis for several weeks (Hauser, 2022).

Clinical manifestations are generally due to demyelination or inflammation of the spinal cord and can be idiopathic or secondary to a neurologic or autoimmune condition. TM results in sensory weakness and autonomic dysfunction at the level of the lesion. In addition to autoimmune disorders and inflammation, other causes include, but are not limited to, infections such as human immunodeficiency virus (HIV), shingles or Lyme disease, and postvaccination. Approximately 50% of those who sustain transverse myelitis have experienced a recent respiratory tract infection.

Acute transverse myelitis has been a concern post COVID-19 due to its neurologic complications. It includes symptoms such as loss of consciousness, convulsions, status epilepticus, and encephalitis, to name a few, and should prompt early diagnosis and management (Alketbi et al., 2020). In patients suffering from any recent infections who present with rapid onset of sensory and motor decline, the provider should consider transverse myelitis as a differential diagnosis with proper diagnosis and treatment. Fever, tachycardia, and tachypnea may indicate infection. In addition to acute weakness and sensory impairments, the patient with TM may present with bowel and bladder changes, including nausea, vomiting, abdominal cramps, constipation, and pseudo-obstruction (Camilleri, 2021). Failure to properly diagnosis and manage the patient who is experiencing acute TM can result in paralysis, autonomic dysfunction, neurogenic bladder, incontinent bowels, and pain that is neuropathic or musculoskeletal in nature (Lim, 2020).

The patient with transverse myelitis may present with a rapid onset of unilateral or bilateral paraplegia of the upper or lower extremities or parathesis that may result in back pain, sphincter dysfunction, and a positive Babinski, depending on the level of the lesion (Sudhakar & Goldsmith, 2022). Clinical deficits may progress 4 hours to 21 days after symptom onset. Autonomic dysfunction in the autonomous nervous system caused by transverse myelitis may result in a lack of functional control and may include orthostatic hypotension, drooling, bladder dysfunction, gastrointestinal dysfunction, and excessive sweating (Xu & Lu, 2019). Common manifestations include neurogenic bladder with urinary incontinence or retention, gastrointestinal disturbances of incontinence or constipation, and sexual dysfunction (Sudhakar & Goldsmith, 2022). Neurogenic bladder is an atypical function of the bladder caused by brain or spinal cord injury or disease, which can lead to upper urinary tract damage (Lee, 2021).

The imaging of choice for diagnosis of suspected acute myelitis is MRI. T2-weighted fast spin-echo and short-tau inversion recovery (STIR) offer high sensitivity when viewing the spinal cord for lesions (Alketbi et al., 2020; Lim, 2020). CT may be necessary to properly diagnose bowel involvement. Immunoglobulin G antibodies may help determine neuromyelitis optica as the etiology. Basic laboratory tests should include blood cultures, a metabolic panel, and a complete blood count. A lumbar puncture may be helpful for detecting the cause of acute TM, specifically to reveal CSF pleocytosis and collect a CSF autoimmune panel (Moreno-Escobar et al., 2021). Additional testing should aim to detect infections and should include assessments of antinuclear antibodies, the erythrocyte sedimentation rate, immunoglobulin levels, anti-double-stranded DNA antibodies, and SS-A antibody to detect Sjogren disease, to name a few (Lim, 2020). Serologic testing for various viruses that could precede TM should include assessments for HIV, cytomegalovirus, Lyme disease, West Nile virus, Zika virus, poliovirus, hepatitis, and most recently known offender, COVID-19, as previously indicated (Lim, 2020). A thorough history, physical examination, and testing must be done to eliminate possible causes of acute TM, prior to diagnosing TM as idiopathic, and to prevent misdiagnosis. Acute TM has been confused with Guillain-Barre syndrome in the acute phase, as symptoms of weakness and in some cases autonomic dysfunctions present similarly (Chandrashekhar & Dimachkie, 2022). Table 20.6 lists the inclusion and exclusion criteria that must be considered when diagnosing idiopathic acute TM (Lim, 2020).

TABLE 20.6 Inclusion and Exclusion Criteria Necessary When Diagnosing Idiopathic Acute Transverse Myelitis

• Development of sensory, motor, or autonomic dysfunction attributable to the spinal cord • Bilateral signs or symptoms (although not necessarily symmetric) • Clearly defined sensory level • Exclusion of extraaxial compressive etiology by neuroimaging (MRI or myelography; CT of spine not adequate) • Inflammation within the spinal cord demonstrated by CSF pleocytosis or elevated IgG index or gadolinium enhancement. If no inflammatory criterion is met at symptom onset, repeated MRI and lumbar puncture evaluation between 2 and 7 days after symptom onset meet criteria. • Progression to nadir between 4 h and 21 days after the onset of symptoms (if patient awakens with symptoms, symptoms must become more pronounced from point of awakening)	• History of previous radiation to the spine within the last 10 years • Clear arterial distribution clinical deficit consistent with thrombosis of the anterior spinal artery • Abnormal flow voids on the surface of the spinal cord consistent with AVM • Serologic or clinical evidence of connective tissue disease (e.g., sarcoidosis, Behçet disease, Sjögren syndrome, SLE, mixed connective tissue disorder) • CNS manifestations of syphilis, Lyme disease, HIV, HTLV-1, mycoplasma, other viral infection (e.g., HSV-1, HSV-2, VZV, EBV, CMV, HHV-6, enteroviruses) • Brain MRI abnormalities suggestive of multiple sclerosis • History of clinically apparent optic neuritis

AVM, Arteriovenous malformation; *CMV*, cytomegalovirus; *CNS*, central nervous system; *CSF*, cerebrospinal fluid; *CT*, computed tomography; *EBV*, Epstein-Barr virus; *HHV*, human herpes virus; *HIV*, human immunodeficiency virus; *HSV*, herpes simplex virus; *HTLV-1*, human T-lymphotropic virus 1; *IgG*, immunoglobulin G; *MRI*, magnetic resonance imaging; *SLE*, systemic lupus erythematosus; *VZV*, varicella-zoster virus.
Modified from Transverse Myelitis Consortium Working Group. Proposed diagnostic criteria and nosology of acute transverse myelitis. *Neurology*. 2002;59:499–505.

Treatment

Treatment of acute TM and idiopathic TM should begin with high-dose IV glucocorticoids, specifically methylprednisolone (30 mg/kg up to 1000 mg daily) or dexamethasone (120 to 200 mg daily) (Greenberg, 2022; Moreno-Escobar et al., 2021). Intravenous glucocorticoids may be initiated alone or in addition to plasma exchanges (Greenberg, 2022). Recommendations for the treatment of aggressive TM in patients with systemic lupus erythematosus include intravenous cyclophosphamide (800 t0 1200 mg/m^2 as a single pulse dose) (Greenberg, 2022). Treatment of acute TM due to a secondary cause should be directed at the underlying cause.

Hemodynamic monitoring and management of underlying comorbidities should be initiated. Special attention should be given to airway management if the patient sustained acute TM in addition to bladder control. A Foley catheter should be placed in the patient experiencing symptoms of neurogenic bladder. Placing the patient on fall precautions, seizure precautions, and aspiration precautions are preventive measures to avoid further complications for the geriatric patient in the acute care setting. Frequent neurologic management and physical assessment of the patient should be performed.

In addition to a neurologic consult, consultations with a physical therapist, occupational therapist, and case manager are important when caring for the geriatric patient in the acute care setting. Due to deconditioning and possible chronic neurologic deficits that may exist or may be perceived, preparing the patient for reentry into the home, rehabilitation center, or skilled nursing facility is warranted. Interprofessional collaboration remains vital to improve the safety and outcomes of the geriatric patient.

Sepsis

Definitions

Sepsis: A life-threatening systemic syndrome that causes organ dysfunction and is caused by an infection (Alderman, et al., 2022).

Systemic inflammatory response syndrome (SIRS): Characterized as two or more inflammatory response symptoms that may or may not be triggered by an infection (Keeley et al., 2017; Makic et al., 2018).

Sepsis is the leading cause of death in adult intensive care units (ICUs) and is associated with more than 850,000

TABLE 20.7 Criteria for Systemic Inflammatory Response Syndrome

☐	Temperature <36°C (96.8 °F) or >38°C (100.4 °F) (1 point)
☐	Heart rate >90 beats/min (1 point)
☐	Respiratory rate >20 breaths/min or $PaCO_2$ <32 mm Hg (1 point)
☐	WBC <4000/mm^3, or WBC >12,000/mm^3, or WBC bands >10% (1 point)

WBC, White bood count.
From Bone, R. C., Balk, R. A., Cerra, F. B., Dellinger, R. P., Fein, A. M., Knaus, W. A., Schein, R. M. H., & Sibbald, W. J. (1992). Definitions for sepsis and organ failure and guidelines for the use of innovative therapies in sepsis. *Chest*, *101*(6), 1644–1655. https://doi.org/10.1378/chest.101.6.1644

emergency department visits and a mortality rate as high as 40% (Berg & Gerlach, 2018; Napolitano, 2018; Wang et al., 2017). Due to multiple comorbidities, the aging population is more at risk of morbidity and mortality related to sepsis. Most sepsis diagnoses occur in adults older than age 65 (Rowe & McKoy, 2017). By 2060 the number of adults older than age 65 is projected to double to 98 million (Department of Health and Human Services [DHHS], 2015). In 2016, the Third International Consensus Definitions for Sepsis and Septic Shock (Sepsis-3) task force defined sepsis as "a life-threatening organ dysfunction caused by a dysregulated host response to infection" (Singer, 2016). The Surviving Sepsis Campaign: International Guideline for Management of Sepsis and Septic Shock 2021 recommends using the systemic inflammatory response syndrome (SIRS) criteria (Table 20.7), the Modified Early Warning Score (MEWS) (Fig. 20.6), or the National Early Warning Score (NEWS) 2 (Table 20.8) as a single screening tool for sepsis or septic shock (Evans et al., 2021). Use of the SIRS screening (see Table 20.7) has been found to be significantly superior to the SOFA (Kalil et al., 2022).

Patients with known infection or who are predisposed to infection are at risk of sepsis. This includes patients who are immunocompromised, such as those diagnosed with HIV, cancer, or who are taking immunosuppressive medications. Other patients who are at increased risk of sepsis in the acute care setting are those with central lines, Foley catheters, and older adults, as previously mentioned, with multiple comorbidities. Patients diagnosed with sepsis should have any intravascular access devices that could be the source of infection removed promptly (Evans et al., 2021).

Systemic inflammatory response syndrome (SIRS) is characterized as two or more inflammatory response symptoms that may or may not be triggered by an infection (Keeley et al., 2017; Makic et al., 2018). SIRS criteria consist of having two or more of the following: a temperature >38°C or <36°C, a respiratory rate >20 breaths per minute, a heart rate >90 per minute, or a white blood cell count

CASE STUDY 20.6

Mr. Y is an 80-year-old male who presents with a chronic cough that has worsened over the past week. Upon physical examination you discover that he has rhonchi throughout his lung fields with increased tactile fremitus. He is confused and has a temperature of 101.3°, blood pressure of 94/48, a heart rate of 114, and a respiratory rate of 26. What are your differential diagnoses for Mr. Y, and how will you manage his care?

Early Warning Score = Sum of All Points

Points	3	2	1	0	1	2	3
SBP	≤ 90	91–100	101–110	111–219			≥ 220
Temp (°F)	≤ 95		95.1–96.8	96.9–100.4	100.5–102.2	≥ 102.3	
HR	≤ 40		41–50	51–90	91–110	111–130	≥ 131
RR	≤ 8		9–11	12–20		21– 24	≥ 25
O_2 Sat	≤ 91%	92–93%	94–95%	≥ 96%			
FiO2				Room Air		Suppl O_2	
Alertness				Awake, alert			Altered*

* Altered = stuporous, lethargic, obtunded, unresponsive, or comatose.

• **Fig. 20.6** Modified Early Warning Score (MEWS). (From Barnett, W. R., Radhakrishnan, M., Macko, J., Hinch, B. T., Altorok, N., & Assaly, R. [2021]. Initial MEWS score to predict ICU admission or transfer of hospitalized patients with COVID-19: A retrospective study. *Journal of Infection, 82*[2], 282–327. https://doi.org/10.1016/j.jinf.2020.08.047.)

TABLE 20.8 The National Early Warning Score 2 (NEWS2)

	3	2	1	0	1	2	3
Pulse (bpm)	≤ 40		41–50	51–90	91–110	111–130	≥131
BR (bpm)	≤8		9–11	12–20		21–24	≥25
T (ºC)	≤35		35.1–36	36.1–38	38.1–39	≥39.1	
SBP (mm Hg)	≤90	91–100	101–110	111–219			≥220
SpO_2 (%) Scale 1	≤91	92–93	94–95	≥96			
SpO_2 (%) Scale 2	≤83	84–85	86–87	88–92 ≥93 air	93–94 Oxygen	95–96 Oxygen	≥97 Oxygen
Air oxygen		Oxygen		Air			
AVPU (scale)				A			V, P, U

AVPU, Alert, verbal, pain, unresponsive; *BR*, breathing rate; *SBP*, systolic blood pressure; SpO_2, oxygen saturation; *T*, temperature.
In patients with hypercapnic respiratory insufficiency, scale 2 should be used to weight the oxygen saturation score.
Each category is graded 0–3. Scores for each category are added together to give a total. Composite scores of greater than 5 (or 3 in any one parameter) trigger an urgent medical review. A score of over 7 triggers a review by a critical care outreach team or medical response team.
From Martín-Rodríguez, F., Sanz-Garcia, A., Guijarro, L., Ortega, G., Perez, Marta, Villamor, M., et al. (2020). Comorbidity-adjusted NEWS predicts mortality in suspected patients with COVID-19 from nursing homes: Multicentre retrospective cohort study. *Journal of Advanced Nursing, 78*. https://doi.org/10.1111/jan.15039)

of $>12x10^9$/L or $<4 \times 10^9$/L (Keeley et al., 2017). Note the clinical calculator in Table 20.7 (Bone et al., 1992). Although SIRS is a pro-inflammatory state, 10% to12% of patients with sepsis may not meet the SIRS criteria. Geriatric patients are less likely to present with fever and often may be hypothermic or normothermic. The geriatric patient is also less likely to present with tachycardia (Alderman et al., 2022). Meeting the criteria for SIRS in the presence of infection meets the diagnosis of sepsis.

The clinical signs of sepsis are directly related to the origin of infection and the system. Early detection of sepsis and the cause of infection are vital to the survival of the patient. Patients who are septic may exhibit generalized symptoms, which include, but are not limited to, fever, chills, rigors, dyspnea on exertion or at rest, chest pain, fatigue, malaise, confusion, fainting, nausea, vomiting, diarrhea, oliguria, flank pain, myalgia, and generalized pain. Initial symptoms are generally related to the origin of infection (Alderman et al., 2022).

The adult gerontology acute care provider or physician assistant managing the patient with a likely diagnosis of sepsis must complete a through history and physical examination to find the culprit of infection. Additionally, initiating appropriate diagnostics, including appropriate laboratory testing, should be directed at diagnosing and managing the infection. When unsure of the site of infection, the provider can turn to basic diagnostics such as chest radiography to determine a respiratory source, two sets of blood cultures (one from invasive lines and one peripherally), the baseline complete blood count, a complete metabolic panel, a urinalysis and culture, a sputum culture, an influenza test, and a test for COVID-19. Biomarkers of sepsis include C-reactive protein, procalcitonin, adrenomedullin, and, most historically used, lactate (Rello et al., 2017). Lactate is a biomarker of hypoperfusion, and increases have been associated with organ dysfunction and mortality. Patients with a lactate reading of >4 mmol/l with organ dysfunction, hypoperfusion, and infection are in septic shock (Rello et al., 2017).

Other diagnostic testing is specific to the patient's symptoms and physical examination findings. Patients for whom GI is the source of infection will benefit from a FAST ultrasound and likely a CT. Lumbar puncture may be necessary when meningitis is suspected. MRI of the brain or spine may also be indicated. Patients suspected of cardiovascular involvement will require not only a baseline ECG but possibly an echocardiogram. Testing should be completed for both infectious and noninfectious illnesses that may present as sepsis (Evans et al., 2021).

Treatment

The goal of managing sepsis is to diagnosis and initiate treatment as soon as possible, within 1 hour of recognition. As sepsis and septic shock are medical emergencies, the Surviving Sepsis Campaign International Guideline for Management of Sepsis and Septic Shock 2021 strongly recommend that treatment and fluid resuscitation begin immediately. Crystalloids are considered the first-line fluid for resuscitation (Evans et al., 2021). Intensive fluid resuscitation and broad-spectrum antibiotics are vital for the effective management of septic shock (Rello et al., 2017). In addition, a response to organ failure that results in continued hypoperfusion may require vasopressors, oxygen, mechanical ventilation, transfusion, or packed red blood cells (Rello et al., 2017). Although various vasopressors may be used based on the patient's cardiovascular history, in general norepinephrine is recommended as the first-line agent over other vasopressors (Evans et al., 2021).

When a diagnosis of sepsis is made, empiric broad-spectrum antibiotics (gram positive and gram negative) should be initiated immediately to cover all likely pathogens. However, adequate diagnosis of the infectious pathogen, laboratory findings, and data will later aid in narrowing antimicrobial therapy. Therefore, blood cultures should be drawn from separate sites prior to the administration of antibiotics, if possible. Evidence supports starting antibiotics early, preferably within 1 hour, to decrease sepsis-related morbidity and mortality (Rello et al., 2017). Adults with known methicillin-resistant Staphylococcus aureus (MRSA), with a history of MRSA, or with a high suspicion of having MRSA should be managed with empirical antibiotics with MRSA coverage rather than those without (Evans, et al., 2021).

Although the Surviving Sepsis Campaign does not strongly recommend antifungals and antivirals, they may be initiated in consultation with an infectious disease specialist. Corticosteroid therapy has shown favorable results in patients with systemic inflammation; however, the benefits of steroids to treat sepsis remain uncertain. Steroids may be utilized based on consultation with and at the discretion of the intensivist and ICU team (Myer & Dries, 2022). Providers should keep in mind the impact steroids have on inflammatory process when monitoring the white blood cell count for improvement in leukocytosis. The acute care provider should collaborate with the doctor of pharmacy (PharmD) to ensure appropriate dosing of antibiotic therapy in the geriatric patient and any patient with compromised renal function.

The patient with sepsis requires closes hemodynamic monitoring. Central venous pressure monitoring is an important indicator of fluid resuscitation and should be done continuously. Central venous pressure (CVP) is an excellent indicator of volume resuscitation in the patient diagnosed with sepsis, so this factor should also be closely monitored. Other hemodynamic monitors include but are not limited to, mean arterial pressure (MAP) and central venous oxyhemoglobin saturation ($SvcO_2$). The goals of the MAP should be ≥ 65 mm Hg, CVP >8 mm Hg, and $SvcO_2$ >70%. Glycemic control and prevention of hypoglycemia are also important in the management of sepsis (Cecconi et al., 2018). Insulin therapy should be initiated for glucose levels ≥ 180 mg/dL (10 mmol/L) (Evans et al., 2021). Venous thromboembolism prophylaxis should be initiated with low-molecular-weight heparin when not contraindicated (Evans et al., 2021).

In patients who have sepsis-induced acute respiratory distress syndrome (ARDS) and are mechanically ventilated, the goal of prone ventilation should be more than 12 hours daily. Providers are also recommended to use a low tidal volume strategy of 6 mL/kg rather than a high tidal volume strategy of >10 mL/kg (Evans et al., 2021). The upper limit goals for plateau pressures should be 30 cm H_2O over higher plateau pressures (Evans et al., 2021).

Special Considerations for the Geriatric Patient Experiencing Sepsis

The geriatric patient faces more challenges with sepsis than does the younger patient and is at an increased risk for morbidity and mortality. One of the primary challenges is the rate of comorbidities that come with the aging body. This includes frailty as the human body ages. Another risk is the compromised immune system of the older adult, which makes the patient more vulnerable to infection and sepsis. The older patient may not present with the same expected clinical signs as the younger adult. For instance, a high temperature is not necessarily a finding in the geriatric patient who is septic. A geriatric patient who is septic may present with a hypothermic temperature or a low normothermic temperature. It is important to complete a thorough evaluation of the geriatric patient to identify sepsis and the source of infection and to begin treatment as soon as possible to prevent morbidity and mortality, both of which are increased in the geriatric patient. Additionally, the older adult may often present with confusion, an early sign of infection. Infection in the older patient often originates in the genitourinary system as a urinary tract infection or in the lungs as pneumonia when no other obvious source is present.

As with all inpatient care, interprofessional collaboration among the intensivist, the acute care provider, and the acute care team is vital to ensure that the geriatric patient survives sepsis with minimal long-term effects and to decrease the patient's length of stay in the intensive care unit and hospital. The interprofessional approach helps to ensure patient safety, positive outcomes, and an increased quality of life after discharge.

Trauma

CASE STUDY 20.7

Mr. G. P. is a 69-year-old male who lives alone and presents to the emergency room with a laceration to the forehead after sustaining a fall. He takes warfarin daily and is bleeding excessively from the head laceration. The bleeding has been stabilized and sutures placed. However, G.P. reports dizziness and informs you this is his third fall this month. How should you, as the acute care provider, proceed, as the patient also complains of abdominal pain and reports black, tarry stools?

The geriatric population is at increased risk of falls, injury, and trauma. The risk of trauma increases with age and is the leading cause of disability, hospitalizations, and admissions to long-term care facilities, further increasing the risks of morbidity and mortality in the older population (Gioffre-Florio, 2018). Among adults ages 65 years and older, falls remain the leading cause of injury. In 2018 more than 950,000 hospitalizations and nearly 32,000 deaths among geriatric patients were related to injuries from falls (Moreland, et. al, 2020). Trauma and deaths related to falls continue to increase within the aging population, particularly among individuals ages 85 years and older (Burns et al., 2018). For these reasons it is important to perform a falls risk assessment on all geriatric patients and encourage measures for fall prevention. The United States spends an estimated $50 million annually to address falls related to the geriatric population (Florence et al., 2018). To provide health care providers with clinical guidelines to prevent falls, the Center for Disease Control's Injury Center developed the Stopping Elderly Accidents, Deaths, and Injuries (STEADI) initiative (Florence et al., 2018). This initiative focuses on the following:

1. Screening older patients to identify their fall risk
2. Assessing at-risk patients to identify their modifiable fall risk factors
3. Intervening by using effective strategies to reduce the number of fall risk factors

Appropriate screening, assessment, and intervention are important to reduce the risks of falls in the geriatric population, which ultimately will reduce traumatic events related to falls.

Although falls are common in the geriatric patient population, trauma is not limited to falls. Traumatic injuries of any kind in the older adult should be triaged and assessed appropriately to prevent increased morbidity and mortality. This includes trauma from motor vehicle accidents, blunt chest wall trauma, wounds, and trauma resulting in intubation or the need for emergent surgery. Geriatric individuals are also at risk for various traumas after being involved in a motor vehicle accident, such as spinal trauma, hip and limb fractures, abdominal trauma, and traumatic head injuries. Older adults are more at risk of poor outcomes after a traumatic injury than are younger adults. Evidence shows that geriatric patients admitted to level I trauma centers who require intubation or who have preexisting congestive heart failure have an increased risk of postinjury morbidity. Although age and rib fractures showed a correlation with posttraumatic mortality (Sawa et al., 2018), other factors associated with postinjury morbidity included diabetes mellitus, cardiopulmonary disease, chronic obstructive pulmonary disease, protein calorie malnutrition, and the use of ambulatory assist devices (Sawa et al., 2018).

Thorough assessment of the geriatric patient is important. Older patients who experience trauma are often undertriaged, as tools to assess levels of trauma are often indicated for one specific traumatic event (Alshibani et al., 2021). For this reason, the geriatric patient who has experienced a fall, minor car accident, or any trauma-related event, no matter the severity, should receive a thorough comprehensive examination and close observation. The geriatric patient occasionally presents differently than the adult patient due to age-related physiologic and anatomic changes (Alshibani et al., 2021). Patients ages 55 years and older are less likely to present with the same vital signs as younger patients. For instance, the systolic blood pressure, heart rate, and respiratory rate may be significantly lower than they would be in a younger patient, and the parameters normally identified as signs of shock may differ as well (Alshibani et al., 2021). These differences may be due to the medications older adults take to manage other comorbidities. Differences may also be noted in the Glasgow Coma Scale (Alshibani et al., 2021). For these reasons, a comprehensive geriatric assessment (CGA) should be completed within 24 hours of admission of an older patient who has experienced trauma (Fisher et al., 2017). The CGA is vital for assessing older adults when addressing how to positively impact outcomes and decrease mortality and morbidity based on the evidence (Conroy & Thomas, 2021). Additionally, the time up and go (TUG) can also be used as an indicator to predict functional decline in older patients following minor trauma (Eagles et al., 2016).

Older adult patients who have experienced trauma should be monitored closely and admitted for observation even if the overall presentation appears normal due to the drastic decline and delay or misrepresentation of how posttraumatic symptoms may surface. The delayed physiologic response of the geriatric patient should always be considered after any traumatic event, including what is considered a minor fall. The TUG assessment can be used to measure mobility and indicate the possibility of a subsequent fall. For this reason, continued fall and risk assessments should be performed.

Of the major traumatic injuries experienced by older adults, over 70% are traumatic brain injuries (Griffiths & Kumar, 2017). Older patients are less likely to be transferred to a trauma center and, unfortunately, have a delay in obtaining a CT compared to younger adults (Griffiths & Kumar, 2017). This delay of care should not be an issue for the older adult. In fact, older adults are generally frailer and at risk of poor outcomes; for this reason, care of the older adult who has experienced a traumatic brain injury should be expedited. Approximately 5% of adults ages 60 years and older receive neurosurgical interventions, which take four times as long as those of younger adults (Trauma Audit and Research Network, 2017).

If there is unexplained trauma not associated with a specific accident or fall, the geriatric patient should be assessed for elder abuse (Schuur & Cooper, 2018). The primary survey and assessment of the patient who has experienced trauma should always begin with the ABCs: airway, breathing, and circulation (Walls et al., 2018a, 2018b) (Fig. 20.7). Critical evaluation of the patient's airway, breathing, and circulation is vital to survival. Protecting the patient's airway, ensuring adequate ventilation, and evaluating the patient for signs of shock should be priority, in addition to ongoing assessments, when managing the geriatric patient who has experienced trauma. Monitoring hemodynamic parameters and continued examination for internal bleeding are also crucial.

Patients with insufficient respiratory effort, a GCS score less than or equal to 8, or who are vomiting or actively bleeding may need an artificial airway. Inadequate ventilation should be suspected and addressed in posttrauma patients who exhibit cyanosis, difficulty breathing, decreased oxygen saturation, tachypnea, labored breathing, or unequal breath sounds. A patient's circulation is in question with hypotension, tachycardia, decreased capillary refill, or mottled extremities and further indicate signs of shock (Walls et al., 2018a, 2018b).

The algorithm in Fig. 20.7 provides special considerations based on the mechanism of injury for blunt and penetrating trauma.

A FAST exam is always warranted when injury to the internal organs or bleeding is suspected in the abdominal cavity. Other radiographic evaluations may consist of a chest x-ray and CT of the affected or suspected area of injury. Standard laboratory testing should be completed, which includes, but is not limited to, a complete metabolic panel, a complete blood count, and a coagulopathy panel. For patients with previous diagnoses of diabetes mellitus, congestive heart failure, or other comorbidities, appropriate laboratory testing should be completed to manage the patient adequately. An electrocardiogram should be performed on all geriatric patients following traumatic events, minor or major. It is important to detect if myocardial infarction is a result or cause of the traumatic injury so as to manage the patient appropriately and prevent reoccurrence. Other cardiac markers may also be indicated.

Treatment upon primary survey and assessment of the posttrauma patient should consist of managing the patient to the point of protecting the airway, ensuring adequate ventilation, and treating shock. Proper airway and ventilation should be managed to maintain an oxygen saturation of 92% or greater. This may include a binasal cannula, face mask ventilation, high-flow oxygen, a nonrebreather, or intubation.

Vital signs and neurologic checks should be monitored frequently, because the geriatric patient's status may drastically change at any time. Trauma patients should be placed on supplemental oxygen with large bore intravenous (IV) access for the administration of IV fluids and possible blood products if needed. Crystalloids may be used for fluid resuscitation, and for emergent need of blood, O-positive should be used if the geriatric patient's blood type is not available.

For patients exhibiting signs of shock, fluid resuscitation and ensuring there is no active bleeding are priorities for correcting hypovolemic or hemorrhagic shock. Hypovolemic shock is a reduction of intravascular volume that lowers preload and causes the body to compensate by increasing stroke volume, heart rate, and oxygen consumption (Lier et al., 2018). Hypovolemic hemorrhagic shock impairs circulation and affects multiple organ systems. Identifying the source of bleeding and early massive transfusion should be initiated for patients in shock (Cannon, 2018). For patients with severe hemorrhage, rapid control of all sites of hemorrhage is crucial. Definitive hemostasis should be achieved as soon as possible to ensure survival. A type and cross for compatible transfusions should be performed at the first indication of blood loss, hemorrhage, or severe anemia. As previously indicated, O-positive should be administered in emergent situations and when there is a need for an immediate transfusion. Acute care providers should be careful not to under-resuscitate. Crystalloid infusions should be limited to less than 3 liters in the first 6 hours (Cannon, 2018). Laboratory monitoring should include a chemistry, complete metabolic panel, complete blood count, and a coagulopathy panel. Frequent laboratory monitoring of the hematocrit and hemoglobin should be performed post transfusion and if there is any sudden change in the patient's status. Additional laboratory monitoring should be completed when indicated. For patients with acute bleeding, massive-transfusion protocols provide universal donor products such as packed red blood cells, platelets, plasma, and cryoprecipitate to increase the rate of survival (Cannon, 2018). Acute care providers should follow the hospital's massive-transfusion protocol when available.

Special Considerations for the Geriatric Patient Who Experiences Trauma

Geriatric patients who experience trauma are at risk of increased morbidity and mortality due to multiple comorbidities as

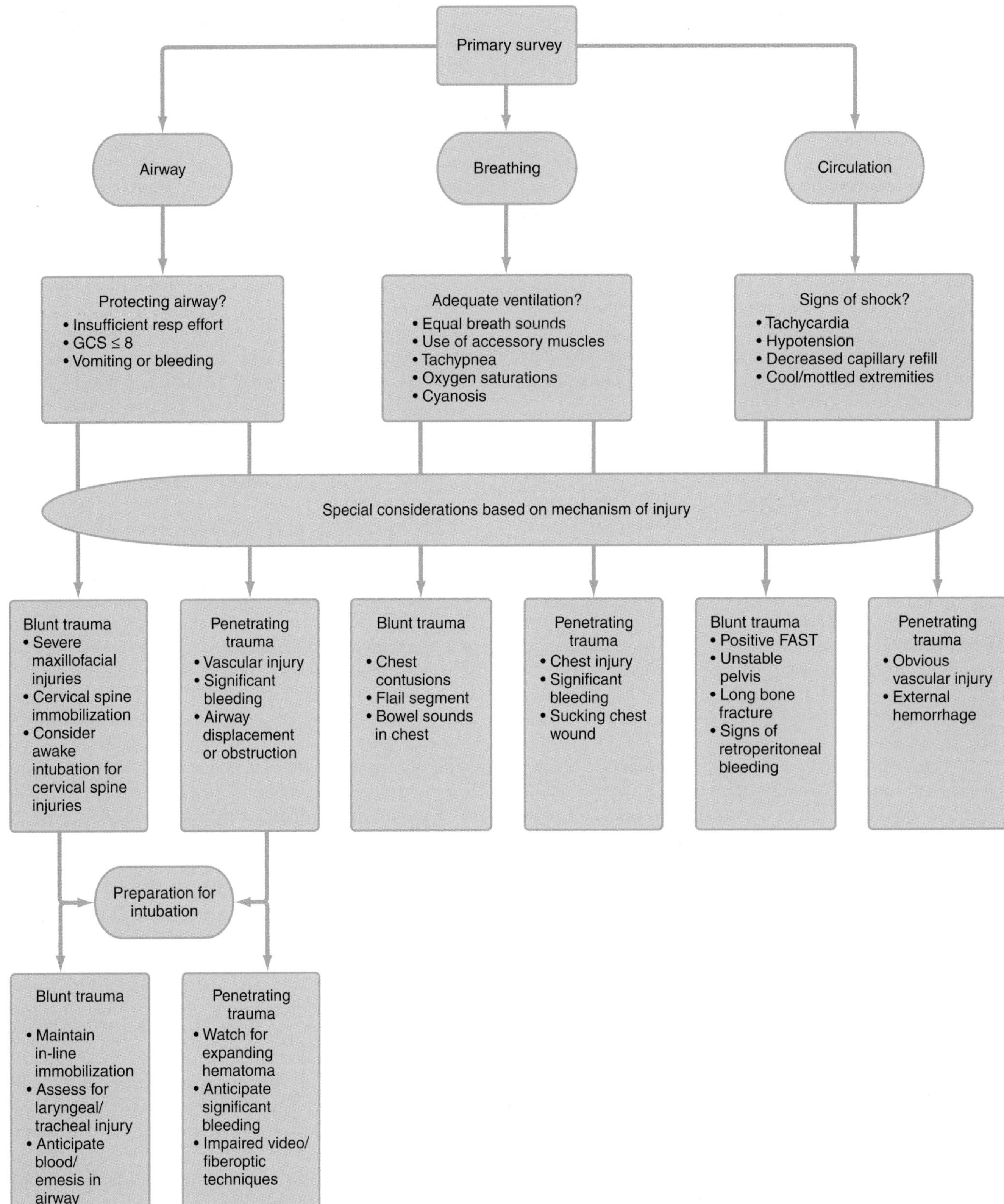

• **Fig. 20.7** Algorithm for Evaluating the ABCs of Patients Who Experienced Trauma. (From Walls, R. M., Hockberger, R. S., Gausche-Hill, M., Bakes, K. M., Gross, E., & Martel, M. [2018]. Multiple trauma. In *Rosen's emergency medicine: Concepts and clinical practice* [pp. 287–300]. Elsevier.)

well as physiologic and anatomic changes associated with age. This in turn increases one's hospital length of stay and decreases positive long-term outcomes. For this reason, older adults should not receive a delay in care post minor or major traumatic events or injuries. Fall prevention and screenings should be initiated in the inpatient and outpatient settings to decrease the risk for and to prevent falls. Comprehensive geriatric examinations should be performed annually or when indicated to ensure the older adult is assessed appropriately and to see to it that any deficits or needs are identified.

The acute care provider has the responsibility to verify that the patient or the patient's power of attorney has specified life-saving measures or any limitations to heroic measures documented in the patient's chart. More important, the acute care provider should ensure that the legally documented requests are followed. The acute care provider should discuss with the patient, family, surgeon, and patient-care team any end-of-life measures regarding intubation, cardiopulmonary resuscitation, transferring the patient to a trauma center, and consulting palliative care or hospice (Schuur & Cooper, 2018).

Interprofessional Collaboration and Disposition

In collaboration with the interprofessional team, the acute care provider should ensure that discharge planning begins upon admission to the inpatient setting. General consults should involve a geriatric specialist, a physical therapist, an occupational therapist, a pharm D, a case manager, and a social worker. Discharge planning consists of a thorough comprehensive geriatric assessment along with an evaluation by a physical therapist, an occupational therapist, and social services to ensure the geriatric patient is appropriately dispositioned upon discharge. The input of a pharm D is vital to decrease the risks of polypharmacy and eliminate medications that may increase the risk of falls or reinjury for the geriatric patient. Ensuring that all needs of the older adult are met is vital to prevent falls, posttraumatic injuries, or surgery. Prolonged hospitalization can negatively impact the older adult's baseline abilities to function independently, including the activities of daily living. Returning to "normal" can be particularly challenging postoperatively if sedatives, prolonged bed rest, decreased ambulation, or delirium was a major factor during the patient's hospital stay. Returning to normal for the geriatric patient can be challenging and take more time than expected. Conversations with the patient's family members and support system should begin early upon hospital admission to ensure the geriatric patient has a positive outcome post trauma.

Key Points

- The immediate diagnosis and management of myocardial infarction (MI) are vital to decrease morbidity and mortality in the older adult patient.
- Interprofessional collaboration is key in the treatment and disposition of the older adult patient who has suffered an MI.
- Patients over the age of 70 are nearly twice as likely to experience hemorrhagic stroke with the use of fibrinolytics.
- Patient and family education play an important role in preventing the reoccurrence of occlusion and acute coronary syndrome (ACS).
- An accurate diagnosis of stroke is vital when managing older patients with comorbidities that may mimic stroke.
- Special considerations should be taken when managing the older adult who has experienced a cerebrovascular attack (CVA).
- Discharge planning should begin upon hospital admission and include an interprofessional team approach.
- Surgical consult should be initiated to manage bowel obstruction in the older adult patient.
- Patients ages 80 and older who have emergent exploratory laparotomies have an increased risk of mortality.
- Surgical intervention includes appropriate bowel preparation and preoperative broad-spectrum antibiotics.
- Potential complications in the older adult patient further decrease quality of life and increase mortality.
- The goals of treatment for the older adult patient who sustained a hip fracture are to minimize pain, restore mobility with complete weight-bearing ambulation, decrease mortality, and improve quality of life.
- Rehabilitation should be coordinated in collaboration with the patient, the interprofessional team, and the patient's family to achieve optimal recovery.
- Transverse myelitis should be considered in patients who are suffering from any recent infections and are positive for the rapid onset of sensory and motor decline.
- Common manifestations include a neurogenic bladder with urinary incontinence or retention, gastrointestinal disturbances of incontinence or constipation, and sexual dysfunction.
- The imaging of choice for a diagnosis of suspected acute myelitis is an MRI.
- Treatment of acute transverse myelitis (TM) and idiopathic TM should begin with high-dose IV gluco-corticoids.
- Treatment of acute TM due to a secondary cause should be directed at the underlying cause.
- The goal of managing sepsis is to diagnosis and initiate treatment as soon as possible.
- Intensive fluid resuscitation and broad-spectrum antibiotics are vital for the effective management of septic shock.
- Older adult patients face more challenges with sepsis and have an increased risk for mortality.

- The older patient may not present with the same expected clinical symptoms as the younger adult.
- Older patients are often undertriaged following traumatic events due to anatomic and physiologic changes.
- A comprehensive geriatric assessment should be performed on all older adult patients who experience any traumatic event, no matter the severity.
- Fluid resuscitation and ensuring there is no active bleeding are priorities for correcting hypovolemic or hemorrhagic shock.
- Older adult patients who experience trauma are at risk for increased morbidity and mortality.
- Fall prevention and screenings should be initiated to decrease the risk for and to prevent falls.

More information about tools and Interprofessional Education Collaborative (IPEC) competencies mentioned in this chapter can be found in Appendix 1: Tools and Appendix 2: IPEC Competencies.

References

Aben, H. P., Luijten, L., Jansen, B. P. W., Visser-Meily, J. M. A., Spikman, J. M., Biessels, G. J., & de Kort, P. L. M. (2020). Absence of an infarct on MRI is not uncommon after clinical diagnosis of ischemic stroke. *Journal of Stroke and Cerebrovascular Diseases, 29*(8), 104979. https://doi.org/10.1016/j.jstrokecerebrovasdis.2020.104979.

Adam, A., Dixon, A. K., Gillard, J. H., Schaefer-Prokop, C., Rovera, A., Cremer, S., & Sundgren, P. (2021). Inflammatory and metabolic disease. In *Grainger & Allison's diagnostic radiology: A textbook of medical imaging* (pp. 1498–1549) (7th ed.). Elsevier.

Alderman, E., Ananthakrishnan, A., Baron, T., Barth, B., Bernstein, J., & Bhatt, D. (2022, March 24). Sepsis clinical overview. *ClinicalKey.* https://www.clinicalkey.com/.

AlKetbi, R., AlNuaimi, D., AlMulla, M., AlTalai, N., Samir, M., Kumar, N., & AlBastaki, U. (2020). Acute myelitis as a neurological complication of covid-19: A case report and MRI findings. *Radiology Case Reports, 15*(9), 1591–1595. https://doi.org/10.1016/j.radcr.2020.06.001.

Alshibani, A., Singler, B., & Conroy, S. (2021). Towards improving prehospital triage for older trauma patients. *Zeitschrift Für Gerontologie Und Geriatrie, 54*(2), 125–129. https://doi.org/10.1007/s00391-021-01844-4.

Amarenco, P. (2020). Transient ischemic attack. *New England Journal of Medicine, 382*(20), 1933–1941.

American Academy of Physician Assistants (AAPA). (2022, January 31). *Competencies for the physician assistant profession.* https://www.aapa.org/career-central/employer-resources/employing-a-pa/competencies-physician-assistant-profession/.

American Association of Colleges of Nursing (AACN). (2021). *AACN scope and standards for adult-gerontology and pediatric acute care nurse practitioners.* Aacn.org. https://www.aacn.org/nursing-excellence/standards/aacn-scope-and-standards-for-adult-gerontology-and-pediatric-acute-care-nurse-practitioners.

American College of Cardiology (ACC) American Heart Association (AHA)/Society for Cardiovascular Angiography & Interventions (SCAI). (2022). Correction to 2021: Guideline for coronary artery revascularization: A report of the American College of Cardiology/American Heart Association joint committee on clinical practice guidelines. *Circulation, 145*(11). https://doi.org/10.1161/cir.0000000000001060.

American Stroke Association (ASA). (2021). *Stroke symptoms.* www.stroke.org. https://www.stroke.org/en/about-stroke/stroke-symptoms.

Anderson, D. R., Morgano, G. P., Bennett, C., Dentali, F., Francis, C. W., Garcia, D. A., Kahn, S. R., Rahman, M., Rajasekhar, A., Rogers, F. B., Smythe, M. A., Tikkinen, K. A. O., Yates, A. J., Baldeh, T., Balduzzi, S., Brożek, J. L., Ikobaltzeta, I. E., Johal, H., Neumann, I., Wiercioch, W., Yepes-Nuñez, J. J., Schünemann, H. J., & Dahm, P. (2019). American Society of Hematology 2019 guidelines for management of venous thromboembolism: Prevention of venous thromboembolism in surgical hospitalized patients. *Blood Advances, 3*(23), 3898–3944. https://doi.org/10.1182/bloodadvances.2019000975. PMID: 31794602; PMCID: PMC6963238.

Andreotti, F., Rocca, B., Husted, S., Ajjan, R. A., ten Berg, J., Cattaneo, M., Collet, J. -P., De Caterina, R., Fox, K. A. A., Halvorsen, S., Huber, K., Hylek, E. M., Lip, G. Y. H., Montalescot, G., Morais, J., Patrono, C., Verheugt, F. W. A., Wallentin, L., Weiss, T. W., & Storey, R. F. (2015). Antithrombotic therapy in the elderly: Expert position paper of the European Society of Cardiology Working Group on thrombosis. *European Heart Journal, 36*(46), 3238–3249. https://doi.org/10.1093/eurheartj/ehv304.

Antman, E. M., & Loscalzo, J. (2018). ST-segment elevation myocardial infarction. In J. Jameson, A. S. Fauci, D. L. Kasper, S. L. Hauser, D. L. Longo, & J. Loscalzo (Eds.), *Harrison's principles of internal medicine* (20th ed.). McGraw Hill. https://accessmedicine-mhmedical-com.ezproxy.uthsc.edu/content.aspx?bookid=2129§ionid=192130008.

A-Rahim, Y., & Falchuk, M. (2021, October 14). Bowel preparation before colonoscopy in adults. J. R. Saltzman & K. M. Robson, (Eds.). *UpToDate.* https://www-uptodate-com.ezproxy.uthsc.edu/contents/bowel-preparation-before-colonoscopy-in-adults.

Aroor, S., Goldstein, L., & Singh, R. (2017). Be-fast (balance, eyes, face, arm, speech, time): Reducing the proportion of strokes missed using the fast mnemonic. *Stroke, 48*(2), 479–481. https://pubmed.ncbi.nlm.nih.gov/28082668/.

Baiu, I., & Hawn, M. T. (2018). Small bowel obstruction. *Journal of the American Medical Association, 319*(20), 2146. https://doi.org/10.1001/jama.2018.5834.

Barkley, T. W. (2021). *Practice considerations for adult-gerontology acute care nurse practitioners* (3rd ed.). Barkley and Associates. https://www.npcourses.com/ebook/practice-considerations-agacnp-3rd-edition/.

Benjamin, E. J., Blaha, M. J., Chiuve, S. E., Cushman, M., Das, S. R., Deo, R., de Ferranti, S. D., Floyd, J., Fornage, M., Gillespie, C., Isasi, C. R., Jiménez, M. C., Jordan, L. C., Judd, S. E., Lackland, D., Lichtman, J. H., Lisabeth, L., Liu, S., Longenecker, C. T., Mackey, R. H., Matsushita, K., Mozaffarian, D., Mussolino, M. E.,

Nasir, K., Neumar, R. W., & Muntner, P. (2017). Heart disease and stroke statistics—2017 update: A report from the American Heart Association. *Circulation.* https://pubmed.ncbi.nlm.nih.gov/28122885/.

Berg, D., & Gerlach, H. (2018). Recent advances in understanding and managing sepsis. *F1000Research*, *7*, 1570. https://doi.org/10.12688/f1000research.15758.1.

Bhatt, D. L., Lopes, R. D., & Harrington, R. A. (2022). Diagnosis and treatment of acute coronary syndromes: A review. *Journal of the American Medical Association*, *327*(7), 662–675. https://doi.org/10.1001/jama.2022.0358. Erratum in Journal of the American Medical Association, May 3, 2022, 327(17), 1710. PMID: 35166796.

Burns, E., & Kakara, R. (2018). Deaths from falls among persons aged ≥65 years—United States, 2007–2016. *Morbidity and Mortality Weekly Report*, *67*(18), 509–514. https://doi.org/10.15585/mmwr.mm6718a1.

Camargo, E., Ding, M., Zimmerman, E., & Silverman, S. (2017). Cerebrovascular disease. In J. B. Halter, J. G. Ouslander, S. Studenski, K. P. High, S. Asthana, M. A. Supiano, & C. Ritchie (Eds.), *Hazzard's geriatric medicine and gerontology* (7th ed.). McGraw Hill. https://accessmedicine-mhmedical-com.ezproxy.uthsc.edu/content.aspx?bookid=1923§ionid=144523594.

Catena, F., Di Saverio, S., Coccolini, F., Ansaloni, L., De Simone, B., Sartelli, M., & Van Goor, H. (2016). Adhesive small bowel adhesions obstruction: Evolutions in diagnosis, management and prevention. *World Journal of Gastrointestinal Surgery*, *8*(3), 222. https://doi.org/10.4240/wjgs.v8.i3.222.

Cecconi, M., Evans, L., Levy, M., & Rhodes, A. (2018). Sepsis and septic shock. *The Lancet*, *392*(10141), 75–87. https://doi.org/10.1016/s0140-6736(18)30696-2.

Centers for Disease Control and Prevention (CDC), National Center for Health Statistics Underlying Cause of Death 1999–2020 on CDC WONDER Online Database. (2021). http://wonder.cdc.gov/ucd-icd10.html.

Centers for Medicate and Medicaid Services. (2021). *Hospital readmissions reduction program.* https://www.cms.gov/Medicare/Medicare-Fee-for-Service-Payment/AcuteInpatientPPS/Readmissions-Reduction-Program.

Chandrashekhar, S., & Dimachkie, M. (2021). Guillain-Barré syndrome in adults: Pathogenesis, clinical features, and diagnosis: Evidence-based clinical decision support. *UpToDate*. https://www.uptodate.com/home.

Chang, K. J., Marin, D., Kim, D. H., Fowler, K. J., Camacho, M. A., Cash, B. D., Garcia, E. M., Hatten, B. W., Kambadakone, A. R., Levy, A. D., Liu, P. S., Moreno, C., Peterson, C. M., Pietryga, J. A., Siegel, A., Weinstein, S., & Carucci, L. R. (2020). ACR appropriateness criteria® suspected small-bowel obstruction. *Journal of the American College of Radiology*, *17*(5), 305–314. https://doi.org/10.1016/j.jacr.2020.01.025.

Conroy, S., & Thomas, M. (2021). Urgent care for older people. *Age and Ageing*, *51*(1). https://doi.org/10.1093/ageing/afab019.

De Filippo, M., & Capasso, R. (2016). Coronary computed tomography angiography (CCTA) and cardiac magnetic resonance (CMR) imaging in the assessment of patients presenting with chest pain suspected for acute coronary syndrome. *Annals of Translational Medicine*, *4*(13), 255. https://doi.org/10.21037/atm.2016.06.30. PMID: 27500156; PMCID: PMC4958724.

Dellinger, R. P., & Parrillo, J. E. (2019). *Critical care medicine. [electronic resource]: principles of diagnosis and management in the adult* (5th ed.). Elsevier.

Department of Health and Human Services (DHHS). (2015). *Administration on aging: A profile of aging Americans.* ACL Administration for Community Living. https://acl.gov/about-acl/administration-aging.

Di Carli, M. F., Kwong, R. Y., & Solomon, S. D. (2018). Noninvasive cardiac imaging: Echocardiography, nuclear cardiology, and magnetic resonance/computed tomography imaging. In J. Jameson, A. S. Fauci, D. L. Kasper, S. L. Hauser, D. L. Longo, & J. Loscalzo (Eds.), *Harrison's principles of internal medicine* (20th ed). McGraw Hill. https://accessmedicine-mhmedical-com.ezproxy.uthsc.edu/content.aspx?bookid=2129§ionid=192280465.

Dippel, D. W. J., Roozenbeek, B., Kerkhoff, H., Lingsma, H. F., van der Lugt, A., van Es, A. C. G., Rozeman, A. D., Moudrous, W., Vermeij, F. H., Venema, E., Duvekot, M. H. C., Alblas, K. C. L., Mulder, L. J. M. M., Wijnhoud, A. D., Maasland, L., van Eijkelenburg, R. P. J., Biekart, M., Willeboer, M. L., Buijck, B., & Roozenbeek, B. (2021). Comparison of eight prehospital stroke scales to detect intracranial large-vessel occlusion in suspected stroke (PRESTO): A prospective observational study. *The Lancet Neurology*, *20*(3), 213–221. https://doi-org.ezproxy.uthsc.edu/10.1016/S1474-4422(20)30439-7.

Dove, J. H., & Jenkins, D. R. (2022). Hip fracture. In J. G. Levins (Ed.), *Ferri's clinical advisor 2022* (pp. 763. e2–763. e6). Elsevier.

Eagles, D., Perry, J. J., Sirois, M. -J., Lang, E., Daoust, R., Lee, J., Griffith, L., Wilding, L., Neveu, X., & Emond, M. (2016). Timed up and go predicts functional decline in older patients presenting to the emergency department following minor trauma. *Age and Ageing*, *6*(2), 214–218. https://doi.org/10.1093/ageing/afw184.

Elsevier. (2022, February 10). *Clinical overview Elsevier point of care femoral neck fracture. Clinical Keys.* https://doi.org/10.1016/j.jcot.2022.101917.

Evans, L., Rhodes, A., Alhazzani, W., Antonelli, M., Coopersmith, C. M., French, C., Machado, F. R., Mcintyre, L., Ostermann, M., Prescott, H. C., Schorr, C., Simpson, S., Wiersinga, W. J., Alshamsi, F., Angus, D. C., Arabi, Y., Azevedo, L., Beale, R., Beilman, G., & Levy, M. (2021). Surviving sepsis campaign: International guidelines for management of sepsis and septic shock 2021. *Intensive Care Medicine*, *47*(11), 1181–1247. https://doi.org/10.1007/s00134-021-06506-y.

Federle, M. P., & Lau, J. N. (2018). Small bowel obstruction. *Imaging in abdominal surgery* (pp. 222–225). Elsevier.

Ferri, F. F. (2021). *Ferri's Clinical Advisor 2022.* Elsevier.

Fihn, S. D., Gardin, J. M., Abrams, J., Berra, K., Blankenship, J. C., Dallas, A. P., Douglas, P. S., Foody, J. A. M., Gerber, T. C., Hinderliter, A. L., King, S. B., Kligfield, P. D., Krumholz, H. M., Kwong, R. Y. K., Lim, M. J., Linderbaum, J. A., Mack, M. J., Munger, M. A., Prager, R. L., & Williams, S. V. (2012). 2012 ACCF/AHA/ACP/AATS/PCNA/SCAI/STS guideline for the diagnosis and management of patients with stable ischemic heart disease. *Circulation*, *126*(25). https://doi.org/10.1161/cir.0b013e318277d6a0.

Fisher, J. M., Bates, C., & Banerjee, J. (2017). The growing challenge of major trauma in older people: A role for comprehensive geriatric assessment. *Age and Ageing*, *46*(5), 709–712. https://doi.org/10.1093/ageing/afx035.

Florencc, C. S., Bergen, G., Atherly, A., Burns, E., Stevens, J., & Drake, C. (2018). Medical costs of fatal and nonfatal falls in older adults. *Journal of the American Geriatrics Society*, *66*(4), 693–698. https://doi.org/10.1111/jgs.15304.

Fornari, M. J., & Lawson, S. L. (2021). Pediatric blunt abdominal trauma and point-of-care ultrasound. *Pediatric Emergency Care*,

37(12), 624–629. https://doi.org/10.1097/PEC.0000000000002573. PMID: 34908375.

Foschi, M., Padroni, M., Abu-Rumeileh, S., Abdelhak, A., Russo, M., D'Anna, L., & Guarino, M. (2022). Diagnostic and prognostic blood biomarkers in transient ischemic attack and minor ischemic stroke: An up-to-date narrative review. *Journal of Stroke and Cerebrovascular Diseases, 31*(3), 106292. https://doi.org/10.1016/j.jstrokecerebrovasdis.2021.106292.

Garatti, A., Castelvecchio, S., Canziani, A., Santoro, T., & Menicanti, L. (2018). CABG in patients with left ventricular dysfunction: indications, techniques and outcomes. *Indian Journal of Thoracic and Cardiovascular Surgery, 34*(Suppl. 3), 279–286. https://doi.org/10.1007/s12055-018-0738-8.Epub2018Oct17.PMID:33060950; PMCID: PMC7525418.

Gioffrè-Florio, M., Murabito, L. M., Visalli, C., Pergolizzi, F. P., & Famà, F. (2018). Trauma in elderly patients: A study of prevalence, comorbidities and gender differences. *Giornale Di Chirurgia–Journal of Surgery, 39*(1), 35. https://doi.org/10.11138/gchir/2018.39.1.035.

Giugliano, R. P., Cannon, C. P., & Braunwald, E. (2018). Non-ST-segment elevation acute coronary syndrome (non-ST-segment elevation myocardial infarction and unstable angina). In J. Jameson, A. S. Fauci, D. L. Kasper, S. L. Hauser, D. L. Longo, & J. Loscalzo (Eds.), *Harrison's principles of internal medicine* (20th ed.). McGraw Hill. https://accessmedicine-mhmedical-com.ezproxy.uthsc.edu/content.aspx?bookid=2129§ionid=192029959.

Global Burden of Disease (GBD) 2016 Lifetime Risk of Stroke Collaborators, Feigin, V. L., Nguyen, G., Cercy, K., Johnson, C. O., Alam, T., Parmar, P. G., Abajobir, A. A., Abate, K. H., Abd-Allah, F., Abejie, A. N., Abyu, G. ,Y., Ademi, Z., Agarwal, G., Ahmed, M. B., Akinyemi, R. O., Al-Raddadi, R., Aminde, L. N., Amlie-Lefond, C., Ansari, H., & …Roth, G. A. (2018). Global, regional, and country-specific lifetime risks of stroke, 1990 and 2016. *New England Journal of Medicine, 379*(25), 2429–2437. https://doi.org/10.1056/NEJMoa1804492. PMID: 30575491; PMCID: PMC6247346.

Global Burden of Disease (GBD) 2019 Stroke Collaborators. (2021). Global, regional, and national burden of stroke and its risk factors, 1990–2019: A systematic analysis for the Global Burden of Disease Study 2019. *Lancet Neurology*, 795–820. https://doi.org/10.3410/f.735332959.793586164.

Goldberger, A.L. and Mirvis, D.M. (2021). Basic principles of electrocardiographic interpretation. UpToDate.com

Golla, G., & Satya, M. (2022, January 1). Myocardial infarction clinical overview. *ClinicalKey.* https://www-clinicalkey-com.ezproxy.uthsc.edu/#!/content/derived_clinical_overview/76-s2.0-B9780323755702006196.

Greenberg, B. (2022). Transverse myelitis. *UpToDate.* https://www.uptodate.com/home

Griffiths, R., & Surendra Kumar, D. (2017). Major trauma in older people: Implications for anaesthesia and Intensive Care Medicine. *Anaesthesia, 72*(11), 1302–1305. https://doi.org/10.1111/anae.14027.

Halter, J. B., Ouslander, J. G., Studenski, S., High, K. P., Asthana, S., Supiano, M. A., Ritchie, C. S., Binder, E. F., Orwig, D., & Magaziner, J. (2017). Hip fractures. *Hazzard's geriatric medicine and gerontology.* McGraw-Hill Education.

Heidenreich, P. A. (2022, April 1). 2022 AHA/ACC/HFSA guideline for the management of heart failure: A report of the American College of Cardiology/American Heart Association Joint Committee on Clinical Practice Guidelines. *Circulation.* https://www.ahajournals.org/doi/10.1161/CIR.0000000000001063.

Huedebert, A., Rengarajan, A., Fritz, C., Noé, J., Wang, X., & Crees, Z. (Eds.). (2020). *The Washington manual® of medical therapeutics* (36th ed.). Wolters Kluwer Health/Lippincott Williams & Wilkins. https://online.statref.com/document/okbn_W8Zvm_TjVWQO53FBN.

Hobson, R. P., Britton, R., Davidson, S., Sir, Ralston, S., Penman, I. D., & Strachan, M. W. J. (2018). *Davidson's principles and practice of medicine* [electronic resource] (23rd ed.). Elsevier.

Huda, S., Whittam, D., Bhojak, M., Chamberlain, J., Noonan, C., & Jacob, A. (2019). Neuromyelitis optica spectrum disorders. *Clinical Medicine (London), 19*(2), 169–176. https://doi.org/10.7861/clinmedicine.19-2-169. PMID: 30872305; PMCID: PMC6454358.

Humphries, M. D., Welch, P., Hasegawa, J., & Mell, M. W. (2021). Correlation of patient activation measure level with patient characteristics and type of vascular disease. *Annals of Vascular Surgery, 73*, 55–61. https://doi.org/10.1016/j.avsg.2020.11.019. Epub 2020 Dec 29. PMID: 33385528; PMCID: PMC8882319.

Husted, S., James, S., Becker, R. C., Horrow, J., Katus, H., Storey, R. F., Cannon, C. P., Heras, M., Lopes, R. D., Morais, J., Mahaffey, K. W., Bach, R. G., Wojdyla, D., & Wallentin, L. (2012). Ticagrelor versus clopidogrel in elderly patients with acute coronary syndromes. *Circulation: Cardiovascular Quality and Outcomes, 5*(5), 680–688. https://doi.org/10.1161/circoutcomes.111.964395.

Interprofessional Education & Collaboration (IPEC). (2016). Core competencies. *LibGuides at USA.* https://libguides.southalabama.edu/c.php?g=884029&p=6352403.

Jacobs, D. O. (2022). Acute intestinal obstruction. In J. Loscalzo, A. Fauci, D. Kasper, S. Hauser, D. Longo, & J. Jameson (Eds.), *Harrison's principles of internal medicine* (21st ed.). McGraw Hill. https://accesspharmacy-mhmedical-com.ezproxy.uthsc.edu/content.aspx?bookid=3095§ionid=265428768.

Joshi, P. H., & de Lemos, J. A. (2021). Diagnosis and management of stable angina: A review. *Journal of the American Medical Association, 325*(17), 1765–1778. https://doi.org/10.1001/jama.2021.1527. PMID: 33944871.

Kalil, A. C., Johnson, D. W., Lisco, S. J., & Sun, J. (2017). Early Goal-Directed Therapy for Sepsis: A Novel Solution for Discordant Survival Outcomes in Clinical Trials. *Critical care medicine, 45*(4), 607–614. https://doi.org/10.1097/CCM.0000000000002235.

Kass, J., & Goldsmith, C. (2022, January 1). Stroke, secondary prevention. *ClinicalKey.* https://www.clinicalkey.com/.

Keeley, A., Hine, P., & Nsutebu, E. (2017). The recognition and management of sepsis and septic shock: A guide for non-intensivists. *Postgraduate Medical Journal, 93*(1104), 626–634. https://doi.org/10.1136/postgradmedj-2016-134519.

Kwok, C. S., Hulme, W., Olier, I., Holroyd, E., & Mamas, M. A. (2017). Review of early hospitalisation after percutaneous coronary intervention. *International Journal of Cardiology, 227*, 370–377. https://doi-org.ezproxy.uthsc.edu/10.1016/j.ijcard.2016.11.050.

Lange, R., & Mukherjee, D. (2020). Acute coronary syndrome: Unstable angina and non–ST elevation myocardial infarction. *Goldman-Cecil medicine* (pp. 379–388). Elsevier.

Lee, J. K. (2021 Jann). Neurogenic Bladder Management. *Radiol Technol, 92*(3), 281–295. PMID: 33472879.

Levine, G. N., Parekh, M., Litvak, P., Martini, S., & Kent, T. (2023). Ischemic Stroke. *Cardiology secrets* (6th ed., pp. 482–492). Elsevier.

Lier, H., Bernhard, M., & Hossfeld, B. (2018). Hypovolämisch-hämorrhagischer Schock [Hypovolemic and hemorrhagic shock]. *Anaesthesist, 67*(3), 225–244. German. https://doi.org/10.1007/s00101-018-0411-z.PMID:29404656.

Long, B., Robertson, J., & Koyfman, A. (2019). Emergency medicine evaluation and management of small bowel obstruction: Evidence-based recommendations. *Journal of Emergency Medicine, 56*(2), 166–176. https://doi.org/10.1016/j.jemermed.2018.10.024.

Lopes, R. D., Heizer, G., Aronson, R., Vora, A. N., Massaro, T., Mehran, R., Goodman, S. G., Windecker, S., Darius, H., Li, J., Averkov, O., Bahit, M. C., Berwanger, O., Budaj, A., Hijazi, Z., Parkhomenko, A., Sinnaeve, P., Storey, R. F., Thiele, H., & Alexander, J. H. (2019). Antithrombotic therapy after acute coronary syndrome or PCI in atrial fibrillation. *New England Journal of Medicine, 380*(16), 1509–1524. https://doi.org/10.1056/nejmoa1817083.

Loscalzo, J., Fauci, A. S., Kasper, D. L., Hauser, S. L., Longo, D. L., Jameson, J. L., & Harrison, T. R. (2018). Diseases of the spinal cord. *Harrison's principles of internal medicine*. Essay. McGraw Hill.

Lowenstern, A., Alexander, K. P., Hill, C. L., Alhanti, B., Pellikka, P. A., Nanna, M. G., Mehta, R. H., Cooper, L. S., Bullock-Palmer, R. P., Hoffmann, U., & Douglas, P. S. (2020). Age-related differences in the noninvasive evaluation for possible coronary artery disease: Insights from the prospective multicenter imaging study for evaluation of chest pain (PROMISE) trial. *JAMA Cardiology, 5*(2), 193–201. https://doi.org/10.1001/jamacardio.2019.4973.

Madhavan, M., Gersh, B., Alexander, K., et al. (2018). Coronary artery disease in patients ≥80 years of age. *Journal of the American College of Cardiology, 71*(18), 2015–2040. https://doi.org/10.1016/j.jacc.2017.12.068.

Magee, D. J., & Manske, R. (2021). Head and face. *Orthopedic physical assessment* (pp. 73–163). Saunders Elsevier.

Makic, M. B., & Bridges, E. (2018). CE: Managing sepsis and septic shock: Current guidelines and definitions. *American Journal of Nursing, 118*(2), 34–39. https://doi.org/10.1097/01.naj.0000530223.33211.f5.

Mark, P. B., Jhund, P. S., Walters, M. R., Petrie, M. C., Power, A., White, C., Robertson, M., Connolly, E., Anker, S. D., Bhandari, S., Farrington, K., Kalra, P. A., Tomson, C. R. V., Wheeler, D. C., Winearls, C. G., McMurray, J. J. V., Macdougall, I. C., & Ford, I. (2021). Stroke in hemodialysis patients randomized to different intravenous iron strategies: A prespecified analysis from the pivotal trial. *Kidney360, 2*(11), 1761–1769. https://doi.org/10.34067/kid.0004272021.

Martín-Rodríguez, F., López-Izquierdo, R., del Pozo Vegas, C., Sánchez-Soberón, I., Delgado-Benito, J. F., Martín-Conty, J. L., & Castro-Villamor, M. A. (2020). Can the prehospital national early warning SCORE 2 identify patients at risk of in-hospital early mortality? A prospective, Multicenter Cohort Study. *Heart & Lung, 49*(5), 585–591. https://doi.org/10.1016/j.hrtlng.2020.02.047.

Maung, A. A., Johnson, D. C., Piper, G. L., Barbosa, R. R., Rowell, S. E., Bokhari, F., Collins, J. N., Gordon, J. R., Ra, J. H., & Kerwin, A. J. (2012). Evaluation and management of small-bowel obstruction. *Journal of Trauma and Acute Care Surgery, 73*(5), 362–369. https://doi.org/10.1097/ta.0b013e31827019de.

Mehta, A., Fifi, J. T., Shoirah, H., Singh, I. P., Shigematsu, T., Kellner, C. P., De Leacy, R., Mocco, J., & Majidi, S. (2021). National trends in utilization and outcome of endovascular thrombectomy for acute ischemic stroke in elderly. *Journal of Stroke and Cerebrovascular Diseases, 30*(2), 105505. https://doi.org/10.1016/j.jstrokecerebrovasdis.2020.105505.

Mirvis, D., & Goldberger, A. (2021). Electrocardiography. *Braunwald's heart disease: A textbook of cardiovascular medicine* (pp. 141–174). Elsevier.

Mohammadian, M., Shah, D., Santana, M., Elkattawy, S., & Jesani, S. (2022). Levine's sign points to spontaneous coronary artery dissection in a healthy young male. *Cureus, 14*(5), e24893. https://doi.org/10.7759/cureus.24893. PMID: 35698691; PMCID: PMC9186000.

Mora, S., Shufelt, C. L., & Manson, J. E. (2022). Whom to treat for primary prevention of atherosclerotic cardiovascular disease: The aspirin dilemma. *JAMA Internal Medicine, 182*(6), 587–589. https://doi.org/10.1001/jamainternmed.2022.1365.

Moreland, B., Kakara, R., & Henry, A. (2020). Trends in nonfatal falls and fall-related injuries among adults aged ≥65 years—United States, 2012–2018. *Morbidity and Mortality Weekly Report, 69*(27), 875–881. https://doi.org/10.15585/mmwr.mm6927a5.

Moreno-Escobar, M. C., Kataria, S., Khan, E., Subedi, R., Tandon, M., Peshwe, K., Kramer, J., Niaze, F., & Sriwastava, S. (2021). Acute transverse myelitis with dysautonomia following SARS-COV-2 infection: A case report and review of literature. *Journal of Neuroimmunology, 353*, 577523. https://doi.org/10.1016/j.jneuroim.2021.577523.

Morris, R. J., & Roberts, C. H. (2020). Haematological effects of intermittent pneumatic compression for deep vein thrombosis prophylaxis. *Thrombosis and Haemostasis, 120*(6), 912–923. https://doi.org/10.1055/s-0040-1710016. PMID: 32359225.

Myer, B., & Dries, D. J. (2022). Steroids and sepsis. *Air Medical Journal, 41*(1), 6–10. https://doi.org/10.1016/j.amj.2021.09.002.

Napolitano, L. M. (2018). Sepsis 2018: Definitions and guideline changes. *Surgical Infections, 19*(2), 117–125. https://doi.org/10.1089/sur.2017.278.

Newland, P., Lorenz, R., & Oliver, B. J. (2020). Patient activation in adults with chronic conditions: A systematic review. *Journal of Health Psychology, 26*(1), 103–114. https://doi.org/10.1177/1359105320947790.

Nguyen, M. H., & Lui, S. K. (2020). Holistic management of older patients with hip fractures. *Orthopaedic Nursing, 39*(3), 183–191. https://doi.org/10.1097/nor.0000000000000656.

Oza, R., Rundell, K., & Garcellano, M. (2017). Recurrent ischemic stroke: Strategies for prevention. *American Family Physician, 96*(7), 436–440. PMID: 29094912.

Peters, A. E., & Keeley, E. C. (2017). Patient engagement following acute myocardial infarction and its influence on outcomes. *American Journal of Cardiology, 120*(9), 1467–1471. https://doi.org/10.1016/j.amjcard.2017.07.037.

Pollack, C. V., Amin, A., Wang, T., Deitelzweig, S., Cohen, M., Slattery, D., Fanikos, J., DiLascia, C., Tuder, R., & Kaatz, S. (2020). Contemporary NSTEMI management: The role of the hospitalist. *Hospital Practice, 48*(1), 1–11. https://doi.org/10.1080/21548331.2020.1701329.

Powers, W. J., Rabinstein, A. A., Ackerson, T., Adeoye, O. M., Bambakidis, N. C., Becker, K., Biller, J., Brown, M., Demaerschalk, B. M., Hoh, B., Jauch, E. C., Kidwell, C. S., Leslie-Mazwi, T. M., Ovbiagele, B., Scott, P. A., Sheth, K. N., Southerland, A. M., Summers, D. V., & Tirschwell, D. L. (2019). Correction to: Guidelines for the early management of patients with acute ischemic stroke: 2019 update to the 2018 guidelines for the early management of acute ischemic stroke: A guideline for healthcare professionals from the American Heart Association/American Stroke Association. *Stroke, 50*(12), 440–441. https://doi.org/10.1161/str.0000000000000215.

Price, T. G. (2020). Bowel obstruction. In J. E. Tintinalli, O. Ma, D. M. Yealy, G. D. Meckler, J. Stapczynski, D. M. Cline, & S. H. Thomas (Eds.), *Tintinalli's emergency medicine: A comprehensive study guide* (9th ed.). McGraw Hill. https://accessmedicine-mhmedical-com.ezproxy.uthsc.edu/content.aspx?bookid=2353§ionid=204498674.

Reddy, S. R., & Cappell, M. S. (2017). A systematic review of the clinical presentation, diagnosis, and treatment of small bowel obstruction. *Current Gastroenterology Reports, 19*(6), 28. https://doi.org/10.1007/s11894-017-0566-9.

Rello, J., Valenzuela-Sánchez, F., Ruiz-Rodriguez, M., & Moyano, S. (2017). Sepsis: A review of advances in management. *Advances in Therapy, 34*(11), 2393–2411. https://doi.org/10.1007/s12325-017-0622-8.

Riemen, A. H. K., & Hutchison, J. D. (2016). The multidisciplinary management of hip fractures in older patients. *Orthopaedics and Trauma, 30*(2), 117–122. https://doi.org/10.1016/j.mporth.2016.03.006.

Ross, A. B., Lee, K. S., Chang, E. Y., Amini, B., Bussell, J. K., Gorbachova, T., Ha, A. S., Khurana, B., Klitzke, A., Mooar, P. A., Shah, N. A., Singer, A. D., Smith, S. E., Taljanovic, M. S., & Kransdorf, M. J. (2019). ACR appropriateness criteria®: Acute hip pain-suspected fracture. *Journal of the American College of Radiology, 16*(5), 18–25. https://doi.org/10.1016/j.jacr.2019.02.028.

Rowe, T. A., & McKoy, J. M. (2017). Sepsis in older adults. *Infectious Disease Clinics of North America, 31*(4), 731–742. https://doi.org/10.1016/j.idc.2017.07.010.

Sandoval, Y., Apple, F. S., & Smith, S. W. (2018). High-sensitivity cardiac troponin assays and unstable angina. *European Heart Journal: Acute Cardiovascular Care, 7*(2), 120–128. https://doi.org/10.1177/2048872616658591. PMID: 27388716.

Sawa, J., Green, R. S., Thoma, B., Erdogan, M., & Davis, P. J. (2018). Risk factors for adverse outcomes in older adults with blunt chest trauma: A systematic review. *Canadian Journal of Emergency Medicine, 20*(4), 614–622. https://doi.org/10.1017/cem.2017.377.

Singer, M. (2016, February 23). Consensus definitions for sepsis and septic shock. *Journal of the American Medical Association, 315(8),* 801–810. https://jamanetwork.com/journals/jama/fullarticle/2492881.

Smith, D. A., Kashyap, S., & Nehring, S. M. (2021). Bowel obstruction. *Stat Pearls.* https://www.ncbi.nlm.nih.gov/books/NBK441975/.

ten Broek, R. P. G., Krielen, P., Di Saverio, S., Coccolini, F., Biffl, W. L., Ansaloni, L., Velmahos, G. C., Sartelli, M., Fraga, G. P., Kelly, M. D., Moore, F. A., Peitzman, A. B., Leppaniemi, A., Moore, E. E., Jeekel, J., Kluger, Y., Sugrue, M., Balogh, Z. J., Bendinelli, C., & van Goor, H. (2018, June 19). Bologna guidelines for diagnosis and management of adhesive small bowel obstruction (ASBO): 2017 update of the evidence-based guidelines from the World Society of Emergency surgery asbo working group–World Journal Of Emergency Surgery. *BioMed Central.* https://doi.org/10.1186/s13017-018-0185-2.

Trauma Audit and Research Network. (2017). *Major trauma in older people.* https://www.tarn.ac.uk/content/downloads/3793/Major%20Trauma%20in%20Older%20People%202017.pdf.

Walls, R. M., Hockberger, R. S., Gausche-Hill, M., Bakes, K. M., Gross, E., & Martel, M. (2018a). Multiple trauma. In *Rosen's emergency medicine: Concepts and clinical practice* (pp. 287–300). Elsevier.

Walls, R. M., Hockberger, R. S., Gausche-Hill, M., Bakes, K. M., Thomas, J., & Brady, W. (2018b). Acute coronary syndrome. In *Rosen's emergency medicine: Concepts and clinical practice* (pp. 891–928) (9th ed.). Elsevier.

Wang, H. E., Jones, A. R., & Donnelly, J. P. (2017). Revised national estimates of emergency department visits for sepsis in the United States. *Critical Care Medicine, 45*(9), 1443–1449. https://doi.org/10.1097/ccm.0000000000002538.

Weisbord, S. D., Gallagher, M., Jneid, H., Garcia, S., Cass, A., Thwin, S.-S., Conner, T. A., Chertow, G. M., Bhatt, D. L., Shunk, K., Parikh, C. R., McFalls, E. O., Brophy, M., Ferguson, R., Wu, H., Androsenko, M., Myles, J., Kaufman, J., Palevsky, P. M., & Weisbord, S. D. (2018). Outcomes after angiography with Sodium Bicarbonate and Acetylcysteine. *New England Journal of Medicine, 378*(7), 603–614. https://doi-org.ezproxy.uthsc.edu/10.1056/NEJMoa1710933.

Wenger, N., & Engberding, N. (2017). Faculty opinions recommendation of 2013 ACCF/AHA guideline for the management of st-elevation myocardial infarction: A report of the American College of Cardiology Foundation/American Heart Association task force on practice guidelines. *Faculty opinions–post-publication peer review of the biomedical literature.* https://doi.org/10.3410/f.718180330.793537123.

Winn, H. R., Youmans, J. R., Yaeger, K., Hardigan, T., & Mocco, J. (2022). Acute medical management of ischemic and hemorrhagic stroke. In *Youmans and Winn neurological surgery* (8th ed., pp. 3219–3222). Elsevier. https://www-clinicalkey-com.ezproxy.uthsc.edu/#!/content/book/3-s2.0-B9780323661928004055?indexOverride=GLOBAL.

Xu, X., & Le, W. (2019). Exercise and Parkinson's disease. In S.-Y. Yau (Ed.), *International review of neurobiology*, 147, (pp. 45–74). Academic Press. https://www.sciencedirect.com/science/article/pii/S0074774219300236.

21 Long-Term Care

SHARON WOODS, BS, MPAS, PA-C

OBJECTIVES

Student Learning Objectives

After completing this chapter, the student should be able to do the following:

1. Define long-term care, and compare and contrast the common sites of care, costs associated with care, and funding strategies for care.
2. Discuss global and national aging trends, population predictions, and disease projections for the coming decades.
3. Describe the concept of care transitions and the differences between the common sites of care for the older adult, including community-based outpatient care, Programs of All-Inclusive Care for the Elderly (PACE), assisted living, short-term rehabilitation facilities, and long-term care facilities.
4. Discuss the role of the nurse practitioner (NP)/physician assistant (PA) and other members of the multidisciplinary care team in providing care for the older adult in a long-term care setting.
5. Summarize the guidelines for the NP/PA caring for the older adult in a long-term care facility, including documentation guidelines and quality measures for data collection.

Practitioner Objectives

After completing this chapter, the practitioner should be able to do the following:

1. Critically analyze data and evidence-based medicine to evaluate global and national aging trends.
   - *NP competency: Scientific foundation competency*
   - *PA competency: Medical knowledge competency*
2. Understand the concept of care transitions in the older adult, and identify common sites of long-term care.
   - *NP competency: Health care delivery system competency*
   - *PA competency: Systems-based practice*
3. Create effective, therapeutic, and ethically sound relationships with patients, and foster collaborative relationships with the multidisciplinary team in the long-term care setting.
   - *NP competency: Leadership competencies*
   - *PA competency: Patient care, interpersonal, and communication skills*
4. Understand the legal and regulatory requirements associated with long-term care as well as understanding funding sources and payment systems that provide for patient care of the older and disabled adult.
   - *NP competency: Policy competency*
   - *PA competency: Professionalism, systems-based practice*

Introduction

Long-Term Care

Definition

The National Institute of Aging (NIA) defines long-term care as services or support for individuals' personal or health needs to allow them to live independently and safely when they can no longer perform these activities by themselves. Note that the definition does not specify where this type of care or support occurs or who is providing the support. This is because there is no standard service location for long-term care or defined caregivers. Today's long-term care is an all-encompassing endeavor aimed to support an increasingly frail and aging population in a spectrum of care locations by a team of highly trained care staff.

Using this broad definition, long-term care can consist of a variety of services intended to keep an older adult supported in the community and may consist of home-based support and assistance with personal tasks of everyday life, often referred to the activities of daily living (ADLs). These include activities such as bathing, grooming, dressing, and incontinence care. ADL assistance is often provided by unpaid family members in a private home, by personal care assistants (PCAs), or in a spectrum of care locations by a team of trained staff members. Depending on one's needs, an older adult may need additional support in other areas involving other tasks that do not necessarily involve personal care or hygiene but remain vitally important in order for them to remain independent in the community. These can include such tasks as meal preparation or meal delivery, medication management (including dispensing and proper administration of all medications), grocery shopping, housework, and transportation. These activities are referred to as instrumental activities of daily living (IADLs) (Table 21.1).

Additional IADLs that have not been validated but are relevant in today's society and reflect the impact of technology in modern life include the ability to use a cellphone or smartphone, the ability to use a computer or the Internet, and the ability to manage and keep a schedule.

It is necessary for the clinician to make a careful assessment of each older adult's functional ability as it pertains to the individual ADL and IADL, and this should be

CASE STUDY

RT is an 88-year-old female with a past medical history of mild cognitive impairment, hypertension, macular degeneration, and osteoporosis. She was admitted to the emergency department (ED) after falling at home. She has been living alone in her own home and uses a four-wheeled walker for mobility. She has some extra help at home in the form of Meals on Wheels, who provide one hot meal per day on weekdays, and she cooks microwave dinners at night. She has a personal care assistant (PCA) 14 hours per week for personal care support for 2 hours per day. The PCA helps her get dressed in the morning and assists with bathing and personal hygiene. Despite this, she is alone at night and alone for many hours during the day. She has one son who helps as often as he can, but he works full time and is unable to hire 24-hour support for her due to the excessive costs. The ED workup revealed a right intertrochanteric hip fracture, and she was admitted to the hospital. She underwent operative repair by an orthopedics practitioner, but her hospital course was complicated by postoperative delirium secondary to a urinary tract infection (UTI), which prolonged her hospital stay.

She was evaluated by physical and occupational therapists as part of her discharge plan, and it was determined that it would be unsafe for her to return to her prior living situation due to her increased need for assistance with ambulation and activities of daily living. Several new medications were added to her regimen during the hospitalization. She was referred to a short-term rehabilitation facility where she received 20 days of inpatient physical and occupational therapy and daily nursing supervision from a comprehensive rehabilitative team approach. While she was at rehab, her son became concerned about her cognitive state, as she was not as sharp as before. She underwent a formal cognitive evaluation by a speech language pathologist who noted new deficits in several cognitive domains. It was determined that she was not safe to return home due a combination of medical and physical care needs, and she was referred to an assisted living facility (ALF), her next level of care.

Once at the ALF, her son was quickly faced with the high cost of financing her care and was forced to sell her home to cover the costs. Although it was reassuring for him and his mother to have some assistance with tasks such as managing her medications and structured meals, there were still significant portions of the day where she was left unattended and her cognition slowly worsened. While at the ALF, she suffered a series of falls due to her increasingly unsteady gait, and she often forgot to use her walker. She was transferred several times from the assisted living facility to the hospital ED for evaluation of confusion and altered mental status, and she underwent a variety of tests each time she was transferred. She was sent back to the facility many times with recommendations for changes in her medications to assist with her increasing confusion, but often the workups were unrevealing. One winter evening, RT was found on the grounds of the facility, laying in a snowbank after having gone missing for several hours. She was admitted again to the hospital with hypothermia and several wounds related to frostbite. Once she was stabilized, she was transitioned to a locked dementia unit of the skilled nursing facility (SNF) for long-term care.

At the SNF, RT had difficulty with restlessness and agitation, in part due to advancement of her dementia but also likely due to pain from her wounds and the inability to ambulate due to her unsteady gait and recurrent falls. Months later, she ultimately succumbed to sepsis, after transitioning to a palliative care and hospice unit within her long-term care facility.

TABLE 21.1 Example of Activities of Daily Living

Activities of Daily Living (ADL)	Instrumental Activities of Daily Living (IADL)
Bathing	Using the telephone
Dressing yourself	Shopping at a store
Getting in and out of bed/chair	Plan and fix meals
Using the toilet	Clean your house
Feeding yourself	Manage finances and pay bills
Walking	Taking medicine correctly
	Able to use transportation services - drive, taxi, bus, etc.

periodically assessed during routine examinations. An individual's need for ADL/IADL assistance can help determine one's need for additional support such as PCA services in the home, an inpatient level of care, and reimbursement for payment of services. A formal ADL assessment, often performed by an occupational therapist, assesses a patient's ability to complete tasks and whether the patient requires an assistant to complete the tasks safely. A patient is described as follows:

Independent: Able to perform a task or complete an ADL by him or herself (with or without an assistive device as indicated) without physical or verbal assistance from others.

Needs some assistance: The level of assistance required to safely complete the task can range from setup help only, to supervision, limited assistance, extensive assistance, or maximal assistance.

Dependent: Physically or cognitively unable to contribute effort toward completion of task and a helper had to contribute all of the effort needed to complete the task.

Care Providers

Current data suggest that the 80% of at home care is provided by unpaid family members who provide on average 20 hours per week of personal care activities (LongTermCare.gov, 2019). Two-thirds of these caregivers are women; additionally, 14% of the caregivers themselves are age 65 or older. Home-based care can also be provided by personal care assistants (PCAs) or home health aides (HHAs). PCAs can be paid family members or someone the client privately hires to assist with ADL tasks such as meal preparation, bathing, grooming, mobility, and providing companionship. Home health aides provide similar services but undergo more extensive training and can provide more complex services such as monitoring vital signs and assisting with wound management.

Home-based support may include a skilled nursing component when ordered by a licensed provider (medical doctor [MD], doctor of osteopathic medicine [DO], nurse practitioner [NP], physician assistant [PA]). Skilled nursing visits are generally short term and may be accompanied by physical therapy, occupational therapy, or speech therapy depending on the medical indication.

The Interprofessional Care Team

The concept of the interprofessional care team is not unique to the practice of geriatrics and gerontology; however, it is championed by leaders in the field as a highly effective care strategy for older adults. Using input and oversight from practitioners across many domains, the interprofessional care team seeks to provide a coordinated, comprehensive, and integrated care plan for those entrusted in their care while prioritizing the older adult's personal goals of care.

The interprofessional care team begins with the primary care provider (PCP), who may be a physician or an advanced practice provider (MD/DO/NP/PA). The PCP may be a geriatrician or a provider with additional training in geriatrics whose main role is to coordinate and manage all aspects of the older adult's care, taking input from other providers and consultants on the team who are working with their patient. The typical interprofessional care team also includes members from the nursing and direct care staffs (certified nursing aide, personal care attendant, home health aide, etc.) as well as routine oversight by pharmacists, social workers, case managers, and registered dietitians with expertise in the care of older adults. Depending on an individual's need, other professionals may be involved, including physical or occupational therapists and speech language pathologists when rehabilitation services are indicated.

Demographics and Aging Trends

Global Trends

An overall decline in regional fertility rates coinciding with a rise in life expectancy has given rise to the picture of an aging global population. The percentage of the world's population living in what was deemed a high-fertility country decreased from nearly 25% in 1975–1980 to 8% in 2010–2015 (Department of Economic and Social Affairs, 2019). By the 2030s, two-thirds of the world's population is expected to live in countries with fertility rates below the replacement level—that is, the level at which a given generation can exactly replace itself. Although there are clear regional and geographic distinctions and trends, data presented from the *World Population Prospects: The 2019 Revision* (Department of Economic and Social Affairs, 2019) depict a larger percentage of adults ≥60 years old in the coming decades. In fact, it is anticipated that by 2050, one in six adults worldwide will be over the age of 65. Aging is considered to be a strong risk factor for chronic disease and with this older, sicker population comes associated increases in health care costs and an increased utilization of health care and economic resources. With this changing demographic, there will be unanticipated social, economic, and environmental considerations to address in the years to come.

In 2018, adults ≥ age 60 accounted for 25% of the global population in more developed regions and 10.6% of the population in less developed regions, and it is expected to surpass 1 billion in 2019 (Department of Economic and Social Affairs, 2019). These numbers showed tremendous growth over the preceding decades with the global proportion of older adults more than tripling in developed regions from 1950 to 2018 (from 94 to 316 million) and more than quintupling (from 108 to 675 million) in less developed regions. Countries with the highest proportion of older adults include China (235.4 million), India (130.1 million), and the United States (71.8 million). Aging trends can also be viewed through median age, the age that divides the population into half younger and half older. Since 1950, the global median age has risen from 23.6 years to 29.6 years in 2015 and is projected to be 36.1 by 2050 (Fig. 21.1).

Factors linked to global aging trends include global decreases in fertility rates and in increased life expectancy at birth (Department of Economic and Social Affairs, 2019). In 2015–2020 the global fertility rate dropped to half the value of the 1950–1955 rate of 5 children per woman to 2.5 live births per woman in 2019. With these declining fertility rates, each generation of parents is only expected to replace itself with an equivalent number of children who survive into adulthood without a net increase in overall population. The result is zero population growth. In 2018 there were 128 countries whose total fertility rates were at or below the replacement level of 2.1, with expectations that these trends will continue in the coming years (US Census Bureau, 2019).

National Trends

The US population is rapidly aging, triggered by the aging baby boomer generation (those born between 1946 through 1964). Data from the US Census Bureau predict that by 2030 one in five Americans will be ≥65 years old (US Census Bureau, 2019). The aging US population is growing more diverse as well, with the minority population expected to surpass the white, non-Hispanic population in total numbers by 2044. Data recently published by the National Center for Health Statistics (NCHS) reported that the US birth rate in 2018 had decreased by 2% from 2017, recording the lowest number of births in 32 years (Centers for Disease Control and Prevention, 2019). This continued a trend, as it reflected the fourth year in a row of declining birth rates for the United States, which kept its total fertility rate below the replacement level, where it has been since 1971.

Life expectancy at birth had risen globally by 4.8 years from the 2000–2018 time period, but life expectancy for both males and females decreased in 27 out of 29 countries across Europe, Chile, and the United States from 2019 to 2020 due mainly to the COVID-19 pandemic (Aburto et al., 2021). Increased mortality for adults over age 60 due to

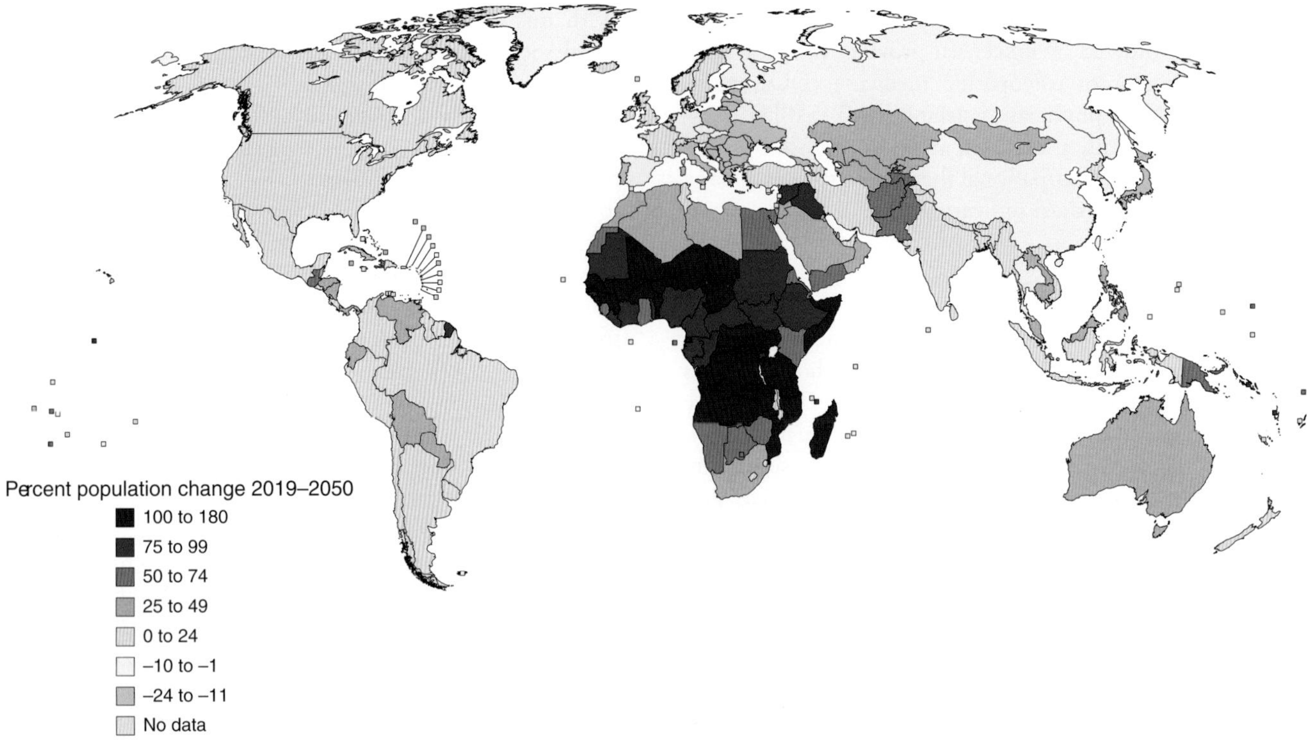

The designations employed and the presentation of material on this map do not imply the expression of any opinion whatsoever on the part of the Secretariat of the United Nations concerning the legal status of any country, territory, city or area or of its authorities, or concerning the delimitation of its frontiers or boundaries. Dotted line represents approximately the Line of Control in Jammu and Kashmir agreed upon by India and Pakistan. The final status of Jammu and Kashmir has not yet been agreed upon by the parties. Final boundary between the Republic of Sudan the Republic of South Sudan has not yet been determined. A dispute exists between the Governments of Argentina and the United Kingdom of Great Britain and Northern Ireland concerning sovereignty over the Falkland Islands (Malvinas).
Note: Countries or areas with surface area less than 30,000 km^2 are shown with squares coloured according to their statistical values.

• **Fig. 21.1** Changes in Total Population Between 2019 and 2050, According to the Medium-Variant Projection (From https://population.un.org/wpp/Publications/Files/WPP2019_DataBooklet.pdf.)

COVID-19 led to a reduction in total US life expectancy by 1.5 years to a low of 78.8 years for the period January 2020–December 2020. (Arias, 2021). We have yet to understand the full impact of the COVID-19 pandemic on global or national life expectancy due regional and national variations in testing and inconsistencies in tracking and identification of COVID-19–related deaths. Prior to the COVID-19 epidemic, global and national studies demonstrated that geographic disparities in life expectation are prevalent and continue to influence population statistics. Socioeconomic factors such as educational level, median household income, nutrition and obesity levels, physical activity status, as well as other contributors including race, ethnicity, and behavioral and metabolic risk factors have been shown to influence variations in life expectancy by as many as 20 years by regional county in the United States (Dwyer-Lindgren, 2017). These same factors, can have global impacts on life expectancy and population trends and are thought to play a role in the disproportional impact of COVID-19 on certain populations and communities (Fig. 21.2).

Financing American Health care

Funding for health care in the United States is a complicated, constantly evolving system. In 1965, the US Congress passed Title XVIII, known initially as the Social Security Act, which was legislation intended to improve health care for the older adult. Medicare's original intent was to provide health care for older adults who at the time had little or no coverage or whose costs for care greatly exceeded their younger cohorts. In time, it has expanded to include eligibility for younger patients with permanent disabilities, added optional payments to health maintenance organizations (HMOs), and provided coverage to beneficiaries with certain life-threatening medical conditions such as end-stage renal disease and amyotrophic lateral sclerosis. In later decades payments were expanded for some self-administered medications, services such as physical and speech therapy, chiropractic care, and selected hospice benefits. Over the ensuing decades, these programs have

SAFETY ALERT

Addressing modifiable risk factors at each health care visit can help optimize quality of life and life expectancy. These topics can include the following:

- Diet and nutrition
- Exercise and physical activity levels
- Obesity and weight management
- Tobacco cessation
- Clinical preventive services
- Immunizations

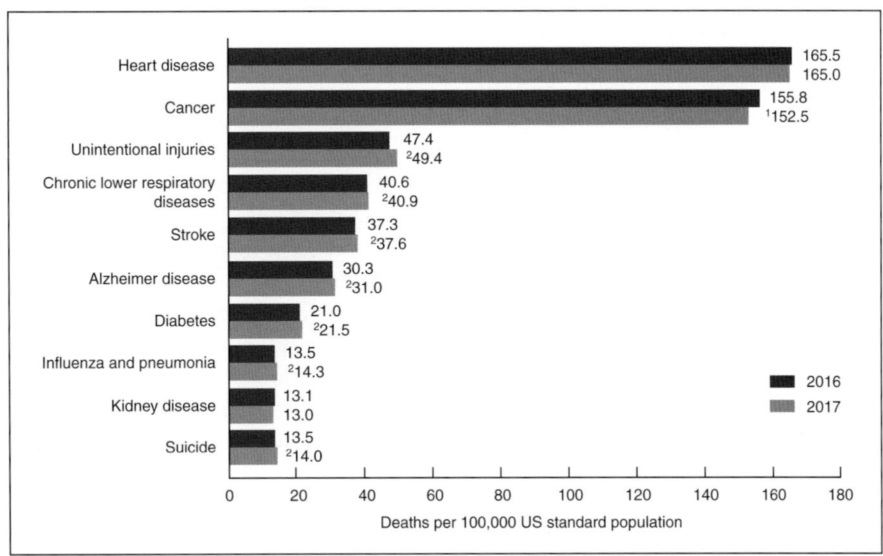

• **Fig. 21.2** National Center for Health Statistics (NCHS) National Vital Statistics System (From Murphy, S. L., Xu, J. Q., Kochanek, K. D., & Arias, E. [2018]. Mortality in the United States, 2017. NCHS Data Brief, no 328. National Center for Health Statistics.)

evolved into the current programs known as Medicare and Medicaid and other individual insurance plans that seek to provide the care for those who need it at as they age or become disabled (Social Security Association, 2017).

Medicare, a federal insurance program run by the Centers for Medicare & Medicaid Services (CMS), is a division of the US Department of Health and Human Services (HHS) and was previously known as the Health Care and Financing Administration. Medicare is funded by a combination of a payroll taxes paid by both employers and employees, beneficiary premium surtaxes, and revenue from the US Treasury Department. All people age 65 or older who have been legal US residents for at least 5 years are eligible for Medicare. In addition, people with certain disabilities and who are under the age of 65 may be eligible if they are receiving Social Security Disability Insurance (SSDI).

As it was originally enacted, Medicare paid health care professionals and organizations using two separate fee-for service (FFS) plans, using predetermined amounts to pay for health care and health care–related expenses. However, costs have escalated and are expected to reach $1.1 trillion in 2026. Legislation has sought to change the reimbursement structure to both rein in costs while shifting the focus toward preventive care and health care maintenance.

Medicare Comprises Four Components

Medicare Part A

Often considered hospital insurance (HI), Part A covers such things as hospital admissions, skilled nursing home care, and home health care and hospice services following a qualifying 3-day hospital admission. Older Americans and their spouses who have Medicare taxes taken out of their paychecks for at least 10 years (40 quarters) are eligible for coverage for Part A once they reach age 65. Medicare Part A is generally funded by a 2.5% payroll tax on employers and workers.

Regarding hospital benefits, Part A generally covers the first 60 days of the hospitalization with the beneficiary being responsible for a one-time deductible. The maximum number of hospitals days covered per calendar year is 90. On days 61 to 90, the beneficiary is responsible for a coinsurance payment per day for the remainder of the hospital stay. The beneficiary is also given a "lifetime reserve" of 60 additional days to be used in one's lifetime. A new pool of 90 days of coverage, with new copays begins after 60 days of continuous nonuse of inpatient benefits.

It is important to note that Medicare Part A does not cover custodial care, long-term care, or nonskilled care. Custodial or nonskilled care is defined as any nonmedical care that can be provided by a nonlicensed caregiver and includes activities such as bathing, dressing, cooking, and laundry and homemaking services. There is often much confusion in the lay community as to what defines skilled care versus custodial or nonskilled care. Skilled care is routinely provided by a nurse or licensed physical, occupational, or speech therapist. Care is delivered by these providers as part a treatment plan ordered by an MD/NP or PA, usually following an acute medical illness or change of medical status. Once a patient has reached a plateau or is no longer actively making progress toward a rehabilitation or medical goal, she or he may transition to custodial care services, which are then provided by a nonlicensed caregiver and are thus no longer covered by Medicare.

Medicare Part B

Part B insurance is considered optional, and eligible participants may "opt out" of enrolling in Part B initially, if covered under another plan that provides similar care. Part B covers outpatient services including physician, nurse practitioner, and physician assistant charges; durable medical equipment (DME) such as mobility aides (walkers, canes, etc.); or prosthetics, laboratory tests, and most professionally administered prescription medications. It also provides coverage for vaccinations. It uses regional insurance companies, or *carriers*, to pay for these services.

At age 65, if eligible for Part A, then participants can enroll in Part B and must pay premiums for this, which are usually deducted from Social Security payments. It is important to note that neither Part A nor Part B covers the cost of homemaking services, routine dental or podiatry care, hearing aids, eyeglasses, or care abroad. There are other limitations. Part B is partially funded by premiums paid by Medicare enrollees and US Treasury revenue.

Medicare Part C

Part C insurance is also known as Medicare Advantage (MA) and is considered an alternative plan for those who elect not to enroll in traditional Medicare plans A, B, or D. Participants select a managed care plan offered from private insurers whose coverage and benefits are at least comparable to benefits under standard Medicare Parts A, B, and C but at fixed monthly payments using a select network of providers. Part C or Medicare Advantage plans must provide at minimum what is covered by Medicare Part A and Part B and can offer additional benefits such as lower out-of-pocket costs with set copays, transportation services, and other extra benefits.

Medicare Part D

Part D was established in 2003 as part of Medicare reform and is open to all Medicare beneficiaries to cover some outpatient prescription medication costs. Participants may purchase from a selection of several options of prescription coverage plans with variations in premiums, deductibles, copays, and formularies. There are annual coverage maximums beyond which the enrollee is responsible for costs, often referred to as the *donut hole* or *coverage gap*, for which enrollees often purchase additional policies to close these gaps. Part D is also partially funded by premiums paid by Medicare enrollees and US Treasury revenue.

Hospice

To receive hospice benefits under Medicare, an individual must be eligible for Medicare A and be certified by a physician to be terminally ill and within 6 months or less from death. A patient may receive hospice medical benefits under Medicare Part A or hospice medication benefits under Part D.

Services covered by Medicare for a patient on hospice can include the following:

- Doctor services
- Nursing care
- Medical equipment (like wheelchairs or walkers)
- Medical supplies (like bandages and catheters)
- Prescription drugs for hospice-related diagnoses
- Hospice aide and homemaker services
- Physical and occupational therapy
- Speech-language pathology services
- Social worker services
- Dietary counseling
- Grief and loss counseling for the patient and the patient's family
- Short-term inpatient care (for pain and symptom management)
- Short-term respite care

Services not covered by Medicare for a patient on hospice include the following:

- Treatment intended to cure any illness
- Medications or prescriptions *not* related to the terminal illness
- Room and board for most inpatient care
- Any care not set up by the patient's hospice provider, including outpatient care (Centers for Medicare & Medicaid Services, 2020)

Medigap

Medigap is a supplemental plan that is purchasable and designed to fill gaps in coverage from Parts A and B. Because traditional Medicare does not cover all of a patient's expenses, many older adults purchase these plans to help with additional out-of-pocket costs, which can include co-insurance, deductibles, preventive care, and care in foreign countries. People often use the terms *Medigap* and *Medicare supplemental insurance* interchangeably, and it is important to remember that these plans are bought by a Medicare recipient to supplement any gaps in coverage from traditional Medicare. A participant must carry Medicare Part A and Part B also in order to be eligible for a Medigap or supplemental plan. It is important to note that Medigap generally does not cover long-term care, hearing aids, eyeglasses, dental expenses, some prescriptions, or private duty nursing.

Medicaid

Medicaid is a joint state and federal program of health insurance for those with low incomes and limited savings. Criteria for admission varies from state to state. Patients who qualify for both Medicare and Medicaid are said to be dual eligible, and at that point Medicaid can begin to cover some of the Part B premiums, deductibles and other costs. Medicaid provides benefits and services such as fixed rates for generic drugs and name-brand prescriptions, dental care, and long-term custodial care. In 2016, over 70% Medicaid dollars were spent on long-term care expenditures.

Long-Term Care Insurance

Long-term care insurance is a costly and rarely utilized option in the United States for older adults, and less than 5% of adults over the age of 45 carry such policies (Kaiser Family Foundation, 2014). Operating on the principle of experience rating, long-term care insurance charges older adults an ever-increasing premium as they age, making these policies often unobtainable to those who are often less able to cover the financial costs. In addition, these policies often require large deductibles be met (measured in nursing home days) before they begin to provide coverage and usually reimburse using low fixed daily rates, which do not cover all costs incurred. For example, a typical policy may require a 90-day deductible be met before paying a daily reimbursement rate, in addition to ongoing payment of the premium. The daily reimbursement rate is often far below total daily costs, making the policies financially unattractive to older adults.

Nurse Practitioner/Physician Assistant Role

Medicare traditionally reimburses providers based on volume of patients seen, known as the fee-for-service model. Based on this reimbursement model, all providers, MDs, DOs, NPs, and PAs alike, were incentivized to maximize the number of patients seen in a day. To improve quality and reduce costs, the passage of the Affordable Care Act in 2010 sought to shift the focus of care from volume of patients seen to the value of services provided. A greater emphasis was placed on clinical outcomes while attempting to streamline costs. Payments for services rendered during an illness or course of treatment now are bundled, rather than individualized, reducing the duplication of services, eliminating costs, and aligning care goals.

Both current and anticipated shortages in physicians specializing in both primary care and geriatrics have placed both NPs and PAs in a position to bridge the gap by providing high-quality, value-based care to our older adults in all settings of the long-term care spectrum. Other direct incentives such as increased federal funding for graduate nursing education programs and National Health Service Corps funding for loan reimbursement are bringing more advanced practice clinicians into the fields of long-term care.

Care Transitions

Older adult patients with chronic health care needs frequently engage with the health care system at multiple delivery points. This may expose them to multiple providers or points of access within the system, which can promote fragmented care. Care transitions occur when a patient travels from one location of care to another or from one provider to another. These care transitions can be particularly vulnerable periods of time for the older adult and are often associated with uncertainty and risk. Examples of care transitions include community-dwelling older adults who transfer to the hospital for an acute illness or exacerbation of a chronic problem. From the hospital, these patients may be discharged back home or to an extended care facility for a rehabilitation stay before going home. Another broad category of care transition involves the transfer of nursing home residents or those involved in end-of-life care to an acute care hospital for the evaluation and management of an acute issue.

Each transfer of care is an opportunity for the patient to be evaluated by a different provider and possibly multiple other team members who may make changes to the patient's medical plan, adjust medications, or prescribe a different course of treatment. These care transitions often add layers of complexity and confusion for both the patient and family and can contribute to polypharmacy, increase the risk of medication errors, add to communication misunderstandings between patients and providers, and contribute to patient readmission rates. Nearly one in five Medicare beneficiaries discharged from the hospital, or 2.6 million seniors, are readmitted to the hospital within 30 days of discharge often because of these factors, costing more than $26 billion annually (Jencks, 2009).

Effective care coordination and communication among providers are key factors for achieving successful transitional care and thereby minimizing unnecessary hospital readmissions, medication escalations, and fragmentations in care. Factors that have been studied and have been associated with lower readmission rates include performance of medication reconciliation or medication reviews with each entry into a new health care site as well as education and counseling with both the patient and the caregivers (Mueller, 2012). This includes a comprehensive review of all outpatient medication lists as they compare with any medications or treatments that have been added, changed, or discontinued during the course of treatment in the new service location. Timely medical follow-up after a care transition serves as an opportunity for the provider to assess both the patient and the caregiver's understanding of new medications or treatment regimens and to provide any education or additional interventions as needed. These medication reviews have been shown to reduce actual and potential adverse drug events (Mueller, 2012).

SAFETY ALERT

Factors Associated With Patient Safety in Care Transitions

- Communication between providers
- Medication reconciliation
- Early follow-up with the receiving provider after discharge

Care Models

Community-Based Care/Outpatient Care

The hallmarks of any effective outpatient care program for the older adult population are a recognition of the need for a comprehensive approach to the patient with multiple chronic medical conditions, timely preventive services, and a focus on optimal function. Many traditional primary care practices lack the expertise in dealing with the complexities of the geriatric patient who often has two or more long-term health conditions, sensory or functional impairments, and physical or mental health conditions. This concept of multiple comorbidities or multimorbidity is common in the geriatric population.

More than two-thirds of Medicare beneficiaries over the age of 65 have two or more chronic medical conditions, and more than half have four or more (Partnership for Solutions, 2004). The impact of multimorbidity is broad and has far-reaching implications. People with multiple medical conditions are often more likely to be diagnosed with new diagnoses that contribute to escalations in clinical care, increasing care complexity, and rising health care costs. Two-thirds of Medicare beneficiaries with multimorbidity account for 96% of all Medicare expenditures (Partnership for Solutions, 2004). Multimorbidity is associated with higher risks of adverse clinical outcomes and increased usage of health care resources such as emergency department visits, avoidable inpatient admissions, and nursing home placement in the older adult population (Boyd, et al., 2012).

Geriatrics in Primary Care

In most traditional primary care practices, the practitioner is taught to tailor management of a disease process or condition utilizing traditional practice guidelines. The high prevalence of multimorbidity in the geriatric patient has required primary care clinicians who serve this patient population to reevaluate the traditional disease-focused approach to patient care. For a patient with multiple competing clinical entities, strict adherence to clinical practice guidelines has been shown to increase health care costs, contribute to polypharmacy, and, at times, give competing recommendations to patients. The traditional disease-focused practice guidelines or care models often force clinicians to adhere to strict care protocols that may be conflicting, costly, and often at odds with the patient's goals or functional status. The American Geriatrics Society recommends that the approach to geriatrics in primary care should involve "person-centered" care (American Geriatrics Society, 2016) (Box 21.1)—that is, care that displays knowledge of the individual based on his or her preferences and goals. This is accomplished by paying particular attention to the individual's medical conditions while ensuring his or her optimal overall function given each person's unique circumstances. A provider must appreciate the possibly fluctuating and evolving health status of the older patient while being mindful of possible shifting priorities as they relate to the patients' personal goals of care and quality of life as they advance along in their health care journey.

One approach to manage geriatrics in the outpatient setting is modeled after the pediatric concept of the patient-centered medical home (PCMH) model of practice. Using this concept, the primary care clinician develops a personalized plan of care for the patient, while building partnerships with other medical staff and clinicians, family, and team members in order to improve the health and well-being of the PCMH members. The PCMH model of care also embraces the concept of the multidisciplinary care team by incorporating input from multiple care members from a variety of disciplines. Each team member contributes to the care plan of the individual patient with a common goal of ensuring the patient's personalized goals are met while acknowledging the patient's unique personal circumstances. Embracing the philosophy of the Affordable Care Act's goal of measurable outcomes and value-driven care, the PCMH model encourages communication between clinicians and the clients they serve in order to create strong relationships and individualized care plans. This team-based primary care model has been associated with reduced health care costs and utilization of services among chronically ill patients (Meyers, 2018). The main concept of the PCMH includes the premise that the primary care provider (PCP) (often a NP or PA) along with a community of resources, can provide efficient, higher-quality, and lower-cost care for an individual patient than a series of fragmented, unconnected, high-cost interactions with the health care system. Evidence has shown that team-based care has reduced unplanned hospitalizations and emergency room visits in the most vulnerable (sicker) patients (Meyers, 2018).

• BOX 21.1 American Geriatrics Society: Key Component of Geriatric Care

Focus on Function

- Focus on managing chronic diseases
- Identify and manage psychological and social aspects of care
- Respect patient dignity and autonomy
- Respect cultural and spiritual beliefs
- Be sensitive to the patient's financial condition
- Promote wellness
- Listen and communicate effectively
- Take a patient-centered approach to care and a customer approach to service
- Maintain a realistic attitude of optimism and hope
- Use a team approach to care

From the American Geriatrics Society. www.geriatricscareonline.org/toc/person-centered-care-a-definition-and-essential-elements/CL020

Locations for Care

A clinician caring for older adults is often tasked with determining whether or not a patient is living safely in the appropriate environment. This is a complicated clinical scenario, one that must be balanced by weighing the older adult's desire for independence along with several other factors such as functional status, including mobility and ADL status, the level and availability of family and social support, and financial considerations. Individuals may move across a spectrum of locations (Fig. 21.3) as their care needs change. When using the patient-centered approach to care, the clinician must be aware of community, outpatient, and inpatient support options that are available within one's local network. There is evidence to support the use of an enhanced network of support systems to keep frail older adults in their homes as a method of avoiding unnecessary hospitalizations. Research has demonstrated that through the use of extended medical and community support systems and communication with primary care providers, it is

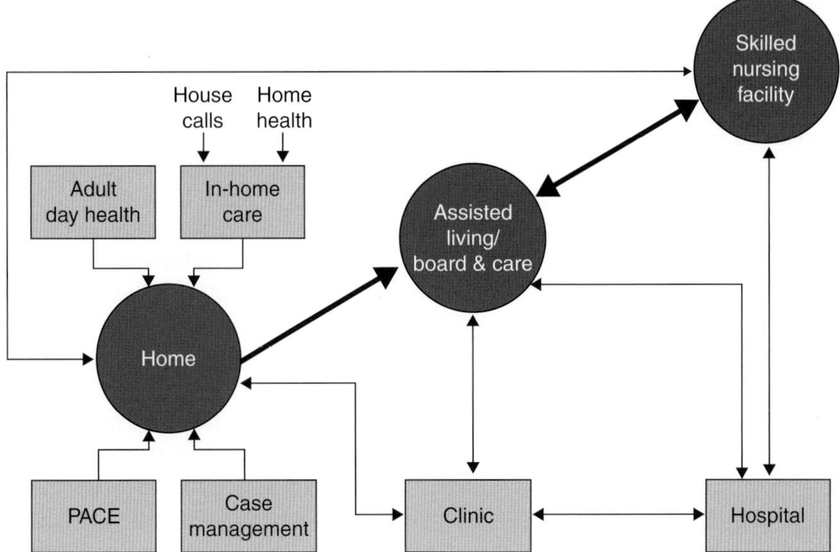

Sites of long-term care. A diagrammatic representation of the locations in which elders live (circles), with thick arrows showing the directions in which elders move from location to location. The thin arrows identify those medical services available to elders living in different sites and the medical/service centers to which elders travel (squares).

• **Fig. 21.3** Sites of Long-Term Care (From Long-Term Care, Nursing Home, & Rehabilitation, Williams, B. A., Chang, A., Ahalt, C., Chen, H., Conant, R., Landefeld, C., Ritchie, C., Yukawa, & M. [2014]. Current diagnosis & treatment: Geriatrics (2nd ed). https://accessmedicine.mhmedical.com/ViewLarge.aspx?figid=53376549&gbosContainerID=0&gbosid=0&groupID=0.)

possible to reduce unplanned hospitalizations and unnecessary emergency room visits in frail older adults with multiple long-term health conditions (Chapman, 2018).

Home-Based Care

A common entry point into the complicated world of long-term care may involve the addition of home services to an older adult's care plan. These services are often added following an acute hospitalization or in response to a change in medical or functional status and can include the addition of skilled nursing support or skilled physical, occupational, or speech therapists. Although the goal of such support is often to return patients to prior level of function, it can also allow older adults to stay in their homes longer, if safe to do so. Additional caregivers such as patient care assistants (PCAs) or home health aides (HHA) may be necessary to assist with both ADLs and household tasks. An increasing number of medical practices are now offering medical home visits, or "house calls," for both routine health care checkups and urgent visits for older adults. These home visits are generally supplemental to one's standard primary, office-based care but can provide medical oversight for both routine matters and urgent issues when transportation and impaired mobility may impact one's ability to leave her or his residence.

Adult Day Care

Adult day care programs represent an increasingly popular option for part-time care and support outside of the home environment. These nonresidential centers, also known as adult day centers, are designed to provide varying levels of care and support for adults who need some degree of supervision or socialization during the day. Adult day programs can vary in programs and services offered, but in general all provide an opportunity for socialization, recreational activities, meals, snacks, and transportation for adults who need more supervision, increased opportunities for socialization, or structured care outside the home. A facility is designated an adult day health care program (ADHC) if it also provides onsite medical support as well as rehabilitation services and can be used as part of the overall rehabilitation care plan following a hospitalization if needed. Structured programs for those with dementia or cognitive impairment have been shown to both improve older adults' quality of life as well as reduce caregiver stress, allowing for predictable respite periods during caregiving (Zarit, 2014).

Program of All-Inclusive Care (PACE)

The Program of All-Inclusive Care for the Elderly (PACE) is a care model developed in San Francisco in 1973, born from a desire to keep the city's immigrant population in their homes rather than placing them in nursing facilities (National Pace Association, 2019b). Charged with this task, community leaders developed a comprehensive program of outpatient services, including medical oversight, physical and occupational therapy, transportation services, socialization, and adult day support. This community-based program, originally called On Lok

Senior Health Services, Cantonese for "peaceful happy abode," quickly began receiving Medicaid reimbursement for its services and rapidly grew in scope and intent. The PACE model was expanded in 1986 through funding from the Robert Wood Johnson Foundation for six additional sites using Medicare and Medicaid waivers, and in 1997 the Balanced Budget Act gave PACE a provider benefit under Medicaid.

Today, there are more than 250 PACE centers in the United States. The PACE program's intent is to coordinate the care of each enrollee to allow the person to continue to live in the community as long and as independently as possible. The program provides all the medical support and coordination of services the individual needs through a multidisciplinary team approach while ensuring a high level of coordinated care.

PACE participants are appointed a primary care provider (MD/DO/NP/PA) who acts as the center point for care coordination. The PCP will then interact with other members of the multidisciplinary care team, including nurses, social workers, therapists, drivers, PCAs, and many others whose primary goal is to provide preventive and supportive care for the client and to respond to the changing needs of the client as situations arise.

PACE is funded through a monthly bundled payment from Medicare and/or Medicaid for each client; this acts as a lump sum payment to the program that covers all services that the client may need, including medical visits, transportation, skilled nursing visits, medications, hospital visits, and other costs. This includes all hospital-related and procedure costs.

To be eligible for PACE, a patient must be 55 or older, live in a PACE service area, and be certified by the state to need a nursing home level of care at the time of admission to the program. About 7% of PACE participants do reside in a nursing home If a participant does require a nursing home level of care, it is paid for by PACE, who then continues to coordinate the individual's care.

Statistics reveal that the average PACE participant is female (75%), 76 years old, and has 7.9 medical conditions, the majority of which are chronic, such as diabetes, congestive heart failure, chronic obstructive pulmonary disease, and psychiatric disorders (National Pace Association, 2019a). Almost half of PACE participants (47%) carry a diagnosis of dementia. Over 90% live in the community and obtain enhanced support from the program. If nursing home support is required, they do not need to disenroll from the program; it is covered by PACE in certain facilities that contract with the organization.

Assisted Living

Definition

Broadly defined, assisted living (AL) consists of a system of housing and limited care systems designed for older adults (and other generally disabled adults) who need some assistance with activities of daily living but do not meet the criteria for a nursing home level of care. The National Assisted Living Workgroup, tasked by the US Senate Special Council on Aging in 2003, defined assisted living as a state-regulated and monitored residential long-term care option that provides or coordinates oversight and services to meet residents' individualized needs (Center For Excellence in Assisted Living, 2003). The goal is for the resident to maintain independence for as long as possible while providing a network of support for that patient to make this achievable.

Services provided in assisted living facilities vary widely and are regulated by individual state laws (National Center for Assisted Living, 2019). These generally include basic functions such as the provision of meals (two to three hot meals per day), assistance with certain activities of daily living (bathing, dressing, grooming, toileting), housekeeping, laundry services, recreation and social activities, as well as transportation. Other possible services include medication management (medication prefill or prompted medication reminders), access to onsite medical services or onsite nursing support (occasional versus 24-hour support), and variances in the number of personal care hours per day/week provided. Residents may elect to receive the services they feel will optimize individual autonomy, privacy, choice, dignity, and aging in place in a homelike environment. Some of these ancillary services may be purchased for an additional monthly fee.

Assisted living costs vary by state, geographic location, size of unit, and extent of services provided. The national average cost for a one-bedroom unit is $119/day or $3628/month and is not covered by Medicare (National Center for Assisted Living, 2019). Specialty units, such as dementia care units, cost more. The average assisted living resident needs help with 4.5 IADLs, and four-fifths need assistance with housework, laundry, medications, transportation, and meal preparation. Fifty-four percent use walking devices (such as a walker or cane) and 31% have urinary incontinence (National Center for Assisted Living, 2019). Most assisted living residents pay out of pocket or use private financial resources to cover the costs of assisted living.

Rehabilitation/Subacute/Acute Rehabilitation

Following a hospitalization, it is often necessary to determine whether a patient can safely return home or if a period of rehabilitation is necessary. The purpose of rehabilitation is to enhance and restore functional ability as well as quality of life to those with physical impairments or disabilities. Because the population is aging, adults over age 65 are the fastest segment of the population requiring rehabilitation services. Rehabilitation can take place in a variety of settings (Box 21.2). The determination of what services an individual requires and where best to receive these services is often a task fulfilled by the interdisciplinary care team.

Rehabilitation can begin in the acute care hospital with assessments by the physical, occupational, or speech therapist and can include such services as

• BOX 21.2 Rehabilitation Settings

- Acute hospital (transitional care unit within the hospital)
- Inpatient rehabilitation facility (IRF or acute rehab)
- Long-term acute care hospital (LTACH)
- Skilled nursing facility (subacute rehab unit or SNF, often embedded in a long-term care facility)
- Veteran's Association (VA)–affiliated rehabilitation programs
- Home health care
- Outpatient rehabilitation

SAFETY ALERT

Members of the Multidisciplinary Team

- Medical provider
- Nurse
- Physical therapist
- Occupational therapist
- Speech therapist
- Physical medicine and rehabilitation provider
- Social worker
- Nurse case manager
- Dietitian
- Orthotist/prosthetist
- Psychologist
- Recreational therapist
- Others whose goal is to evaluate the patient's overall function and make recommendations for a safe disposition based on the individual's overall care needs

mobilization, dysphagia therapy, and ADL assessments. In virtually all settings, a patient may receive the basics of rehabilitation services. This may include at a minimum, physical therapy, occupational therapy, and speech and language therapy. These basic rehabilitation services are available to both hospital level patients, patients receiving rehabilitation in skilled nursing facilities or other inpatient facilities, outpatient rehabilitation facilities or through various home agencies. For hospitalized patients that are determined to need care after the acute hospitalization, choosing the appropriate location for this postacute care can be a challenging process. Even among specialists within the multidisciplinary care team there appears to be a lack of consensus regarding criteria for referrals to each care location. In the postacute settings, each site differs in the types of services offered as well as the number of therapy hours provided. There are also differences in the levels of medical and nursing support available as well as reimbursement factors that come into play when choosing a locale for the patient. Facilities that are hospital based or are closer to larger medical centers may allow patients greater access to rehabilitation sub-specialization in the fields of Wound Management, Amputee Care, Orthopedic Rehabilitation, Stroke Rehabilitation, Traumatic Brain Injury and Spinal Cord Injury amongst others.

SAFETY ALERT

Members of the Multidisciplinary Team

- Medical provider (geriatrician, NP/PA)
- Nursing
- Physical therapist
- Occupational therapist
- Speech therapist
- Physical medicine and rehabilitation provider
- Social worker
- Nurse case manager
- Dietitian
- Orthotist/prosthetist
- Psychologist
- Recreational therapist
- Others whose goal is to evaluate the patient's overall function and make recommendations for a safe disposition based on the individual's overall care needs

Overview of Geriatric Rehabilitation, Multidisciplinary Team

Disability, or the inability to carry out a basic functional activity, is commonly associated with the aging process. Nearly one in four older adults receiving Medicare has at least one health care–related disability (Manton, 2008). The inability to perform ADLs without assistance can affect one's ability to live independently and can have negative impacts on an older adult's quality of life (Manton, 2008). The goal of geriatric rehabilitation, or any rehabilitation program, is to optimize function while recognizing a patient's individual medical and functional limitations. This is a reinforcement of the patient-centered approach to care during the rehabilitation process.

Disability in the older adult comes in many forms. It may be present as an acute process, such as difficulty walking, aphasia, and dysphagia following a new stroke, or it may be more insidious in onset, such as months of unintended weight loss and chronic pain without a clear inciting event leading to a slow decline in function over a period of time. Both examples require a comprehensive assessment that is best performed by a multidisciplinary care team with the expertise to address this special population.

Geriatric rehabilitation programs are often led by a team of providers whose primary goal is to perform a comprehensive assessment of the individual, regardless of the setting in which the rehabilitation is taking place. Most inpatient rehabilitation programs occur at either inpatient rehabilitation facilities (IRFs) or skilled nursing facilities (SFNs; also known as subacute rehabilitation facilities), although other locations are possible. Older adults are often referred for inpatient rehabilitation following an acute hospitalization. Hospitalized patients are assessed by an inpatient physical therapist/occupational therapist and speech-language pathologist (SLP), if indicated, as well as other consultants who help the inpatient care teams determine whether or not a patient will require a postacute rehabilitation. Therapy services for many older adults begins during these acute hospitalizations, often even in the emergency department. Patients who are deemed safe enough to return home can then receive home care services and will begin a course of either home or outpatient rehabilitation. Once home, their care is generally followed by the primary care provider or a geriatrician who coordinates their outpatient services. Patients who need more care and supervision, as determined by these inpatient therapy assessments, are recommended for an inpatient postacute rehabilitation stay following their acute hospitalization. These determinations regarding post-hospital sites of care are often referred to as determinations of disposition.

Postacute rehabilitation programs vary in locale and the number of therapy and nursing hours per day the patient receives; however, each program's goal is to optimize the patient's level of function using a personalized approach to care. All postacute rehabilitation programs operate using the multidisciplinary care team approach and usually provide perform the following services:

- Comprehensive assessment of the patient's impairment on admission
- Assessment of ADLs
- Cognitive assessment
- Speech, language, swallowing function evaluation
- Gait, balance, transfers assessment
- Equipment and wheelchair evaluation (durable medical equipment)
- Kitchen and homemaking evaluation
- Assessment of support services, community resources
- Home evaluation

Some facilities offer specialized assessment programs tailored to certain disorders, including neuromuscular/stroke rehabilitation, orthopedic rehabilitation, amputee care, orthotics and prosthetics assessment, neuropsychiatric and behavioral health programs, access to driving evaluations, and specialized wound and pain management programs. The multidisciplinary care team meets often and regularly to discuss each patients' progress toward functional goals and discharge. Prior to discharge there is often a family meeting to discuss discharge planning and next steps in order to make care transitions smooth and without disruptions in care.

Nursing Home Care

Historically, nursing facilities provided nursing or custodial care to older adults with cognitive or functional impairments. In today's changing demographic, the role of the nursing facility has expanded to involve caring for the medically complex younger patient as well as the older patient with multimorbidity who needs more thorough medical oversight. These patients require more involvement from providers who are skilled in caring for this challenging population and who are more readily available for frequent interaction.

Facilities differ in the type and number of services offered as well as the type of residents they serve. They are often described as levels 1 through IV, reflecting the types and intensity of services provided, and include the following:

- *Level I intensive nursing and rehabilitative care facility:* Provides continuous skilled nursing care and an organized program of restorative services.
- *Level II skilled nursing care facility:* Provides continuous skilled nursing care and meaningful availability of restorative services and other therapeutic services.
- *Level III supportive nursing care facility:* Provides routine nursing and periodic availability of skilled nursing, restorative, and other therapeutic services as indicated.
- *Level IV resident care facility:* Provides or arranges for a supervised supportive, protective living environment and support services incident to old age for residents who are having difficulty caring for themselves and who do not require level II or III nursing care or other medically related services on a regular basis.

Nursing Home Population in the United States

According to CMS data, there are nearly 16,000 Medicare- and Medicaid-certified nursing facilities in the United States, with 1.65 million available beds (Harrington, Nursing Facilities, Staffing, Residents and Facilities Deficiencies, 2009–2016, 2017). Currently the percentage of Americans over the age of 65 who are nursing home residents is small, about 2.6% or 1.4 million, but the numbers have grown since the early 2000s. The percentage of adults younger than age 65 residing in long-term care facilities has increased 8% to 15%, and the percentage of those over the age of 85 has increased by 38% to 43%. Nursing home residents have a high prevalence of functional disability, defined as requiring assistance in one or more activities of daily living. Current data suggest that 90% require assistance in three or more ADLs, and one in four require assistance in five or more ADLs (Harrington, Nursing Facilities, Staffing, Residents and Facilities Deficiencies, 2009–2016, 2017). Multiple comorbidities are also prevalent, with two-thirds of residents meeting the definition of multimorbidity.

Factors associated with nursing home placement include advancing age, poor social and family support including lack of spouse or children, and lower income status. Widowed or divorced and never-married adults have higher risks of long-term care admission (Harrington, Nursing Facilities, Staffing, Residents and Facilities Deficiencies, 2009–2016, 2017). Substantial race and ethnic variations in nursing home admissions are noted as well, with under usage in certain minorities. Blacks and Hispanics tend to stay in their communities longer; however, they are more impaired upon admission. Older Black individuals with a coexisting mental health diagnosis were also noted to have higher rates of nursing home admission (Yu, 2018).

Care in nursing facilities is highly regulated on both the state and federal levels to ensure proper care of the residents by utilizing a mandated, interdisciplinary team approach. Membership in the interdisciplinary team can vary depending on facility and patient needs. Table 21.2

provides an overview of nursing facility interdisciplinary care team members and their roles. The goal of the interdisciplinary team is to optimize care and coordinate all aspects of the resident's medical, psychological, social, and functional life.

Federal regulations and governance of nursing facilities were overhauled with the passage of the Omnibus Reconciliation Act (OBRA) of 1987, which contained the Nursing Home Reform Act. OBRA was initiated, in part, due to long-standing concerns from the public regarding poor-quality care in facilities, specifically the lack of focus on the quality of life for the resident. OBRA also addressed several areas of concern, specifically the usage of chemical and physical restraints in nursing facilities, the high-frequency of urinary catheter usage, and pressure ulcer development among residents. The passage of OBRA resulted in a stronger federal government role in facility inspection, staff training, improved assessment of resident needs, and

TABLE 21.2 Interdisciplinary Care Team in Nursing Facilities

Provider	Scope of Practice
Medical director	Physician leadership, patient care-clinical leadership, quality control, education; Omnibus Reconciliation Act (OBRA) required.
Attending primary care physician	Initial patient care, admissions, discharges, periodic assessments.
Nurse practitioner	Advanced practice RN: Provides all aspects of medical care to residents, including performance of admissions, discharges, periodic assessments; part of physician-NP team.
Physician assistant	Health care provider: Provides all aspects of medical care to residents, including performance of admissions, discharges, periodic assessments; part of physician-PA team.
Registered nurse	Works directly with the patient and family, frequently interacting with the patient and performing assessments, administering medication, performing procedures, documenting progress and changes in status.
Licensed practical nurse	Provides direct patient care, often reports directly to the RN. Performs tasks such as wound care and medication administration as per state guidelines.
Certified nursing assistant	Provides hands-on, direct personal care for the residents, including all assistance with activities of daily living (ADLs). Works under the supervision of the nurse.
Registered nurse assessment coordinator	Coordinates the completeness of Minimum Data Set (MDS) and other federally mandated paperwork in order to maintain compliance.
Director of nursing	Oversees and supervises the nursing staff to ensure compliance and high-quality patient care, adherence to standards, and completion of requirements.
Nursing home administrator	Managing officer of the facility; controls the day-to-day functions. Responsible for compliance with all regulations and rules.
Social worker	Facilities with >120 residents are required to employ a full-time social worker to assist with activities such as patient advocacy, mental health referrals, and counseling and discharge planning.
Dietitian	Plans food, oversees nutrition for residents, supervises meal preparations, performs nutrition screenings, assesses diet-related concerns.
Physical therapist	Evaluates and treats patients with physical difficulties or impairments in function to optimize strength, flexibility, and motor control and to reduce pain or other functional limitations.
Occupational therapist	Evaluates and treats patients with difficulties in activities of daily living to promote optimum levels of function
Speech therapist	Performs a variety of tasks, such as evaluates and treats dysphagia as well as language and cognitive dysfunction. May perform swallowing assessments and make dietary recommendations.
Recreational therapist	Provides therapeutic programs that offer art, music, dance, sports, games, culture, and craft activities for residents appropriate to their abilities.
Consultant pharmacist	Reviews and manages medication regimens of residents.

From Fenstemacher, P. A., & Winn, P. (2016). *Post-acute and long-term care medicine: A pocket guide* (2nd ed.). Humana Press. Material adapted from the Bureau of Labor and Statistics, May 2013. www.bls.gov/oes/current/oes291141.htm

an improved regulatory process by adopting the geriatric assessment method championed by the geriatric community and promoting or mandating the application of a process of assessing residents based on the model of the comprehensive geriatric assessment.

Based on OBRA influences, nursing facilities are now heavily focusing on quality of life and quality of care for each resident, as these factors are a major component of an annual state survey conducted by federal regulators.

Data Collection

Each resident admitted to a skilled nursing facility undergoes a comprehensive screening assessment in order to gauge their medical, functional, and nursing needs. These assessments are performed by members of the multidisciplinary care team and include such screening tools as the Minimum Data Set (MDS) and Resident Assessment Instrument (RAI). The MDS is federally mandated to be completed on admission to a facility, and it must be updated quarterly, annually, and anytime there is a significant change in status or condition. The MDS evaluates areas such as ADLs status, mobility, continence, behavioral concerns, pain, falls, language and communication ability, and the level of assistance, if any, needed with each area. The facility MDS coordinator enters this information into a database; it is then entered into the state database where it is transmitted to national CMS databases for further review. From there, CMS determines a per diem pay rate for the facility based on the resident's unique resource utilization group (RUG). State surveyors also use this information to determine individual facility quality measures.

In the fall of 2014, Congress passed the Improving Medicare Post-Acute Care Transformation Act of 2014, or the IMPACT Act, in a further effort to both standardize patient assessment data and improve quality-of-care outcomes. Briefly, this legislation requires that all patients with Medicare A as well as some residents with managed Medicare plans who are admitted to a rehabilitation facility or are receiving home rehabilitation undergo specific functional assessments completed by their providers with respect to their overall function, self-care, and mobility. Falls and skin breakdown are also assessed if applicable. The MDS coordinator of the admitting facility will perform a "first 3-day" usual performance assessment using data collected from nursing assistants as well as data from physical and occupational therapists involved in the patient's care. This information is entered into a specific section of the MDS call the GG code. This initial assessment's purpose is to serve as a functional baseline as the patient begins the rehabilitation process and is then repeated at discharge to determine functional trends and monitor overall progress.

Nursing facilities are highly regulated on both the state and federal levels and undergo rigorous inspection to ensure appropriate care standard adherence. Despite this, nearly one in five facilities in the United States is citied annually for deficiencies that caused actual harm or placed residents in immediate jeopardy (Harrington, Nursing Facilities, Staffing, Residents and Facilities Deficiencies, 2009 Through 2015, 2015). The aim of the Department of Health and Human Services (DHHS) National Nursing Home Quality Initiative is to improve care in both short-stay facilities and long-term facilities, and the department has posted each facility's quality measures on its website so that they are available to the public. These "report cards" offer a concise report of each facilities status, but a more complete report of each individual facility's state survey is available to residents and families at both the individual facility and the state DHHS office. The availability of this data has helped improve transparency between the facility and its residents, helped the public make better informed decisions regarding placement of their loved ones, and motivated providers to improve care delivered to their patients.

CMS additionally created the Nursing Home Five Star Quality Rating System whose intent was to help consumers compare facilities using an easy-to-recognize one-to-five star rating system. It also allows consumers and residents to identify areas of concern within a facility and organize questions to administration should they be necessary. Facilities receiving one star are said to be of below average quality, whereas those receiving five stars are considered to be of above average quality. Savvy consumers and facilities alike are using a facility's star rating as a marketing strategy as well as a primary motivation for placement decisions (Centers for Medicare & Medicaid Services, 2019). Stars are distributed to a facility based on nursing home performance in several key domains, including the following:

- *Health inspections:* Outcomes of the annual state inspection as well as the number and severity of any deficiencies identified during the survey as well as the last three annual surveys. Thirty-six months of complaint investigations are also taken into consideration. Data from health inspections, fire safety inspections, and any incidents or complaints and their resolutions are included.
- *Staffing:* Staffing ratios including RN hours per resident per day, total nurse staffing hours per resident per day (RN/licensed practical nurse/nursing assistant), and physical therapy hours available.
- *Quality measures:* Data based on MDS collected information and other claims-based data.

SAFETY ALERT

The IMPACT Act

- Requires collection of data across all postacute sites, including inpatient rehabilitation facilities, skilled nursing facilities, long-term acute care hospitals, and home health aides
- Assesses functional mobility, ADLs, and other key areas such as falls and skin breakdown
- Tracks whether a patient is independent, needs some assistance, or is dependent with an activity

• BOX 21.3 Centers for Medicare & Medicaid Services (CMS) Quality Measures Based on the Minimum Data Set (MDS), April 2019

Measures for Long-Stay Residents (Defined as Residents Who Are in the Nursing Home for Greater Than 100 Days) That Are Derived From MDS Assessments

- Percentage of residents whose need for help with activities of daily living has increased
- Percentage of residents whose ability to move independently worsened
- Percentage of high-risk residents with pressure ulcers
- Percentage of residents who have/had a catheter inserted and left in their bladder
- Percentage of residents with a urinary tract infection
- Percentage of residents who self-report moderate to severe pain
- Percentage of residents experiencing one or more falls with major injury
- Percentage of residents who received an antipsychotic medication

Measures for Long-Stay Residents That Are Derived From Claims Data

- Number of hospitalizations per 1000 long-stay resident days
- Number of outpatient emergency department (ED) visits per 1000 long-stay resident days

Measures for Short-Stay Residents That Are Derived From MDS Assessments

- Percentage of residents who made improvement in function
- Percentage of skilled nursing facility (SNF) residents with pressure ulcers that are new or worsened
- Percentage of residents who self-report moderate to severe pain
- Percentage of residents who newly received an antipsychotic medication

Measures for Short-Stay Residents That Are Derived From Claims Data

- Percentage of short-stay residents who were rehospitalized after a nursing home admission
- Percentage of short-stay residents who have had an outpatient emergency department (ED) visit
- Rate of successful return to home and community from a skilled nursing facility (SNF)

From https://www.cms.gov/NursingHomeQualityInits/25_NHQIMDS30.asp

Star ratings related to quality measures include CMS data collected, such as measures and outcomes related to the percentage of residents who appropriately receive the influenza vaccination, the usage of antipsychotic medications among residents, the incidence of pressure ulcers, and other functional related data as noted in Box 21.3. In April 2019, an updated version of quality measures was added to the CMS collection data with additional focused areas of surveillance and monitoring.

As part of the passage of the Nursing Home Reform Act of 1987, language was included to further protect the residents' dignity, enable them to pursue proper care and optimal quality of life. From this evolved the Nursing Home Residents Bill of Rights, which are often prominently displayed in any long-term care facility (Box 21.4).

• BOX 21.4 Resident Bill of Rights

Nursing home residents have certain rights and protections under the law. The nursing home must list and give all new residents a copy of these rights.

These resident rights include, but are not limited to the following:

- The right to be treated with dignity and respect.
- The right to be informed in writing about services and fees before you enter the nursing home.
- The right to manage your own money or to choose someone else you trust to do this for you.
- The right to privacy, and to keep and use your personal belongings and property as long as it doesn't interfere with the rights, health, or safety of others.
- The right to be informed about your medical condition, medications, and to see your own doctor. You also have the right to refuse medications and treatments.
- The right to have a choice over your schedule (for example, when you get up and go to sleep), your activities, and other preferences that are important to you.
- The right to an environment more like a home that maximizes your comfort and provides you with assistance to be as independent as possible (Medicare.gov).

From cms.gov/medicare/Your_Resident_Rights_and_Protections_section.pdf

Medical Care in Long-Term Care Facilities

The medical care of each resident admitted to a long-term care facility is tightly regulated by state and federal guidelines and is routinely reevaluated to ensure safety standards are upheld Individual state guidelines may be viewed under the individual State Department of Public Health websites. Every aspect of care is accounted for to ensure a person-centered approach to care, as well as to protect these frail individuals who may not be able to speak for themselves.

Each resident is assigned an attending physician upon admission. The attending physician is responsible for the continuous medical care and periodic reevaluation throughout the resident's stay. The physician may be part of a team of providers that includes a nurse practitioner or physician assistant who shares a care relationship for the resident in the facility, and this is designated upon admission. All providers and care teams must be designated and posted in the chart along with contact information available to the facility.

Every resident must have a complete physical examination and medical evaluation including the development of a care plan upon admission to the facility. This comprehensive evaluation includes information such as the following:

- Primary diagnosis
- Other diagnoses/conditions
- Pertinent findings (including vital signs, weight)
- Past medical history
- Significant special conditions, limitations
- Prognosis
- Assessment of function (including ambulation status, ADL status, continence of bowel and bladder)
- Cognitive assessment
- Treatment plan, including the following:
  - Medications
  - Special treatments (wounds, dressings, topical, etc.)
  - Restorative services (physical therapy, occupational therapy, speech-language pathology)
  - Dietary needs
  - Ambulation and activity orders
  - Preventive or maintenance measures
  - Short-term goals
  - Long-term goals
- Other considerations upon admission
  - Advance directives, code status
  - Health care proxy

Each resident or his or her designee/next of kin has the right to determine which health care providers are involved in the resident's care. Additional services that are routinely required include the following:

- *Dental services:* A complete annual dental examination is part of each resident's plan of care, as well as periodic reevaluation as per the dentist's recommendation
  - This includes prophylactic, therapeutic, and emergency care.
  - Consultant documentation should be recorded in the patient record.
  - Consultant notes/recommendations and treatment plans are coordinated with the MD/DO/PA/NP care team.
- *Podiatry services:* Access to proper footwear, and foot care as needed
  - Consultant documentation should be recorded in the patient record.
  - Consultant notes/recommendations and treatment plans are coordinated with the MD/DO/NP/PA care team.
- *Ancillary services:* Access to optometry and audiology
  - Consultant documentation should be recorded in the patient record.
  - Consultant notes/recommendations and treatment plans are coordinated with the MD/DO/NP/PA care team.
- *Diagnostics:* Access to the laboratory and radiology departments, ECG, and so on as per facility
  - Diagnostics should be documented and recorded in the patient record.
  - Diagnostics are coordinated with the MD/DO/NP/PA care team.

SAFETY ALERT

Provider documentation is exceptionally important in the long-term care facility because not only do these documents serve as the primary source of medical information but, it is important to note, facilities use these documents as a source of material for MDS data collection. Inaccuracies in the medical record can have far-reaching implications for MDS data collection and facility staffing and reimbursement.

Providers must list all current medical conditions with a corresponding appropriate billing code, and all prescribed medications must have a corresponding accurate diagnosis in order to adhere to facility and state standards of care.

Documentation Guidelines

The timing of completion of the initial physical examination and medical care plan is also closely regulated along with required periodic reassessments of the residents (Health, 1994). These guidelines also vary according to the type and level of the facility as documented by individual state regulations.

Level I facilities, often referred to intensive skilled nursing and rehabilitative facilities, are facilities or units that provides continuous skilled nursing care and an organized program of rehabilitation services in addition to the minimum, basic care and services.

Level II facilities provide continuous skilled nursing care, rehabilitation services, and other therapeutic services to residents who have the potential for improvement or restoration to a stabilized condition or who have a deteriorating condition requiring skilled care. Level II facilities may care for adults or have specialized programs for children.

Level III facilities provide routine nursing services (as well as skilled nursing on a periodic basis), rehabilitation, and other therapeutic services in addition to the minimum, basic care and services. Residents residing in a level III facility only require supportive nursing care, supervision, and observation.

Level IV facilities are often referred to as rest homes. Residents of a rest home require a supervised, supportive, and protective living environment and some support services but do not require the nursing, medical, or rehabilitative support provided by the other types of facilities. (Health, 1994)

All level I and level II facilities require that the medical care plan must be completed and recorded in the chart within 5 days prior to admission or up to 48 hours after admission. Level III and level IV facilities require completion within 14 days prior to admission and up to 72 hours following admission. If the patient's attending physician completes the physical exam and care plan in the office within the allowed time frame prior to nursing home admission and continues to be the resident's attending physician at the nursing facility, no additional examination or care plan is necessary. However, if the admission physical examination is completed by an NP or PA, the admission physical examination and medical care plan must be reviewed and cosigned by the attending physician within 10 days for level I and level II facilities and within 30 days for level III and level IV facilities.

Each resident is required to undergo periodic reevaluations, which involve repeat physical examinations and reevaluation of the medical care plan. These reevaluations can be alternately performed by the MD or advanced practitioner provider working with the resident according to the following schedule:

Level II facilities: Every 30 days following admission a resident must be reexamined and reevaluated, including a review of the medical care plan with any necessary revisions. Visits may be alternated by the physician, physician-nurse practitioner, or physician-physician assistant team. If after 90 days following admission the attending physician, physician-nurse practitioner, or physician-physician assistant team feels it is unnecessary to see the patient with this frequency, an alternate schedule of visits can be implemented with documentation in the medical record. At no time may the alternate schedule of visits be greater than 60 days between visits.

Level III facilities: Every 60 days following admission a resident must be reexamined and reevaluated, including a review of the medical care plan with any necessary revisions. Visits may be alternated by the physician, physician-nurse practitioner, or physician-physician assistant team. If after 90 days following admission the attending physician, the physician-nurse practitioner, or physician-physician assistant team feels it is unnecessary to see the patient with this frequency, an alternate schedule of visits can be implemented with documentation in the medical record. At no time may the alternate schedule of visits be greater than 90 days between visits.

Level IV facilities: Every 6 months following admission a resident must be reexamined and reevaluated, including a review of the medical care plan with any necessary revisions, except for community support residents who must be seen every 3 months unless the physician documents that they may be seen less frequently.

If the periodic reevaluations and visits are performed by a nurse practitioner or physician assistant, the supervising physician is required to perform an onsite review and evaluation of the patient and write a progress note confirming that she or he has personally evaluated the patient, reviewed the medical care plan put forth by the NP/PA, and participated in any revisions as indicated. This must occur at least every 6 months for level I and level II patients and at least every 12 months for level III and level IV patients.

Key Points

- Long-term care is a system of services and support for older and disabled adults to enable them to live independently and safely when they can no longer perform these activities by themselves. Services may be provided by a multidisciplinary team of workers in a variety of care locations.
- Statistics reveal a globally and nationally aging population with ever-increasing health care utilization and rising economic costs.
- The American health care system is a complex, evolving system comprised of Medicare and Medicaid as well as other programs that cover some, but not all, costs for older adults.
- Care models for the older adult can include outpatient primary care, home-based services, PACE programs, assisted living, inpatient rehabilitation facilities, and long-term care facilities.
- Long-term care facilities are highly regulated on both the state and federal levels to ensure patient safety and care standards are upheld.

More information about tools and Interprofessional Education Collaborative (IPEC) competencies mentioned in this chapter can be found in Appendix 1: Tools and Appendix 2: IPEC Competencies.

References

Aburto, J. M., Scholey, J., Kashnitsky, I., Zhang, L., Rahal, C., Missov, T., & Kashyap, R. (2021). Quantifying impacts of the COVID-19 though life expectancy losses: A population level study of 29 countries. *International Journal of Epidemiology.*

American Geriatrics Society Expert Panel on Person-Centered Care, (2016). Person-centered care: A definition and essential elements. *Journal American Geriatrics Society*, 15–18.

Arias, E., & Tejada-Vera, B. (2021). *Provisional life expectancy estimates for January 2020 through June 2020, Vital Statistics Rapid Release.* US Department of Health and Human Services, Centers For Diease Control and Prevention, National Center for Health Statistics, National Vital Statistics System.

Boyd, C. M., McNabney, M. K., Brandt, N., et al. (2012). Guiding principles for the care of older adults with multimorbidity: An approach for clinicians. *Journal American Geriatrics Society*, E1–E25.

Center For Excellence in Assisted Living. (2003, April). *A Report to the US Senate Special Committee on Aging.* https://www.theceal.org/assisted-living.

Centers for Disease Control and Prevention, N. C., (2019). *Vital Statistics Rapid Release: Births: Provisional Data for 2018.* National Center for Health Statistics. Centers for Disease Control and Prevention.

Centers for Medicare & Medicaid Services. (2019, April). Design for nursing home compare five-star quality rating system: Technical users' guide. https://www.cms.gov/Medicare/Provider-Enrollment-and-Certification/CertificationandComplianc/downloads/usersguide.pdf

Centers for Medicare & Medicaid Services, M. H. (2020, June 27). https://www.medicare.gov/Pubs/pdf/02154-medicare-hospice-benefits.pdf

Chapman, H. F. (2018). Okay to stay? A new plan to help people with long-term conditions remain in their own homes. *Primary Health Care and Research & Development*, 1–6.

Department of Economic and Social Affairs. (2019). *World Population Propspects: 2019 Highlights.* http://esa.un.org/wpp.

Dwyer-Lindgren, L., & Bertozzi-Villa, A. (2017). Inequalities in life expectancy among US counties, 1980 to 2014. *JAMA Internal Medicine*, 1003–1011.

Harrington, C., & Carrillo, H. (2015). Nursing facilities, staffing, Residents and facilities deficiencies, 2009 through 2015. *The Henry J. Kaiser Family Foundation.*

Harrington, C., Carrillo, H. (2017, July). *Nursing facilities, staffing, Residents and facilities deficiencies, 2009–2016.* https://www.kff.org/medicaid/report/nursing-facilities-staffing-residents-and-facility-deficiencies-2009-through-2016/

Jencks, S. M. (2009). Rehospitalizations among patients in the Medicare Fee-for-Service Program. *New England Journal of Medicine*, 1418–1428.

Kaiser Family Foundation (2014). Kaiser Family Foundation. www.kff.org

LongTermCare.Gov. (2019). What is long-term care (LTC) and who needs it? www.longtermcare.acl.gov/the-basics/who-will-provide-your-care.html

Manton, K. G., & Gu, X. (2008). Cohort changes in active life expectancy in the US elderly population: Experience from the 1982–2004 national long term care survey. *Journals of Gerontology Series B: Psychological Sciences and Social Sciences*, S269–S281.

Massachusetts Department of Public Health, (1994). *105 CMR 150:000 licensing of long term care facilities.* State of Massachusetts.

Meyers, D. C. (2018). Association of team-based primary care with health care utilization and costs among chronically ill patients. *JAMA Internal Medicine.*

Mueller, S. K. -B. (2012). Hospital-based medication reconciliation practices: A systematic review. *Archives of Internal Medicine, 172*, 1057.

National Center for Assisted Living. (2019). https://www.ahcancal.org/ncal/advocacy/regs/Pages/AssistedLivingRegulations.aspx

National Pace Association. (2019a). https://www.npaonline.org/policy-and-advocacy/pace-facts-and-trends-0

National Pace Association. (2019b). wnapaonline.org/pace-you

Partnership for Solutions. (2004). Chronic conditions: Making the case for ongoing care. September 2004 update. http://www.partnershipforsolutions.org/DMS/files/chronicbook2004.pdf

Social Security Association, (2017). *Facts & figures about Social Security.* Office of Reseasch, Evaluation and Statistics.

US Census Bureau. (2019). www.census.gov.census.gov/topics/population.html.

Yu, K., Miller, N. A., & Huey-Ming, H. (2018). Race and mental health disorders' impact on older patients' nursing home admissions upon hospital discharge. *Archives of Gerontology and Geriatrics*, 269–274.

Zarit, S. H. (2014). Daily stressors and adult day service use by family caregivers: Effects on depressive symptoms, positive mood, and dehydroepiandrosterone-sulfate. *American Journal of Geriatric Psychiatry, 22*(12), 1592–1602.

22

Palliative Care and Hospice

RORY B. FARRAND, MS, MA, MSN, APRN-BC AND LORIE L. WEBER, MS, PA-C

OBJECTIVES

Student Learning Objectives

After completing this chapter, the student should be able to do the following:

1. Describe primary palliative, secondary (specialist) palliative, and hospice care.
2. Discuss outcomes of palliative care.
3. Identify components of serious illness communication, goals-of-care discussion, and portable order for life-sustaining treatment (POLST) completion.
4. Discuss common symptoms and interventions used in palliative care.

Practitioner Objectives

After completing this chapter, the practitioner should be able to do the following:

1. Demonstrate serious illness communication skills to elicit patient wishes, values, and goals for care.
2. Choose prognostication tools to evaluate the progression of serious illness and to formulate a plan of care that aligns with patient and family values.
3. Collaborate with an interdisciplinary team, and analyze palliative interventions for adults with serious illness.

Overview

We can thank advances in medical care and technology for contributing to the longevity of the US population. Yet despite these medical advances, adults facing serious illness or end-stage disease can suffer burdensome symptoms and distress. Ultimately, all of us will face the end of our lives and the challenges associated with this process. Addressing patient suffering and offering holistic interventions to lessen distress are the foundations of palliative care. This chapter introduces palliative care as a medical specialty and details the benefits it provides to seriously ill individuals. It will explain how to identify and manage common symptoms associated with chronic disease and serious illness and understand palliative domains of care beyond the physical. By the conclusion of this chapter, readers will appreciate how specialty palliative care and hospice care provide additional holistic layers of support for patients and families experiencing complex medical issues and at the end of life.

Interprofessional Collaboration

Managing patients with serious illness is complex, and patient-centered care requires a variety of interdisciplinary health care professionals for best outcomes (Meier & McCormick, 2020). Although the patient's illness or condition is managed by disease-focused medical providers, the goal of the palliative provider is to lend support based on the patient's total needs. This means in addition to physical, psychological, and existential elements, it is necessary to address factors such as social determinants of health so as to treat the patient holistically.

Disadvantaged people age 65 and older with chronic disease, especially near the end of life, experience increased hardship (Enclara Pharmacia, 2021). Low income can result in residential plumbing or air conditioning issues that interfere with patients being comfortable in their home or require patients to choose between paying for medications or paying for food. Low health literacy can result in misunderstanding regarding instructions or a deep-seated distrust of the medical system, which can delay or thwart interventions for the seriously ill or dying patient (Enclara Pharmacia, 2021).

The Healthy People 2030 project (Office of Disease Prevention and Health Promotion, 2020) studies five key social determinants of health (SDOH): economic stability, neighborhoods and built environments, access to health care and health care quality, social and community context, plus education access and quality. The initiative aims to promote and track improvement in the health and well-being of US citizens. When palliative team resources are limited, providers may need to rely on community partners to assist in supporting patients in these SDOH domains such as collaborating with peer support group specialists to accompany patients to medical appointments or promote adherence to medical recommendations, enrolling in subscription medication delivery services or in-home counseling/monitoring of medications, identifying transportation vendors to help patients get to medical appointments, using transitional care management programs to follow up emergency room visits or hospital discharges including transition to skilled facilities, obtaining home-delivered meals, and connecting patients and families to 24-hour behavioral health crisis teams, as well as to faith-based community visitations (Center for Medicare and Medicaid Services, 2020a). More information for community resources can be found at www.CMS.gov.

Palliative Care

There are many definitions of palliative care. Nearly all include the goal of alleviating physical discomfort, psychosocial despair, and existential distress that can accompany serious illness. According to the Center to Advance Palliative Care (CAPC), palliative care is specialized medical care that focuses on providing relief from the symptoms and stress of an illness and improving the quality of life for both the patient and family. It is important to remember that palliative care can be provided to patients anytime in their disease trajectory and in conjunction with treatments to manage their illnesses. Whether the goal is curative, restorative, or comfort focused, palliative care is attentive to what the patient values and needs rather than the prognosis (Center to Advance Palliative Care, 2019).

Primary and Secondary (Specialist) Palliative Care

There are two types of palliative care: primary and secondary/specialist. Primary palliative care refers to the basic skills and competencies required of all physicians and other health care professionals: managing uncomplicated pain and symptoms, treating anxiety and depression, incorporating cultural and spiritual aspects into care, initiating advance care planning, and coordinating services among interdisciplinary professionals (Quill & Abernethy, 2013). Primary care clinicians are on the front line of care for older adults because they are responsible for integrated services, including personal health needs, and for ensuring ongoing relationships with the patient and family over time.

Despite their best intentions, primary care clinicians are not always the individuals managing care in serious illness or end-of-life situations, especially if an older adult spends much of that time in acute or long-term care. Although the best people to have goals-of-care conversations about complex symptom management, disease trajectory, prognosis, or life expectancy should be the clinicians who know the patient best, many times they do not have the opportunity due to the amount of time patients spend away from the primary care practice due to illness, debility, limited access to transportation, or other reasons (Institute of Medicine, 2015).

About 60% of patients who would benefit from palliative care could receive this care from a primary care provider (Connor et al., 2020). There is considerable similarity and overlap in the skill sets of geriatric primary care and palliative care practices: use of excellent communication skills, involvement of the patient-family unit, identification and articulation of goals for care, advocating for an integrated care delivery model, and use of a holistic approach that addresses psychosocial, spiritual, and cultural concerns (Voumard et al., 2018). However, as health care continues to become more complex and fragmented, our systems face a crisis in how to best manage the care of seriously ill older adults. Most of the average population does not understand what palliative care is, much less how to access it; therefore deferring the provision of palliative care to specialists runs the risk of people who need this care being unable to receive it (Webb & Casarett, 2017). Despite the increasing likelihood of patients being referred to a specialist for care of specific conditions or illnesses, patients in general prefer to see their primary care physician despite perceptions that specialists are more competent in care for that specific medical condition. Additionally, if patients fail to grasp the importance of the specialty referral, if they feel overwhelmed or confused about how to navigate the health care system, or if, due to disparities common to certain socioeconomic, racial, and ethnic groups, they avoid the referral altogether, many patients who could benefit from palliative care are unlikely to receive it (Kelley & Morrison, 2015).

For all of these reasons, compounded by the fact that the number of Medicare beneficiaries is projected to significantly increase from 54 million beneficiaries to 80 million by 2030 (Medicare Payment Advisory Commission, 2015), it is safe to assume that the need for palliative care by this population will only increase (National Quality Forum, 2012). Sadly, between workforce shortages for palliative care personnel and increasing growth of at-risk populations, the support of primary clinicians being able to provide basic palliative care is going to be instrumental for meeting the care needs of an aging population. It is important, however, for primary care clinicians to be aware of their limitations: many office-based clinical providers are unfamiliar with the specifics of care for advanced serious illness or end-of-life care, they may not feel comfortable with complex pain or symptom management, or perhaps they are simply overbooked and do not have adequate time to engage in thoughtful, progressive conversations about wishes, values, and what matters to a person as she or he approaches the end of life. In some instances, secondary palliative care clinicians—that is, specialist clinicians and organizations that provide consultation and specialty care—are engaged instead.

An Arizona survey found that less than 40% of physician participants routinely initiated conversation about medical care preferences or end-of-life discussions with their patients (Fischler & Fagan, 2018). Participants in the study identified barriers to these discussions as patient expectations, lack of readiness, and family discord; additional barriers identified by other studies (Howard et al., 2018; Lum & Sudore, 2016) are found in Table 22.1.

These studies found survey participants were in favor of receiving additional training in palliative care skills such as pain management, completion of medical orders for life-sustaining treatment, and end-of-life discussions to confidently integrate palliative care into their practices.

Primary care providers should be aware of available community resources, recognize when they can meet the palliative

TABLE 22.1 Barriers to Initiating Serious Illness or End-of-Life Discussion

Medical Providers	Patient and Family
Uncertain of patient/family reaction; timing	Fear of dying process
Having enough time to conduct discussion	Concern about abandonment
Legalities and experience in discussions	Conflict, finances, psychosocial issues
Difficulty with prognostication	Understanding prognosis

Data from Howard, M., Bernard, C., Klein, D., Elston, D., Tan, A., Slaven, M., . . . Heyland, D. (2018). Barriers to and enablers of advance care planning with patients in primary care: Survey of health care providers. *Canadian Family Physician/Medecin de Famille Canadien, 64*(4), e190–e198. https://pubmed.ncbi.nlm.nih.gov/29650621/; Lum, H., & Sudore, R. (2016). Advance care planning and goals of care communication in older adults with cardiovascular disease and multi-morbidity. *Clinical Geriatric Medicine, 32*(2), 247–260. https://doi.org/10.1016/j.cger.2016.01.011

TABLE 22.2 Primary Versus Specialty Palliative Care Skill Set

Primary	Specialty
Identification of symptoms & basic management: • Pain, depression, anxiety, dyspnea, etc.	Management of refractory symptoms: • Pain as well as other disease specific symptoms
Basic discussion about: • Disease trajectory • Prognosis • Goals for care • Suffering • Code status	Management of complex aspects of illness: • Depression, anxiety • Anticipatory grief or existential distress
	Assist with conflict resolution between: • Patient/family • Patient/treatment teams Regarding goals care or treatment options
	Addressing futile treatment options (risk versus benefit): • Cardiopulmonary resuscitation (CPR) • Nutrition/hydration • Withdrawal of life-sustaining treatments

Data from Quill, T. E., & Abernethy, A. P. (2013). Generalist plus specialist palliative care: Creating a more sustainable model. *New England Journal of Medicine, 368*, 1173–1175. https://doi.org/10.1056/NEJMp1215620

care needs of their patients, and recognize when they should consider referral to a palliative care specialist (Swami & Case, 2018). To better explain this concept, clinicians can review primary palliative care skills versus specialist palliative care skills (Table 22.2) (Quill & Abernethy, 2013), the main delineation being that specialist palliative care providers often have advanced training in symptom management, goals-of-care conversations, and managing pain or other symptoms in cases of advanced serious illness and at the end of life.

Palliative care is not standardized across all care settings. The services vary according to geographic location and resources available within the local health care system (Meier, 2019). Ideally, palliative care is provided by an interdisciplinary team, which includes medical providers (physicians, nurse practitioners, physician assistants), nurses, social workers, spiritual counselors, and others to meet the needs of patients and families.

The Role of the Nurse Practitioner and Physician Assistant in Palliative Care

Nurse practitioners (NPs) and physician assistants/associates (PAs) are well suited for the field of palliative care. They both receive advanced training that focuses on holistic, person-centered care and are accustomed to collaborative work across health care specialties. Both NPs and PAs maintain professional competencies that demonstrate the knowledge, skills, attitudes, and clinical experiences required for clinical practice. The competencies that serve the NP or PA provider in a palliative care can be found in Table 22.3.

While honing professional competencies, NPs and PAs are trained to be sensitive and responsive to patients regardless of race, religion, sexual orientation, or status. They are skilled in recognizing and managing their own personal bias to earn the trust of each patient. All providers have personal biases, but some biases are easy to recognize, whereas others are outside of our awareness (Curseen, 2019). The judgment made on a subconscious level stemming from personal beliefs or experiences of which we are unaware is implicit bias. It is important to be aware that implicit bias has the potential to subvert patient trust and is especially high when dealing with the complexities of serious illness or end of life. To mitigate this risk, all providers can ensure patient-centered care is delivered in a compassionate and respectful way by recognizing and managing their own thoughts and emotions. (Curseen, 2019). Consider the patient/primary care provider (PCP) encounter described in the case study, and assess this scenario for bias.

Could implicit bias be at play in the physician's initial response to the request for hospice in this case? Could gender, ethnicity, or culture have contributed to this bias? While reading about the case, what might one imagine the physician looked like? The scenario never did reveal any details of the PCP. Therefore, whatever characteristics that were imagined were the result of implicit bias at work. Everyone operates from unconscious beliefs that normally develop throughout the course of life, based on personal experiences.

TABLE 22.3 Palliative Care Competencies for NPs and PAs

Patient Care	MedicalKnowledge	InterpersonalSkills	Professionalism
Patient- and family-centered approaches	Pain and symptom treatment	Compassionate communication	Provide informed consent
Comprehensive assessments	Activities of daily living (ADLs) and frailty	Elicit patient goals of care	Manage personal bias
Able to address both physical and emotional diagnoses	Risks and benefits of treatments	Interdisciplinary collaboration and care provision across specialties to achieve best outcomes	Medical ethics: Committed to ethical principles pertaining to patient autonomy, relevant laws
Focus on patient satety	Prognostication	End-of-life conversations	Accountable for respectful and inclusive care with integrity
Incorporate social determinants of health (SDOH) into plans of care	Focus on holistic, evidence and value-based care	Effective, adaptive and compassionate exchanges with others	Demonstrates emotional resilience and flexibility

Data from *Competencies for the Physician Assistant (PA) Profession*. (2020). From the Pennsylvania Art Education Association. paea.org. https://paeaonline.org/wp-content/uploads/imported-files/competencies-for-the-pa-profession-060520.pdf; National Organization of Nurse Practitioner Faculties (NONPF). (2017). *Nurse practitioner core competencies*. https://cdn.ymaws.com/www.nonpf.org/resource/resmgr/competencies/2017_NPCoreComps_with_Curric.pdf

CASE STUDY

Buck, an 82-year-old man, had a long history of congestive heart failure (CHF), chronic obstructive pulmonary disease (COPD), and smoking. Over the past 10 years, he had suffered from dyspnea and fatigue despite maximum treatment with antibiotics, steroids, BiPAP, and oxygen. In addition, Buck endured chronic hip pain secondary to arthritis. His disease continued to progress with several hospitalizations resulting in little improvement or symptomatic relief. It became clear to Buck that he was nearing the end of life, and he wanted to elect hospice care to focus on comfort instead of continuing certain medications and treatments. He had a good life and knew of others who passed away peacefully with hospice care. He felt he was ready. Buck made an appointment with his primary care provider (PCP) to discuss his decision to stop his medical treatments and seek comfort-only measures.

To his surprise, Buck was met with resistance to his request for hospice and his decision to discontinue curative medical care. His PCP insisted that there was more they could do, and that it was not time to surrender to death. Buck realized a very frank conversation with his PCP was needed to convey why he had come to his decision. Although his physician had been involved in Buck's life for years, he did not understand the pain that Buck experienced as he had watched his wife endure 4 years of long-term care while in a vegetative state; Buck knew he did not want the same fate and knew that he needed to convey this perspective to his physician. Together, Buck and the physician undertook the conversation regarding the decline in his health: they discussed how easily fatigued and dyspneic Buck felt, even at rest these days; they reviewed Buck's risk of suffering a stroke and discussed probabilities for survival if that were to happen. Having completed an advance directive many years prior, Buck now confirmed his choices for no cardiopulmonary resuscitation/mechanical ventilation, reiterated his desire to avoid any intervention except comfort measures as his illness continued, and expressed to his physician that he wanted to allow a natural death.

Finally, after his PCP explored other possible underlying concerns and determined Buck was making an informed decision with full capacity, a hospice evaluation was ordered. With his hospice team in place, Buck's mood elevated, and he was relieved when his chronic hip pain was remedied by aggressive pain management. He informed family members that he was gladly receiving hospice service and anticipated a fast decline. Four months later, Buck was admitted to a hospice inpatient unit for symptomatic control at the end of life and said goodbye to his daughter and loved ones. In the inpatient unit he soon became comatose and died on the fourth day of his stay.

To manage these biases, clinicians must intentionally tune into their own physical sensations and thoughts in a nonjudgmental way to determine where implicit bias might be at work. By paying attention, providers can train themselves to pause and become aware there is a choice in how to respond in every scenario. By exploring alternative responses rather than verbalizing one's unexamined thought, providers can deliver better patient-centered care. Another option to manage implicit bias is seeking the opinion of other professionals knowledgeable about a particular case the provider may find challenging (Curseen, 2019).

Benefits and Outcomes of Palliative Care

Many studies show that referring seriously ill patients for palliative care consults and intervention results in numerous

• BOX 22.1 Beneficial Outcomes of Early Palliative Care

- Pain and symptom relief
- Decreased emotional or spiritual suffering
- Improved patient and family satisfaction
- Reduced ICU length of stay
- Reduced hospital readmissions
- Lower hospital costs
- Earlier hospice referrals

Data from Meier, E. A., Gallegos, J. V., Thomas, L. P., Depp, C. A., Irwin, S. A., & Jeste, D. V. (2016). Defining a good death (successful dying): Literature review and a call for reasearch and public dialogue. *American Journal of Geratric Psychiatry: Official Journal of the American Association for Geriatric Psychiatry, 24*(4), 261–271. https://doi.org/10.1016/j.jagp.2016.01.135; Rogers, J., Patel, C., Mentz, R., Granger, B., Steinhauser, K., Fiuzat, M., Adams, P., Speck, A., Johnson, K., Krishnamoorthy, A., Yang, H., Anstrom, K., Dodson, G., Taylor, D. Jr., Kirchner, J., Mark, D., O'Connor, C., & Tulsky, J. (2017). Palliative care in heart failure: The PAL-HF randomized, controlled clinical trial. *Journal of the American College of Cardiology, 70*(3), 331–341. https://doi.org/10.1016/j.jacc.2017.05.030

beneficial outcomes (CAPC, 2019; Oluyase et al., 2021). On satisfaction surveys, patients and families give high marks for early palliative symptom relief and patient support (Kavalieatos et al., 2016), whereas a study of patients with heart failure and concurrent palliative care demonstrated psychosocial and spiritual improvements with depression, anxiety, and spiritual dilemmas (Rogers et al., 2017).

Overall, the most beneficial aspect of primary palliative care is addressing the patient's personal well-being and goals while seeking medical management of disease. The CAPC is dedicated to improving patient care and health outcomes through promoting evidence-based palliative care training for health care professionals (CAPC, 2019), as well as defining and measuring the quality of palliative care interventions while supporting research on the impacts of palliative care (CAPC, 2019). Major benefits of palliative care are listed in Box 22.1.

Serious Illness Communication

Recognizing which patients would benefit from palliative intervention is key to delivering care and outcomes the patient perceives to be beneficial (Meier & McCormick, 2020). When medical providers focus solely on lab values, medications, and interventions rather than seeking to understand patient priorities, discordant care can occur. Skilled serious illness communication is needed to make sure providers ask, listen, and understand what the patient really wants (Severson, 2020).

Ariadne Labs, developers of the Serious Illness Care program (Ariadne Labs, 2021), have promoted training and education aimed to help providers establish trust and to elicit a patient's understanding and concerns regarding their illness. The crux of the work is a structured communication tool (the Serious Illness Conversation guide) developed from best practices in having conversations with seriously ill patients and families. When providers use this tool to engage with patients and their families, patients report better communication with their providers, feel they can better plan for the future, and feel that their medical care is enhanced, which reduces suffering. This intentional and standardized approach to serious illness communication is extremely effective for clinicians and patients alike: clinicians report increased satisfaction in their roles and less anxiety around having serious illness conversations, whereas patients and family feel closer to their clinician by being able to articulate their goals and to avoid unnecessary or unwanted treatments. The guide can be downloaded from the Ariadne Labs website.

Some patients and families want the option to try all treatments available and may worry they will not receive it. The use of the term *palliative care* may give them the impression that they are being asked to forgo curative treatment (Meier & McCormick, 2020). Trends in the field of palliative care show an increase in use of the term *supportive care*, which may more clearly describe how palliative care can be a benefit and thus may help patients and families accept a palliative consultation. It is important to communicate with patients that the objective of primary palliative care is to relieve the burdens facing both the patient and family whether they are seeking aggressive, life-sustaining treatments or comfort-only care.

Serious illness communication requires authentic inquiry, listening, and understanding to reduce misinformation, anxiety, suffering, and distrust (Pope, 2021). Skill is required to effectively communicate with patients and families facing serious illness, and some studies have found that less than 30% of clinicians routinely discuss what matters to the patient (Ariadne Labs, 2021). Federal law protects patient autonomy or the rights of patients to make medical choices free from coercion, with helpful advice and suggestions from health care professionals (Siamak, 2021). Therefore, it is important that medical providers encourage patients to share in the decisions regarding their medical care.

Training and experience are both helpful when conveying disappointing news, explaining the risks and benefits of medical interventions, and discovering what patients' value most given their current prognosis (Severson, 2020). But even in the absence of either, responding with empathy when strong emotions are expressed during these conversations increases the quality of care for the patient and family. Basic elements for having a serious illness conversation and eliciting the goals patients have for their care are outlined in Box 22.2 (Ariadne Labs, 2021; LeBlanc & Tulsky, 2020; Silveira, 2021), as well as some online resources for training. Following these basic elements or seeking training in standardized serious illness communication helps instill trust and accuracy when initiating advance care planning or deciding on medical interventions to manage a life-threatening situation (Severson, 2020).

• BOX 22.2 Elements of Serious Illness Communication and Goals-of-Care Discussion

1. Consider timing and seek permission to discuss patient understanding of illness.
2. Inquire if another person should be involved in discussions or decision making.
3. Focus on what the patient considers the best quality of life in view of the prognosis.
4. Assess what the patient would be willing to endure for more time or to achieve a personal goal.
5. Ask if there is a trusted person to speak for the patient if she or he is unable to do so.
6. Confirm that the conversation/values are documented and communicated with loved ones.

Vital Talk, https://www.vitaltalk.org/

Ariadne Labs, https://www.ariadnelabs.org/serious-illness-care/

Center for Advancing Palliative Care–Communication training, https://www.capc.org/training/communication-skills/

Data from Ariadne Labs. (2021). *Serious illness care*. ariadnelabs.org. https://www.ariadnelabs.org/serious-illness-care/; LeBlanc, T. W., & Tulsky, J. (2020). Discussing goals of care. *UpToDate*(R). https://www.uptodate.com/contents/discussing-goals-of-care; Silveira, M. (2021). Advance care planning and advance directives. *UpToDate*. https://www.uptodate.com/contents/advance-care-planning-and-advance-directives?search=advance-care-planning-and-%20Advance-directive&source=search_result&selectedTitle=1~150&usage_type=default&display_rank=1

• BOX 22.3 Types of Advance Directives

Living will
Health care proxy
Durable health care power of attorney
Medical power of attorney

Data from Siamak, N. (2021). *Advance medical directives (living will, power of attorney, and health-care proxy)* and MedicineNet: https://www.medicinenet.com/advance_medical_directives/article.htm

Advance Directives

The likelihood of experiencing serious illness and chronic disease increases with a person's age. Often patients look to their primary provider for guidance with what lies ahead (American Medical Association, 2017). Advance directives (ADs) and portable orders for life-sustaining treatment (POLSTs) are legal documents used to help ensure medical care aligns with the patients' values (National POLST, 2021). An AD is a document used to record a person's values and preferences for medical care and appoint a representative or surrogate to guide care if needed (Silveira, 2021). This document is encouraged for everyone age 18 and older. It can be filled out at home and becomes legal once signed and witnessed by one other adult who is not related by family (Silveira, 2021).

There are many advantages for adults to complete an AD. Besides giving people the peace of mind that comes from knowing they have expressed their values for medical care in hypothetical situations, an AD can relieve loved ones of the burden of making tough medical decisions (Carr & Luth, 2017). For instance, if a person experiences a life-threatening medical event and is not able to speak or his or her own behalf, an AD is activated and guides the surrogate to make medical decisions based on the person's documented preferences. The surrogate's job is to voice and confirm the patient preferences when medical decisions are required. As an example, an 88-year-old man appoints his 22-year-old granddaughter to be his surrogate in his advance directive. Later, he suffers a life-threatening stroke and is found not breathing and unresponsive. At the hospital he is placed on total life-support to keep his body functioning until his family is notified and the AD is produced. The AD clearly documents that when the prognosis is poor, health care providers are to refrain from prolonging life with artificial means. Initially, the family members are divided regarding his wishes but look to the surrogate for the decision to sustain or withdraw life support. Although this is a difficult situation, the AD is clear and the surrogate need only honor the documented preference of her grandfather to the best of her ability.

Complying with some ADs can be challenging. For example, ambiguity can occur when an AD was completed during a period of health, without regard to future illness or a potential poor prognosis; additionally, if the risks and benefits of specific treatment options were not clarified at the time the AD was completed, patients may make a choice that has an outcome that they were not expecting (Carr & Luth, 2017). People who complete ADs often do so years prior to a life-threatening medical event and without information from a medical provider. Also, if a surrogate believes there was a change in the patient's values over time, ambiguity can also occur. It makes sense, then that best practice for AD integrity is to regularly update the document and communicate any changes with the surrogate/family when a patient's prognosis or personal preferences for care change over the life span.

Types of acceptable ADs can vary from state to state, and most can be easily found online (Siamak, 2021). Examples of variations in ADs can be found in Box 22.3. Most ADs are honored even when activated in a state other than the state of origin. However, providers need to be aware that slight differences can exist. To avoid state law violations, providers must research unfamiliar ADs prior to implementation of medical preferences (Pope, 2021). Research shows that despite medical provider reimbursement for advance care planning, less than 40% of adults in the United States have completed an AD and appointed a surrogate to speak for them if they become incapacitated (Yadav et al., 2017).

Portable Order for Life-Sustaining Treatment (POLST)

An alternative such as the National POLST is another option for patients to document medical care preferences when illness is advanced. According to National POLST (2021), "A POLST form is a portable medical order communicating patient treatment preferences" (p. 5). The completion of this document is voluntary and may be advantageous for patients wanting added confidence that their wishes for care will be honored when a prognosis is poor and the probability of requiring aggressive medical intervention to preserve life is high. The intent of a POLST is to provide actionable orders for health care providers to initiate, withhold, or apply time-limited interventions for patients who may or may not want life-sustaining intervention (National POLST, 2021).

The National POLST differs from an advance directive in that completion of a POLST form requires informed consent and consideration of the patient's current prognosis. It is only appropriate for patients with a 1-to-2-year prognosis and requires periodic review or updating to maintain accordance with the patient's health status and preferences (National POLST, 2021). Outside of the hospital, a POLST clearly communicates and provides medical orders for emergency medical technicians to attempt or withhold treatment such as cardiopulmonary resuscitation (CPR) or intubation or patient transfers in life-threatening situations. In the hospital, a POLST communicates patient preference to medical providers and guides care related to resuscitation, intensive care unit (ICU) utilization, medical interventions, and discharge planning (National POLST, 2021; Severson, 2020).

A POLST is the best option for seriously ill patients with preferences for medical treatments in emergencies. Patients experiencing a medical crisis without a POLST may not have time to discuss treatment preferences or consult advance directives; in this situation, medical providers and families must make decisions about implementing or withholding life-sustaining treatments. These critical decisions may or may not reflect the type of care the patient would want. If a medical crisis occurs when patient wishes are unknown, the default is to do everything to sustain life (Severson, 2020).

Both POLSTs and ADs express a person's preferences for medical care. However, advance directives omit informed consent or the process of analyzing and understanding the risks and benefits of treatment options in the context of a person's current health status (Shah et al., 2020). Advance directives focus on future or hypothesized medical situations, whereas a POLST focuses on the immediate medical needs of the patient (National POLST, 2021). The responsibility to provide informed consent and confirm that a patient understands the risks and benefits of any medical intervention belongs to a licensed medical provider (Shah et al., 2020). The purpose of a National POLST (2021) is to bridge the gaps between patient values for care and the actual medical treatments administered. It is not necessary for a patient to have both a POLST and an advance directive. Each one is valid by itself. However, if a patient does have a POLST and an advance directive, they should align and be updated together to avoid misunderstanding by providers, surrogates, or family when critical medical decisions are needed (National POLST, 2021).

Completion of a National POLST (2021) begins with a goals-of-care discussion. These ongoing discussions consider the patient's life history, values, goals, and current prognosis to ensure all parties understand the patient's desires for medical care, including treatment risks and benefits (LeBlanc & Tulsky, 2020). Clinicians need to understand that the reason for initiating a goals-of-care discussion needs to be clear because the phrase "goals of care" is not standardized among health care professionals and its use can be misinterpreted (Klement & Marks, 2020). As an example, a referring provider asks a palliative team to consult with a cancer patient for a goals-of-care discussion. Without communicating directly with the palliative care team, the referring provider intended to use the palliative care consultant's expertise in eliciting code status and ICU utilization preferences from the patient. However, when the palliative care consultant asked if the the patient understood the illness and care preferences, the discussion turned to avoiding suffering and future hospitalization. From there, a hospice benefits discussion ensued. When the palliative care consultant later recommended referral to hospice, the referring provider was flummoxed.

Miscommunication of intent for the goals-of-care discussion is one illustration of the potential for confusing patients and subverting beneficial treatments. To alleviate goals-of-care miscommunication, the clinicians can use a two-step process intended to help standardize communication between the patient and the care teams (Klement & Marks, 2020). The first step is to establish a shared understanding of the primary goal for medical treatment. Three generalized goals considered in step 1 are cure, life-prolongation, or comfort. Once a mutual goal has been identified in collaboration with the patient/surrogate, step 2 consists of five categories to further clarify the patient's preferences for achieving the mutual goal. These categories include preferences to address patient functional ability, survival, family matters, cognition, and certitude. For example, a terminal patient whose goal is life prolongation for an upcoming event (such as a wedding or graduation) may choose treatments to maintain her or his current functional status of mobility and alertness. However, if a medical crisis jeopardizes the patient care goal, modalities such as ICU admission and other life-sustaining treatments may become part of the life-prolonging care plan until the crisis has passed, after which time a reassessment of the goals of care and a new care plan would be appropriate.

The language used during serious illness conversation is crucial, and failure to clarify the *intent* of a goals-of-care discussion can further complicate the patient's understanding of the prognosis and ensuing care plan (Klement & Marks, 2020). Therefore, seeking additional training in interdisciplinary and serious illness communication can enhance the quality of the goals-of-care discussion and POLST completion (National POLST, 2021). In the absence of additional training (as well as in addition to), decision aids have been shown to be helpful with facilitating goal setting discussions (Hyden et al., n.d). See Table 22.4.

TABLE 22.4 Online Decision-Making Aids

A Decision Aid to Prepare Patients and Their Families About CPR https://vimeo.com/48147363
A Decision Aid for Left Ventricular Assist Device (LVAD) https://patientdecisionaid.org/LVAD/
Advance Care Planning: Should I Have Artificial Hydration and Nutrition? https://www.healthwise.net/ohridecisionaid/Content/StdDocument.aspx?DOCHWID=tu4431
Advance Care Planning: Should I Stop Treatment That Prolongs My Life? https://www.healthwise.net/ohridecisionaid/Content/StdDocument.aspx?DOCHWID=tu1430
Making Choices: Feeding Options for Patients with Dementia https://vimeo.com/51776155
The Plan Well Guide for Healthcare Professionals https://planwellguide.com/for-health-care-professionals/

Data from Hyden, K., Gelfmin, L., Dionne-Odom, N., Smith, C., & Coats, H. (n.d.). Update in hospice and palliative care. *Journal of Palliative Medicine, 23*(2), 165–169. https://doi.org/10.1089/jpm.2019.0500; Patient Decision Aids. (2020). The Ottawa Hospital Research Institute. https://decisionaid.ohri.ca/AZlist.html

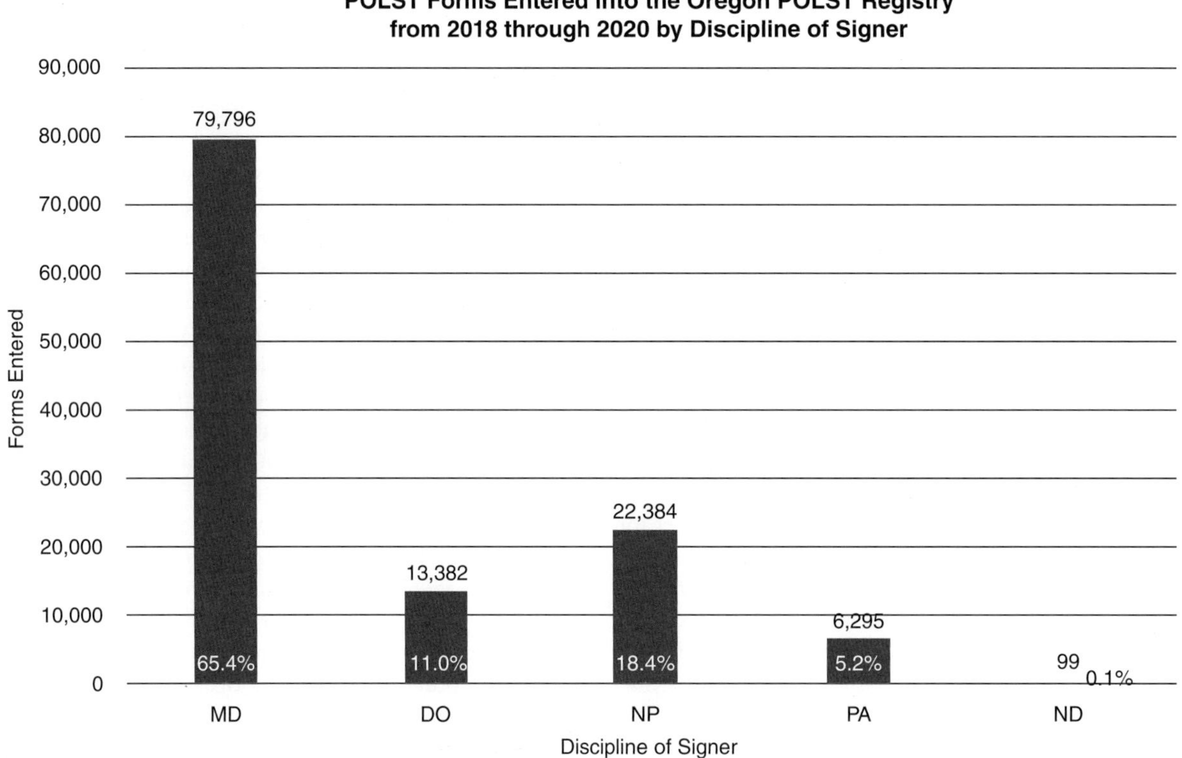

• **Fig. 22.1** Comparison of Medical Providers Completing Oregon Portable Orders for Life-Sustaining Treatment (POLSTs). *MD*, Medical doctor; *DO*, doctor of osteopathic medicine; *NP*, nurse practitioner; *PA*, physician assistant; *ND*, naturopathic doctor. (From Oregon POLST Registry.)

POLST Form Completion

Training on the proper way to complete the document is key to aligning patient wishes with immediate care needs no matter which licensed medical provider completes a POLST form. NPs are second only to medical doctors in completing the Oregon POLST form (Tolle & Ferrell, 2021); of note, NPs doubled the number of POLSTs completed between 2011 to 2018 and were involved in the completion of 21% of the registry POLST forms in Oregon (Fig. 22.1). Both NPs and PAs have been welcomed by the National POLST to participate in the POLST process and advocate for patient concordant care (National POLST, 2021).

The standardized National POLST form has four main parts: (A) cardiopulmonary resuscitation orders, (B) initial treatment orders, (C) additional instructions or orders, and (D) medically assisted nutrition orders (National POLST,

2021). Part A focuses on cardiopulmonary resuscitation (CPR). There are two choices for the patient to consider: either attempt resuscitation (CPR) or do not attempt resuscitation (DNR). Patients must be informed that part A only pertains to a situation in which the patient is found to have no pulse and is not breathing; it does not pertain when a patient is *in jeopardy of* cardiopulmonary arrest (National POLST, 2021). For those wishing to forgo CPR when pulse and breathing are absent, the DNR is an appropriate choice. With a DNR order in place, no defibrillator or chest compression should be used when the patient is found without a pulse and is not breathing (Severson, 2020). Part B covers initial treatment orders that would apply to a patient who is breathing and has a pulse. The three options for initial treatment orders include full treatment, selective treatment, or comfort-focused treatment. Full treatment requires the patient's agreement to receive all appropriate medical and surgical interventions necessary to attempt prolongation of life. These treatments include intensive care, CPR, mechanical ventilation, use of a left ventricular assist device (LVAD), and other life-sustaining medications and interventions as needed (National POLST, 2021).

A patient who chooses "attempt CPR" in part A is required to select full treatment in part B so that chances of prolonging life after the initiation of CPR is maximized. In contrast, all three part B initial treatment options are available for patients who select DNR in part A (National POLST, 2021). For example, when full treatment is selected by a patient who also selects DNR, the patient is attempting to avoid cardiac arrest or respiratory failure with aggressive treatment before the loss of pulse or breathing. In this situation, if full treatment interventions fail and the patient decompensates into cardiopulmonary arrest, then at this time, no attempt at CPR would be implemented per the DNR order (National POLST, 2021).

Part B also offers selective treatments and comfort-focused care. The selective treatment option is intended to avoid intensive care and provide patients with basic care such as antibiotics or intravenous (IV) fluid replacement. The comfort-focused option would provide orders to allow natural death while managing pain and symptoms as needed. No matter what treatment choices are selected on the POLST form, all patients will receive treatment for pain and burdensome symptoms (Rich, 2001).

Part C of the POLST form allows for writing in orders such as dialysis or use of blood products (National POLST, 2021). Some patients may opt for time-limited trials of life-sustaining interventions. These time trials can benefit a patient with a potential for recovery when prognosis is uncertain. Depending on the severity of the illness, time trials lasting between 3 to 15 days can provide better predictability for patient prognosis and positive outcomes (Vink et al., 2018).

Part D addresses medically assisted nutrition, such as feeding tubes or IV nutrition. Progression of serious illness and end stage disease can cause loss of appetite and cachexia. Eventually all forms of nutrition, including medically assisted intervention, will prove futile near the end of life and can become burdensome for the body to manage (American Academy of Hospice and Palliative Medicine, 2013). Discussion about benefits and burdens of medically assisted nutrition is especially important for patients at risk for advanced dementia or stroke. These conditions often incapacitate the patient and leave family and surrogates to make complex and difficult decisions to either supplement or withhold medical nutrition (Severson, 2020).

POLST Pitfalls

Misunderstandings and misinterpretation of POLST selections can result in discordant care for the patient. Two major sources of POLST discordance are incomplete or contradictory treatment selections on the POLST form and misinterpretation of POLST orders resulting in medical errors in care delivery (National POLST, 2021). According to at least one study, contradictory and incomplete selections were recorded on more than 7000 POLST documents (Moss et al., 2017). Further concern about POLST quality arose from a 2015 study of emergency physicians and personnel revealing emergency care providers varied significantly in their interpretation of POLST documentation (Mirarchi et al., 2015). The authors found concordant care only when the POLST specified full treatment (e.g., CPR). Conversely, when the POLST indicated comfort measures only and do not resuscitate (DNR), 10% of the emergency personnel still indicated they would initiate CPR, which suggested that the survey participants did not interpret or honor the POLST accurately (Mirarchi et al., 2015). In contrast, another study found some provider participants in their study withheld CPR when POLST orders called for full life-saving treatment; thus caution is necessary, and appropriate education and training for clinicians must be provided to improve and maintain quality POLST utilization (Moss et al., 2017).

Completing the POLST form is only initiated with permission from the patient and after thorough consultation with the patient and/or surrogate or family member when the patient lacks capacity to make decisions (National POLST, 2021). A compassionate conversation is necessary to ensure all essential components are discussed and to guarantee quality completion of the POLST form. These components include prognosis and a goals-of-care discussion, prior to treatment selection, summarization, signatures, and review (National POLST, 2021).

Treatment Options

The National POLST (2021) process requires a medical provider to share the risks and benefits of procedures or treatment within the context of the patient's current medical condition. For example, patients need to be informed that selecting "attempt CPR" in part A of the POLST form will enable emergency providers to use defibrillation, intubation, intensive care, and often continued mechanical ventilation until stabilized. It also requires patients receive personalized information about the probability of survival and likely outcome of treatment options.

Seven in ten sudden cardiac arrest events happen at home without the benefit of hospital CPR and advanced life-support (Sudden Cardiac Arrest Foundation, 2019). The likelihood of the 1-year survival of a patient who has experienced an in-hospital cardiac arrest with a full cardiopulmonary resuscitation attempt is up to 13.4%. However, chances of achieving good functional status for this same patient drops to a likelihood of 8.4% (Schluep et al., 2018). After patients/surrogates receive information regarding the likely outcome of life-sustaining interventions and select which they value most on the POLST form, it is time to confirm the patient's understanding and validate the POLST. This is the time the providers confirm that they understand the patient's values and which treatments the patient does or does not want (National POLST, 2021). After summarization is complete, it is time to validate the POLST with signatures.

When preparing to sign the POLST, the order in which the patient and provider choose to sign is important. The patient should sign first because his or her signature acknowledges that the POLST process was voluntary and treatment options and goals of care were discussed with a medical provider (Severson, 2020). Other professionals involved in the care of the patient, such as social workers, nurses, and chaplains, often assist the clinician with the POLST form. There is a box on the backside of the POLST to identify which person provided the assistance (National POLST, 2021).

Once the patient or surrogate/representative signs the POLST form, it is then appropriate for the medical provider to sign (Severson, 2020). The provider's signature confirms that the orders reflect the patient's wishes to the best of the provider's knowledge and validates the POLST as a medical order (National POLST, 2021). Next, the medical provider uploads the POLST form into the patient medical record, including the summation of the goals-of-care discussion. A copy of the National POLST (2021) form is printed on bright pink paper and is given to the patient/surrogate to place on the refrigerator or headboard of the patient's bed. National POLST (2021) recommends states participate in a POLST registry to ensure the most recent and updated POLST is electronically accessible to medical personnel when needed.

Review and Updating

Patients with advanced serious illness can expect to experience changes in their medical condition or preferences for care over time. Without regular review, any advance directive, including POLSTs, can be at risk of providing discordant care (National POLST, 2021). A 2018 study found that patients made several changes to their POLSTs as disease progressed and health status declined, with preferences changing from selective interventions to comfort-focused treatment in 85% of reviewed cases (Hopping-Winn, et al., 2018). "While advance care planning and the POLST form provide invaluable tools for recording patients' wishes, our study highlights a need to track patients' wishes as they evolve over time and a need for ongoing, real-time conversations about goals of care, even after a POLST is completed" (p. 541).

Because a POLST is a medical order, it is crucial that regular review and updates produce POLST orders that are relevant to the immediate status and preferences of the patient. In addition to patient-initiated and regularly scheduled reviews, significant events to trigger a POLST review should include when a patient transfers between settings of care, after changes in a patient's medical condition or prognosis, or if there are changes in patient wishes, goals, or preferences for medical interventions (National POLST, 2021; Severson, 2020).

When an update is made to the National POLST (2020) form, the current form must be voided/destroyed, and a new POLST form completed. The new POLST follows the same process as the original and is distributed with notification to surrogates and family. POLST registries can ensure the updated POLST is valid and immediately accessible electronically, avoiding confusion when several versions of the POLST form exist from the past (National POLST, 2021). For best practice, remember to inquire if the patient has an advance directive and, if so, that document needs to be updated to reflect the new POLST choices or be invalidated to avoid confusion or discordant care (Severson, 2020). Remember, patient wishes and goals can change with fluctuations in health status or life circumstances. This necessitates that providers initiate review and update the POLST regularly with patients/surrogates. This review can also prompt discussions about end-of-life care, and a POLST is often used when patients enroll into hospice service (National POLST, 2021).

Palliative Symptom Management

As noted earlier in the chapter, pain and symptom management is an essential proficiency for all providers but becomes of paramount importance when caring for patients with serious or terminal illnesses. Although being pain-free is a priority for patients living with serious and advanced illnesses, older persons may reside in several different settings and reports vary regarding the prevalence of pain among those diagnosed with a serious or life-limiting illness: specific diagnoses, age, frailty and other comorbid conditions all may be contributing factors to both whether or not an older adult experiences pain as well as the severity or frequency of pain. Pain is most associated with individuals with a cancer diagnosis, as it has been reported that between 20% and 50% of patients receiving treatment for cancer and up to 80% of patients (whose cancer is considered advanced) experience pain (American Cancer Society, 2019). Within groups of people who suffer from pain, certain subpopulations are more likely to be undertreated: older adults, minorities, women, and children. Pain is often one of the primary reasons palliative care clinicians are consulted within hospital settings, as almost 75% of patients with advanced cancer seen in the hospital complain of un- or poorly treated pain at the time of their admission, and sadly for many patients, pain continues even after curative treatments are concluded. Patients diagnosed with conditions such as HIV and certain neuromuscular or cardiovascular disorders (conditions that are not primarily characterized by pain symptoms) may have pain nonetheless, and these are the patients who may find their pain poorly understood and thus untreated. Most patients admitted to hospice or palliative care are older adults, who are already more likely to have existing persistent pain syndromes such as lumbago or osteoarthritis. Poorly treated pain in the geriatric patient can lead to depression, decreased socialization, insomnia, and loss of functional capacity, whereas poorly treated pain at the end of life may actually hasten death by increasing physiologic stress, potentially negatively modulating the immune response, decreasing mobility (putting patients at increased risk for thromboembolic events or pneumonia), and increasing the work of breathing/myocardial oxygen requirements, not to mention the loss of one's will to live. The Hospice and Palliative Nurses Association hold the position that "nurses and other health care providers must advocate for effective, efficient and safe pain and symptom management to alleviate suffering for every patient receiving end-of-life care regardless of their age, disease, history of substance misuse or site of care" (Coyne et al., 2018, p. 3). Along with decreasing the quality of life, for these reasons alone it is incumbent for clinicians who care for older adult patients or those with advanced illnesses to conduct a thorough evaluation of patients for the presence of pain and to ensure that treatment modalities regarding pain relief are adequate and ongoing.

Pain in Palliative Care

Although global and national organizations all have slightly varying definitions for palliative care, fundamentally they each state that palliative care refers to patient- and family-centric care that aims to optimize the patient's quality of life by anticipating, preventing, and alleviating real and perceived suffering. Few would argue that one of the greatest causes of human suffering is the experience of pain. However, as pain is a multifaceted and complex unpleasant sensory experience that exists whenever the person experiencing it *says* it does, many clinicians find pain, and especially chronic pain, difficult to manage. Pain accompanies many diseases as they progress into more advanced stages, and thus it is an essential component of palliative care. Palliative care clinicians, though experts in pain management, can also feel intimidated by pain management, especially early in their career. As pain control is critical to the management of suffering, it is a necessary skill that all palliative care clinicians need to master.

Pain is not simply experienced in relation to actual or potential tissue damage. There are many different types and ways in which a person can experience pain. The International Association for the Study of Pain (IASP) website lists more than 20 different words to describe pain, characterized primarily by an individual's perception of the sensations it creates or by the primary drivers of the sensation.

Basic Pain Management for the Seriously Ill

Management of pain begins with a comprehensive, multidisciplinary assessment. Some basic pain assessment questions such as "How does the patient describe the pain?" and "How does the pain affect the patient's affect, mood, or ability to function?" are enough to get started, but as pain is generally conceptualized along a continuum of duration, additional, more detailed questions are required. Clinicians distinguish between acute pain (associated with injury/tissue damage, or a disease process and of relatively brief duration) and persistent or chronic pain (lasting months, years, or lifelong and negatively affects a person's functioning or well-being). In addition to duration, pain is also classified by pathophysiologic terms that assist clinicians in determining the appropriate treatment, as the pain management intervention works to interrupt the specifics of those pathways. These terms include *nociceptive pain* (visceral or somatic pain that arises from the stimulation of pain receptors), *neuropathic pain* (caused by stimulation of the peripheral or central nervous system), *mixed/unspecified pain*, and *pain due to psychological disorders*.

Barriers to Effective Pain Management

Many barriers exist both within the health care landscape as well as in the community that sometimes make effective pain management difficult; these include barriers faced by the professional community, the health care system itself, and barriers raised by the patient/family or society. Fortunately, many of these barriers have been identified, and NPs and PAs are in key positions to work collaboratively with patients and professionals to clarify misconceptions about pain and its management.

Importantly, NPs and PAs must be cognizant of creating a culture in their practice where pain can be reported and therefore addressed. Both older adults and their families have numerous misconceptions about the nature of pain and available therapies; oftentimes family members are the source of the misinformation and have the ability to influence a patient's report of pain or adherence to the therapeutic intervention. The NP and PA must ensure that education and counseling about pain and its relief focus on some of these barriers.

Patient-specific barriers include the idea that pain is a part of aging and must simply be endured, difficulty in expressing pain due to cognitive function or impaired mental status, fear of the side effects of pain medications (including fears about addiction), as well as the ability of family members to downplay the severity of pain or even to dissuade patients from taking medication for pain relief.

Barriers about pain assessment and treatment are not limited to the patient population. Perhaps surprisingly, there are health professionals who also practice with myths and misconceptions about pain in older adults, which unfortunately result in the reduced use of effective medications. Nursing home residents, who experience the most pain, are often deprived of relief because they are unable to communicate pain, already appear withdrawn, or the severity of the pain experienced by the resident is underestimated by the care team. Residents with cognitive impairment are even more likely to be undertreated for pain, even though their self-report is just as valid as pain reports from cognitively intact older adults.

Lack of understanding and knowledge about various assessment tools and the efficacy of pain medications is the primary challenge for nurses and other members of the care team. Especially in this era, unfounded concerns about addiction, physical dependence, or abuse

of medication generally stem from a misunderstanding of the actual definitions of these terms. Other barriers that impact health professionals, as well as barriers that can be found at the health system level, are identified in Table 22.5.

Comprehensive Assessment for Pain

All patients experiencing pain should have a comprehensive (multidisciplinary) pain assessment. However, there are numerous factors that complicate the pain assessment process in older adults. First is an understanding of the distinction between acute and chronic pain: acute pain always serves a biologic purpose and is associated with physiological and autonomic responses, is typically well described and localized, and generally subsides with, or without, treatment. In contrast, chronic pain never serves a biologic purpose, is rarely associated with physiologic or autonomic responses, is poorly localized and described, and rarely resolves on its own. Sadly, chronic pain can be progressive and debilitating, leading to depression and altered mental states. However, the lack of these observable phenomena (in contrast to acute pain) may lead the clinical treatment team to doubt whether the pain is present. Older adults become conditioned to not feeling heard or believed when they report pain, so they cease commenting on it, creating a vicious cycle of progressive pain and suffering.

The American Geriatrics Society (American Geriatrics Society Panel on Persistent Pain in Older Persons, 2002; American Geriatrics Society Panel on Pharmacological Management of Persistent Pain in Older Persons, 2009) recommends that providers use a comprehensive pain assessment

TABLE 22.5 Barriers to Effective Pain Management

Health Care/Professional Barriers	
Lack of identification of pain or limited understanding of global nature of pain, including both physical as well as psychosocial, spiritual/existential contributing factors	Relief not viewed as of primary importance in patient's care
Perceived lack of time to conduct thorough assessment	Poor continuity of care (among providers and across transitions)
Poor communication among members of treatment team	Prejudice or bias toward patient/caregivers with pain histories, drug abuse, or inability to accept patient's reports of pain as credible
Inadequate knowledge of available assessments or lack of awareness of available validated tools for pain assessment (whether patient is verbal or nonverbal)	Fear of doing harm: Causing adverse effects, development of addiction, concern about diversion behaviors
Fear of legal issues	Personal hubris; discomfort with asking a specialist for assistance with pain management
Health Care System Barriers	
Systems that fail to hold professionals accountable for pain assessment and treatment	Lack of culturally or clinically appropriate tools for adequate pain assessment
Restrictive formularies, cost prohibitions (either at the facility level or patient's insurer), or limited access to opioids that could provide effective treatment	Lack of access to specialists, whether pain management or palliative care providers; limited education regarding appropriate, effective, and safe opioid prescribing practices
Lack of institutional policies regarding pain assessment/treatment	Fear of regulatory scrutiny regarding pain management (e.g., opioid prescribing)
Family/Societal Barriers	
Patient/family/caregiver unable to accurately report symptoms (e.g., cognitively impaired patients, lack of common language to describe symptoms)	Patient fearful of bothering family, staff to obtain pain relief
Cultural or age-related stoicism resulting in downplaying pain report	Fear of not being believed or fear of being seen as "drug seeking"
Perception that pain is a normal part of aging and that nothing can be done about it	Fear of side effects, drug-dependence or addiction, or abuse

and collect a detailed pain history. A newer assessment tool, the Clinically Aligned Pain Assessment (CAPA) Tool for Pain, provides a more comprehensive way to for clinicians to assess pain (by taking into consideration personal comfort [pain is intolerable, tolerable with discomfort, totally manageable], changes in pain [getting worse, the same, better], pain control [inadequate, partially effective, fully effective], and the effects of pain on function and sleep); this approach aims to improve treatment options and provide better outcomes (Vitelli et al., 2020). The CAPA tool helps patients describe their unique pain *experience*, in contrast to more commonly used pain assessment tools like the numeric rating scale, which are unilateral and do not fully capture all the domains of an individual's pain experience. Although the CAPA tool shows improvement in pain assessment by evaluating pain across multiple dimensions, pain assessment in palliative care should also consider how pain affects a patient's (or sometimes, even a caregiver's) emotional state, how the person's history or attitudes/belief shape the experience of pain, behavioral cues or changes that indicate pain is present, how a person's sociocultural background impacts the expression of and coping with pain, and, finally, the impact of the environment on the same (Table 22.6). Various questions can be used to evaluate a patient's experience of pain, and these approaches should take into consideration a variety of interrelated factors.

Multidisciplinary pain assessment is not a one and done activity, but a continuous process to formulate an ongoing plan of care to ensure that the patient is able to function at his or her highest level (with or without ongoing medication). Comprehensive assessments include a detailed history (noting pain characteristics, intensity, and its effects on the patient's functioning), history of previous treatments (both pharmacologic and nonpharmacologic) for the pain, previous substance abuse, thorough physical examination (including both painful areas and referred pain areas), psychosocial and cultural assessment, and an appropriate diagnostic workup to determine the cause of the pain. Patients should be screened for pain upon any transition of care (between home and hospital, hospital to nursing care, etc.) as well as if there is a change in the patient's report of pain or a change to the pain treatment plan. Remember, pain assessments/reassessments and treatment plans should be individualized and documented so that all multidisciplinary team members will have a thorough understanding of the patient's pain issue, as well as the role each team member can play in its treatment or resolution. If a positive impact on the quality of life is one of the overarching goals of palliative care, then the multifactorial perspective of pain management is foundational to the provision of this care to patients and their families.

Because pain is subjective, sensory factors of the pain experience are often used to explain both the cause and character of an individual's pain. Patients should be asked to describe their pain with words (Table 22.7) as well as to use words that help to measure the quality, intensity, location, temporal pattern, and aggravating as well as alleviating factors. Many clinicians rely on the mnemonic "OPQRST" to help capture all these components (Box 22.4); use of these qualifiers facilitates the clinician's understanding of the patient's experience of his or her pain and can help to optimize pain treatment as well as monitor the responses to/outcomes of pain treatment.

TABLE 22.6 Pain Assessment Questions

Physical	• What is causing the pain? • How does the patient describe the experience of his or her pain?
Affective	• Does the patient's emotional state or affect impact her or his perception of pain? • Is the pain impacting the patient's mood?
Cognitive	• What is the patient's past experience with (this) pain or pain treatment? • Does the patient's knowledge or attitude affect his or her report of pain?
Behavioral	• Is the patient demonstrating pain behavior (nonverbal cues, etc.)? • What does the patient do that worsens (or improves) the pain?
Sociocultural	• Is the patient's pain/pain report impacted by sociological or cultural factors?
Environmental	• Does the environment contribute to the expression of pain?

Pain Assessments for Nonverbal or Cognitively Impaired Patients

Although patient self-report is the gold standard of pain assessment, it is critically important to note that simply because a patient cannot verbally express his or her pain, that does not mean that pain is absent. Pain assessment in nonverbal or cognitively impaired patients remains an

TABLE 22.7 Pain Descriptors

Neuropathic	Numb, burning, radiating, shooting, electrical, tingling, pins and needles
Visceral (poorly localized)	Gnawing, cramping, squeezing, deep, pressure, bloating, stretching, pulling
Somatic (well-localized)	Throbbing, aching, dull, sore
Psychological	All over, all encompassing, everywhere

imperative for palliative care clinicians and for their partners in care so as to avoid undertreatment (McGuire et al., 2016). Astute observations of the patient's behaviors, in addition to soliciting input from family or caregivers, then become the proxy for a patient's self-report of pain. See Table 22.8.

It cannot be emphasized enough that the absence of certain behaviors indicates that a patient is pain-free. Inability to speak or communicate, either due to illness or another reason, obviously impacts the acquisition of information necessary to form treatment decisions, but this factor alone should not become a barrier to effective management. For nonverbal or cognitively impaired patients with a serious/life-limiting illness or a known condition likely to cause pain (e.g., osteoarthritis, spinal stenosis, decubiti, etc.), it is best to assume that underlying conditions are likely still painful and to continue interventions based on previous treatment history. Likewise, a new onset of negative behaviors in a cognitively impaired patient or even an onset of delirium should include a high index of suspicion for pain as the cause, unless another factor (new medication, infection, etc.) proves otherwise.

Concern about the undertreatment of pain in this population has contributed to the development of several tools (Table 22.9, not a comprehensive list) that can be used by the multidisciplinary team. Although there is not a single tool that is recommended across clinical settings, the ones outlined in Table 22.9 all take stock in the observation of patient behaviors; clinicians should be familiar with at least several to ensure that nonverbal or cognitively impaired patients have their pain behaviors captured or recognized. Close partnership with family or caregivers who know the patient best and who can attest as to the variation from routine or normal behavior will be critical when relying on tools like these.

• BOX 22.4 Mnemonic Device to Describe Pain

O	Onset: When did it begin?
P	Provocation/palliation: What makes it worse? What makes it better?
Q	Quality: What is the nature of the pain?
R	Radiation: Is the pain localized, or does it radiate to other parts of the body?
S	Severity: How bad is it? (scale 0–10, mild/moderate/severe)
T	Temporal: Is there a time of day that it is better or worse?

Devising Treatment Plans for Pain

Once the presence of pain has been determined, the clinical team should seek to devise the most appropriate treatment plan. Fortunately, most patients obtain relief with existing therapies, whether those are pharmacologic agents, interventional techniques, or a combination of the two. Pain relief is most effective when the skills of the full multidisciplinary team are utilized in combination with strengths inherent within the patient and family relationship. Working alongside physicians, nurse practitioners and physician assistants bring a sound understanding of pharmacotherapy, which is of utmost importance in determining the most effective course of treatment for a patient's pain. In addition to matching the drug class to the likely etiology of pain/pain pathway, this understanding allows for close monitoring of adverse effects that may be related to the use (or misuse) of the medication, as well as due to drug/drug or drug/disease interactions. NPs' and PAs' responsibilities in pain management include not only prescribing but educating the patient, family, and the other members of the multidisciplinary team on these adverse or untoward outcomes so that every interaction with the patient includes multiple sets of eyes keen to scan for any of these issues.

Lastly, providers must be sure to involve the patients themselves in setting goals for pain management. Total absence of pain may be unattainable, so the provider can

TABLE 22.8 Possible Pain Behavior in Nonverbal or Cognitively Impaired Patients

Behavior Category	Example Pain Behavior
Facial expression	Pinched expression, grimace, frown, sad/frightened expression, wrinkled or furrowed brow, closed/clenched eyelids, clenched jaw
Bodily movement	Jittery, restless, agitated, pacing, fidgeting, rocking, constant shifting of position, withdrawal
Protective mechanism	Rubbing/massaging affected body part, bracing, guarding, splinting, grabbing side rails/chair arms during movement
Vocalization or verbalization	Moaning, groaning, crying out, sighing, whining, screaming, heavy breathing; phrases such as "help me," "don't touch me," or cursing, praying, verbally abusive
Mental status change(s)	Depression, confusion, irritability, distress, sadness
Changes in activity pattern, routines or interpersonal interaction	Decreased engagement, appetite, changes in sleep pattern (usually lack of), changes in ambulation, resistance to care

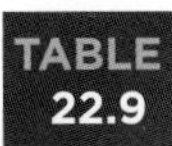

TABLE 22.9 Examples of Pain Assessment Tools for Nonverbal or Cognitively Impaired Patients

Tool	Comments
Abbey Pain Scale	Assesses pain in late-stage patients with dementia in nursing homes by monitoring six behavioral indicators (vocalization, facial expression, change in body language, behavioral change, physiologic change, physical change)
Assessment of Discomfort in Dementia Protocol (ADD)	Expands on items from the Discomfort Scale for Dementia of Alzheimer type to include more overt symptoms in order to improve recognition and treatment of pain/discomfort in patients who are unable to report their internal state
Checklist of Nonverbal Pain Indicators (CNPI)	Rates the absence or presence of pain behaviors both at rest and with movement
Pain Assessment in Advanced Dementia (PAINAD)	Assesses pain in patients with advance dementia through clinician observation of five parameters (breathing, negative vocalization, facial expression, body language and consolability)

Adapted from McGuire, D. B., Snow Kaiser, K., Haisfield-Wolfe, M., & Iyamu, F. (2016). Pain assessment in noncommunicative adult palliative care patients. *The Nursing Clinics of North America, 51*(3), 397–431. https://doi.org/10.1016/j.cnur.2016.05.009

ask the patient, "What is an acceptable level for pain relief, on a zero to ten scale?" In some cases, perhaps the goal is not a number on a scale but a functional (or enjoyable) activity, such as being able to get up from a chair without pain or being able to walk in the garden for 20 minutes each day. Understanding what matters to the patient and how the pain has impacted his or her ability to participate in certain aspects of life will help the provider to maximize the impact of pain intervention.

Matching Drug Class to Pain

A basic and widely used protocol to pain management is illustrated by the World Health Organization's (WHO) pain ladder (Fig. 22.2), which begins with the lower levels of pharmacologic therapy and suggests interventions at each step, beginning with the use of mild nonopioid medications and advancing up the ladder through adjuvant medications before reaching the middle and top levels where opioids are introduced in response to moderate-severe pain.

The treatment plan should consider the type of pain (somatic, visceral, neuropathic) and begin with a drug that matches that pain type; many classes of medications may be suitable to manage the pain even though their initial use was intended for something else. The secondary consideration to choosing the drug class is whether the medication is safe for that patient; whereas acetaminophen should be considered as adjunct to any chronic pain regimen, patients with renal insufficiency or liver dysfunction should expect reduced total daily dosage. Similarly, patients with reduced renal function or those with bleeding disorders should use caution or entirely avoid the use of nonsteroidal antiinflammatory drugs (NSAIDs). The ready availability of these over-the-counter medications coupled with their mixed formulations also put patients at risk for accidental overdoses if clinicians do not take a careful or detailed history of all medications being taken by that patient. The last consideration for choice of medication is whether the drug offers the lowest risk but will effectively treat the patient's pain.

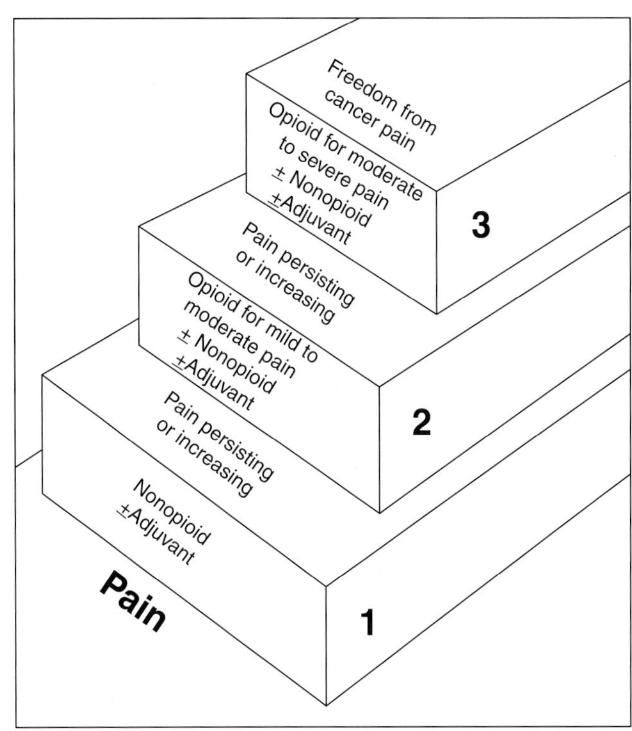

• **Fig. 22.2** World Health Organization's Pain Ladder. (From Long-Term Care, Nursing Home, & Rehabilitation. Williams BA, Chang A, Ahalt C, Chen H, Conant R, Landefeld C, Ritchie, C, Yukawa M. *Current Diagnosis & Treatment: Geriatrics*, 2e; 2014.)

Patient Factors That Influence Prescribing Decisions

Once the specific medication has been determined, clinicians must now consider the safest route for delivery of the medication: the environment in which the patient is at the time the medication will be delivered (home, hospital, or other facility), the person administering the medication (the patient, caregiver, or clinician), clinical conditions (swallowing difficulty, tremors, manual dexterity, hand-eye coordination), as well as cognitive status, mood, or any other issues that may prevent an individual from properly administering his or her medication. As noted in Table 22.10, analgesic medications come in a variety of formulations: oral, enteral, buccal, rectal, transdermal, and parenteral (intravenous [IV], intramuscular [IM], subcutaneous [SC]). Opioids have the most robust options when choosing routes for administration. First, and whenever possible, the oral route is the easiest to use and is available across settings of care. If rapid dose finding is required and the patient is in a monitored setting, IVs can provide rapid relief. In nonhospital settings, the subcutaneous route is an option. Although convenient for a few reasons (it reduces the number of doses that is taken daily), the use of transdermal delivery for opioids is only recommended after the patient has been stabilized on the dosage of the medication (not for the opioid naïve), and for patients who require long-term management, including those with cognitive or physical impairments.

In the home setting, the clinician should consider the cost and availability of medications before settling on the final medication formulation. Medications that are costly, require prior authorization to be covered, or are not routinely stocked in the pharmacy can be a barrier to a patient obtaining adequate and timely pain relief. Additionally, the clinician must educate support staff or caregivers to ensure that they understand the method to deliver the medication including the proper route of administration, timing of doses, and the difference between adverse effects and expected side effects. Side effects, which can be common but bothersome, are easily managed in most circumstances.

Pharmacologic Management of Pain in Seriously Ill Patients or at End of Life

One of the most challenging aspects of providing pain management stems from difficult pain syndromes such as bone pain, pain crises, or refractory pain at the end of life. As described previously, these are the circumstances where specialist palliative care (whether alone or from within hospice) is required. Many clinicians think that the only options for pain management in seriously ill patients are opioids, when in fact nonopioids, and co-analgesics are frequently deployed to great effect (Wood et al., 2018). As a pharmacologic class, however, opioid analgesics are incredibly useful to manage pain associated with advanced disease; they are nonspecific and act by decreasing one's perception of pain throughout the nervous system, regardless of the pathophysiology of the pain. Attention to the destructive "opioid epidemic" has led experienced and novice providers alike to view opioid medications with a healthy dose of caution; however, that cautious behavior can sometimes lead to the undertreatment of pain (Zhang et al., 2021). It is therefore essential for clinicians to clearly understand safe and appropriate prescribing principles to ensure that the most effective medication is provided, at the safest lowest dose, for the shortest amount of time (when possible).

Critical to ensuring safe prescribing practice is a deep understanding of the distinctions for the following clinical conditions: tolerance, physical dependence, addiction, pseudo-addiction, and pseudo-tolerance (Box 22.5). This is important, as patients' clinical responses to different opioids are varied and individualized, and close monitoring of a patient's response is necessary in order to ascertain if the intended outcomes have been reached (i.e., pain relief without sedation, adverse result, or intolerable side effects). Like how patients respond differently to antidepressant therapy, some patients may require trials of different medications, doses or formulations to ensure that the most effective drug, dose and route of delivery and desired outcomes are achieved.

Opioid Trials and Prescribing

Many older persons experience chronic pain, and opioid therapy can be appropriate in this population to manage chronic moderate to severe pain that is not responsive to nonopioid options. Centrally acting opioids (such as morphine) or opioid-agonists show a propensity for the μ–receptor, and morphine is generally considered the gold standard of the opioid family and is used as a measure for dose equivalence for equianalgesic purposes (Table 22.11). Short-acting opioids (either alone or in combination with acetaminophen) can be titrated to provide pain relief from mild-to-moderate acute pain, but as previously noted, these combination products should be prescribed only on a short-term basis and care should be taken to avoid overuse or acetaminophen hepatotoxicity. If longer-acting medications are necessary after a trial of short-acting medications has been evaluated or if the patient has persistent chronic pain, the clinician may consider converting to a longer-acting formulation.

By and large, morphine, as compared to other medications such as meperidine (Demerol) and propoxyphene (active agent in Darvocet), is preferred when treating older persons, primarily due to the accumulation of toxic metabolites in some other medications (such as those mentioned); however, morphine is not for the opioid naïve. "Start low, and go slow, but GO!" is a helpful phrase when prescribing opioids for chronic pain in this population. Understanding pharmacodynamics is critical if the clinician is to be aware of the timing of analgesic peak effects and the overall expected duration of the therapy, thereby avoiding both breakthrough pain (or end-of-dose failure) and overtreatment. In some older adult patients, the peak effect may be heightened or the duration extended due to changes in metabolic function that normally breaks down these medications. Many clinicians feel comfortable starting with a trial of short-acting opioids at half of the usual starting dose. This option allows for longer dosing intervals until the patient's response to the medication has been evaluated.

A word about the use of transdermal fentanyl in this population: it should never be used in patients not already tolerant to opioid medications, although it is frequently

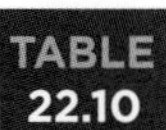

TABLE 22.10 Analgesic Considerations in the Older Patient

Medication Type	When to Use	When to Avoid (Use With Caution)
Acetaminophen *Note:* Has no antiinflammatory properties	• Mild to moderate somatic and visceral pain as a single agent or combined with an opioid • Treats fever, headache, muscle, and general pain • Oral, liquid, rectal, and intravenous formulations • Does not affect platelets	• Patients with liver impairment (monitor liver function test (LFTs) • Narrow therapeutic ratio: NTI 4 g/24 h with close monitoring or 3 g/24 h unmonitored. Minor increases above recommended doses pose serious risk to hepatic necrosis or death.
Nonsteroidal antiinflammatory analgesics (NSAIDs)* Note: Celecoxib is the only remaining Cox-2 inhibitor on the US market, but it has not demonstrated greater analgesic efficacy or safety compared to other NSAIDs	• Mild to moderate somatic and visceral pain as a single agent or combined with an opioid • Indicated when treating inflammatory states in the musculoskeletal system • Oral, liquid, topical and intravenous formulations • Long-term use must carefully weigh benefits versus risk (longer therapy and higher doses increase risk of toxicity)	Increased risk of toxicity or other serious adverse events are possible for patients with preexisting bleeding risk (namely to gastrointestinal tract), patients with low platelet count, patients with prior history of gastritis • If taking in presence of other anticoagulants such as enoxaparin or warfarin • Patients with renal dysfunction, patients with diabetes (due to greater risk for renal dysfunction); older adult patients with CrCl <30 ml/min; patients with congestive heart failure (risk of cardiotoxicity as well as renal failure) • Patients already taking antiinflammatory product such as corticosteroid (due to increased risk of bleeding)
Opioids Notes: Specific drug choice and dosing must be considered in presence of underlying organ dysfunction (liver/kidney) Common side effects are manageable by most patients (constipation, nausea, sedation) but require attention by prescribing clinician Abrupt discontinuation after longer-term use should be avoided; tapered approach is necessary	• Moderate to severe pain as a single agent or combined with acetaminophen or NSAID • Effective for somatic, visceral, and neuropathic pain types • Mainstay for moderate to severe pain caused by malignancies • Diverse formulations: oral, liquid, transbuccal, transdermal, rectal, subcutaneous, intravenous allowing for administration even if traditional routes are compromised or unavailable • Does not impact platelets, renal or liver function, or gastric mucosa	• Patients taking opioids for persistent noncancer pain without additional underlying serious illness should consider pain specialist for management
Antiepileptics *Note:* Drug-drug interactions exist but usually are well tolerated by patients	• Moderate to severe neuropathic pain, as single agent or combined with other drugs (e.g., pregabalin, gabapentin) • Mainstay for treatment of neuropathic pain • Available only via oral formulations • Side effects are manageable	• Patients with renal failure or renal insufficiency (older adults) should be monitored and dose adjustments are necessary • Patients who are fall risks or with gait abnormalities, due to side effects of sedation, confusion, ataxia, and edema
Antidepressants *Notes:* Delirium can be side effect; selective serotonin-reuptake inhibitors have not been shown to have specific pain-relieving properties	• Moderate to severe pain as a single agent or combined with other drugs (includes tricyclic antidepressants and serotonin norepinephrine reuptake inhibitors) • Mainstay for patients with neuropathy *and* mood disorders • Available in oral formulation only	• Patients with underlying cardiac disease due to anticholinergic properties (QT prolongation) • Patients who are fall risks due to side effects of sedation and orthostasis • Patients with gastroparesis (due to anticholinergic side effects of constipation, urinary retention)

(Continued)

TABLE 22.10 Analgesic Considerations in the Older Patient—cont'd

Medication Type	When to Use	When to Avoid (Use With Caution)
Corticosteroids	• Moderate to severe somatic and visceral pain as a single agent or combined with other drugs • May be used as multipurpose analgesic for bone pain, capsular pain, headaches due to elevated intracranial pressure, pain caused by tumor compression (e.g., bowel obstruction) • Shown to improve appetite, sense of well-being, and fatigue (useful in cancer patients receiving treatment) • Formulations include oral, liquid, intravenous, rectal, subcutaneous and depot intramuscular injection	• Patients already taking NSAID or at risk for gastrointestinal bleed • Side effects may appear early so use with caution if already at risk for agitation, delirium, hyperglycemia, fluid retention, hypertension, and increased risk of infection • Long-term use may see patients develop adrenal insufficiency, myopathy, hyperglycemia, gastrointestinal bleed, avascular necrosis, osteoporosis or bone fractures, increased risk of infection
Topical agents (capsaicin)	• Mild-to-moderate pain from arthritis, herpes zoster, diabetic neuropathy • Reduces inflammation and hypersensitivity accompanying many neuralgias by depleting nerve terminals of substance • Initial applications may increase pain but it subsides after repeated applications; compliance may be improved by concurrent use of topical anesthetic	• Avoid applying over broken skin/open areas • Careful application and hand-washing after use are necessary to avoid transferring agent to unwanted areas (e.g., mucous membranes, eyes, etc.)

• BOX 22.5 Definitions of Clinical Conditions Relating to Patients' Responses to Opioids

Addiction: A primary, chronic, neurobiologic disease characterized by behaviors that include impaired control over drug use, compulsive use, continue use despite harm, and craving for the drug

Physical dependence: A state of adaptation that manifests as a drug-class specific set of withdrawal symptoms occurring from abrupt withdrawal, discontinuation, cessation, rapid-dose reduction, or introduction of an antagonist

Pseudo-addiction: Mistaken assumption of addiction in a patient who is legitimately seeking relief from pain

Pseudo-tolerance: Misunderstanding of increasing need for drug being caused by tolerance, rather than progression of illness or other (related or not) disease factors (e.g., tumor growth or spread)

Tolerance: A state of adaptation whereby continued exposure to a drug leads to diminution of the drug's effects over time

deployed in long-term care facilities due to its ease of use (72-hour delivery of medication, ability to be placed where patients may not be able to access it, useful for patients who cannot take oral medications, etc.). Patients should be tolerating a daily dose of at least 30 to 40 mg of short-acting opioid medication prior to initiating the lowest dose of a transdermal fentanyl patch. Many clinicians do not grasp the equianalgesic conversion between other opioid preparations or may not understand that it should be used for only continuous, steady-state pain (not for episodic bouts of pain due to movement or other aggravating factors). If supplemented with only acetaminophen or NSAIDs alone, patients with rheumatoid arthritis (RA), osteoarthritis (OA), bony metastases, or other conditions may not obtain adequate relief. As such, most patients using fentanyl are supplemented with other opioid preparations that are short acting.

As noted earlier, pain assessment is not a one and done activity; this is especially true after the initiation of pain relief therapies. Behavioral indicators such as improved function, mood, or appetite may signify a positive response. Ongoing monitoring for how the patient is responding to the therapy is critical and must also include an assessment for side effects, both expected and not.

Lastly, a word on one the most common and significant side effects of opioids: constipation. Unlike other initial adverse effects from opioids (sedation, nausea), patients do *not* develop tolerance to the effects of opioids on the bowel. Untreated constipation can lead to additional pain, vomiting, restlessness, or delirium, as discussed in the following section. Therefore, clinicians should be sure to prescribe a bowel regimen at the same time and throughout the duration of time that they prescribe the opioid narcotic. The regimen should include both mild laxatives as well as stool softeners. Softeners alone are unable to alleviate opioid-induced constipation.

TABLE 22.11 **Opioid Prescribing Recommendations for the Older Adult**

Opioid	Route of Administration	Dose Equivalent to 10 mg of IV Morphine	Starting Dose in Older Patients	Duration of Effect (in Hours)
Morphine	IV PO	10 30	0.5–2 mg 5–10 mg	3–4 3–4
Sustained-release morphine	PO	30	15–30 mg	8–12
Oxycodone	PO	20	5–10 mg	3–4
Sustained-release oxycodone	PO	20	10–20 mg	8–12
Codeine	PO	200	15–30 mg	1–2
Hydromorphone	IV PO	1.5 7.5	0.5–1 mg 0.5–1 mg	3–4 3–4
Fentanyl	IV	0.25	0.5–1 mg	3–4
Transdermal fentanyl	TD	0.25	12.5 mcg/hr	72

IV, Intravenous; *PO*, oral; *TD*, transdermal.

Management of Other Symptoms

Pain is not the only symptom experienced by seriously ill patients. Table 22.12 presents some of the more common symptoms, although it is not an exhaustive list. Many similar symptoms exist across a variety of different conditions, such as anorexia and fatigue in heart failure or COPD patients, as well as in patients actively receiving treatment for cancer. Depression and anxiety may increase as a person's functional status declines; patients fear becoming a burden on their loved ones. Although many other similar examples exist, for the most part, the condition in which the patient is experiencing the symptom is of little importance.

A variety of tools can be referenced to quantify the severity of symptoms, such as the Edmonton Symptom Assessment System-Revised (ESAS-R) or the Memorial Symptom Assessment Scale (MSAS), which allow patients to quantify the severity of their symptoms on a numeric scale and are easily employed in the clinical setting. Generally, the tools are intended to collect "symptom" information, which is the experience of the patient and her or his response to the occurrence, in contrast to signs, which are observable by the clinical professional. As noted in the earlier discussion of the concept of total pain, suffering has four domains: physical, emotional, social, and spiritual/existential. As in the evaluation of pain, the assessment of nonpain symptoms should include severity, timing, exacerbating factors, and effect on quality of life—not only the physical component, but also the emotional upset and mental or spiritual anguish that may accompany it. Unrelieved suffering is demoralizing and demeaning. Suffering patients can lose the will to live, become depressed or withdrawn, and will decline more rapidly.

A hallmark of palliative care, in contrast to hospice, is that patients can continue to seek curative treatments while also obtaining relief from their bothersome symptoms. For patients receiving palliative care, it is important to not overlook symptom management while focusing on cure or disease modifying therapies. To achieve the best outcomes, identification of the underlying pathophysiology or mechanism that leads to the symptom will determine the best course of treatment. For example, a patient who has anxiety due to dyspnea should have the shortness of breath addressed first, then the anxiety (Albert, 2017). Other principles of symptom control include anticipation of predictable complications of advanced disease states (e.g., bowel obstruction in colorectal cancer patients) or complications of palliative treatments (e.g., side effects of opioids), evaluation and support for psychosocial difficulties (e.g., poor home support, low income, and expensive medications), and assurance that the patient's care goals drive even symptom management decisions (e.g., clarity of mind versus relief of pain).

Dyspnea

Dyspnea, or the sensation of feeling short of breath, is a common symptom, particularly in patients with pulmonary disease or congestive heart failure; however, dyspnea has been reported in varying amounts in patients with other illnesses, such as cerebrovascular disease and cancer (Albert, 2017). This is a bothersome symptom for patients as it diminishes functional status, social activities, and quality of life; if left untreated it can negatively impact the will to live. Typically, patients report symptoms as chronic or progressively worsening and interspersed with acute episodes, which though unpredictable are not unexpected. Many clinicians may say the patient "looks dyspneic"; however, patient self-report is the only accurate measure of dyspnea, regardless of whether or not the patient measures it as hypoxic.

TABLE 22.12 Nonpain Symptoms at End of Life

Symptom	Assessment and Treatment Options	Pharmacologic Options
Dyspnea	• Address underlying cause when possible • Reduce the need for exertion, reposition, improve air circulation, and avoid triggers • Opioid (lower doses than needed for pain) and oxygen are mainstays	• Morphine oral: 2.5–10 mg every 3–4 h • Morphine IV or SC: 2.5–10 mg every 3–4 h • Oxycodone oral: 2.5–10 mg every 3–4 h
Fatigue	• Address underlying cause when possible • Rest, energy conservation techniques, and proper spacing of activities • Steroids and psychostimulants provide short-term improvements but caution with side effects	• Dexamethasone 2–20 mg • Methylphenidate 2.5–15 mg q a.m. and noon
Anorexia	• Corticosteroids and megestrol acetate have significant risks • Involve patient in in meal planning, make dietary changes, avoid foods with strong or unpalatable odors • Offer easy-to-swallow, sweet foods or soft/pureed foods	• Dexamethasone 2–4 mg/qd • Megestrol acetate 400 mg elixir qd (20 ml of 40 mg/ml)
Nausea	• Multiple efferent pathways that can cause nausea, match drug class to likely pathway • Antiemetics, prokinetics are viable options	• Scopolamine 1 or 2 1.5-mg patch every 72 h • Haloperidol 0.5–2 mg oral or IV every 4–8 h • Metoclopramide 5–20 mg oral or IV every 6 h • Ondansetron 4–8 mg oral or IV every 4–8 h
Depression	• Selective serotonin-reuptake inhibitors (SSRIs) may take too long to demonstrate effect, especially at end of life • Methylphenidate has shorter time to efficacy and may have good results for patients with anergia or anhedonia	• Methylphenidate start with 2.5 mg daily, usual dose 5–10 mg daily
Delirium	• Treat reversible causes • Use caution when adding medications	• Haloperidol 0.5–1 mg oral, SC or IV every 30 min, titrate to effect (NTI 3 mg/24 h) • Olanzapine 2.5–5 mg daily • Risperidone 0.5 mg twice daily

IV, Intravenous; *SC*, subcutaneous.

Detailed explanation of the physiology and pathophysiology of dyspnea is outside the scope of this chapter but simply put, the sensory cortex receives input or commands from peripheral chemoreceptors and mechanoreceptors in the body as well as taking in data from both the motor cortex and the medulla. Dyspnea occurs if the degree of motor output required is perceived to be unsustainable or disproportionate to the sensory information received.

Generalized treatment measures include reducing the need for exertion, repositioning, improving air circulation, and avoiding triggers that make the symptom worse (strong odors, fumes, smoke, pets). Primary symptomatic treatment of dyspnea includes both oxygen and opioids. Oxygen may act to improve dyspnea both by correcting hypoxemia and through direct stimulation of the trigeminal nerve; however, many patients may report improvement in the sensation of dyspnea even if not hypoxemic, so there may be a placebo effect as well. Opioids reduce the subjective sensation of dyspnea by decreasing respiratory drive, metabolic rate, and ventilatory requirements, and likely also from analgesic effects to pain (lessening pain-induced respiratory drives) and the anxiolytic effects of opioids. As with pain management, opioids should be chosen based on previous opioid exposure and ease for administration, among other factors. Other medications such as benzodiazepines and bronchodilators play a role in the treatment of dyspnea for patients with concomitant anxiety and airflow obstruction, respectively.

Fatigue

Fatigue can be defined as an unpleasant symptom that incorporates total body feelings ranging from tiredness to exhaustion, creating an overall condition that interferes with individuals' ability to function to their normal capacity. Primary fatigue is thought to be related to the condition/illness itself (cancer produces chemicals and hormones that lead to feelings of tiredness or other complex problems), whereas secondary fatigue stems from the sequelae of the primary illness (depression, insomnia, infection, anemia, medication side effects, etc.). Many patients with serious advanced illness report fatigue as a significant symptom, and it can be one of the most complex symptoms that cancer patients experience (Henson et al., 2020).

Fatigue is easily assessed by direct questioning about patients' ability to complete simple physical activities related to activities of daily living, but cognitive abilities such as reading or other leisure activities can be impacted as well. The inability to do these things has a profound impact on quality of life for both patients and caregivers. Health professionals often underrecognize this negative impact, perhaps worsened by a poor understanding of the pathophysiology and treatment of fatigue. When there is a correctable cause of fatigue, such as dehydration, anemia, depression, or medications, these sources should be addressed first; but, of course, where there is no clear etiology, clinicians may feel at a loss of what to suggest. Rest, energy conservation techniques, and proper spacing of activities can be a start, and the use of both steroids and psychostimulants (methylphenidate) has been the major pharmacologic therapy for fatigue. Some clinicians may consider tricyclic antidepressants, but their adverse effects may outweigh the benefit; caution is advised in the geriatric population.

Anorexia

Anorexia, defined by progressive weight loss, lipolysis, loss of organ and skeletal protein, and a profound loss of appetite, is another commonly reported symptom in patients with both life-threatening illnesses and progressive chronic illnesses. Anorexia may develop in response to certain conditions or disease states (gastritis, peptic ulcers, tumors) as well as from other causes like pain, fatigue, nausea, or depression. Treatments for primary illnesses (chemotherapy or radiation therapy) as well as certain drugs can also be contributing factors to the development of anorexia. Whereas treatments aimed at alleviating pain, nausea, or depression may improve appetite, pharmacologic treatment of anorexia can be difficult in the older adult patient for a variety of reasons.

Corticosteroids, often the first-line treatment for cancer-related anorexia, is not a good long-term option due to the side effects. Megestrol acetate, a progesterone analog, may stimulate appetite; however, as with corticosteroids, megestrol's common side effects (adrenal insufficiency, hyperactivity, edema, hot flashes, and gastrointestinal side effects) coupled with reports of deep venous thrombosis and fatal pulmonary emboli may cause clinicians to steer clear of this option. Most pharmacologic options do not work for very long, and all have short durations of action plus (some very serious) side effects. Treatment for anorexia, then, may be limited to activities such as patient involvement in meal planning, dietary changes to include patients' favorite foods, avoidance of foods with strong or unpalatable odors, or easy-to-swallow, sweet foods such as puddings and ice creams, or soft/pureed foods.

Nausea and Vomiting

Nausea is the unpleasant sensation of impending vomiting and can accompany vomiting or occur independently. The two symptoms can be associated with autonomic signs (hypersalivation, pallor, cold sweats, decreased respiratory rate, or diarrhea), or they can exist alone. Nausea and vomiting are not the same, nor are they interchangeable, and are caused by a variety of stimuli or inputs; both nausea and vomiting are complex physiologic processes and can be very bothersome for some patients.

Although the experience of nausea and vomiting is unpleasant, vomiting at least can also lead to dehydration or electrolyte imbalances, thus the treatment of nausea and vomiting should initially attempt to correct these conditions. When possible, the causative agent should be removed but sometimes that is not possible. It is critical to attempt to determine the cause to create the most appropriate treatment protocol, as the symptoms may have myriad etiologies such as disturbances arising from the central nervous or endocrinologic systems as well as iatrogenic, obstructive, and mucosal causes. Medications and therapeutic agents are also common causes of acute nausea or vomiting, but often those diminish over exposure and time.

VOMIT (Box 22.6) is an acronym some may find helpful for considering the etiology of nausea/vomiting based on inputs possibly driving the symptom, which would then suggest appropriate treatment options. Antiemetics act on the central nervous system to repress nausea. The major categories of antiemetics are anticholinergic agents, histamine blockers, phenothiazines, and serotonin 5-HT antagonists. Antidopaminergic agents, such as haloperidol and metoclopramide have both antiemetic and prokinetic properties. For refractory nausea, anticholinergic medications, corticosteroids, or cannabinoids are sometimes added, though they should be used with caution as they can cause delirium (Albert, 2017). Nonpharmacologic options include measures to enhance gastric emptying or to decrease gastric distention, reduction of noxious or associated stimuli, acupuncture, cognitive-behavioral therapy to promote muscle relaxation and reverse autonomic arousal, and gingerroot.

Depression

Being diagnosed with a serious, advanced, or terminal illness is a significant, life-changing event. Both in the immediate

• BOX 22.6 VOMIT Acronym for Potential Causes of and Treatments for Nausea or Vomiting

Vestibular (cholinergic, histaminic receptors): *Scopolamine, Promethazine*

Obstruction of bowel by constipation (cholinergic, histaminic, likely 5HT3 receptors): *Senna*

Dys**M**otility of upper gut (cholinergic, histaminic, 5HT3 and 5HT4 receptors): *Metoclopramide*

Infection, **I**nflammation (cholinergic, histaminic, 5HT3, NK1 receptors): *Promethazine (e.g., for labyrinthitis), Prochlorperazine*

Toxins stimulating the chemoreceptor trigger zone (dopamine 2, 5HT3 receptors): *Haloperidol, Ondansetron, Prochlorperazine*

aftermath as well as during treatment, it is not uncommon for patients to experience depression or sadness. As referenced in the previous sections, unmanaged or poorly managed pain or other symptoms (as well as a predisposition to the condition) can lead to depression; however, spiritual or existential concerns, unresolved personal issues, or fear of the unknown after death can also lead to depression symptoms.

Simply asking, "Are you depressed?" has been validated as a good screening tool in terminally ill (or imminently dying) patients; however, treating depression in the terminally ill patient can be difficult. With adequate responses to selective serotonin-reuptake inhibitors (SSRIs) taking up to 6 weeks to attain, this time frame may not be tenable for patients or for families. When patients have significant anergia or anhedonia and their prognoses are very short, methylphenidate has been used and has been found to be particularly helpful when patients have, for example, unresolved business to attend to or families who want to say goodbye.

Delirium

Delirium is a common problem in patients who are dying, and the etiology of delirium is often multifactorial. As with delirium in the geriatric patient who is not dying, delirium is not a distinct disease state, so clinicians must consider medications, infections, organ failure, electrolyte imbalances, CNS pathology, or drug/alcohol withdrawal among the possible causes. Many medications, too numerous to list here, can contribute to the onset of delirium, and there should be a high index of suspicion when delirium occurs within the temporal occurrence of newly prescribed meds. Delirium can present clinically as restlessness, confusion, disorientation, hallucinations, delusions, and emotional lability, among other symptoms. In addition to short onset (as contrasted with dementia), another hallmark of delirium is its fluctuating state, which can make it difficult for clinicians to assess. Detailed input from other care providers and family become critical to ensure that delirium is diagnosed and effectively treated. There are a few assessment tools that can assist with diagnosis, including the Confusion Assessment Method and the Delirium Rating Scale. Other tools for assessing cognition may not capture the fluctuations of the mood, activity, or actions of the patient with delirium.

Management of delirium via pharmacology can be problematic, as the commonly prescribed medications have, like most medications prescribed to the older adult, significant side effect risk profiles. However, delirium is often very disconcerting to both patient and caregivers alike, so prompt attention and immediate mitigation must occur after the onset of delirium. Benzodiazepines may cause paradoxical worsening of symptoms and should not be used as a first-line treatment; thus clinicians often use antipsychotic medications as the mainstay of treatment (Albert, 2017). Behavioral management should always be included in delirium management: provision of a quiet, nonstimulating environment, good lighting that approximates natural circadian rhythms, and a variety of reorienting tools such as clocks or calendars can help. Clinicians must be cognizant that competency can be impacted during a patient's delirious state. Patients may not make sound choices regarding their own care during this time, so frequent reassessments regarding competency is appropriate.

Additional Domains of Palliative Care: Psychosocial, Spiritual, Existential, and Cultural

When patients are first diagnosed with a serious, life-limiting illness, it would stand to reason that most clinicians' initial thoughts turn to either disease management though curative treatments or symptom management if patients focus more on quality of life. But from the patient or family perspective, often the first thing that is experienced is not a physical symptom, but an emotional one: shock, anger, disbelief, fear, or grief. These reactions to hearing a serious illness diagnosis, as much as the sequelae of the illness itself, impact the patient or family's quality of life. Although the disease and management of it are a necessary and important focus in palliative care, psychosocial well-being and care should not be undervalued in any way.

Psychosocial Aspects of Care

Palliative care's holistic approach to whole-person or whole-family care includes regular assessment and intervention of these other aspects of the human experience and how they affect a particular patient/family's journey. Interestingly, psychosocial issues can manifest as physical symptoms, which hearkens back to the concept of total pain conceptualized by Dame Cicely Saunders and underscores the need for comprehensive interdisciplinary assessments to ensure that all of a person's struggles and suffering are addressed.

Many palliative care teams rely on social workers to evaluate and support patients' nonphysical needs to determine appropriate plans of care. These team members study past and current health situations, family structure and roles, patterns of communication, and decision making in the family, social supports, and mental health functioning among other areas of consideration. Social workers consider the immediate and extended environment as part of the landscape of the patient and family, which impacts and supports (or detracts) from the patient's total health. Assessments may include a traditional evaluation of mental health as well as a review of overall functioning and coping styles, an assessment of the extent of the patient's connectedness to family and social networks, and a review of other social determinants of health. When one or more of these aspects are broken or problematic, the palliative care social worker can develop plans of care to repair and support the patient and family toward optimizing health and function to the greatest extent possible. The role of the social worker, then, can be that of counselor, advocate, community liaison and resource finder, educator, or healer. The skills that palliative care social workers bring regarding working with families and groups are possibly some of the most important on the interdisciplinary team.

Spiritual and Existential Aspects of Care

Examples and interventions of spiritual and existential distress can be found in Table 22.13 and Table 22.14. Spirituality is an awareness and connection to a higher power or divine presence, a harmonious relationship or a connection with self, nature, or community that enables people to discover the essence of their being. Spirituality can include religious beliefs, rituals, and practices, but it does not always include participation in organized religion. When events such as a serious illness or terminal diagnosis happen in a person's life, this can rock the foundation of

TABLE 22.13 Spiritual Distress

Symptoms	Interventions
Feelings of fear, hopelessness, or guilt	Being present with the patient and family
Anger at God or higher power	Listening with sensitivity and openness
Feelings of emptiness or loss of direction	Honoring and respecting the patient's faith traditions
Questions: "Where is Allah?" "Why hasn't God taken me yet?" "What have I done to deserve this?"	Encouraging patients to tell their story
Feeling of disconnection from God or higher power	Helping the patient to finish incomplete tasks that may be causing anxiety, such as making a phone call, writing a letter, or journaling
Physical pain that is unrelieved after extensive and appropriate pharmacologic intervention(s) or pain that is unspecified or frequently changes location	Encouraging practice of spiritual rituals such as meditation, scripture reading, or prayer
Insomnia or increased shortness of breath	Offering to contact the patient's priest, pastor, rabbi, imam, spiritual adviser, or chaplain
Fear of death/dying	
Depression, restlessness, anxiety, emotional outbursts, or fatigue	
Expressing desire for forgiveness	
Declination of assistance with hygiene or basic care needs	
Power struggles with family members	
Sudden change or rejection of previous religious practices, faith, or rituals	

TABLE 22.14 Existential Distress

Symptoms	Interventions
Inner turmoil due to individual's confrontation with existence or end of existence	Due to feelings of loss of control, providing ways the patient and family can maintain some kind of control
Feelings of hopelessness, burden to others, loss of sense of identity/dignity	Providing active listening and presence to combat the feelings of isolation
Suffering that extends beyond physical pain	Encouraging patients to let people in or to forge closer bonds with those they care about
Issues related to identity, personal integrity, or an unfulfilled past	Helping the patient face reality and understanding that they have the ability to create meaning out of a distressing/suffering event
Alienation and isolation	Exploring what the concepts of death, freedom/responsibility, or isolation means to the patient
Profound loneliness, intolerable emptiness, sadness—this is known as existential loneliness	Helping the patient find hope through meaning
Loss of meaning	Discussing and embracing meaningful events that have occurred in the patient's life

someone's entire belief system; the person may be said to be experiencing spiritual distress. In some cases, these disruptions may cause patients to question everything that they know or believe. During these periods of questioning or distress, the palliative care interdisciplinary team seeks to help the patient find or restore a sense of meaning and purpose. Spiritual distress can be so profound that it throws a patient into a depression and may exacerbate physical symptoms of illness, such as headaches, feelings of nausea, or pain.

Part of the goal of holistic person/family-centered care is to assist our seriously ill patients in finding meaning and purpose in their life, receive love and forgiveness, and complete any unfinished tasks, including saying goodbye to families and loved ones. For some, the objective may be a reconciliation with the individual's God or a higher power, or creating a sense of self-acceptance and inner peace, which will ultimately lead to a good death.

Existentialism is concerned with human existence, finding self, and the meaning of life through free will, choice, and personal responsibility. Existentialism stresses that a person's judgment is the determining factor for what is to be believed. In short, this means that within the context of existentialism, there is no essential human existence or human nature. Belief in free will, personal accountability, and responsibility, rather than abiding by religious or secular world values, determines a person's nature; what makes up a life is the result of one's choices; there is nothing external on which to cast blame if the way one's life events unfold end up being unsatisfying.

When one deeply contemplates his or her existence or the end of one's existence, the individual may come to believe that there was no meaning or purpose to life, which may lead to a sense of alienation and isolation in the world, along with a heightened awareness of mortality. For some, these feelings may be accompanied by a sense of demoralization and despair and may even manifest as or exacerbate existing physical symptoms. Contemplation of death (both in theory and one's own), isolation, meaninglessness, and freedom are profound topics, and depending on how a patient processes these concepts, some patients may find themselves intellectually stuck, or they may find a path to move forward to new levels of thought, acceptance, and functioning.

Both religious or nonreligious/nonspiritual persons may experience existential distress, and in contrast to nearly all the other symptoms discussed in this chapter, there are no pharmacologic interventions to deploy. Providing the patient and family with support may be best accomplished through listening or being present. Difficulties may stem from an inability to reconcile/make peace with the major existential fears or concepts mentioned previously. Although nonreligious/nonspiritual patients may decline the offer of a palliative care chaplain, these members of the interdisciplinary team remain excellent resources to help a patient through this process.

Cultural Aspects of Care

What is culture? Is it race, ethnicity, religion, language, or history? The answer encompasses these aspects and more, including attitudes and beliefs, traditions and social customs, cuisine, music, and the social dynamics of a group of people. One aspect of culture that is often not mentioned is how these components interact, impact, and influence a person or family's perception of their health, wellness, death, and dying. To provide good care, in general, clinicians need to ensure that they understand these components of a person's background or culture. There are many terms that can be used when discussing culturally competent care; they include *cultural awareness, cultural sensitivity*, and others, the exploration of which is beyond the scope of this chapter. As palliative care is frequently underutilized by many culturally diverse communities, to improve outcomes, reduce health disparities, and achieve equitable health care, clinicians should delve more deeply into the subject—both in general and in terms of how the cultural background of the patient, in particular, will affect her or his care (Givler et al., 2021).

Living in and practicing in a culturally, ethnically, and religiously diverse society affords us the opportunity to interact with different types of people on any given day. Although no one can be well versed in every iteration of a culture or language/dialect, practitioners can certainly take steps to develop cultural awareness or sensitivity, especially when providing palliative care and care for persons at the end of life. Many articles discuss the critical importance of culturally appropriate approaches to pain and palliative care (Givler et al., 2021), as well as in general practice (Swihart et al., 2021). Patients and families bring their own experiences, history, attitudes, or biases into the exam room every day, and it is our job to set aside our own and to seek to understand and learn through curiosity and listening. We must be comfortable asking questions to patients, and in some cases to extended family members, so that as interdisciplinary professionals we tear down barriers that culturally diverse persons' experience in order to provide appropriate, person- and family-centered care.

It would be remiss to neglect to mention lesbian, gay, bisexual, transgender, queer, intersex, and asexual older persons, their partners or caregivers, and the need to provide compassionate care for this population of adults. Although more attention has been levied on the unique palliative care needs of LGBTQIA+ older persons and their caregivers, this group has been generally misunderstood and mistreated by health care systems, including during times serious illness or when facing the end of life. Additionally, there is a relative dearth of research and guides to assist professionals, but this is changing (Cloyes et al., 2018; National Hospice and Palliative Care Organization Diversity Advisory Council, 2021).

Although the additional domains of palliative and end-of-life care just covered may seem naturally aligned with the work of social workers or chaplains, our patients and families only want to feel assured that they are receiving the best care possible. All dimensions of the human experience (physical, psychosocial, spiritual, existential, cultural, and religious) become the responsibility of each member of the interdisciplinary team. This applies not only to palliative care providers, but providers across the board should acknowledge and respect patient/family beliefs, rituals, attitudes, and biases. Every person, and how each one has lived and will experience the end of their life, is unique. Palliative care clinicians understand that the best way to determine how to provide for the holistic care needs of patients and families starts with listening and asking. It never hurts to always be open to ideas, beliefs, and customs that differ from one's own experience.

Prognostication

Prognostication is the prediction of the probability that an individual will succumb to a particular outcome over time; in palliative care and hospice, that outcome is generally death from an illness or injury. We prognosticate for a variety of reasons. Patients and families want information about life expectancy to help plan realistically for their futures and to be sure that treatment paths align with their preferences regarding goals of care (curative versus comfort oriented). Additionally, whereas many clinicians are moving away from an outdated model of reactive care toward proactive care, prognostication also supports value-based care and cost effectiveness. Clinicians need to determine life expectancy so they can decide if therapeutic interventions have enough time to be of a benefit to the patient. This is the lag time to benefit (LtB) ratio. If a particular screen or treatment has an LtB ratio that is greater than a patient's life expectancy, then clinicians must consider not making a recommendation in support of that option. An example would be depression in terminally ill patients. If an SSRI takes 1 to 2 months to reach its full therapeutic effect, then a patient whose life expectancy is less than 30 days is not likely to experience the benefit of the treatment before death (Table 22.15).

An Art and a Science

Although clinical judgment can correlate with survival times, a hallmark study indicated that the tendency is toward overestimation of survival by a factor of 5.3 (Christakis & Lamont, 2000), and the reasons for this stem from fewer years of tenure as a physician, type of specialty (e.g., oncologic practice versus other types of specialties), and duration of the physician/patient relationship, with accuracy *worsening* the longer the length of the physician/patient relationship. The only group more overly optimistic than health care providers are patients and families. These errors regarding overestimation in survivability of a condition or disease state are generally made at the most critical time in patients' lives; this leads to late referrals to hospice, with many patients receiving less than 1 month of the benefit. Prognostication has not been considered important and thus is not routinely taught in medical and nursing classes, although it is a core clinical skill for providers in geriatric clinical practice and should be an integral part of every medical decision. Many clinicians find this to be one of the most difficult aspects of their jobs, as prognostication is not merely the prediction but also communication about the information. This challenging task is one of the main reasons that primary care and specialists refer to palliative care.

"Would I be surprised if this patient died in the next year?" Curiously, this simple question has been validated as a tool that correlates with mortality (White et al., 2017). But surprise aside, skillful prognostication is both an art and science In addition to a clinician's gut impression, there are myriad factors that come into play when thinking about a patient's prognosis, such as if the illness has been maximally treated or is terminal, the degree of symptom burden, comorbid conditions, functional status, psychosocial and spiritual factors, and other considerations.

TABLE 22.15 Lag Time to Benefit (LtB)

Time Frame	Considerations
Life expectancy < LtB	Intervention potentially harmful, consider not recommending
Life expectancy = LtB	Equal risk and benefit, preference should determine recommendation
Life expectancy > LtB	Intervention potentially beneficial, consider recommending

Tools We Can Use

Generally, when clinicians examine the pathways or trajectories leading to death, there are four predominant patterns (Lunney et al., 2003). These generally align with disease categories and occur with the following frequency: sudden death (10%), cancer (25%), organ failure (40%) and frailty (25%) (Fig. 22.3). Understanding these typical disease trajectories are important but only a piece of the puzzle when it comes to making estimates of survival. Functional status has been shown to be one of the key factors in determining prognosis, especially for geriatric oncology patients (Morishima et al., 2020), thus it has been incorporated into several tools commonly used for helping to suggest prognosis. Analysis of prospective, longitudinal data showed that an increase in the number of activities of daily living (ADLs) in which a person demonstrated dependency negatively correlated with time of survival, although these varied by time and which of the four patterns of death was reviewed. Regardless, many tools used by palliative care clinicians for prognosis incorporate functional status as an integral aspect of the tool; however, any tool should be used in conjunction with disease-specific clinical predictors of survival (Stone et al., 2021). A patient's functional dependence should be considered along with other factors such as nutritional and cognitive status, gender, age, and the number of hospitalizations or additional complications (falls with fracture, pneumonia, sepsis, etc.) experienced within the past year when determining prognosis.

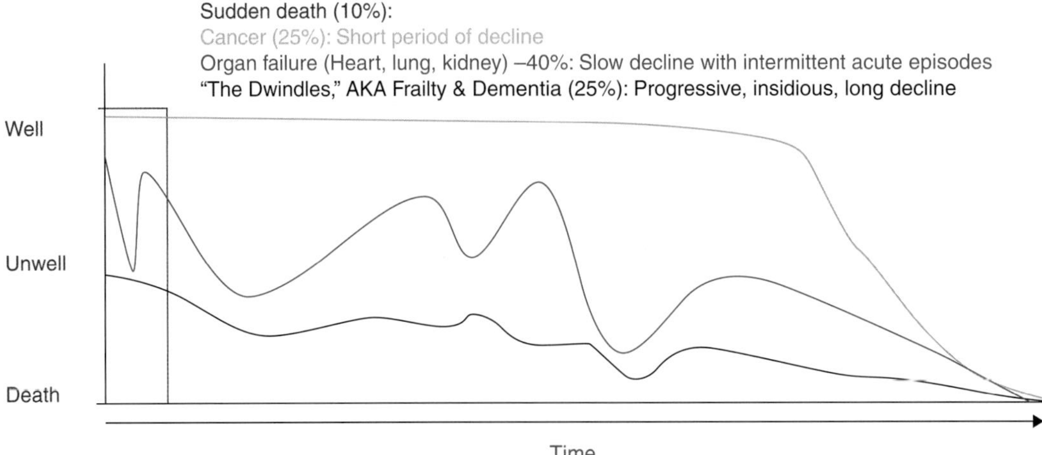

• **Fig. 22.3** End-of-Life Disease Trajectories and Prognostications. (Adapted from Lunney, J. R., Lynn, J., Foley, D. J., Lipson, S., & Guralnik, J. M. [2003]. Patterns of functional decline at the end of life. *Journal of the American Medical Association, 289*[18], 2387–2392. https://doi.org/10.1001/jama.289.18.2387.)

National and local coverage determinations (LCDs) establish eligibility for hospice and will be covered elsewhere in this chapter; however, they often incorporate biometric models of prognostication such as New York Heart Association (NYHA) classes for heart failure, the BODE index (body mass index [B], degree of obstruction [O], dyspnea [D], and exercise capacity [E]) for pulmonary disease, the Model for End-Stage Liver Disease (MELD) score for liver disease, the Eastern Cooperative Oncology Group (ECOG) for cancer, and the Functional Assessment Staging Tool (FAST) for Alzheimer-type dementia (not validated for any other type of dementia). Although generally not part of the LCDs, hospice and palliative clinicians may use the Palliative Prognostic Score (PaP), Palliative Prognostic Index (PPI), or the Palliative Performance Scale (PPS). Another tool is the Mortality Risk Index, which is based on the Minimum Data Set (MDS) used with nursing facility patients. It covers several risk factors and assigns points; once again, functional status is heavily weighted among the components. The higher the score, the greater likelihood of death within 12 months (Mitchell et al., n.d.).

The Most Important Part of Prognosis: Communication

Disease-specific clinical performance indicators, function status, or other inputs combined with provider experience are the essential components to an informed prognosis. The last component of prognostication is communication of this information to affected stakeholders: other clinicians but most important the patient and family. As discussed previously, cultural or religious factors will influence what, when, how, and with whom this information is shared. The role of the NP or PA on the team may be to deliver the message, so confirming that the patient/family is ready to hear this is a critical first step. Setting the stage for critical conversations, such as using the SPIKES protocol and ensuring the appropriateness of place and time, was covered earlier. SPIKES is an acronym for presenting distressing information in an organized manner to patients and families. The SPIKES protocol provides a step-wise framework for difficult discussions such as when cancer recurs or when palliative or hospice care is indicated. Each letter represents a phase in the six-step sequence.

Prognostic information should be presented as a range, such as months to a year, weeks to months, or days to weeks. No matter to whom this information is directed, do not use euphemisms or give false hope. Speak in a straightforward but sincere and empathic tone, stressing nonabandonment and commitment to ongoing support. Likely, this information will be met with strong emotion, even if expected, so be sure to allow for silence and contemplation. When the patient or family is ready, move on to what this information means as it relates to the patient's goals of care or readiness for transition to hospice. Communicating a patient's prognosis is never easy, but it is an essential skill and requires time, effort, and attention to nuances of both verbal and nonverbal communication to ensure compassionate delivery of the information.

Complex Palliative Care Issues

Sometimes despite best efforts for aggressive pain and symptom management, some patients at the end of life develop serious complications that if not promptly recognized and treated can cause extreme suffering for the patient and distress for the family or caregivers. Those urgent syndromes can include superior vena cava obstruction, pleural or pericardial effusions, hemoptysis, spinal cord compression, or hypercalcemia. Sometimes the symptoms are insidious, whereas for others the onset appears suddenly. The responsibility of NPs and PAs who care for patients nearing or at the end of life is to be able to recognize and intervene if any of these syndromes develop and to provide both education and support to patients and families alike. Where the cause is reversible, the clinician should aim to eliminate the cause;

when it is not, it is incumbent on the clinician to understand treatment, including supportive care, and any options that may be appropriate or available.

Many times, the syndromes noted previously respond to palliative interventions, but at other times, even in supportive care settings, sometimes the symptom burden is so great that additional interventions are required to ensure that the patient is not suffering. As addressed previously, symptoms at the end of life can include pain, dyspnea, nausea/vomiting, and delirium, not to forget other forms of suffering, whether psychiatric or spiritual/existential. Suffering is generally multifactorial, with patients experiencing physical, emotional, and existential crises at the same time.

Palliative Sedation

Clinicians supporting patients at the end of life do not have a consensus on what constitutes a "good death" (Meier et al., 2016), although a report by the Committee on Care at the End of Life (Institute of Medicine [US] Committee on Care at End of Life, 1997, p. 6) defines it as "one that is free from avoidable death and suffering for patients," and in theory this is likely something upon which many can agree. Although sedation is understood and accepted prior to surgical procedures, sedation at the end of life, known as terminal or palliative sedation, has yet to gain similar levels of acceptance and is generally considered to be a last resort. Within the hospice and palliative communities, most practitioners identify physical symptoms as the impetus for palliative sedation, although a small minority may consider existential suffering as the reason. Regardless of the cause of the suffering, both the American Academy of Hospice and Palliative Medicine (AAHPM) and the Hospice and Palliative Nurses Association (HPNA) have published position statements on the practice (American Academy of Hospice and Palliative Medicine, 2014; Hospice and Palliative Nurses Association, 2016). The consensus between these organizations is that each patient's circumstance must be thoroughly assessed and maximally treated first, the safest and most efficacious medications to reduce suffering or a lower level of consciousness must be used, and the goal is always to relieve refractory suffering (not to hasten death).

Medical Assistance in Dying

Although the goal of palliative sedation is relief of suffering, there is some chance that NPs and PAs may be approached by patients or families for a discussion on medical assistance in dying (MAiD). As of this writing, 10 US jurisdictions have a provision for this by having enacted death with dignity laws, generally modeled after Oregon's act, which has been hailed as successful due to the robust certification requirements as well as safeguards to prevent misuse. The protections in the statutes are designed to ensure that the decision about MAiD is an autonomous desire of the patient to ensure that the patient is fully informed regarding all aspects of the request and is able to ingest the lethal medications independently. Advocates for the practice cite respect for patient autonomy, relief of suffering, and safe medical practice, which requires a health care professional. Those against MAiD list concerns regarding depression in advanced illness, suicide contagion, and the idea that the practice would introduce a slippery slope for physicians (Dugdale et al., 2019). For most clinicians, MAiD queries will trigger a referral to a specialty palliative care consult service, as members of the interdisciplinary team are trained to manage these conversations with sensitivity and compassion. As note previously, both AAHPM and HPNA have positions available for review.

Withdrawal or Withholding of Life-Sustaining Therapies

Everyone will eventually die, and only less than 10% of those deaths will occur suddenly (Lunney et al., 2003). More than 90% of us will succumb after a prolonged illness. Although death should be expected given these facts, many families have little to no actual experience with death and as such have created an exaggerated sense of the dying process, namely as an overly medical event. However, dying is a physical, psychological, social, and spiritual event. When viewed in this way, the patient and family are a continued unit of care with the goals of the hospice and palliative care teams focused on optimizing patient comfort, dignity, choice, acceptance, final tasks, saying goodbye, and life closure. All aspects of care intensify, and needs frequently change; thus the interdisciplinary team must remain focused on helping the patient achieve a dignified death and to learn what the family needs to care for the patient up to and including the moment of death as well as how to approach the time that follows. As much as we may try to prepare for death, the time cannot be predicted, as signs and symptoms are merely a guideline. In general, dying is a natural process of the slowing of all bodily functions, which may occur over days and weeks or may come on only hours or minutes prior to death.

Although spiritual and existential issues were discussed earlier, it is common for patients and families to express fears about dying, abandonment, the unknown, pain, and anguish. It can be difficult to watch a loved one demonstrate increased weakness and fatigue, lose their appetite, reject food or fluids, appear to waste away, experience changes in bladder or bowel function, have pain, or begin to have delusions or hallucinations. Many of these symptoms are manageable with supportive care, coupled with education for the caregivers/families regarding what to expect of the dying process. However, despite education that certain experiences are to be expected as serious illnesses advance and the patient moves closer to death, this reality is often difficult when it moves from theoretic concepts to actual events. Patients and families alike may request treatments to prolong the patient's life, even when sometimes those life-sustaining treatments (LSTs) may cause additional discomfort, suffering, or have a low probability of extending the patient's life span.

Many people may believe that discussion of withdrawal of LSTs occurs only after neurologic death has been declared. Today, discussions about treatments and the desire for or preference to avoid certain interventions/treatments occur before significant events transpire, in the form of advance care planning (ACP) conversations, which should be a regular component of the practice of any clinician working with the geriatric population; the importance of POLST completion was discussed previously. Decisions about limiting treatments may be initiated by clinicians working with the patient or family; however, caregivers acting as surrogate decision makers are usually the ones to make the actual decision about when to withhold or withdraw therapy. When the time comes, the patient is many times too ill to participate in the discussion, ergo this is the critical reason for every adult with capacity to execute an advance care plan, review it regularly (at least annually or upon a change in condition), and to share this plan with both family members and practitioners.

Part of the reason for an advance care directive is to state not only what a person wants to transpire if his or her were to stop but also what the person will not tolerate. Patients can elect a time-limited trial of certain interventions, such as mechanical ventilation for a period but to discontinue it if the condition is prolonged or unlikely to improve (Vink et al., 2018). Although some clinicians think it is helpful to explain the details of what cardiopulmonary resuscitation (CPR) entails or to articulate the low probability of survival after a cardiac event, a more thoughtful practice would be to focus the conversation on a patient's goals or values and to only introduce recommendations that would support that outcome. For example, if the focus is on comfort above all else, then the placement of a feeding tube or the initiation of CPR is not likely to produce that desired effect.

Although the following interventions are by no means inconsequential therapies, patients and families may be more comfortable with accepting blood products, hemodialysis, vasopressors, total parenteral nutrition, antibiotics, IV fluids, and tube feedings; in contrast, patients and families may have strong opinions regarding initiating or withholding interventions such as CPR and mechanical ventilation. For many people, emotionally there is a distinction between withdrawal (removing an intervention) and withholding (never initiating it at all), although when viewing these terms through an ethical lens, the distinction does not exist.

Strangely, discussions with families regarding withdrawal or withholding of artificial feeding or hydration can be quite difficult. For many families and cultures, sharing of food and drink equates to caring; often families are not aware that loss of appetite and reduced intake are normal aspects of the dying process. There is a sense that lack of food or water is causing the patient's decline and that additional caloric intake will improve the patient's energy level or strength, or even heal them in some way. There remains a misconception that aspiration can be avoided by feeding tube placement, and often the family has not considered that nutrition administered in this way is both invasive and uncomfortable (not to mention does not achieve the intended result of avoiding aspiration). Families are also generally unaware of the consequences of IV hydration in the terminal patient, which stem from the body's increasing difficulty with proper mobilization or the incorporation of introduced fluids. Additionally, increased urine output may require placement of a Foley catheter (again, an invasive procedure that can be painful and increase discomfort), an increase in oropharyngeal secretions or edema/third spacing, as well as increases in nausea/vomiting. Some death with dignity advocates believe that terminal dehydration results in the release of certain chemicals (ketones), which act as an anesthetic, supporting the concept of a good death. Regardless of this perspective, discussions with families about food and fluids need to be delivered compassionately and should focus on the risks and benefits of any provision of artificial nutrition or hydration (American Academy of Hospice and Palliative Medicine, 2013).

Practitioners not routinely accustomed to seeing dying and death daily may feel less comfortable discussing all of the options that can be considered life-sustaining treatment; often this is the impetus for a referral to the specialist palliative care team. Families often have specific concerns and misconceptions about the process, which can incorporate historic experience as well as cultural or religious beliefs, and they may express concerns that by withholding or withdrawing LSTs they are hastening death. When faced with this situation, clinicians can address concerns by focusing on the goals of the treatment rather than the therapy itself and by gently reminding the family that the underlying illness is the cause of death—not the stopping of the machine. Other concerns that families may express include statements indicating that their interpretation of religious teachings means that they are prohibited from discontinuing LSTs or a fear that discontinuation of treatment will lead to intractable pain or suffering. In these latter two scenarios, the clinician may inquire about the family's religious beliefs to open a dialogue, perhaps with the support of a palliative care chaplain, that will help them to explore and understand their feelings more deeply. Regarding worries of pain and suffering, often the duration of time between discontinuation of LSTs and death is short, but providing reassurance that symptoms will be well controlled both before and after the machine is turned off can help helpful.

When preparing to discuss the limitations of LSTs, the clinician must ensure that the team has a good understanding of legal and regulatory parameters at both the state and local hospital levels. It is important to be well versed in the condition and prognosis of the patient, as this reassures families that the team cares enough to know the details about their loved one. The clinician should have a clear understanding of how clinical teams maintain comfort and dignity during the process and, above all, ensure that all parties involved have coordinated with the members of the extended clinical team to plan the process and content of the discussion. Again, as with discussing goals of care and prognosis, preparation is key.

The participants in the discussion are of critical importance and extended family may have different levels of understanding of the critical or terminal nature of the illness (or the lack of further benefit from the treatment/therapy), so it is necessary to ascertain the amount of knowledge regarding the patient's situation from everyone who is present; some education may be required in order for everyone to be on the same page. Rather than launching into the discussion, invite the participants to discuss the treatment plan, and when permission has been granted, explain the basis for the decision to discontinue or to forgo additional treatment. Keep the focus on the stated goals, values, wishes, and preferences of the patient; here is where referencing the patient's advance care plan or medical orders for life-sustaining treatment is helpful. Reminding the family that they are merely carrying out the stated wishes or values of the patient helps to remove the guilt that many families feel when having to make a critical decision about withholding or withdrawing treatment. Finally, ensure that the group who is involved understands that the decision to discontinue life-sustaining treatments or therapies does *not* equate to discontinuing all care. Supportive care, such as aggressive pain and symptom management, as well as other types of support such as playing music, massage therapy, having visits from loved ones, and a host of other complementary or alternative medicine interventions to maintain comfort, can continue as long as the patient lives (Zeng et al., 2018).

An important component of the entire process is to be aware of and respond to the reaction of the family present; many times, this will be a strong emotion. This is natural and to be expected, as discussion about limiting or discontinuing therapy forces an awareness of the nearness of death. Emotions should be acknowledged and responded to before attempting to have any further discussion, which demonstrates both care and concern on behalf of the clinician, but also because during times of strong emotional feelings, executive functioning processes in the frontal lobe decrease. Anticipate questions and be open to additional perspectives or philosophies; the goal would be to find consensus about what the patient would have wanted, rather than to create or exacerbate existing family conflicts. Clinicians are not expected to always have all the answers, but families want to know that the health care provider will seek out necessary information and return to share it with them.

If the decision to withhold or withdraw treatment has been made, it becomes paramount to review exactly what happens next. Sometimes timing is an issue, as families may decide to delay so that out-of-town relatives can arrive and say goodbye or to arrange for services that must happen quickly after death according to religious law. The responsibility of the clinician is to support and reduce the feelings of stress or pressure that timing issues may raise. Families may request support from their religious or spiritual communities, so being aware of these preferences and needs is also very important. Describe the process using compassionate language, so the family understands what happens when the treatment is withheld or withdrawn; however, be clear that it is up to the family to decide if they want to be present or not during that process.

Many families do not have direct experience with death, and their imaginations have created a frightening picture that is often quite different from the reality. If they give permission to talk about it, have them describe what they expect and then help them to understand what happens during the dying process. Simple and straightforward descriptions, including what they may observe regarding vital signs on the monitors or hear (such as noises from respiratory secretions, snoring, etc.) will help set realistic expectations and alleviate some of their fears. Again, summarize and check for understanding regarding all aspects of these conversations; do not be surprised if these conversations take several sessions before all involved parties have a clear understanding of the situation, prognosis, or decision.

A word regarding ethical or legal concerns: withdrawal or withholding LSTs may give rise to fears for both providers (who worry about liability) and families (who worry about ethical issues) alike. As noted earlier, there is not a legal distinction between withholding and withdrawing therapy. These decisions are generally made in a clinical setting, and it is unusual that courts need to get involved. When patients die after clinicians and families uphold their wishes to withhold or withdraw therapy, these deaths are considered neither suicide nor homicide, and providers are not liable. Ethically, decisions to withdraw or withhold LSTs should take risk/benefit burdens into consideration as well as respecting that everyone with full mental capacity has a right to make a choice that aligns with his or her personal morals and values. By respecting individual autonomy, clinicians must be prepared for times when patients will refuse care when it seems too early to stop or, conversely, may demand ongoing aggressive care when it seems inappropriate to continue or the proposed therapy is unlikely to produce the intended result (often life prolongation). When in doubt or when these issues are not clear, palliative care and hospice teams often find additional professional support by incorporating the hospital or other facility's experts in ethics as extended members of the interdisciplinary team.

Let this statement be reiterated here, as it is extremely important: patients' wishes, preferences and goals can and will change with fluctuations in health status or life circumstances. As an illness progresses or personal circumstances change (including the ability of someone to provide care), providers must review that patient's wishes regarding the goals of his or her care, which will include conversations around withholding or withdrawing life-sustaining treatments. In many cases this prompts discussions about end-of-life care transitions, such as hospice care.

Hospice

Hospice service is a philosophy of care that focuses on comfort rather than a cure for terminally ill patients with a 6-month prognosis (CMS, 2020b, 2020c). In contrast to palliative care outside of hospice (which can be administered along with curative treatments), hospice is a standardized and Medicare/insurance-recognized palliative care option for patients who, when eligible, can elect to focus on comfort rather than cure. Hospice is the most well-established program providing expert palliative interventions with the goal of comfort and support for the patient and loved ones through the end of life. Ninety percent of hospice patients receive this service through the Medicare hospice benefit (CMS, 2020b, 2020c).

Hospice care is a unique comprehensive benefit that brings expert palliative care to patients wherever they call home. As part of the benefit (CMS, 2020b), hospice professionals teach and support family or loved ones willing to care for the patient by instructing them on how to provide the day-to-day caregiving tasks. Hospice professionals do not move into the home. The routine level of hospice care provides 24/7 registered nurse (RN) phone consultation and medications for pain and symptoms management, regularly scheduled clinical visits, plus medical equipment such as a hospital bed or oxygen and other supplies needed to care for the patient. For help with personal care such as bathing and grooming, a trained hospice aide will come to the home and provide care. For management of psychosocial-spiritual needs, hospice professionals and volunteers are scheduled for home visits. These services and more are part of the Medicare hospice benefit with minimal to no out-of-pocket cost to the patient or family for supplies or medications required for comfort related to the terminal/certifying illness (CMS, 2020b, 2020c).

History of Hospice

Today's modern hospice differs greatly from the first hospice originating in Europe around the 14th century. The word *hospice* comes from the Latin word *hospes*, which translates to "guest or traveler." Between the 14th and 19th centuries, care of the dying moved from small homes to large hostels where religious and volunteers tended to the needs of the dying (Lutz, 2011). As the concept of hospice progressed into the 20th century, a British nurse and social worker named Cicely Saunders dedicated herself to the practice of administering to the dying. She also became a hospice physician during the interim of her career.

Dr. Saunders contributed new understanding about the dying patient and the process of death. She discovered that when a patient's physical, emotional, and spiritual issues were addressed, the patient experienced improved relief throughout the dying process. The approach espoused by Dr. Saunders was novel, as she insisted the best method to care for the dying had a holistic focus. It was through the work of Dr. Saunders that the hospice concept was modernized. In 1967, she was credited with establishing the first modern hospice, which utilized her multidisciplinary approach to alleviating suffering for the dying (Lutz, 2011).

In the United States, Dr. Saunders' holistic approach to care was increasingly valued for its humane treatment of the dying coupled with its ability to reduce the costs of futile medical treatments. Thus in 1982, the US Congress established the Medicare hospice benefit for Medicare recipients with the full complement of team-based, end-of-life care we know today (Lutz, 2011).

Eligibility

Medicare limits the hospice benefits to patients who are near the end stage of disease with a 6-month prognosis if the disease runs its normal course. According to Medicare (CMS, 2020b, 2020c), only a hospice physician, together with the patient's medical provider if available, can certify a patient with a terminal prognosis of 6 months or less. An evaluation of the patient for hospice eligibility is conducted at no cost to the patient when a referral is made for evaluation. There is no obligation for the patient to elect the benefit (CMS, 2020b, 2020c).

To confirm hospice eligibility and determine the terminal diagnosis, the hospice physician/medical director analyzes the patient's medical history, current physical status, and lab or imaging studies. This assessment is then compared with specific hospice disease criteria, known as local coverage determinants, to select the hospice terminal diagnosis to report to Medicare (CMS, 2020d). For example, if a patient has stage 4 lung cancer and end-stage heart disease, both disorders may meet the hospice criteria for a terminal prognosis of 6 months or less. However, only one of the conditions will be reported as the hospice terminal diagnosis. The diagnosis chosen is the one most likely to result in death the soonest, whereas the other disease is documented as secondary or supportive of the terminal prognosis. In this example, the end-stage heart failure would be listed as the hospice terminal diagnosis, with the lung cancer listed as secondary (CMS, 2020d). See Fig. 22.4 for causes of US mortality (Centers for Disease Control (CDC), 2019). Examples of patient comorbidities that can be used to support the clinical judgment for a terminal prognosis include weight loss, decreased functional status, recurrent infection, or multiple comorbidities per local coverage determinants (CMS, 2020d).

Once hospice eligibility is confirmed, the hospice philosophy, benefits, and limitations are explained to the patient or the patient's surrogate/representative. Most patients who agree to hospice support are acknowledging their mortality and focusing their attention on the meaning of their life. This can be a valuable time of reflection and healing for the patient and family. Steinhauser et al. (2000) identify five top priorities of patients near the end of life: retention of mental capacity or awareness, a sense of peace, not being a burden to others, identification of a purpose and a sense of feeling complete or satisfied with life. After confirming that the patient or surrogate/family understands the hospice program, the informed consent form is signed attesting to the agreement to forgo curative treatment in favor of comfort-only measures with hospice. Next, the election statement is signed, which alerts Medicare to begin hospice coverage.

Once the hospice admission is completed, the hospice team is then responsible for all medical care related to

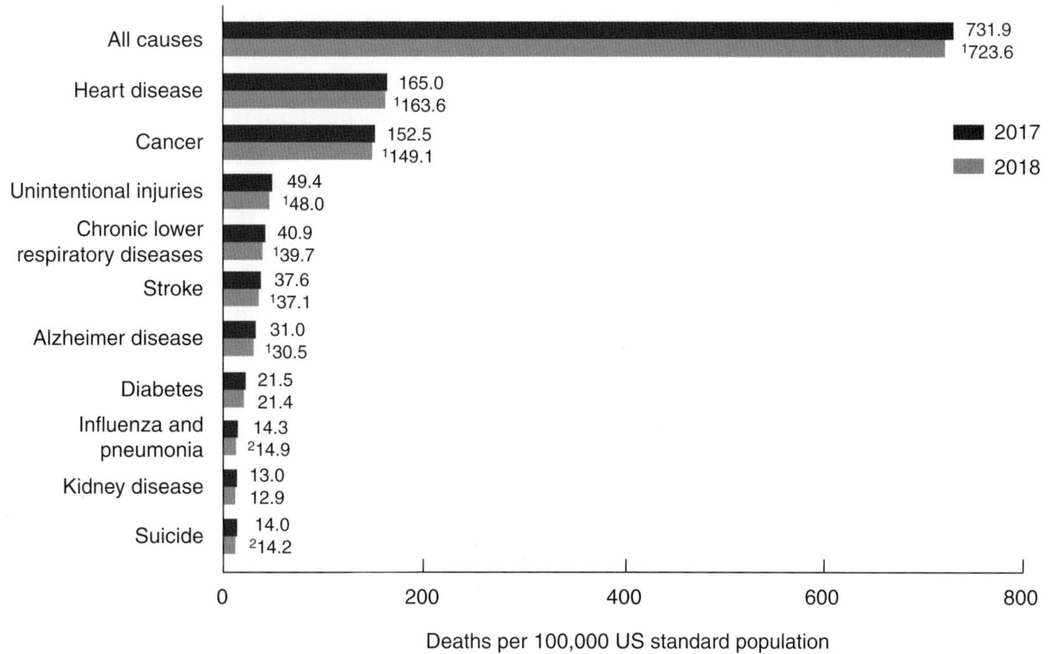

• **Fig. 22.4** Leading Causes of Death in the United States, 2017–2018. (From the Centers for Disease Control [CDC]. [2019]. *Leading causes of death.* cdc.gov. https://www.cdc.gov/nchs/fastats/leading-causes-of-death.htm.)

the certifying terminal diagnosis for the patient until the patient's death or live discharge. It is important to understand that in the event another medical issue occurs that is not associated with the hospice terminal diagnosis, the patient's original Medicare/Medicaid benefit would be available to cover this care (CMS, 2020b, 2020c). For example, if a hospice patient with a terminal diagnosis of kidney disease falls and fractures a wrist, the original Medicare part A or B would cover the cost of fracture care while the patient remains on hospice. However, for Medicare to cover this new medical issue, the hospice team must make the arrangements and coordinate the care or risk nonpayment (CMS, 2020b, 2020c). Few medical services are not covered by the hospice benefit. Those not covered by hospice include room and board for patients who reside in assisted or skilled nursing facilities and medications not necessary to relieve symptoms at the end of life (CMS, 2020b, 2020c).

The Medicare hospice program (CMS, 2020c) is divided into two consecutive 90-day benefit periods and an unlimited subsequent 60-day period until the death or live discharge of the patient. A live discharge most commonly occurs when a patient's prognosis improves to a point where he or she no longer meets hospice eligibility requirements (CMS, 2020b, 2020c). Recertification by the hospice medical director and a face-to-face assessment of the patient is required to confirm a prognosis of 6 months or less. This recertification must be completed at the start of each benefit period after the first 90 days so the patient can continue to receive hospice care (CMS, 2020c). A patient also has the option of revoking or switching to another hospice. This also is rare and may occur if a patient/family decides to retry curative treatment, is unhappy with the hospice program, or move to another city/state (CMS, 2020b, 2020c). In instances where the safety of the hospice staff is placed at risk, the hospice can discharge a patient from service if a resolution cannot be found (CMS, 2020b, 2020c).

Hospice Care Team

The Medicare hospice benefit requires that a patient and family are offered services from an established team of interdisciplinary professionals to meet their end-of-life needs (CMS, 2020b, 2020c). The hospice interdisciplinary team consists of a hospice physician, nurse case manager, hospice aide, social worker, chaplain, and trained volunteer. In addition, specialized services such as those of a nutritionist or skilled therapist (physical or occupational) can also be assigned to meet the palliative needs of the patient. All hospice interventions are implemented and managed through the RN case manager with the hospice interdisciplinary team as written in the patient care plan (CMS, 2020b, 2020c).

Hospice physician/medical directors ensure the treatment and services provided to the patient and family are effective and that the patient's medical status is progressively declining. Sometimes a patient's status improves to the point of lengthening the prognosis to greater than 6 months. When this occurs, a well-developed discharge plan is initiated over the course of several weeks so the patient and family can adjust and establish a new plan to care for their loved one. Live discharge due to an improved patient prognosis occurs about 5% to 10% of the time (CMS, 2020b, 2020c; National Hospice and Palliative Care Organization [NHPCO], 2020). According to the Medicare hospice benefit, should the patient's condition begin to deteriorate once again after discharge, the patient can be reevaluated for hospice eligibility and be readmitted if the 6-month prognosis is determined by the hospice physician (CMS, 2020b, 2020c).

Nurse case managers have an extensive role that implements and manages the plan of care for the patient. They meet with the patient and family often. The frequency of these home visitsdepends on the needs of the patient. The goal of the RN is to assess and create a care plan that addresses patient symptoms and supports the patient's functional status in accordance with her or his quality-of-life goals (CMS, 2020c). RNs also coordinate all other professional and team visits with the patient and family. They are responsible for providing all appropriate medication, supplies, equipment, and personal care via a trained hospice aide for palliation (CMS, 2020b, 2020c).

Every 2 weeks, the RN case manager meets with the hospice medical director and team in an interdisciplinary team (IDT) meeting to review the effectiveness of the care plan (CMS, 2020c). Collaboration during the IDT meeting improves interdisciplinary communication and problem solving for patient and family issues. For example, if a patient displays signs of severe suffering despite aggressive pain medication, alternative intervention such as a psychosocial or spiritual evaluation can be key to identifying the source of the suffering and address the issue. Whole-person care with interdisciplinary collaboration is essential to solving complex end-of-life issues for some patients and families. This biweekly update of the care plan is part of the hospice conditions of participation for Medicare certification and reimbursement and improves the quality of care (CMS, 2020b, 2020c).

Most hospice services are provided wherever a patient calls home, but there are three other levels of care from which patients and families can benefit should patient symptoms or caregiver burden become too overwhelming (CMS, 2020b, 2020c; NHPCO, 2020). Continuous home care is utilized when there is a significant symptom burden. This service provides in-home RN and hospice aid coverage to resolve brief periods of crisis while keeping the patient home. General in-patient care requires transferring the patient to a hospice inpatient unit or skilled nursing facility for 24-hour RN monitoring and is utilized during end-of-life crises/complex situations or when aggressive pain or symptom management is not feasible in the patient's home. Finally, respite care is available, which provides a 5-day transfer of the patient to a skilled care facility to give the family/caregiver a rest or to cover during a caregiver's absence.

Hospice social workers (SWs) and chaplains attend to the social, psychological, and spiritual needs of the patient and loved ones. These hospice professionals are trained to integrate patient well-being, family dynamics, and the practical responsibilities that accompany the dying process (CMS, 2020b). They personally counsel family discord and use community resources to help the patient and family navigate responsibilities such as funeral planning, wills, insurance, caregiving needs, and much more. Spiritual care, bereavement support, and volunteer visits are core elements available to the hospice patient and family as well. These services are offered to the patient and family at the time of admission and throughout the course of enrollment; grief and bereavement support is available to the surviving family members for over 13 months after the patient's death (CMS, 2020b, 2020c).

Most patients electing hospice are covered by Medicare, with 5% of patients using private insurance or philanthropic funds (CMS, 2020c; NHPCO, 2020). Both for-profit and nonprofit hospice organizations participate with the conditions of the Medicare hospice benefit to receive reimbursement. These organizations all comply with the standards and requirements set by Medicare. Patients may prefer one hospice over another and have a right to enroll in the hospice of their choice (CMS, 2020c; NHPCO, 2020). For complaints of hospice care, patients or families can file the complaint with the Medicare Beneficiary and Family-Centered Care Quality Improvement Organization (BFCC-QIO). These professionals review complaints, "quick appeals," and quality-of-care issues for Medicare recipients (CMS, 2020b, 2020c).

Role of the Nurse Practitioner or Physician Assistant in Hospice Care

The roles of NPs and PAs in hospice are new and evolving. Medicare has been challenged to modernize its regulations to keep pace with the needs of hospice beneficiaries and an increased influx of admissions. With an aging US population and a physician shortage forecast, NPs and PAs can be a solution to increased hospice demand. Changes to Medicare regulations have increased the utilization of NPs and PAs in hospice. For example, Medicare now recognizes both NPs and PAs as attending providers when patients who elect hospice declare them as their attending provider (American Academy of Physician Assistants (AAPA), 2018; CMS, 2020c). This choice/declaration by the patient or surrogate must occur at the time of hospice enrollment. Once this designation is established, it enables NPs and PAs to be reimbursed for oversight of the hospice plan of care and to provide primary care for the patient should a medical concern arise outside the hospice diagnosis (American Academy of Physician Assistants [AAPA], 2018; CMS, 2020c). For example, if a hospice patient with a diagnosis of end-stage cancer falls and fractures a wrist, the attending NP or PA provider can treat and bill for the fracture using Medicare part A or B. This is allowed because the wrist fracture is not part of the hospice diagnosis, yet it is still part of standard care per Medicare (CMS, 2020b, 2020c).

When compared, the roles of NPs and PAs in terms of the Medicare hospice benefit have some disparities. For example, PAs are not permitted to perform the face-to-face exams for patient recertification and cannot place some medication orders (American Academy of Physician Assistants [AAPA], 2018; CMS, 2020b, 2020c). This barrier stems from the omission of PAs in the original Medicare hospice statues and provisions. This omission predated the expansive growth of the PA profession and is not due to the training or ability of the PA to provide complex symptom management and end-of-life care (Boucher & Nix, 2016). In addition to the PA medical model of training, PAs also receive training in palliative care, hospice, serious illness communication, advance care planning, POLST, and pain management (ARC-PA, 2020). Modernization of the Medicare hospice benefit is an ongoing challenge for PA advocates (Boucher & Nix, 2016).

Summary

When palliative interventions become part of serious illness care, patients and families report increased quality of life (Meier & McCormick, 2020). Hospitals, accountable care organizations (ACOs), and payment models are evolving to extend palliative care services to patients earlier in the course of their disease. As providers of palliative care move upstream earlier in the course of serious illness and if palliative care is available everywhere, more people will have access to the care they want; subsequent benefits of having access to care include fewer futile interventions, less discordant care, and less suffering (Meyers, 2018). Expanding the traditional boundaries of hospice and palliative specialty care to include quality telehealth and community-based care may be the next step in advocating for patients aged 65 and older.

Key Points

- Palliative care is the practice of alleviating the physical discomfort, psychosocial despair, and existential distress that can accompany serious illness.
- Primary palliative care is composed of skills that all practitioners should have and includes managing uncomplicated pain and symptoms, treating anxiety and depression, incorporating cultural and spiritual aspects into care, initiating advance care planning, and coordinating services between interdisciplinary professionals.
- Secondary (specialist) palliative care is practiced by an interdisciplinary team of clinicians with additional training; these clinicians are skilled in having more complicated goals of care/serious illness conversations, have experience in the provision of complex pain and symptom management, provide support and management of patient/family conflicts, utilize tools to address ethical dilemmas, understand how to support uniquely complicated end-of-life syndromes, and provide appropriate transitions to other settings of care (including hospice).
- Palliative care can be integrated into the plan of care for any patient experiencing suffering due to serious illness or chronic disease.
- The beneficial outcomes of palliative care include higher patient satisfaction, lower health care costs, and better treatment outcomes.
- The training of both NPs and PAs is conducive for communicating with serious illness patients and working on interdisciplinary palliative care teams.
- Palliative care training is available for NPs and PAs to advance their skills in delivering patient concordant care in primary, specialty, and hospital settings.

More information about tools and Interprofessional Education Collaborative (IPEC) competencies mentioned in this chapter can be found in Appendix 1: Tools and Appendix 2: IPEC Competencies.

References

Albert, R. H. (2017). End-of-life care: Managing common symptoms. *American Family Physician, 95*(6), 356–361.

American Academy of Hospice and Palliative Medicine. (2013, September 13). *Statement on artificial nutrition and hydration near the end of life*. http://aahpm.org/positions/anh.

American Academy of Hospice and Palliative Medicine. (2014). *Statement on palliative sedation*. http://aahpm.org/positions/palliative-sedation.

American Academy of Physician Assistants (AAPA). (2018). *New law permits PAs to provide hospice care to Medicare patients*. https://www.aapa.org/news-central/2018/02/new-law-permits-pas-provide-hospice-care-medicare-patients/.

American Geriatrics Society Panel on Persistent Pain in Older Persons. (2002). The management of persistent pain in older persons. *Journal of the American Geriatrics Society, 50*(6 Suppl.), S205–S224. https://doi.org/10.1046/j.1532-5415.50.6s.1.x.

American Geriatrics Society Panel on Pharmacological Management of Persistent Pain in Older Persons. (2009). Pharmacological management of persistent pain in older persons. *Journal of the American Geriatrics Society, 57*(8), 1331–1346. https://doi.org/10.1111/j.1532-5415.2009.02376.x.

American Medical Association. (2017). *Code of medical ethics 5.1 advance care planning*. https://policysearch.ama-assn.org/policyfinder/detail/advance%20directive?uri=%2FAMADoc%2FEthics.xml-E-5.1.xml.

ARC-PA. (2020). *Accreditation review commission on education for physician assistants* (5th ed.). http://www.arc-pa.org/accreditation/standards-of-accreditation/.

Ariadne Labs. (2021). *Serious illness care*. https://www.ariadnelabs.org/serious-illness-care/.

Boucher, N., & Nix, H. (2016). The benefits of expanded physician assistant practice in hospice and palliative medicine. *Journal of the American Academy of Physician Assistants, 29*, 38–43. https://doi.org/10.1097/01.JAA.0000490948.25684.

Carr, D., & Luth, E. (2017). Advance care planning: Contemporary issues and future directions. *Innovation in Aging, 1*(1), igx012. https://www.ncbi.nlm.nih.gov/pmc/articles/PMC6177019/#CIT0001.

Center for Medicare and Medicaid Services (CMS). (2020a). *Care coordination to help manage chronic disease*. https://www.cms.gov/About-CMS/Agency-Information/OMH/equity-initiatives/ccm/patient-resources.

Center for Medicare and Medicaid Services (CMS). (2020b). *Medicare hospice benefit*. https://www.medicare.gov/Pubs/pdf/02154-Medicare-Hospice-Benefits.PDF.

Center for Medicare and Medicaid Services (CMS). (2020c). Chapter 9: Coverage of hospice services under hospital insurance. In *Medicare hospice policy manual*. https://www.cms.gov/Regulations-and-Guidance/Guidance/Manuals/Downloads/bp102c09.pdf.

Center for Medicare and Medicaid Services (CMS). (2020d). Coverage guidance. In Local coverage determinations for hospice. https://www.cms.gov/medicare-coverage-database/view/lcd.aspx?lcdid=33393&ver=5&keyword=hospice%20diagnosis&keywordType=starts&areaId=all&docType=NCA,CAL,NCD,MEDCAC,TA,MCD,6,3,5,1,F,P&contractOption=all&sortBy=relevance&bc=1 https://www.capc.org/the-case-for-palliative-care/. https://www.capc.org/the-case-for-palliative-care/.

Centers for Disease Control and Prevention (CDC). (2019). *Leading causes of death*. https://www.cdc.gov/nchs/fastats/leading-causes-of-death.htm.

Christakis, N. A., & Lamont, E. B. (2000). Extent and determinants of error in doctors' prognoses in terminally ill patients: Prospective cohort study. *BMJ (Clinical Research Ed.), 320*(7233). https://doi.org/10.1136/bmj.320.7233.469.

Cloyes, K. G., Hull, W., & Davis, A. (2018). Palliative and end-of-life care for lesbian, gay, bisexual and transgender (LGBT) cancer patients and their caregivers. *Seminars in Oncology Nursing, 34*(1). https://doi.org/10.1016/j.soncn.2017.12.003.

Competencies for the physician assistant (PA) profession. (2020). From the Pennsylvania Art Education Association. https://paea-online.org/wp-content/uploads/imported-files/competencies-for-the-pa-profession-060520.pdf.

Connor, S., Centeno, C., Garralda, E., Clelland, D., & Clark, D. (2020). Estimating the number of patients receiving specialized palliative care globally in 2017. *Journal of Pain and Symptom Management, 61*(4), 812–816.

Coyne, P., Mulvenon, C., & Paice, J. A. (2018). American Society for Pain Management Nursing and Hospice and Palliative Nurses Association position statement: Pain Management at the End of life. *American Society for Pain Management Nursing, 19*(1 [February]), 3–7.

Curseen, K. (2019). *Implicit bias and its impact on palliative care (part one and two)*. https://www.capc.org/blog/palliative-pulse-palliative-pulse-june-2017-implicit-bias-and-palliative-care-part-1/.

Dugdale, L. S., Lerner, B. H., & Callahan, D. (2019). Pros and cons of physician aid in dying. *Yale Journal of Biology and Medicine, 92*(4), 747–750.

Enclara Pharmacia. (2021, January 18). *Hospices and the five social determinants of health*. https://enclarapharmacia.com/hospices-social-determinants-of-health.

Fischler, R. S., & Fagan, T. C. (2018, March). *End of life care survey of Arizona physicians*. https://azpulse.org/end-of-life-survey-of-arizona-physicians/.

Givler, A., Bhatt, H., & Maani-Fogelman, P. A. (2021). The importance of cultural competence in pain and palliative care. In *StatPearls*. https://www.ncbi.nlm.nih.gov/books/NBK493154/.

Henson, L. A., Maddocks, M., Davidson, M., Hicks, S., & Higginson, I. J. (2020, Mar). Palliative care and the management of common distressing symptoms in advanced cancer: Pain, breathlessness, nausea and vomiting, and fatigue. *Journal of Clinical Oncology, 38*(9), 905–914. https://doi.org/10.1200/JCO.19.00470.

Hopping-Winn, J., Mullin, L., March, M., Caughey, M., Stern, M., & Jarvie, J. (2018). The progression of end-of-life wishes and concordance with end-of-life care. *Journal of Palliative Medicine, 21*(4), 541–545. https://doi.org/10.1089/jpm.2017.0317.

Hospice and Palliative Nurses Association. (2016). Value, policy, and position statements. https://advancingexpertcare.org/position-statements/.

Howard, M., Bernard, C., Klein, D., Elston, D., Tan, A., Slaven, M., & Heyland, D. (2018). Barriers to and enablers of advance care planning with patients in primary care: Survey of health care providers. *Canadian Family Physician/Medecin de Famille Canadien, 64*(4), e190–e198. https://pubmed.ncbi.nlm.nih.gov/29650621/.

Hyden, K., Gelfmin, L., Dionne-Odom, N., Smith, C., & Coats, H. (n.d.). Update in hospice and palliative care. *Journal of Palliative Medicine*, 23(2), 165–169. https://doi.org/10.1089/jpm.2019.0500.

Institute of Medicine (US) Committee on Care at End of Life. (1997). In M. J. Field & C. K. Cassel, *Approaching death: Improving care at the end of life*. National Academies Press.

Institute of Medicine. (2015). *Dying in America: Improving quality and honoring individual preferences near the end of life*. The National Academies Press. https://doi.org/10.17226/18748.

Kavalieatos, D., Corbelli, J., Zhang, Di, Dionne-Odom, N., Ernecoff, N. C., Hanmer, J., Hoydich, Z. P., Ikejiani, D. Z., Klein-Fedyshin, M., Zimmermann, C., Morton, S. C., Arnold, R. M., Heller, L., Schenker, Y., & Zhang, D. (2016). Association between palliative care and patient and caregiver outcomes: A systematic review and meta-analysis. *Journal of the American Medical Association, 316*(20), 2104–2114. https://doi.org/10.1001/jama.2016.16840.

Kelley, A. S., & Morrison, R. S. (2015). Palliative care for the seriously ill. *New England Journal of Medicine, 373*(8), 747–755. https://doi.org/10.1056/NEJMra1404684.

Klement, A., & Marks, S. (2020). The pitfalls of utilizing "goals of care" as a clinical buzz phrase: A case study and proposed solution. *Palliative Medicine Reports*, 216–220. http://online.liebertpub.com/doi/10.1089/pmr.2020.0063.

LeBlanc, T. W., & Tulsky, J. (2020). Discussing goals of care. *UpToDate(R)*. https://www.uptodate.com/contents/discussing-goals-of-care.

Lum, H., & Sudore, R. (2016). Advance care planning and goals of care communication in older adults with cardiovascular disease and multi-morbidity. *Clinical Geriatric Medicine, 32*(2), 247–260. https://doi.org/10.1016/j.cger.2016.01.011.

Lunney, J. R., Lynn, J., Foley, D. J., Lipson, S., & Guralnik, J. M. (2003). Patterns of functional decline at the end of life. *Journal of the American Medical Association, 289*(18), 2387–2392. https://doi.org/10.1001/jama.289.18.2387.

Lutz, S. (2011). The history of hospice and palliative care. *Current Problems in Cancer, 35*(6), 304–309. https://doi.org/10.1016/j.currproblcancer.2011.10.004.

McGuire, D. B., Snow Kaiser, K., Haisfield-Wolfe, M., & Iyamu, F. (2016). Pain assessment in noncommunicative adult palliative care patients. *Nursing Clinics of North America, 51*(3), 397–431. https://doi.org/10.1016/j.cnur.2016.05.009.

Medicare Payment Advisory Commission. (2015). *Report to the Congress: Medicare and the health care delivery system*. https://www.medpac.gov/wp-content/uploads/import_data/scrape_files/docs/default-source/reports/jun21_medpac_report_to_congress_sec.pdf.

Meier, D. (2019). *State-by-state access to hospital palliative care*. https://media.capc.org/recorded-webinars/slides/CAPCWebinar_ReportCard_Final.pdf.

Meier, D., & McCormick, E. (2020). Benefits, services and models of subspecialty palliative care. *UpToDate*. https://www.

uptodate.com/contents/benefits-services-and-models-of-subspecialty-palliative-care?search=primary%20palliative%20care%20table%201&topicRef=2199&source=related_link.

Meier, E. A., Gallegos, J. V., Thomas, L. P., Depp, C. A., Irwin, S. A., & Jeste, D. V. (2016). Defining a good death (successful dying): Literature review and a call for research and public dialogue. *American Journal of Geriatric Psychiatry: Official Journal of the American Association for Geriatric Psychiatry, 24*(4), 261–271. https://doi.org/10.1016/j.jagp.2016.01.135.

Meyers, K. (2018). *As boundaries blur, "palliative care everywhere" is the goal.* California: Health Care Foundation blog. https://www.chcf.org/blog/as-boundaries-blur-palliative-care-every where-is-the-goal/.

Mirarchi, F., Doshi, A., Zerkle, S., & Clooney, T. (2015). TRIAD VI: How well do emergency physicians understand physician orders for life sustaining treatment (POLST) forms? *Journal of Patient Safety, 11*(1), 1–8. https://doi/10.1097/PTS.0000000000000165.

Mitchell, S. L., Kiely, D. K., Hamel, M. B., Park, P. S., Morris, J. N., & Fries, B. E. (n.d.). Estimating prognosis for nursing home residents with advanced dementia. *Journal of the American Medical Association, 291*(22), 2734–2740. https://doi.org/10.1001/jama.291.22.2734.

Morishima, T., Sato, A., Nakata, K., & Miyashiro, I. (2020). Geriatric assessment domains to predict overall survival in older cancer patients: An analysis of functional status, comorbidities, and nutritional status as prognostic factors. *Cancer Medicine, 9*(18), 5839–5850. https://doi.org/10.1002/cam4.3205.

Moss, A., Zive, D., Falkenstine, E., & Dunithan, C. (2017). The quality of POLST completion to guide treatment: A 2-state study. *Journal of the American Medical Directors Association, 18*(9), 810.e5–810. https://doi/.org/10.1016/j.jamda.2017.05.01.

National Hospice and Palliative Care Organization (NHPCO). (2020). *Facts and figures.* https://www.nhpco.org/factsfigures/.

National Hospice and Palliative Care Organization Diversity Advisory Council. (2021). *LGBTQ+ resource guide.* https://www.nhpco.org/new-hospice-and-palliative-care-resource-guide-for-lgbtq-communities.

National Organization of Nurse Practitioner Faculties (NONPF). (2017). *Nurse practitioner core competencies.* https://cdn.ymaws.com/www.nonpf.org/resource/resmgr/competencies/2017_NPCoreComps_with_Curric.pdf.

National POLST. (2021). *National POLST form: Guide for professionals.* https://polst.org/wp-content/uploads/2021/03/2021.03-Form-Guide.pdf.

National Quality Forum. (2012, April). *Palliative care and end-of-life care: A consensus report.* https://www.qualityforum.org/Publications/2012/04/Palliative_Care_and_End-of-Life_Care%e2%80%94A_Consensus_Report.asp.

Office of Disease Prevention and Health Promotion. (2020). *Social determinants of health.* https://health.gov/healthypeople/objectives-and-data/browse-objectives#social-determinants-of-health.

Oluyase, A. O., Higginson, I. J., Yi, D., Gao, W., Evans, C. J., Grande, G., Todd, C., Costantini, M., Murtagh, F., & Bajwah, S. (2021). Hospital-based specialist palliative care compared with usual care for adults with advanced illness and their caregivers: A systematic review. PMID: 34057828.

Patient Decision Aids. (2020). The Ottawa Hospital Research Institute. https://decisionaid.ohri.ca/AZlist.html.

Pope, T. (2021). Legal aspects in palliative and end of life care in the Unites States. *UpToDate.* https://www.uptodate.com/contents/legal-aspects-in-palliative-and-end-of-life-care-in-the-united-states?search=legal-aspects-in-Palliative-and-end-of-life-care-in-the-united-states&source=search_result&selectedTitle=1~150&usage_type=default&display_rank=1.

Prabhakar, A., & Smith, T. J. (2021, March). *Palliative Care Network of Wisconsin.* https://www.mypcnow.org/fast-fact/total-pain/.

Quill, T. E., & Abernethy, A. P. (2013). Generalist plus specialist palliative care: Creating a more sustainable model. *New England Journal of Medicine,* 1173–1175. https://doi.org/10.1056/NEJMp1215620.

Reid, M. C., Eccleston, C., & Pillemer, K. (2015). Management of chronic pain in older adults. *BMJ (Clinical Research ed.), 350,* h532. https://doi.org/10.1136/bmj.h532.

Rich, B. (2001). Physicians' legal duty to relieve suffering. *Western Journal of Medicine, 175*(3), 151–152. https://doi.org/10.1136/ewjm.175.3.151.

Rogers, J., Patel, C., Mentz, R., Granger, B., Steinhauser, K., Fiuzat, M., Adams, P., Speck, A., Johnson, K., Krishnamoorthy, A., Yang, H., Anstrom, K., Dodson, G., Taylor, D. Jr., Kirchner, J., Mark, D., O'Connor, C., & Tulsky, J. (2017). Palliative care in heart failure: The PAL-HF randomized, controlled clinical trial. *Journal of the American College of Cardiology, 70*(3), 331–341. https://doi.org/10.1016/j.jacc.2017.05.030.

Schluep, M., Gravesteijn, B., Stolker, R., Endeman, H., & Hoeks, E. (2018). One-year survival after in-hospital cardiac arrest: A systematic review and meta-analysis. *Resuscitation, 32,* 90–100. https://doi.org/10.1016/j.resuscitation.2018.09.001.

Severson, S. (2020). Communicating serious illness and introduction to POLST: Train the trainer. *Arizona Hospital and Home Care Association.* https://www.azhha.org/arizonapolst_forms

Shah, P., Thornton, I., & Hipskind, J. (2020, March 30). *Informed consent.* https://www.ncbi.nlm.nih.gov/books/NBK430827.

Siamak, N. (2021). *Advance medical directives (living will, power of attorney, and health-care proxy).* https://www.medicinenet.com/advance_medical_directives/article.htm.

Silveira, M. (2021). Advance care planning and advance directives. *UpToDate.* https://www.uptodate.com/contents/advance-care-planning-and-advance-directives?search=advance-care-planning-and-%20Advance-directive&source=search_result&selectedTitle=1~150&usage_type=default&display_rank=1.

Steinhauser, K., Christakis, N., Clipp, E., McNeilly, M., McIntyre, L., & Tulsky, J. (2000). Factors considered important at the end of life by patients, family, physicians and other care providers. *Journal of the American Medical Association, 284*(19), 2476–2482. https://doi.org/10.1001/jama.284.19.2476.

Stone, P., Vickerstaff, V., Kalpakidou, A., Todd, C., Griffiths, J., Keeley, K., & Omar, R. Z. (2021). Prognostic tools or clinical predictions: Which are better in palliative care. *PLOS ONE, 16*(4), e0249763. https://doi.org/10.1371/journal.pone.0249763.

Sudden Cardiac Arrest Foundation. (2019). *Sudden cardiac arrest.* https://jtbfoundation.org/sudden-cardiac-arrest/.

Swami, M., & Case, A. A. (2018). Effective palliative care: What is involved? *Oncology, 32*(4), 180–187.

Swihart, D. L., Yarrarapu, S., & Martin, R. L. (2021). Cultural religious competence in clinical practice. *In StatPearls* PMID: 2963026.

Tolle, S., & Ferrell, B. (2021). *Becoming more inclusive of our NP and PA colleagues.* https://www.youtube.com/watch?v=tnqjLFLupaQ

Vink, E., Azoulay, E., Caplan, A., Kompanje, E., & Bakker, J. (2018). Time-limited trial of intensive care treatment: An overview of current literature. *Intensive Care Medicine, 44,* 1369–1377. https://doi.org/10.1007/s00134-018-5339-x.

Vitelli, M., Holloway, D., Tellson, A., Nguyen, H., Estimon, K., Linthicum, J., & Huddleston, P. (2020). Surgical patients' and registered nurses' satisfaction and perception of using the Clinically

Aligned Pain Assessment (CAPA(c)) Tool for pain assessment. *Journal of Vascular Nursing, 38*(3), 118–131.

Voumard, R., Rubli Truchard, E., Benaroyo, L., Borasio, G. D., Bula, C., & Jox, R. J. (2018). Geriatric palliative care: A view of its concept, challenges and strategies. *BMC Geriatrics, 18*(220).

Webb, J. A., & Casarett, D. (2017). A prescription for population-based palliative care education. *Generations, 41*(1), 68–73.

White, N., Kupeli, N., Vickerstaff, V., & Stone, P. (2017). How accurate is the "surprise question" at identifying patients at end of life? A systematic review and meta-analysis. *BMC Medicine*, 15. https://doi.org/10.1186/s12916-017-0907-4.

Wood, H., Dickman, A., Star, A., & Boland, J. W. (2018, Feb). Updates in palliative care: Overview and recent advancements in the pharmacological management of cancer pain. *Clin Med (London), 18*(1), 17–22.

Yadav, K., Gabler, N., Cooney, E., Kent, S., Kim, J., Herbst, N., & Courtright, K. (2017). Approximately one in three US adults completes any type of advance directive for end-of-life care. *Health Affairs (Project Hope), 36*(7), 1244–1251. https://doi.org/10.1377/hlthaff.2017.0175.

Zeng, Y. S., Wang, C., Ward, K. E., & Hume, A. (2018). Complementary and alternative medicine in hospice and palliative care: A systematic review. *Journal of Pain and Symptom Management, 56*(5), 781–794 e4. https://doi.org/10.1016/j.jpainsymman.2018.07.016.

Zhang, H., Paice, J., Portenoy, R., Bruera, E., Carrington Reid, M., & Bao, Y. (2021). Prescription opioids dispenses to patients with cancer with bone metastasis: 2011–2017. *The Oncologist* https://doi.org/10.1002/onco.13898.

Appendix 1

Tools

Chapter 1

ADAM Questionnaire

Androgen Deficiency in the Aging Male (ADAM) Questionnaire

This basic questionnaire about symptoms of low testosterone can be very useful for men to describe the kind and severity of their low testosterone symptoms.

1. Do you have a decrease in libido (sex drive)? Yes No
2. Do you have a lack of energy? Yes No
3. Do you have a decrease in strength and/or endurance? Yes No
4. Have you lost height? Yes No
5. Have you noticed a decreased "enjoyment of life"? Yes No
6. Are you sad and/or grumpy? Yes No
7. Are your erections less strong? Yes No
8. Have you noticed a recent deterioration in your ability to play sports? Yes No
9. Are you falling asleep after dinner? Yes No
10. Has there been a recent deterioration in your work performance? Yes No

If you answer Yes to number 1 or 7 or if you answer Yes to more than 3 questions, you may have low testosterone.

From Morley, J. (2000). Validation of a screening questionnaire for androgen deficiency in aging males. *Metabolism, 49*(9), 1239–1242.

Chapter 2

Rapid Estimate of Adult Literacy in Medicine—Short Form (REALM-SF)

Rapid Estimate of Adult Literacy in Medicine—Short Form (REALM-SF)

The Rapid Estimate of Adult Literacy in Medicine—Short Form (REALM-SF) is a 7-item word recognition test to provide clinicians with a valid quick assessment of patient health literacy. The REALM-SF has been validated and field tested in diverse research settings and has excellent agreement with the 66-item REALM instrument in terms of grade-level assignments.

REALM-SF Score Sheet

Patient ID #: ______________ Date: ______________ Examiner Initials: ___________

Behavior _____

Exercise _____

Menopause _____

Rectal _____

Antibiotics _____

Anemia _____

Jaundice _____

TOTAL SCORE ______

Administering the REALM-SF

Suggested Introduction

"Providers often use words that patients don't understand. We are looking at words providers often use with their patients in order to improve communication between health care providers and patients. Here is a list of medical words.

Starting at the top of the list, please read each word aloud to me. If you don't recognize a word, you can say 'pass' and move on to the next word."

Interviewer: Give the participant the word list. If the participant takes more than 5 seconds on a word, say "pass" and point to the next word. Hold this scoring sheet so that it is not visible to the participant.

Scores and Grade Equivalents for the REALM-SF

Score	Grade Range
0	Third grade and below; will not be able to read most low-literacy materials; will need repeated oral instructions, materials composed primarily of illustrations or audio or videotapes.
1–3	Fourth to sixth grade; will need low-literacy materials, may not be able to read prescription labels.
4–6	Seventh to eighth grade; will struggle with most patient education materials; will not be offended by low-literacy materials.
7	High school; will be able to read most patient education materials.

(Davis, T., Crouch, M., & Long, S. (1993). *Rapid estimate of adult literacy in medicine (REALM)*. Shreveport, LA: LSU Med Ctr From U.S. Department of Health & Human Services. https://www.ahrq.gov/professionals/quality-patient-safety/quality-resources/tools/literacy/index.html#rapid. (The REALM-SF was developed with AHRQ funding, independently of REALM. To obtain permission to use the REALM, contact Dr. Terry Davis at tdavis1@lsuhsc.edu.)

REALM-SF Validation study: Arozullah, A. M., Yarnold, P. R., Bennett, C. L., et al. (2007). Development and validation of a short-form, rapid estimate of adult literacy in medicine. Medical Care, *45*(11), 1026–1033. PMID: 18049342.

Short Test of Functional Health Literacy in Adults (TOFUL-A)

The Short Test of Functional Health Literacy in Adults (TOFHLA) provides a complete estimate of patients' functional health literacy. This test takes approximately 7 minutes to complete.

Data from Baker, D. W., Williams, M. V., Parker, R. M., Gazmararian, J. A., & Nurss, J. (1999). Development of a brief test to measure functional health literacy. *Patient Education and Counseling, 38*(1), 33–42. https://doi.org/10.1016/s0738-3991(98)00116-5. PMID: 14528569.

Chapter 3

Short Test of Functional Health Literacy in Adults (TOFUL-A)

(See Appendix 1, Chapter 2)

Rapid Estimate of Adult Literacy in Medicine—Short Form (REALM-SF)

(See Appendix 1, Chapter 2)

Chapter 4

Aid to Capacity Evaluation

Used to determine if a person has the mental capacity to understand the medical problem, treatment, consequences of the treatment, and consequences of refusing treatment.

Capacity to Consent to Treatment Instrument

The capacity to consent to treatment requires the ability to understand and retain information, to use this information as part of the decision-making process, and to make free choices. This capacity is specific to a particular decision and can be unstable.

Data from Moye, J., Karel, M. J., Guerra, R., & Azar, A. (2004). Capacity to consent to treatment: Empirical comparison of three instruments in older adults with and without dementia. *Gerontologist 44*(2), 166–175. https://doi.org/10.1093/geront/44.2.166

Elder Abuse Screening Tools for Health Care Professionals

Screening Tools

At the Elder Mistreatment Symposium convened by the Centers for Medicare and Medicaid Services in 2013, three screening tools (presented in table below) were identified for increased use in practice for the screening of elder mistreatment. These tools were identified for their ability to assess multiple types of abuse, for the specifications of the measure, and for the focus of each tool when combined (McMullen et al., 2014). These tools are intended to be used by trained professionals in health care settings.

Assessment Items Administration Psychometrics Setting Elder Abuse Suspicion Index (EASI)	6	Completed by health care professional to assess risk, neglect, verbal, psychological, emotional, financial, physical, and sexual abuse over a 12-month period; 2 minutes to complete	Sensitivity: 0.77 Specificity: 0.44	Validated in family practices and ambulatory care settings
Hwalek-Sengstock Elder Abuse Screening Test (H-S/EAST)	6	Self-report or interview by a professional	Construct and predictive validity, weak item reliability, but good cross-cultural adaptation	Suitable in emergency or outpatient setting
Vulnerability Tt Abuse Screening Scale (VASS)	12	Self-report of dependency, dejection, coercion, and vulnerability	Moderate ranges of reliability and moderate to good construct validity	N/A

Other Elder Abuse Screening Tools With Psychometrics

- Brief Elder Screen for the Elderly (BASE) (Reis et al., 1993)
- Caregiver Abuse Screen (CASE) (Reis & Namiash, 1995)
- Elder Assessment Instrument (EAI) (Fulmer & O'Maliey, 1987)
- Expanded Indicators of Abuse (E-IOA) (Cohen et al., 2006)
- Geriatrics Mistreatment Scale (GMS) (Giraldo-Rodriguez & Rosas-Carrasco, 2013)
- Indicators of Abuse (IOA) (Reis & Nahmiash, 1998)
- Older Adult Financial Exploitation Measure (OAFEM) (Conrad et al., 2010)
- Screening Tools and Referral Protocol Stopping Abuse Against Older Ohioans: A Guide for Service Providers (Bass et al., 2001)
- Self-disclosure tool (Cohen et al., 2007)
- Signs of abuse inventory (Cohen, 2011)

Without Psychometrics

- Case Detection Guidelines (Rathbone-McCuan, 1980)
- Elder Abuse and Neglect Protocol (Tomita, 1983)
- Health, Attitudes towards aging, Living arrangements, and Finances (H.A.L.F.) (Ferguson & Beck, 1983)
- Screening Protocols for the Identification of Abuse and Neglect in the Elderly (Johnson, 1981)

Burnett et al., 2014.
From National Center on Elder Abuse, Elder Abuse Screening Tools for Healthcare Professionals, 2016, https://ncea.acl.gov/NCEA/media/Publication/Elder-Abuse-Screening-Tools-for-Healthcare-Professionals.pdf
McMullen, T., Schwartz, K., Yaffe, M., & Beach, S. II.6 Elder Abuse and Its Prevention: Screening and Detection. Institute of Medicine and National Research Council. 2014. Elder Abuse and Its Prevention: Workshop Summary. Washington, DC: The National Academies Press. doi: 10.17226/18518.
National Academies of Sciences, Engineering, and Medicine. 2014. Elder Abuse and Its Prevention: Workshop Summary. Washington, DC: The National Academies Press. https://doi.org/10.17226/18518.
For full references, see original source in table.

Elder Abuse Suspicion Index (EASI)

EASI Questions
Q.I–Q.5 asked of patient; Q.6 answered by doctor
Within the past 12 months:

(1) Have you relied on people for any of the following: bathing, dressing, shopping, banking, or meals?	Yes	No	Did not answer
(2) Has anyone prevented you from getting food, clothes, medication, glasses, hearing aids, or medical care, or from being with people you wanted to be with?	Yes	No	Did not answer
(3) Have you been upset because someone talked to you in a way that made you feel shamed or threatened?	Yes	No	Did not answer
(4) Has anyone tried to force you to sign papers or to use your money against your will?	Yes	No	Did not answer
(5) Has anyone made you afraid, touched you in ways that you did not want, or hurt you physically?	Yes	No	Did not answer
(6) Doctor: Elder abuse may be associated with findings such as poor eye contact, withdrawn nature, malnourishment, hygiene issues, cuts, bruises, inappropriate clothing, or medication compliance issues. Did you notice any of these today or in the last 12 months?	Yes	No	Not sure

The EASI was developed* to raise a doctor's suspicion about elder abuse to a level at which it might be reasonable to propose a referral for further evaluation by social services, adult protective services, or equivalents. While all six questions should be asked, a response of "yes" on one or more of questions 2–6 may establish concern. The EASI was validated* for asking by family practitioners of cognitively intact seniors seen in ambulatory settings.

*Table from The University of Iowa: https://medicine.uiowa.edu/familymedicine/sites/medicine.uiowa.edu.familymedicine/files/wysiwyg_uploads/EASI.pdf. (From Mark J. Yaffe, Christina Wolfson, Maxine Lithwick & Deborah Weiss (2008) (EASI)©, Journal of Elder Abuse & Neglect, 20:3, 276-300, https://doi.org/10.1080/08946560801973168). The Elder Abuse Suspicion Index (EASI) was granted copyright by the Canadian Intellectual Property Office (Industry Canada) February 21, 2006. (Registration # 1036459). Mark J. Yaffe, MD McGill University, Montreal, Canada mark.vaffe@)mcgill.ca Maxine Lithwick, MSW CSSS Cavendish, Montreal, Canada maxine.lithwick.cvd@)ssss.gouv.qc.ca Christina Wolfson, PhD McGill University, Montreal, Canada Christina.wolfson@mcgill.ca

HWALEK-SENGSTOCK ELDER ABUSE SCREENING TEST (H-S/EAST)

Read the questions and write in the answers. A response of "no" to items 1, 6, 12, and 14; a response of "someone else" to item 4; and a response of "yes" to all others is scored in the "abused" direction.

1. Do you have anyone who spends time with you, taking you shopping or to the doctor?
2. Are you helping to support someone?
3. Are you sad or lonely often?
4. Who makes decisions about your life—like how you should live or where you should live?
5. Do you feel uncomfortable with anyone in your family?
6. Can you take your own medication and get around by yourself?
7. Do you feel that nobody wants you around?
8. Does anyone in your family drink a lot?
9. Does someone in your family make you stay in bed or tell you you're sick when you know you're not?
10. Has anyone forced you to do things you didn't want to do?
11. Has anyone taken things that belong to you without your OK?
12. Do you trust most of the people in your family?
13. Does anyone tell you that you give them too much trouble?
14. Do you have enough privacy at home?
15. Has anyone close to you tried to hurt you or harm you recently?

From Neale, A. V., Hwalek, M. A., Scott, R. O., & Stahl, C. (1991). Validation of the Hwalek-Sengstock elder abuse screening test. *Journal of Applied Gerontology, 10*(4), 406–415.

MacArthur Competence Assessment Tool for Treatment (MacCAT-T)

The MacArthur Competence Assessment Tool for Treatment (MacCAT-T) is a semistructured interview that assists clinicians in assessing a patient's competence to consent to treatment.

Data from Grisso, T., Appelbaum, P. S., Hill-Fotouhi, C. (1997). The MacCAT-T: A clinical tool to assess patients' capacities to make treatment decisions. *Psychiatric Services, 48*(11),1415–1419. https://doi.org/10.1176/ps.48.11.1415. PMID: 9355168

MacArthur Competence Assessment Tool for Clinical Research (MacCAT-CR)

The MacCAT-CR provides a structured format for capacity assessment that can typically be administered in 15 to 20 minutes.

Data from Appelbaum, P. S., & Grisso, T. (2001). *MacArthur competence assessment tool for clinical research (MacCAT-CR).* Professional Resource Press/Professional Resource Exchange.

Vulnerability to Abuse Screening Scale (VASS)

Purpose: To identify older women at risk of elder abuse through a self-report instrument.

Instructions: Questionnaire can be mailed to subjects with instructions to answer "yes" or "no."

1.	Are you afraid of anyone in your family?	Yes	No
2.	Has anyone close to you tried to hurt you or harm you recently?	Yes	No
3.	Has anyone close to you called you names or put you down or made you feel bad recently?	Yes	No
4.	Do you have enough privacy at home?	Yes	No
5.	Do you trust most of the people in your family?	Yes	No
6.	Can you take your own medication and get around by yourself?	Yes	No
7.	Are you sad or lonely often?	Yes	No
8.	Do you feel that nobody wants you around?	Yes	No
9.	Do you feel uncomfortable with anyone in your family?	Yes	No
10.	Does someone in your family make you stay in bed or tell you you're sick when you know you're not?	Yes	No
11.	Has anyone forced you to do things you didn't want to do?	Yes	No
12.	Has anyone taken things that belong to you without your OK?	Yes	No

From University of Iowa, https://medicine.uiowa.edu/familymedicine/sites/medicine.uiowa.edu.familymedicine/files/wysiwyg_uploads/VASS.pdf.

Schofield, M. J., & Mishra, G. D. (2003). Validity of self-report screening scale for elder abuse: Women's Health Australia Study. *Gerontologist, 43*(1), 110–120, Table 1.

Chapter 5

The ADAM Questionnaire

(See Appendix 1, Chapter 1)

Montreal Cognitive Assessment (MoCA)

MONTREAL COGNITIVE ASSESSMENT (MOCA)

NAME :
Education : Date of birth :
Sex : DATE :

VISUOSPATIAL / EXECUTIVE

E End
A
5
B
2
1 Begin
D
4
3
C

[ ]

Copy cube [ ]

Draw CLOCK (Ten past eleven) (3 points)

[ ] Contour [ ] Numbers [ ] Hands

POINTS __/5

NAMING

[ ] [ ] [ ] __/3

MEMORY

Read list of words, subject must repeat them. Do 2 trials. Do a recall after 5 minutes.

	FACE	VELVET	CHURCH	DAISY	RED
1st trial					
2nd trial					

No points

ATTENTION

Read list of digits (1 digit/ sec.).
Subject has to repeat them in the forward order [ ] 2 1 8 5 4
Subject has to repeat them in the backward order [ ] 7 4 2
__/2

Read list of letters. The subject must tap with his hand at each letter A. No points if ≥ 2 errors
[ ] FBACMNAAJKLBAFAKDEAAAJAMOFAAB __/1

Serial 7 subtraction starting at 100 [ ] 93 [ ] 86 [ ] 79 [ ] 72 [ ] 65
4 or 5 correct subtractions: 3 pts, 2 or 3 correct: 2 pts, 1 correct: 1 pt, 0 correct: 0 pt __/3

LANGUAGE

Repeat : I only know that John is the one to help today. [ ]
The cat always hid under the couch when dogs were in the room. [ ] __/2

Fluency / Name maximum number of words in one minute that begin with the letter F [ ] ____(N ≥ 11 words) __/1

ABSTRACTION

Similarity between e.g., banana – orange = fruit [ ] train – bicycle [ ] watch – ruler __/2

DELAYED RECALL

Has to recall words WITH NO CUE	FACE [ ]	VELVET [ ]	CHURCH [ ]	DAISY [ ]	RED [ ]	Points for UNCUED recall only
Optional: Category cue						
Optional: Multiple choice cue						

__/5

ORIENTATION

[ ] Date [ ] Month [ ] Year [ ] Day [ ] Place [ ] City __/6

www.mocatest.org

Normal ≥ 26/30

TOTAL __/30
Add 1 point if ≤ 12 yr edu

- Montreal Cognitive Assessment (MoCA) (© Z. Nasreddine MD. www.mocatest.org.)

Chapter 6

CAGE Screening Tool

CAGE Questionnaire

- Have you ever felt you should **C**ut down on your drinking?
- Have people **A**nnoyed you by criticizing your drinking?
- Have you ever felt bad or **G**uilty about your drinking?
- Have you ever had a drink first thing in the morning to steady your nerves or to get rid of a hangover (**E**ye opener)?

Item responses on the CAGE are scored 0 or 1, with a higher score an indication of alcohol problems A total score of 2 or greater is considered clinically significant.
Developed by Dr. John Ewing, founding director of the Bowles Center for Alcohol Studies, University of North Carolina at Chapter Hill. Ewing, J A. (1984). Detecting alcoholism: The CAGE questionnaire. *Journal of the American Medical Association, 252*(14), 1905–1907.

Clock Drawing

Clock Drawing Test

Clock Drawing ID:__________ Date:______________

• Clock Drawing (From Freedman, M. I., Leach, L., Kaplan, E., Winocur, G., Shulman, K. J., Delis, D. C. [Eds.]. [1994]. *Clock drawing*. Oxford University Press.)

Elder Abuse Suspicion Index (EASI)

(See Appendix 1, Chapter 4)

Edmonton Frail Scale (EFS)

The Edmonton Frail ScaleScoring

NAME:______________________________
d.o.b :__________________ **DATE :**__________________

Frailty domain	Item	0 point	1 point	2 points
Cognition	Please imagine that this pre-drawn circle is a clock. I would like you to place the numbers in the correct positions then place the hands to indicate a time of 'ten after eleven'	No errors	Minor spacing errors	Other errors
General health status	In the past year, how many times have you been admitted to a hospital?	0	1-2	≥2
	In general, how would you describe your health?	'Excellent' 'Very good' 'Good'	"Fair"	'Poor'
Functional independence	With how many of the following activities do you require help? (meal preparation, shopping, transportation, telephone, housekeeping, laundry, managing money, taking medications)	0-1	2-4	5-8
Social support	When you need help, can you count on someone who is willing and able to meet your needs?	Always	Sometimes	Never
Medication use	Do you use five or more different prescription medications on a regular basis?	No	Yes	
	At times, do you forget to take your prescription medications?	No	Yes	
Nutrition	Have you recently lost weight such that your clothing has become looser?	No	Yes	
Mood	Do you often feel sad *or* depressed?	No	Yes	
Continence	Do you have a problem with losing control of urine when you don't want to?	No	Yes	
Functional performance	I would like you to sit in this chair with your back and arms resting. Then, when I say 'GO', please stand up and wait at a safe and comfortable pace to the mark on the floor (approximately 3 m away), return to the chair and sit down"	0-10 s	11-20s	One of: >20s, or patient unwilling or requires assistance.
Totals	Final score is the sum of column totals			

Total /17
0-5 = Not Frail
6-7 = Vulnerable
8-9 = Mild Frailty
10-11 = Moderate Frailty
12-17 = Severe Frailty
Administered by:
(From Edmonton Frail Scale (EFS). https://edmontonfrailscale.org/new-index#:~:text=The%20Edmonton%20Frail%20Scale%20is%20a%20multidimensional%20frailty,frailty%20in%20terms%20that%20are%20meaningful%20to%20clinicians.)

Elder Assessment Instrument (EAI)

Purpose: To be used as a comprehensive approach for screening suspected elder abuse victims in all clinical settings.
Instructions: There is no "score" for this instrument. A patient should be referred to social services if the following exists: (1) if there is any positive evidence without sufficient clinical explanation, (2) whenever there is a subjective complaint by the older adult of elder mistreatment, or (3) whenever the clinician deems there is evidence of abuse, neglect, exploitation, or abandonment.

1. General Assessment	Very Good	Good	Poor	Very Poor	Unable to Assess
a. Clothing					
b. Hygiene					
c. Nutrition					
d. Skin integrity					

Additional Comments:

2. Possible Abuse Indicators	No Evidence	Possible Evidence	Probable Evidence	Definite Evidence	Unable to Assess
a. Bruising					
b. Lacerations					
c. Fractures					
d. Various stages of healing of any bruises or fractures					
e. Evidence of sexual abuse					
f. Statement by older adult related to abuse					

Additional Comments:

3. Possible Neglect Indicators	No Evidence	Possible Evidence	Probable Evidence	Definite Evidence	Unable to Assess
a. Contractures					
b. Decubiti					
c. Dehydration					
d. Diarrhea					
e. Depression					
f. Impaction					
g. Malnutrition					
h. Urine burns					
i. Poor hygiene					
j. Failure to respond to warning of obvious disease					
k. Inappropriate medications (over/under)					
l. Repetitive hospital admissions due to probable failure of health care surveillance					
m. Statement by older adult related to neglect					

Additional Comments:

From Fulmer, T. (2003). Elder abuse and neglect assessment. *Journal of Gerontological Nursing*, *29*(6), 4–5. Reprinted by permission: SLACK, Incorporated, Thorofare, New Jersey

Faces Pain Scale

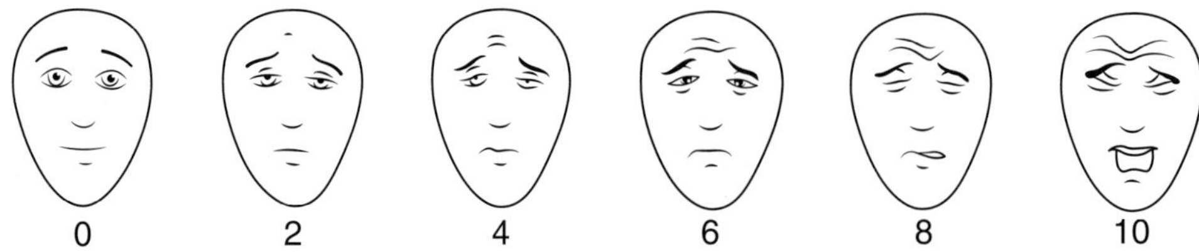

Faces Pain Scale - Revised, ©2001, International Association for the Study of Pain

• Faces Pain Scale (©2001, International Association for the Study of Pain. https://www.iasp-pain.org/resources/faces-pain-scale-revised/.)

Frailty Index for Elders (FIFE)

Item	Circle	Response	
1.	Do you need help getting in or out of bed?	Yes	No
2.	Do you need help with washing or bathing?	Yes	No
3.	Without wanting to, have you lost or gained 10 pounds in the last 6 months?	Yes	No
4.	Do you have tooth or mouth problems that make it hard to eat?	Yes	No
5.	Do you have a poor appetite and quickly feel full when you eat?	Yes	No
6.	Did your physical health or emotional problems interfere with your social activities?	Yes	No
7.	Would you say your health is fair or poor?	Yes	No
8.	Do you get tired easily?	Yes	No
9.	Were you hospitalized in the last 3 months?	Yes	No
10.	Did you visit an emergency room for a health problem in the past 3 months?	Yes	No

Scoring:
A score of 0 indicates no frailty
A score of 1–3 indicates frailty risk
A score of 4 or greater indicates frailty

From Tocchi, C., Dixon, J., Naylor, M., Jeon, S., McCorkle, R. (2014). Development of a frailty measure for older adults: The frailty index for elders. *Journal of Nursing Measurement, 22*(2), 223–40. https://doi.org/10.1891/1061-3749.22.2.223. PMID: 25255675.

Hwalek-Sengstock Elder Abuse Screening Test (H-S/East)

(See Appendix 1, Chapter 4)

Kayser-Jones Brief Oral Health Status Examination (BOHSE)

Resident's Name　　　　Date
Examiner's Name　　　　TOTAL SCORE

Category	Measurement	0	1	2
Lymph nodes	Observe and feel nodes	No enlargement	Enlarged, not tender	Enlarged and tender
Lips	Observe, feel tissue and ask resident, family or staff (e.g., primary caregiver)	Smooth, pink, moist	Dry, chapped, or red at corners	White or red patch, bleeding or ulcer for 2 weeks
Tongue	Observe, feel tissue and ask resident, family or staff (e.g., primary caregiver)	Normal roughness, pink and moist	Coated, smooth, patchy, severely fissured or some redness	Red smooth white or red patch: ulcer for 2 weeks
Tissue inside cheek, floor, and roof of mouth	Observe, feel tissue and ask resident, family or staff (e.g., primary caregiver)	Pink and moist	Dry, shiny, rough red, or swollen	White or red patch, bleeding, hardness: ulcer for 2 weeks
Gums between teeth and/or under artificial teeth	Gently press gums with lip of tongue blade	Pink, small indentations; firm, smooth and pink under artificial teeth		Swollen or bleeding gums redness at border around 7 or more teeth, loose teeth: generalized redness or sores under artificial teeth
Saliva (effect on tissue)	Touch tongue blade to center of tongue and floor of mouth	Tissues moist, saliva free flowing and watery	Tissues dry and sticky	Tissues parched, red, no saliva
Condition of natural teeth	Observe and count number of decayed or broken teeth	No decayed or broken teeth/roots	1–3 decayed or broken teeth/roots	4 or more decayed or broken teeth roots: fewer than 4 teeth in either jaw
Condition of artificial teeth	Observe and ask patient, family or staff (e.g., primary caregiver)	Unbroken teeth, worn most of the time	1 broken/missing tooth, or worn for eating or cosmetics only	More than 1 broken or missing tooth, or either denture missing or never worn
Pairs of teeth in chewing position (natural or artificial)	Observe and count pairs of teeth in chewing position	12 or more pairs of teeth in chewing position	8–11 pairs of teeth in chewing position	0–7 pairs of teeth in chewing position
Oral cleanliness	Observe appearance of teeth or dentures	Clean, no food particles tartar in the mouth or on artificial teeth	food particles/tartar in one or two places in (the mouth or on artificial teeth	Food particles, tartar in most places in the mouth or on artificial teeth

Upper dentures labeled: Yes　No　None　Lower dentures labeled: Yes　No　None
Is your mouth comfortable? Yes　No　If no, explain:
Additional comments:

From Kayser-Jones, J., Bird, W. F., Paul, S. M., Long, L., & Schell, E. S. (1995). An instrument to assess the oral health status of nursing home residents. *Gerontologist, 35*(6), 814–824, Figure 2, p. 823.

Lawton Instrumental Activities of Daily Living Scale

Lawton Instrumental Activities of Daily Living Scale

A. Ability to Use Telephone
1. Operates telephone on own initiative; looks up and dials numbers................1
2. Dials a few well-known numbers......................1
3. Answers telephone, but does not dial............1
4. Does not use telephone at all.............0

B. Shopping
1. Takes care of all shopping needs independently............1
2. Shops independently for small purchases.....0
3. Needs to be accompanied on any shopping trip........................0
4. Completely unable to shop.........................0

C. Food Preparation
1. Plans, prepares, and serves adequate meals independently...................1
2. Prepares adequate meals if supplied with ingredients...............................0
3. Heats and serves prepared meals or prepares meals but does not maintain adequate diet..0
4. Needs to have meals prepared and served................................0

D. Housekeeping
1. Maintains house alone with occasion assistance (heavy work)... 1
2. Performs light daily tasks such as dishwashing, bed making...........................1
3. Performs light daily tasks, but cannot maintain acceptable level of cleanliness..........1
4. Needs help with all home maintenance tasks..........................1
5. Does not participate in any housekeeping tasks.....................0

E. Laundry
1. Does personal laundry completely.............1
2. Launders small items, rinses socks, stocking, etc......1
3. All laundry must be done by others..........0

F. Mode of Transportation
1. Travels independently on public transportation or drives own car.........1
2. Arranges own travel via taxi, but does not otherwise use public transportation........1
3. Travels on public transportation when assisted or accompanied by another.........1
4. Travel limited to taxi or automobile with assistance of another............0
5. Does not travel at all.................0

G. Responsibility for Own Medications
1. Is responsible for taking medication in correct dosages at correct time.............1
2. Takes responsibility if medication is prepared in advance in separate dosages.....0
3. Is not capable of dispensing own medication...........0

H. Ability to Handle Finances
1. Manages financial matters independently (budgets, writes checks, pays rent and bills, goes to bank); collects and keeps track of income..................1
2. Manages day-to-day purchases, but needs help with banking, major purchases, etc. 1
3. Incapable of handling money..............0

Scoring: For each category, circle the item description that most closely resembles the client's highest functional level (either 0 or 1).

From Lawton, M. P., & Brody, E. M. (1969). Assessment of older people: Self-maintaining and instrumental activities of daily living. *Gerontologist*, 9(3), 179–186.

Malnutrition Screening Tool

Malnutrition Screening Tool (MST)

STEP 1: Screen with the MST

1 Have you recently lost weight without trying?

No	0
Unsure	2

If yes, how much weight have you lost?

2-13 lb	1
14-23 lb	2
24-33 lb	3
34 lb or more	4
Unsure	2

Weight loss score:

2 Have you been eating poorly because of a decreased appetite?

No	0
Yes	1

Appetite score:

Add weight loss and appetite scores

MST SCORE:

STEP 2: Score to determine risk

MST = 0 OR 1
NOT AT RISK

Eating well with little or no weight loss

If length of stay exceeds 7 days, then rescreen, repeating weekly as needed.

MST = 2 OR MORE
AT RISK

Eating poorly and/or recent weight loss

Rapidly implement nutrition interventions. Perform nutrition consult within 24-72 hrs, depending on risk.

STEP 3: Intervene with nutritional support for your patients at risk of malnutrition.

Notes:

Ferguson, M et al. *Nutrition* 1999 15:458-464

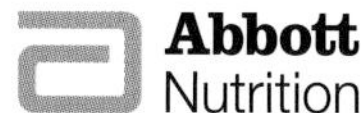

• Malnutrition Screening Tool (In Cameron, J. L., & Cameron, A. M. [2023]. *Current surgical therapy* [14th ed.]. Elsevier.)
From Ferguson, M., et al. [1999]. Development of a valid and reliable malnutrition screening tool for adult acute hospital patients. *Nutrition, 15*, 458–464.

Mini-Cog

(See Chapter 6)

Mini-Cog©

Instructions for Administration & Scoring

ID:__________ Date: ______________

Step 1: Three Word Registration

Look directly at person and say, "Please listen carefully. I am going to say three words that I want you to repeat back to me now and try to remember. The words are [select a list of words from the versions below]. Please say them for me now." If the person is unable to repeat the words after three attempts, move on to Step 2 (clock drawing).

The following and other word lists have been used in one or more clinical studies.[1-3] For repeated administrations, use of an alternative word list is recommended.

Version 1	Version 2	Version 3	Version 4	Version 5	Version 6
Banana	Leader	Village	River	Captain	Daughter
Sunrise	Season	Kitchen	Nation	Garden	Heaven
Chair	Table	Baby	Finger	Picture	Mountain

Step 2: Clock Drawing

Say: "Next, I want you to draw a clock for me. First, put in all of the numbers where they go." When that is completed, say: "Now, set the hands to 10 past 11."

Use preprinted circle (see next page) for this exercise. Repeat instructions as needed as this is not a memory test. Move to Step 3 if the clock is not complete within three minutes.

Step 3: Three Word Recall

Ask the person to recall the three words you stated in Step 1. Say: "What were the three words I asked you to remember?" Record the word list version number and the person's answers below.

Word List Version: ________ Person's Answers: ______________ ______________ ______________

Scoring

Word Recall: ______ (0-3 points)	1 point for each word spontaneously recalled without cueing.
Clock Draw: ______ (0 or 2 points)	Normal clock = 2 points. A normal clock has all numbers placed in the correct sequence and approximately correct position (e.g., 12, 3, 6 and 9 are in anchor positions) with no missing or duplicate numbers. Hands are pointing to the 11 and 2 (11:10). Hand length is not scored. Inability or refusal to draw a clock (abnormal) = 0 points.
Total Score: ______ (0-5 points)	Total score = Word Recall score + Clock Draw score. A cut point of <3 on the Mini-Cog™ has been validated for dementia screening, but many individuals with clinically meaningful cognitive impairment will score higher. When greater sensitivity is desired, a cut point of <4 is recommended as it may indicate a need for further evaluation of cognitive status.

• Mini-Cog Used with permission of the author S. Borson soob@uw.edu).

Clock Drawing

ID:__________ Date:______________

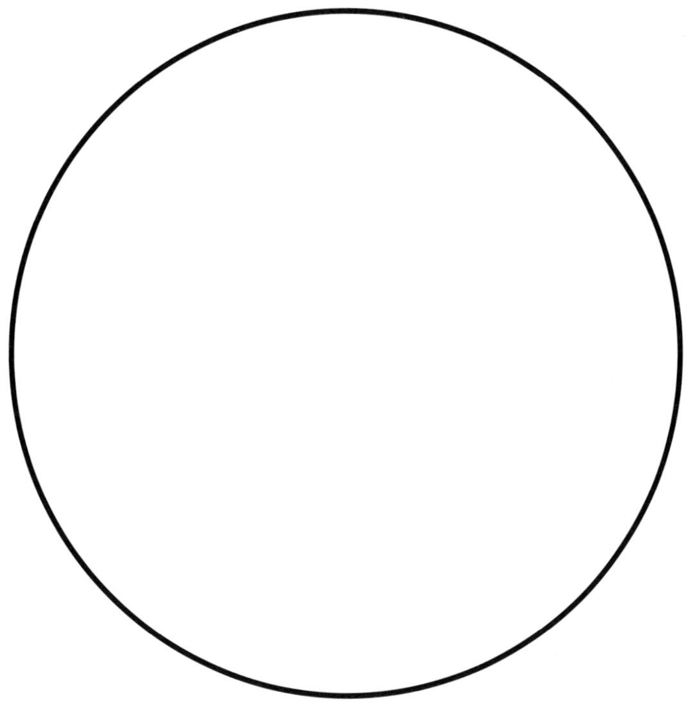

References

1. Borson S, Scanlan JM, Chen PJ et al. The Mini-Cog as a screen for dementia: Validation in a population based sample. J Am Geriatr Soc 2003;51:1451–1454.

2. Borson S, Scanlan JM, Watanabe J et al. Improving identification of cognitive impairment in primary care. Int J Geriatr Psychiatry 2006;21: 349–355.

3. Lessig M, Scanlan J et al. Time that tells: Critical clock-drawing errors for dementia screening. Int Psychogeriatr. 2008 June; 20(3): 459–470.

4. Tsoi K, Chan J et al. Cognitive tests to detect dementia: A systematic review and meta-analysis. JAMA Intern Med. 2015; E1-E9.

5. McCarten J, Anderson P et al. Screening for cognitive impairment in an elderly veteran population: Acceptability and results using different versions of the Mini-Cog. J Am Geriatr Soc 2011; 59: 309-213.

6. McCarten J, Anderson P et al. Finding dementia in primary care: The results of a clinical demonstration project. J Am Geriatr Soc 2012; 60: 210-217.

7. Scanlan J & Borson S. The Mini-Cog: Receiver operating characteristics with the expert and naive raters. Int J Geriatr Psychiatry 2001; 16: 216-222.

• Mini-Cog (Used with permission of the author S. Borson soob@uw.edu).

Montreal Cognitive Assessment (MoCA©)

(See Appendix 1, Chapter 5)

OARS Multidimensional Functional Assessment Questionnaire

This instrument assesses functional status and use of services in frail older adults. This tool was developed by the Duke University Older Americans Resources and Services (OARS) program. This can evaluate the cost-effectiveness of service programs on the functional status of older persons.

Patient Health Questionnaire (PHQ-9)

(See Chapter 6)

Patient Health Questionnaire (PHQ-9)

Patient Name: ____________________ Date: ______________

	Not at All	Several Days	More Than Half the Days	Nearly Every Day
1. Over the *last 2 weeks*, how often have you been bothered by any of the following problems?				
a. Little interest or pleasure in doing things.	☐	☐	☐	☐
b. Feeling down, depressed, or hopeless.	☐	☐	☐	☐
c. Trouble falling/staying asleep, sleeping too much.	☐	☐	☐	☐
d. Feeling tired or having little energy.	☐	☐	☐	☐
e. Poor appetite or overeating.	☐	☐	☐	☐
f. Feeling bad about yourself or that you are a failure or have let yourself or your family down.	☐	☐	☐	☐
g. Trouble concentrating on things, such as reading the newspaper or watching television.	☐	☐	☐	☐
h. Moving or speaking so slowly that other people could have noticed. Or the opposite, being so fidgety or restless that you have been moving around a lot more than usual.	☐	☐	☐	☐
i. Thoughts that you would be better off dead or of hurting yourself in some way.	☐	☐	☐	☐

2. If you checked off any problem on this questionnaire so far, how difficult have these problems made it for you to do your work, take care of things at home, or get along with other people?	Not Difficult at All	Somewhat Difficult	Very Difficult	Extremely Difficult

Scoring: Add up all checked boxes on PHQ-9
For every ✓ Not at all = 0; Several days = 1; More than half the days = 2; Nearly every day = 3
Interpretation of Total Score

Total Score	Depression Severity
1–4	Minimal depression
5–9	Mild depression
10–14	Moderate depression
15–19	Moderately severe depression
20–27	Severe depression

Saint Louis University Mental Status (SLUMS)

VAMC
SLUMS EXAMINATION

Questions about this assessment tool? E-mail aging@slu.edu

Name ________________________________ Age ____________

Is the patient alert? ______________ Level of education ______________

__/1	(1) **1. What day of the week is it?**
__/1	(1) **2. What is the year?**
__/1	(1) **3. What state are we in?**
	4. Please remember these five objects. I will ask you what they are later. Apple Pen Tie House Car
__/3	**5. You have $100 and you go to the store and buy a dozen apples for $3 and a tricycle for $20.** (1) **How much did you spend?** (2) **How much do you have left?**
__/3	**6. Please name as many animals as you can in one minute.** (0) 0–4 animals (1) 5–9 animals (2) 10–14 animals (3) 15+ animals
__/5	**7. What were the five objects I asked you to remember? 1 point for each one correct.**
__/2	**8. I am going to give you a series of numbers and I would like you to give them to me backwards. For example, if I say 42, you would say 24.** (0) 87 (1) 648 (1) 8537
__/4	**9. This is a clock face. Please put in the hour markers and the time at ten minutes to eleven o'clock.** (2) Hour markers okay (2) Time correct
__/2	(1) **10. Please place an X in the triangle.** (1) Which of the above figures is largest?
__/8	**11. I am going to tell you a story. Please listen carefully because afterwards, I'm going to ask you some questions about it.** Jill was a very successful stockbroker. She made a lot of money on the stock market. She then met Jack, a devastatingly handsome man. She married him and had three children. They lived in Chicago. She then stopped work and stayed at home to bring up her children. When they were teenagers, she went back to work. She and Jack lived happily ever after. (2) **What was the female's name?** (2) **What work did she do?** (2) **When did she go back to work?** (2) **What state did she live in?**

________ **TOTAL SCORE**

SCORING		
High School Education		**Less than High School Education**
27–30	Normal	25–30
21–26	Mild Neurocognitive Disorder	20–24
1–20	Dementia	1–19

CLINICIAN'S SIGNATURE ____________ DATE ____________ TIME ____________

SH Tariq, N Tumosa, JT Chibnall, HM Perry III, and JE Morley. The Saint Louis University Mental Status (SLUMS) Examination for detecting mild cognitive impairment and dementia is more sensitive than the Mini-Mental Status Examination (MMSE) - A pilot study. Am J Geriatr Psych 14:900-10, 2006.

• Saint Louis University Mental Status (SLUMS) (From Tariq, S. H., Tumosa, N., Chibnall, J. T., Perry, M. H., III, & J. E. Morley. [2006]. The Saint Louis University mental status [SLUMS] examination for detecting mild cognitive impairment and dementia is more sensitive than the minimental status examination [MMSE]: A pilot study. *American Journal of Geriatric Psychiatry, 14*, 900–910.)

Tobacco, Alcohol, Prescription Medication, and Other Substance Use (TAPS) Tool

National Institute on Drug Abuse (NIDA) Clinical Trials Network

(See Chapter 6)

TOBACCO, ALCOHOL, PRESCRIPTION MEDICATION, AND OTHER SUBSTANCE USE (TAPS) TOOL

National Institute on Drug Abuse (NIDA) Clinical Trials Network

TAPS Tool Part 1

General instructions: The TAPS Tool Part 1 is a 4-item screening for tobacco use, alcohol use, prescription medication misuse, and illicit substance use in the past year. Question 2 should be answered only by males and Question 3 only be females. Each of the four multiple-choice items has five possible responses to choose from. Check the box to select your answer.

Segment
Visit number

1. In the PAST 12 MONTHS, how often have you used any tobacco product (for example, cigarettes, e-cigarettes, cigars, pipes, or smokeless tobacco)?
   [] Daily or Almost Daily [] Weekly [] Monthly [] Less Than Monthly [] Never
2. In the PAST 12 MONTHS, how often have you had 5 or more drinks containing alcohol in one day? One standard drink is about 1 small glass of wine (5 oz), 1 beer (12 oz), or 1 single shot of liquor. (Note: This question should only be answered by males.)
   [] Daily or Almost Daily [] Weekly [] Monthly [] Less Than Monthly [] Never
3. In the PAST 12 MONTHS, how often have you had 4 or more drinks containing alcohol in one day? One standard drink is about 1 small glass of wine (5 oz), 1 beer (12 oz), or 1 single shot of liquor. (Note: This question should only be answered by females.)
   [] Daily or Almost Daily [] Weekly [] Monthly [] Less Than Monthly [] Never
4. In the PAST 12 MONTHS, how often have you used any drugs including marijuana, cocaine or crack, heroin, methamphetamine (crystal meth), hallucinogens, ecstasy/MDMA?
   [] Daily or Almost Daily [] Weekly [] Monthly [] Less Than Monthly [] Never
5. In the PAST 12 MONTHS, how often have you used any prescription medications just for the feeling, more than prescribed or that were not prescribed for you? Prescription medications that may be used this way include: opiate pain relievers (for example, OxyContin, Vicodin, Percocet, Methadone), medications for anxiety or sleeping (for example, Xanax, Ativan, Klonopin), medications for ADHD (for example, Adderall or Ritalin).
   [] Daily or Almost Daily [] Weekly [] Monthly [] Less Than Monthly [] Never

TAPS Tool Part 2

General instructions: The TAPS Tool Part 2 is a brief assessment for tobacco, alcohol, and illicit substance use and prescription medication misuse in the PAST 3 MONTHS ONLY. Each of the following questions and subquestions has two possible answer choices—either yes or no. Check the box to select your answer.

1. In the PAST 3 MONTHS, did you smoke a cigarette containing tobacco? [] Yes [] No
   If "Yes," answer the following questions:
   a. In the PAST 3 MONTHS, did you usually smoke more than 10 cigarettes each day?
      [] Yes [] No
   b. In the PAST 3 MONTHS, did you usually smoke within 30 minutes after waking?
      [] Yes [] No
2. In the PAST 3 MONTHS, did you have a drink containing alcohol? [] Yes [] No
   If "Yes," answer the following questions:
   a. In the PAST 3 MONTHS, did you have 4 or more drinks containing alcohol in a day?*
      (Note: This question should only be answered by females.) [] Yes [] No
   b. In the PAST 3 MONTHS, did you have 5 or more drinks containing alcohol in a day?*
      (Note: This question should only be answered by males.) [] Yes [] No
      *One standard drink is about 1 small glass of wine (5 oz), 1 beer (12 oz), or 1 single shot of liquor.
   c. In the PAST 3 MONTHS, have you tried and failed to control, cut down, or stop drinking? [] Yes [] No
      In the PAST 3 MONTHS, has anyone expressed concern about your drinking? [] Yes [] No
3. In the PAST 3 MONTHS, did you use marijuana (hash, weed)? [] Yes [] No
   If "Yes," answer the following questions:
   a. In the PAST 3 MONTHS, have you had a strong desire or urge to use marijuana at least once a week or more often? [] Yes [] No
   b. In the PAST 3 MONTHS, has anyone expressed concern about your use of marijuana? [] Yes [] No
4. In the PAST 3 MONTHS, did you use cocaine, crack, or methamphetamine (crystal meth)? [] Yes [] No
   If "Yes," answer the following questions:
   a. In the PAST 3 MONTHS, did you use cocaine, crack, or methamphetamine (crystal meth) at least once a week or more often? [] Yes [] No
   b. In the PAST 3 MONTHS, has anyone expressed concern about your use of cocaine, crack, or methamphetamine (crystal meth)? [] Yes [] No

5. In the PAST 3 MONTHS, did you use heroin? [ ] Yes [ ] No
   If "Yes," answer the following questions:
   a. In the PAST 3 MONTHS, have you tried and failed to control, cut down, or stop using heroin? [ ] Yes [ ] No
   b. In the PAST 3 MONTHS, has anyone expressed concern about your use of heroin? [ ] Yes [ ] No
6. In the PAST 3 MONTHS, did you use a prescription opiate pain reliever (for example, Percocet, Vicodin) not as prescribed or that was not prescribed for you? [ ] Yes [ ] No
   If "Yes," answer the following questions:
   a. In the PAST 3 MONTHS, have you tried and failed to control, cut down, or stop using an opiate pain reliever? [ ] Yes [ ] No
   b. In the PAST 3 MONTHS, has anyone expressed concern about your use of an opiate pain reliever? [ ] Yes [ ] No
7. In the PAST 3 MONTHS, did you use a medication for anxiety or sleep (for example, Xanax, Ativan, or Klonopin) not as prescribed or that was not prescribed for you? [ ] Yes [ ] No
   If "Yes," answer the following questions:
   a. In the PAST 3 MONTHS, have you had a strong desire or urge to use medications for anxiety or sleep at least once a week or more often? [ ] Yes [ ] No
   b. In the PAST 3 MONTHS, has anyone expressed concern about your use of medication for anxiety or sleep? [ ] Yes [ ] No
8. In the PAST 3 MONTHS, did you use a medication for ADHD (for example, Adderall, Ritalin) not as prescribed or that was not prescribed for you? [ ] Yes [ ] No
   If "Yes," answer the following questions:
   a. In the PAST 3 MONTHS, did you use a medication for ADHD (for example, Adderall, Ritalin) at least once a week or more often? [ ] Yes [ ] No
   b. In the PAST 3 MONTHS, has anyone expressed concern about your use of a medication for ADHD (for example, Adderall or Ritalin)? [ ] Yes [ ] No
9. In the PAST 3 MONTHS, did you use any other illegal or recreational drug (for example, ecstasy/molly, GHB, poppers, LSD, mushrooms, special K, bath salts, synthetic marijuana ("spice"), whip-its, etc.)? [ ] Yes [ ] No
   If "Yes," answer the following question:
   In the PAST 3 MONTHS, what were the other drug(s) you used?
   Comments:

Trail Making Test (TMT), Parts A and B

Instructions: Both parts of the Trail Making Test consist of 25 circles distributed over a sheet of paper. In Part A, the circles are numbered 1–25, and the patient should draw lines to connect the numbers in ascending order. In Part B, the circles include both numbers (1–13) and letters (A–L); as in Part A, the patient draws lines to connect the circles in an ascending pattern, but with the added task of alternating between the numbers and letters (i.e., 1-A-2-B-3-C, etc.). The patient should be instructed to connect the circles as quickly as possible, without lifting the pen or pencil from the paper. Time the patient as he or she connects the "trail." If the patient makes an error, point it out immediately and allow the patient to correct it. Errors affect the patient's score only in that the correction of errors is included in the completion time for the task. It is unnecessary to continue the test if the patient has not completed both parts after five minutes have elapsed.

Step 1: Give the patient a copy of the Trail Making Test Part A worksheet and a pen or pencil.
Step 2: Demonstrate the test to the patient using the sample sheet (Trail Making Part A–SAMPLE).
Step 3: Time the patient as he or she follows the "trail" made by the numbers on the test.
Step 4: Record the time.
Step 5: Repeat the procedure for Trail Making Test Part B.

Scoring: Results for both TMT A and B are reported as the number of seconds required to complete the task; therefore, higher scores reveal greater impairment.

	Average	Deficient	Rule of Thumb
Trail A	29 seconds	>78 seconds	Most in 90 seconds
Trail B	75 seconds	>273 seconds	Most in 3 minutes

Corrigan, J. D., & Hinkeldey, M. S. (1987). Relationships between parts A and B of the trail making test. *Journal of Clinical Psychology, 43*(4), 402–409; Gaudino, E. A., Geisler, M. W., & Squires, N. K. (1995). Construct validity in the trail making test: What makes part B harder? *Journal of Clinical and Experimental Neuropsychology, 17*(4), 529–535; Lezak, M. D., Howieson, D. B., & Loring, D. W. (2004). *Neuropsychological assessment* (4th ed.). Oxford University Press; Reitan, R. M. (1958). Validity of the trail making test as an indicator of organic brain damage. *Perceptual and Motor Skills, 8*, 271–276.

Trail Making Test Part A

Patient's Name: ______________________________ Date: ____________________

17 21 15 22 20 19 16 18 4 5 13 24 14 6 7 1 8 10 2 3 9 11 25 23 12

Trail Making Test Part A – *SAMPLE*

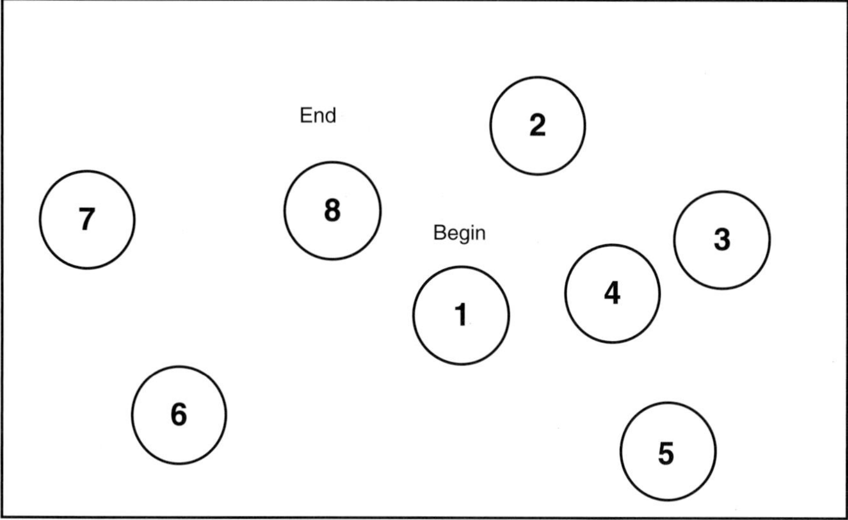

Trail Making Test Part B

Patient's Name: ______________________________ Date: ____________________

8 I 10
9 4 D
B
H
3
7 1
12
C
G
5
J
2
L A
6
E
F
11
K

Trail Making Test Part B – *SAMPLE*

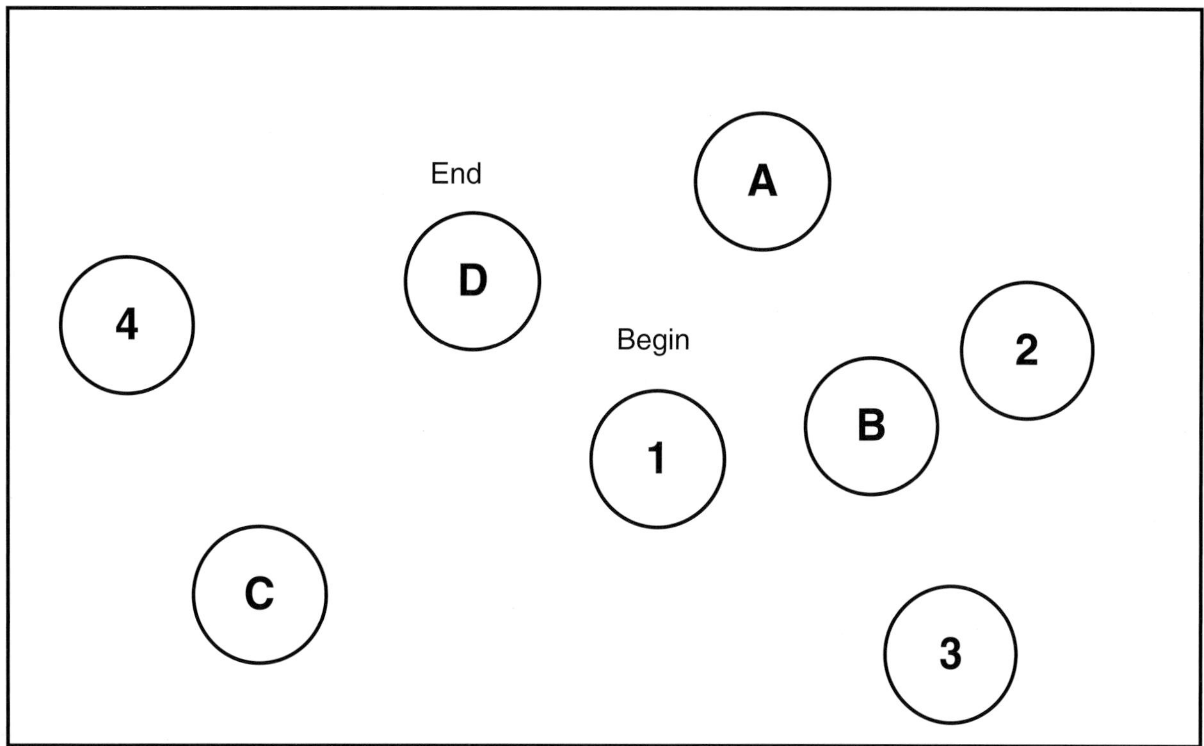

• Trail Making Test A (TMT-A) (From Barncord, S. W., & Wanlass, R. L. [2001]. The symbol trail making test: Test development and utility as a measure of cognitive impairment. *Applied Neuropsychology, 8*, 99–103. From University of South Dakota. http://apps.usd.edu/coglab/schieber/psyc423/pdf/IowaTrailMaking.pdf

Vulnerable Elder Survey-13 (VES-13)

VES-13

1. Age ______________________

> **SCORE:** *1 POINT FOR AGE 75-84*
> *3 POINTS FOR AGE ≥ 85*

2. In general, compared to other people your age, would you say that your health is:

☐ Poor,* *(1 POINT)*
☐ Fair,* *(1 POINT)*
☐ Good,
☐ Very good, or
☐ Excellent

> **SCORE:** *1 POINT FOR FAIR or POOR*

3. How much difficulty, <u>on average</u>, do you have with the following physical activities:

	No Difficulty	A little Difficulty	Some Difficulty	A Lot of Difficulty	Unable to Do
a. stooping, crouching or kneeling?.........	☐	☐	☐	☐*	☐*
b. lifting, or carrying objects as heavy as 10 pounds?..	☐	☐	☐	☐*	☐*
c. reaching or extending arms above shoulder level?	☐	☐	☐	☐*	☐*
d. writing, or handling and grasping small objects?..	☐	☐	☐	☐*	☐*
e. walking a quarter of a mile?	☐	☐	☐	☐*	☐*
f. heavy housework such as scrubbing floors or washing windows?............................	☐	☐	☐	☐*	☐*

> **SCORE:** *1 POINT FOR EACH* RESPONSE IN Q3a THROUGH f.* <u>*MAXIMUM OF 2 POINTS*</u>.

4. Because of your health or a physical condition, do you have any difficulty:

a. shopping for personal items (like toilet items or medicines)?

☐ YES→ Do you get help with shopping? ☐ YES* ☐ NO
☐ NO
☐ DON'T DO→ Is that because of your health? ☐ YES* ☐ NO

b. managing money (like keeping track of expenses or paying bills)?

☐ YES→ Do you get help with managing money? ☐ YES* ☐ NO
☐ NO
☐ DON'T DO→ Is that because of your health? ☐ YES* ☐ NO

.... *Continued*

c. walking across the room? USE OF CANE OR WALKER IS OK.

☐ YES→ Do you get help with walking? ☐ YES* ☐ NO
☐ NO
☐ DON'T DO→ Is that because of your health? ☐ YES* ☐ NO

d. doing light housework (like washing dishes, straightening up, or light cleaning)?

☐ YES→ Do you get help with light housework? ☐ YES* ☐ NO
☐ NO
☐ DON'T DO→ Is that because of your health? ☐ YES* ☐ NO

e. bathing or showering?

☐ YES→ Do you get help with bathing or showering? ☐ YES* ☐ NO
☐ NO
☐ DON'T DO→ Is that because of your health? ☐ YES* ☐ NO

SCORE: *4 POINTS FOR ONE OR MORE* RESPONSES IN Q4a THROUGH Q4e*
.

• Vulnerable Elder Survey-13 (VES-13) (From Saliba, S., Elliott, M., Rubenstein, L. A., Solomon, D. H., et al. [2001]. *Journal of the American Geriatric Society, 49*, 1691–1699. Image used with permission-Copyright 2001 RAND.)

Yesavage Geriatric Depression Scale (GDS)

(See Chapter 6)

Yesavage Geriatric Depression Scale (GDS)–Short Form

Circle the answer that best describes how you felt over the *past week*.

1. Are you basically satisfied with your life? Yes No
2. Have you dropped many of your activities and interests? Yes No
3. Do you feel that your life is empty? Yes No
4. Do you often get bored? Yes No
5. Are you in good spirits most of the time? Yes No
6. Are you afraid that something bad is going to happen to you? Yes No
7. Do you feel happy most of the time? Yes No
8. Do you often feel helpless? Yes No
9. Do you prefer to stay at home, rather than going out and doing things? Yes No
10. Do you feel that you have more problems with memory than most? Yes No
11. Do you think it is wonderful to be alive now? Yes No
12. Do you feel worthless the way you are now? Yes No
13. Do you feel full of energy? Yes No
14. Do you feel that your situation is hopeless? Yes No
15. Do you think that most people are better off than you are? Yes No

Scoring Instructions

Instructions: Score 1 point for each bolded answer; a score of 5 or more suggests depression.

From Sheikh, J. I., & Yesavage, J. A. (1986). Geriatric depression scale: Recent evidence and development of a shorter version. *Clinical Gerontology, 5*, 165–172.

Chapter 7

Beers Criteria

The American Geriatric Society Beers Criteria aims to guide older people and health professionals away from potentially harmful treatments while helping health care providers to assess quality of care.

Data from the American Geriatrics Society (AGS). (2019). American Geriatrics Society 2019 Updated AGS Beers Criteria® for potentially inappropriate medication use in older adults. *Journal of the American Geriatrics Society, 67*(4), 674–694. https://doi.org/10.1111/jgs.15767

Exercise Assessment and Screening for You (EASY) Preexercise Program Questionnaire

EASY Question 1	Do you have pains, tightness, or pressure in your chest during physical activity (walking, climbing stairs, household chores, similar activities)?
EASY Question 2	Do you currently experience dizziness or lightheadedness?
EASY Question 3	Have you ever been told that you have high blood pressure?
EASY Question 4	Do you have pain, stiffness, or swelling that limits or prevents you from doing what you want or need to do?
EASY Question 5	Do you fall, feel unsteady, or use an assistive device while standing or walking?
EASY Question 6	Is there a reason not mentioned why you would be concerned about starting an exercise program?

From Resnick, B. (2008). A proposal for a new screening paradigm and tool called exercise assessment and screening for you (EASY). *Journal of Aging and Physical Activity, 16*(2), 215–233.

Pines Burnout Measure

PINES BURNOUT MEASURE: SHORT VERSION

When you think about your work overall how often do you feel the following?

1	2	3	4	5	6	7
Never	Almost	Rarely	Sometimes	Often	Very often	Always

Tired
Disappointed with people
Hopeless
Trapped
Helpless
Depressed
Physically weak/sickly
Worthless/like a failure
Difficulties sleeping
"I've had it"

To calculate your burnout score, add your responses to the 10 items and divide by 10.

Score between 0 and 2.4 = you have little or no burnout
A score of 2.5 to 3.4 = you are at risk for burnout.
Score of 3.5 or higher = you are burned out with high burnout being in the 4.5 to 5.4 range and very high burnout in the 5.5 or higher range.

From Malach-Pines, A. (2005). The burnout measure, short version. *International Journal of Stress Management, 12*(1), 78–88. https://doi.org/10.1037/1072-5245.12.1.78

Chapter 10

Alcohol Use Disorder Identification Test-Consumption Questionnaire AUDIT-C

ALCOHOL USE DISORDER IDENTIFICATION TEST-CONSUMPTION QUESTIONNAIRE (AUDIT-C)

General Instructions

The Alcohol Use Disorders Identification Test-Concise (AUDIT-C) is a brief alcohol screening instrument. Please give a response for each question.

Segment: __

Visit Number: __

1. How often do you have a drink containing alcohol?
   - ☐ Never
   - ☐ 2–3 times a week
   - ☐ Monthly or less
   - ☐ 4 or more times a week
   - ☐ 2–4 times a month
2. How many standard drinks containing alcohol do you have on a typical day?
   - ☐ 1 or 2
   - ☐ 7 to 9
   - ☐ 3 to 4
   - ☐ 10 or more
   - ☐ 5 to 6
3. How often do you have six or more drinks on one occasion?
   - ☐ Daily or almost daily
   - ☐ Less than monthly
   - ☐ Weekly
   - ☐ Never
   - ☐ Monthly

From Bush, K., Kiviahan, D. R., et al. (1998). The AUDIT alcohol consumption questions (AUDIT-C): An effective brief screening test for problem drinking. Ambulatory Care Quality Improvement Project (ACQUIP). *Archives of Internal Medicine, 158*, 1789–1795..)

The CAGE Screening Tool

(See Appendix 1, Chapter 6)

Cannabis Use Disorder Identification Test-Short Form (CUDIT-R)

Please answer the following questions about your cannabis use. Select the response that is most correct for you in relation to your cannabis use over the last six months. This questionnaire was designed for self-administration and is scored by adding each of the 8 items. Questions 1–7 are scored on a 0–4 scale. Question 8 is scored 0, 2, or 4.

1. How often do you use cannabis?
   Never (0 points)
   Monthly or less (1 point)
   2–4 times a month (2 points)
   2–3 times a week (3 points)
   4 or more times a week (4 points)
2. How many hours were you "stoned" on a typical day when you were using cannabis?
   Less than 1 (0 points)
   1 or 2 (1 point)
   3 or 4 (2 points)
   5 or 6 (3 points)
   7 or more (4 points)
3. How often during the last 6 months did you find that you were not able to stop using cannabis once you had started?
   Never (0 points)
   Less than monthly (1 point)
   Monthly (2 points)
   Weekly (3 points)
   Daily or almost daily (4 points)
4. How often during the last 6 months did you fail to do what was normally expected from you because of using cannabis?
   Never (0 points)
   Less than monthly (1 point)
   Monthly (2 points)
   Weekly (3 points)
   Daily or almost daily (4 points)

5. How often in the past 6 months have you devoted a great deal of your time to getting, using, or recovering from cannabis?
   Never (0 points)
   Less than monthly (1 point)
   Monthly (2 points)
   Weekly (3 points)
   Daily or almost daily (4 points)
6. How often during the last 6 months have you had a problem with your memory or concentration after using cannabis?
   Never (0 points)
   Less than monthly (1 point)
   Monthly (2 points)
   Weekly (3 points)
   Daily or almost daily (4 points)
7. How often do you use cannabis in situations that could be physically hazardous, such as driving, operating machinery, or caring for children?
   Never (0 points)
   Less than monthly (1 point)
   Monthly (2 points)
   Weekly (3 points)
   Daily or almost daily (4 points)
8. Have you ever thought about cutting down, or stopping, your use of cannabis?
   Never (0 points)
   Yes, but not in the past 6 months (2 points)
   Yes, during the past 6 months (4 points)

Scores of 8 points or more indicate hazardous cannabis use. Scores of 12 or more indicate a possible cannabis use disorder and it would be a good idea to explore this more with an expert.

From Adamson, S. J., Kay-Lambkin, F. J., et al. (2010). The cannabis use disorders identification test–revised (CUDIT-R). *Drug and Alcohol Dependence, 110*, 137–143.

Elder Abuse Suspicion Index

(See Appendix 1, Chapter 4)

Katz Index of Independence in Activities of Daily Living and Instrumental Activities of Daily Living Scale

The Katz Index of Independence in Activities of Daily Living, (Katz ADL), is used to assess functional status as a measurement of the client's ability to perform activities of daily living independently. Clinicians typically use the tool to assess function and detect problems in performing activities of daily living and to plan care accordingly. (See Chapter 6)

Malnutrition Universal Screening Tool (MUST)

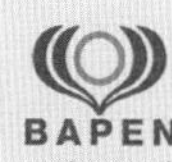

Step 1 + **Step 2** + **Step 3**

Step 1 – BMI score

BMI kg/m²	Score
>20 (>30 Obese)	= 0
18.5-20	= 1
<18.5	= 2

Step 2 – Weight loss score

Unplanned weight loss in past 3-6 months

%	Score
<5	= 0
5-10	= 1
>10	= 2

Step 3 – Acute disease effect score

If patient is acutely ill **and** there has been or is likely to be no nutritional intake for >5 days
Score 2

If unable to obtain height and weight, see reverse for alternative measurements and use of subjective criteria

Acute disease effect is unlikely to apply outside hospital. See 'MUST' Explanatory Booklet for further information

Step 4

Overall risk of malnutrition

Add Scores together to calculate overall risk of malnutrition
Score 0 Low Risk Score 1 Medium Risk Score 2 or more High Risk

Step 5

Management guidelines

0
Low Risk
Routine clinical care
- Repeat screening
  Hospital – weekly
  Care Homes – monthly
  Community – annually
  for special groups
  e.g., those >75 yrs

1
Medium Risk
Observe
- Document dietary intake for 3 days
- If adequate – little concern and repeat screening
  - Hospital – weekly
  - Care Home – at least monthly
  - Community – at least every 2-3 months
- If inadequate – clinical concern – follow local policy, set goals, improve and increase overall nutritional intake, monitor and review care plan regularly

2 or more
High Risk
Treat*
- Refer to dietitian, Nutritional
- Set goals, improve and increase
- Monitor and review care plan
  Hospital – weekly
  Care Home – monthly
  Community – monthly

* Unless detrimental or no benefit is expected from nutritional support e.g., imminent death.

All risk categories:
- Treat underlying condition and provide help and advice on food choices, eating and drinking when necessary.
- Record malnutrition risk category.
- Record need for special diets and follow local policy.

Obesity:
- Record presence of obesity. For those with underlying conditions, these are generally controlled before the treatment of obesity.

Re-assess subjects identified at risk as they move through care settings

See The 'MUST' Explanatory Booklet for further details and The 'MUST' Report for supporting evidence.

• Malnutrition Universal Screening Tool (MUST) (MUST is reproduced here with the kind permission of BAPEN (British Association for Parenteral and Enteral Nutrition). For further information on 'MUST' see www.bapen.org.uk. Copyright© BAPEN 2012.)

Nutritional Risk Screening—2002 (NRS-2002)

Table 1 Initial Screening

		Yes	No
1	Is BMI <20.5?		
2	Has the patient lost weight within the last 3 months?		
3	Has the patient had a reduced dietary intake in the last week?		
4	Is the patient severely ill? (e.g., in intensive therapy)		

Yes: If the answer is "Yes" to any question, the screening in Table 2 is performed.
No: If the answer is "No" to all questions, the patient is re-screened at weekly intervals. If the patient e.g., is scheduled for a major operation, a preventive nutritional care plan is considered to avoid the associated risk status.

Table 2 Final Screening

Impaired Nutritional status		Severity of Disease (≈ Increase in Requirements)	
Absent Score 0	Normal Nutritional Status	Absent Score 0	Normal Nutritional Requirements
Mild Score 1	Wt loss >5% in 3 mths or food intake below 50–75% of normal requirement in preceding week	Mild Score 1	Hip fracture* Chronic patients, in particular with acute complications: cirrhosis* COPD* *Chronic hemodialysis, diabetes, oncology*
Moderate Score 2	Wt loss >5% in 2 mths or BMI 18.5–20.5 + impaired general condition or food intake 25–60% of normal requirement in preceding week	Moderate Score 2	Major abdominal surgery* Stroke* *Severe pneumonia, hematologic malignancy*
Severe Score 3	Wt loss >5% in 1 mth (>15% in 3 mths) or BMI <18.5 + impaired general condition or food intake 0–25% of normal requirement in preceding week	Severe Score 3	Head injury* Bone marrow transplantation* *Intensive care patients (APACHE> 10).*
Score:	+	**Score**	**= Total score**

Age if > 70 years: Add 1 to total score above = Age adjusted total score

Score >3: The patient is nutritionally at-risk and a nutritional care plan is initiated.
Score<3: Weekly re-screening of the patient. If the patient e.g., is scheduled for a major operation, a preventive nutritional care plan is considered to avoid the associated risk status.

NRS-2002 is based on an interpretation of available randomized clinical trials. *Indicates that a trial directly supports the categorization of patients with that diagnosis. Diagnoses shown in italics are based on the prototypes given below. Nutritional risk is defined by the present nutritional status and risk of impairment of present status, due to increased requirements caused by stress metabolism of the clinical condition.

A nutritional care plan is indicated in all patients who are (1) severely undernourished (score = 3), or (2) severely ill (score = 3), or (3) moderately undernourished + mildly ill (score 2 +1), or (4) mildly undernourished + moderately ill (score 1 + 2).Prototypes for severity of disease

Score = 1: a patient with chronic disease, admitted to hospital due to complications. The patient is weak but out of bed regularly. Protein requirement is increased, but can be covered by oral diet or supplements in most cases.
Score = 2: a patient confined to bed due to illness, e.g., following major abdominal surgery. Protein requirement is substantially increased, but can be covered, although artificial feeding is required in many cases.
Score = 3: a patient in intensive care with assisted ventilation etc. Protein requirement is increased and cannot be covered even by artificial feeding.

Protein breakdown and nitrogen loss can be significantly attenuated.

From Kondrup, J., Rasmussen, H. H., Hamberg, O., & Stanga, Z., An Ad Hoc ESPEN Working Group. (2003). Nutritional risk screening (NRS 2002): A new method based on an analysis of controlled clinical trials. *Clinical Nutrition, 22*(3), 321–336. https://doi.org/10.1016/s0261-5614(02)00214-5. PMID.

Opioid Risk Tool (ORT)

This tool should be administered to patients upon an initial visit prior to beginning opioid therapy for pain management. A score of 3 or lower indicates low risk for future opioid abuse, a score of 4 to 7 indicates moderate risk for opioid abuse, and a score of 8 or higher indicates a high-risk tor opioid abuse.

Mark Each Box That Applies	Female	Male
Family History of Substance Abuse		
Alcohol	1	3
Illegal drugs	2	3
Rx drugs	4	4
Personal History of Substance Abuse		
Alcohol	3	3
Illegal drugs	4	4
Rx drugs	5	5
Age 16–45 years	1	1
History of preadolescent sexual abuse	3	0
Psychological Disease		
ADD, OCD, bipolar, schizophrenia	2	2
Depression	1	1
Scoring totals		

Questionnaire developed by Lynn R. Webster, MD, to asses risk of opioid addiction.
ADD, Attention deficit disorder; *OCD*, obsessive-compulsive disorder.
(From Webster, L. R., & Webster, R. (2005). Predicting aberrant behaviors in opioid-treated patients: Preliminary validation of the opioid risk too. *Pain Medicine, 6*(6), 432; In Cheatle, M., Compton, P., Dhingra, L., Wasser, T., & O'Brien, C. P. (2019). Development of the revised opioid risk tool to predict opioid use disorder in patients with chronic nonmalignant pain. *Journal of Pain. 20*(7), 842–851.)

Patient Health Questionnaire (PHQ-9)

(See Appendix 1, Chapter 6)

STOP-BANG Questionnaire

Yes	No	Snoring?
		Do you snore loudly (loud enough to be heard through closed doors or your bed partner elbows you for snoring at night)?
Yes	No	Tired?
		Do you often feel tired, fatigued, or sleepy during the daytime (such as falling asleep during driving or talking to someone)?
Yes	No	Observed?
		Has anyone observed you stop breathing or choking gasping during your sleep?
Yes	No	Pressure?
		Do you have or are being treated for high blood pressure?
Yes	No	Body mass index more than 35 kg/m^2?
Yes	No	Age older than 50 years?
Yes	No	Neck size large (measured around Adam's apple) for male, is your shirt collar 17 inches or larger?
Yes	No	Sex = male?

For general population, OSA–low risk: yes to 0-2 questions; OSA–intermediate risk: yes to 3-4 questions; or OSA–high risk: yes to 5-8 questions, yes to 2 or more of 4 STOP questions+male sex, yes to 2 or more of 4 STOP questions+BMI>35 kg/m2, or yes to 2 or more of 4 STOP questions+neck circumference 16 inches/40 cm.

In Cooney, M., & Quinlan-Colwell, A. (2021). *Assessment andltimodal management of pain: An integrative approach*. Elsevier. Property of University Health Network. Please use "About Us" for more information. http://www.stopbang.ca. Permission obtained from University Health Network.Modified from Chung, F., Yegneswaran, B., Liao, P., Chung, S. A., Vairavanathan, S., Islam, S.,... & Shapiroet, C. M. (2008). STOP Questionnaire: A tool to screen patients for obstructive sleep apnea. *Anesthesiology, 108*, 812; Chung, F. (2012). High STOP-BANG scores indicate a high probability of obstructive sleep apnea. *British Journal of Anaesthesia, 108*(5), 768–775; and Chung, F., Yang, Y., Brown, R., & Liao, P. (2014). Alternative scoring models of STOP-Bang questionnaire specificity to detect undiagnosed obstructive sleep apnea. *Journal of Clinical Sleep Medicine, 10*, 951–958.From Avitsian, R., & Galway, U. (2015). Assessment and management of obstructive sleep apnea for ambulatory surgery. *Advances in Anesthesia, 33*(1), 61–75.
OSA, Obstructive sleep apnea.

The Tobacco, Alcohol, Prescription medication, and other Substance use (TAPS) Tool NIDA Clinical Trials Network

(See Appendix 1, Chapter 6)

Yesavage Geriatric Depression Scale (GDS)

(See Appendix 1, Chapter 6)

Chapter 11

Activities-Specific Balance Confidence (ABC) Scale

0% 10 20 30 40 50 60 70 80 90 100%
No Confidence Completely Confident
How confident are you that you will not lose your balance or become unsteady when you...

1. walk around the house? __%
2. walk up or down stairs? __%
3. bend over and pick up a slipper from the front of a closet floor?__%
4. reach for a small can off a shelf at eye level? __%
5. stand on your tip toes and reach for something above your head? __%
6. stand on a chair and reach for something? __%
7. sweep the floor? __%
8. walk outside the house to a car parked in the driveway? __%
9. get into or out of a car? __%
10. walk across a parking lot to the mall?__%
11. walk up or down a ramp? __%
12. walk in a crowded mall where people rapidly walk past you?___%
13. are bumped into by people as you walk through the mall? ___%
14. step onto or off of an escalator while you are holding onto a railing? ___%
15. step onto or off an escalator while holding onto parcels such that you cannot hold onto the railing? ___%
16. walk outside on icy sidewalks?___%

From Powell, L. E., & Myers, A. M. (1995). The activities-specific balance confidence (ABC) scale. *Journals of Gerontology Series A Biological Sciences and Medical Sciences, 50*(1), M28–M34. Used with permission of University of Waterloo–California.

CONFUSION ASSESSMENT METHOD (CAM) ALGORITHM

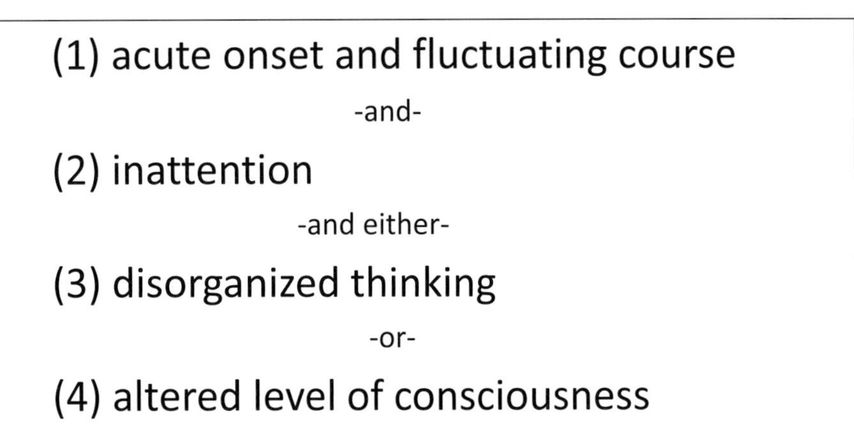

(1) acute onset and fluctuating course
-and-
(2) inattention
-and either-
(3) disorganized thinking
-or-
(4) altered level of consciousness

[Score based on cognitive testing. See details at:
[https://www.deliriumcentral.org/]

Falls Efficacy Scale–I (International)

	Not at All Concerned 1	Somewhat Concerned 2	Fairly Concerned 3	Very Concerned 4
1. Cleaning the house (e.g., sweep, vacuum, dust)				
2. Getting dressed or undressed				
3. Preparing simple meals				
4. Taking a bath or shower				
5. Going to the shop				
6. Getting in or out of a chair				
7. Going up or down stairs				
8. Walking around in the neighborhood				
9. Reaching for something above your head or on the ground				
10. Going to answer the telephone before it stops ringing				
11. Walking on a slippery surface (e.g., wet or icy)				
12. Visiting a friend or relative				
13. Walking in a place with crowds				
14. Walking on an uneven surface (e.g., reeky ground, poorly maintained pavement)				
15. Walking up or down a slope				
16. Going out to a social event (e.g., religious service, family gathering, or club meeting)				
Subtotal				
TOTAL				/64

From Yardley, L., Beyer, N., et al. (2005). Development and initial validation of the falls efficacy scale-international (FES-I). *Age and Ageing, 34*(6), 614–619. https://doi.org/10.1093/ageing/afi196

Mini-Cog©

(See Appendix 1, Chapter 6)

Montreal Cognitive Assessment (MoCA©)

(See Appendix 1, Chapter 5)

Morse Fall Scale

Risk Factor	Scale	Score
History of falls	Yes	25
	No	0
Secondary diagnosis	Yes	15
	No	0
Ambulatory aid	Furniture	30
	Crutches/cane/walker	15
	None/bed rest/wheelchair/nurse	0
IV/heparin lock	Yes	20
	No	0
Gait/transferring	Impaired	20
	Weak	10
	Normal/bed rest/immobile	0
Mental status	Forgets limitations	15
	Oriented to own ability	0
To obtain the Morse Fall Score, add the score from each category.		
Morse Fall Score High risk		45+
Moderate risk		25–44
Low risk		0–24

In Crawford, R., & Yoost, B. (2016). *Fundamentals of nursing: Active learning for collaborative practice*, Elsevier. From Morse, J. M., Black, C., Oberle, K., et al. (1989). A prospective study to identify the fall-prone patient. *Social Science & Medicine, 28*(1), 81–86.

Nutritional Health Checklist

The National Health Service (NHS) continuing health care checklist is a screening tool that can be used in a variety of settings to help practitioners identify individuals who may need a referral for a full assessment of eligibility for NHS continuing health care.

Data from The Nutrition Screening Initiative, American Academy of Family Physicians, July 2001, https://www.gov.uk/government/publications/nhs-continuing-healthcare-checklist

St. Thomas Risk Assessment Tool in Falling Elderly (STRATIFY)

	Yes	No
1. Did the patient present to the hospital with a fall or has he/she fallen on the ward since admission?	1	0
2. Is the patient agitated?		
3. Is the patient visually impaired to the extent that everyday function is affected?	1	0
4. Is the patient in need of especially frequent toileting?	1	0
5. Does the patient have a combined transfer and mobility score of 3 or 4?	1	0

Transfer score: Choose **one** of the following options which best describes the patient's level of capability when transferring from a bed to a chair:
- 0 = Unable
- 1 = Needs major help
- 2 = Needs minor help
- 3 = Independent

Mobility score: Choose **one** of the following options which best describes the patient's level of mobility:
- 0 = Immobile
- 1 = Independent with the aid of a wheelchair
- 2 = Uses walking aid or help of one person
- 3 = Independent

Combined score (transfer + mobility):____________
Total score from questions 1–5: ___________
0 = Low risk
1 = Moderate risk
2 or above = High risk

Table from the Agency for Healthcare Research and Quality, https://www.ahrq.gov/patient-safety/settings/hospital/fall-prevention/toolkit/stratify-scale.html

Tinetti Balance and Gait Assessment Tool

Task

1. Sitting balance
   0 = Leans or slides in chair
   1 = Steady and safe
2. Arises
   0 = Unable without help
   1 = Able, but uses arm to help
   2 = Able to arise in one attempt
3. Attempts to arise
   0 = Unable without help
   1 = Able, but requires more than one attempt
   2 = Able to arise in one attempt
4. Immediate standing balance (first 5 seconds)
   0 = Unsteady (e.g., staggers, moves feet, marked trunk sway)
   1 = Steady, but uses walker or cane or grabs another object for support
   2 = Steady without walker, cane, or other support
5. Standing balance
   0 = Unsteady
   1 = Steady, but has a wide stance (i.e., medial heels 4 inches apart) or uses a cane, walker, or other support
   2 = Narrow stance without support
6. Nudge (with subject at maximum position with feet as close together as possible; examiner pushes lightly on subject's sternum three times with palm of the hand)
   0 = Begins to fall
   1 = Staggers, grabs, but catches self
   2 = Steady

Tinetti Balance and Gait Assessment Tool

7. Eyes closed (at maximum position as in #6)
   0 = Unsteady
   1 = Steady

8. Turn 360 degrees
   0 = Discontinuous steps
   1 = Continuous steps 0 = Unsteady (e.g., grabs, staggers)
   2 = Steady

9. Sit down
   0 = Unsafe (e.g., misjudges distance, falls into chair)
   1 = Uses arms or does not use a smooth motion
   2 = Safe, smooth motion

In Yeager, J. J., & Meiner, S. E. (2019). *Gerontologic nursing* (6th ed). Elsevier. From Fortinsky, R., Iannuzzi-Sucich, M., Baker, D., Gottschalk, M., King, M., Brown, C., & Tinetti, M. (2004). Fall-risk assessment and management in clinical practice: Views from healthcare providers. *Journal of the American Geriatrics Society, 52*(9), 1522–1526. https://doi.org/10.1111/j.1532-5415.2004.52416.x. Reprinted with permission, Mary E. Tinetti, M.D. © Copyright 2006. From Tinetti, M. E., Williams, T. F., & Mayewski, R. (1986). Fall risk index for elderly patients based on number of chronic disabilities. *American Journal of Medicine, 80*, 429–434.

Timed Up and Go Test (TUG)

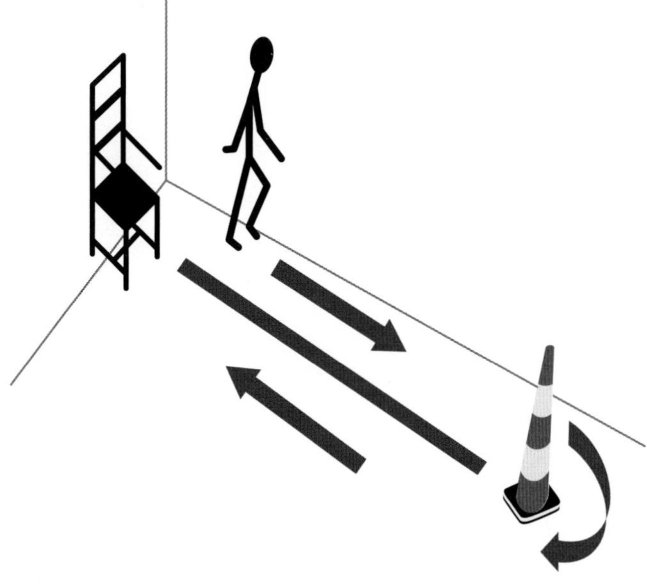

• Timed Up and Go Test (TUG) (From Chen, M. S., Lin, T. C., & Jiang, B.C. [2015]. Aerobic and resistance exercise training program intervention for enhancing gait function in elderly and chronically ill Taiwanese patients. *Public Health, 129*[8],1114–1124.)

The Saint Louis University Mental Status (SLUMS©)

(See Appendix 1, Chapter 6)

Trauma -Specific Frailty Index

TRAUMA-SPECIFIC FRAILTY INDEX

Comorbidities

- Cancer history
- Coronary heart disease
- Dementia

Daily Activities

- Help with grooming
- Help managing money
- Help doing household work
- Help toileting
- Help walking

Health Attitude

- Feel less useful
- Feel sad
- Feel effort to do everything
- Falls
- Feel lonely
- Function, sexually active
- Nutrition, albumin

From Joseph, B., Pandit, V., Zangbar, B., et al. (2014). Validating trauma-specific frailty index for geriatric trauma patients: A prospective analysis. *Journal of the American College of Surgeons, 219*(1), 10–17e1. https://doi.org/10.1016/j.jamcollsurg.2014.03.020

Yesavage Geriatric Depression Scale (GDS)

(See Appendix 1, Chapter 6)

Chapter 13

COPD Assessment Test (CAT)

Patient-completed questionnaire assessing globally the impact of COPD (cough, sputum, dyspnea, chest tightness) on health status.

European Heart Rhythm Association (EHRA) Symptom Guide

EHRA Score	Symptoms	Description
1	None	
2a	Mild	Normal daily activity not affected
2b	Moderate	Normal daily activity not affected, but patient troubled by symptoms
3	Severe	Normal daily activity affected
4	Disabling	Normal daily activity discontinued

From Wynn, G. J., Todd, D. M., Webber, M., Bonnett, L., McShane, J., Kirchhof, P., & Gupta, D. (2014). The European Heart Rhythm Association symptom classification for atrial fibrillation: Validation and improvement through a simple modification. *EP Europace, 16*(7), 965–972. https://doi.org/10.1093/europace/eut395. With permission of the European Heart Rhythm Association.

Chapter 14

CURB-65

A Point Is Applied for Each Item Present	
C	Confusion
U	Urea plasmatic > 44 mg/dL (BUN > 19.6 mg/dL)
R	Respiratory rate ≥ 30 bpm
B	Systolic BP < 90 mm Hg or diastolic BP ≤ 60 mm Hg
65	Age ≥ 65 years old
Score	Stratification
0 or 1	Low mortality (0.7%–2.1%). Possible outpatient treatment
2	Intermediate mortality (9.2%). Consider hospital treatment
3	High mortality (14.5%). Hospital admission.
4–5	Mortality of > 40%. Admission. Consider intensive care unit

From The British Thoracic Society. (1987). Community-acquired pneumonia in adults in British hospitals in 1982-1983: A survey of aetiology, mortality, prognostic factors and outcome. *Quarterly Journal of Medicine, 62*(239), 195–220.

Laboratory Risk Indicator for Necrotizing Fasciitis (LRINEC)

C-reactive protein	<15 mg/dL (150 mg/L) 0		
	≥15 mg/dL (150 mg/L) +4		
White blood cell count (×10000/μL	<15 0	15–25 +1	>25 +2
Hemoglobin (g/dL)	>13.5 0		
	11–13.5 +1		
	<11 +2		
Sodium (mEq/L)	≥135 0		<135 +2
Creatinine	≤1.6 mg/dL (141 μmol/L) 0		
	>1.6 mg/dL (141 μmol/L) +2		
Glucose	≤180 mg/dL (10 mmol/L) 0		
	>180 mg/dL (10mmol/L) +1		

From Wong, C. H., Khin, L. W., Heng, K. S., et al. (2004). The LRINEC (Laboratory Risk Indicator for Necrotizing Fasciitis) score: A tool for distinguishing necrotizing fasciitis from other soft tissue infections. *Critical Care Medicine*, 32(7), 1535–1541.

Pneumonia Severity Index (PSI)

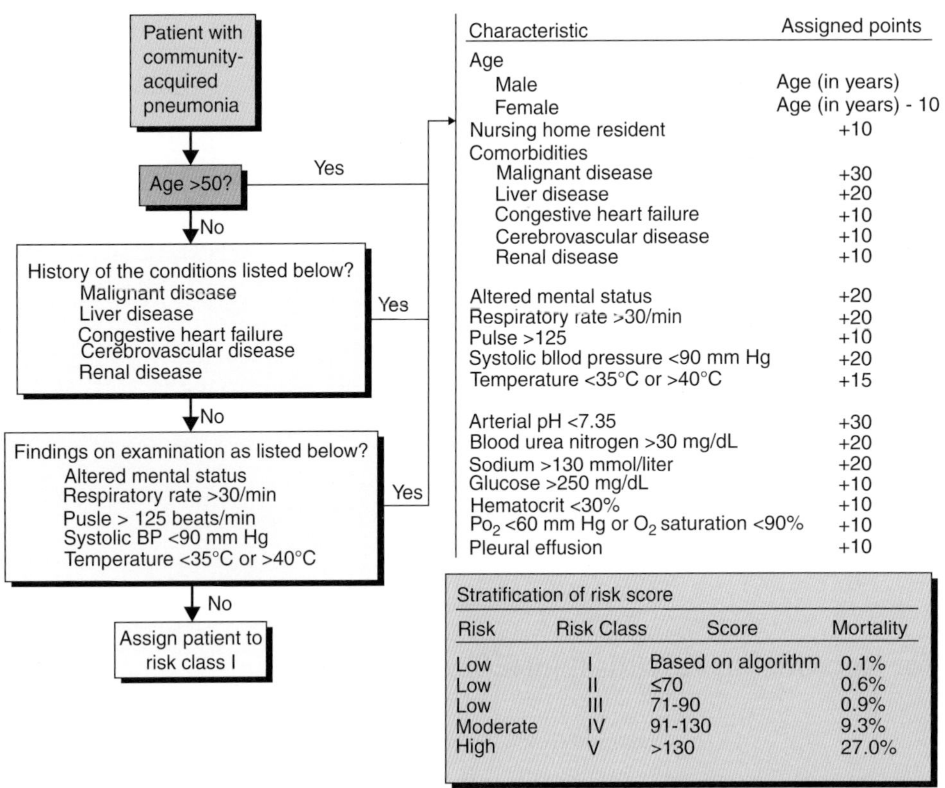

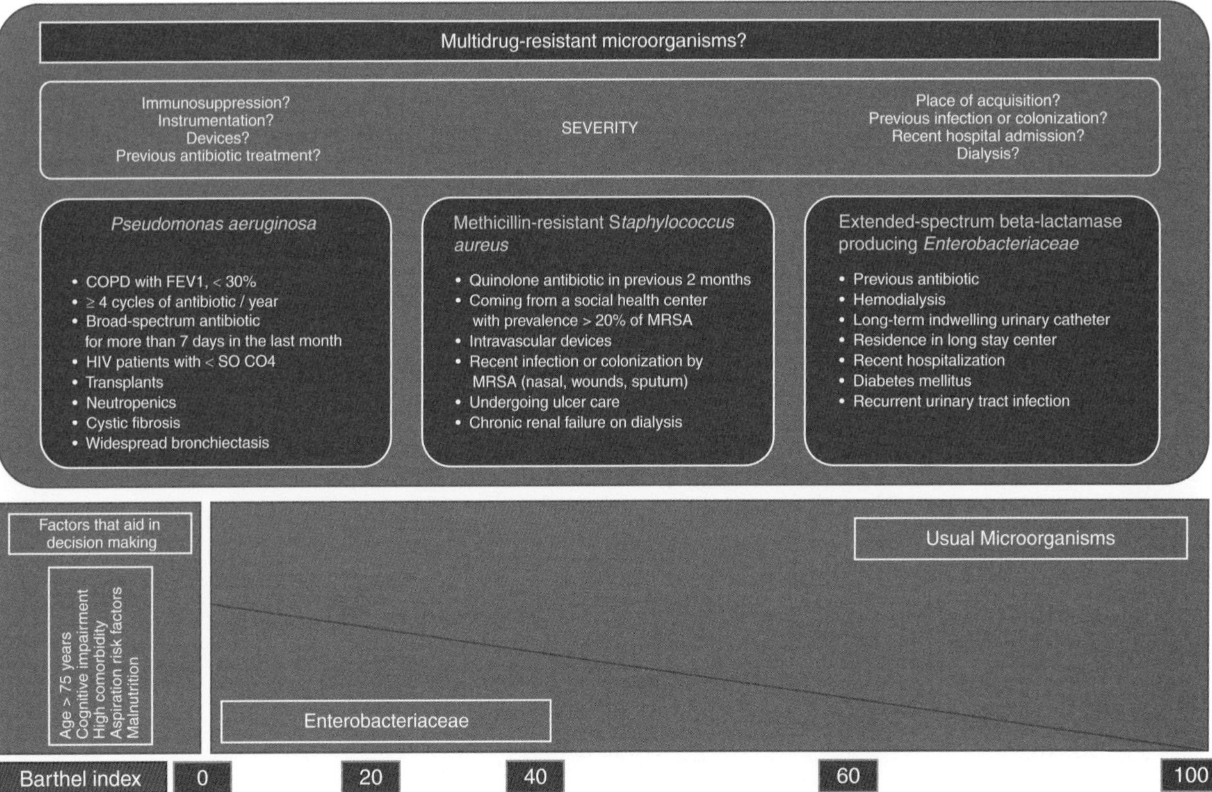

• The pneumonia severity index (PSI) ([A] From Sellke, F. W., et al. [2016]. *Sabiston & Spencer surgery of the chest*, [9th ed.]. Elsevier. [B] From Sellke, F. W., et al. [2016]. *Sabiston & Spencer surgery of the chest*, [9th ed.]. Elsevier; Halter, J. B., Ouslander, J. G., Studenski, S., High, K. P., Asthana, S., Supiano, M. A., Ritchie, C., & Hazzard, W. R., Woolard, N. F. [2021] *Hazzard's geriatric medicine and gerontology* [7th ed.]. www.accessmedicine.com. Copyright McGraw Hill Education. All rights reserved.)

Chapter 15

Health Assessment Questionnaire (HAQ)

The STANFORD HEALTH ASSESSMENT QUESTIONNAIRE©
Stanford University School of Medicine, Division of Immunology & Rheumatology

<u>HAQ Disability Index:</u>
In this section we are interested in learning how your illness affects your ability to function in daily life. Please feel free to add any comments on the back of this page.

Please check the response which best describes your usual abilities OVER THE PAST WEEK:

	Without ANY difficulty 0	With SOME difficulty 1	With MUCH difficulty 2	UNABLE to do 3
DRESSING & GROOMING				
Are you able to:				
-Dress yourself, including tying shoelaces and doing buttons?	☐	☐	☐	☐
-Shampoo your hair?	☐	☐	☐	☐
ARISING				
Are you able to:				
-Stand up from a straight chair?	☐	☐	☐	☐
-Get in and out of bed?	☐	☐	☐	☐
EATING				
Are you able to:				
-Cut your meat?	☐	☐	☐	☐
-Lift a full cup or glass to your mouth?	☐	☐	☐	☐
-Open a new milk carton?	☐	☐	☐	☐
WALKING				
Are you able to:				
-Walk outdoors on flat ground?	☐	☐	☐	☐
-Climb up five steps?	☐	☐	☐	☐

Please check any AIDS OR DEVICES that you usually use for any of these activities:

☐ Cane
☐ Walker
☐ Crutches
☐ Wheelchair

☐ Devices used for dressing (button hook, zipper pul long-handled shoe horn, etc.)
☐ Built up or special utensils
☐ Special or built up chair
☐ Other (Specify:_____________)

Please check any categories for which you usually need HELP FROM ANOTHER PERSON:

☐ Dressing and Grooming
☐ Arising

☐ Eating
☐ Walking

Please check the response which best describes your usual abilities **OVER THE PAST WEEK:**

	Without ANY difficulty 0	With SOME difficulty 1	With MUCH difficulty 2	UNABLE to do 3
HYGIENE				
Are you able to:				
-Wash and dry your body?	☐	☐	☐	☐
-Take a tub bath?	☐	☐	☐	☐
-Get on and off the toilet?	☐	☐	☐	☐
REACH				
Are you able to:				
-Reach and get down a 5-pound object (such as a bag of sugar) from just above your head?	☐	☐	☐	☐
-Bend down to pick up clothing from the floor?	☐	☐	☐	☐
GRIP				
Are you able to:				
-Open car doors?	☐	☐	☐	☐
-Open jars which have been previously opened?	☐	☐	☐	☐
-Turn faucets on and off?	☐	☐	☐	☐
ACTIVITIES				
Are you able to:				
-Run errands and shop?	☐	☐	☐	☐
-Get in and out of a car?	☐	☐	☐	☐
-Do chores such as vacuuming or yardwork	☐	☐	☐	☐

Please check any AIDS OR DEVICES that you usually use for any of these activities:

☐ Raised toilet seat
☐ Bathtub seat
☐ Jar opener (for jars previously opened)
☐ Bathtub bar
☐ Long-handled appliances for reach
☐ Long-handled appliances in bathroom
☐ Other (Specify:__________)

Please check any categories for which you usually need HELP FROM ANOTHER PERSON:

☐ Hygiene
☐ Reach
☐ Gripping and opening things
☐ Errands and chores

We are also interested in learning whether or not you are affected by pain because of your illness.

How much pain have you had because of your illness IN THE PAST WEEK:

PLACE A VERTICAL (|) MARK ON THE LINE TO INDICATE THE SEVERITY OF THE PAIN

No Pain **Severe Pain**

0 ______________________________ **100**

Considering all the ways that your arthritis affects you, rate how you are doing on the following scale by placing a vertical mark on the line.

Very Well **Very Poor**

0 ______________________________ **100**

• Health Assessment Questionnaire (HAQ) (From Bruce, B., & Fries, J. F. [2003]. The Stanford health assessment questionnaire: Dimensions and practical applications. *Health and Quality of Life Outcomes, 1*, 20. https://doi.org/10.1186/1477-7525-1-20.) The Stanford Health Assessment Questionnaire, Copyright Stanford University School of Medicine, Division of Immunology & Rheumatology.)

Chapter 16

36-Item Short Survey (SF-36)

The 36-Item Short Form (SF-36) is a set of generic, coherent, and easily administered quality-of-life measures. These measures rely on patient self-reporting and have been widely used.

Data from RAND. RAND® is a registered trademark. ©1994–2022 RAND Corporation. https://www.rand.org/health-care/surveys_tools/mos/36-item-short-form.html

Health Assessment Questionnaire-II (HAQ-II)

A short, 10-item questionnaire that is for patients with rheumatological diseases. It allows the healthcare provider to assess the patients disability or physical function in these patients.

Symptom Severity Scale (SSS)

1. How severe is the hand or wrist pain that you have at night?
   - I do not have hand or wrist pain
   - Mild pain
   - Moderate pain
   - Severe pain
   - Very severe pain
2. How often did hand or wrist pain wake you up during a typical night in the past two weeks?
   - Never
   - Once
   - Two to three times
   - Four or five times
   - More than five times
3. Do you typically have pain in your hand or wrist during the daytime?
   - I never have pain during the day
   - I have mild pain during the day
   - I have moderate pain during the day
   - I have severe pain during the day
   - I have very severe pain during the day
4. How often do you have hand or wrist pain during the daytime?
   - Never
   - Once or twice a day
   - Three to five times a day
   - More than five times a day
   - The pain is constant
5. How long, on average, does an episode of pain last during the daytime?
   - I never get pain during the day
   - Less than 10 minutes
   - 10 to 60 minutes
   - Greater than 60 minutes
   - The pain is constant throughout the day
6. Do you have numbness (loss of sensation) in your hand?
   - No
   - I have mild numbness
   - I have moderate numbness
   - I have severe numbness
   - I have very severe numbness
7. Do you have weakness in your hand or wrist?
   - No weakness
   - Mild weakness
   - Moderate weakness
   - Severe weakness
   - Very severe weakness
8. Do you have tingling sensations in your hand?
   - No tingling
   - Mild tingling
   - Moderate tingling
   - Severe tingling
   - Very severe tingling
9. How severe is numbness (loss of sensation) or tingling at night?
   - I have no numbness or tingling at night
   - Mild
   - Moderate
   - Severe
   - Very severe
10. How often did hand numbness or tingling wake you up during a typical night during the past two weeks?
    - Never
    - Once
    - Two or three times
    - Four or five times
    - More than five times
11. Do you have difficulty with the grasping and use of small objects such as keys or pens?
    - No difficulty
    - Mild difficulty
    - Moderate difficulty
    - Severe difficulty
    - Very severe difficulty

Table from Demino, C., & Fowler, J. R. (2020). Diagnostic value of ultrasound in CTS in diabetic versus nondiabetic populations. *Journal of Hand Surgery Global Online, 2*(5), 267–271. https://doi.org/10.1016/j.jhsg.2020.06.001. Erratum in *Journal of Hand Surgery Global Online, 3*(6), 373–374, November 17, 2021. PMID: 35415520; PMCID: PMC8991754, Figure 2.

Chapter 17

Balducci Frailty Criteria

Frailty Criteria	Characteristics
Age	≥85 y
ADLs	Dependence for 1 or more
Comorbidity	3 or more
Geriatric syndromes	One or more of the following: • Delirium • Dementia • Depression • Osteoporosis • Incontinence • Falls • Neglect and abuse • Failure to thrive

ADLs, Activites of daily living.
From Pal, S. K., Katheria, V., & Hurria, A. (2010), Evaluating the older patient with cancer: Understanding frailty and the geriatric assessment. *CA: A Cancer Journal for Clinicians, 60*, 120–132. https://doi.org/10.3322/caac.20059; Balducci, L., & Extermann, M. (2000). Management of the frail person with advanced cancer. *Critical Reviews in Oncology/Hematology, 33*, 143–148.

Cancer and Aging Research Group (CARG): Chemotoxicity Calculator

The Chemo-Toxicity Calculator is a prechemotherapy assessment that captures sociodemographics, tumor/treatment variables, laboratory test results (hemoglobin, creatinine clearance), and geriatric assessment variables (function, comorbidity, cognition, psychological state, social activity/support, and nutritional status).

Data from https://www.mycarg.org/?page_id=2405.

Chemotherapy Risk Assessment Scale for High-Age Patients (CRASH)

Predictors	0 Points	1 Point	2 Points
Hematologic score			
Diastolic Blood Pressure (BP)	≤72	>72	
Independent Activities of Daily Living (IADL)	26–29	10–25	
Lactate Dehydrogenase (LDH) (if ULN 618 U/L; otherwise, 0.74 /LULN)	0–459		>459
Chemotox	0–0.44	0.45–0.57	>0.57
Nonhematologic score			
ECOG PS (Eastern Cooperative Oncology Group Performance Status)	0	1–2	3–4
MMS (mini mental health status)	30		<30
MNA Mini Nutrtional Assessment	28–30		<28
Chemotox	0–0.44	0.45–0.57	>0.57

Adapted from Extermann, M., Boler, I., Reich, R. R., et al. (2012). Predicting the risk of chemotherapy toxicity in older patients: The Chemotherapy Risk Assessment Scale for High-Age Patients [CRASH] score. *Cancer, 118*(13), 3377–3386.

Distress Thermometer

The Distress Thermometer is a scale represented on a visual graphic of a thermometer that ranges from 0 (no distress) to 10 (extreme distress). Patients use the Distress Thermometer to indicate their level of distress.

Electronic Rapid Fitness Assessment (eRFA)

The electronic Rapid Fitness Assessment (eRFA) is a questionnaire developed at Memorial Sloan Kettering and used by all the doctors on the Geriatrics Service to gauge and understand an older patient's level of fitness.

Data From Shahrokni, A., Tin, A., Downey, R. J., et al. (2017). Electronic rapid fitness assessment: A novel tool for pre-operative evaluation of the geriatric oncology patient. *Journal of the National Comprehensive Cancer Network, 15*(2), 172–179. https://doi.org/10.6004/jnccn.2017.0018

Fried Frailty Criteria

Abnormalities	Frailty Scale
Involuntary weight loss of 10 lbs or more in the last 6 months	Fit (no abnormalities)
Reduced grip strength	Pre-frail (2 abnormalities or less)
Difficulty initiating movements	Frail (3 or more abnormalities)
Reduced walking speed	
Fatigue	

Categories of Frailty:

- Fit: No abnormalities.
- Pre-Frail: 2 abnormalities or less.
- Frail: 3 or more abnormalities.

From Fried, L. P., Tangen, C. M., Walston, J., et al. Cardiovascular Health Study Collaborative Research Group. (2001). Frailty in older adults: Evidence for a phenotype. *Journals of Gerontology Series A Biological Sciences and Medical Sciences, 56*(3), M146–M56.

Patient Health Questionnaire-2 (PHQ-2)

The PHQ-2 inquires about the frequency of depressed mood and anhedonia over the past two weeks. The PHQ-2 includes the first two items of the PHQ-9.

- The purpose of the PHQ-2 is to screen for depression in a "first-step" approach.
- Patients who screen positive should be further evaluated with the PHQ-9 to determine whether they meet criteria for a depressive disorder.

Over the **last 2 weeks**, how often have you been bothered by the following problems?	Not at all	Several days	More than half the days	Nearly every day
1. Little interest or pleasure in doing things	○ 0	○ +1	○ +2	○ +3
2. Feeling down, depressed or hopeless	○ 0	○ +1	○ +2	○ +3

PHQ-2 score obtained by adding score for each question (total points)

Interpretation:

- A PHQ-2 score ranges from 0-6. The authors identified a score of 3 as the optimal cutpoint when using the PHQ-2 to screen for depression.
- If the score is 3 or greater, major depressive disorder is likely.
- Patients who screen positive should be further evaluated with the PHQ-9, other diagnostic instruments, or direct interview to determine whether they meet criteria for a depressive disorder.

Operating Characteristics of PHQ-2 as a Screener for Depressive Disorders in 580 Patients Who Had an Independent Mental Health Professional Interview

Major Depressive Disorder (7% Prevalence)			
PHQ-2 Score	Sensitivity	Specificity	Positive Predictive Value (PPV*)
1	97.6	59.2	15.4
2	92.7	73.7	21.1
3	82.9	90.0	38.4
4	73.2	93.3	45.4
5	53.7	96.8	56.4
6	26.8	99.4	78.6

Any Depressive Disorder (18% Prevalence)			
PHQ-2 Score	Sensitivity	Specificity	Positive Predictive Value (PPV*)
1	90.6	65.4	36.9
2	82.1	80.4	48.3
3	62.3	95.4	75.0
4	50.9	97.9	81.2
5	31.1	98.7	84.6
6	12.3	99.8	92.9

Notes:

- *Because the PPV varies with the prevalence of depression, the PPV will be higher in settings with a higher prevalence of depression and lower in settings with a lower prevalence.

• Patient Health Questionnaire-2 (PHQ-2) (Image Copyright 2022 National HIV Curriculum–The University of Washington. Created from Kroenke, K., Spitzer, R. L., & Williams J. B. W. [2003]. The patient health questionnaire-2: Validity of a two-item depression screener. *Medical Care, 41*, 1284–1292.)

Patient Health Questionnaire (PHQ-9)

(See Appendix 1, Chapter 6)

Yesavage Geriatric Depression Scale (GDS)

(See Appendix 1, Chapter 6)

Chapter 18

Abnormal Involuntary Movement Scale (AIMS)

Instructions: Complete the examination procedure before making ratings. Circle score for each item.

Patient Name:	Date:	None	Minimal, May Be Extreme Normal	Mild	Moderate	Severe
Facial and Oral Movements						
1. Muscles of Facial Expression e.g., movements of forehead, eyebrows, periorbital area, cheeks; include frowning, blinking, smiling, grimacing		0	1	2	3	4
2. Lips and Perioral Area e.g., puckering, pouting, smacking		0	1	2	3	4
3. Jaw e.g., biting, clenching, chewing, mouth opening, lateral movement		0	1	2	3	4
4. Tongue Rate only increases in movement both in and out of mouth, NOT inability to sustain movement		0	1	2	3	4
Extremity Movements						
5. Upper (arms, wrists, hands, fingers) Include choreic movements (i.e., rapid, objectively purposeless, irregular, spontaneous); athetoid movements (i.e., slow, irregular, complex, serpentine). DO NOT include tremor (i.e., repetitive, regular, rhythmic).		0	1	2	3	4
6. Lower (legs, knees, ankles, toes) e.g., lateral knee movement, foot tapping, heel dropping, foot squirming, inversion and eversion of Foot		0	1	2	3	4

Patient Name:	Date:	None	Minimal,	Mild	Moderate	Severe
Trunk Movements						
7. Neck, shoulders, hips		0	1	2	3	4
e.g., rocking, twisting, squirming, pelvic gyrations						
Global Judgments						
8. Severity of abnormal movements		0	1	2	3	4
9. Incapacitation due to abnormal movements		0	1	2	3	4
10. Patient's awareness of abnormal movements (rate only		0	1	2	3	4
patient's report)						
0 = not aware; 1 = aware, no distress; 2 = aware, mild						
distress; 3 = aware, moderate distress; 4 = aware.\,						
severe distress						
Dental Status						
11. Current problems with teeth and/or dentures?		No	Yes			

AIMS Examination Procedure

Either before or after completing the Examination Procedure, observe the patient unobtrusively, at rest (e.g., in the waiting room). The chair to be used in this examination should be a hard, firm one without arms.

1. Ask the patient whether there is anything in his/her mouth (i.e., gum, candy, etc.) and if there is, remove it.
2. Ask patient about the current condition of his/her teeth. Do teeth bother patient now?
3. Ask the patient whether he/she notices any movements in mouth, face, hands, or feet. If yes, ask to describe and to what extent they currently bother patient or interfere with his/her activities.
4. Have patient sit in chair with hands on knees, legs slightly apart, and feet flat on floor. (Look at entire body for movements while in this position.)
5. Ask patient to sit with hands hanging unsupported: if male, between legs; if female and wearing a dress, hanging over knees. (Observe hands or other body areas.)
6. Ask patient to open mouth. (Observe tongue at rest within mouth.) Do this twice.
7. Ask patient to protrude tongue. (Observe abnormalities of tongue movement.) Do this twice.
8. Ask patient to tap thumb, with each finger as rapidly as possible for 10 to 15 seconds; first with right hand, then with left hand. (Observe facial and leg movements.)
9. Flex and extend patient's left and right arms (one at a time).
10. Ask patient to stand up. (Observe in profile. Observe all body areas again, hips included.)
11. Ask patient to extend both arms outstretched in front with palms down. (Observe trunk, legs, and mouth,)
12. Have patient walk a few paces, turn, and walk back to chair. (Observe hands and gait.) Do this twice.

From Maryland Department of Health. (n.d.). https://mmcp.health.maryland.gov/pap/docs/Abnormal%20Involuntary%20Movement%20Scale.pdf. Adapted from Guy, W. (1976). *ECDEU Assessment manual for psychopharmacology–revised* (DHEW PublNo ADM 76-338), US Department of Health, Education and Welfare.

Adult Manifest Anxiety Scale–Elderly Version (AMAS-E)

The Adult Manifest Anxiety Scale-Elderly Version (AMAS-E) is a multidimensional measure of chronic, manifest anxiety designed specifically for the older adult population, ages 60 and older.

Data from Lowe, P. A., & Reynolds, C. R. (2006) Examination of the psychometric properties of the adult manifest anxiety scale–elderly version scores. *Educational and Psychological Measurement, 66*(1), 93–115. https://doi.org/10.1177/0013164405278563

The Alcohol Use Disorder Identification Test-Consumption questionnaire AUDIT-C

(See Appendix 1, Chapter 10)

Ask Suicide-Screening Questions (ASQ)

Ask the patient:

1. **In the past few weeks, have you wished you were dead?** ❍ Yes ❍ No
2. **In the past few weeks, have you felt that you or your family would be better off if you were dead?** ❍ Yes ❍ No
3. **In the past week, have you been having thoughts about killing yourself?** ❍ Yes ❍ No
4. **Have you ever tried to kill yourself?** ❍ Yes ❍ No

   If yes, how? ____________________

   When? ____________________

If the patient answers **Yes** *to any of the above, ask the following acuity question:*

5. **Are you having thoughts of killing yourself right now?** ❍ Yes ❍ No

   If yes, please describe: ____________________

Next steps:

- If patient answers "No" to all questions 1 through 4, screening is complete (not necessary to ask question #5). No intervention is necessary (*Note: Clinical judgment can always override a negative screen).
- **If patient answers "Yes" to any of questions 1 through 4, or refuses to answer, they are considered a positive screen.** Ask question #5 to assess acuity:
  - ☐ **"Yes"** to question #5 = **acute positive screen** (imminent risk identified)
    - **Patient requires a STAT safety/full mental health evaluation. Patient cannot leave until evaluated for safety.**
    - Keep patient in sight. Remove all dangerous objects from room. Alert physician or clinician responsible for patient's care.
  - ☐ **"No"** to question #5 = **non-acute positive screen** (potential risk identified)
    - **Patient requires a brief suicide safety assessment to determine if a full mental health evaluation is needed. Patient cannot leave until evaluated for safety.**
    - Alert physician or clinician responsible for patient's care.

Provide resources to all patients

- 24/7 National Suicide Prevention Lifeline 1-800-273-TALK (8255) En Español: 1-888-628-9454
- 24/7 Crisis Text Line: Text "HOME" to 741-741

asQ Suicide Risk Screening Toolkit NATIONAL INSTITUTE OF MENTAL HEALTH (NIMH) NIH 7/1/2020

• Ask Suicide-screening Questions (ASQ) (From The National Institute of Mental Health [NIMH]. https://www.nimh.nih.gov/sites/default/files/documents/research/research-conducted-at-nimh/asq-toolkit-materials/asq-tool/screening_tool_asq_nimh_toolkit.pdf.)

Brief Carroll Depression Rating Scale (BCDRS)

Date of Visit:

Visit Number:

Patient Initials: Hospital Reg. No.
F M L

Complete *ALL* the following statements by *CIRCLING* YES or NO, based on how you have felt during *the past few days*.

1.	I feel just as energetic as always	Yes	No
2.	I am losing weight	Yes	No
3.	I have dropped many of my interests and activities	Yes	No
4.	Since my illness I have completely lost interest in sex	Yes	No
5.	I am especially concerned about how my body is functioning	Yes	No
6.	It must be obvious that I am disturbed and agitated	Yes	No
7.	I am still able to carry on doing the work I am supposed to do	Yes	No
8.	I can concentrate easily when resind the papers	Yes	No
9.	Getting to sleep takes me more than half an hour	Yes	No
10.	I am restless and fidgety	Yes	No
11.	I wake up much earlier than I need to in the morning	Yes	No
12.	Dying is the best solution for me	Yes	No
13.	I have a lot of trouble with dizzy and faint feelings	Yes	No
14.	I am being punished for something bad in my past	Yes	No
15.	My sexual interest is the same as before I got sick	Yes	No
16.	I am miserable or often feel like crying	Yes	No
17.	I often wish I were dead	Yes	No
18.	I am having trouble with indigestion	Yes	No
19.	I wake up often in the middle of the night	Yes	No
20.	I feel worthless and ashamed about myself	Yes	No
21.	I am so slowed down that I need help with bathing and dressing	Yes	No
22.	I take longer than usual to fall asleep at night	Yes	No
23.	Much of the time I am very afraid but don't know the reason	Yes	No
24.	Things which I regret about my life are bothering me	Yes	No
25.	I get pleasure and satisfaction from what I do	Yes	No
26.	All I need is a good rest to be perfectly well again	Yes	No
27.	My sleep is restless and disturbed	Yes	No
28.	My mind is as fast and alert as always	Yes	No
29.	I feel that life is still worth living	Yes	No
30.	My voice is dull and lifeless	Yes	No
31.	I feel irritable or jittery	Yes	No
32.	I feel in good spirits	Yes	No
33.	My heart sometimes beats faster than usual	Yes	No
34.	I think my case is hopeless	Yes	No
35.	I wake up before my usual time in the morning	Yes	No
36.	I still enjoy my meals as much as usual	Yes	No

Brief Carroll Depression Rating Scale (BCDRS)

37. I have to keep pacing around most of the time	Yes	No
38. I am terrified and near panic	Yes	No
39. My body is bad and rotten inside	Yes	No
40. I got sick because of the bad weather we have been having	Yes	No
41. My hands shake so much that people can easily notice	Yes	No
42. I still like to go out and meet people	Yes	No
43. I think I appear calm on the outside	Yes	No
44. I think I am as good a person as anybody else	Yes	No
45. My trouble is the result of some serious internal disease	Yes	No
46. I have been thinking about trying to kill myself	Yes	No
47. I get hardly anything done lately	Yes	No
48. There is only misery in the future for me	Yes	No
49. I worry a lot about my bodily symptoms	Yes	No
50. I have to force myself to eat even a little	Yes	No
51. I am exhausted much of the time	Yes	No
52. I can tell that I have lost a lot of weight	Yes	No

From Carroll, B. J., & Feinberg, M., et al. (1981). The Carroll rating scale for depression. I. Development, reliability and validation. *British Journal of Psychiatry, 138*, 194–200.

The CAGE Screening Tool

(See Appendix 1, Chapter 6)

Clinical Institute Withdrawal Assessment (CIWA) for Alcohol

Patient:____________ Date:_________ Time________(24-hour clock, midnight = 00.00)

Pulse or heart rate, taken for one minute:______________ Blood pressure:____________

NAUSEA AND VOMITING—Ask "Do you feel sick to your stomach? Have you vomited?" Observation.
0 no nausea and no vomiting
1 mild nausea with no vomiting
2
3
4 intermittent nausea with dry heaves
5
6
7 constant nausea, frequent dry heaves and vomiting

TREMOR—Arms extended and figures spread apart. Observation.
0 no tremor
1 not visible, but can be felt fingertip to fingertip
2
3
4 moderate, with patient's arms extended
5
6
7 severe, even with arms not extended

TACTILE DISTURBANCES—Ask "Have you any itching, pins and needles sensations, any burning, any numbness, or do you feel bugs crawling on or under your skin?" Observation.
0 none
1 very mild itching, pins and needles, burning or numbness
2 mild itching, pins and needles, burning or numbness
3 moderate itching, pins and needles, burning or numbness
4 moderately severe hallucinations
7 continuous hallucinations

AUDITORY DISTURBANCES—Ask "Are you more aware of sounds around you? Are they harsh? Do they frighten you? Are you hearing anything that is disturbing to you? Are you hearing things you know are not there?" Observation.
1 very mild harshness or ability to frighten
2 mild harshness or ability to frighten
3 moderate harshness or ability to frighten
4 moderately severe hallucinations
5 severe hallucinations
6 extremely severe hallucinations
7 continuous hallucinations

PAROXYSMAL SWEATS—Observation.
0 barely perceptible sweating, palms moist
2
3
4 beads of sweat obvious on forehead
5
6
7 drenching sweats

VISUAL DISTURBANCES—Ask "Does the light appear to be too bright? Is its color different? Does it hurt your eyes? Are you seeing anything that is disturbing to you? Are you seeing things you know are not there? Observation.
0 not present
1 very mild sensitivity
2 mild sensitivity
3 moderate sensitivity
4 moderately severe hallucinations
5 severe hallucinations
6 extremely severe hallucinations
7 continuous hallucinations

ANXIETY—Ask "Do you feel nervous?" Observation.
0 no anxiety, at ease
1 mild anxious
2
3
4 moderately anxious, or guarded, so anxiety is inferred
5
6
7 equivalent to acute panic states as seen in severe delirium or acute schizophrenic reactions

HEADACHE, FULLNESS IN HEAD—Ask "Does your head feel different? Does it feel like is a band around your head?" Do not rate for dizziness or light headedness. Otherwise, rate severity.
0 not present
1 very mild
2 mild
3 moderate
4 moderately severe
5 severe
6 very severe
7 extremely severe

AGITATION -- Observation.
0 normal activity
1 somewhat more than normal activity
2
3
4 moderately fidgety and restless
5
6
7 paces back and forth during most of the interview, or constantly thrashes about

ORIENTATION AND CLOUDING OF SENSORIUM—Ask "What day is this? Where are you? Who am I?
0 oriented and can do serial additions
1 cannot do serial additions or is uncertain about date
2 disoriented for date by no more than 2 calendar days
3 disoriented for date by more than 2 calendar days
4 disoriented for place/or person

Total **CIWA-Ar** Score____________
Rater's initial____________
Maximum possible score 67

The **CIWA-Ar** is not copyrighted and may be reproduced freely. This assessment for monitoring withdrawal symptoms requires approximately 5 minutes to administer. The maximum score is 67 (see instrument). Patients scoring less than 10 do not usually need additional medication for withdrawal.

From Sullivan, J. T., Sykora, K., et al. (1989). Assessment of alcohol withdrawal: The revised clinical institute withdrawal assessment for alcohol scale (CIWA-Ar). *British Journal of Addiction 84*, 1353–1357.

Geriatric Anxiety Inventory (GAI)

I worry a lot of the time.
I find it difficult to make a decision.
I often feel jumpy.
I find it hard to relax.
I often cannot enjoy things because of my worries.
Little things bother me a lot.
I often feel like I have butterflies in my stomach.
I think of myself as a worrier.
I can't help worrying about even trivial things.
I often feel nervous.
My own thoughts often make me anxious.
I get an upset stomach due to my worrying.
I think of myself as a nervous person.
I always anticipate the worst will happen.
I often feel shaky inside.
I think that my worries interfere with my life.
My worries often overwhelm me.
I sometimes feel a great knot in my stomach.
I miss out on things because I worry too much.
I often feel upset.

Adapted from Pachana, N. A., Byrne, G. J., Siddle, H., Koloski, N., Harley, E., & Arnold, E. (2007). Development and validation of the geriatric anxiety inventory. *International Psychogeriatrics, 19*(1),103–114. https://doi.org/10.1017/S1041610206003504; with permission.

Geriatric Anxiety Scale (GAS-10)

Below is a list of common symptoms of anxiety or stress. Please read each item in the list carefully. Indicate how often you have experienced each symptom during the PAST WEEK, INCLUDING TODAY by checking under the corresponding answer.

	Not at All (0)	Sometimes (1)	Most of the Time (2)	All of the Time (3)
1. I was irritable.				
2. I felt detached or isolated from others.				
3. I felt like I was in a daze.				
4. I had a hard time sitting still.				
5. I could not control my worry.				
6. I felt restless, keyed up, or on edge.				
7. I felt tired.				
8. My muscles were tense.				
9. I felt like I had no control over my life.				
10. I felt like something terrible was going to happen to me.				

GAS-10 Scoring Instructions

Items 1 through 10 are summed to provide a Total Score. Each item ranges from 0 to 3.Score distribution for GAS-10 (N = 556)

Raw	T-Score	Percentile	Descriptive Category
1	42	21	Minimal
2	44	30	Minimal
3	46	34	Minimal
4	48	45	Minimal
5	51	53	Minimal
6	53	63	Minimal
7	55	70	Mild
8	57	75	Mild
9	59	82	Mild
10	61	90	Moderate
12	66	95	Severe
14	70	98	Severe
16	74	99	Severe
18	79	99	Severe
24	92	99	Severe
30	104	99	Severe

From Segal, D. L., June, A., Payne, M., Coolidge, F. L., & Yochim, B. (2010). Development and initial validation of a self-report assessment tool for anxiety among older adults: The geriatric anxiety scale. *Journal of Anxiety Disorders, 24*, 709–714; Mueller, A. E., Segal, D. L., Gavett, B., Marty, M. A., Yochim, B., June, A., & Coolidge, F. L. (in press). Geriatric anxiety scale: Item response theory analysis, differential item functioning, and creation of 10-item short form (GAS-10). *International Psychogeriatrics*.

Mini-Cog©

(See Appendix 1, Chapter 6)

Montreal Cognitive Assessment (MoCA©)

(See Appendix 1, Chapter 5)

Patient Health Questionnaire-2 (PHQ-2)

(See Appendix 1, Chapter 17)

Yesavage Geriatric Depression Scale (GDS)

(See Appendix 1, Chapter 6)

Chapter 21

Instrumental Activities of Daily Living Scale

(See Appendix 1, Chapter 6)

The Lawton Instrumental Activities of Daily Living Scale

(See Appendix 1, Chapter 6)

Minimum Data Set (MDS)

Data collection tool used by CMS in the nursing home setting: The Minimum Data Set (MDS) 3.0 Resident:
From https://www.cms.gov/Medicare/Quality-Initiatives-Patient-Assessment-Instruments/NursingHomeQualityInits/MDS30RAIManual

NIH Stroke Scale

NIH STROKE SCALE

Patient Identification. ___ ___-___ ___ ___-___ ___ ___

Pt. Date of Birth ___ ___/___ ___/___ ___

Hospital ______________________(___ ___-___ ___)

Date of Exam ___ ___/___ ___/___ ___

Interval: [ ] Baseline [ ] 2 hours post treatment [ ] 24 hours post onset of symptoms ±20 minutes [ ] 7–10 days
[ ] 3 months [ ] Other ______________________________(___ ___)

Time: ___ ___:___ ___ [ ]am [ ]pm

Person Administering Scale ___________________________________

Administer stroke scale items in the order listed. Record performance in each category after each subscale exam. Do not go back and change scores. Follow directions provided for each exam technique. Scores should reflect what the patient does, not what the clinician thinks the patient can do. The clinician should record answers while administering the exam and work quickly. Except where indicated, the patient should not be coached (i.e., repeated requests to patient to make a special effort).

Instructions	Scale Definition	Score
1a. Level of Consciousness: The investigator must choose a response if a full evaluation is prevented by such obstacles as an endotracheal tube, language barrier, orotracheal trauma/bandages. A 3 is scored only if the patient makes no movement (other than reflexive posturing) in response to noxious stimulation.	0 = **Alert;** keenly responsive. 1 = **Not alert**; but arousable by minor stimulation to obey, answer, or respond. 2 = **Not alert**; requires repeated stimulation to attend, or is obtunded and requires strong or painful stimulation to make movements (not stereotyped). 3 = Responds only with reflex motor or autonomic effects or totally unresponsive, flaccid, and areflexic.	______
1b. LOC Questions: The patient is asked the month and his/her age. The answer must be correct – there is no partial credit for being close. Aphasic and stuporous patients who do not comprehend the questions will score 2. Patients unable to speak because of endotracheal intubation, orotracheal trauma, severe dysarthria from any cause, language barrier, or any other problem not secondary to aphasia are given a 1. It is important that only the initial answer be graded and that the examiner not "help" the patient with verbal or non-verbal cues.	0 = **Answers** both questions correctly. 1 = **Answers** one question correctly. 2 = **Answers** neither question correctly.	______
1c. LOC Commands: The patient is asked to open and close the eyes and then to grip and release the non-paretic hand. Substitute another one step command if the hands cannot be used. Credit is given if an unequivocal attempt is made but not completed due to weakness. If the patient does not respond to command, the task should be demonstrated to him or her (pantomime), and the result scored (i.e., follows none, one or two commands). Patients with trauma, amputation, or other physical impediments should be given suitable one-step commands. Only the first attempt is scored.	0 = **Performs** both tasks correctly. 1 = **Performs** one task correctly. 2 = **Performs** neither task correctly.	______
2. Best Gaze: Only horizontal eye movements will be tested. Voluntary or reflexive (oculocephalic) eye movements will be scored, but caloric testing is not done. If the patient has a conjugate deviation of the eyes that can be overcome by voluntary or reflexive activity, the score will be 1. If a patient has an isolated peripheral nerve paresis (CN III, IV, or VI), score a 1. Gaze is testable in all aphasic patients. Patients with ocular trauma, bandages, pre-existing blindness, or other disorder of visual acuity or fields should be tested with reflexive movements, and a choice made by the investigator. Establishing eye contact and then moving about the patient from side to side will occasionally clarify the presence of a partial gaze palsy.	0 = **Normal.** 1 = **Partial gaze palsy;** gaze is abnormal in one or both eyes, but forced deviation or total gaze paresis is not present. 2 = **Forced deviation,** or total gaze paresis not overcome by the oculocephalic maneuver.	______

NIH STROKE SCALE

Patient Identification. ___ ___-___ ___ ___-___ ___ ___

Pt. Date of Birth ___ ___/___ ___/___ ___

Hospital ______________________(___ ___-___ ___)

Date of Exam ___ ___/___ ___/___ ___

Interval: [ ] Baseline [ ] 2 hours post treatment [ ] 24 hours post onset of symptoms ±20 minutes [ ] 7–10 days
[ ] 3 months [ ] Other ______________________________(___ ___)

3. Visual: Visual fields (upper and lower quadrants) are tested by confrontation, using finger counting or visual threat, as appropriate. Patients may be encouraged, but if they look at the side of the moving fingers appropriately, this can be scored as normal. If there is unilateral blindness or enucleation, visual fields in the remaining eye are scored. Score 1 only if a clear-cut asymmetry, including quadrantanopia, is found. If patient is blind from any cause, score 3. Double simultaneous stimulation is performed at this point. If there is extinction, patient receives a 1, and the results are used to respond to item 11.	0 = **No visual loss.** 1 = **Partial hemianopia.** 2 = **Complete hemianopia.** 3 = **Bilateral hemianopia** (blind including cortical blindness).	______
4. Facial Palsy: Ask — or use pantomime to encourage — the patient to show teeth or raise eyebrows and close eyes. Score symmetry of grimace in response to noxious stimuli in the poorly responsive or non-comprehending patient. If facial trauma/bandages, orotracheal tube, tape or other physical barriers obscure the face, these should be removed to the extent possible.	0 = **Normal** symmetrical movements. 1 = **Minor paralysis** (flattened nasolabial fold, asymmetry on smiling). 2 = **Partial paralysis** (total or near-total paralysis of lower face). 3 = **Complete paralysis** of one or both sides (absence of facial movement in the upper and lower face).	______
5. Motor Arm: The limb is placed in the appropriate position: extend the arms (palms down) 90 degrees (if sitting) or 45 degrees (if supine). Drift is scored if the arm falls before 10 seconds. The aphasic patient is encouraged using urgency in the voice and pantomime, but not noxious stimulation. Each limb is tested in turn, beginning with the non-paretic arm. Only in the case of amputation or joint fusion at the shoulder, the examiner should record the score as untestable (UN), and clearly write the explanation for this choice.	0 = **No drift;** limb holds 90 (or 45) degrees for full 10 seconds. 1 = **Drift;** limb holds 90 (or 45) degrees, but drifts down before full 10 seconds; does not hit bed or other support. 2 = **Some effort against gravity;** limb cannot get to or maintain (if cued) 90 (or 45) degrees, drifts down to bed, but has some effort against gravity. 3 = **No effort against gravity;** limb falls. 4 = **No movement.** UN = **Amputation** or joint fusion, explain: ________________ **5a. Left Arm** **5b. Right Arm**	 5a. ______ 5b. ______
6. Motor Leg: The limb is placed in the appropriate position: hold the leg at 30 degrees (always tested supine). Drift is scored if the leg falls before 5 seconds. The aphasic patient is encouraged using urgency in the voice and pantomime, but not noxious stimulation. Each limb is tested in turn, beginning with the non-paretic leg. Only in the case of amputation or joint fusion at the hip, the examiner should record the score as untestable (UN), and clearly write the explanation for this choice.	0 = **No drift;** leg holds 30-degree position for full 5 seconds. 1 = **Drift;** leg falls by the end of the 5-second period but does not hit bed. 2 = **Some effort against gravity;** leg falls to bed by 5 seconds, but has some effort against gravity. 3 = **No effort against gravity;** leg falls to bed immediately. 4 = **No movement.** UN = **Amputation** or joint fusion, explain: ______________ **6a. Left Leg** **6b. Right Leg**	 6a. ______

NIH STROKE SCALE

Patient Identification. ___ ___-___ ___ ___-___ ___ ___

Pt. Date of Birth ___ ___/___ ___/___ ___

Hospital ______________________(___ ___-___ ___)

Date of Exam ___ ___/___ ___/___ ___

Interval: [ ] Baseline [ ] 2 hours post treatment [ ] 24 hours post onset of symptoms ±20 minutes [ ] 7–10 days
[ ] 3 months [ ] Other ______________________________(___ ___)

		___
7. Limb Ataxia: This item is aimed at finding evidence of a unilateral cerebellar lesion. Test with eyes open. In case of visual defect, ensure testing is done in intact visual field. The finger-nose-finger and heel-shin tests are performed on both sides, and ataxia is scored only if present out of proportion to weakness. Ataxia is absent in the patient who cannot understand or is paralyzed. Only in the case of amputation or joint fusion, the examiner should record the score as untestable (UN), and clearly write the explanation for this choice. In case of blindness, test by having the patient touch nose from extended arm position.	0 = **Absent.** 1 = **Present in one limb.** 2 = **Present in two limbs.** UN = **Amputation** or joint fusion, explain: ______________	___
8. Sensory: Sensation or grimace to pinprick when tested, or withdrawal from noxious stimulus in the obtunded or aphasic patient. Only sensory loss attributed to stroke is scored as abnormal and the examiner should test as many body areas (arms [not hands], legs, trunk, face) as needed to accurately check for hemisensory loss. A score of 2, "severe or total sensory loss," should only be given when a severe or total loss of sensation can be clearly demonstrated. Stuporous and aphasic patients will, therefore, probably score 1 or 0. The patient with brainstem stroke who has bilateral loss of sensation is scored 2. If the patient does not respond and is quadriplegic, score 2. Patients in a coma (item 1a=3) are automatically given a 2 on this item.	0 = **Normal;** no sensory loss. 1 = **Mild-to-moderate sensory loss;** patient feels pinprick is less sharp or is dull on the affected side; or there is a loss of superficial pain with pinprick, but patient is aware of being touched. 2 = **Severe to total sensory loss;** patient is not aware of being touched in the face, arm, and leg.	___
9. Best Language: A great deal of information about comprehension will be obtained during the preceding sections of the examination. For this scale item, the patient is asked to describe what is happening in the attached picture, to name the items on the attached naming sheet and to read from the attached list of sentences. Comprehension is judged from responses here, as well as to all of the commands in the preceding general neurological exam. If visual loss interferes with the tests, ask the patient to identify objects placed in the hand, repeat, and produce speech. The intubated patient should be asked to write. The patient in a coma (item 1a=3) will automatically score 3 on this item. The examiner must choose a score for the patient with stupor or limited cooperation, but a score of 3 should be used only if the patient is mute and follows no one-step commands.	0 = **No aphasia;** normal. 1 = **Mild-to-moderate aphasia;** some obvious loss of fluency or facility of comprehension, without significant limitation on ideas expressed or form of expression. Reduction of speech and/or comprehension, however, makes conversation about provided materials difficult or impossible. For example, in conversation about provided materials, examiner can identify picture or naming card content from patient's response. 2 = **Severe aphasia;** all communication is through fragmentary expression; great need for inference, questioning, and guessing by the listener. Range of information that can be exchanged is limited; listener carries burden of communication. Examiner cannot identify materials provided from patient response. 3 = **Mute, global aphasia;** no usable speech or auditory comprehension.	___
10. Dysarthria: If patient is thought to be normal, an adequate sample of speech must be obtained by asking patient to read or repeat words from the attached list. If the patient has severe aphasia, the clarity of articulation of spontaneous speech can be rated. Only if the patient is intubated or has other physical barriers to producing speech, the examiner should record the score as untestable (UN), and clearly write an explanation for this choice. Do not tell the patient why he or she is being tested.	0 = **Normal.** 1 = **Mild-to-moderate dysarthria;** patient slurs at least some words and, at worst, can be understood with some difficulty. 2 = **Severe dysarthria;** patient's speech is so slurred as to be unintelligible in the absence of or out of proportion to any dysphasia, or is mute/anarthric. UN = **Intubated** or other physical barrier, explain:________________________	___

NIH STROKE SCALE

Patient Identification. ___ ___-___ ___ ___-___ ___ ___

Pt. Date of Birth ___ ___/___ ___/___ ___

Hospital ____________________(___ ___-___ ___)

Date of Exam ___ ___/___ ___/___ ___

Interval: [ ] Baseline [ ] 2 hours post treatment [ ] 24 hours post onset of symptoms ±20 minutes [ ] 7–10 days [ ] 3 months [ ] Other ______________________________(___ ___)

11. Extinction and Inattention (formerly Neglect): Sufficient information to identify neglect may be obtained during the prior testing. If the patient has a severe visual loss preventing visual double simultaneous stimulation, and the cutaneous stimuli are normal, the score is normal. If the patient has aphasia but does appear to attend to both sides, the score is normal. The presence of visual spatial neglect or anosagnosia may also be taken as evidence of abnormality. Since the abnormality is scored only if present, the item is never untestable.	0 = **No abnormality.** 1 = **Visual, tactile, auditory, spatial, or personal inattention** or extinction to bilateral simultaneous stimulation in one of the sensory modalities. 2 = **Profound hemi-inattention or extinction to more than one modality;** does not recognize own hand or orients to only one side of space.	_____

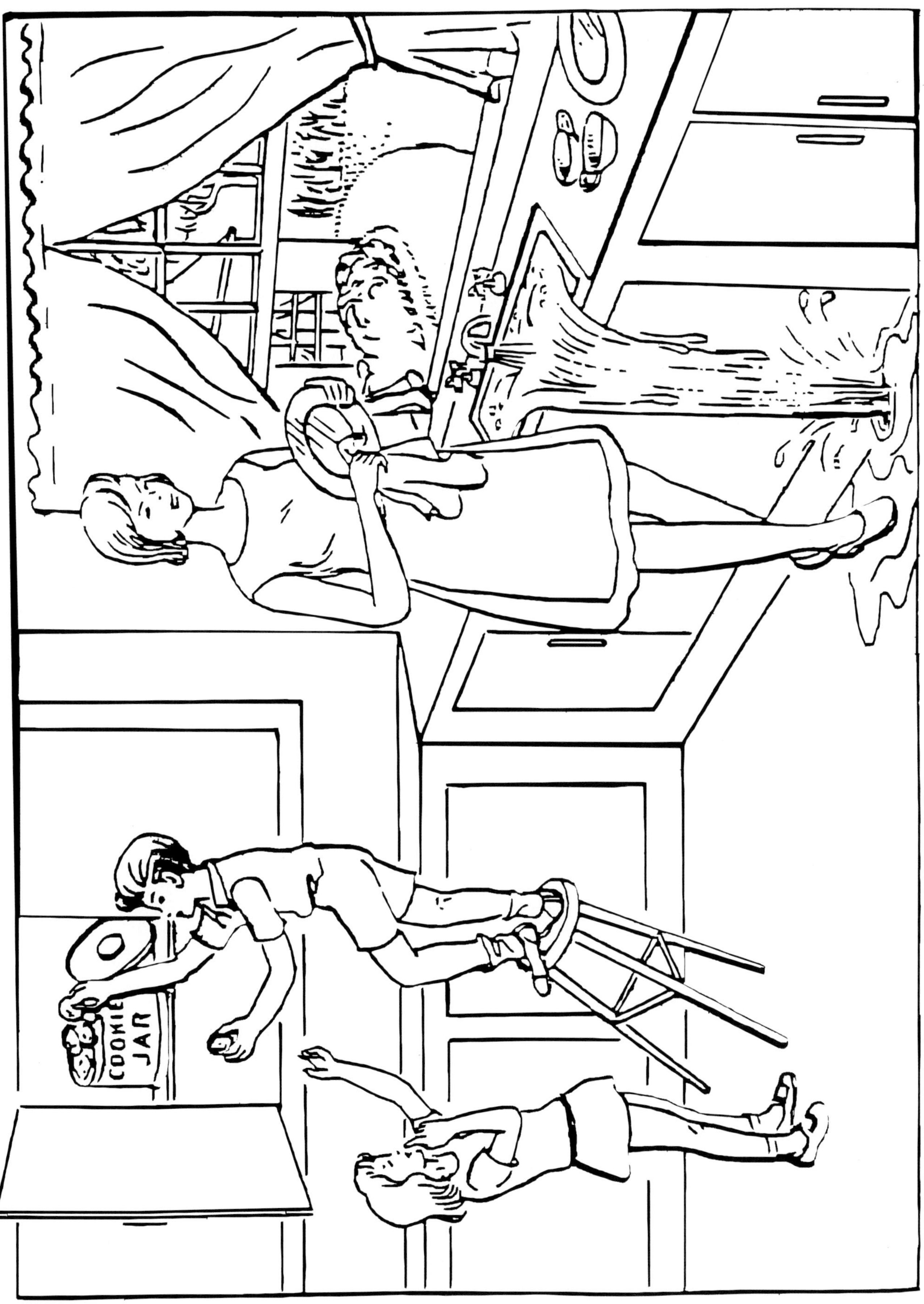
COOKIE
JAR

You know how.

Down to earth.

I got home from work.

Near the table in the dining room.

They heard him speak on the radio last night.

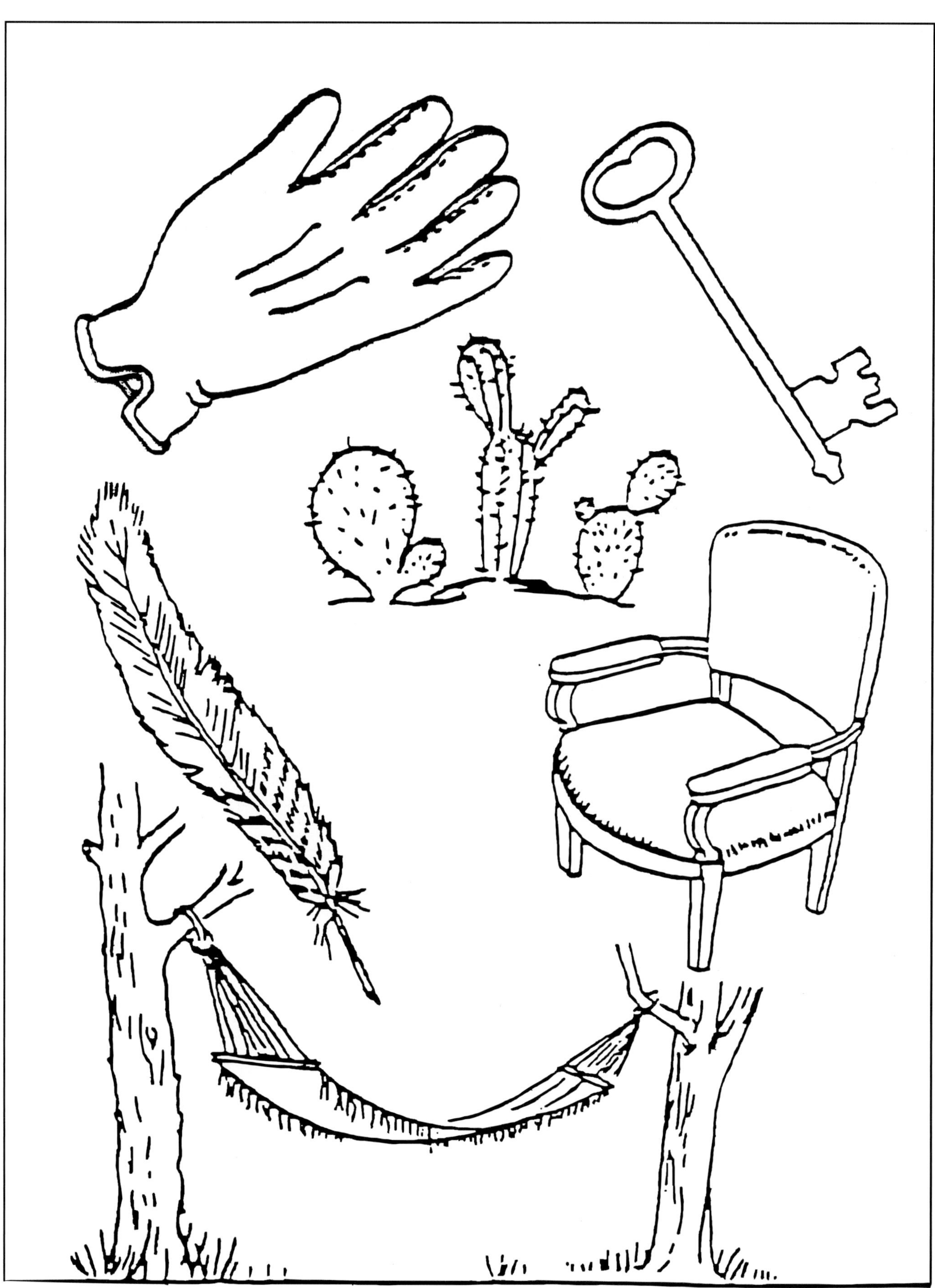

MAMA

TIP – TOP

FIFTY – FIFTY

THANKS

HUCKLEBERRY

BASEBALL PLAYER

- NIH Stroke Scale (From National Institutes of Health. https://www.stroke.nih.gov/documents/NIH_Stroke_Scale.pdf.)

Resident Assessment Instrument (RAI)

The Resident Assessment Instrument (RAI) helps nursing home staff in gathering definitive information on a resident's strengths and needs, which must be addressed in an individualized care plan. Interdisciplinary use of the RAI promotes this emphasis on quality of care and quality of life.

Data from https://www.cms.gov/Medicare/Quality-Initiatives-Patient-Assessment-Instruments/NursingHomeQualityInits/MDS30RAIManual

Chapter 22

Abbey Pain Scale

Vocalization Whimpering, crying	Absent 0 Mild +1 Moderate +2 Severe +3
Facial expression Tense, frowning, grimacing, frightened	Absent 0 Mild +1 Moderate +2 Severe +3
Body language Fidgeting, rocking, guarding, withdrawn	Absent 0 Mild +1 Moderate +2 Severe +3
Physiological changes Temp, pulse or BP elevations, diaphoresis, flushing/pallor	Absent 0 Mild +1 Moderate +2 Severe +3
Physical changes Skin tears, Pressure sores, arthritis, contractures, previous injuries	Absent 0 Mild +1 Moderate +2 Severe +3

From Abbey, J., Piller, N., De Bellis, A., Esterman, A., Parker, D., Giles, L., & Lowcay, B. (2004). The Abbey pain scale: A 1-minute numerical indicator for people with end-stage dementia. *International Journal of Palliative Nursing, 10*(1), 6–13.

Assessment of Discomfort in Dementia Protocol (ADD)

Complete for (a) observed behavioral changes; *OR* (b) if behavior/pain symptoms are coded on the MDS (Sections E4A or J2a). Report appropriate sections to the prescriber.

Resident's Name: Date:

Behavioral Symptoms: Circle all that apply

Facial Expressions	Irritability, confusion, withdrawal, agitation, aggressiveness
Body Language	Tense, wringing hands, clenched fists, restless, rubbing/holding body part, hyper or hypoactive, guarding body part, noisy breathing
Voice	Moaning, mumbling, chanting, grunting, whining, calling out, screaming, crying, verbally aggressive
Behavior	Change in appetite, sleep, mobility, gait, function, participation, exiting, wandering, elopement, physically aggressive, socially inappropriate or disruptive, resists cares

Other

(Check when completed) All basic needs met (toileting, thirst, hunger, glasses & hearing aids in place)

Steps of the ADD Protocol

Step 1: Assessment	+	–	N/A	Notes: Assess, RX, and Response
↑ BP, P, sweating				
↑ T				
Eyes, Nose, Mouth				
Skin				
Heart/Lungs				
Abdomen				
BM/Rectal Check				
Extremities				
Multistix Urine				
Other S&S				

Step 2: ✓'d R/T Current of Past Hx of Pain	✓if done	Notes: Assess, RX, and Response
Step 3: If Steps 1 and 2 Are Negative ASSESS • Environmental press • Pacing of activity/stimulation • Meaningful human interaction and INTERVENE • Nonpharmacological Rx's		
Step 4: If unsuccessful, medicate with non-narcotic analgesic per written order	✓ if done	
Step 5: If symptoms persist, consult with physician/other health professional or medicate with prn psychotropic per written order		

Nurse's Signature: Date:

*If new nursing/medical intervention initiated, complete below:

Evaluate effectiveness of new nursing and/or medical intervention on behavioral symptoms. (Be specific)

Plan of Care Updated (if appropriate)

Nurse's Signature: Date:

MDS, Minimum data set.

 From Kovach, C. R., Noonan, P. E., Griffie, J., Muchka, S., & Weissman, D. E. (2002). The assessment of discomfort in dementia protocol. *Pain Management Nursing, 3*(1), 16–27.

Checklist of Nonverbal Pain Indicators (CNPI)

Pain Scale for Cognitively Impaired, Nonverbal Adults

Checklist of Nonverbal Pain Indicators (CNPI)

Indicators:	With Movement	At Rest
Vocal Complaints (non-verbal expression of pain demonstrated by moans, groans, grunts, cries, gasps, sighs)		
Facial Grimaces and Winces Furrowed brow, narrowed eyes, tightened lips, dropped jaw, clenched teeth, distorted expression)		
Bracing (clutching or holding onto bed/chair, caregiver, or affected area during movement)		
Restlessness (constant or intermittent shifting of position, rocking, intermittent hand motions, inability to keep still)		
Rubbing (massaging affected area)		
Vocal Complaints (verbal expression of pain using words, e.g., “ouch” or “that hurts,” cursing during movement or exclamation of protest, e.g., “stop” or “that’s enough”)		
Total Score		

In Cooney, M., & Quinlan-Colwell, A. (2021). *Assessment and multild assessment and multimodal management of pain: An integrative approach*. Elsevier; From Feldt, K. S. (2000). The checklist of nonverbal pain indicators (CNPI). *Pain Management Nursing, 1*(1), 13–21.

Confusion Assessment Method (CAM)

(See Appendix 1, Chapter 11)

Edmonton Symptom Assessment System-Revised (ESAS-R)

Please circle the number that best describes how you feel NOW:

No pain	0	1	2	3	4	5	6	7	8	9	10	Worst possible pain
No tiredness *(Tiredness = lack of energy)*	0	1	2	3	4	5	6	7	8	9	10	Worst possible tiredness
No drowsiness *(Drowsiness = feeling sleepy)*	0	1	2	3	4	5	6	7	8	9	10	Worst possible drowsiness
No nausea	0	1	2	3	4	5	6	7	8	9	10	Worst possible nausea
No lack of appetite	0	1	2	3	4	5	6	7	8	9	10	Worst possible lack of appetite
No shortness of breath	0	1	2	3	4	5	6	7	8	9	10	Worst possible shortness of breath
No depression *(Depression = feeling sad)*	0	1	2	3	4	5	6	7	8	9	10	Worst possible depression
No anxiety *(Anxiety = feeling nervous)*	0	1	2	3	4	5	6	7	8	9	10	Worst possible anxiety
Best well-being *(well-being = how you feel overall)*	0	1	2	3	4	5	6	7	8	9	10	Worst possible well-being
No ________ *Other problem (for example, constipation)*	0	1	2	3	4	5	6	7	8	9	10	Worst possible ________

Patient name: ________________

Date: ________________

Time: ________________

Please mark on these pictures where it is that you hurt:

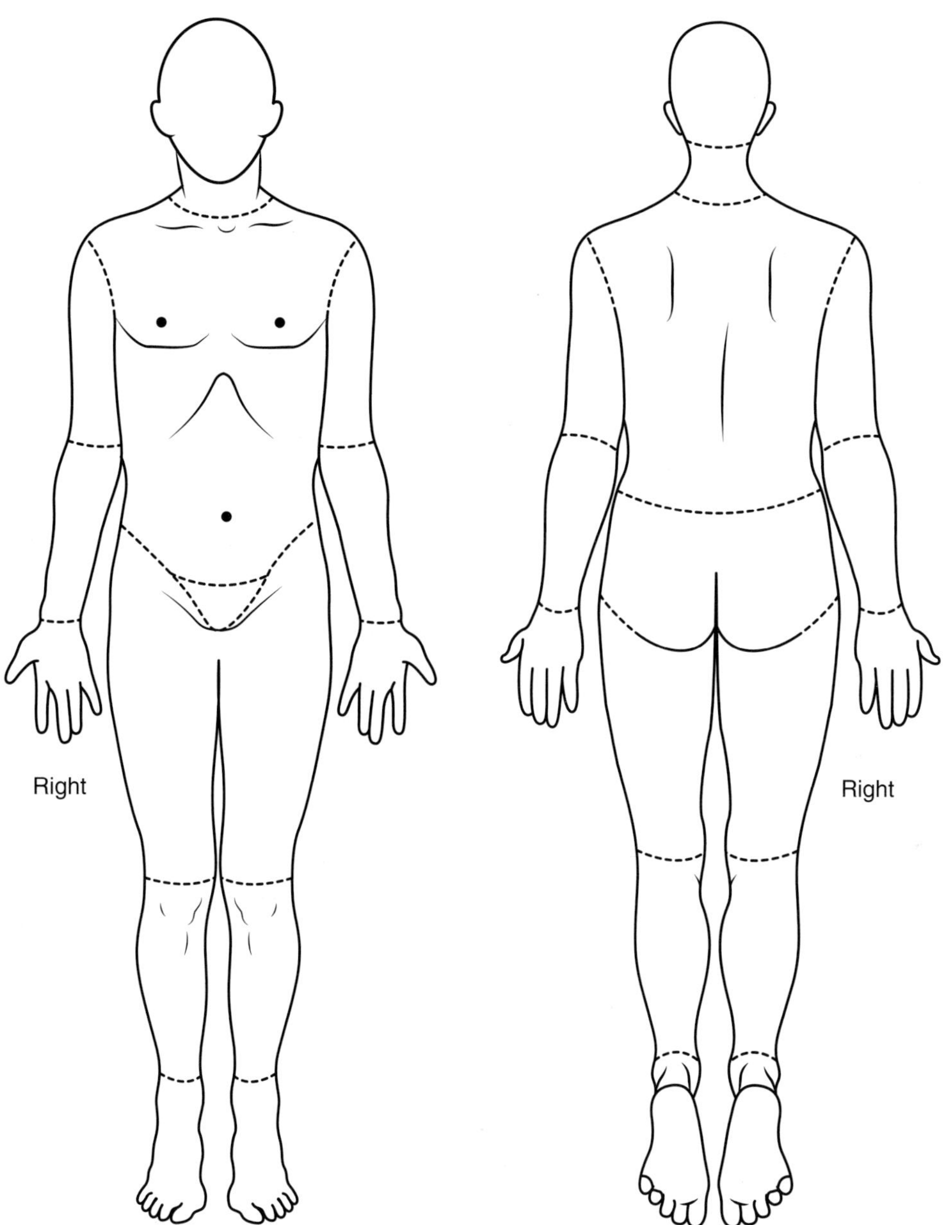

Side B

• Edmonton Symptom Assessment System-Revised (ESAS-R) (From Watanabe, S. M., Nekolaichuk, C., Beaumont, C., et al. [2011]. A multicenter study comparing two numerical versions of the Edmonton symptom assessment system in palliative care patients. *Journal of Pain and Symptom Management, 41*[2], 456–468.)

Eastern Cooperative Oncology Group (ECOG) Performance Status Scale

Grade	ECOG Performance Status
0	Fully active, able to carry on all pre-disease performance without restriction
1	Restricted in physically strenuous activity but ambulatory and able to carry out work of a light or sedentary nature, e.g., light house work, office work
2	Ambulatory and capable of all selfcare but unable to carry out any work activities; up and about more than 50% of waking hours
3	Capable of only limited selfcare; confined to bed or chair more than 50% of waking hours
4	Completely disabled; cannot carry on any selfcare; totally confined to bed or chair
5	Dead

From Ecog-ACRIN: https://ecog-acrin.org/resources/ecog-performance-status/. Oken, M. M., Creech, R., Tormey, D., et al. (1982). Toxicity and response criteria of the Eastern Cooperative Oncology Group. *American Journal of Clinical Oncology, 5*, 649–655.

Functional Assessment Staging Tool for Alzheimer-Type Dementia (FAST)

Stage 1: Normal edit	Shows no functional decline.
Stage 2: Normal older adult	Shows personal awareness of some functional decline
Stage 3: Early Alzheimer's disease	Demonstrates noticeable deficits in demanding job situations
Stage 4: Mild Alzheimer's disease	Requires assistance in complicated tasks such as handling finances or planning parties
Stage 5: Moderate Alzheimer's disease	Requires assistance in choosing proper attire
Stage 6: Moderately severe Alzheimer's disease	Requires assistance dressing, bathing and toileting Experiences urinary and fecal incontinence
Stage 7: Severe Alzheimer's disease	Speech ability declines to about a half dozen intelligible words Demonstrates progressive loss of abilities to walk, sit up, smile, and hold up head

From Sclan, S. G., & Reisberg, B. (1992). Functional assessment staging (FAST) in Alzheimer's disease: Reliability, validity, and ordinality. *International Psychogeriatrics, 4*(Suppl. 1), 55–69. Table from Touhy, T. A. (2022). *Ebersole & Hess' toward healthy aging: Human needs and nursing response* (10th ed.). Elsevier.

Model for End-Stage Liver Disease (MELD) Score

Dialysis at least twice in the past week Or CVVHD for ≥24 hours in the past week	No	Yes
Creatinine Cr >4.0 mg/dl is automatically assigned a value of 4.0	Norm: 0.7 – 1.3	mg/dL ⇋
Bilirubin	Norm: 0.3 – 1.9	mg/dL ⇋
INR	Norm: 0.8 – 1.2	
Sodium	Norm: 136 – 145	mEq/L ⇋

CVVHD, Continuous veno-venous hemodialysis.

 Table from https://www.mdcalc.com/calc/78/meld-score-model-end-stage-liver-disease-12-older, For End-Stage Liver Disease (12 and older)–MDCalc.

Memorial Symptom Assessment Scale (MSAS)

MEMORIAL SYMPTOM ASSESSMENT SCALE

Name   Date

Section 1

Instructions: We have listed 24 symptoms below. Read each one carefully. If you have had the symptom during this past week, let us know how OFTEN you had it, how SEVERE it was usually, and how much it DISTRESSED or BOTHERED you by circling the appropriate number. If you DID NOT HAVE the symptom, make an "X" in the box marked "DID NOT HAVE."

DURING THE PAST WEEK Did you have any of the following symptoms?	DID NOT HAVE	IF YES How OFTEN did you have it?				IF YES How SEVERE was it usually				IF YES How much did it DISTRESS or BOTHER you?				
		Rarely	Occasionally	Frequently	Almost Constantly	Slight	Moderate	Severe	Very Severe	Not at All	A Little Bit	Somewhat	Quite a Bit	Very Much
Difficulty concentrating		1	2	3	4	1	2	3	4	0	1	2	3	4
Pain		1	2	3	4	1	2	3	4	0	1	2	3	4
Lack of energy		1	2	3	4	1	2	3	4	0	1	2	3	4
Cough		1	2	3	4	1	2	3	4	0	1	2	3	4
Feeling nervous		1	2	3	4	1	2	3	4	0	1	2	3	4
Dry mouth		1	2	3	4	1	2	3	4	0	1	2	3	4
Nausea		1	2	3	4	1	2	3	4	0	1	2	3	4
Feeling drowsy		1	2	3	4	1	2	3	4	0	1	2	3	4
Numbness/tingling in hands/feet		1	2	3	4	1	2	3	4	0	1	2	3	4
Difficulty sleeping		1	2	3	4	1	2	3	4	0	1	2	3	4
Feeling bloated		1	2	3	4	1	2	3	4	0	1	2	3	4
Problems with urination		1	2	3	4	1	2	3	4	0	1	2	3	4
Vomiting		1	2	3	4	1	2	3	4	0	1	2	3	4
Shortness of breath		1	2	3	4	1	2	3	4	0	1	2	3	4
Diarrhea		1	2	3	4	1	2	3	4	0	1	2	3	4
Feeling sad		1	2	3	4	1	2	3	4	0	1	2	3	4
Sweats		1	2	3	4	1	2	3	4	0	1	2	3	4
Worrying		1	2	3	4	1	2	3	4	0	1	2	3	4
Problems with sexual interest or activity		1	2	3	4	1	2	3	4	0	1	2	3	4
Itching		1	2	3	4	1	2	3	4	0	1	2	3	4
Lack of appetite		1	2	3	4	1	2	3	4	0	1	2	3	4
Dizziness		1	2	3	4	1	2	3	4	0	1	2	3	4
Difficulty swallowing		1	2	3	4	1	2	3	4	0	1	2	3	4
Feeling irritable		1	2	3	4	1	2	3	4	0	1	2	3	4

Section 2										
INSTRUCTIONS: We have listed 8 symptoms below. Read each one carefully. If you have had the symptom during this past week, let us know how SEVERE it was usually and how much it DISTRESSED or BOTHERED you by circling the appropriate number. If you DID NOT HAVE the symptom, make an "X" in the box marked "DID NOT HAVE."										
<u>DURING THE PAST WEEK,</u> Did you have any of the following symptoms?	DID NOT HAVE	<u>IF YES</u> How SEVERE was it usually?				<u>IF YES</u> How much did it DISTRESS or BOTHER you?				
		Slight	Moderate	Severe	Very Severe	Not at All	A Little Bit	Somewhat	Quite a Bit	Very Much
Mouth sores		1	2	3	4	0	1	2	3	4
Change in the way food tastes		1	2	3	4	0	1	2	3	4
Weight loss		1	2	3	4	0	1	2	3	4
Hair loss		1	2	3	4	0	1	2	3	4
Constipation		1	2	3	4	0	1	2	3	4
Swelling of arms or legs		1	2	3	4	0	1	2	3	4
"I don't look like myself"		1	2	3	4	0	1	2	3	4
Changes in skin		1	2	3	4	0	1	2	3	4
IF YOU HAD ANY OTHER SYMPTOMS DURING THE PAST WEEK, PLEASE LIST BELOW AND INDICATE HOW MUCH THE SYMPTOM HAS DISTRESSED OR BOTHERED YOU.										
Other:						0	1	2	3	4
Other:						0	1	2	3	4
Other:						0	1	2	3	4

• Memorial Symptom Assessment Scale (MSAS) (From Portenoy, R. K., Thaler, H. T., Kornblith, A. B., et al. [1994]. The memorial symptom assessment scale: An instrument for the evaluation of symptom prevalence, characteristics and distress. *European Journal of Cancer, 30A*[9],1326–1336. Image from NPCRC.org.)

New York Heart Association (NYHA) Classes Heart Failure

Class	Patient Symptoms
I	No limitation of physical activity. Ordinary physical activity does not cause undue fatigue, palpitation, dyspnea (shortness of breath).
II	Slight limitation of physical activity. Comfortable at rest. Ordinary physical activity results in fatigue, palpitation, dyspnea (shortness of breath).
III	Marked limitation of physical activity. Comfortable at rest. Less than ordinary activity causes fatigue, palpitation, or dyspnea.
IV	Unable to carry on any physical activity without discomfort. Symptoms of heart failure at rest. If any physical activity is undertaken, discomfort increases.

Class	Objective Assessment
A	No objective evidence of cardiovascular disease. No symptoms and no limitation in ordinary physical activity.
B	Objective evidence of minimal cardiovascular disease. Mild symptoms and slight limitation during ordinary activity. Comfortable at rest.
C	Objective evidence of moderately severe cardiovascular disease. Marked limitation in activity due to symptoms, even during less-than-ordinary activity. Comfortable only at rest.
D	Objective evidence of severe cardiovascular disease. Severe limitations. Experiences symptoms even while at rest.

For Example:

- A patient with minimal or no symptoms but a large pressure gradient across the aortic valve or severe obstruction of the left main coronary artery is classified:
  - Function Capacity I, Objective Assessment D
- A patient with severe anginal syndrome but angiographically normal coronary arteries is classified:
  - Functional Capacity IV, Objective Assessment A

From The American Heart Association: https://www.heart.org/en/health-topics/heart-failure/what-is-heart-failure/classes-of-heart-failure. Adapted from Dolgin, M., Fox, A. C., Gorlin, R., Levin, R. I., New York Heart Association. Criteria Committee. (1994). *Nomenclatures and criteria for diagnosis of diseases of the heart and great vessels* (9th ed.). Lippincott Williams and Wilkins; Original source: Criteria Committee, New York Heart Association, Inc. (1964). *Diseases of the heart and blood vessels: Nomenclature and criteria for diagnosis* (6th ed., p. 114). Little, Brown and Co.

Pain Assessment in Advanced Dementia (PAINAD)

Instructions: Observe the patient for five minutes before scoring his or her behaviors. Score the behaviors according to the following chart. Definitions of each item are provided on the following page. The patient can be observed under different conditions (e.g., at rest, during a pleasant activity, during caregiving, after the administration of pain medication).

Behavior	0	1	2	Score
Breathing Independent of vocalization	• Normal	• Occasional labored breathing • Short period of hyperventilation	• Noisy labored breathing • Long period of hyperventilation • Cheyne-Stokes respirations	
Negative vocalization	• None	• Occasional moan or groan • Low-level speech with a negative or disapproving quality	• Repeated troubled calling out • Loud moaning or groaning • Crying	
Facial expression	• Smiling or inexpressive	• Sad • Frightened • Frown	• Facial grimacing	
Body language	• Relaxed	• Tense • Distressed pacing • Fidgeting	• Rigid • Fists clenched • Knees pulled up • Pulling or pushing away • Striking out	
Consolability	• No need to console	• Distracted or • reassured by voice or touch	• Unable to console, distract, or reassure	

TOTAL SCORE

Scoring: The total score ranges from 0–10 points. A possible interpretation of the scores is 1–3 = mild pain; 4–6 = moderate pain; 7–10 = severe pain. These ranges are based on a standard 0–10 scale of pain, but have not been substantiated in the literature for this tool.

PAINAD Item Definitions

Breathing

1. Normal breathing is characterized by effortless, quiet, rhythmic (smooth) respirations.
2. Occasional labored breathing is characterized by episodic bursts of harsh, difficult, or wearing respirations.
3. Short period of hyperventilation is characterized by intervals of rapid, deep breaths lasting a short period of time.
4. Noisy labored breathing is characterized by negative-sounding respirations on inspiration or expiration. They may be loud, gurgling, wheezing. They appear strenuous or wearing.
5. Long period of hyperventilation is characterized by an excessive rate and depth of respirations lasting a considerable time.
6. Cheyne-Stokes respirations are characterized by rhythmic waxing and waning of breathing from very deep to shallow respirations with periods of apnea (cessation of breathing).

Negative Vocalization

1. None is characterized by speech or vocalization that has a neutral or pleasant quality.
2. Occasional moan or groan is characterized by mournful or murmuring sounds, wails, or laments. Groaning is characterized by louder than usual inarticulate involuntary sounds, often abruptly beginning and ending.
3. Low level speech with a negative or disapproving quality is characterized by muttering, mumbling, whining, grumbling, or swearing in a low volume with a complaining, sarcastic, or caustic tone.
4. Repeated troubled calling out is characterized by phrases or words being used over and over in a tone that suggests anxiety, uneasiness, or distress.
5. Loud moaning or groaning is characterized by mournful or murmuring sounds, wails, or laments in much louder than usual volume. Loud groaning is characterized by louder than usual inarticulate involuntary sounds, often abruptly beginning and ending.
6. Crying is characterized by an utterance of emotion accompanied by tears. There may be sobbing or quiet weeping.

Facial Expression

1. Smiling or inexpressive. Smiling is characterized by upturned corners of the mouth, brightening of the eyes, and a look of pleasure or contentment. Inexpressive refers to a neutral, at ease, relaxed, or blank look.
2. Sad is characterized by an unhappy, lonesome, sorrowful, or dejected look. There may be tears in the eyes.
3. Frightened is characterized by a look of fear, alarm, or heightened anxiety. Eyes appear wide open.
4. Frown is characterized by a downward turn of the corners of the mouth. Increased facial wrinkling in the forehead and around the mouth may appear.
5. Facial grimacing is characterized by a distorted, distressed look. The brow is more wrinkled, as is the area around the mouth. Eyes may be squeezed shut.

Body Language

1. Relaxed is characterized by a calm, restful, mellow appearance. The person seems to be taking it easy.
2. Tense is characterized by a strained, apprehensive, or worried appearance. The jaw may be clenched. (Exclude any contractures.)
3. Distressed pacing is characterized by activity that seems unsettled. There may be a fearful, worried, or disturbed element present. The rate may be faster or slower.
4. Fidgeting is characterized by restless movement. Squirming about or wiggling in the chair may occur. The person might be hitching a chair across the room. Repetitive touching, tugging, or rubbing body parts can also be observed.
5. Rigid is characterized by stiffening of the body. The arms and/or legs are tight and inflexible. The trunk may appear straight and unyielding. (Exclude any contractures.)
6. Fists clenched is characterized by tightly closed hands. They may be opened and closed repeatedly or held tightly shut.
7. Knees pulled up is characterized by flexing the legs and drawing the knees up toward the chest. An overall troubled appearance. (Exclude any contractures.)
8. Pulling or pushing away is characterized by resistiveness upon approach or to care. The person is trying to escape by yanking or wrenching him- or herself free or shoving you away.
9. Striking out is characterized by hitting, kicking, grabbing, punching, biting, or other form of personal assault.

Consolability

1. No need to console is characterized by a sense of well-being. The person appears content.
2. Distracted or reassured by voice or touch is characterized by a disruption in the behavior when the person is spoken to or touched. The behavior stops during the period of interaction, with no indication that the person is at all distressed.
3. Unable to console, distract, or reassure is characterized by the inability to soothe the person or stop a behavior with words or actions. No amount of comforting, verbal or physical, will alleviate the behavior.

From Warden, V., Hurley, A. C., & Volicer, L. (2003). Development and psychometric evaluation of the pain assessment in advanced dementia (PAINAD) scale. *Journal of the American Medical Directors Association, 4*(1), 9–15.

Palliative Prognostic Index (PPI)

The PPI relies on the assessment of performance status using the Palliative Performance Scale (PPS, oral intake, and the presence or absence of dyspnea, edema, and delirium).

Performance Status/Symptoms	Partial Score
Palliative Performance Scale	
10–20	4
30–50	2.5
>60	0
Oral Intake	
Mouthfuls or less	2.5
Reduced by more than mouthfuls	1
Normal	0
Edema	
Present	1
Absent	0
Dyspnea at Rest	
Present	3.5
Absent	0
Delirium	
Present	4
Absent	0

Scoring

PPI score > 6 = survival shorter than 3 weeks
PPI score > 4 = survival shorter than 6 weeks
PPI score < 4 = survival more than 6 weeks

From Stone, C., Tierman, E., & Dooley, B. (2008). Prospective validation of the palliative prognostic index in patients with cancer. *Journal of Pain and Symptom Management, 35*(6), 617–622. Copyright (2008).

Palliative Prognostic Score (PaP)

The PaP uses the Karnofsky Performance Score (KPS) and five other criteria to generate a numerical score from 0 to 17.5 to predict 30-day survival (higher scores predict shorter survival).

Performance Status/Symptoms	**Partial Score**
Dyspnea	
No	0
Yes	1
Anorexia	
No	0
Yes	1
KPS	
≥50	0

Performance Status/Symptoms	Partial Score
30–40	0
10–20	2.5
Clinical Prediction of Survival (Weeks)	
>12	0
11–12	2.0
9–10	2.5
7–8	2.5
5–6	4.5
3–4	6.0
1–2	8.5
Total WBC	
Normal (4800–8500 cell/mm3)	0
High (8501–11,000 cell/mm3)	0.5
Very high (>1000 cell/rnir.3)	1.5
Lymphocyte Percentage	
Normal (20.0%–40.0%)	0
Low (12.0%–19.9%)	1.0
Very low (0–11.9%)	2.5
Risk Groups	Total Score
A. 30-day survival probability >70%	0–5.5
B. 30-day survival probability 30–70%	5.6–11.0
C. 30-day survival probability <30%	11.1–17.5

From Maltoni, M., Nanni, O., Pirovano, M., Scarpi, E., Indelli, M., Martini, C., et al. (1999). Successful validation of the palliative prognostic score in terminally ill cancer patient. *Journal of Pain and Symptom Management, 17*(4), 240–247.
PaP score = Dyspnea score + Anorexia score + KPS score + CPS score + Total WBC score + Lymphocyte percentage score.

Appendix 2: IPEC Competencies

CORE COMPETENCIES FOR INTERPROFESSIONAL COLLABORATIVE PRACTICE: 2016 UPDATE

Competency-Based Interprofessional Education: Definitional Framework

Operational Definitions

Interprofessional education:
"When students from two or more professions learn about, from and with each other to enable effective collaboration and improve health outcomes" (WHO 2010).

Interprofessional collaborative practice:
"When multiple health workers from different professional backgrounds work together with patients, families, [careers], and communities to deliver the highest quality of care" (WHO 2010).

Interprofessional teamwork:
The levels of cooperation, coordination and collaboration characterizing the relationships between professions in delivering patient-centered care.

Interprofessional team-based care:
Care delivered by intentionally created, usually relatively small work groups in health care who are recognized by others as well as by themselves as having a collective identity and shared responsibility for a patient or group of patients (e.g., rapid response team, palliative care team, primary care team, andoperating room team).

Professional competencies in health care:
Integrated enactment of knowledge, skills, values, and attitudes that define the areas of work of a particular health profession applied in specific care contexts.

Interprofessional competencies in health care:
Integrated enactment of knowledge, skills, values, and attitudes that define working together across the professions, with other health care workers, and with patients, along with families and communities, as appropriate to improve health outcomes in specific care contexts.

The 2011 charge to the expert panel was to identify individual-level inter professional competencies for future health professionals in training that are specifically relevant to the pre-licensure/pre-credentialed student. The expert panel also identified eight reasons why it is important to agree on a set of core competencies across the professions, which still hold true today. They are needed to:

1. Create a coordinated effort across the health professions to embed essential content in all health professions education curricula.
2. Guide professional and institutional curricular development of learning approaches and assessment strategies to achieve productive outcomes.
3. Provide the foundation for a learning continuum in interprofessional competency development across the professions and the lifelong learning trajectory.
4. Acknowledge that evaluation and research work will strengthen the scholarship in this area.
5. Prompt dialogue to evaluate the "fit" between educationally identified core competencies for interprofessional collaborative practice and practice needs/demands.
6. Find opportunities to integrate essential interprofessional education content consistent with current accreditation expectations for each health professions education program.
7. Offer information to accreditors of educational programs across the health professions that they can use to set common accreditation standards for interprofessional education and to know where to look in institutional settings for examples of implementation of those standards.
8. Inform professional licensing and credentialing bodies in defining potential testing content for interprofessional collaborative practice.

Interprofessional Collaboration Domain

Recognizing that educators and IPE development teams have used the 2011 competencies extensively for curriculum design and mapping, the original structure is retainedin this 2016 update. The two changes are to present Interprofessional Collaborationas a domain in and of itselfand to better integrate population health competencies. The first change flows from the work of Englander et al. (2013). Instead of depicting four domainswithin interprofessional collaborative practice (values/ethics, roles/responsibilities, interprofessional communication, teams and teamwork), the four topical areas fall under the single domain of interprofessional collaboration in which four corecompetencies and related sub-competencies now reside.The second change responds to shifts inthe health system since the 2011 report was released, most prominently the increased focus on the Triple Aim and implementation of the Patient Protection and Affordable Care Act in 2010.

Interprofessional Collaboration Competency Domain

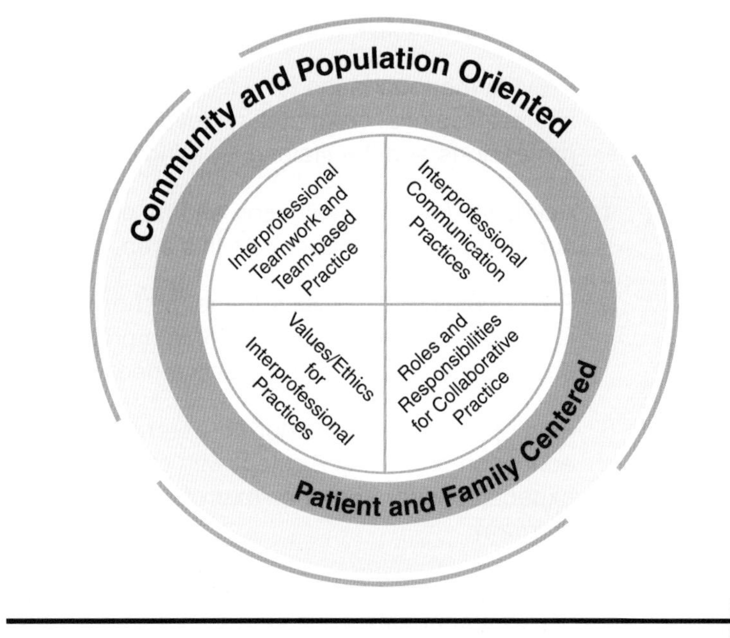

CORE COMPETENCIES FOR INTERPROFESSIONAL COLLABORATIVE PRACTICE: 2016 UPDATE

Four Core Competencies

The core competencies and sub-competencies feature the following desired principles: patient and family centered (hereafter termed "patient centered"); community and population oriented; relationship focused; process oriented; linked to learning activities, educational strategies, and behavioral assessments that are developmentally appropriate for the learner; able to be integrated across the learning continuum; sensitive to the systems context and applicable across practice settings; applicable across professions; stated in language common and meaningful across the professions; and outcome driven.

NOTE: The 2016 updates to the competencies and sub-competencies appear in bold.

Competency 1

Work with individuals of other professions to maintain a climate of mutual respect and shared values. (Values/Ethics for Interprofessional Practice)

Competency 2

Use the knowledge of one's own role and those of other professions to appropriately assess and address the health care **needs of patients** and **to promote and advance the health of populations.** (Roles/Responsibilities)

Competency 3

Communicate with patients, families, communities, **and professionals in health and other fields** in a responsive and responsible manner that supports a team approach to the **promotion and** maintenance of health and the **prevention and** treatment of disease. (Interprofessional Communication)

Competency 4

Apply relationship-building values and the principles of team dynamics to perform effectively in different team roles to **plan, deliver, and evaluate** patient/population-centered care **and population health programs** and policiesthat are safe, timely, efficient, effective, and equitable. (Teams and Teamwork)

IPEC Core Competencies for Interprofessional Collaborative Practice

Work with individuals of other professions to maintain a climate of mutual respect and shared values. (Values/Ethics for Interprofessional Practice)

Values/Ethics Sub-competencies:

VE1.	Place interests of patients and populations at center of interprofessional health care delivery **and population health programs and policies, with the goal of promoting health and health equity across the life span.**
VE2.	Respect the dignity and privacy of patients while maintaining confidentiality in the delivery of team-based care.
VE3.	Embrace the cultural diversity and individual differences that characterize patients, populations, and the **health team**.
VE4	Respect the unique cultures, values, roles/responsibilities, and expertise of other health professions **and the impact these factors can have on health outcomes**.
VE5	Work in cooperation with those who receive care, those who provide care, and others who contribute to or support the delivery of prevention and health services **and programs**.
VE6	Develop a trusting relationship with patients, families, and other team members (CIHC, 2010).
VE7.	Demonstrate high standards of ethical conduct and quality of care in contributions to team-based care.
VE8	Manage ethical dilemmas specific to interprofessional patient/ population centered care situations.
VE9.	Act with honesty and integrity in relationships with patients, families, **communities**, and other team members.
VE10.	Maintain competence in one's own profession appropriate to scope of practice.

CORE COMPETENCIES FOR INTERPROFESSIONAL COLLABORATIVE PRACTICE: 2016 UPDATE

Use the knowledge of one's own role and those of other professions to appropriately assess and address the health care needs **of patients** and **to promote and advance the health of populations.** (Roles/Responsibilities)

Roles/Responsibilities Sub-competencies:

RR1.	Communicate one's roles and responsibilities clearly to patients, families, **community members**, and other professionals.
RR2.	Recognize one's limitations in skills, knowledge, and abilities.
RR3.	Engage diverse professionalswho complement one's own professional expertise, as well as associated resources, to develop strategies to meet specific **health and healthcare** needs **of patients and populations**.
RR4.	Explain the roles and responsibilities of other providers and how the team works together to provide care, **promote health, and prevent disease**.
RR5.	Use the full scope of knowledge, skills, and abilities of **professionals from health and other fields** to provide care that is safe, timely, efficient, effective, and equitable.
RR6.	Communicate with team members to clarify each member's responsibility in executing components of a treatment plan or public health intervention.
RR7.	Forge interdependent relationships with other professions **within and outside of the health system** to improve care and advance learning.
RR8.	Engage in continuous professional and interprofessional development to enhance team performance **and collaboration**.
RR9.	Use unique and complementary abilities of all members of the team to optimize **health and** patient care.
RR10.	**Describe how professionals in health and other fields can collaborate and integrate clinical care and public health interventions to optimize population health.**

CORE COMPETENCIES FOR INTERPROFESSIONAL COLLABORATIVE PRACTICE: 2016 UPDATE

Communicate with patients, families, communities, and professionals in health and other fields in a responsive and responsible manner that supports a team approach to the promotion and maintenance of health and the prevention and treatment of disease. (Interprofessional Communication)

Interprofessional Communication Sub-competencies:

CC1.	Choose effective communication tools and techniques, including information systems and communication technologies, to facilitate discussions and interactions that enhance team function.
CC2.	**Communicate** information with patients, families, **community members**,and **health team** members in a form that is understandable, avoiding discipline-specific terminology when possible.
CC3.	Express one's knowledge and opinions to team members involved in patient care **and population health improvement** with confidence, clarity, andrespect, working to ensure common understanding of information, treatment, care decisions, **and population health programs and policies.**
CC4.	Listen actively, and encourage ideas and opinions of other team members.
CC5.	Give timely, sensitive, instructive feedback to others about their performance on the team, responding respectfully as a team member to feedback from others.
CC6.	Use respectful language appropriate for a given difficult situation, crucial conversation, or conflict.
CC7.	Recognize how one's uniqueness (experience level, expertise, culture, power, and hierarchy within the **health** team) contributes to effective communication, conflict resolution, and positive interprofessional working relationships (University of Toronto, 2008).
CC8.	Communicate the importance of teamwork in patient-centered **care and population health programs and policies.**

CORE COMPETENCIES FOR INTERPROFESSIONAL COLLABORATIVE PRACTICE: 2016 UPDATE

Apply relationship-building values and the principles of team dynamics to perform effectively in different team roles to **plan, deliver,and evaluate** patient/population-centered care **and population health programs and policies** that are safe, timely, efficient, effective, and equitable. (Teams and Teamwork)

Team and Teamwork Sub-competencies:

TT1.	Describe the process of team development and the roles and practices of effective teams.
TT2.	Develop consensus on the ethical principles to guide all aspects of **team work**.
TT3.	**Engage health and other professionals** in shared patient-centered **and population-focused** problem-solving.
TT4.	Integrate the knowledge and experience of **health and** other professions to inform **health and** care decisions, while respecting patient and community values and priorities/preferences for care.
TT5.	Apply leadership practices that support collaborative practice and team effectiveness.
TT6.	Engage self and others to constructively manage disagreements about values, roles, goals, and actions that arise among **health and other** professionals and with patients**, families, and community members.**
TT7.	Share accountability with other professions, patients, and communities for outcomes relevant to prevention and health care.
TT8.	Reflect on individual and team performance for individual, as well as team, performance improvement.
TT9.	Use process improvement to increase effectiveness of interprofessional teamwork and team-based **services, programs, and policies.**
TT10.	Use available evidence to inform effective teamwork and team-based practices.
TT11.	Perform effectively on teams and in different team roles in a variety of settings.

Taken from IPEC: Core Competencies for Interprofessional Collaborative Practice: 2016 Update

Index

E

S

T

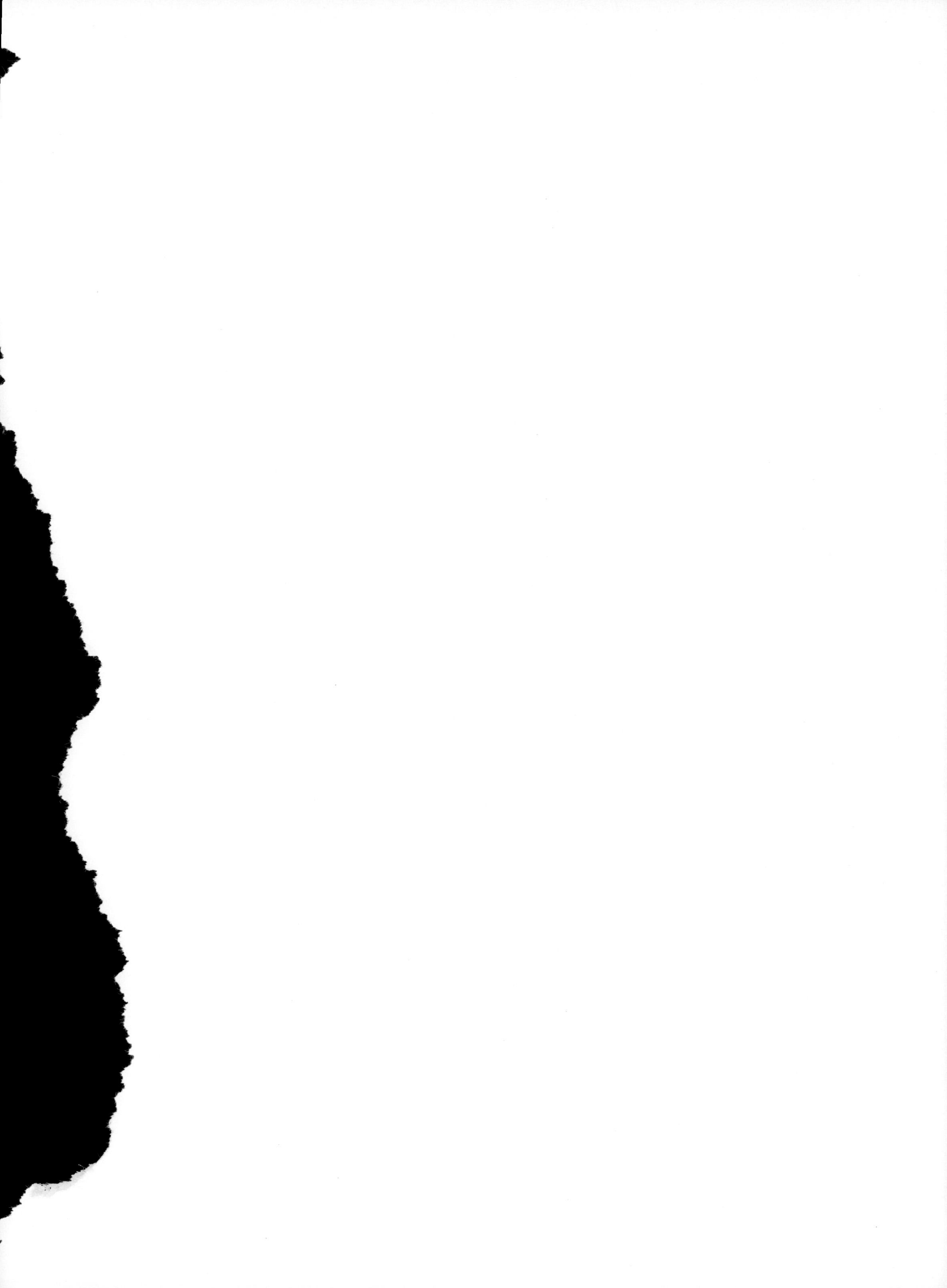

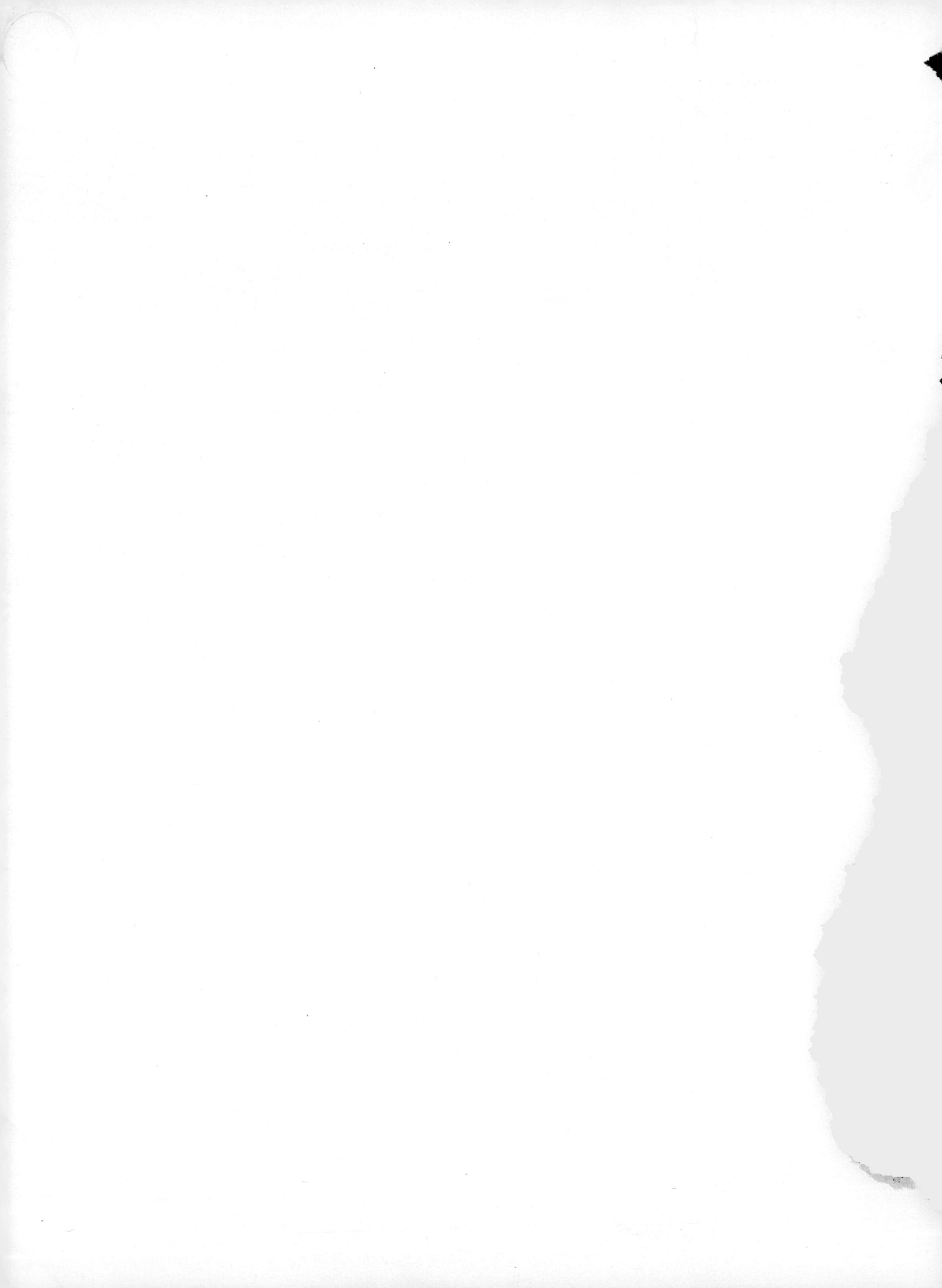